Pleural Disease

LUNG BIOLOGY IN HEALTH AND DISEASE

Executive Editor

Claude Lenfant

Former Director, National Heart, Lung, and Blood Institute
National Institute of Health
Bethesda, Maryland

For information on volumes 25–182 in the *Lung Biology in Health and Disease* series, please visit www.informahealthcare.com

The opinions expressed in these volumes do not necessarily represent the views of the National Institutes of Health.

Pleural Disease
Second Edition

edited by
Demosthenes Bouros
Democritus University of Thrace
Alexandroupolis, Greece

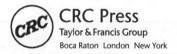

CRC Press
Taylor & Francis Group
Boca Raton London New York

CRC Press is an imprint of the
Taylor & Francis Group, an **informa** business

CRC Press
Taylor & Francis Group
6000 Broken Sound Parkway NW, Suite 300
Boca Raton, FL 33487-2742

First issued in paperback 2019

© 2010 by Taylor & Francis Group, LLC
CRC Press is an imprint of Taylor & Francis Group, an Informa business

No claim to original U.S. Government works

ISBN-13: 978-1-4200-7738-4 (hbk)
ISBN-13: 978-0-367-38456-2 (pbk)

Library of Congress Cataloging-in-Publication Data

Pleural disease / edited by Demosthenes Bouros. – 2nd ed.
    p. ; cm. – (Lung biology in health and disease ; 229)
    Includes bibliographical references and index.
    ISBN-13: 978-1-4200-7738-4 (hb)
    ISBN-10: 1-4200-7738-4 (hb)   1. Pleura–Diseases.   I. Bouros,
Demosthenes.   II. Series: Lung biology in health and disease ; v. 229.
    [DNLM: 1. Pleural Diseases.   2. Pleura.   3. Thoracoscopy.
W1 LU62 v.229 2009 / WF 700 P7266 2009]
    RC751.P535 2009
    616.2'5–dc22

                                 2009034900

Visit the Taylor & Francis Web site at
http://www.taylorandfrancis.com

and the CRC Press Web site at
http://www.crcpress.com

Introduction

"Attempt the end, and never stand in doubt; Nothing's so hard, but search will find out."

Robert Herrick (1591–1694)
"Hesperides"

In 2004, the series of monographs Lung Biology in Health and Disease introduced the first edition of *Pleural Disease*, edited by Professor Demosthenes Bouros. Today, only five years later, we are presenting an updated and revised edition of this volume.

Some may ask "Why so soon?" The answer is found in the first sentence of the editor's Preface: "The second edition of *Pleural Disease* updates our knowledge on frequent, but usually neglected, diseases of the everyday clinical practice."

We know that both Aristotle (384–322 BC) and Galen (AD 129–200) had identified and described a "structure," a membrane as it is called now, surrounding the lungs and that others in between had described pleurisy. However, it appears that we had to wait until the 16th to 17th centuries to see an emergence of interest in this membrane on the part of the pioneer clinical investigators of the time (1).

Today, we know a great deal about diseases of the pleura, but it would seem that this knowledge has not fully reached the medical practice. Professor Bouros calls them "neglected diseases." Since the first edition of this monograph, many investigators have brought new information that could—not to say should—become useful diagnostic and therapeutic tools in medical practice. To paraphrase Robert Herrick, fundamental and clinical scientists are "attempting the end" and they know that "search will find out."

We are not at the end yet, but much needs to be communicated and this is the goal of this second edition of *Pleural Disease*. The readers will see some new chapters and meet some new contributors. It is hoped that this is the presentation of the critical assessment of what we know and what works will benefit the medical community and their patients.

It is with gratitude to the editor and the many experts from several countries who have contributed that I am pleased to present this new edition to our readership.

Claude Lenfant, MD
Vancouver, Washington, U.S.A.

Reference

1. Yernault JC. The history of pleural disease. In: Bouros D, ed. *Pleural Disease.* 1st ed. London and New York: Taylor & Francis, 2004:1–21.

Preface

The second edition of *Pleural Disease* updates our knowledge on frequent, but usually neglected, diseases of the everyday clinical practice. As it was stated in the first edition, it is estimated that about 25% of the consultations of a pulmonary service concern pleural diseases. Various medical specialties are dealing with their diagnosis and treatment, including pneumonologists, thoracic surgeons, radiologists, internists, pediatricians, pathologists and oncologists. However, only a few scientists and clinicians with their excellent and continuous work contributed to the advancement of our understanding of basic and clinical aspects of the health and diseased pleura.

The second edition features the current molecular approaches, interventional applications, biomarkers, proteomics, translational medicine, pleural malignancies, new diagnostic approaches, clinical manifestations, and treatment methodologies. All chapters have been updated to include recent advances in clinical medicine and basic science, while some other more classical ones have been omitted to have a more concise book. New chapters have been added that represent the current state of the art presentation of all aspects of pleural diseases by world leading authorities. Authors from all continents and renowned medical schools contributed to this 45 chapter book, combining the international approach to current diagnosis and treatment of pleural diseases, both benign and malignant. Newer techniques, like medical thoracoscopy, pleural lavage, intrapleural fibrinolytics, image-guided small bore catheters, video-assisted thoracoscopic surgery (VATS), pleuroperitoneal shunt and extrapleural pneumonectomy are presented in detail.

Recent advances in physiology, pathophysiology, imaging and interventional medicine of the pleura are presented by experts. One of the assets of the book is the state of the art description of the application of the interventional techniques for the diagnosis and treatment of the pleural diseases. They include pleural thoracentesis and closed biopsy, chest tube insertion, pleural lavage, medical thoracoscopy and VATS are presented by leading authorities.

A critical assessment of the various diagnostic tests and the importance of clinical evaluation in the differential diagnosis of a pleural effusion are presented in detail.

A great deal of the book is dedicated to pleural infection. A number of experts present their experience in the diagnosis and management of parapneumonic and surgical pleural infections both from the medical and surgical point of view. Tuberculous pleuritis continues to be a major health problem in developing countries and a frequent diagnostic problem in the clinical practice.

Malignant pleural effusions, primary or metastatic, are an important cause of morbidity. The various aspects of this condition are presented in some extent both from the clinical and the surgical point of view. The current understanding and management of mesothelioma and the benign asbestos-related pleural disease is professionally presented, as well as recent advances for other frequent diseases, including pneumothorax, and hemothorax.

I hope that physicians, thoracic surgeons, radiologists, pediatricians, and students will find the new book useful in their everyday clinical and research practice.

Demosthenes Bouros

Contributors

Gerald F. Abbott   Rhode Island Hospital, Providence, Rhode Island, U.S.A.

Michael G. Alexandrakis   University of Crete Medical School, University Hospital of Heraklion, Heraklion, Crete, Greece

Katerina M. Antoniou   Department of Thoracic Medicine Medical School, University of Crete, Heraklion, Crete, Greece

Veena B. Antony   University of Florida School of Medicine, Gainesville, Florida, U.S.A.

Philippe Astoul   Département des Maladies Respiratoires, Unité d'Oncologie Thoracique—Hôpital Sainte-Marguerite, Marseille, France

Robert P. Baughman   University of Cincinnati, Cincinnati, Ohio, U.S.A.

Michael H. Baumann   Division of Pulmonary and Critical Care Medicine, University of Mississippi Medical Center, Jackson, Mississippi, U.S.A.

Chris Bolliger   Respiratory Research Unit, Faculty of Health Sciences, University of Stellenbosch, Cape Town, South Africa

Philippe Bonniaud   Department of Pulmonary Disease and Intensive Care, University Medical Center—Hôpital du Bocage, Faculté de Médecine—Université de Bourgogne, Dijon, France

Demosthenes Bouros   Democritus University of Thrace Medical School, and University Hospital of Alexandroupolis, Alexandroupolis, Greece

Philippe Camus   Department of Pulmonary Disease and Intensive Care, University Medical Center—Hôpital du Bocage, Faculté de Médecine—Université de Bourgogne, Dijon, France

Clio Camus   Department of Pulmonary Disease and Intensive Care, University Medical Center—Hôpital du Bocage, Faculté de Médecine—Université de Bourgogne, Dijon, France

Biswajit Chakrabarti   Aintree Chest Centre, University Hospital Aintree, Liverpool, U.K.

Iain Crossingham   Manchester Royal Infirmary, Manchester, U.K.

Kristina Crothers   University of Washington School of Medicine, Seattle, Washington, U.S.A.

Peter D. O. Davies   The Cardiothoracic Centre, Liverpool NHS Trust, Liverpool, U.K.

Antoine Delage   Departement Multidisciplinaire de Pneumologie, Institut Universitaire de Cardiologie et de Pneumologie de Quebec—Hôpital Laval, Quebec, Canada

Andreas Diacon   Respiratory Research Unit, Faculty of Health Sciences, University of Stellenbosch, Cape Town, South Africa

Dean M. Donahue   Harvard Medical School, Division of Thoracic Surgery, Massachusetts General Hospital, Boston, Massachusetts, U.S.A.

Pierre-Emmanuel Falcoz   Université Louis Pasteur and Hôpitaux Universitaires de Strasbourg, Strasbourg, France

Marios E. Froudarakis   Department of Pneumonology, Democritus University of Thrace Medical School, Alexandroupolis, Greece

Dimitris Georgopoulos   University of Crete and University Hospital of Heraklion, Heraklion, Crete, Greece

E. Brigitte Gottschall   National Jewish Health and University of Colorado Denver, and Colorado School of Public Health and School of Medicine, Denver, Colorado, U.S.A.

Kostas I. Gourgoulianis   University of Thessaly, Larissa, Greece

Elpis Hatziagorou   Aristotelian University of Thessaloniki, Hippokration General Hospital, Thessaloniki, Greece

Demondes Haynes   Division of Pulmonary and Critical Care Medicine, University of Mississippi Medical Center, Jackson, Mississippi, U.S.A.

John E. Heffner   Providence Portland Medical Center, Portland, Oregon, U.S.A.

Joost P. J. J. Hegmans   Department of Pulmonary Medicine, Erasmus MC, Rotterdam, The Netherlands

Laurence Huang   University of California, San Francisco, California, U.S.A.

Philippe G. Jorens   Antwerp University Hospital, Edegem, Antwerp, Belgium

Marc A. Judson   Division of Pulmonary, Critical Care, Allergy and Sleep Medicine, Medical University of South Carolina, Charleston, South Carolina, U.S.A.

Ok-Hwa Kim Department of Radiology, Ajou University Medical Center, Suwon, South Korea

Epaminondas N. Kosmas 3rd Department of Pulmonary Medicine, Chest Diseases Hospital "Sotiria", Voula, Athens, Greece

Georgios Kouliatsis University Hospital of Alexandroupolis, Alexandroupolis, Greece

Despina S. Kyriakou University of Thessaly Medical School, University Hospital of Larissa, Larissa, Thessaly, Greece

Y. C. Gary Lee Department of Medicine & Lung Institute of Western Australia, University of Western Australia and Sir Charles Gairdner Hospital, Perth, Australia

Marc Licker Département d'Anesthésiologie, Hôpitaux Universitaires Genevois, Geneva, Switzerland

Richard W. Light Vanderbilt University, Nashville, Tennessee, U.S.A.

Katerina Malagari Medical School of University of Athens, Athens, and Department of Radiology, Attikon University Hospital, Haidari, Athens, Greece

Gian Pietro Marchetti Divisione di Pneumologia, Spedali Civili di Brescia, Brescia, Italy

Eugene J. Mark Harvard Medical School and Massachusetts General Hospital, Boston, Massachusetts, U.S.A.

Charles-Hugo Marquette Service de Pneumologie, Oncologie Thoracique et Soins Intensifs Respiratoires, Hôpital Pasteur, Centre Hospitalier Universitaire de Nice, France

Gilbert Massard Université Louis Pasteur and Hôpitaux Universitaires de Strasbourg, Strasbourg, France

Douglas J. Mathisen Harvard Medical School, Division of Thoracic Surgery, Massachusetts General Hospital, Boston, Massachusetts, U.S.A.

Theresa C. McLoud Department of Radiology, Massachusetts General Hospital, Boston, Massachusetts, U.S.A.

Ioanna Mitrouska University of Crete and University Hospital of Heraklion, Heraklion, Crete, Greece

John F. Murray University of California, San Francisco, California, U.S.A.

Lee S. Newman National Jewish Health and University of Colorado Denver, and Colorado School of Public Health and School of Medicine, Denver, Colorado, U.S.A.

Kyung Joo Park Department of Radiology, Ajou University Medical Center, Suwon, South Korea

Ioannis Pneumatikos Critical Care Department, University Hospital of Alexandroupolis, Democritus University Thrace, Alexandroupolis, Greece

Vlasis S. Polychronopoulos 3rd Chest Department, Sismanogleion General Hospital, Athens, Greece

José M. Porcel Department of Internal Medicine, Arnau de Vilanova University Hospital, Lleida, Spain

Udaya B. S. Prakash Pulmonary and Critical Care, Mayo Clinic College of Medicine, Mayo Clinic, Rochester, Minnesota, U.S.A.

Luis Puente-Maestu Hospital Universitario Gregorio Marañón, Madrid, Spain

Lesek Purek Centre Valaisan de Pneumologie, Réseau Santé Valais, Montana, Switzerland

Francisco Rodriguez-Panadero Unidad Médico-Quirúrgica de Enfermedades Respiratorias, Hospital Universitario Virgen del Rocío, Sevilla, Spain

Charis Roussos Critical Care Department, Evangelismos Hospital, National and Capodistrian University of Athens, Athens, Greece

Steven A. Sahn Division of Pulmonary, Critical Care, Allergy and Sleep Medicine, Medical University of South Carolina, Charleston, South Carolina, U.S.A.

Arnaud Scherpereel Service de Pneumologie et Oncologie Thoracique—Hôpital Calmette, Centre Hospitalier Universitaire de Lille, France

Patrique Segers Academic Medical Center, Amsterdam, The Netherlands

Nikolaos M. Siafakas Department of Thoracic Medicine Medical School, University of Crete, Heraklion, Crete, Greece

Georgios T. Stathopoulos Department of Critical Care and Pulmonary Services, General Hospital "Evangelismos", School of Medicine, University of Athens, Athens, Greece

Charlie Strange Medical University of South Carolina, Charleston, South Carolina, U.S.A.

David J. Sugarbaker Harvard Medical School, Brigham & Women's Hospital, Boston, Massachusetts, U.S.A.

Gian Franco Tassi Divisione di Pneumologia, Spedali Civili di Brescia, Brescia, Italy

Pascal Thomas   Université de Marseille, Hôpital Sainte Marguerite, Marseille, France

Michael Toumbis   Chest Diseases Hospital of Athens "Sotiria", Athens, Greece

John N. Tsanakas   Aristotelian University of Thessaloniki, Hippokration General Hospital, Thessaloniki, Greece

Jean Marie Tschopp   Centre Valaisan de Pneumologie, Réseau Santé Valais, Montana, Switzerland

Paul E. Van Schil   Antwerp University Hospital, Edegem, Antwerp, Belgium

Johny A. Verschakelen   University Hospitals, Gasthuisberg, Leuven, Belgium

Victoria Villena   Hospital Universitario 12 de Octubre, Madrid, Spain

Athol U. Wells   Royal Brompton Hospital, London, U.K.

Mark Woodhead   Manchester Royal Infirmary, Manchester, U.K.

Cameron D. Wright   Harvard Medical School and Massachusetts General Hospital, Boston, Massachusetts, U.S.A.

Sotirios Zarogiannis   University of Thessaly, Larissa, Greece

Lambros Zellos   Harvard Medical School, Brigham & Women's Hospital, Boston, Massachusetts, U.S.A.

Contents

1
Physiology of the Pleura

SOTIRIOS ZAROGIANNIS and KOSTAS I. GOURGOULIANIS
University of Thessaly, Larissa, Greece

The pleura consist of two membranes: the visceral covering the lung and the parietal pleura covering the diaphragm and the chest wall. Between these two membranes there is a potential space named pleural space, which is filled with a thin film of fluid, called pleural fluid. The pleural fluid is a filtrate of the parietal pleura capillaries. The main function of the pleural fluid is to eliminate friction forces (acting as a lubricant) allowing extensive movement of the lung to the chest wall during respiratory movements. The visceral pleura also contributes to the shape of the lung, provides a limit to expansion, and contributes to the work of deflation (1,2). Pleural space also provides a protecting mechanism against the development of pneumothorax and alveolar edema. During edema, excess fluid could escape the lung by entering the pleural space (3). The continuous submesothelial tissue with the connective tissue of the lung parenchyma prevents the overdistension of alveoli at the pleura surface (4).

I. Functional Anatomy

After development from the embryonic mesoderm, the pleural mesothelia differentiate into the visceral and the parietal pleura by the third week of gestational age. By nine weeks, the pleural cavity has become separated from pericardial space.

Pleural membranes have some histological similarities and important anatomical differences. Pleura consists of five layers: (a) the mesothelium, (b) a layer of submesothelial connective tissue, (c) a thin layer of elastic tissue, (d) a second layer of connective tissue containing blood and lymph vessels and nerves, and (e) a fibroelastic layer adherent to the underlying tissue (absent in the visceral pleura of small mammals). The submesothelial connective tissue layer of the parietal is thicker than its visceral pleura (5).

The visceral pleura lacks innervation, and its blood supply is more complex than parietal pleura. Mammals are divided into two categories in relation to thickness and blood supply of the visceral pleura (6). One is the mammals with thin visceral pleura that are supplied with blood from the pulmonary circulation (i.e., dogs, cats, rabbits) and the other is the mammals with thick visceral pleura that are supplied with blood from the bronchial systemic circulation (i.e., man, sheep, pigs). In both categories, the blood is drained by the pulmonary veins (7). The parietal pleura is supplied with blood by intercostal arteries (systemic circulation) and is innervated by the intercostals nerves (8). In mammals with thick visceral pleura, therefore, both pleurae have a systemic circulation, although the visceral circulation may have a slightly lower pressure because of its drainage into a lower pressure venous system (9).

Pleural lymphatics are connected to the pleural cavity via lacunas or stomas in the mesothelial surface of the parietal pleura. These stomas are numerous in the lower portion of the mediastinal and costal pleura, and over the diaphragmatic portion of parietal pleura. Efferent lymphatic vessels from parietal pleura drain to parasternal and paravertebral nodes, whereas the lymphatics drain into tracheobronchial nodes (10). The lymphatic network is very rich within the parietal pleura. Lymphatics of the visceral do not communicate with the pleural cavity and are parts of the pulmonary lymphatic system (11).

The pleural membranes are lined with a single cell layer of mesothelial cells flat or cuboidal in shape with a maximum body thickness of 4 μm and a maximum diameter of 40 μm. Mesothelial cells synthesize and secrete several macromolecules of the pleural matrix, such as elastin, fibronectin, glycoproteins (rich in hyaluronan) and collagen, and phagocytose particles and neutrophil chemotactic factors. Both visceral and parietal mesothelial cells present microvilli protruding into the pleural space. Microvilli are more dense over the visceral pleura than the parietal pleura and in the caudal regions than in the cranial regions (12). Additionally, in a recent study of our group, it was demonstrated that in the diaphragmatic parietal pleura, the mesothelial cells are more crowded with a greater ratio of cuboidal/flat and a denser microvillous surface compared to the costal parietal pleura (13) and this result is in agreement with previous studies (14). Microvilli increase the area for metabolic functions and are covered with glucoproteins rich in hyaluronan, enmeshed among them (5). Mesothelial cells connect to each other with tight junctions (14,15) and are provided with all the morphological features relevant to active transmembrane and transcellular transport (16).

II. Pleural Fluid Pressure and Dynamics

The parietal and visceral pleurae are separated by a thin layer, about 20 μm, of fluid. Normally, pleural fluid volume is 0.1 mL/kg of body weight—approximately 10 mL in a healthy adult man. Despite the small volume of fluid present in the pleural space, the rate of pleural fluid filtration and reabsorption exceeds 1 L/day. Glucose concentration in pleural fluid is similar to that in plasma, whereas the concentration of macromolecules such as albumin is lower than their concentration in the blood (17,18).

Movement of fluid within pleural membranes is based on the balance of hydrostatic and oncotic pressures between the microvasculature and the pleural space (19,20). Fluid exchange across the pleural membranes is described by Starling's law:

$$\text{Fluid movement} = L \times S[(P_{cap} - P_{pl}) - \sigma(\Pi_{cap} - \Pi_{pl})],$$

where P and Π are the hydrostatic and osmotic pressures, respectively, within the capillaries (cap) and pleural space (pl); L is the hydraulic conductivity of the membrane; S is the surface area; and σ is the osmotic coefficient for proteins (Fig. 1). At the parietal pleura, there is fluid filtration from systemic capillaries into the adjacent interstitium and from the latter across the mesothelium to pleural space. The actual pleural pressure in humans is approximately -5 cm H_2O at functional residual capacity and -30 cm H_2O at total lung capacity. According to this model of pressure gradients, net transmembrane Starling pressure moves fluid from pleural space to visceral pleura and then to pulmonary capillaries (21,22). In species with thin visceral pleura where blood supply occurs from the pulmonary circulation, thus even lower hydrostatic pressures exist, the net gradients further favor pleural fluid absorption through the visceral pleura (23).

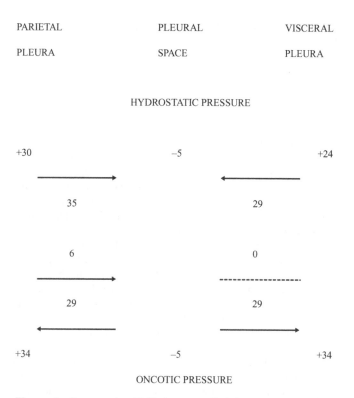

Figure 1 Pressures (cm H$_2$O) that normally influence the movement of fluid in and out of the pleural space.

Recently, there have been conflicting data concerning the entry and exit of pleural fluid normally. Pressure gradients are not the only explanation of the fluid turnover. The pleural space is analogous to any interstitial space of the body. Because intrapleural pressure is lower than interstitial pressure, this pressure difference constitutes a gradient for fluid movement into, but not out of, the pleural cavity. The normal protein concentration (10 g/L) in pleural fluid is low, which implies sieving of the proteins across a high–pressure gradient such as from the high-pressure systemic vessels. Additionally, erythrocytes instilled into pleural space are absorbed intact and in almost the same proportion as the fluid and protein. Pleural mesothelium also exhibits electrolyte-transport activity both in visceral and parietal pleura, as well as in transcytosis of proteins. Thus, lymphatic drainage via the lymphatic stomas of the parietal pleura, solute-coupled liquid absorption on both parietal and visceral pleura, contributes additionally to the exit of pleural fluid from the pleural space (7,16,24–26).

III. Pleural Lymphatic Flow

Lymphatics have a large capacity for absorption. When fluid was instilled into the pleural space of awake sheep, the exit rate increased to about 30 times the baseline exit rate

(27). Our previous data showed that about 1 out of 4 women had pleural effusion during labor and possibly in the third trimester of pregnancy (28). The conditions of labor appear to favor the development of pleural effusion. We speculate that obstruction of lymphatic stomas of parietal pleura during Valsalva maneuvers is the main reason for this phenomenon. Other minor reasons are the increased pressure in systemic circulation, the decreased oncotic pressures, and possible changes in hormonal status. According to Starling's equation, all these pressure changes increase the fluid influx into the pleural cavity. Additionally, the lymphatics lose their large capacity for absorption, which results in the accumulation of fluid during labor (28,29).

The ability of the lymphatics of the diaphragm to drain fluid at subatmospheric pressure has been demonstrated in spontaneously breathing rabbits. Lymphatic flow is based on an intrinsic mechanism (myogenic activity of the lymphatic wall) and an extrinsic mechanism (movement of the tissues surrounding the lymph channels) (30). Labor seems to influence the extrinsic mechanism and to decrease dramatically the pleural fluid efflux.

A recent study from our research group showed that amiloride increased the transepithelial resistance of only parietal pleura, although ouabain, an inhibitor of the Na^+–K^+ pump and nitroprusside sodium, a nitric oxide donor, had the same effect on parietal and visceral pleura. This amiloride effect is most serious in the basolateral, diaphragmatic membrane, than in the apical pleural membrane (31). Amiloride is a drug known to impair smooth muscle contractility (32). Negrini et al. estimated that about 40% of total pleural lymphatic flow depends on an intrinsic mechanism (9,11). Our data are in agreement with Negrini et al. because the amiloride effect occurred only in sites with stomas (parietal pleura, especially diaphragmatic) (33,34). The real increase in parietal pleura resistance is from 20 to about 22 $\Omega \cdot cm^2$. This small increase of parietal resistance may induce difficulties in pleural fluid exit (31,35). In conjunction with the previously mentioned findings, another study of our group investigating the effects of estrogen on the transepithelial resistance of parietal and visceral pleura, concluded that high estrogen concentrations (such as those encountered during pregnancy) decrease the ionic transporting capacity of both pleurae due to rapid release of nitric oxide, preventing further absorption of excess pleural liquid through electrolyte transportation across the mesothelium (36).

Lymphatics represent a regulatory system. Lymphatics have the ability to increase flow when pleural fluid or pressure increases. If the lymphatic conductance decreases significantly (labor) and the filtration coefficient is normal, only a small increase in pleural fluid results (benign postpartum pleural effusion). If the filtration coefficient increases significantly (inflammation), the lymphatic conductance increases lymph flow to maximum. When the filtration rate exceeds the maximum flow rate, lymphatic drainage is insufficient to counterbalance filtration rates, which results in pleural fluid accumulation (parapneumonic pleural effusion) (37).

However, recent experimental data regarding in vivo studies in rabbits with provoked small (0.12 mL/kg) and large (2.4 mL/kg) hydrothoraces containing labeled albumin and dextran revealed that under physiological conditions, the lymphatic drainage through the stomata does not represent the main route for pleural protein and liquid absorption. In fact 39% and 64% of the overall labeled albumin and dextran was removed through lymphatic stomata in small and large hydrothoraces, respectively (38). Moreover, the studies on rabbit sternal pericardium provided evidence of an additional pathway of macromolecular removal from the mesothelium, through transcytosis. These data highlighted the role of transcytosis in pleural protein removal from the pleural cavity (16). The above imply that in physiologic state, Starling forces and lymphatic drainage through parietal stomata are not sufficient in order to explain a rather multifactorial phenomenon like pleural fluid absorption.

IV. Water and Ion Transportation

Nearly 30 years ago, D'Angelo and colleagues were the first that provided evidence for a small, active transport of Na^+ from the serosal to the interstitial side of the dog parietal pleura in vitro (39). In early 1990s, Zocchi et al. provided indirect evidence to support active electrolyte transport by mesothelial cells. They showed the occurrence of solute-coupled liquid absorption from the pleural cavity of rabbits using inhibitors for the Na^+/Cl^-, Na^+/H^+, Cl^-/HCO_3^- double exchange or for the Na^+-K^+ pump (40,41).

Our experiments in sheep showed active transport across both visceral and parietal pleurae (31)—more specifically, an increase in the transepithelial electrical resistance when (a) ouabain, an inhibitor of Na^+-K^+ pump, was added to the mucosal surface of visceral pleura; (b) amiloride, an inhibitor of Na^+ channels and Na^+/H^+ exchanger, was added to the serosal solution in parietal pleura; and (c) sodium nitroprusside, a nitric oxide donor, was added to the serosal surface of parietal pleura and to the serosal or mucosal solutions of visceral pleura. We suggest the occurrence of two kinds of cells in the pleural mesothelium. The first type has double exchanger or Na^+ channels on the serosal side. These cells should transport Na^+ (and hence water) out of the pleural space. The second kind of cell is likely to be provided by the Na^+-K^+ pump on the serosal side and would be involved in recycling K^+. Nitric oxide increases resistance. This phenomenon suggests an effect on either pleural mesothelium or endothelium of lymphatic stomas or both (42,43).

Recent studies of our group have demonstrated that the parietal pleural mesothelium of sheep and humans (mammals with thick visceral pleura) does not have a uniform electrophysiological profile and active transport capacity (13,44). More specifically, in sheep, the costal parietal pleura represents a more "leaky" mesothelium than the diaphragmatic parietal pleura (13) and exhibits a greater electrical activity as shown from studies with inhibitors of Na^+ transport, such as adrenaline, amiloride, and morphine (45–47). In humans, it was found that the caudal parietal pleura is a more "leaky" membrane compared to cranial and mediastinal parietal pleura. Moreover, it exhibits greater electrical activity as shown with Na^+ (amiloride) and Na^+-K^+ pump (ouabain) inhibitors (44). Additionally, human costal parietal pleura has been found to become more permeable to ions when glucose and pH levels drop from normal (48).

Lately, more direct evidence were provided regarding solute transporters (Na^+–glucose cotransporter—SGLT1, and Na^+-K^+ pump) in both visceral and parietal pleurae in mammals with thin (rabbits) as well as with thick (lamb, sheep, humans) visceral pleura, strengthening the theory that liquid removal from the pleural space occurs in both pleurae by solute coupled liquid absorption in series with Starling forces, with lymphatic drainage from parietal stomata and transcytosis (49,50).

Because pleural fluid is filtered and reabsorbed through the parietal pleura, a useful description of pleural fluid turnover can be attempted by a model considering four compartments, capillaries parietal or visceral, interstitium, pleural space, and mesothelial cells parietal or visceral, separated by two resistances—endothelium of capillaries and mesothelium of pleura and an outflow lymphatic system draining from parietal pleura. Most experiments showed that the Starling mechanism determines flow production through the endothelium of capillaries.

V. Pathophysiology

For pleural fluid accumulation, either the entry rate of liquid must increase to more than 30 times that of normal to exceed the lymphatic removal capacity, or the exit rate of fluid must decrease, or both rates must change. The increase in capillary filtration leads to hypooncotic pleural effusion (transudate). More transudates result from congestive heart failure and were thought to originate from the pleural capillaries. In these patients with interstitial pulmonary edema, fluid may come from the pulmonary interstitium across the leaky visceral pleura. When interstitial edema is formed, interstitial pressure increases from -10 to about 6 cm H_2O. Over a three-hour period, no fluid flux occurred across the visceral pleura to the pleural cavity. This finding is in agreement with the clinical observation that pulmonary edema is rarely complicated with pleural effusion. These data suggest that pleural effusion in interstitial edema is the final status when liquid influx exceeds lymphatic drainage (16,51). Other transudates, from nephrotic syndrome or pulmonary atelectasis, may be formed because of pressure changes across the pleural capillaries.

Hyperoncotic fluid (exudates) occurs when the protein permeability is increased. Exudates arise from injured capillaries due to inflammation or malignancy. Although many clinicians are unsure about the role of lymphatics in pleura physiology, the disturbances of the lymphatic system (benign postpartum pleural effusion, yellow nail syndrome), the infiltration of draining parasternal lymph nodes (malignancies), and elevation of the systemic venous pressure into which the lymph drains (heart failure) are causes of pleural fluid accumulation (23).

Acknowledgment

We thank Professor P.A. Molyvdas for his useful comments.

References

1. Gray SW, Skandalakis JE. Development of the pleura. In: Chretien J, Bignon DJ, Hirsh A, eds. The Pleura in Health and Disease. New York, NY: Marcel Dekker, 1985:3–18.
2. Albertine KH, Wiener-Kronish JP, Staub NC. The structure of the parietal pleura and its relationship to pleural liquid dynamics in sheep. Anat Rec 1984; 208:401–409.
3. Wiener-Kronish JP, Matthay MA. Pleural effusions associated with hydrostatic and increased permeability pulmonary edema. Chest 1988; 93:852–858.
4. Miserocchi G, Agostoni E. Contents of the pleural space. Respir Physiol 1971; 30:208–218.
5. Wang NS. Anatomy of the pleura. Clin Chest Med 1998; 19:229–240.
6. Mc Laughlin RF, Tyler WS, Canada RO. A study of the subgross pulmonary anatomy of various mammals. Am J Anat 1961; 108:149–159.
7. Albertine KH, Wiener-Kronish JP, Roos PI, et al. Structure, blood supply, and lymphatic vessels of the sheep's visceral pleura. Am J Anat 1982; 165:277–294.
8. Light RW. Anatomy of the pleura. In: Pleural Diseases. 4th ed. Philadelphia, PA: Lippincott, Williams & Wilkins, 2001:1–7.
9. Negrini D, Mukenge S, Del Fabbro M, et al. Distribution of diaphragmatic lymphatic stomata. J Appl Physiol 1991; 70:1544–1549.

10. Wang NS. The performed stomas connecting the pleura cavity and the lymphatics in the parietal pleura. Am Rev Respir Dis 1975; 111:12–20.
11. Negrini D, Del Fabbro M, Gonano C, et al. Distribution of diaphragmatic lymphatic lacunae. J Appl Physiol 1993; 74:1779–1784.
12. Wang NS. The regional differences of pleural mesothelial cells in rabbits. Am Rev Respir Dis 1974; 110:623–633.
13. Zarogiannis S, Hatzoglou C, Stefanidis I, et al. Comparison of the electrophysiological properties of the sheep isolated costal and diaphragmatic parietal pleura. Clin Exp Pharm Physiol 2007; 34:129–131.
14. Mariassy TA, Wheeldon EB. The pleura: A combined light microscopic, scanning, and transmission electron microscopic study of the pleura. Exp Lung Res 1983; 4:293–313.
15. Staub NC, Wiener-Kronish JP, Albertine KH. Transport through the pleura: Physiology of normal liquid and solute exchange in the pleural space. In: The Pleura in Health and Disease. New York, NY: Marcel Dekker, 1977:169–193.
16. Agostoni E, Zocchi L. Pleural liquid and its exchanges. Respir Physiol Neurobiol 2007; 159:311–323.
17. Agostoni E, Zocchl L. Solute-coupled liquid absorption from the pleural space. Respir Physiol 1990; 81:19–27.
18. Albertine KH, Wiener-Kronish JP, Staub NC. The structure of the parietal pleura and its relationship to pleural liquid dynamics in sheep. Anat Rec 1984; 208:401–409.
19. D'Angelo E, Helsler N, Agostoni E. Acid-base balance of pleural liquid in dogs. Respir Physiol 1979; 37:137–149.
20. Kinasewitz GT, Fishman AP. Influence of alterations in starling forces on visceral pleural fluid movement. J Appl Physiol 1981; 51:671–677.
21. Kinasewitz GT, Groome LJ, Marshall RP, et al. Permeability of the canine visceral pleura. J Appl Physiol 1983; 55:121–130.
22. Payne DK, Kinasewitz GT, Gonzalez E. Comparative permeability of canine visceral and parietal pleura. J Appl Physiol 1988; 65:2558–2564.
23. Light RW. Physiology of the pleural space. In: Pleural Diseases. 4th ed. Philadelphia, PA: Lippincott, Williams & Wilkins, 2001:8–20.
24. Engelberg J, Radin J. Tracheal-vascular and vascular-pleural potential in the rat lung. Respir Physiol 1977; 30:253–263.
25. Fromter I, Diamond JM. Route of passive ion permeation in epithelia. Nat New Biol 1972; 235:9–13.
26. Gourgoulianis KI, Hatzoglou CH, Molyvdas PA. The major route for absorption of fluid from the pleural space. 2002; 35:97–98.
27. Leak LV, Rahil K. Permeability of the diaphragmatic mesothelium: The ultrastructural basis for "stomata". Am J Anat 1978; 151:557–564.
28. Gourgoulianis KI, Karantanas AH, Diminikou G, et al. Benign postpartum pleural effusion. Eur Respir J 1995; 8:1748–1750.
29. Tsilibary EC, Wissing SL. Lymphatic absorption from peritoneal cavity: Regulation of patent of mesothelial stoma. Microvasc Res 1983; 25:22–39.
30. Miserocchi G. Effect of diaphragmatic contraction or relaxation on size and shape of lymphatic stomata on the peritoneal surface in anesthetized rabbits. Proc Physiol Soc 1989; 417: 132P.
31. Hatzoglou CH, Gourgoulianis KI, Molyvdas PA. Effects of SNP ouabain and amiloride on electrical potential profile of isolated sheep pleura. J Appl Physiol 2001; 90:1565–1569.
32. Ding JW, Dickie J, O'Brodovich H, et al. Inhibition of amiloride-sensitive sodium-channel activity in distal lung epithelial cells by nitric oxide. Am J Physiol Lung Cell Mol Physiol 1998; 274:L378–L387.
33. Diamond JM. Transport of salt and water in rabbit and guinea pig gall bladder. J Gen Physiol 1964; 48:1–14.

34. Lewis SA, Diamond JM. Na$^+$ transport by rabbit urinary bladder, a tight epithelium. J Membr Biol 1976; 28:1–40.

35. Lucky J, Chen XJ, Brown LA, et al. Nitric oxide inhibits lung sodium transport through a cGMP-mediated inhibition of epithelial cation channels. Am J Physiol Lung Cell Mol Physiol 1998; 274:L475–L484.

36. Hatzoglou C, Gourgoulianis KI, Hatzoglou A, et al. Rapid effects of 17-β estradiol and progesterone on sheep visceral and parietal pleurae via a nitric oxide pathway. J Appl Physiol 2002; 93:752–758.

37. Kim K, McElroy Critz A, Crandall E. Transport of water and solutes across sheep visceral pleura. Am Rev Respir Dis 1979; 120:883–892.

38. Bodega F, Agostoni E. Contribution of lymphatic drainage through stomata to albumin removal from pleural space. Respir Physiol Neurobiol 2004; 142:251–263.

39. D'Angelo E, Helsler N, Agostoni E. Acid-base balance of pleural liquid in dogs. Respir Physiol 1979; 37:137–149.

40. Zocchi L, Agostoni E, Cremaschi D. Electrolyte transport across the pleura of rabbits. Respir Physiol 1991; 86:125–138.

41. Zocchi L, Agostoni E, Cremaschi D. Liquid volume, Na$^+$ and mannitol concentration in hypertonic mannitol-ringer hydrothorax. Respir Physiol 1992; 89:341–351.

42. Guo V, Duvall MD, Crow JP, et al. Nitric oxide inhibits Na$^+$ absorption across cultured alveolar type II monolayers. Am J Physiol Lung Cell Mol Physiol 1998; 274:L369–L377.

43. Basset G, Bouchonnet F, Crone C, et al. Potassium transport across rat alveolar epithelium: Evidence for an apical Na$^+$–K$^+$ pump. J Physiol (Lond) 1988; 400:529–543.

44. Kouritas VK, Hatzoglou C, Foroulis CN, et al. Human parietal pleura present electrophysiology variations according to location in pleural cavity. Interact Thorac CardioVasc Surg 2008; 7:544–547.

45. Zarogiannis S, Hatzoglou C, Stefanidis I, et al. Effect of adrenaline on transmesothelial resistance of isolated sheep pleura. Respir Physiol Neurobiol 2006; 150:165–172.

46. Zarogiannis S, Hatzoglou C, Stefanidis I, et al. Adrenergic influence on the permeability of sheep diaphragmatic parietal pleura. Respiration 2007; 74:118–120.

47. Vogiatzidis K, Hatzoglou C, Zarogiannis S, et al. μ-Opioid influence on the transmesothelial resistance of isolated sheep pleura and parietal pericardium. Eur J Pharm 2006; 530:276–280.

48. Kouritas VK, Hatzoglou C, Foroulis CN, et al. Low glucose level and low pH alter the electrochemical function of human parietal pleura. Eur Respir J 2007; 30:354–357.

49. Sironi C, Bodega F, Porta C, et al. Expression of Na$^+$–glucose cotransporter (SGLT1) in visceral and parietal mesothelium of rabbit pleura. Respir Physiol Neurobiol 2007; 159: 68–75.

50. Sironi C, Bodega F, Porta C, et al. Na$^+$–glucose cotransporter is also expressed in mesothelium of species with thick visceral pleura. Respir Physiol Neurobiol 2008; 161:261–266.

51. Miserocchi G, Negrini D, Gonado C. Direct measurement of interstitial pulmonary pressure in in-situ lungs with intact pleural space. J Appl Physiol 1990; 69:2168–2174.

2
Pathophysiology of the Pleura

VEENA B. ANTONY
University of Florida School of Medicine, Gainesville, Florida, U.S.A.

I. Defense Mechanisms of the Pleura

The pleura is a monolayer of mesothelial cells intricately connected with the underlying lung and tissues through a network of balancing cellular and humoral factors that allow for host defense of the pleural space. The pleural membrane not only serves as a barrier function, but also has multiple other defense mechanisms that are focused on maintaining the homeostatic balance of the pleural space. Because the pleura encircles a closed potential space, it does not interface with the external environment as does the lung (1). Changes in the delicate homeostatic balance of the pleural space can be initiated by the presence of foreign cells, proteins, or microbes. Even the presence of air in the pleural space changes this balance.

Innate immunity of the pleura is seen early during inflammation, within the first few hours following an insult to the pleural space (2). A significant proportion of the innate immunity of the pleura is provided by the pleural mesothelial cell, a multipotent cell that completely lines the pleural space. The pleural mesothelial cell must not only recognize the offending organism, but it must also initiate the process of responses and coordinate the perpetuation of the inflammatory changes. These responses may differ, depending on the invading microbe or cell. Malignant cells must be recognized as foreign in spite of their development of multiple factors that allow them to present themselves as innocuous and allow them to enter the pleural space as a Trojan horse.

The free surface of the mesothelium is covered by glycoconjugates, which consist of pleural mesothelial cell–associated sialomucins (3). These are strong anionic sites that coat the pleural surface with a negative charge and act to repulse the presence of abnormal particles and organisms. Thus, not only do these glycoproteins mechanically repel (because of their strong negative charge) the opposing pleural membrane, but they also provide a second level of mechanical repulsion to invading cells, microbes, and particulates (4). The presence of these sialomucins on the surface of the mesothelium allows it to function mechanically as "Teflon" rather than "Velcro." Epithelial surfaces that have been stripped of their sialomucins are far more susceptible to damage. Mesothelial cells also have multiple pattern recognition receptors, which recognize the carbohydrate residual of microbial metabolism. The innate immune system of the mesothelial cell also recognizes pathogen-associated molecular patterns, which then can initiate multiple levels of defense mechanisms (5). Some of these pattern recognition receptors include CD14, integrins, and the mannose receptor. The inflammatory responses initiated by the pleural mesothelial cell include release of chemokines to recruit neutrophils, mononuclear cells, and lymphocytes, and the release of factors such as interleukin (IL)-1, IL-6, and interferons, which function as co-stimulators of T cells. T-cell–independent mesothelial responses following phagocytosis of asbestos particles, microbes, etc., lead to the release of IL-12 and tumor necrosis factor (TNF)-α. These cytokine responses perpetuate the proinflammatory loop.

Acquired immunity is the specific immune system of lymphocytes, both T and B lymphocytes, that allows for expression of distinct antigenic receptors (6). Activated–T lymphocytes orchestrate specific immune responses in the pleural space. Mesothelial cells contribute to the cytokines that allow for an undifferentiated T cell to become a T-helper (Th)1- or Th2-type cell that leads to different responses in the pleural space (7). Thus, the defense mechanisms of the pleura include functions starting from providing a mechanical barrier to invasion as well as a sophisticated, multilayered, and coordinated system of cytokines and recruited cells.

II. Cytokine Networks in the Pleural Space

Cytokines are polypeptide structures with multiple biological functions and are key ingredients for the process of initiation, perpetuation, and resolution of the inflammatory response of the pleura. Cytokines do not act alone, but form a multitiered, connecting network that establishes communication between cells and allows for an orchestrated inflammatory cascade of events critical to the inflammatory response (8). The accumulation of inflammatory cells and fluid in the pleural space is a classic response of pleural inflammation. The mesothelial cell is known to produce multiple chemokines from the chemokine family (9). The chemokine family is named according to the location of the amino-terminal cystine residue with a C, C-C, C-X-C, or CCXXXC motif. Pleural mesothelial cells are known to release chemokines from all the member family groups. The C-X-C chemokines, such as IL-8, have been well characterized. These chemokines are critical for neutrophil chemotactic and activating properties. The C-X-C chemokines themselves include those that contain an amino acid residue that precedes the first N-terminal cysteine residue. These amino acids are GLU-LEUARG, otherwise known as the ELR motif. The presence or absence of the GLULEU-ARG (ELR) motif appears to be critical and is defined by logical activities noted among the C-X-C chemokines. The factors that lack the ELR motif are not potent neutrophil chemotaxins and also have angiostatic properties, while those containing an ELR motif, such as IL-8, are chemotactic for neutrophils and are also angiogenic (10). The C-C group of chemokines is defined by the position of the first two end-terminal cysteines. These include macrophage inflammatory protein-1α, β, γ; MCP-1, 2, 3, and 4; and RANTES. The C chemokine lymphotaxin is important for the recruitment of lymphocytes to the pleural space. Mesothelial cells have also been described to produce fractalkine.

A. Cytokine Networks During Acute Infections

A characteristic feature of parapneumonic effusions is the accumulation of neutrophils and mononuclear phagocytes. IL-8, an 8.3 kDa protein, is found in significant quantities in pleural fluids obtained from patients who develop parapneumonic effusions. The pleural fluid from both patients with uncomplicated parapneumonic effusions as well as empyema is chemotactic for neutrophils and contains higher levels of IL-8 when compared to pleural effusions of patients with malignancy, tuberculosis, or heart failure (11). In patients with uncomplicated parapneumonic effusions, a significantly higher correlation of neutrophil to chemokine level is seen with epithelial neutrophil–activating protein-78 (ENA-78) than with IL-8. This chemokine is also known to have specific chemotactic activity for neutrophils. Broaddus et al. (12), using an endotoxin model for pleurisy, demonstrated that inhibition of neutrophil entry into the pleural space was mediated by antibodies to rabbit IL-8. Other early mediators released by mesothelial cells include IL-1β and TNF-α. The early responses of the pleural mesothelial cell in acute inflammation lead to a widening of the inflammatory changes with the recruitment of several phagocytic cells that may themselves release cytokines and thus communicate with the resident mesothelial cell. In the exudative stage of parapneumonic effusions, the pleural fluid is still free flowing. However, during the fibrinopurulent stage, as there is further movement of inflammatory cells and bacteria into the pleura space, other cytokine networks appear to be initiated.

Pleural mesothelial cells release growth factors such as platelet-derived growth factor, transforming growth factor (TGF)-β, and fibroblast growth factor. These factors are known to be mitogenic for fibroblasts and are also angiogenic. The goal appears to be walling off of the pleural space in a fibrous peel for the development of new capillaries and revascularization of the injured mesothelium. This allows for an increased influx of inflammatory cells into the area to prevent further spread of the infection to other areas. In effect, the pleural space is transformed into an abscess cavity.

B. Cytokine Networks in Granulomatous Disease of the Pleura

Tuberculosis is a classic example of a pleural granulomatous response. This includes the development of cytokine networks that drive the Th1/Th2 responses. Early during the course of granulomatous disease there is a neutrophil predominant response (13), but the most persistent response is that of mononuclear phagocytes that engulf mycobacteria, resulting in a coalescing of mononuclear cells into granulomas. Mesothelial cells release members of the C-C chemokine family, including MCP-1. MCP-1 is a protein member of the supergene family that has been demonstrated in tuberculous pleural fluids. These fluids have also been described to contain MIP-1α, a specific chemokine for monocytes. Interferon (IFN)-γ, a critical cytokine for the recruitment of mononuclear cells, is also present in pleural fluids of patients with granulomatous inflammation (14). Mesothelial cells produce IL-12, which drives the Th response towards the Th1 cytokines, including IL-4. Neutralization of the IFN-γ response in the pleural space causes abrogation of the development of granulomas. IFN-γ augments cytokine and chemokine production by local cells and allows for a significant increase in MCP-1 and MIP-1 production by mesothelial cells.

Interferon-γ upregulates microbicidal, phagocytic, and T–cell–activating functions as well as nitric oxide release by mesothelial cells (15). Nitric oxide is part of a microbicidal mechanism of mesothelial cells that results in the killing of mycobacteria as well as increased production of other oxidants such as H_2O_2 and superoxide anion. IFN-γ itself is regulated by other cytokines such as TNF-α, which synergize with IFN-γ in macrophage activation. IL-12 also functions with TNF-α, IL-1β, IL-15, and IL-18 to achieve optimal IFN-γ expression. In patients with human immunodeficiency (HIV) infection, there is a disruption of the cytokine network in the pleural space with disastrous results for the patients. Cytokines such as IL-10 are present in significant quantities in the pleural fluid of patients with disseminated tuberculosis and can prevent critical Th1-type responses from functioning. This leads to poor granuloma formation and dissemination of the disease.

III. Changes in Pleural Cell Populations

The pleural mesothelial cell is the single most common cell of the pleural space. It is also the primary cell that initiates responses to noxious stimuli (16,17). The mesothelial cell is a metabolically active cell that maintains a dynamic state of homeostasis in the pleural space until provoked. It is actively phagocytic and is capable of producing several cytokines, as mentioned above (8). Mesothelial cells are ciliated, and have multiple tight intercellular adherens junctions as well as focal adhesions that anchor the mesothelial cell onto the extracellular membrane via integrins (7). When injured, mesothelial cells respond via proliferation and chemotaxis to cover areas of denuded extracellular matrix. This proliferative and chemotactic response is mediated in part by an autocrine response to the production of chemokines in the local area of injury. Mesothelial cells also maintain both juxtacrine and paracrine communications between cells to allow for a rapid response during inflammation.

A. Neutrophils

Neutrophils are the first cells to respond during inflammation (18). Neutrophils are produced in the bone marrow, where they evolve from pluripotent stem cells that also give rise to other cells of the granulocytic series, including eosinophils. During inflammation, these cells move from the vascular compartment into the pleural space and form the first line of inflammatory-cell defense against invading organisms or particulates such as asbestos (19). A significantly large number of neutrophils are found in the lung vasculature. During inflammation, neutrophils move out of the vascular compartment and into the pleural space using the adhesion molecule ICAM-1 on mesothelial surfaces to interdigitate with the CD11/CD18 ligands on their surfaces (20). The primary function of neutrophils in the pleural space is phagocytosis and bacterial killing (21). They have potent antibacterial defense mechanisms such as release of oxidants and proteases (6,22). Neutropenic animals with empyema are unable to clear bacteria and develop disseminated disease. The eventual fate of neutrophils in the pleural space during acute inflammatory events such as empyema is unclear. Neutrophils are cleared from the pleural space by macrophages that engulf apoptotic cells. Mesothelial cells regulate the process of apoptosis of neutrophils via production of granulocyte-macrophage colony–stimulating factor (GM-CSF), thus manipulating the life span of the neutrophil in the pleural space (23–26).

B. Lymphocytes

The mesothelial cell releases several chemokines, which are directed at lymphocytes. Both B- and T-cell lymphocytes are found during inflammatory disease. Lymphocytes are common in granulomatous disease, while both T and B lymphocytes are found in malignant pleural effusions and in effusions caused by abnormal of immune responses such as lupus erythematosus and rheumatoid disease (26). Pleural fluid from patients with tuberculosis contains natural killer (NK) cells as well as gamma–delta T cells, which are critical for responses against mycobacteria. The T lymphocytes are divided into CD4 and CD8 lymphocytes. The CD4 lymphocytes predominate in diseases such as tuberculosis, while CD8 lymphocytes predominate in diseases such as lymphoma. Activated T lymphocytes release multiple cytokines, including IFN-γ and a host of other cytokines (27). CD8 T lymphocytes can function as specific cytotoxic cells, while NK cells can regulate B-cell function. B-cell immunoglobulin production is displayed on its surface as an IgM molecule. They can exhibit specific markers and make immunoglobulins with specificity for a single antigen.

C. Pleural Fibroblasts

Pleural fibroblasts, though not present in large numbers under normal conditions, are often exposed to the environment of the pleural space when there is denudation of the mesothelium. The pleural fibroblast is a spindle-shaped elongated cell with a large oval nucleus with one or more nucleoli. The cytoplasm consists of abundant rough endoplasmic reticulum with well-developed Golgi apparatus and numerous mitochondria. Fibroblasts are known to produce collagen and can release several cytokines such as chemokines, which can then perpetuate the inflammatory process. The proliferation of fibroblasts is determined by the environment that is present in the pleural milieu. Potent mitogens for fibroblasts include PDGF, FGF, and EGF. Inhibitors of fibroblast growth include PGE2, which can also be produced by pleural mesothelial cells (28). IFN-γ may have either an inhibitory or a stimulatory effect on the growth of pleural fibroblasts. Fibroblasts derived from different tissue sites display distinct morphological, structural, and functional characteristics. Pleural fibroblasts appear to have specific functions and demonstrate specific behavior in response to injury of the overlying extracellular matrix and cells (29).

D. Malignant Cells

The presence of malignant cells in the pleural space is abnormal. Certain malignant cells demonstrate a greater predilection for the pleural space than elsewhere. Cancers of the lung, breast, stomach, and ovary following metastasis are seen in greater frequency in the pleural space than at other sites. The presence of a malignant cell in the pleural space indicates that the malignant cell has overcome the pleural defense mechanisms to localize in the pleural space. Malignant cells have a large armamentarium of mechanisms whereby they can present themselves as innocuous cells to the mesothelial cellular environment (30). Malignant cells may use a host of factors such as receptors for CD44 (31), whose ligand is hyaluron, which is produced in significant quantities by the pleural mesothelial cell to interdigitate with the mesothelial cell (32). This allows for proteolytic digestion of large molecular weight hyaluron, leaving smaller fragments, which are both chemotactic for the malignant cells and angiogenic.

Angiogenesis is critical for the ability of the malignant cells to develop an environment surrounded by blood vessels through which it is fed and can grow. Malignant cells can produce multiple cytokines including VEGF and bFGF, which are angiogenic and increase the permeability of the tissues around it to allow for growth of new capillaries, leading to vascularization of the pleural surface. This leads to the eventual seeding of the pleural surface and independent growth of the tumor by eluding the defense mechanisms of the pleura. Malignant cells can also produce autocrine growth factors. Mesothelin, a mesothelioma-derived biomarker, has predictive and prognostic implications (33).

IV.   Pleural Effusion Formation During Inflammation

One of the signatures of an inflammatory process in the pleural space is the development of an exudative pleural effusion. Whether it is a movement of leukocytes from the vascular compartment into the pleural space or malignant cells moving from the vascular or lymphatic space, a critical barrier provided by the mesothelial monolayer has been breached. Individual pleural mesothelial cells are linked together into a tight membrane by connecting intracellular proteins at key areas called adherens junctions. Pleural mesothelial cell adherens junction transmembrane, cell-to-cell connecting, homophilic proteins are responsible for maintaining pleural barrier function. Activation of the pleural mesothelial monolayer by malignant cells, bacteria, or cytokines causes a breach in the integrity of the pleura and results in altered shape, gap formation between mesothelial cells, and leakage of protein, fluids, and movement of phagocytic cells out into the pleural space. Vascular permeability factor (VPF) (34), also commonly known as vascular endothelial growth factor (VEGF), is upregulated in mesothelial cells when they are activated. VEGF has been found in large quantities in parapneumonic effusions as well as malignant pleural effusions. VEGF is a 35–45 kDa dimeric polypeptide expressed in several isoforms resulting from alternative mRNA splicing of a single gene and is now recognized to be a pivotal permeability and angiogenic factor mediating neovascularization under many conditions (35). VEGF is also known to play a central role in the formation of ascites in animal models. Adherens junction proteins, namely cadherins and catenins, are transmembrane proteins that function as a zipper between cells, allowing a change in permeability to occur via signaling mechanisms that lead to contraction of the intracellular actin cytoskeletal filaments leading to gap formation between cells (36). A major cadherin in pleural mesothelial cells is neural cadherin (n-cadherin). When adherens junctions are stabilized as in tightly confluent cells, the majority of n-cadherin loses tyrosine phosphorylation and combines with plakoglobin and actin (37). However, when cells have weakened junctions, n-cadherin is heavily phosphorylated in tyrosine, and there is decreased expression of β-catenin as well (38). Thus, n-cadherin and β-catenin are critical determinants of mesothelial paracellular permeability. This interaction is a dynamic one, since this permeability is also reversible. VEGF induces tyrosine phosphorylation of adherens junction proteins to allow paracellular permeability. During the formation of a pleural effusion, not only can cells migrate via the interaction of surface ligands for intercellular molecules expressed on mesothelial cells, but this also allows proteins of high molecular weight to leak across the pleural membrane. Exposure of pleural mesothelial monolayers to malignant cells or organisms leads to a rapid drop-off in electrical resistance across the pleural membrane and a transfer of protein.

V.   Resolution of Pleural Inflammation

The resolution of a pleural inflammatory process is dependent on multiple factors, but primarily on the neutralization of the inciting agent. In infections secondary to bacteria, mycobacteria, viruses, etc., death of the organism and eventual clearance of the bacterial cell products from the pleural space are associated with resolution. However, in diseases such as malignant pleural effusions, this may not occur on its own without the use of chemotherapeutic options. For example, in diseases such as metastatic small-cell carcinoma, chemotherapy can cause a rapid decrease and resolution of malignant pleural effusions, while in diseases such as mesothelioma or non–small-cell lung cancer, effective resolution of the pleural effusion is much more difficult. Interestingly, the pleural mesothelial cell plays a role during the process of resolution of acute inflammatory diseases such as empyema. GM-CSF is known to prolong the life span of leukocytes by inhibition of apoptosis (23). GM-CSF is found in high levels in parapneumonic effusions and in empyema (24). Mesothelial cells are also shown to undergo apoptosis when stimulated with live bacteria, but not with dead organisms.

Inflammation of the pleural surface may resolve with fibrosis or without fibrosis. The cytokine networks that move the resolution of inflammation towards fibrosis are not clear. However, it is apparent that resolution without fibrosis requires regeneration of a normal mesothelial surface following injury and denudation, while repair with fibrosis involves the production and proliferation of fibroblasts.

VI. Therapeutic Strategies Based on Pathophysiology of Pleural Disease

A. Gene Therapy

Gene therapy in the pleural space uses exogenous cDNA to manipulate the mesothelial cell to achieve a certain therapeutic effect. Gene therapy has been used in the pleural space primarily to counteract mesothelioma. Gene therapy against mesothelioma has used both viral-based vectors, such as adenovirus or adeno-associated virus-based systems, as well as non–viral-based systems. These include liposomes where cationic lipids are mixed with neutral lipids, which combine with DNA. The rationale for the administration of a replication-deficient recombinant adenovirus that has been genetically engineered to contain the herpes simplex virus thymidine kinase gene, is the hope that delivery of this gene into the pleural cavity of patients with mesothelioma would transduce the tumor cells enabling them to express viral thymidine kinase and convey sensitivity to the nontoxic antiviral drug ganciclovir. Phase 1 studies of both this drug as well as the γ-interferon gene have been partially successful, and the outcomes of these studies are as yet unclear and undergoing further clarification (39).

B. Pleurodesis

Pleurodesis implicates the obliteration of the pleural space and the absence of defining surfaces between the parietal and visceral pleurae. All pleurodesis agents aim at initiating an inflammatory response that eventually results in the development of pleural fibrosis. Talc has been demonstrated to cause release of several fibroblast growth factors by the pleural mesothelial cells. These include bFGF, PDGF, and TGF-β (40). Initiation of an inflammatory response that allows for the directed movement of the inflammation to resolve with fibrosis has been the goal. Interestingly, if malignant disease is advanced to the point where the pleural mesothelial surface is covered by malignant deposit so that the talc or other sclerosing agent has little interaction with the normal pleural mesothelial surface, the fibrotic response has been found to be attenuated with decreases in the amount of pleural fluid fibroblast growth factors. This finding emphasizes the important role played by the mesothelial cell in the process of pleural fibrosis.

References

1. Wang N. Mesothelial cells in situ. In: Chretien J, Bignon J, Hirsch A, eds. The Pleura in Health and Disease. New York, NY: Marcel Dekker, 1985:23–42.
2. Medzhitov R, Janeway CA Jr. Innate immunity: Impact on the adaptive immune response. Curr Opin Immunol 1997; 9:4–9.
3. Ohtsuka A, Yamana S, Murakami T. Localization of membrane-associated sialomucin on the free surface of mesothelial cells of the pleura, pericardium, and peritoneum. Histochem Cell Biol 1997; 107:441–447.
4. Sassetti C, Van Zante A, Rosen SD. Identification of endoglycan, a member of the CD34/podocalyxin family of sialomucins. J Biol Chem 2000; 275:9001–9010.
5. Gorbach S, Bartlett J, Blacklow N. Infectious diseases. In: Gorbach S, Bartlett J, Blacklow N, eds. Host Factors. Philadelphia, PA: Saunders, 1992:37.
6. Burton DR, Woof JM. Human antibody effector function. Adv Immunol 1992; 51:1–84.
7. Mohammed KA, Nasreen N, Ward MJ, et al. Induction of acute pleural inflammation by *Staphylococcus aureus*. I. CD4+ T cells play a critical role in experimental empyema. J Infect Dis 2000; 181:1693–1699.
8. Jonjic N, Peri G, Bernasconi S, et al. Expression of adhesion molecules and chemotactic cytokines in cultured human mesothelial cells. J Exp Med 1992; 176:1165–1174.
9. Antony VB, Hott JW, Kunkel SL, et al. Pleural mesothelial cell expression of C-C (monocyte chemotactic peptide) and C-X-C (interleukin 8) chemokines. Am J Respir Cell Mol Biol 1995; 12:581–588.
10. Strieter RM, Koch AE, Antony VB, et al. The immunopathology of chemotactic cytokines: The role of interleukin-8 and monocyte chemoattractant protein-1. J Lab Clin Med 1994; 123:183–197.
11. Antony VB, Godbey JB, Kunkel SL, et al. Recruitment of inflammatory cells to the pleural space chemotactic cytokinesis IL-8 and MCP-1 in human pleural fluids. J Immunol 1993; 15:7216–7233.
12. Broaddus VC, Boylan AM, Hoeffel JM, et al. Neutralization of IL-8 inhibits neutrophil influx in a rabbit model of endotoxin-induced pleurisy. J Immunol 1994; 152:2960–2967.
13. Antony VB, Sahn SA, Antony AC, et al. Bacillus Calmette-Guerin-stimulated neutrophils release chemotaxins for monocytes in rabbit pleural spaces and in vitro. J Clin Invest 1985; 76:1514–1521.
14. Ellner JJ, Barnes PF, Wallis RS, et al. The immunology of tuberculous pleurisy. Semin Respir Infect 1988; 3:335–342.
15. Owens MW, Milligan SA, Grisham MB. Nitric oxide synthesis by rat pleural mesothelial cells: Induction by growth factors and lipopolysaccharide. Exp Lung Res 1995; 21:731–742.
16. Chen JY, Chiu JH, Chen HL, et al. Human peritoneal mesothelial cells produce nitric oxide: Induction by cytokines. Perit Dial Int 2000; 20:772–777.
17. Owens MW, Grisham MB. Nitric oxide synthesis by rat pleural mesothelial cells: Induction by cytokines and lipopolysaccharide. Am J Physiol 1993; 265:L110–L116.
18. Malech H. Phagocytic cells: Egress from marrow and diapedesis. In: Gallin JI, Goldstein IM, Snyderman R, eds. Inflammation: Basic Principles and Clinical Correlates. New York, NY: Raven Press, 1988:297–308.
19. Broaddus VC, Yang L, Scavo LM, et al. Asbestos induces apoptosis of human and rabbit pleural mesothelial cells via reactive oxygen species. J Clin Invest 1996; 98:2050–2059.
20. Nasreen N, Hartman D, Mohammed K, et al. Talc induces pleural mesothelial cell expression of proinflammatory cytokines and intracellular adhesion molecule-1 (ICAM-1). Am J Respir Crit Care Med 1998; 158:971–978.
21. Spitznagel J. Non-oxidative antimicrobial reactions of leukocytes. Contemp Top Immunobiol 1984; 14:283.
22. Ganz T, Selsted ME, Szklarek D, et al. Defensins. Natural peptide antibiotics of human neutrophils. J Clin Invest 1985; 76:1427–1435.

23. Cox G, Gauldie J, Jordana M. Bronchial epithelial cell-derived cytokines (G-CSF and GM-CSF) promote the survival of peripheral blood neutrophils in vitro. Am J Respir Cell Mol Biol 1992; 7:507–513.
24. Nasreen N, Mohammed KA, Sanders KL, et al. Differential expression of C-phos, C-June, and apoptosis in pleural mesothelial cells exposed to *Stap. aureus*. Am J Respir Crit Care Med 2001; 163:A772.
25. Payne CM, Glasser L, Tischler ME, et al. Programmed cell death of the normal human neutrophil: An in vitro model of senescence. Microsc Res Tech 1994; 28:327–344.
26. Sahn SA. State of the art. The pleura. Am Rev Respir Dis 1988; 138:184–234.
27. Mantovani A, Garlanda C. Novel pathways for negative regulation of inflammatory cytokines centered on receptor expression. Dev Biol Stand 1999; 97:97–104.
28. Hott JW, Godbey SW, Antony VB. Mesothelial cell modulation of pleural repair: Thrombin stimulated mesothelial cells release prostaglandin E2. Prostaglandins Leukot Essent Fatty Acids 1994; 51:329–335.
29. Rennard S, Jaurand M, Bignon J, et al. Connective tissue matrix of the pleura. In: Chretien J, Bignon J, Hirsch A, eds. The Pleura in Health and Disease, Vol. 5. New York, NY: Marcel Dekker, 1985:69–85.
30. Antony VB. Pathogenesis of malignant pleural effusions and talc pleurodesis. Pneumologie 1999; 53:493–498.
31. Ponta H. The CD44 protein family. Int J Biochem Cell Biol 1998; 30:299–305.
32. Bourguignon LY, Lokeshwar VB, Chen X, et al. Hyaluronic acid-induced lymphocyte signal transduction and HA receptor (GP85/CD44)-cytoskeleton interaction. J Immunol 1993; 151:6634–6644.
33. Robinson BW, Musk AW, Lake RA, Malignant mesothelioma. Lancet 2005; 366:397–408.
34. Becker PM, Alcasabas A, Yu AY, et al. Oxygen-independent upregulation of vascular endothelial growth factor and vascular barrier dysfunction during ventilated pulmonary ischemia in isolated ferret lungs. Am J Respir Cell Mol Biol 2000; 22:272–279.
35. Thickett DR, Armstrong L, Millar AB. Vascular endothelial growth factor (VEGF) in inflammatory and malignant pleural effusions. Thorax 1999; 54:707–710.
36. Corada M, Liao F, Lindgren M, et al. Monoclonal antibodies directed to different regions of vascular endothelial cadherin extracellular domain affect adhesion and clustering of the protein and modulate endothelial permeability. Blood 2001; 97:1679–1684.
37. Blankesteijn WM, van Gijn ME, Essers-Janssen YP, et al. Betacatenin, an inducer of uncontrolled cell proliferation and migration in malignancies, is localized in the cytoplasm of vascular endothelium during neovascularization after myocardial infarction. Am J Pathol 2000; 157:877–883.
38. Antony VB, Loddenkemper R, Astoul P, et al. Management of malignant pleural effusions. Eur Respir J 2001; 18:402–419.
39. Dejana E. Endothelial adherens junctions: Implications in the control of vascular permeability and angiogenesis. J Clin Invest 1996; 98:1949–1953.
40. Antony V, Kamal M, Godbey S, et al. Talc induced pleurodesis: Role of basic fibroblast growth factor (bFGF). Eur Respir J 1997; 10:403S.

3
Respiratory Function in Pleural Effusion

IOANNA MITROUSKA and DIMITRIS GEORGOPOULOS
University of Crete and University Hospital of Heraklion, Heraklion, Crete, Greece

The pleural space is approximately 10 to 20 μm wide and encompasses the area between the mesothelium of the parietal and visceral pleura (the two layers of the pleura) (1). The pleural space actually contains a tiny amount of fluid (0.3 mL/kg body mass) with a low concentration of protein (~1 g/dL). The surface pressure of the visceral pleura together with alveolar pressure set the transpulmonary pressure, while the surface pressure of the parietal pleura sets the transthoracic pressure (2). These surface pressures usually differ from the pleural liquid pressure due to the presence of contacts between the lung and chest wall and the additional distortions that result (3,4). In upright humans, the vertical gradient of pleural surface pressure is approximately 0.25 cm H_2O/cm height, whereas within the liquid column the gradient is somewhat greater (~1 cm H_2O/cm height) (5). In normal humans, the difference between surface and liquid pleural pressure is relatively small in the bottom of the lung and increases higher up, with liquid pressure becoming more negative than surface pressure.

The pressures of the pleural space are important determinants of the mechanical properties of the lung and chest wall, and thus, of the total respiratory system (6). This is because the distending pressure of the lung and chest wall is critically dependent on the relevant pressures of the pleural space (7). Any distortion of the pressures of pleural space affects the distending pressures of the lung and chest wall and thus the relevant volumes, which in turn influences the gas exchange properties of the lung via several mechanisms (8). It follows that pleural effusion, which alters both the liquid and surface pleural pressures affects the mechanical properties of the respiratory system as well as the gas exchange properties (9).

Interpretation of the effects of pleural effusion on the respiratory system is rather complicated for several reasons. First, it is difficult to find and study patients with "pure" pleural effusion without lung disease. Second, the validity of esophageal pressure measurement in patients with pleural disease is questionable (10,11). Indeed, in the presence of pleural effusion, esophageal pressure might not reflect pressure of the pleural space, and thus the calculation of transpulmonary and transthoracic pressures may be misleading. In which case measuring mechanical properties of respiratory system is complicated. Third, data from studies that use animal models of pleural effusion may not be applicable in humans, because there are considerable differences in pleural anatomy between species (12). All these factors should be taken into account when the effects of pleural effusion on respiratory system function are considered.

I. Theoretical Considerations

A pure increase in the amount of fluid in the pleural space causes an increase in pleural pressure (surface and liquid). This increase results in an alteration in distending pressures of chest wall and lung. The distending pressure of the chest wall increases while that of the lung decreases. As a result, all else being the same, the volume of chest wall and lung is increased and decreased, respectively (13). It follows that with pleural effusion an uncoupling between the volume of lung and chest wall occurs; the volume of chest wall is no longer equal with that of the lung, a situation that is broadly similar to that encountered in pneumothorax. The differences between these two conditions are mainly due to the enhanced gravitational gradient of pleural pressure due to the presence of liquid and the fact that the pleural effusion usually does not occupy the entire pleural space, creating local alteration in pleural pressure. Nevertheless, although above the effusion normal pleural pressure may apply, there would still be a tendency toward chest wall enlargement because of the rib cage stability, which would be opposed by the lung elastic recoil. Theoretical considerations predict that pleural effusion should cause a restrictive ventilatory defect characterized by a reduction in vital capacity, functional residual capacity, and total lung capacity.

Accumulation of fluid in the pleural space may also affect the function of respiratory muscles mainly because of an increase in chest wall volume. The force–length relationship of respiratory muscles dictates that for a given neural activation the pressure developed by the muscles decreases with a decrease in their length (14). An increase in chest wall volume decreases the length of inspiratory muscles, mainly that of the diaphragm, and increases the length of expiratory muscles. It follows that with pleural effusion, all else being the same, for a given neural activation, pressure developed by the inspiratory and expiratory muscles should decrease and increase, respectively.

The above analysis is oversimplified because it ignores the secondary effect of pleural effusion on the pressure–volume (P–V) curve of the chest wall and lung and the interaction between the two hemithoraces. However, it is useful as a framework to explain the animal and human data regarding the effects of pleural effusion on respiratory system.

Gas exchange properties of the lung may be also affected by pleural effusion. The decrease in functional residual capacity (FRC) may force the lung volume at the end of expiration to operate near or even below the closing volume, a situation clearly associated with hypoxemia (15–18). This should be further aggravated by assuming the supine position (15–17,19). Finally, under certain circumstances large pleural effusion may impede the filling of the right heart, and by decreasing the cardiac output an exaggerated effect of ventilation/perfusion inequalities and right to left shunt on PO_2 occurs (20–22).

II. Respiratory System Mechanics

The effect of pleural effusion on respiratory system mechanics may be studied either by instillation of fluid into the pleural space or by removing fluid from pleural space. Obviously, the first method is used in animals, while the second is the only practical way to study pleural effusion effects in humans (23–30).

Animal data indicate that a pure increase in the amount of fluid in the pleural space causes an increase and a decrease in the chest wall and lung volumes, respectively.

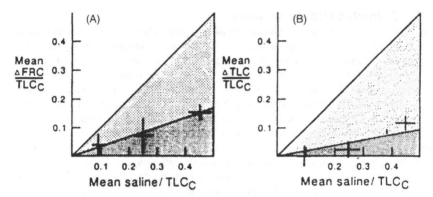

Figure 1 Changes in lung volume with saline effusions in a dog model of pleural effusion. (A) Decrease in functional residual capacity as a function of saline volume added to pleural space (mean±SD). The change in FRC and the volume of saline were expressed as a fraction of control total lung capacity (Δ FRC/TLCc and saline/TLC$_c$, respectively). (B) Similar graph for mean decrease in total lung capacity (Δ TLC/TLC$_c$) as a function of saline volume added to pleural space (saline/TLC$_c$). Line delineating stippled area, line of identity. Because sum of decrease in lung volume and increase in chest wall volume must equal added saline volume, light stippled area represents increase in chest wall volume for each value of saline. Increase of chest wall volume would be overestimated by amount equal to volume of intrathoracic blood displaced by addition of saline. Decrease in lung volume is about one-third and increase in chest wall volume is about two-thirds the added saline volume. Note change in lung volume is about one-fifth the volume of saline added. *Source*: From Ref. 27.

Krell and Rodarte (27) have shown in head-up dogs that lung volume decreased by about one-third the saline volume added to the pleural space at FRC and one-fifth at total lung capacity (TLC) (Fig. 1). Consequently, chest wall volume increased by two-thirds at FRC and four-fifths at TLC. The pressure–volume curve showed an apparent increase in lung elastic recoil and a decrease in chest wall elastic recoil with the addition of saline. These authors further showed that the reduction in lung volume was mainly due to a reduction in lower lobe with minimal change in upper lobe volume. As a result, an increase of the vertical gradient in regional lung volumes with increasing effusion volumes was observed. These results indicate that pleural effusion produces a nonuniform alteration in pleural pressure, which in turn affects the regional lung and chest wall volumes.

The static changes induced by pleural effusion may also alter the dynamic properties of respiratory system. Dechman et al. (25) infused normal saline into the pleural space of dogs and using multiple regression analysis calculated dynamic elastance and resistance of respiratory system, lung, and chest wall. Pleural effusion caused a marked increase in respiratory system elastance and resistance due to alteration in dynamic properties of the lung, while the dynamic elastance and resistance of the chest wall decreased. Similar results have been observed by Sousa et al. in rats (29). The changes in dynamic properties of the lung were partially reversed by deep inflation, suggesting that airway closure may be an important determinant of these alterations (25). These secondary effects of pleural effusion on lung function should be considered when therapy is planned for patients.

Several studies in humans have examined the effects of pleural effusion on respiratory system function (8,23–27). The interpretation of the results, however, is complicated mainly due to the underlying lung diseases. Indeed, it has been found that pleural effusion is not always associated with an increase in pleural pressure. Light et al. (31) measured directly pleural pressure in a large number of patients with pleural effusion and observed values between -21 and $+8$ cm H_2O. In a subsequent study, the same group showed that the increase in vital capacity as a result of removing an amount of pleural fluid was related to the initial value of pleural pressure as well as with its change during aspiration; a markedly negative initial pressure or a large change during aspiration was associated with a relatively small increase in vital capacity (VC) (28). These results presumably may be explained by the underlying disease, which caused a poorly compliant lung. Pleural thickening and the resulting low chest wall compliance may also underlie the observed changes in some patients. These findings have also been confirmed by other investigators (24,32).

Notwithstanding the difficulties in separating the effects of pleural effusion from those of the underlying diseases, several studies have shown that aspiration of pleural fluid is associated with increases in static lung volume, which are less than the volume of fluid removed (24,26,32). This observation indicates that pleural effusion causes a decrease in lung volume and a chest wall expansion in accordance with the theoretical prediction. Estenne et al. (32) measured respiratory mechanics two hours after removal a mean fluid volume of 1800 mL and observed that mean total lung capacity, vital capacity, and FRC increased by 640, 300, and 460 mL, respectively. They also demonstrated that the static pressure–volume curve of the lung was shifted upward and to the left, so for a given lung volume elastic recoil pressure was lower after thoracentesis (Fig. 2). Therefore, it appears that pleural effusion may alter the lung compliance. Decompression of the lung with reopening of some air spaces and a decrease in the surface tension of the alveolar lining fluid layer due to breathing at higher lung volumes are the most plausible mechanisms that mediate the change in lung compliance. Gilmartin et al. (26) studied seven patients for 24 hours after removal of pleural fluid (0.8–2.5 L) and observed that in addition to static lung volume increase, FEV_1 was also increased. Furthermore, they analyzed the forced flow–volume curves and the obtained information indicated that the lung emptied slightly faster in the presence of effusion. Indeed, the time constant of forced expiration derived from the slope of expired volume–flow relationship was significantly less before aspiration. The authors explained this finding by accepting that pleural effusion reduces the number of functioning compliant lung units, while airway size remains inappropriate large for the reduced lung volume. This assumption is in accordance with the results of Estenne et al. (32), who found that pleural effusion has an effect on lung compliance. Animal data also indicate that pleural effusion, apart from the changes in static lung volume, may also have secondary effects on lung mechanics (27).

In a landmark study, Anthonisen and Martin (23) used ^{133}Xe gas distribution and studied regional lung volume and ventilation in patients with small-to-moderate sized pleural effusion and no evidence of other respiratory system disease. Although regional lung volume at the base with the effusion was reduced, lung expansion at the site of effusion did not differ from that of the other side. These results suggest that at least with small-to-moderate sized pleural effusion, the lung may actually float on the effusion rather

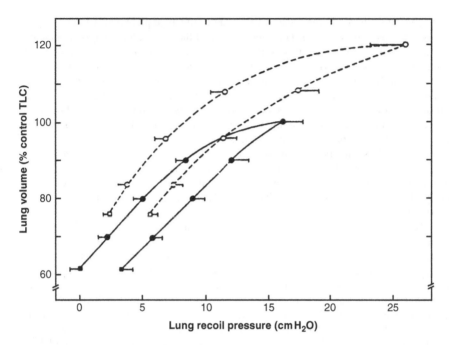

Figure 2 Static inspiratory and expiratory pressure–volume curve of the lung before (*closed circles*) and after (*open circles*) thoracentesis. Lung volume was expressed as a percentage of total lung capacity (TLC) before thoracentisis. The squares indicate the position of functional residual capacity. Each bar represents ±SE. *Source*: From Ref. 32.

than be compressed. It appears that the amount of pleural effusion may be a critical factor for the observed change in respiratory system mechanics.

III. Respiratory Muscles

The effect of pleural effusion on respiratory muscle function has been studied by Estenne et al. (32). They measured minimal pleural pressure–volume curves obtained during static maximal inspiratory efforts at different volumes before and after removal of pleural fluid and found that for a given lung volume, pleural pressure was approximately 20 cm lower after thoracentesis (Fig. 3). This finding indicates that either the power of inspiratory muscles increased or their efficiency improved. The authors estimated the change in chest wall volume following the fluid aspiration and observed that if minimal pleural pressure was related to chest wall volume, the pressures generated by the inspiratory muscles before and after thoracentesis fall on the same curve (Fig. 4). These results strongly suggest that pleural effusion, by increasing the chest wall volume, decreases the length of inspiratory muscles and thus reduces their effectiveness. The effects of pleural effusion on expiratory muscles are not known, but according to the above results, it is reasonable to conclude that in the presence of pleural effusion the efficiency of expiratory muscles would probably be increased.

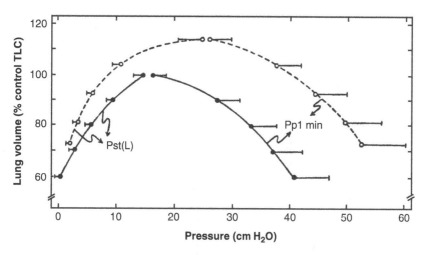

Figure 3 Pressure–volume of lung recoil pressure [Pst(L)] and maximal static inspiratory pleural pressure (Pp1 min) versus lung volume, before (*closed circles*) and after (*open circles*) thoracentesis. Lung volume was expressed as a percentage of total lung capacity (TLC) before thoracentesis. Each bar represents ±SE. *Source*: From Ref. 32.

IV. Gas Exchange

Although pleural effusion is thought to contribute to hypoxemia (33), studies in humans have demonstrated contradictory results (34). Oxygenation has been shown to improve, remain unchanged, or even worsen after thoracentesis (34,35). The underlying lung disease and the occurrence of interstitial edema due to reexpansion of the lung after thoracentesis complicates the interpretation of these results. In an attempt to resolve this issue, Nishida et al. (18) created graded increasing bilateral pleural effusion in anesthetized pigs. At each pleural volume, intravascular volume was altered to normal, low, or high to investigate the interaction between oxygenation, hemodynamics, and pleural effusion. They observed that pleural effusion caused an acute decrease in PaO_2 the magnitude of which depended on the volume of pleural effusion. The hypoxemia was mainly due to calculated intrapulmonary right-to-left shunt, which increased proportionally to the volume of the instilled pleural fluid (Fig. 5). At highest volume of pleural effusion, mixed venous O_2 was reduced, and this may also contribute to hypoxemia, particularly in the presence of increased shunt. All these changes were reversed by aspirating the pleural fluid without any evidence of hysteresis. The intravascular volume status did not appear to influence PaO_2 significantly. Although this model has several limitations, these data suggest that even moderately sized pleural effusions may be an important contributor to arterial hypoxemia, particularly in the presence of respiratory failure. It is possible that under these circumstances removal of the pleural fluid either by thoracentesis or by using negative fluid balance could have potential benefits in term of oxygenation. Talmor et al. (36) inserted a chest tube in a subset of mechanically ventilated patients with acute respiratory failure and pleural effusion who had a poor response to positive end-expiratory pressure (PEEP) and observed that oxygenation and respiratory system compliance improved immediately after chest tube drainage. These results should be interpreted with caution, however. The risk:benefit

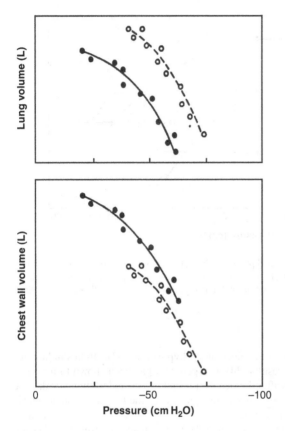

Figure 4 Proposed mechanism of the more negative pleural pressures generated by the inspiratory muscles after removal of 1500 mL of pleural fluid. Total lung capacity increased by 350 mL after fluid removal. *Closed circles* represent data obtained before thoracentesis; *open circles* represent data obtained after thoracentesis. In the top panel, pleural pressures are expressed as a function of lung volume; in the bottom panel, they are expressed as a function of total chest wall volume. *Source*: From Ref. 32.

ratio of this procedure is not well established. Furthermore, several studies in patients with acute respiratory distress syndrome (ARDS) have shown that mortality, the main outcome variable, is not related to the level of hypoxemia (37). It has been suggested that improvement in oxygenation may be a cosmetic effect. At present, insertion of a chest tube is not recommended as routine procedure in these patients. In selected patients with large pleural effusion and refractory hypoxemia, in whom other measures to increase oxygenation have failed, chest tube drainage may be beneficial.

Agusti et al. (38) used the multiple inert gas elimination technique (MIGET) (39) to study the distribution of ventilation–perfusion ratios as well as the effects of thoracentesis in patients with pulmonary effusion. The results of this study showed that

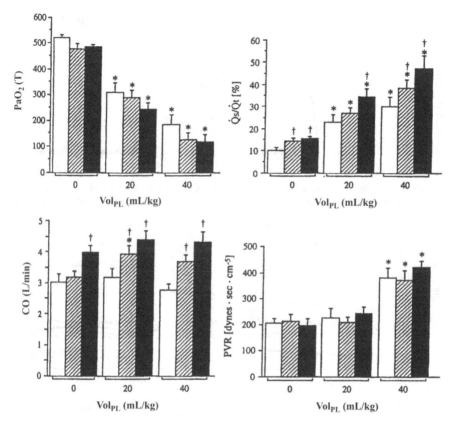

Figure 5 Effects of intrapleural volume (Vol_{PL}) and intravascular volume (Vol_{vasc}) on PaO_2 (*top left*), calculated intrapulmonary shunt (Qs/Qt) (*top right*), cardiac output (CO) (*bottom left*), and pulmonary vascular resistance (PVR) (*bottom right*) in a pig model of pleural effusion. Open bars, low Vol_{vasc}; hatched bars, normal Vol_{vasc}; solid bars, high Vol_{vasc}. *$p < 0.05$ vs. $Vol_{PL} = 0$ mL/kg. †$p < 0.05$ vs. low Vol_{vasc}. *Source*: From Ref. 18.

the intrapulmonary shunt was the main mechanism underlying arterial hypoxemia, in line with the animal data (18). Withdrawing approximately 700 mL of pleural fluid caused a significant decrease in pleural pressure (from 3.6 to −7.1 cm H_2O) without a significant effect on PaO_2, shunt, and alveolar–arterial difference for PO_2 (Figs. 6 and 7). A significant, although small, increase in blood flow perfusing low V/Q' units was observed after thoracentesis, indicating that either some degree of lung reexpansion or acute interstitial pulmonary edema occurred as a result of pleural pressure decrease. Nevertheless, despite the relatively large pleural fluid drainage, the changes in gas exchange properties of the lung were quite small, suggesting that the effects of pleural effusion on oxygenation indices are longlasting, possibly due to delayed pulmonary volume reexpansion after fluid drainage (24,40,41) with or without the coexistence of ex vacuo pulmonary edema (41–43).

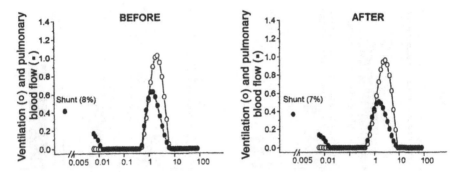

Figure 6   Distribution of ventilation–perfusion (VA/Q) ratios in representative patient, before (*left panel*) and after (*right panel*) thoracentesis studied with the MIGET technique. *Source*: From Ref. 38.

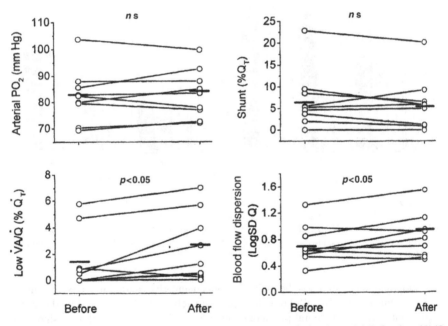

Figure 7   Individual (*open circles*) and mean (*solid bars*) values of arterial PaO_2, low VA/Q ratios, shunt, and blood flow dispersion before and 30 minutes after draining pleural effusion by thoracentesis. *Source*: From Ref. 38.

The effect of pleural effusion on cardiac function, although beyond the scope of this review, deserves some comments. It has been shown in dogs that large pleural effusion may compromise the right heart function by inducing diastolic collapse of the right ventricle, which is associated with a decrease in cardiac output (44). This condition is similar to cardiac tamponade. This may aggravate hypoxemia, particularly in the presence of increased right-to-left shunt. It is of interest to note that this complication may occur when pleural pressure is about 4 cm H_2O, a value frequently seen in patients (21). Indeed, compromised cardiac function documented by echocardiography has been reported in patients with large pleural effusion (22). Therapeutic thoracentesis may be lifesaving in these patients by increasing both cardiac output and oxygenation (32).

V. Conclusion

The accumulation of pleural fluid causes a restrictive ventilatory effect. Pure pleural effusion is associated with chest wall volume expansion, and this reduces the efficiency of inspiratory muscles. Drainage of pleural fluid usually results in an increase in static lung volume, which is considerably less that the amount of aspirated fluid. Pleural effusion is invariably associated with hypoxemia due to an increase in right-to-left shunt, effect that an at least in humans, is not readily reversible upon fluid aspiration.

References

1. Light RW. Anatomy of the pleura. In: Light RW, ed. Pleural Diseases. Vol. 1. Philadelphia, PA: Lippincot Williams & Wilkins, 2001:1–7.
2. Light RW. Physiology of the pleural space. In: Light RW, ed. Pleural Diseases. Vol. 1. Philadelphia: Lippincot Williams & Wilkins, 2001:8–20.
3. Agostoni E. Mechanics of the pleural space. Resp Physiol 1972:57–128.
4. Lee KF, Olak J. Anatomy and physiology of the pleural space. Chest Surg Clin North Am 1994; 4:391–403.
5. Milic-Emili J, Henderson JAM, Dolovich MB, et al. Regional distribution of inspired gas in the lung. J Appl Physiol 1966; 21:749–759.
6. Fenn WO. The pressure–volume diagram of the breathing mechanism. In: W BM, ed. Respiratory Physiology in Aviation: Rundolph Field. USAF School of Aviation Medicine, 1954: 19–27.
7. Ward ME RC, Macklem PT. Respiratory mechanics. In: Murray JF, ed. Textbook of Respiratory Medicine. Vol. 1. Philadelphia, PA: WB Saunders, 1994:90–138.
8. Lai-Fook SJ, Rodarte JR. Pleural pressure distribution and its relationship to lung volume and interstitial pressure. J Appl Physiol 1991; 70:967–978.
9. Agostoni E, D'Angelo E. Pleural liquid pressure. J Appl Physiol 1991; 71:393–403.
10. Milic-Emili JMJ, Turner JM, Glauser EM. Improved technique for estimating pleural pressure from esophageal balloons. J Appl Physiol 1964; 19:207–211.
11. Villena V, Lopez-Encuentra A, Pozo F, et al. Measurement of pleural pressure during therapeutic thoracentesis. Am J Respir Crit Care Med 2000; 162:1534–1538.
12. Tenney SMBDF. Comparative mammalian respiratory control. In: Cherniak NSWJ, ed. The Respiratory System. Vol. 2. Bethesda, MD: American Physiological Society, 1986: 833–855.
13. Agostoni EHER. Static behavior of the respiratory system. A FP, ed. Handbook of Physiology. Vol. 3. Bethesda, MD: American Physiological Society, 1986:113–130.
14. Younes M, Riddle W. A model for the relation between respiratory neural and mechanical outputs. I. Theory. J Appl Physiol 51:963–978.
15. Craig DB, Wahba WM, Don HF, et al. "Closing volume" and its relationship to gas exchange in seated and supine positions. J Appl Physiol 1971; 31:717–721.
16. Blair EHJ. The effect of change in body position on lung volume and intrapulmonary gas mixing in normal subjects. J Clin Invest 1955; 34:383–398.
17. Kaneko K, Milic-Emili J, Dolovich MB, et al. Regional distribution of ventilation and perfusion as a function of body position. J Appl Physiol 1966; 21:767–777.

18. Nishida O, Arellano R, Cheng DC, et al. Gas exchange and hemodynamics in experimental pleural effusion. Crit Care Med 1999; 27:583–587.
19. Neagley SR, Zwillich CW. The effect of positional changes on oxygenation in patients with pleural effusions. Chest 1985; 88:714–717.
20. Negus RA, Chachkes JS, Wrenn K. Tension hydrothorax and shock in a patient with a malignant pleural effusion. Am J Emerg Med 1990; 8:205–207.
21. Kisanuki A, Shono H, Kiyonaga K, et al. Two-dimensional echocardiographic demonstration of left ventricular diastolic collapse due to compression by pleural effusion. Am Heart J 1991; 122:1173–1175.
22. Kaplan LM, Epstein SK, Schwartz SL, et al. Clinical, echocardiographic, and hemodynamic evidence of cardiac tamponade caused by large pleural effusions. Am J Respir Crit Care Med 1995; 151:904–908.
23. Anthonisen NR, Martin RR. Regional lung function in pleural effusion. Am Rev Respir Dis 1977; 116:201–207.
24. Brown NE, Zamel N, Aberman A. Changes in pulmonary mechanics and gas exchange following thoracocentesis. Chest 1978; 74:540–542.
25. Dechman G, Sato J, Bates JH. Effect of pleural effusion on respiratory mechanics, and the influence of deep inflation, in dogs. Eur Respir J 1993; 6:219–224.
26. Gilmartin JJ, Wright AJ, Gibson GJ. Effects of pneumothorax or pleural effusion on pulmonary function. Thorax 1985; 40:60–65.
27. Krell WS, Rodarte JR. Effects of acute pleural effusion on respiratory system mechanics in dogs. J Appl Physiol 1985; 59:1458–1463.
28. Light RW, Stansbury DW, Brown SE. The relationship between pleural pressures and changes in pulmonary function after therapeutic thoracentesis. Am Rev Respir Dis 1986; 133: 658–661.
29. Sousa AS, Moll RJ, Pontes CF, et al. Mechanical and morphometrical changes in progressive bilateral pneumothorax and pleural effusion in normal rats. Eur Respir J 1995; 8: 99–104.
30. van Noord JA, Demedts M, Clement J, et al. Effect of rib cage and abdominal restriction on total respiratory resistance and reactance. J Appl Physiol 1986; 61:1736–1740.
31. Light RW, Jenkinson SG, Minh VD, et al. Observations on pleural fluid pressures as fluid is withdrawn during thoracentesis. Am Rev Respir Dis 1980; 121:799–804.
32. Estenne M, Yernault JC, De Troyer A. Mechanism of relief of dyspnea after thoracocentesis in patients with large pleural effusions. Am J Med 1983; 74:813–819.
33. Mattison LE, Coppage L, Alderman DF, et al. Pleural effusions in the medical ICU: Prevalence, causes, and clinical implications. Chest 1997; 111:1018–1023.
34. Dobyns EL. Pleural effusions and hypoxemia. Crit Care Med 1999; 27:472.
35. Chang SC, Shiao GM, Perng RP. Postural effect on gas exchange in patients with unilateral pleural effusions. Chest 1989; 96:60–63.
36. Talmor M, Hydo L, Gershenwald JG, et al. Beneficial effects of chest tube drainage of pleural effusion in acute respiratory failure refractory to positive endexpiratory pressure ventilation. Surgery 1998; 123:137–143.
37. Luhr OR, Karlsson M, Thorsteinsson A, et al. The impact of respiratory variables on mortality in non-ARDS and ARDS patients requiring mechanical ventilation. Intensive Care Med 2000; 26:508–517.
38. Agusti AG, Cardus J, Roca J, et al. Ventilation–perfusion mismatch in patients with pleural effusion: Effects of thoracentesis. Am J Respir Crit Care Med 1997; 156:1205–1209.
39. Evans JW, Wagner PD. Limits on V A/Q distributions from analysis of experimental inert gas elimination. J Appl Physiol 1977; 42:889–898.
40. Perpina M, Benlloch E, Marco V, et al. Effect of thoracentesis on pulmonary gas exchange. Thorax 1983; 38:747–750.

41. Doerschuk CM, Allard MF, Oyarzun MJ. Evaluation of reexpansion pulmonary edema following unilateral pneumothorax in rabbits and the effect of superoxide dismutase. Exp Lung Res 1990; 16:355–367.
42. Trapnell DH, Thurston JG. Unilateral pulmonary oedema after pleural aspiration. Lancet 1970; 1:1367–1369.
43. Brandstetter RD, Cohen RP. Hypoxemia after thoracentesis. A predictable and treatable condition. JAMA 1979; 242:1060–1061.
44. Vaska K, Wann LS, Sagar K, et al. Pleural effusion as a cause of right ventricular diastolic collapse. Circulation 1992; 86:609–617.

4

Imaging of the Pleura

THERESA C. MCLOUD
Department of Radiology, Massachusetts General Hospital, Boston, Massachusetts, U.S.A.

GERALD F. ABBOTT
Rhode Island Hospital, Providence, Rhode Island, U.S.A.

KATERINA MALAGARI
Medical School of University of Athens, Athens, and Department of Radiology,
Attikon University Hospital, Haidari, Athens, Greece

I. Introduction

A variety of imaging techniques can be used to evaluate the pleura and the pleural space. Standard radiographs are the most common. Sonography, computed tomography, and magnetic resonance imaging (MRI) have assumed an increasing and important role in the diagnosis of pleural disease. This chapter will discuss a variety of diffuse and focal pleural processes and the contribution of each of these imaging techniques to diagnosis and management of pleural disease.

II. Pleural Effusion

Pleural effusions develop when an imbalance occurs in the rates of pleural fluid production and resorption. Clinically, pleural effusions are classified as transudates or exudates by analysis of their specific gravity and determination of their protein and lactic acid dehydrogenase (LDH) content (1). Transudates are commonly bilateral and develop due to physical factors that affect the rate of pleural fluid formation and resorption (e.g., increased hydrostatic pressure, decreased osmotic pressure). Exudates occur when the pleura is pathologically altered with associated impairment of lymph flow or increase in permeability.

Pleural effusion has many causes, the most frequent being (in order of decreasing incidence) left ventricular failure (CHF), pneumonia, malignancy, pulmonary embolism, cirrhosis, pancreatitis, collage vascular disease, and tuberculosis.

On chest radiographs of erect subjects, a moderate-size pleural effusion typically manifests as a homogeneous lower-zone opacity with a well-defined curvilinear upper border and concave surface abutting the lung. Free pleural fluid may extend into the interlobar fissures and produce opacities that vary with the shape and orientation of the fissure and the direction of the X-ray beam (2). Focal collections within fissures may form mass-like opacities ("pseudotumor") (Fig. 1). Incomplete interlobar fissures may manifest as curvilinear sharp interfaces in the presence of pleural effusions (3) (Fig. 2). Focal accumulation of fluid at the lateral aspect of the minor fissure produces the thorn

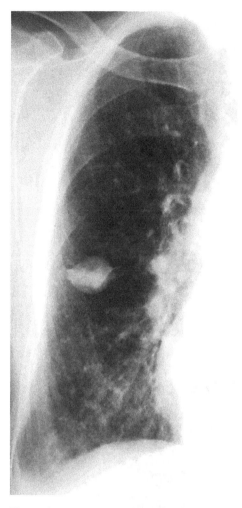

Figure 1   Pseudotumor. PA chest radiograph (detail) demonstrates an elliptical opacity in the right hemithorax with tapering medial and later margins that merge with the minor fissure.

sign, formed by converging concave interfaces extending medially from the lateral pleural surface to form a thorn-like point (4).

Small effusions may not be apparent on PA and lateral radiographs. Lateral decubitus views may detect as little as 5 mL of fluid (5). Ultrasonography and CT are also more sensitive than the chest radiograph in detecting small pleural effusions and may reveal septations and loculations suggestive of an exudate. Transudates are typically anechoic on ultransonography and without associated pleural thickening. Exudates are often associated with pleural thickening and ultrasonography may also demonstrate septation, stranding, and adjacent parenchymal lung disease. CT may be useful in detecting and characterizing effusions as free or loculated, differentiating pleural from parenchymal

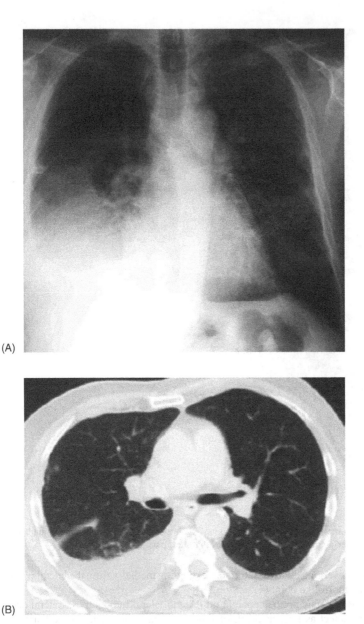

(A)

(B)

Figure 2 Incomplete interlobar fissures. (**A**) PA radiograph demonstrates a right pleural effusion that obscures the lower half of the hemithorax and forms a sharply defined curvilinear interface in the perihilar region. (**B**) CT (lung window) shows pleural effusion extending into an incomplete interlobar fissure.

disease, and facilitating percutaneous biopsy (5,6). Sonography facilitates all the above and offers the ability to guide for thoracocentesis (7).

Large effusions may opacity the entire hemithorax and characteristically produce contralateral shift of the mediastinal structures (Fig. 3). Right-sided large pleural effusions may present a mediastinal convex opacity to the left on frontal plain films that corresponds

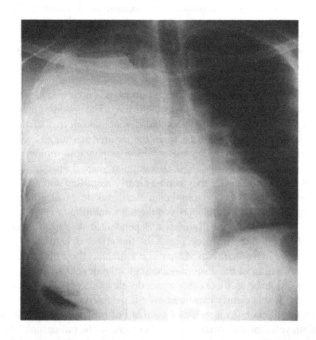

(A)

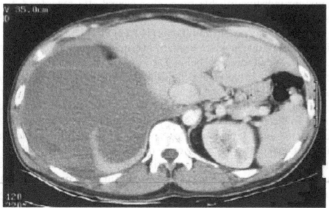

(B)

Figure 3 Hemothorax. (**A**) PA radiograph demonstrates opacification of the right hemithorax with shift of the mediastinal structures to the contralateral side, inferomedial displacement of the right mainstem bronchus, and inferolateral displacement of gas within the hepatic flexure of the colon. (**B**) CT demonstrates a large pleural effusion that inverts the right hemidiaphragm.

with a herniation of the azygoesophageal recess to the left side (8). Large, left-sided pleural effusion may invert the diaphragm, which on plain films is recognized by the displacement of gastric and colonic gaz. Right-sided inversion is infrequent due to the support and resistance from the liver. Inversion of the diaphragm may simulate an abdominal mass, which may lead to paradoxic diaphragmatic movement or pendulum breathing (8,9).

Occasionally, effusions may accumulate in a subpulmonic location and produce unique imaging features. The convex upper edge of a subpulmonic effusion mimics the contour of the hemidiaphragm. The apparent hemidiaphragm appears "elevated" with the peak of its convexity shifted laterally. The fluid is usually mobile and will relocate to the most dependent part of the pleural space on lateral decubitus radiographs (10).

Loculated effusions do not present a gravity-dependent distribution but rather an "atypical" distribution. On plain films, they are better defined when viewed tangentially to the X-ray beam with a well-defined boarder, convex to the lung. The opacities they produce have characteristically greater height than length and different maximum diameters on the frontal and lateral view. When loculated effusions in the fissures are due to heart failure, they come and go, hence resulting in the characterization as phantom tumors. They are best recognized in the lateral view of the chest as lenticular-shaped opacities along the course of the involved fissure(s). On CT, they can be clearly identified and again there is a difference in the posteroanterior and horizontal diameters, and clear margins to the lung are seen with the exception of passive atelectasis of the adjacent lung.

Pleural effusion in the supine position has a dependent distribution layering out posteriorly. On plain films, a hazy diffuse opacity of the affected hemithorax is seen that does not obliterate the lung markings. Other signs include the obliteration of the diaphragmatic contour, blunting of the costophrenic angle, the development of an apical cap (requires at least 500 mL to be seen), or cause a pseudo-elevation of the hemidiaphragm of the affected side. On CT, it is clearly identified even if measuring a few ccs.

Hemothorax usually occurs as a result of trauma but may be a manifestation of coagulopathy, infection, vascular abnormalities, or other causes. The radiographic features of acute hemothorax are indistinguishable from other pleural effusions. On CT, acute collections may show areas of hyperintensity. Subsequently, loculations may form and extensive pleural thickening may occur (fibrothorax) (11,12).

Empyema is defined and diagnosed by a variety of criteria including grossly purulent fluid, positive gram stains or cultures, a pH below 7 or a glucose level less than 40 mg/mL, and a white blood cell count in the pleural fluid greater than 5×10^9 cells/L. Most empyemas are associated with pneumonia, surgery, trauma, or an infectious process occurring below the diaphragm. Empyemas evolve through exudative, fibrinopurulent, and organizing stages. In the early exudative stage, empyemas are indistinguishable from noninfectious pleural effusions. Empyemas that progress to the fibrinopurulent stage tend to form loculations, and ultrasonography often demonstrates septations within such collections. The final, organizing stage is characterized by extensive pleural thickening ("peel"), which encases the lung. In this advanced stage, there may be communication with the lung (bronchopleural fistula) or the fluid may drain through the chest wall (empyema necessitatis) (11,12).

The fibrinopurulent effusions of empyema have a tendency to loculate and will not fall to the most dependent portion of the pleural cavity on radiographs taken in various positions. Such fixed collections typically manifest as oval, lenticular, or round opacities. The margins of these collections are sharply defined when in profile to the X-ray beam, but some margins may be indistinct or imperceptible. Air–fluid levels may be apparent on the chest radiograph if a bronchopleural fistula is present. The appearance of air–fluid levels in abscesses and empyema differ. Typically, a lung abscess is spherical in shape, and if an air–fluid interface is demonstrated within the abscess, it will appear roughly equal in length on orthogonal radiographic views. By contrast, empyemas are often lenticular forming obtuse angles with the chest wall. An air–fluid interface within an empyema will often be disparate in length on orthogonal radiographs, for example, demonstrating a short length on a frontal radiograph and a longer length on a lateral radiograph (13). When multiple air–fluid levels are demonstrated in an empyema, they may extend across lung zones that would normally be interrupted, in the case of parenchymal diseases, by the presence of interlobar fissures (Fig. 4).

Ultrasound and CT are the most useful modalities for demonstrating and characterizing empyema and may be useful in providing guidance for percutaneous drainage. Ultrasound often demonstrates septations within such collections. The septations may be so extensive as to preclude tube thoracostomy (12) (Fig. 5).

CT does not demonstrate septations within an empyema but is a very useful tool in defining the extent of such collections and may help in distinguishing pleural collections from lung abscesses. One of the most useful and specific signs is the demonstration of a "split pleura" which is noted on contrast-enhanced studies. The thickened pleura appears uniform in thickness, with smooth inner and outer margins. The thickened parietal and visceral pleurae brightly enhance and are separated by the pleural fluid collection (Fig. 6).

Pleural effusions can be distinguished from abdominal ascites by several CT criteria. On axial CT images, pleural effusion will lie peripheral to the diaphragm and displace the crus medially; ascites will manifest as fluid density bounded laterally by the diaphragm.

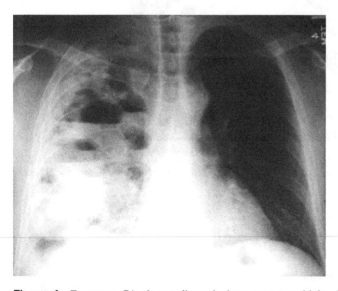

Figure 4 Empyema. PA chest radiograph demonstrates multiple air–fluid levels extending throughout the right hemithorax. The numerous air–fluid levels do not appear to be impeded by interlobar fissures, a feature suggesting their location in the pleural space.

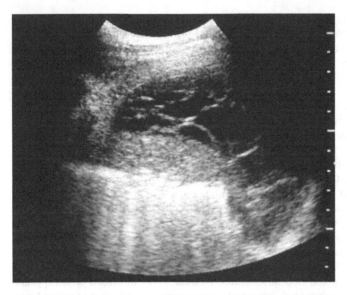

Figure 5   Empyema with septations. Ultrasound demonstrates multiple septations within a loculated empyema.

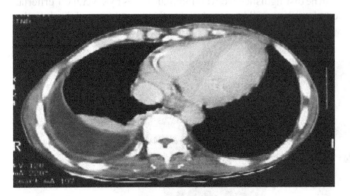

Figure 6   Empyema with "split pleura" sign. Contrast-enhanced CT demonstrates uniformly thickened visceral and parietal pleura separated by a pleural fluid collection in the posterolateral aspect of the right hemithorax.

Furthermore, the surface of the bare area of the liver will be obscured by ascites, but unaffected by pleural effusion (14–17) (Fig. 7).

III.   Pneumothorax

Pneumothorax is an abnormal collection of air in the pleural space. In contradistinction to free pleural effusions, which gravitate to the most dependent portions of the involved thorax, air will rise to the most nondependent portion of the thorax unless pleural adhesions

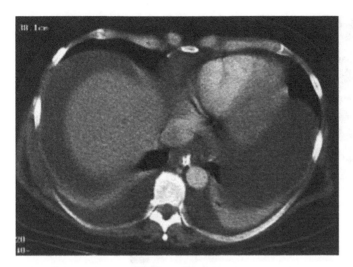

Figure 7 Pleural effusion and ascites. CT demonstrates ascites and bilateral pleural effusions. The pleural effusions, shown in the posterior costophrenic sulci, are "outside" of (posterior to) the hemidiaphragm and displace the diaphragmatic crura anteromedially. Ascites lies "within" the diaphragmatic contours and obscures the hepatic surface.

obliterate the pleural space. In the erect subject, such air collections characteristically manifest as abnormal lucency in the pulmonary apex displacing the sharp well-defined visceral pleural line. Although lung medial to the visceral pleura collapses to a various degree, it presents no increased density unless it loses approximately 90% of its volume (in the absence of a preexisting parenchymal process). This is most likely due to the development of hypoxic vasoconstriction in healthy lung (18). In addition, in large pneumothoraces, the affected hemithorax increases in size since the negative intrapleural pressure does not withhold it and the ipsilateral hemidiaphragm is depressed to a various degree depending on the decrease of the transdiaphragmatic pressure gradient (Figs. 2 and 3).

In films obtained in supine position—most common in the ICU—radiological signs reflect the distribution of free air in the nondependent pleural spaces (19). These include the anterior costophrenic sulcuses, the space between the medial surface of the lung and anterior mediastinum, and the ventral subpulmonic space (19). Due to this anteromedial distribution, the pleural line may not be visualized (not aligned tangentially with the X-ray beam) unless the visceral pleura detachment extends laterally (Fig. 1). Plain film signs of pneumothorax in the supine ICU patient include (a) hyperlucency of the lower hemithorax and hemidiaphragm (air collection in the anterior costophrenic sulcus) associated with an exceptionally sharp diaphragmatic contour (Fig. 3) (19); (b) low position and/or flattening of the hemidiaphragm (air in the anterior costophrenic sulcus) (Figs. 3 and 8) (19); (c) the double diaphragm sign visualized as two interfaces, one cephalad outlining the diaphragmatic dome and the other caudally outlining the anterior attachment of the affected hemidiaphragm (air in the anterior costophrenic sulcus) (Fig. 4) (19); (d) the deep sulcus sign (air in the anterior and lateral costophrenic sulcuses)

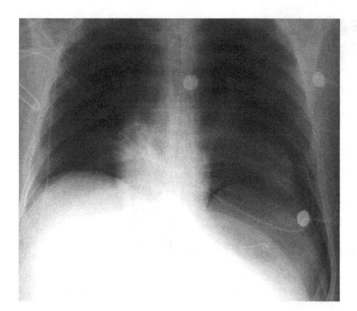

Figure 8 Deep sulcus sign. AP chest radiograph of a supine patient demonstrates abnormal lucency overlying the left hemidiaphragm and extending into the left costophrenic sulcus which appears "deep" in comparison with the contralateral sulcus.

seen as an exceptionally deep lateral costophrenic sulcus (Figs. 4 and 5) (20); (e) a black halo around the cardiac boarder (air anteromedially) (Fig. 6) (19); and (f) the apical fat tag sign (air outlining pericardial fat) (Fig. 1) (21). In this setting, the presence of pneumothorax can be confirmed by decubitus or upright chest radiographs (22). However, in the critically ill cervical spine precautions, skeletal injuries and sedation may not allow performance of decubitus views, especially in the trauma setting.

High-frequency linear ultrasound (US) has been recently introduced for the detection of pneumothorax (23,24). It is a rapid, radiation free, widely available test that can be applied at the bedside and therefore quite suitable for the ICU environment. Sonographic signs of pneumothorax include (*i*) absence of "lung sliding" which refers to the absence of the to-and-fro movement of the visceral and parietal pleurae during respiration; (*ii*) the comet-tail sign or artefact, seen as closely arranged echoes arising from the pleural line spreading downwards; and (*iii*) broadening of the pleural line to a band (Fig. 7) (21–25). It is suggested that thoracic US should be added to the currently performed focused abdominal sonography for trauma—FAST—examination (expanded FAST examination) (26).

> *Atypical pneumothorax* represents pneumothorax assuming a distribution not expected by intrapleural pressures and gravity and in which the lung contour does not preserve its normal shape. Pleural adhesions are the most common cause and may be seen on plain films or CT as linear or band-like structures tethering the partially collapsed lung to the chest wall (Fig. 8) (18).

Tension pneumothorax is a medical emergency that may occur particularly in the mechanically ventilated patient and is present when the intrapleural pressure is positive throughout the respiratory cycle. Radiologically, it is visualized as the combined presence of (a) collapsed lung, (b) contralateral mediastinal shift, (c) flattening or inversion of hemidiaphragm, and (d) enlargement of the ipsilateral hemithorax (27) (Fig. 9). However, the last three of the above signs may be present in most moderate-to-large pneumothoraces due to the release of the effect of negative intrapleural pressure (2). The key radiological feature of tension pneumothorax is lung collapse (18,27); a partially inflated lung indicates

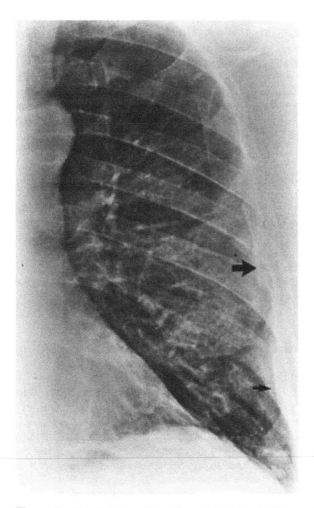

Figure 9 Pleural plaques. PA radiograph (left lung) shows multiple pleural plaques (arrows). They are interrupted, smooth areas of pleural thickening with sharp margins paralleling the chest wall.

that pneumothorax is not under tension with the exception of stiff lungs in adult respiratory distress syndrome (ARDS), extensive pneumonia, and the rare setting in which bronchial obstruction with a valve mechanism coexist. Therefore, in ARDS tension pneumothorax should be considered in any patient whose hemodynamic status deteriorates in the presence of high airway pressures (18,27,28).

A. Radiological Quantitation

A number of methods have been developed based on plain film measurements that apply only to frontal chest roentgenograms with the patient erect (29,30). The only paper that applies in supine frontal views available in ICU has been released by Choi et al. who developed a mathematical formula of quantification using the interpleural distances at the apex and lateral surface of the lung (31). However, in their study, they had no standard of reference such as CT. Overall, all these methods are somehow arbitrary representing only a rough approximation and individual clinical evaluation is needed (32).

Accurate quantitative measurements of pneumothorax can be made by planimetric or volumetric computerized tomography techniques. Visual CT quantification is also feasible and consistent and can be integrated in clinical practice guidelines; using this method in trauma subjects, Wolfman et al. found that pneumothoraces of small or moderate size may be treated conservatively provided that patients are not under assisted ventilation (33). In their paper, pneumothoraces were classified as small when seen as thin collections of air of a maximum 1-cm thickness that extend to no more than four consecutive slices and moderate, defined as air collections of more than 1 cm in thickness not extending beyond the mid coronal line, seen in four or more consecutive slices (33). The value of ultrasound in the assessment of the magnitude of pneumothorax is still restricted to animal models in both ground-based and microgravity conditions (24).

IV. Focal Pleural Disease

Focal pleural abnormalities include asbestos-related pleural plaques, localized pleural tumors, and direct invasion of the pleura by lung carcinoma.

A. Pleural Plaques

Pleural plaques are the most common manifestations of asbestos exposure. They are localized collection of dense collagenous connective tissue (34,35). They serve as a marker of exposure and may be seen with brief or slight exposure.

Generally, plaques do not appear until 20 or more years after initial exposure (36,37). In and of themselves they do not produce any symptoms and they are often incidentally discovered at the time of the chest radiograph. Pleural plaques are usually localized to the posterior and lateral aspects of the pleura. They tend to spare the lung apices and costophrenic angles. They arise from the parietal pleura but occasionally can be seen in the visceral pleura in the interlobar fissures (35,38). In approximately 25% of cases plaques are unilateral (39–41).

The chest radiograph is the principle imaging modality for the detection of asbestos-related pleural plaques. Plaques appear as localized, limited, plateau-like, smooth, and nodular areas of pleural thickening (Fig. 9) (36,32–44). On a posteroanterior (PA) radiograph, a well-developed pleural plaque has either a "profile" or en face presentation

(36–44). A plaque seen in profile appears as a sharply marginated, dense band of soft tissue density, ranging from 1 to 10 mm in thickness, paralleling the inner margin of the lateral thoracic wall. Plaques are usually bilateral, often symmetric, and more prominent in the lower half of the thorax between the 6th and 9th ribs (36,42–44). When seen en face, a pleural plaque appears as a faint, ill-defined, veil-like opacity with irregular edges (36,45).

In addition to the standard PA chest radiograph, oblique views are helpful not only to confirm suspected pleural plaques, but also to detect additional plaques unsuspected on the PA projection (36,46).

Pleural calcification generally does not develop until at least 20 years after exposure to asbestos; however, it is most frequently seen after 30 to 40 years. Calcification usually occurs in localized pleural plaques but may also occur in diffuse pleural thickening. Calcifications can be identified along the chest wall, diaphragm or cardiac border. They are often small and are easily overlooked unless systematically sought after. When viewed en face, they have an irregular unevenly dense pattern likened to the fringe of a holly leaf (Fig. 10) (36,44).

The diagnostic accuracy of radiography in the detection of pleural plaques depends upon the disease prevalence in the sample population and the presence or absence of

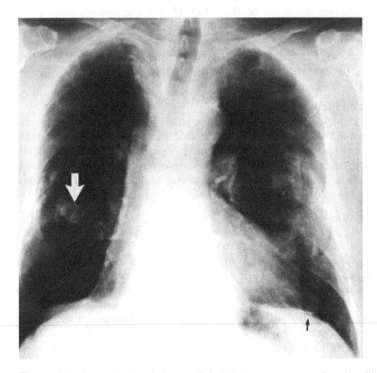

Figure 10 Calcified pleural plaques. Calcified plaques are seen along the diaphragm and chest wall (black arrow). En Face plaques appear as dense geometric opacities superimposed on the lung parenchyma (white arrow).

calcification (35,39,47). With the use of criteria recommended by the International Labor Office (ILO) (48), classification of the pneumoconioses, the sensitivity of radiography for the detection of pleural plaques ranges from 30% to 80% and the specificity ranges from 60% to 80% (35,39,41,49–51). The low specificity of chest radiography in the diagnosis of pleural plaques is related to the difficulty in distinguishing plaques from normal muscle, fat, and companion shadows of the chest wall (11,52). Radiological findings that are suggestive of extrapleural fat are a bilateral location along the mid-lateral chest wall and a symmetric distribution (53).

CT has been shown to be more sensitive in the detection of pleural plaques than standard radiography (54–56). Both the demand for and the cost of CT, as well as the radiation dosage, make it an unrealistic choice as a screening examination in persons who have been exposed to asbestos. However, it can be extremely helpful in differentiating pleural plaques from lung nodules and in resolving equivocal findings on standard radiographs (Fig. 11) (6). The lack of superimposition of structures and the greater contrast resolution of CT and particularly high-resolution CT, allow improved sensitivity in the detection of pleural abnormalities and easy distinction of plaques from extrapleural fat (35). To assess the reliability of CT in detecting discrete pleural lesions, De Raeve et al., using CT, examined 100 asbestos workers with an exposure of more than 10 years and small pleural lesions. They found a good intra-observer agreement (k: 0.68), but fair-to-moderate inter-observer agreement (k: 0.26–0.45) (57). These findings suggest that there is a potential lack of consistency in reporting small pleural abnormalities caused by asbestos exposure.

Pleural plaques on CT appear as circumscribed areas of pleural thickening separated from the underlying rib and extrapleural soft tissues by a thin layer of fat (35).

B. Localized Pleural Tumors

Focal pleural tumors include fibrous tumors of the pleura, lipomas, liposarcomas, and localized invasion of the pleura by lung carcinoma. Occasionally, malignant pleural disease such as malignant mesothelioma and pleural metastases may cause focal abnormalities but they are more commonly associated with diffuse pleural disease. The visualization of bone erosion next to a pleural tumor is diagnostic of malignancy. Most localized pleural tumors with the exception of invasive lung cancer are relatively uncommon.

Fibrous Tumors of the Pleura

Fibrous tumors of the pleura are the most common focal pleural tumors, although they are generally an uncommon neoplasm and account for less than 5% of all pleural tumors (58). These tumors have a peak incidence over the age of 50 and are seen with equal frequency in men and women. They are not related to asbestos exposure (59). Fibrous tumors arise from submesoepithelial mesenchymal cells and from the visceral pleura in about 20% (60,61). Approximately 60% of these tumors are considered benign and 40% are malignant (59). However, both the benign and malignant varieties are associated with long survival after surgical resection (35,59). The malignant variety is characterized by the presence of pleural effusion and occasional chest wall invasion and the tendency to recur after surgical resection. Diagnosis is confirmed by histology; the fibrous acellular nature of these tumors makes the samples obtained by percutaneous biopsy difficult to assess, and surgical sample is imperative (60,61). Approximately 40% of localized pleural fibromas are attached to the visceral pleura by a pedicle (59–61). These tumors may reach

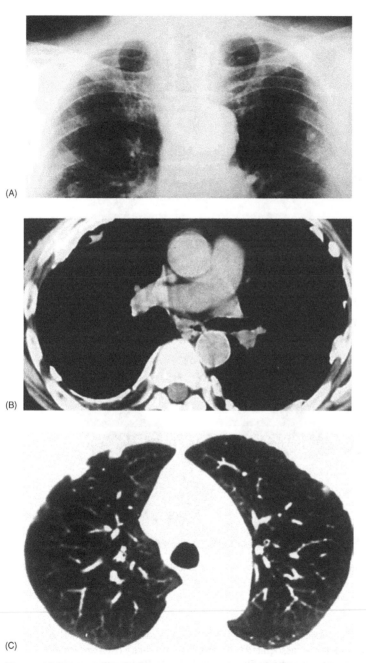

Figure 11   Pleural plaques simulating pulmonary nodules. Patient with long smoking history and asbestos exposure: (**A**) Cone down view of upper thorax demonstrates multiple modular opacities. (**B,C**) CT scan shows multiple plaques seen "en face" on the standard radiograph. Most are calcified.

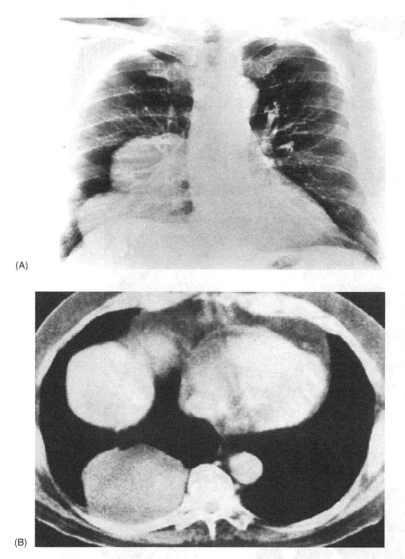

(A)

(B)

Figure 12   Fibrous tumor of the pleura. (**A**) Large elliptical mass filling most of the lower half of the right chest. (**B**) CT demonstrates a partially enhancing mass abutting the pleura but without an obtuse angle with the chest wall.

enormous size and tumors as large as 40 cm have been reported (11,59–61). These tumors may have a high incidence of associated hypertrophic pulmonary osteoarthopathy (60,62) and hypoglycemia is present in 4% to 5% of cases (59–62). Radiographic findings include a well-delineated mass which may form obtuse angles with the chest wall and mediastinum and which displaces the adjacent lung parenchyma (Fig. 12). Frequently the upper edge of the lesion may tend to fade into the lung parenchyma. If the lesion has a pedicle, it may be mobile and change position with different patient posture (11,35,63). These lesions may also occur in the interlobar fissures.

CT findings include a well-delineated often-lobulated soft tissue mass in close relation to the pleural surface (36). Although an obtuse angle of the mass with respect to the pleural surface may not be identified in every case, a smoothly tapering margin is characteristic and may indicate a pleural location (Fig. 12). Calcification is present in 5% of cases. The differential diagnosis of a calcified mass of the pleura also includes metastatic disease from osteosarcoma, chondrosarcoma, mucinous adenocarcinoma, parosteal osteosarcoma, and calcification-ossification of a mesothelioma (64–66). Displacement of adjacent lung parenchyma with compressive atelectasis and bowing of the bronchi and pulmonary vessels around the mass is often noted. Enhancement of the tumor following administration of contrast material is frequent and may be homogenous or heterogenous (67–71). In the malignant variety of this tumor, CT may demonstrate local invasion of the chest wall with associated rib destruction. Larger lesions of 10 cm or greater in diameter are more likely to be malignant.

MRI may be helpful in the diagnosis of these lesions. In cases in which there is a fairly high collagen content, fibrous tumors of the pleura may exhibit low single intensity on both T1- and T2-weighted images and enhancement with intravenously administered gadolinium contrast agent (71) (Fig. 13). This is in contradistinction to most tumors, which will demonstrate increased signal intensity on T2-weighted images because of high water content.

Pleural Lipoma and Liposarcoma

Pleural lipomas and liposarcomas are rare tumors (72–75). Lipomas are usually asymptomatic and are discovered incidentally on chest radiographs. A definitive diagnosis is usually not possible on standard films. However, CT clearly delineates the pleural origin of these lesions and their fatty composition in the majority of cases (−50 to −150 Houndsfield units) (Fig. 14) (76). Benign lipomas have completely uniform fatty density although linear soft tissue strands due to fibrous stroma may be present. On the other hand, thymolipomas, angiolipomas, and teratomas are characterized by islands of soft-tissue density interspersed with fat (77,78). Liposarcomas can be easily differentiated from lipomas by a higher and heterogenous density (79).

Lipomas may be totally intrathoracic, that is, within the ribs, or transmural with extension into the chest wall (72). Pleural lipomas on MR scanning can be identified readily by their signal characteristics. Such lesions are of bright signal intensity on T1-weighted images and also moderately bright on T2-weighted images. However, CT is usually diagnostic, and MRI is not required for diagnosis.

Local Extension of Lung Cancer

Lung cancers that invade the parietal pleura and chest wall are designated as T3 tumors and are potentially resectable. Surgical treatment, however, requires en bloc resection of the pulmonary malignancy and the contiguous chest wall and is associated with slightly increased morbidity and mortality (80). In selecting patients as operative candidates, it may be desirable to determine preoperatively whether chest wall invasion is present. The value of CT scanning in the determination of chest wall invasion is limited. The only CT findings with high positive predictive values are bone destruction adjacent to the lung mass or obvious extension of the mass beyond the ribs into the chest wall (81). Pleural thickening contiguous to the tumor is a nonspecific finding and may be caused by local fibrous adhesions or invasion of the parietal pleura by tumor. Inspiratory and expiratory

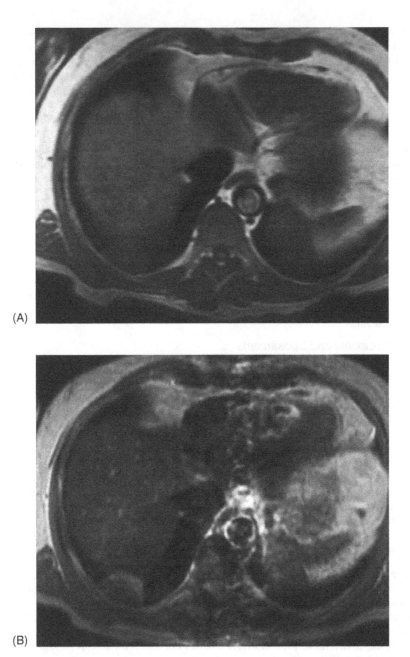

(A)

(B)

Figure 13 (Electronic) MRI fibrous tumor of the pleura. (**A**) T1-weighted image demonstrates a posterior inferior mass of low signal intensity. (**B**) T2-weighted image. The mass exhibits mostly low signal intensity.

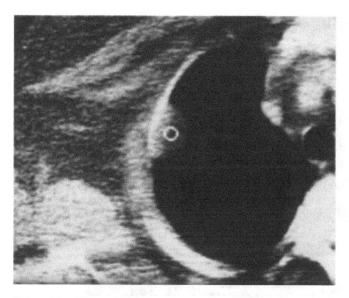

Figure 14 (Electronic) Lipoma. Well-defined peripheral mass of homogenously low attenuation (H.U. = −60).

CT scans have been used to evaluate respiratory shift (i.e., a change in the relative location between the peripheral lung tumor and the chest wall during respiration). The presence of such a shift is a reliable indicator of the lack of parietal pleural invasion by tumor in the lower half of the chest (82). MRI has a slight advantage over CT in the evaluation of chest wall invasion (Fig. 15). T1- and T2-weighted sequences may show direct tumor extension and the yield is improved with the use of gadolinium contrast (83).

Other Rare Conditions

Other causes of localized pleural masses include lymphoma, fibrin bodies, thoracic splenosis, endometriomas, and amyloidomas. Primarily pleural lymphomas are rare and include primary effusion lymphoma (PEL) and pyothorax-associated lymphoma (PAL), and are mostly described as case reports in the literature (84–87). Lymphoma of mucosa-associated lymphoid tissue (EMZL/MALTtype) of primary pleural location has also been reported (85).

V. Diffuse Pleural Disease

Pleural thickening on plain films—when seen tangentially—is visualized as soft tissue opacities adjacent to the ribs or angular blunting of the costophrenic sulci. Apical opacities should be differentiated from an apical cup. In the presence of apical pleural the study of the boarders with the lung are suggestive of the underlying condition. If pleuroparenchymal involvement is present like in tuberculous scaring or fibrobullous chest disease, the boarders to the lung are irregular. Irregular boarders presenting a difference of 1 cm in thickness compared to the contralateral side should raise the suspicion of a Pancoast tumor and further examinations are needed to exclude it.

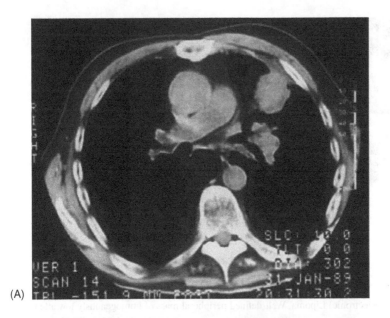

(A)

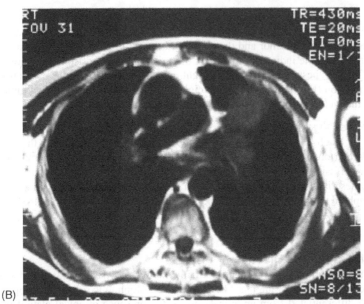

(B)

Figure 15 (Electronic) Lung cancer invading chest wall. (**A**) CT scan demonstrates a peripheral mass with adjacent pleural thickening. CT is indeterminate for chest wall or parietal pleural thickening. (**B**) T1-weighted images demonstrates tongue like extensions of low signal intensity due to tumor invading the extrapleural fat of the chest wall.

A. Fibrothorax

Fibrothorax or diffuse pleural thickening involving most of the pleural space may develop as the result of previous hemothoraces, tuberculous effusions, and other types of empyema, benign asbestos pleurisy, and occasionally other processes.

The definition of diffuse pleural thickening by McLoud et al. (88) is diffuse pleural thickening on chest radiographs as "a smooth, non-interrupted pleural density extending over at least one-fourth of the chest wall" associated or not with costophrenic blunting. On CT scans, Lynch et al. (42) defined diffuse pleural thickening as "a continuous sheet of pleural thickening more than 5-cm wide, more than 8 cm in craniocaudal extent, and more than 3-mm thick." Diffuse pleural thickening is well studied with CT and MRI (89).

Diffuse pleural thickening is often associated with a decrease in volume of the ipsilateral lung. Bilateral pleural thickening may be associated with a severe restrictive defect on pulmonary functioning testing (90).

Diffuse pleural thickening secondary to asbestos exposure is seen less frequently than pleural plaques. It is characterized by uniform homogenous density with smooth contours and frequently by obliteration of the costophrenic angle (Fig. 16) (36,46,91).

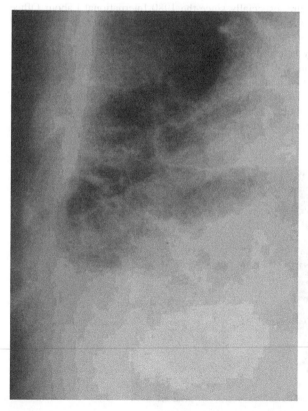

Figure 16 Asbestos pleural thickening. There is diffuse pleural thickening on the right which is smooth and extends to the costophrenic angle. The underlying lung is involved with asbestosis.

Diffuse pleural thickening is most often the result of a previous benign asbestos effusion and as with pleural plaques does not require high levels of exposure (36,92).

Asbestos-related pleural thickening usually involves the visceral pleura and is frequently associated with restrictive lung function (34,93). Gevenois et al. studied with CT-exposed subjects but with subtle signs and found that CT signs could be grouped into three patterns (*i*) septal and intralobular lines, and honeycombing corresponding to pulmonary fibrosis; (*ii*) pleural plaques corresponding to parietal pleural fibrosis; and (*iii*) diffuse pleural thickening, rounded atelectasis, and parenchymal bands corresponding to visceral pleural fibrosis (90). The authors conclude that the association of parenchymal bands and diffuse pleural thickening in the same cluster of findings suggests that parenchymal bands reflect visceral pleural fibrosis rather than interstitial fibrosis. Copley et al. in their study (93) found a reverse relationship of pleural thickening with the FVC, however, the reduced carbon monoxide diffusing capacity of their patients indicates that the reported correlations also bear a component of lung fibrosis (56).

By contrast to pleural plaques, which are considered highly specific for asbestos, pleural thickening is less specific occurring in a number of conditions affecting the pleura. These issues are of great importance when the question is whether pleural disease is a result of occupational exposure, especially since the 1980 International Labour Office (ILO) classification, which did not distinguish between lesions located on the visceral from those on the parietal pleura.

CT may be extremely helpful in both the identification of diffuse pleural thickening and its characterization (Fig. 17). Characteristics of fibrothorax include smoothly contoured pleural thickening without nodularity, thickness of less than 1 cm and lack of involvement of the mediastinal pleura (Fig. 17) (94). CT may also be useful in determining the etiology of fibrothorax. For example, evidence of underlying parenchymal disease is often seen in patients who have had previous tuberculosis (11,35). If pleural

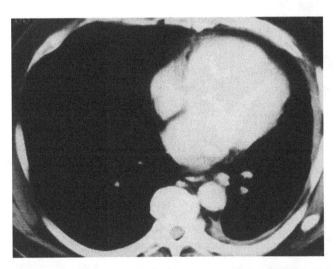

Figure 17   Fibrothorax. CT demonstrates diffuse, smooth pleural thickening with 3 mm in thickness involving the lateral and posterior pleura.

calcification is extensive, it favors previous tuberculosis, hemothorax or empyema. Calcification may be seen in asbestos pleural thickening, but is less common (95). Diffuse asbestos pleural thickening, although most frequently unilateral, may be associated with pleural abnormalities on the opposite side such as pleural plaques.

CT may also be helpful in determining the extent of pleural thickening and to evaluate the underlying parenchyma, particularly in patients with asbestos exposure where the pleural thickening prevents adequate parenchymal lung evaluation (96). CT can eliminate superimposition of opacities, thus allowing better evaluation of the lung parenchyma in the presence of asbestos pleural disease.

B. Pleural Findings Postpleurodesis

Radiological signs of pleurodesis include diffuse pleural thickening and localized effusions. In the pleurodesis group, Avila et al. reported pleural thickening in 65%, effusion in 13%, loculated effusion in 11%, areas of high attenuation in 23%, and mass in 14% (97). Areas of high attenuation were present in all types of pleurodesis (mechanical, 8%; chemical, 13%; talc, 40%). Pleural masses were present in patients who had all types of pleurodesis (mechanical, 10%; chemical, 9%; talc, 24%). The masses commonly enhanced and did not change in size over time. Pleural masses after pleurodesis are difficult to differentiate from mesothelioma (98,99).

C. Pleural Calcification

Pleural calcification virtually always coexists with pleural thickening. It is seen in postinfectious conditions, that is, tuberculous or nontuberculous empyema, hemothorax, asbestos exposure, and calcified metastatic disease from osteosarcoma, chondrosarcoma, mucinous adenocarcinoma, parosteal osteosarcoma, or calcification-ossification of a mesothelioma (65,66). Postempyema calcifications develop in both layers of the pleura. Calcification in asbestos exposure is greater in the diaphragmatic pleura. Empyema-related calcification may be associated with a persistent fluid collection and may be suspected when the two layers of calcification have a distance of more than 2 cm. Re-infection of encapsulated pleural effusions may be suspected when in serial films the distance of the two layers of the pleura increases.

VI. Malignant Pleural Disease

A. Malignant Mesothelioma

Malignant mesothelioma is a rare primary malignant tumor of the pleura. The majority of affected patients (80%) have a history of occupational exposure to asbestos. However, household members and population near to asbestos mines and plants are also at risk for the development of mesothelioma. Occupations with the greatest risk include shipyard work, building construction and demolition, brake-lining manufacture, and heating trades. Approximately 2000 to 3000 new cases of mesothelioma occur in the United States each year (100). There is a latency period of 35 to 40 years after initial exposure for the development of malignant mesothelioma (101). Affected patients are usually in the sixth to eighth decades of life and males are more frequently affected than females by a ratio of approximately 4:1 (102). In a small number of patients, mesothelioma follows radiation therapy, chronic pleural inflammation or exposure to chemical carcinogens (103).

Patients typically present with insidious onset of symptoms, often occurring six to eight months prior to the diagnosis. Patients often complain of chest pain but may also have dyspnea, cough, and weight loss.

Histologically, mesotheliomas are usually divided into three categories: epitheloid, sarcomatoid, and biphasic (mixed). The epitheloid variety is most common and may be difficult to distinguish histologically from metastases to the pleura (104). On gross inspection, tumor involves the parietal pleura more extensively than the visceral layer, often forming sheet-like coalescent tumor masses that may encase the lung and extend into interlobar fissures.

The prognosis of malignant mesothelioma is poor with a median survival of approximately 10 months. Selected patients may undergo extrapleural pneumonectomy, a radical procedure associated with significant morbidity and mortality (105,106). The current staging system for mesothelioma is the International Mesothelioma Interest Group, which defines criteria to assess local extent of the tumor and lymph node involvement (107,108). CT is accurate for most tumor staging and MRI is valuable improving detection of tumor extension to chest wall and diaphragm, while PET is used for evaluation of lymph-node involvement and distant metastasis (109,110).

The characteristic radiographic feature of mesothelioma is unilateral diffuse, irregular, and nodular pleural thickening with or without an associated pleural effusion. Associated asbestos-related pleural disease (e.g., pleural plaques) occurs in 20% to 25% of cases. Mediastinal shift towards the involved hemithorax as a result of tumor encasement and volume loss may be identified. Alternatively, massive tumor bulk and large pleural effusions may produce contralateral shift of the mediastinum. Pleural effusion may obscure tumor masses and be the sole or predominant radiographic finding (Fig. 18).

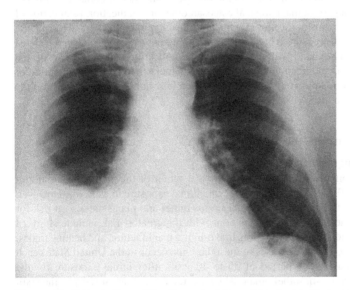

Figure 18 Mesothelioma. PA radiograph. A large right pleural effusion obscures the right lower hemithorax and its underlying involvement by malignant mesothelioma.

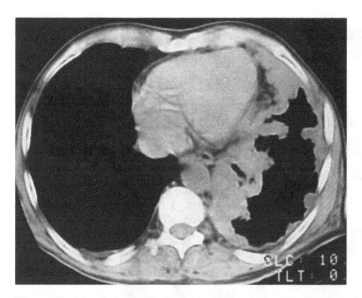

Figure 19 Mesothelioma. CT demonstrates extensive nodular pleural thickening which circumferentially involves the left hemithorax and extends into the medial and lateral aspects of the interlobar fissure anteriorly.

CT better characterizes tumor extent and morphology and may demonstrate focal or diffuse pleural masses, nodular pleural thickening, and fissural involvement. Involvement is typically circumferential with involvement of the mediastinal pleura and characteristically extends into the fissures. The cross-sectional imaging features of malignant mesothelioma are often indistinguishable from metastatic involvement of the pleura (111–113). Lobulated thickening of the pleural that exceeds 1 cm in thickness raises the suspicion of a mesothelioma. Loss of volume of the affected hemithorax is pronounced. Invasion of the chest wall, mediastinum, and diaphragm may be demonstrated by CT, but early invasion is often not apparent or may be underestimated (Fig. 19).

MRI may better characterize the invasive features of mesothelioma. Tumor typically manifests as minimally increased signal on T1-weighted images and moderately increased signal on T2. The multiplanar capabilities of MR may allow better detection and visualization of chest wall, mediastinal, and diaphragmatic extension of tumor and help predict respectability (Fig. 20) (113). Diffuse superficial spread of mesothelioma throughout the pleural space may be difficult to detect by any of the above modalities.

B. Epithelioid Hemangioendothelioma

Epithelioid hemangioendothelioma is a rare malignant tumor of vascular origin that usually arises in bone, liver, soft tissue, or lung. Pleural origin has been less frequently described (114,115). Pleural involvement has the worst prognosis; poor prognostic indicators include symptoms at presentation, lymphangitic spread of tumor, hepatic metastases,

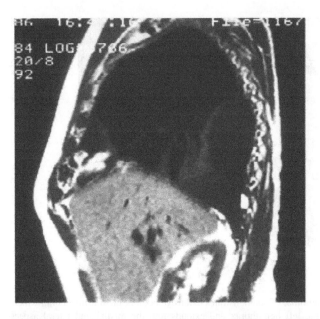

(A)

(B)

Figure 20 Mesothelioma. (**A**) Sagittal MR demonstrates a large mesothelioma posteriorly that does not appear to invade the chest wall or hemidiaphragm. (**B**) Coronal MR of a different patient shows extensive circumferential nodular pleural masses involving the entire right hemithorax and extending into the minor interlobar fissure.

and peripheral lymphadenopathy (114). It affects mostly elderly men. In the series of Crotty et al., the radiological presentation included pleural effusion, diffuse pleural thickening with volume loss of the affected hemithorax similar to those seen in mesothelioma. Signs of invasion of the diaphragm or mediastinal lymphadenopathy and combination thickened interlobular septa suggesting lymphangitic spread of tumor were seen in one-third of their cases (114). At presentation, 50% had multiple pulmonary nodules suggestive of metastatic that enlarged on subsequent examinations.

C. Metastases

Pleural metastases are the most common form of neoplastic involvement of the pleura. Most metastases are adenocarcinomas, typically arising from primary sites in the lung, breast, ovary, and stomach. Lymphomas may also involve the pleura. Metastatic tumor usually involves both the visceral and parietal pleura and often produces malignant pleural effusion (11).

On CT, metastases may manifest as marked thickening and nodularity of the pleura, usually with an associated pleural effusion. In some cases, the effusion may be large and tumor foci may be difficult to identify. Metastases may mimic malignant mesothelioma and the two entities cannot be reliably distinguished by cross-sectional imaging (Figs. 21 and 22) (95).

Finally, certain tumors such as malignant thymoma may produce focal seeding of the pleura. This is usually manifested on CT scanning as localized focal pleural nodules that may be bilateral or unilateral.

The differentiation of malignant from benign pleural thickening provides a challenge for the radiologist. There is overlap of the radiologic manifestations of benign and malignant pleural processes. Leung et al. in a study of 74 consecutive patients with proven diffuse pleural disease demonstrated that CT can play a major role in providing the distinction (94). Features that were helpful in distinguishing malignant from benign pleural disease included (a) circumferential pleural thickening, (b) nodular pleural thickening more than 1 cm in thickness, and (c) mediastinal pleural involvement, all of which occurred more consistently with malignant lesions. These features may be seen in mesothelioma and metastatic pleural disease but are unusual in benign pleural disease. The presence of pleural calcification also is suggestive of a benign process. In this study by Leung et al., calcification was seen in 6 of 35 patients with benign pleural thickening and only in 3 of 39 patients with malignant pleural disease (94). Although calcified pleural plaques may be seen in cases of mesothelioma, they are uncommon.

D. Thoracic Splenosis

Thoracic splenosis is a rare pathologic entity that may mimic pleural neoplasia. Affected patients have a history of thoracoabdominal trauma that ruptures and fragments the spleen. Splenic fragments may implant and grow on the adjacent peritoneal surfaces. With concomitant penetrating trauma to the diaphragm, splenic fragments may implant and grow along pleural surfaces in the lower aspect of the left hemithorax and manifest as multifocal pleural masses ranging in size from 3 to 7 cm (Fig. 23). The diagnosis may be confirmed by radionuclide scans using ^{99m}Tc sulfur colloid (116).

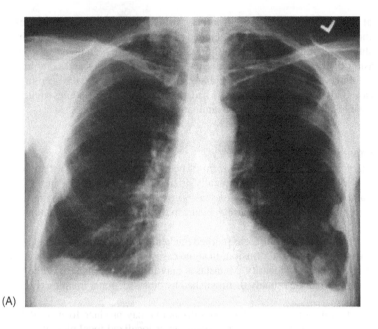

(A)

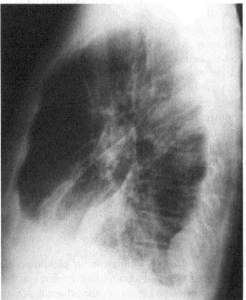

(B)

Figure 21   Pleural metastases (renal cell carcinoma). (**A, B**) PA and lateral radiographs demonstrate multiple areas of nodular pleural thickening that are greater than 1 cm and appear circumferential within the left hemithorax. Involvement of the mediastinal pleural is apparent in the medial aspect of the apical portion of the left hemithorax on the PA view.

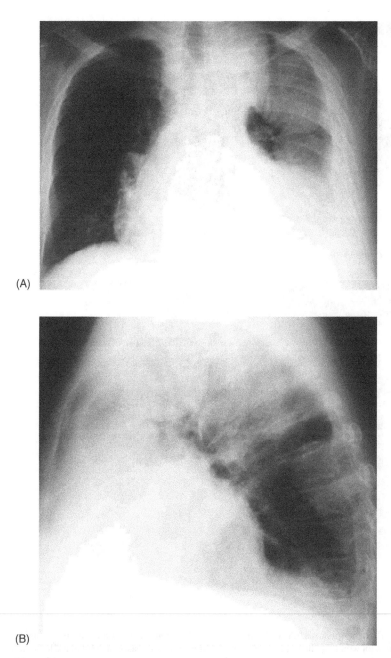

Figure 22 Pleural metastases (lymphoma). (**A, B**) PA and lateral radiographs demonstrate large, contiguous pleural masses in the left hemithorax with marked nodularity and extensive circumferential involvement. (**C**) CT demonstrates the pleural-based configuration of the masses with involvement of the mediastinal pleura and invasion of adjacent mediastinal structures.

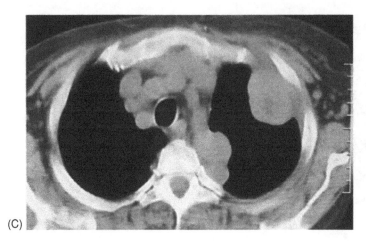

(C)

Figure 22 (*Continued*)

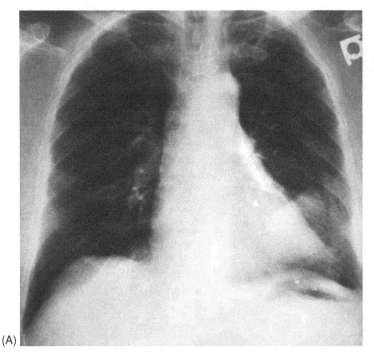

(A)

Figure 23 Thoracic splenosis. (**A, B**) PA and lateral radiographs demonstrate multiple radioden-sities from gunshot wound to the left lower chest. A posterior pleural-based opacity in the lower left hemithorax has incomplete margins on the lateral view, suggesting its extraparenchymal location. (**C**) CT shows two adjacent pleural-based masses posterolaterally in the lower left hemithorax. The diagnosis was confirmed by radionuclide scanning using ^{99m}Tc sulfur colloid (not shown).

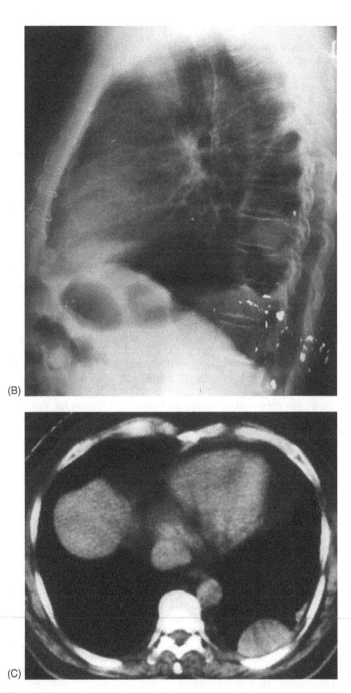

(B)

(C)

Figure 23 (*Continued*)

References

1. Light RW, MacGregor MI, Luchsinger PC, et al. Pleural effusions: The diagnostic separation of transudates and exudates. Ann Intern Med 1972; 77:507–513.
2. Raasch BN, Carsky EW, Lane EJ, et al. Pictorial essay: Pleural effusion; explanation of some typical experiences. Am J Roentgenol 1982; 139:899–904.
3. Heitzman ER. The Lung: Radiologic–Pathologic Correlations, 2nd ed. St Louis, MO: Mosby, 1984.
4. Oestreich AE, Haley C. Pleural effusion: The thorn sign. Chest 1981; 79:365–366.
5. Moskowitz H, Platt RT, Schachar R, et al. Roentgen visualization of minute pleural effusion: An experimental study to determine the minimum amount of pleural fluid visible on a radiograph. Radiology 1973; 109:33–35.
6. McLoud TC, Flowers CD. Imaging the pleura: Sonography, CT and MR imaging. Am J Roentgenol 1991; 156:1145–1153.
7. Yang PC, Luh KT, Chang DB, et al. Value of sonography in determining the nature of pleural effusion: Analysis of 320 cases. Am J Roentgenol 1992; 159:29–33.
8. Pantoha E, Kattan KR, Thomas HA. Some uncommon lower mediastinal densities: A pictorial essay. Radiol Clin North Am 1984; 22:633–646.
9. Mulvey RB. The effect of pleural fluid on the diaphragm. Am J Roentgenol 1965; 84:1080–1085.
10. Friedman RL. Infrapulmonary pleural effusions. Am J Roentgenol Radium Ther Nucl Med 1954; 71:613–623.
11. Fraser RS, Muller NL, Colman N, et al. Diagnosis of Diseases of the Chest, 4th ed. Philadelphia, PA: W. B. Saunders, 1999:2737–2840.
12. Naidich DP, Zerhouni EA, Siegelman SS. Pleura and chest wall. In: Naidich DP, Zerhouni EA, Siegelman SS, eds. Computed Tomography and Magnetic Resonance Imaging of the Thorax, 2nd ed. New York, NY: Raven-Lippincott, 1991:407–471.
13. Stark DD, Federle MP, Goodman PC, et al. Differentiating lung abscess and empyema: Radiography and computed tomography. Am J Roentgenol 1983; 141:163–167.
14. McLoud TC. The pleura and chest wall. In: Haaga JR, Lanzieri CF, Sartoris DJ, Zerhouni Ea, eds. Computed Tomography and Magnetic Resonance Imaging of the Whole Body. St Louis, MO: Mosby, 1994:772–787.
15. Dwyer RA. The displaced crus: A sign for distinguishing between pleural fluid and ascites on computed tomography. J Comput Assist Tomogr 1978; 2:598–599.
16. Griffin DJ, Gross BH, McCrackenn S, et al. Observation on CT differentiation of pleural and peritoneal fluid. J Comput Assist Tomogr 1984; 8:24–28.
17. Halvorsen RA, Fedyshin PJ, Korobkin M, et al. Ascites or pleural effusion? CT differentiation: Four useful criteria. Radiographics 1986; 6:135–149.
18. Armstrong P, Wilson A, Dee P, et al. Imaging of Diseases of the Chest, 4th ed. St Louis, MO: Mosby, 2007.
19. Tocino IM, Miller MH, Fairfax WR. Distribution of pneum othorax in the supine and semirecumbent critically ill adult. AJR Am J Roentgenol 1985; 144(5):901–905.
20. Gordon R. The deep sulcus sign. Radiology 1980; 136;25–27.
21. Lichtenstein D, Meziere G, Biderman P, et al. The comet tail artifact: An ultrasound sign ruling out pneumothorax. Int Care Med 1999; 25:383–388.
22. Chiles C, Ravin CE. Radiographic recognition of pneumothorax in the intensive care unit. Crit Care Med 1986; 14:677–680.
23. Dulchavsky SA, Schwarz KL, Kirkpatrick AW, et al. Prospective evaluation of thoracic ultrasound in the detection of pneumothorax. J Trauma 2001; 50:201–205.
24. Sargsyan AE, Hamilton DR, Nicolaou S, et al. Ultrasound evaluation of the magnitude of pneumothorax: A new concept. Am Surg 2001; 67(3):232–235.

25. Goodman TR, Trail ZC, Phillips AJ, et al. Ultrasound detection of pneumothorax. Clin Radiol 1999; 54:736–739.
26. Phillips GD, Trotman-Dickenson B, Hodson ME, et al. Role of CT in the management of pneumothorax in patients with complex cystic lung disease. Chest 1997; 112(1):275–278.
27. Light RW. Tension pneumothorax. Intensive Care Med 1994; 20(7):468–469.
28. Moss HA, Roe PG, Flower CD. Clinical deterioration in ARDS—An unchanged chest radiograph and functioning chest drains do not exclude an acute tension pneumothorax. Clin Radiol 2000; 55(8):637–639.
29. Collins CD, Lopez A, Mathie A, et al. Quantification of pneumothorax size on chest radiographs using interpleural distances: Regression analysis based on volume measurements from helical CT. AJR Am J Roentgenol 1995; 165(5):1127–1130.
30. Rhea JT, DeLuca SA, Greene RE. Determining the size of pneumothorax in the upright patient. Radiology 1982; 144(4):733–736.
31. Choi BG, Park SH, Yun EH, et al. Pneumothorax size: Correlation of supine anteroposterior with erect posteroanterior chest radiographs. Radiology 1998; 209(2):567–569.
32. Engdahl O, Toft T, Boe J. Chest radiograph—A poor method for determining the size of a pneumothorax. Chest 1993; 103(1):26–29.
33. Wolfman NT, Myers WS, Glauser SJ, et al. Validity of CT classification on management of occult pneumothorax: A prospective study. AJR Am J Roentgenol 1998; 171(5):1317–1320.
34. Schwartz DA. New developments in asbestos-related pleural disease. Chest 1991; 99:191–198.
35. Muller NL. Imaging the pleura. Radiology 1993; 186:297–309.
36. McLoud TC. Asbestos-related diseases: The role of imaging techniques. Postgrad Radiol 1989; 9:65–74.
37. Hillerdal G. Pleural plaques in a health survey material: Frequency, development and exposure to asbestos. Scand J Respir Dis 1978; 59:257–261.
38. Rockoff SD, Kagan E, Schwartz A, et al. Visceral pleural thickening in asbestos exposure: The occurrence and implications of thickened interlobar fissures. J Thorac Imaging 1987; 2: 58–66.
39. Gefter WB, Conant EF. Issues and controversies in the plain-film diagnosis of asbestos-related disorders in the chest. J Thorac Imaging 1988; 3:11–28.
40. Fisher MS. Asymmetric changes in asbestos-related disease. J Can Assoc Radiol 1985; 36:110–112.
41. Withers BF, Ducatman AM, Yang WN. Roentgenographic evidence for predominant left-sided location of unilateral pleural plaques. Chest 1984; 95:1262–1264.
42. Lynch DA, Gamsu G, Aberle DR. Conventional and high resolution computed tomography in the diagnosis of asbestos-related diseases. Radiographics 1989; 9:523–551.
43. Kim KI, Kim CW, Lee MK, et al. Imaging of Occupational Lung Disease 1. Radiographics 2001; 21:1371–1391.
44. Sargent EN, Boswell WD, Ralls PW, et al. Pleural plaques: A signpost of asbestos chest inhalation. Semin Roentgenol 1977; 12:287–297.
45. Anton HC. Multiple pleural plaques, Part III. BJ Radiol 1968; 41:341–348.
46. Sargent EN, Gordonson J, Jacobson G, et al. Bilateral pleural thickening: A manifestation of asbestos exposure. Am J Roentgenol 1978; 131:579–585.
47. Greene R, Boggin C, Jantsch H. Asbestos-related pleural thickening: Effect of threshold criteria on interpretation. Radiology 1984; 152:569–573.
48. International Labour Office. Guidelines for the Use of the ILO International Classification of Radiographics of Pneumoconioses, Revised Edition. International Labour Office Occupational Safety and Health Series, No. 22 (Revised 1980). Geneva, Switzerland: International Labour Office, 1980.

49. Schwartz DA, Fuortes LJ, Galvin JR, et al. Asbestos-induced pleural fibrosis and impaired lung function. Am Rev Resp Dis 1990; 141:321–325.

50. Wain SL, Roggli VL, Foster WL. Parietal pleural plaques, asbestos bodies, and neoplasia: A clinical, pathologic, and roentgenographic correlation of 25 consecutive cases. Chest 1984; 86:707–713.

51. Hourihane DO, Lessog L, Richardson PC. Hyaline and calcified pleural plaques as an index of exposure to asbestos: A study of radiological and pathological features of 100 cases with a consideration of epidemiology. Br Med J 1977; 1:1069–1074.

52. Sargent EN, Boswell WD Jr, Ralls PW, et al. Subpleural fat pads in patients exposed to asbestos: Distinction from non-calcified pleural plaques. Radiology 1984; 152:273–277.

53. Proto AV. Conventional chest radiographs: Anatomic understanding of newer observations. Radiology 1992; 183:593–603.

54. Kreel L. Computed tomography in the evaluation of pulmonary asbestosis. Acta Radiol 1976; 17:405–412.

55. Kreel L. Computed tomography of the lung and pleura. Semin Roentgenol 1978; 131:213–225.

56. Cugell DW, Kamp DW. Asbestos and the Pleura. Chest 2004; 125:1103–1117.

57. De Raeve H, Verschakelen JA, Gevenois PA, et al. Observer variation in computed tomography of pleural lesions in subjects exposed to indoor asbestos. Eur Respir J 2001; 17(5):916.

58. Theros EG, Feigin DS. Pleural tumors and pulmonary tumors: Differential diagnosis. Semin Roentgenol 1977; 12:239–247.

59. England DM, Hockholzer L, McCarthy MJ. Localized benign and malignant fibrous tumors of the pleura: A clinicopathologic review of 223 cases. Am J Surg Pathol 1989; 13:640–658.

60. Truong M, Munden RF, Kemp BL. Localized fibrous tumor of the pleura. Am J Roentgenol 2000; 174:42.

61. Ferretti GR, Chiles C, Choplin RH, et al. Localized benign fibrous tumors of the pleura. Am J Roentgenol 1997; 169:683–686.

62. Briselle M, Mark EJ, Duhersin GR. Solitary fibrous tumors of the pleura: Eight new cases and review of 360 cases in the literature. Cancer 1981; 47:2678–2689.

63. Soulen MC, Greco-Hunt VT, Templeton P. Cases from A3CR2, migratory chest mass. Invest Radiol 1990; 25:209–211.

64. Dedrick CG, McLoud TC, Shepard JO, et al. Computed tomography of localized pleural mesothelioma. Am J Roentgenol 1985; 144:275–280.

65. Sabloff B, Munden RF, Melhem AI, et al. Radiologic–Pathologic conferences of the University of Texas M. D. Anderson Cancer Center: Extraskeletal osteosarcoma of the pleura. Am J Roentgenol 2003; 180:972.

66. Erasmus JJ, McAdams HP, Patz EF Jr, et al. Calcifying fibrous pseudotumor of pleura: Radiologic features in three cases. J Comput Assist Tomogr 1996; 20:763–765.

67. Mendelson DS, Meary E, Bay JN, et al. Localized fibrous pleural mesothelioma: CT findings. Clin Imaging 1991; 15:105–108.

68. Perna V, Rivas F, Morera R, et al. Localized (solitary) fibrous tumors of the pleura: An analysis of 15 patients. Int J Surg 2008; 1 [Epub ahead of print].

69. Lu C, Ji Y, Shan F, et al. Solitary fibrous tumor of the pleura: An analysis of 13 cases. World J Surg 2008; 23 [Epub ahead of print].

70. Chang JC, Su KY, Chao SF, et al. Hypoglycemia in a patient with a huge malignant solitary fibrous tumor of the pleura. Pathol Int 2007; 57(12):791–793.

71. Desser TS. Solitary fibrous tumor of the pleura. J Thoracic Imag 1998; 13:27–35.

72. Buxton RC, Tan CS, Kline NM, et al. Atypical transmural thoracic lipoma. CT diagnosis. J Comput Assist Tomogr 1988; 12:196–198.

73. Epler GR, McLoud TC, Munn CS, et al. Pleural lipoma: Diagnosis by computed tomography. Chest 1986; 90:265–268.

74. Evans AR, Wolstenholte RJ, Shettan SP, et al. Primary pleural liposarcoma. Thorax 1985; 40:554–555.
75. Munk PC, Muller NL. Pleural liposarcoma: CT diagnosis. J Comput Assist Tomogr 1988; 12:709–710.
76. Chalaoui J, Sylvestre J, Dussault RG, et al. Thoracic fatty lesions, some usual and unusual appearances. J Can Assoc Radiol 1980; 32:197–201.
77. Yeh HC, Gordon A, Kirschner PA, et al. Computed tomography and sonography of thymolipoma. Am J Roentgenol 1983; 140:1131–1133.
78. Biondetti PR, Fiore D, Perrin B, et al. Infiltrative angiolipoma of the thoracoabdominal wall. J Comput Assist Tomogr 1982; 6:847.
79. Mendez G, Isilkoff MB, Isilkoff SK, et al. Fatty tumors of the thorax demonstrated by lung CT. Am J Roentgenol 1979; 133:207–212.
80. Piehler J, Pairolere PC, Weiland LH, et al. Bronchogenic carcinoma with chest wall invasion: Factors affecting survival following en bloc resection. Ann Thorac Surg 1986; 34:684–687.
81. Quint Le, Francis IT, Wahl RL, et al. Pre-operative staging of non-small cell carcinoma of the lung: Imaging methods. Am J Roentgenol 1995; 164:1349–1354.
82. Shirakawa T, Fukuda K, Miyamoto Y, et al. Parietal pleural invasion of lung masses: Evaluation with CT performed during deep inspiration and expiration. Radiology 1994; 192: 809–814.
83. Padovant B, Mauroux J, Sekeik L, et al. Chest wall invasion by bronchogenic carcinoma: Evaluation by MR imaging. Radiology 1983; 198:32–37.
84. Alexandrakis MG, Passam FH, Despina SK, et al. Pleural effusions in hematologic malignancies. Chest 2004; 125:1546–1555.
85. Mitchell A, Meunier C, Ouellette D, et al. Extranodal marginal zone lymphoma of mucosa-associated lymphoid tissue with initial presentation in the pleura. Chest 2006; 129:791–794.
86. Ahmad H, Pawade J, Falk S, et al. Primary pleural lymphomas. Thorax 2003; 58:908–909.
87. Hirai S, Hamanaka Y, Mitsui N, et al. Primary malignant lymphoma arising in the pleura without preceding longstanding pyothorax. Ann Thorac Cardiovasc Surg 2004; 10:297–300.
88. McLoud TC, Woods BO, Carrington CB, et al. Diffuse pleural thickening in an asbestos exposed population: Prevalence and causes. Am J Roentgenol 1985; 144:9–18.
89. Weber MA, Bock M, Plathow C, et al. Asbestos-related pleural disease: Value of dedicated magnetic resonance imaging techniques. Invest Radiol 2004; 39(9):554–556.
90. Gevenois PA, de Maertelaer V, Madani A, et al. Asbestosis, pleural plaques and diffuse pleural thickening: Three distinct benign responses to asbestos exposure. Eur Respir J 1998; 11:1021–1027.
91. Jeong YJ, Kim S, Kwak SW, et al. Neoplastic and nonneoplastic conditions of serosal membrane origin: CT findings. Radiographics 2008; 28(3):801–817.
92. McLoud TC, Woods BO, Carrington CB, et al. Diffuse pleural thickening in an asbestos exposed population: Prevalence and causes. Am J Roentgenol 1985; 144:9–18.
93. Copley SJ, Wells AU, Rubens MB, et al. Functional consequences of pleural disease evaluated with chest radiography and CT. Radiology 2001; 220:237–243.
94. Leung AN, Muller NL, Miller RR. CT in differential diagnosis of diffuse pleural disease. Am J Roentgenol 1990; 154:487–492.
95. Friedman AC, Fiel SB, Redeiki PD, et al. Computed tomography of benign pleural and pulmonary parenchymal abnormalities related to asbestos exposure. Semin Ultrasound CT MR 1990; 11:393–408.
96. McLoud TC. The use of CT in the examination of asbestos-exposed persons. Radiology 1988; 169:862–863.
97. Avila NA, Dwyer AJ, Rabel A, et al. CT of pleural abnormalities in lymphangioleiomyomatosis and comparison of pleural findings after different types of pleurodesis. Am J Roentgenol 2006; 186:1007–1012.

98.   Nguyen M, Varma V, Perez R, et al. CT with histopathologic correlation of FDG uptake in a patient with pulmonary granuloma and pleural plaque caused by remote talc pleurodesis. Am J Roentgenol 2004; 182:92–94.

99.   Weiss N, Solomon SB. Talc pleurodesis mimics pleural metastases: Differentiation with positron emission tomography/computed tomography. Clin Nucl Med 2003; 28:811–814.

100. Rusch VW, Piantadaosi S, Holmes EC. The role of exrapleural pneumonectomy in malignant pleural mesothelioma. J Thorac Cardiovasc Surg 1991; 102:1–9.

101. Selikoff IJ, Hammond EC, Seidman H. Latency of asbestos disease among insulation workers in the United States and Canada. Cancer 1980; 46:2736–2740.

102. Pisani RJ, Colby TV, Williams DE. Malignant mesothelioma of the pleura. Mayo Clin Proc 1988; 63:1234–124.

103. Kramer G, Gans S, Rijnders A, et al. Long term survival of a patient with malignant pleural mesothelioma as a late complication of radiotherapy for Hodgkin's disease treated with [90]yttrium-silicate. Lung Cancer 2000; 27:205–208.

104. Roggi VL, Sanfilippo F, Shelburne JD. Mesothelioma. In: Roggli VL, Greenberg SD, Pratt PC, eds. Pathology of Asbestos-Associated Diseases. New York, NY: Little Brown, 1992: 109–153.

105. Aisner J. Current approach to malignant mesothelioma of the pleura. Chest 1995; 107: 332S–344S.

106. Rusch VW. A proposed new international TNM staging system for malignant pleural mesothelioma: From the International Mesothelioma Interest Group. Chest 1995; 108:1122–1128.

107. Patz EF Jr, Rusch VW, Heelan R. The proposed new international TNM staging system for malignant pleural mesothelioma: Application to imaging. AJR Am J Roentgenol 1996; 166:323–327.

108. Wang ZJ, Reddy GP, Gotway MB, et al. Malignant pleural mesothelioma: Evaluation with CT, MR imaging, and PET 1. Radiographics 2004; 24:105–119.

109. Yamamuro M, Gerbaudo VH, Gill RR, et al. Morphologic and functional imaging of malignant pleural mesothelioma. Eur J Radiol 2007; 64(3):356–366.

110. Wechsler RJ, Rao VM, Steiner RM. The radiology of thoracic malignant mesothelioma. Crit Rev Diagn Imaging 1983; 20:283–310.

111. Kawashima A, Libshitz HI. Malignant pleural mesothelioma: CT manifestations in 50 cases. Am J Roentgenol 1990; 155:965–969.

112. Miller BH, Rosado-de-Christenson ML, Mason AC, et al. Malignant pleural mesothelioma: Radiologic–pathologic correlation. Radiographics 1996; 16:613–644.

113. Zervos MD, Bizekis C, Pass HI. Malignant mesothelioma 2008. Curr Opin Pulm Med 2008; 14(4):303–309.

114. Crotty EJ, McAdams PH, Erasmus JJ, et al. Epithelioid hemangioendothelioma of the pleura: Clinical and radiologic features. Am J Roentgenol 2000; 175:1545–1549.

115. Weiss SW, Ishak KG, Dail DH, et al. Epithelioid hemangioendothelioma and related lesions. Semin Diagn Pathol 1986; 3:259–287.

116. Normand J-P, Rioux M, Dumont M, et al. Thoracic splenosis after blunt trauma: Frequency and imaging findings. Am J Roentgenol 1993; 161:739–741.

5
Ultrasonography of the Pleura

OK-HWA KIM and KYUNG JOO PARK
Department of Radiology, Ajou University Medical Center, Suwon, South Korea

I. Introduction

The pleura, a relatively superficial structure, is easily accessible to ultrasonography (US) and has gained its recognition as a highly useful tool in the evaluation of pleural lesions (1–7). Pathological processes that involve the pleura, either directly from isolated pleural disease or indirectly from neighboring pulmonary lesions, manifest as pleural effusion, which is one of the main causes of increased opacity in the hemithorax seen on chest radiography. US easily identifies the cause of the opaque chest on radiography by their acoustic properties and avoids unnecessary diagnostic procedures.

US can also be used to provide imaging guidance for pleural drainage procedures. With US one can determine the depth of the fluid collection and decide on the safest manner to approach for draining fluid. Sonography-guided thoracocentesis or catheter drainage of pleural fluid is a safe, well-tolerated procedure with a high success rate (8,9).

The purpose of this chapter is to summarize the sonographic features of pleural diseases as well as the role of sonography in the therapeutic workup of pleural pathology. We describe the technique of pleural sonography, the characteristic US appearances of pleural effusion, pleural tumors, and give an overview of US-guided diagnostic and therapeutic procedures.

II. Technique of Pleural Ultrasonography

The optimal frequency of the transducer for pleural US varies with the age of the patient. Young children are best imaged with a high resolution 5 to 10 MHz linear-array transducer, whereas adolescents and adults may require 2 to 4 or 4 to 7 MHz sector or linear-array transducer (3,4,9). Either a linear- or a curved-array probe gives a broad view of the near field when used to image through intercostal approach, and an excellent visualization of the pleura/lung interface is obtained with the transducer sweeping along the intercostal spaces. A sector probe is useful for imaging the diaphragmatic pleura by subxiphoid and transdiaphragmatic approaches with liver or spleen as the acoustic window (5,10).

US is performed in the sitting, supine, prone, or decubitus position with the presumed location of the lesion based on the radiographic findings. In the sitting position, the dorsal and lateral costal pleura are visualized, whereas the supine position is preferred for visualizing the ventral costal pleura. Bedridden and intensive care patients are examined by turning them to the oblique position in the bed (5,11).

III.   Normal Pleura and Artifacts of Pleural Ultrasonography

The normal pleura is composed of two membranes comprising the opposed visceral and parietal layers, which are seen as a highly echogenic curvilinear structure [Fig. 1(A)]. Between these two layers there are small hypoechoic inhomogeneities. It is not always possible to visualize sonographically both layers and the hypoechoic space between them (5). The echogenic visceral pleura line moves during respiratory excursions. This has been termed as the "lung sliding" sign (12). Sometimes, the parietal pleura is accompanied by a thin hypoechoic layer and nodular hypoechoic spreading, which represents subpleural fat (7).

At the interphase between the pleura and the ventilated lung tissue, intensive band-like reverberation echoes (comet-tail artifacts) are seen during the breathing movements (6,7) [Fig. 1(A)]. This artifact can be evoked only at the boundary between the visceral pleura and ventilated pulmonary alveoli. Mirror artifacts are commonly seen as duplication of structures external to the pleura projected over the lung because of total reflection of the sound waves at the pleural surface when the US beam strikes the lung surface at certain angles [Fig. 1(B)].

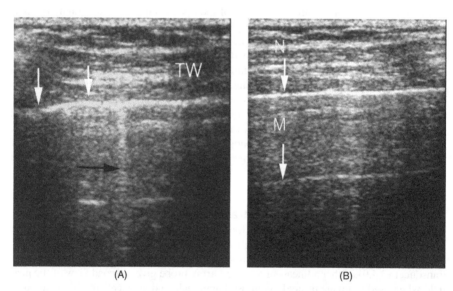

(A)   (B)

Figure 1   Sonographic normal pleura and artifacts. (**A**) Normal pleura and comet-tail artifact. Linear transverse US scan shows highly echogenic band of normal pleura opposed parietal and visceral pleura and interface reflection of aerated lung (arrows), which can be distinguished from the thoracic wall (TW). A vertical reverberation echo, comet-tail artifact (black arrow) evoked at the boundary between the visceral pleural and the ventilated lung is also seen. (**B**) Mirror artifact. Linear transverse US scan shows two echogenic bands, one is normal pleura (N) and the other one is a mirror image (M) of normal pleura in the lung. Duplication of structures outside the pleural space is projected into the lung due to total reflection of sound waves at the lung surface.

IV. Pleural Effusion

The conventional chest radiographic findings of pleural fluid collections are variable and depend on the amount and the age of the fluid collection. These findings range from complete opacification of the hemithorax to less striking but puzzling areas of increased opacity, especially in patients with loculated empyema or associated peripheral pulmonary lesions (3). The presence of pleural fluid may not be identified with chest radiographs when there is extensive pulmonary consolidation or collapse. If there is any doubt whether a pleural effusion exists, US allows easy distinction of pleural fluid from increased opacity due to pulmonary parenchymal lesion (Fig. 2).

On US imaging through an intercostal approach, pleural fluid between the parietal and visceral pleurae is demarcated with a sharp echogenic line delineating the visceral pleura and lung. Sonography can also demonstrate subpulmonic effusion in patients with an apparently elevated hemidiaphragm on plain chest radiographs (Fig. 3), which is particularly useful to detect hemothorax in trauma patients, accurate, and significantly faster than supine and decubitus portable chest radiography (13).

At US, pleural fluid may be characterized as a simple or complicated nature of the fluid. Yang et al. (14) assessed the value of sonography in determining the nature of pleural effusions of various causes. A simple effusion appears as clear anechoic or cloudy hypoechoic fluid that may be transudates or exudates. Transudates are almost always echo-free, whereas about half of the exudates are echogenic (15). Most exudative pleural effusion is of infectious origin, which is known as parapneumonic effusion or empyema (16). Hypoechoic and echogenic fluid may contain diffusely distributed swirling or floating echogenicities that reflects particles in the fluid, for example, cells, protein, fibrin, or blood (5). Homogeneous echogenic effusions may be due to hemorrhagic effusion or empyema.

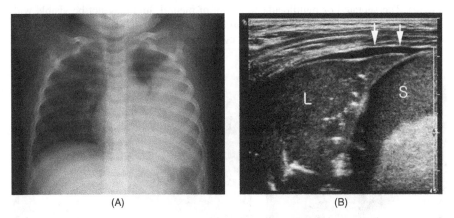

(A) (B)

Figure 2 Sonographic distinction of pleural fluid from pneumonia. (A) Chest radiograph shows an area of increased opacity in the left lower lobe that shows meniscus shape suggesting massive pleural effusion. (B) Linear longitudinal US scan through the intercostal space at the left lower lobe shows scanty amount of hypoechoic effusion (arrows), which is not feasible for aspiration. Most of the opacity shown on the radiography is the echogenic area of pneumonic consolidation (L) and the spleen (S).

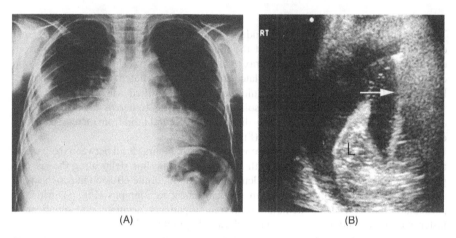

(A)   (B)

Figure 3 Elevated hemidiaphragm due to extensive subpulmonic pleural effusion. (**A**) Chest radiograph shows the elevated right hemidiaphragm associated with pleural effusion along the major fissure. (**B**) Sector oblique longitudinal US scan shows extensive pleural effusion in the subpulmonic and lateral pleural space with collapse of the right lower lobe (L). The right hemidiaphragm (arrow) is not elevated but everted due to subpulmonic effusion.

As exudative fluid collections organize, mobile, linear structures of fibrin bands or to-and-fro motion of septa, which are typical for inflammatory effusions, tend to occur (17). This complicated effusion appears as septated or multiloculated, hypoechoic fluid. In some empyemas, the septa are so profuse that they produce a honeycomb appearance (Fig. 4). The septated or multiloculated nature of pleural fluid may not be visible with computed tomography (CT). The lung could be captured by inflammation and may not slide up and down during the respiratory cycle and no clear demarcation is visualized

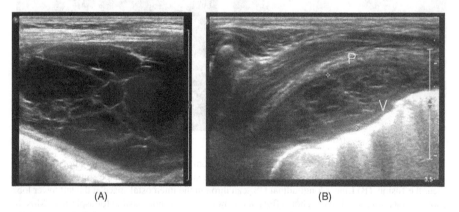

(A)   (B)

Figure 4 Complicated pleural effusion with multiple loculi: (**A**) the pleural space is filled with profusely septated fluid, which has a honeycomb appearance; (**B**) extensive thickening of the parietal (P) and visceral (V) pleura encircles the thickened fluid, which is not amenable for aspiration.

between the lung and pleural components (14). Sonographic findings of thickening of the parietal and visceral pleurae and associated parenchymal lesions in the lung are most likely indicative of empyemas. Septated fluids caused by fibrous strands are mainly observed not only in infected exudative fluid, but also in malignant effusion (18,19), and may rarely be found in patients with tuberculous pleurisy (20,21).

With advance of pleural fluid organization, extensive pleural thickening or fibrothorax may ensue. This appears as echogenic, solid-appearing pleural plaque with or without some loculation of fluid that is predictive of significant difficulties with thoracocentesis (3). US performed with a high-resolution transducer is sensitive in demonstrating the internal derangement about the nature of pleural changes and provides detailed information to determine the planning of therapeutic approaches.

As pleural scars and thickening appear as echogenic rind of pleural plaque, the discrimination between echogenic pleural fluid and solid pleural thickening may be difficult. It is important to determine by the nature of pleural changes whether thoracocentesis is feasible. Characterization of pleural changes with US is very informative in guiding thoracocentesis.

Sonographic differentiation between benign and malignant pleural fluid is possible only if solid nodular structures are visible (15,18). US detection of large, confluent pleural masses greater than 1 cm is indicative of malignant effusion (18). Pleural thickening may occur diffusely in both benign and malignant effusions. According to Leung et al. (22), parietal pleural thickening of more than 1 cm on CT was specific for malignancy in 94%. In benign exudative effusions, associated pleural thickening is usually of less than 1 cm and combined mostly with a lung parenchymal change. Akhan et al. (20) reported thickening of the pleura in one-third of their patients with nonmalignant pleural effusions, especially tuberculous effusions. In almost all cases, thickness was less than 1 cm and decreased with treatment within six months. Therefore, pleural thickening of more than 1 cm should arouse a high suspicion of malignancy.

V. Pleural Tumors

In patients with pleural origin tumors, either primary or metastatic, pleural implants may hide behind pleural fluid collections and go unnoticed on chest radiography. For the further evaluation of pleural masses, either sonography or CT can be used. CT has a distinct advantage in the evaluation of pleural masses, as it can easily evaluate all parts of the pleura including the mediastinal pleura, and thus provide accurate information about the extent of disease and better detect involvement of adjacent structures and pleural-based parenchymal pulmonary involvement (7). Sonography can be useful in finding pleural masses and indicating the origin of the pleural effusion, and guided biopsy by real-time sonographic monitoring increases the chances of obtaining tissue.

Malignant mesotheliomas are usually visualized as diffuse irregular thickenings of the pleura, including localized nodules. Large pleural effusions occur frequently, together with mesotheliomas (5,23,24).

Metastases constitute the overwhelming majority of malignant neoplasms involving the pleura. Metastatic disease to the pleura often causes large pleural effusions that are probably due to impaired lymphatic drainage (18). In some patients, pleural fluid is so profuse that it may mask the tumoral masses on chest radiography. Most pleural metastases are too small to be detected. However, metastases larger than 5 mm in diameter on the

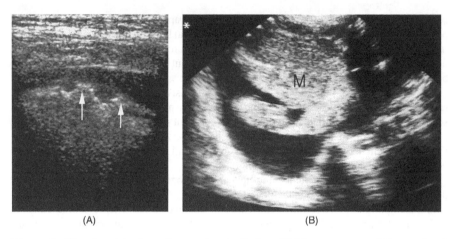

(A)   (B)

Figure 5 Pleural nodules in malignant pleural effusion. (**A**) Linear transverse US scan shows nodular appearance of the visceral pleura (arrows), which is well delineated by hypoechoic pleural effusion. Biopsy showed metastatic squamous cell carcinoma of the pleura. (**B**) Sector transverse US scan shows a massive anechoic effusion containing a bulk of mass (M), metastasis from Wilms tumor.

parietal or diaphragmatic pleura can be detected by sonography. These nodules are round, oval, broad-based, echogenic or moderately echogenic, and well delineated against the pleural effusion (Fig. 5).

VI.   Ultrasonography-Guided Pleural Intervention

It is clear that sonography has important implications in the management of pleural effusion because of its ability to characterize the internal composition of pleural fluid. Diagnostic thoracocentesis can be performed safely at the bedside without imaging guidance if the effusion is reasonably large, extending over several rib spaces on the chest radiograph. When the effusion is smaller than this, associated with underlying pulmonary collapse, or is loculated, aspiration becomes a difficult task. One of the main difficulties for performing unguided pleural aspiration is correctly identifying the level of the hemidiaphragm, thereby avoiding inadvertent subdiaphragmatic puncture of either liver or spleen. If diaphragmatic elevation is suspected on the chest radiograph, ultrasound should be performed (25).

There is still a great deal of controversy around the clinical management of empyema (16). Two main treatment approaches are used: nonoperative in which patients are treated with antibiotics alone or combined with thoracocentesis or tube drainage thoracotomy, and operative where the good of treatment is to evacuate infected debris and reexpand the lung. Sonography is used for guidance of therapeutic thoracocentesis and tube drainage of parapneumonic effusions or empyemas. Sonography clearly shows the extent of fluid collection and, therefore, is an ideal guide for thoracocentesis. Furthermore, it is also an excellent modality as a guide to aspiration and drainage of pleural fluid (26).

Urokinase instillation through the catheter can facilitate the drainage of thoracic empyema. US-guided transcatheter instillation of urokinase can predict the effectiveness of urokinase in the treatment of loculated pleural effusion (27). Urokinase instillation was not effective in patients whose pleural fluid had a honeycomb septation pattern on US or whose parietal pleura was more than 5-mm thick on CT scans (28,29).

Pleurodesis can be performed through sonographically placed small-bore catheters (7–15 Fr) for recurrent malignant pleural effusions or recurrent pneumothoraces with success rates comparable to those seen with large-bore, surgically placed catheters (30,31).

Pneumothorax, the most common complication of pleural taps, is exceedingly rare when the procedure is performed under sonographic control. Pneumothorax rates for guided thoracocentesis have been reported at 2% to 3%, favorable as compared with unguided diagnostic thoracocentesis rates of 9% to 13% (32–34). US-guided placement of large drains also reduces the failure rate. One of the major reasons for failure of catheter drainage is malpositioning of the tube, and complications including laceration of the diaphragm, spleen, and liver. These can be avoided by ultrasound- or CT-guided drainage using catheters of 8 to 14 Fr (25).

Although thoracocentesis or closed pleural biopsy can often establish the diagnosis of pleural malignancy, these methods may not provide enough diagnostic material to confirm the presence of malignancy (35–37). When the pleural disease may be focally involved, real-time US is useful in guiding pleural biopsy of focal or diffuse pleural lesions, particularly when pleural fluid is absent or minimal. Sonography clearly shows thickened pleura or pleural tumors, and the passage of biopsy needles can be monitored. Sonography guidance of the needle biopsy can increase the chances of obtaining tissue with significant pathological changes (35). Sonography-guided core-needle biopsy of possible malignant pleural mesothelioma may become the method of choice owing to its high accuracy and ease of performance (24). US-guided pleural biopsy is a readily available, generally quick and safe procedure with which to establish the diagnosis of pleural malignancy.

In conclusion, pleural US helps to identify the pleural effusion and clarify the nature of effusion. With the detailed sonographic characteristics of pleural fluid, further therapeutic management, the thoracocentesis and/or catheter drainage or surgical intervention, can be determined. Moreover, the detection of pleural tumors can be assessed with US. Under US-guidance biopsy, the chances of obtaining pleural tissues improve the pathologic diagnosis. US of the pleura increases the diagnostic and therapeutic yields in the management of variable pleural diseases.

References

1. Doust BD, Baum JK, Maklad NF, et al. Ultrasonic evaluation of pleural opacities. Radiology 1975; 114:134–140.
2. Lipscomb DJ, Flower CDR, Hadfield JW. Ultrasound of the pleura: An assessment of its clinical value. Clin Radiol 1981; 32:289–290.
3. Kim OH, Kim WS, Kim MJ, et al. US in the diagnosis of pediatric chest diseases. Radiographics 2000; 20:653–671.
4. Tsai TH, Yang PC. Ultrasound in the diagnosis and management of pleural disease. Curr Opin Pulm Med 2003; 9:282–290.
5. Mathis G. Thorax sonography—Part I: Chest wall and pleura. Ultrasound Med Biol 1997; 23:1131–1139.
6. Wernecke K. Sonographic features of pleural disease. AJR Am J Roentgenol 1997; 168:1061–1066.

7.   Wernecke K. Ultrasound study of the pleura. Eur Radiol 2000; 10:1515–1523.
8.   O'Moore PV, Mueller PR, Simeone JF. Sonographic guidance in diagnostic and therapeutic interventions in the pleural spaces. AJR Am J Roentgenol 1987; 149:1–5.
9.   Ben-Ami TE, O'Dpmpvam KC, Yousefzadeh DK. Sonography of the chest in children. Radiol Clin North Am 1993; 31:517–531.
10. McLoud TC, Flower CDR. Imaging the pleura: Sonography, CT, and MR imaging. AJR Am J Roentgenol 1991; 156:1145–1153.
11. Yu CJ, Yang PC, Yang DB, et al. Diagnostic and therapeutic use of chest sonography: Value in critically ill patients. AJR Am J Roentgenol 1992; 159:695–701.
12. Lichtenstein DO, Menu Y. A bedside ultrasound ruling out pneumothorax in the critically ill: Lung sliding. Chest 1995; 108:1345–1348.
13. Ma OJ, Mateer JR. Trauma ultrasound examination versus chest radiography in the detection of hemothorax. Ann Emerg Med 1997; 29:312–315.
14. Yang PC, Luh KT, Chang DB, et al. Value of sonography in determining the nature of pleural effusion: Analysis of 320 cases. AJR Am J Roentgenol 1992; 159:29–33.
15. Reuß J. Sonographic imaging of the pleura: Nearly 30 years experience. Eur J Ultrasound 1996; 3:125–139.
16. Ramnath RR, Heller RM, Ben-Ami T, et al. Implications of early sonographic evaluation of parapneumonic effusions in children with pneumonia. Pediatrics 1998; 101:68–71.
17. Chen KY, Liaw YS, Wang HC, et al. Sonographic septation: A useful prognostic indicator of acute thoracic empyema. J Ultrasound Med 2000; 19:837–843.
18. Görg C, Restrepo I, Schwerk WB. Sonography of malignant pleural effusion. Eur Radiol 1997; 7:1195–1198.
19. Görg C, Schwerk WB, Goerg K, et al. Pleural effusion: An "acoustic window" for sonography of pleural metastases. J Clin Ultrasound 1991; 19:93–97.
20. Akhan O, Demirkazik FB, Özmen MN, et al. Tuberculous pleural effusions: Ultrasonic diagnosis. J Clin Ultrasound 1992; 20:461–465.
21. Chen HJ, Hsu WH, Tu CY, et al. Sonographic septation in lymphocyte-rich exudative pleural effusions. A useful diagnostic predictor for tuberculosis. J Ultrasound Med 2006; 25:857–863.
22. Leung AN, Müller NL, Miller RR. CT in differential diagnosis of diffuse pleural disease. AJR Am J Roentgenol 1990; 154:487–492.
23. Rusch VW. Diagnosis and treatment of pleural mesothelioma. Semin Surg Oncol 1990; 6:279–285.
24. Helio A, Stenwig AE, Solheim OP. Malingant pleural mesothelioma: US-guided histologic core-needle biopsy. Radiology 1999; 21:657–659.
25. Patel MC, Flower CDR. Radiology in the management of pleural disease. Eur Radiol 1997; 7:1454–1462.
26. O'Moore PV, Mueller PR, Simeone JF, et al. Sonographic guidance in diagnostic and therapeutic interventions in the pleural space. AJR Am J Roentgenol 1987; 149:1–5.
27. Park CS, Chung WM, Lim MK, et al. Transcatheter instillation of urokinase into loculated pleural effusion: Analysis of treatment effect. AJR Am J Roentgenol 1996; 167:649–652.
28. Ekingen G, Guvenc BH, Sozubir S, et al. Fibrnolytic treatment of complicated pediatric thoracic empyemas with intrapleural streptokinase. Eur J Cardio thorac Surg 2004; 26:503–507.
29. Toms AP, Tasker AD, Flower CDR. Intervention in the pleura. Eur J Radiol 2000; 34:119–132.
30. Morrison MC, Mueller PR, Lee MJ, et al. Sclerotherapy of malignant pleural effusion through sonographically placed small-bore catheters. AJR Am J Roentgenol 1992; 158:41–43.
31. Seaton KG, Patz EF Jr, Goodman PC. Palliative treatment of malignant pleural effusions: Value of small-bore catheter thoracostomy and doxycycline sclerotherapy. AJR Am J Roentgenol 1995; 164:589–591.
32. Seneff MG, Corwin RW, Gold LH. Complications associated with thoracentesis. Chest 1986; 90:97–100.

33. Collins TR, Sahn SA. Thoracentesis: Clinical value, complications, technical problems, and patient experience. Chest 1987; 91:817–822.
34. Silverman SG, Saini S, Mueller PR. Pleural intervention: Indications, techniques, and clinical applications. Radiol Clin North Am 1989; 27:1257–1266.
35. Yang PC. Ultrasound-guided transthoracic biopsy of the chest. Radiol Clin North Am 2000; 38:323–343.
36. Adams RF, Gleeson FV. Percutaneous image-guided cutting-needle biopsy of the pleura in the presence of a suspected malignant pleural effusion. Radiology 2001; 219:510–514.
37. Heilo A. US-guided transthoracic biopsy. Eur J Ultrasound 1996; 3:141–151.

6
Diagnostic Thoracocentesis and Biopsy

ANDREAS DIACON and CHRIS BOLLIGER
Respiratory Research Unit, Faculty of Health Sciences, University of Stellenbosch,
Cape Town, South Africa

I. Introduction

Diagnostic thoracocentesis (or pleurocentesis) is performed since more than 150 years and remains the first step to be taken in the evaluation of a pleural effusion of unknown origin (1). Thoracocentesis can be combined with closed needle pleural biopsy, a procedure first described in 1955 and refined thereafter (2). The analysis of pleural fluid offers the opportunity of diagnosing the underlying disease directly, or provides valuable information for narrowing the spectrum of possible causes. Moreover, pleural fluid findings may precipitate immediate therapeutic steps in parapneumonic effusion or empyema. Closed needle biopsy, although less often practiced nowadays, is of importance in TB pleurisy and pleural malignancy. Diagnostic thoracocentesis as well as closed needle biopsy are simple and straightforward procedures, and severe complications are rare. This chapter will discuss the technique, indications and contraindications, yield, complications, and limitations of each method. Slight overlap with other chapters may occur where diagnostic yields are dealt with, and the reader is kindly asked to consult the relevant chapters for in-depth information about specific diseases.

II. Indications, Contraindications

A. Diagnostic Thoracocentesis

A diagnostic thoracocentesis to obtain up to 50 mL of pleural fluid is indicated in almost all patients with pleural effusion of unknown origin. If a pleural effusion can be explained by a known medical condition with a high degree of certainty, a watchful waiting strategy may be endorsed. The same is true for expected transudative effusions, since their diagnostic value is limited (3). In all instances where an exudative effusion is likely, analysis of a pleural effusion offers an excellent opportunity to diagnose the underlying disease. In a series of 129 consecutive patients, a definitive diagnosis could be made in 18% of cases with pleural fluid analysis, and a presumptive diagnosis in up to 75% of cases when correlated with clinical findings. Moreover, previously suspected diseases could be excluded in many cases (4).

With closed needle biopsy, a small piece of pleura is obtained for histological and microbiological evaluation. Because of the higher morbidity and the higher cost of needle biopsy, routine use with every thoracocentesis is not generally recommended (5). Since its first description in 1955, closed needle pleural biopsy has been an important diagnostic tool in pleural effusions of unknown origin (2). Its indications have, however, been narrowed to suspected pleural malignancy and TB pleurisy by the ATS in 1989, and the use of closed needle biopsy has decreased further in recent years (6). Since operator experience is crucial for the yield of the method, declining levels of experience may further decrease the effectiveness of the procedure (7). There is ongoing controversy about the role of closed needle biopsy in current practice, due to advances in pleural fluid analysis and revived interest in thoracoscopy (5). We recommend closed needle biopsy when TB pleurisy is suspected, with chemical analysis of adenosine deaminase (ADA) and interferon (INF)-γ remaining inconclusive, or when pleural malignancy is suspected despite repeatedly negative cytology, and thoracoscopy is not available.

There are no absolute contraindications to perform a diagnostic pleurocentesis. If the management of the patient is likely to be influenced by the findings in the pleural fluid, a diagnostic pleurocentesis can also be done in patients with relative contraindications like bleeding diathesis and anticoagulation, while closed needle pleural biopsy is contraindicated in cases with severe coagulopathy. Caution is warranted for both procedures in patients with chest-wall infections, and the risk of transferring the infection into the pleural space at the site of puncture must be individually assessed. In patients with small effusions, ultrasound assistance may be required. Mechanically ventilated patients are at increased risk for pneumothorax, but pleurocentesis can safely be done with ultrasound guidance (8,9). In empyema, closed needle biopsies are rarely indicated, which minimizes the risk of a subcutaneous abscess. A risk–benefit ratio based on clinical grounds should be performed in patients with an unstable medical condition (6).

III. Technique

A. Positioning

Positioning is equal in diagnostic pleurocentesis and closed needle pleural biopsy. It is of utmost importance to take enough time to position patient and operator for a pleural procedure, serving both the patient's comfort and the operator's need for easy access to the pleural puncture or biopsy site. In our experience, the most suitable positioning is with the patient sitting upright on the side of a bed or stretcher, facing away from the investigator with arms crossed and resting on a bedside table. The feet should rest on a footstool. The operating height should be adjusted to accommodate the operating physician, excessive bending over should be avoided, and enough space for the necessary tools to be laid out must be provided (Fig. 1). For patients unable to sit, a puncture can be attempted in the midaxillary line with the head of the bed maximally elevated. Alternatively, a puncture can be tried with the patient lying in a decubitus position with the effusion side down. In both these cases, soft bedding makes access to the most dependent part of the chest difficult, and the patient should be moved to the bedside as far as possible to avoid excessive bulging of the mattress into the working field.

Once a comfortable position for operator and patient is achieved, the site for the puncture must be selected. With the patient in a vertical position, the lowest part of the thorax is usually posterior and pleural fluid can accumulate where puncture can be achieved easiest. The chest radiograph indicates an approximate location, and the definite site is selected with clinical examinations, that is, chest percussion and tactile fremitus. In contrast to the aerated lung above the effusion, the light percussion note becomes dull over the effusion, and the tactile fremitus is lost. The puncture should be attempted one intercostal further down from where fremitus and light percussion note are lost.

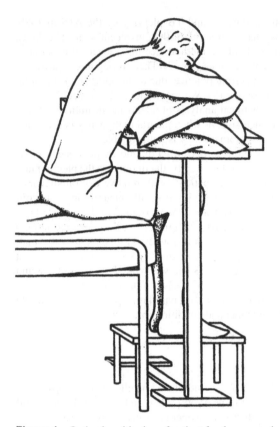

Figure 1   Optimal positioning of patient for thoracentesis.

Puncture site selection is key to success of pleurocentesis. If the clinical technique described above is endorsed, most pleurocentesis attempts failing to produce fluid will be situated too low, as demonstrated in a study reviewing cases of failed thoracocentesis with ultrasound (10). Factors contributing to the wrongful selection of a puncture site in this series of 26 patients were: small effusion with little or no detectable fluid on sonography, blunt costo-phrenic angle on CXR, pleural effusion with multiple loculations, and pulmonary consolidation simulating a large pleural effusion. In challenging situations for puncture site selection, pleural ultrasound may be considered.

Ultrasound is superior to the CXR in identifying pleural fluid collections, which has been proven by several studies more than a decade ago (11–16). However, a reduction of complications or dry taps has not consistently been shown, and cost-effectiveness of ultrasound for routine pleurocentesis has been questioned (14). In the early days, when ultrasound was a stationary and expensive machinery, patients frequently had to be transferred for the examination, causing inconvenience and delay, and were finally punctured by a different physician in a potentially different body position than during the ultrasound examination. In recent years, considerable technical development has taken place and the advent of affordable and transportable ultrasound units has made the technique accessible for the physician at the bedside, and on site sonography by the physician performing the puncture is increasingly popular. A recent study using a mobile ultrasound unit showed excellent yield for obtaining pleural fluid with a very low complication rate in mechanically ventilated patients (9). Despite the lack of recent data, it seems reasonable to recommend ultrasound up front for small effusions and those with the above-mentioned risk constellations. Frequent use of ultrasound for pleural procedures promotes the understanding of how clinical findings are related to anatomic conditions, and increases the level of confidence of the operator. We believe that bedside ultrasound will ultimately be incorporated in training and practice of pulmonary physicians, and that ultrasound should be used liberally whenever available (17–21).

B.   Local Anesthesia and Diagnostic Thoracocentesis

The spot to perform the puncture and eventually the biopsy should be chosen not too close to the spine and just above an easily palpable rib, in order to avoid contact with the intercostal vessels and nerves situated right below the ribs. Local anesthesia is compulsory if pleural biopsy is planned, and of debatable value for straightforward thoracocentesis. In the hands of experienced operators, the trauma of local anesthesia usually matches the one inflicted by the procedure itself, if only one needle is used. Unless the patient is very anxious or the puncture is anticipated to be difficult, for example, in very obese subjects, an experienced operator may also abstain from local anesthesia for diagnostic pleurocentesis only. Since most of the action happens out of the patients view, we find it very useful to keep up a continuous flow of information from operator to patient about the progress of the ongoing procedure.

The puncture should be done perpendicular to the skin, and a puncture pointing upwards must be avoided at all times. We always thoroughly disinfect the selected spot with a wide margin of safety with alcohol. Local anesthesia is performed in three steps: anesthesia of the skin, the rib periostium, and the pleura (Fig. 2). The skin is best punctured with a short 24 G (0.55 mm) needle, and less than 1 mL of lidocaine is usually applied to create a small wheal [Fig. 2(A)]. This needle is then replaced with a 22 G (0.7 mm) needle with 4 cm length, which is inserted through the same spot. With the needle tip in the subcutaneous tissue, the skin is easily moved up and down to adjust for the rib below the planned entry site into the thorax. While moving the needle forward towards the pleural space, small amounts of lidocaine are continuously injected, slowly advancing the needle with frequent aspirations. When the rib periostium is reached, the needle is worked upwards by withdrawing the needle from the rib, moving skin and subcutaneous tissue upwards with the needle inserted, and re-advancing the needle, until it passes over the rib [Fig. 2(B)]. When the pleura is finally punctured, pleural fluid should be aspirated [Fig. 2(C)]. For diagnostic aspiration, the syringe is now changed and the fluid can be aspirated. If a direct puncture without local anesthesia is attempted, a 22-G or 21-G (0.8 mm) needle attached to an empty 20 mL syringe is directly inserted under constant aspiration with the same technique as described above.

If no fluid can be aspirated with a 22-G or 21-G needle inserted all the way (4 cm), the needle is either too short, too far advanced or there is no pleural fluid at the attempted site. The needle should slowly be withdrawn under constant aspiration because a very small rim of effusion can be missed when inserting the needle. If the patient is very obese or muscular, the standard needle should be replaced by a longer one, and the

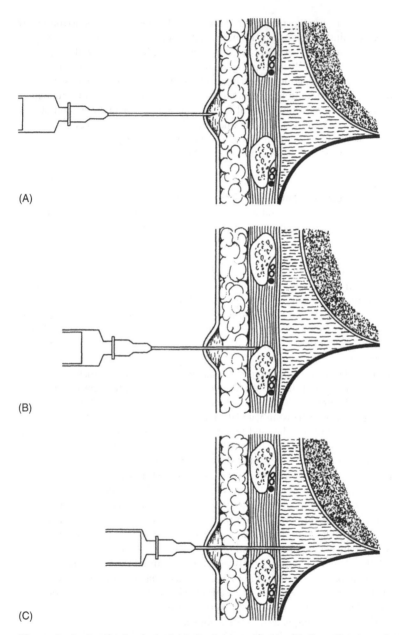

Figure 2   Performing local anesthesia for thoracentesis. Application of local anesthetic to the skin
(**A**), to the upper edge of a rib (**B**), and needle positioned just above a rib within the pleural fluid
(**C**). Note the location of the intercostal neurovascular structures under the rib.

attempt should be repeated. Pleural fluid is almost never too thick to be aspirated through a 21-G or 22-G needle. If air is aspirated, the puncture is probably too high and should be repeated one intercostal space lower, and if no air is aspirated, the puncture was probably too low and should be repeated one intercostal space higher. If the presence of pleural fluid is doubtful and the initial attempt is unsuccessful, a repetition of the puncture with ultrasound assistance should be considered.

C. Needle Types and Technique of Closed Needle Pleural Biopsy

The site for the biopsy is identified in the same way as for diagnostic pleurocentesis. Most needles for pleural biopsy allow for pleural fluid collection as well. Local anesthesia is always needed for closed needle biopsy and is performed as described above. The choice among the several types of needles in use depends on the availability and operator experience.

The Abrams, Cope, and Raja needles are designed for diagnostic fluid aspiration as well as for biopsy of the pleura and the immediate subpleural tissue. For safe use of these needles, a certain amount of pleural effusion is necessary. If no fluid is found on aspiration during local anesthesia, closed needle biopsy should not be attempted (22). The tru-cut needle, in contrast, is designed for core-tissue biopsies of presumed pleural tumors or abundant pleural thickening. No fluid can be aspirated through a tru-cut needle, and fluoroscopy or sonography is mostly used for guidance, especially when no pleural fluid is present.

Abrams Needle

The Abrams needle [Fig. 3(A)] was first described in 1958 as a refinement of the needle described by De Francis in 1955 (2,23). The Abrams needle consists of three parts: a blunt-tipped outer trocar with a notch, an inner cannula with a sharp cutting terminal part, and a solid inner stylet. The biopsy procedure is shown in detail in Figure 4. After a small scalpel skin incision is made, all three parts are introduced together into the pleural space with gentle pressure. Once the needle is believed to be in the pleural space, the stylet is removed and a syringe is attached to the system. After opening the distal notch by rotating the inner cannula, fluid can be aspirated [Fig. 4(A)]. To change syringes, the notch is closed so that no air can enter the pleural space. To take the biopsy, the notch must be in the open position and the knob in the outer trocar is turned away from the upper rib. The needle has to be withdrawn slowly under permanent suction until the notch is hooked at the visceral pleura [Fig. 4(B)]. In this position, it should be possible to still aspirate pleural fluid through the needle, otherwise the needle is probably out of the pleural space and must be repositioned. Finally, the inner trocar is rotated into the closed position to cut off the biopsy specimen [Fig. 4(C)]. The needle is withdrawn with the biopsy specimen contained within it. This procedure should be repeated at least four times.

Cope Needle

The Cope needle [Fig. 3(B)] was first described in 1958 (24). The Cope needle consists of four parts: a large, sharp-tipped outer cannula; an inner trocar with a hooked notch and a blunt tip; a simple hollow trocar; and a solid inner stylet. After the skin incision, the outer cannula is introduced into the pleural space with the hollow trocar and the stylet in place. Fluid can be aspirated with a syringe attached to the outer cannula, after the trocar and the stylet are removed. The inner stylet and cannula can also be directly replaced by

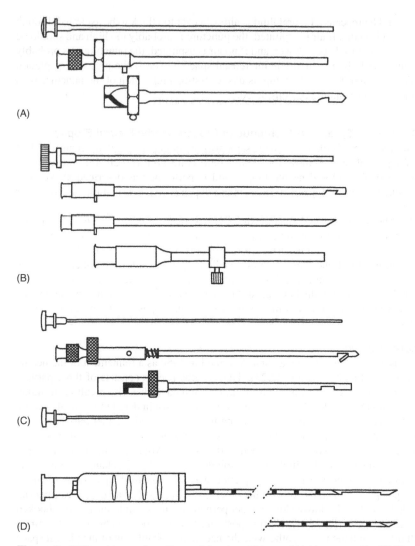

Figure 3   Different types of needles used for pleural biopsy: (**A**) Abrams needle; (**B**) Cope needle; (**C**) Raja needle; (**D**) tru-cut needle in open (top) and closed position (bottom).

the blunt-tipped biopsy trocar with a syringe attached to it. To take a biopsy, the apparatus is withdrawn with the notch directed inferiorly until it hooks at the parietal pleura. The biopsy is taken by advancing the outer sharp cannula toward the pleural space in a gyrating motion. The specimen is then removed with the hooked cannula. This procedure can be repeated until the required number of biopsies is obtained. When using this needle, it is important to occlude the trocar with a syringe, stopcock or the operator's thumb whenever the cannulas are changed to prevent a pneumothorax by air entering the pleural space,

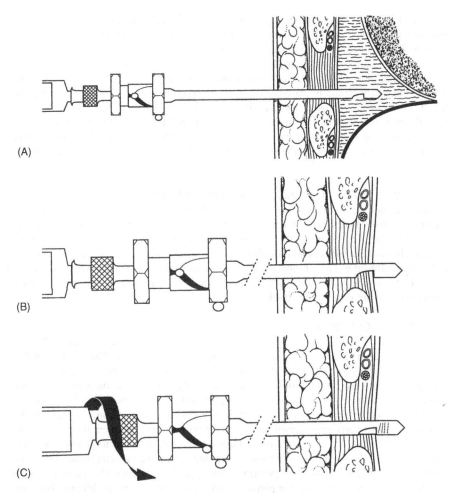

Figure 4 Pleural biopsy with Abrams needle. After introduction into the pleural space, the needle tip with the distal notch open allows for easy aspiration of fluid (**A**). For the biopsy, the visceral pleura is hooked with the notch (**B**) and by closure of the notch the biopsy material is sheared off and transferred into the needle tip (**C**), from where it can be harvested. Note the location of the intercostal neurovascular structures and that the knob on the outer trocar pinpoints the position of the cutting edge inside the thorax.

and the patient should hold his breath at the end of a normal expiration each time. This procedure can be repeated until the required number of biopsies is obtained.

Raja Needle

The Raja needle [Fig. 3(C)], first described in 1989 (25), is a closed system similar to that of the Abrams needle. The Raja needle consists of three parts: a blunt outer cannula with a notch, an inner sharp-tipped cannula with a notch and a biopsy flap, and a solid inner stylet. After a scalpel incision, the two outer parts assembled are inserted into the pleural space connected with a syringe. After entering the pleural space, the inner cannula is slightly moved back until the two notches are in corresponding position and the biopsy flap can deploy into the pleural space. Pleural fluid can be aspirated in this position. To take the biopsy, the flap is turned inferiorly and the needle is withdrawn until the flap is hooked at the parietal pleura. The outer cannula is then withdrawn over the inner cannula, thus forcing the flap with the hooked specimen back into the inner cannula and closing the notch. The apparatus is then removed with the specimen. This procedure can be repeated until the required number of biopsies is obtained. Initial reports by the inventor showed very encouraging results compared to the Abrams needle (26,27). To date, the number of studies with this type of needle is still limited and no conclusive recommendation can be given.

Comparison Between Abrams Needle and Cope Needle

In general, the rate of success with closed needle biopsy seems to be more dependent on the operator's skills than on the needle type used, and diagnostic yields are almost identical (7,28). The blunt tip of the Abrams needle makes insertion somewhat more difficult, but is safer for concomitant therapeutic thoracocentesis because of reduced risk of lacerating the lung. The Abrams needle also seems easier to use and is a closed system, while the Cope needle has the risk of pneumothorax from air entering the pleural space from outside if not properly handled.

The Tru-Cut Needle

The tru-cut needle [Fig. 3(D)] is not a genuine pleural biopsy needle and is generally used to obtain core biopsies from solid tissue material. Different brands and dimensions of this needle are available. Fluid cannot be aspirated with this system, but the needle can be used for conventional pleural biopsy. The tru-cut needle consists of a sharp-tipped, cutting outer cannula, and an inner needle with a sharp tip and a notch. When closed, the notch is hidden in the outer cannula, and one sharp tip is formed by the two components. To take biopsies, the two parts are inserted in the closed position into the pleural cavity or into the tumor. The inner needle is then moved forward so that the tissue to biopsy can bulge into the notch. The specimen is obtained by moving the cutting cannula forward over the inner cannula, which is fixed in its position. To harvest the specimen, the whole needle in the closed position is removed. For pleural biopsy, it is somewhat more difficult than with the other needle types to feel the distal end hooking in the pleura, and the inexperienced operator tends to take biopsies of intercostal tissue rather than of pleura. Because of the sharp tip and the large biopsies that can be obtained, the blind use of this type in dry chests without fluoroscopic or ultrasound guidance is not encouraged (22).

IV. Processing of Material

A. Pleural Fluid

For diagnostic pleurocentesis, it is usually sufficient to tap off 50 mL of pleural fluid. For cytology, it may be suitable to tap off even more, because more cells may be obtained for preparation with cytospin. We carefully note color, viscosity, and smell of the fluid. Fluid pH should be measured with a blood gas machine whenever a parapneumonic effusion or malignancy is suspected. Proposed routine tests performed on the fluid are listed in Table 1.

Table 1 Recommended Routine Tests on Pleural Fluid

Category	Amount (mL)	Specific tests
Hematology	5	Total cell count and differentiation
Chemistry[a]	5	LDH, protein, albumin
Serology[a]		Adenosine deaminase
Microbiology	5	Gram stain
		Aerobic and anaerobic culture
		Tuberculosis stain and culture
		Fungus stain and culture
pH	2	Blood gas machine
Cytology	Remaining amount	

[a] Additional tests may be requested according to the clinical situation and the aspect of the fluid.

Required amounts of fluid and the appropriate tubes for each category may vary in different hospitals. Very helpful, but seldom seen, is a kit of tubes designed for pleural fluid and with a single request form that can contain some useful hints how to order the appropriate test. Since most pleural punctures are done by less experienced and notoriously overworked junior medical staff, such a kit is most welcome and certainly enhances the consistency and usefulness of the tests done. Recent serum values for certain parameters are helpful to interpret the pleural fluid values. A stepwise approach with an initial step to determine whether the fluid is a transudate or an exudate, and more detailed testing done in exudates only would be ideal, but is not realistic in practice. A more in-depth approach to testing of pleural fluid can be found elsewhere in this book.

B. Processing of Closed Needle Biopsy Specimens

Biopsy specimens should be sent for histology in formalin, and at least one sample should be submitted for mycobacterial culture in saline. The ideal number of biopsies for TB pleurisy has been determined to be four in one report, and seven or more biopsy attempts produced at least two specimens containing pleural tissue in another study (29,30). At some institutions, electron microscopy is available, and tissue for workup must be submitted in a specific medium.

V. Complications

In essence, frequency and nature of complications of closed needle biopsy are the same as with diagnostic pleurocentesis. However, lacerations of intercostal vessels are more likely to lead to serious complications due to the cutting character of the devices, and hemothorax as well as arterio-venous fistulas have been described after closed needle biopsy.

Penetration of the lung (aspiration of air) or of an infra-diaphragmatic organ (dry tap) with a thin needle as described above does not necessarily lead to complications. Dry taps are reported in 10% to 13% of attempts for thoracocentesis (4,10,13,31). Pneumothorax is the most frequent complication occurring in 11% to 30% of punctures, and a chest drain is necessary in about 2% of the punctures (4,14,31). A pneumothorax can occur after laceration of the lung with the tip of the needle, and after air has inadvertently entered the pleural space during the procedure. In the latter case, the pneumothoraces tend to be small and stable, while a persistent air leak in the lung will produce an increasing pneumothorax requiring drainage. In closed needle biopsy, the Cope needle as an open system might favor air entry from outside, but pneumothorax is not reported as a significant problem (32). The incidence of pneumothorax seems to be reduced with more experienced operators, and to be increased in patients with underlying COPD (33,34). In our opinion, it is unnecessary to routinely obtain a chest radiograph (CXR) for exclusion of an iatrogenic pneumothorax after each procedure. We routinely repeat percussion and tactile fremitus after the procedure, or repeat the ultrasound when available on site, and check for unexplained alterations of these findings indicating a pneumothorax. We order a CXR only if air was aspirated or if unexplained symptoms occur or if these screening tests fail. This conservative approach is endorsed by the findings of several recent studies (21,35–37).

Very sensitive individuals can suffer a vaso-vagal syncope during the procedure, probably triggered by emotional factors and possibly the penetration of the pleura with the needle, and promoted by the sitting position of the subject. The procedure should then be immediately interrupted and the patient is moved into a supine position. Infection of the pleural space, hemothorax, subdiaphragmatic haematoma, and lacerations of subdiaphragmatic organs are rare, but serious adverse events. Hemothorax has occasionally been reported through laceration of an intercostal artery (38–40). Endorsing the technique described above, which avoids contact with intercostal vessels, and following a sterile approach can prevent most of these complications. Seeding of the needle tract with malignant cells is frequently observed in malignant mesothelioma. Conflicting evidence exists as to whether this can be prevented by local irradiation (41,42).

The use of sonography for puncture site identification seems to reduce the rate of dry taps as well as the rate of complications. The incidence of pneumothorax was only 3% in one study employing ultrasound in 188 patients, and the number of dry taps was reduced in several studies (13,14,16). In a recent large study of 255 pleural procedures, in 205 patients with mostly small effusions, a low incidence of pneumothorax was reported in connection with liberal use of ultrasound (21). The risk for complications is increased in small effusions, loculated pleural effusions, blunt costo-phrenic angles, and lung consolidation (10). It seems therefore reasonable to recommend routine ultrasound for these risk constellations to avoid complications and increase yield of pleural taps (17–19).

VI. Yield of Pleural Thoracocentesis and Biopsy

A. Diagnostic Thoracocentesis

Diagnostic thoracocentesis is an extremely helpful diagnostic tool, though the yield varies with different diseases. In a prospective study of 129 consecutive diagnostic thoracocenteses, a definitive diagnosis could be made in 18%. In 56% of cases, a presumptive diagnosis correlated with clinical findings was possible, while only 26% of the taps remained nondiagnostic (4). Diseases to be diagnosed on the grounds of only pleural fluid findings are listed in Table 2 (43). In many situations, pleural fluid analysis will reveal clues to rule in or out specific diseases, many of which are discussed in separate chapters in this book. Since closed needle biopsy is done mainly in suspected pleural TB and malignancy, we will discuss their relative yield in these selected diseases below. Pleural malignancies and TB pleurisy are dealt with in-depth in the relevant chapters.

Table 2   Diagnoses Established by Pleural Fluid Analysis

Disease	Diagnostic characteristics
Empyema	Pus on aspiration
Malignancy	Malignant cells on cytology
TB pleurisy	Positive AFB stain or culture
Fungal infection	Positive stain or culture
Chylothorax	Elevated triglycerides and cholesterol
Hemothorax	Hematocrit >50% of blood hematocrit
Rheumatoid pleurisy	Typical cytology
Lupus pleurisy	Typical cytology
Esophageal rupture	Very low pH, high amylase

B.   Diagnostic Thoracocentesis and Closed Needle Biopsy in TB Pleurisy

Untreated TB pleurisy usually has a self-limiting course. Nevertheless, the proper identification of the disease is important, because most patients with untreated TB pleurisy will develop some other form of active TB later in their life (44,45). Moreover, the administration of antituberculous therapy dramatically reduces the incidence of subsequent TB (46). With the high prevalence of HIV infection, the number of TB cases is rising in many developing countries, and invasive procedures for the diagnosis of TB pleuritis are not uniformly available and relatively expensive. A simple and cheap diagnostic tool for pleural TB in high-prevalence areas is therefore of substantial epidemiologic interest.

Diagnostic Thoracocentesis in TB Pleurisy

Unfortunately, the diagnostic yield of staining and culture for Mycobacteria in pleural is low. Staining for acid-fast bacilli (AFB) has a sensitivity of only around 20%, and mycobacterial culture of pleural fluid is positive for mycobacteria in around 40% (47,48). These figures may be somewhat higher in HIV patients (49). Polymerase chain reaction (PCR) has shown inconsistent results on pleural fluid, and PCR is expensive and requires expert laboratory staff (50,51). The low yield of all these methods is mainly due to the immunologic nature of TB pleuritis, with only a small number of bacteria present in the pleural fluid.

The best studied and the most widely used alternative test to date is adenosine deaminase (ADA) activity in pleural fluid (52–57). The test has some specificity problems with false positives occurring in bacterial empyema and rheumatic effusions. With a cutoff level of 50 Units, combined with a pleural fluid cell count showing predominant lymphocytosis (>75%), the sensitivity and specificity were 88% and 95%, respectively, in a study on 472 patients with exudative pleural effusions at our institution, which is situated in a high prevalence area for TB pleurisy (54). In the future, commercially available tests for isoenzymes may further increase sensitivity and specificity of AdA on pleural fluid (58). INF-γ in pleural fluid is less well studied, but reported to have similar predictive values as AdA. Discrimination from rheumatoid effusions may be better than with AdA, but INF-γ is expensive and will therefore not be widely available in high-prevalence areas for TB (59,60). It is important to remember that the prevalence of the disease decisively influences the value of these indirect tests on pleural fluid for TB pleurisy. In low-prevalence areas with TB accounting for less than 5% of exudative effusions, even a test with high specificity would still produce an unacceptably high rate of false positives.

Closed Needle Biopsy in TB Pleurisy

The traditional method of choice for the diagnosis of TB pleurisy is closed needle biopsy showing granulomatous inflammation, which is virtually diagnostic for pleural TB (61). In a recent study in 248 patients, closed needle biopsy alone had a yield of about 80% alone, and when added to AFB staining and culture, the overall yield was 91% (48). A slightly better overall sensitivity may be achieved with thoracoscopy, where in contrast to closed needle biopsy the sampling error is reduced by visual identification of the affected pleural regions, but the advantage seems to be minimal (5,62). The popularity of AdA and INF-γ in regions with high incidence of TB pleurisy seems to be responsible for the decreasing use of closed needle pleural biopsy. Yet, replacing pleural biopsy with AdA or INF-γ will result in fewer cultures available for resistance testing. This drawback is debatable, because the diagnosis of TB pleurisy with pleural biopsy relies on the finding of granulomatous tissue on histology rather than on the culture positivity for mycobacteria, and the number of available cultures will only decrease by around 20% when no pleural biopsy is taken (61). Moreover, the resistance to antituberculous drugs depends on regional factors (63). In our opinion, the decision whether to use closed needle pleural biopsy routinely is to be taken locally, based on the availability of pleural fluid tests and local prevalence of TB pleurisy as well as resistance to antituberculous drugs.

C. Diagnostic Thoracocentesis and Closed Needle Biopsy in Malignancy

Malignant pleural effusions are a frequent cause of pleural exudates, mostly from metastatic breast or lung cancer. Prognosis of patients with malignant pleural effusion is poor, and the disease is usually beyond a curable stage. While a certain delay in diagnosis in asymptomatic patients is acceptable, patients with symptomatic effusions should be diagnosed and referred for palliative treatment with pleurodesis to improve quality of life. Closed needle biopsy is not visually controlled and therefore prone to sampling errors in malignant pleural disease, which is not evenly distributed over the parietal pleura.

Malignant Pleural Effusions Due to Metastatic Malignancy

Cytologic evaluation of pleural fluid is an excellent method to diagnose metastatic malignancies to the pleura. The yield of the method will vary with the tumor type, the range of technical examination (cell blocks or smears, use of additional tools like electron microscopy or immuno-histochemistry), the number of successive specimens submitted (the more submitted the higher the percentage of positive results), and the skills of the involved cytologist. While the specificity of a positive result is high, a negative result does not exclude malignancy. Sensitivity varies in published reports from 40% to 87% (47,64–66). After submitting three large-volume specimens, a yield of more than 80% may be expected (67).

In a considerable number of pleural effusions secondary to non–small-cell lung cancer (NSCLC), the pleural fluid may not contain malignant cells, and the pleural effusion is therefore not prohibitive for curative surgery (68). A method with higher sensitivity than pleural fluid cytology might be welcomed in this situation in order to avoid unnecessary exploratory thoracotomies. Unfortunately, closed needle biopsy has a low yield for malignancy. In a study with 281 cases with proven pleural malignancy, closed needle biopsy had a sensitivity of only 43% (64). Increasing the number of biopsy sites as well as the biopsies taken per site does not significantly improve the yield of the method (29,69). In contrast, thoracoscopy under local or general anesthesia establishes the diagnosis of pleural malignancy in 90% of cases, and offers the possibility of effective pleurodesis during the procedure (70–72). In our opinion, the role of closed needle biopsy in suspected malignancy is confined to situations where thoracoscopy is not an option and repeat cytology has failed to produce a diagnosis.

Malignant Effusions Due to Mesothelioma
In the case of mesothelioma, the diagnosis of malignancy can usually be made on cytologic examination of pleural fluid. The distinction between metastatic adenocarcinoma and mesothelioma, however, is difficult, and in about 25% of cases, the diagnosis of mesothelioma cannot be made on cytology alone, although various discriminating cytologic or immuno-histochemical features with good sensitivity and specificity exist (73–78). In addition, the specific diagnosis of mesothelioma has forensic importance in many societies, because compensation can be claimed for mesothelioma associated with asbestos exposure. Traditional closed needle biopsy is usually not diagnostic for mesothelioma (73). Instead, a core-tissue biopsy large enough is best acquired with cutting needle biopsy, thoracoscopy or open surgical biopsy (68,79–82). The yield of these methods is around 90% for mesothelioma (70,71,83).

VII. Limitations
Diagnostic pleurocentesis is a simple, straightforward, and safe procedure. The yield is however limited, because not all pleural diseases feature pleural fluid alterations characteristic enough to allow for definite diagnosis. In our opinion, the potential benefit of diagnostic pleurocentesis is well balanced against the possible harm and discomfort in most situations where an exudative effusion may be expected on clinical grounds.

In contrast, the role of closed needle biopsy in undiagnosed exudative pleural effusions is controversial. The procedure adds little to the diagnostic value of serial pleurocentesis in metastatic malignant disease, and mesothelioma is more readily diagnosed on large tissue biopsies better obtained with different methods. In suspected TB pleurisy, the yield of closed needle biopsy is still comparable to modern biochemical methods and offers the advantage of somewhat higher culture positivity. The usefulness of the technique depends highly on the local availability of operator expertise. We believe that closed needle biopsy still has a strong role in undiagnosed lymphocytic effusions, especially if local operator experience is good and modern biochemical tests are not available.

References
1. Garrison FH. Introduction to the History of Medicine, 4th ed. Philadelphia, PA: W. B. Saunders Co., 1929.
2. De Francis N, Klosk E, Albano E. Needle biopsy of the parietal pleura. NEJM 1955; 252: 948–949.
3. Froudarakis ME. Diagnostic work-up of pleural effusions. Respiration 2008; 75:4–13.
4. Collins TR, Sahn SA. Thoracocentesis. Clinical value, complications, technical problems, and patient experience. Chest 1987; 91:817–822.

5. Baumann MH. Closed needle biopsy: A necessary tool? Pulm Perspect 2000; 17:1–3.
6. Sokolowski JW Jr, Burgher LW, Jones FL Jr, et al. Guidelines for thoracentesis and needle biopsy of the pleura. Position paper of the American Thoracic Society. Am Rev Respir Dis 1989; 140:257–258.
7. Walsh LJ, Macfarlane JT, Manhire AR, et al. Audit of pleural biopsies: An argument for a pleural biopsy service. Respir Med 1994; 88:503–505.
8. Azoulay E. Pleural effusions in the intensive care unit. Curr Opin Pulm Med 2003; 9:291–297.
9. Lichtenstein D, Hulot JS, Rabiller A, et al. Feasibility and safety of ultrasound-aided thoracentesis in mechanically ventilated patients. Intensive Care Med 1999; 25:955–958.
10. Weingardt JP, Guico RR, Nemcek AA Jr, et al. Ultrasound findings following failed, clinically directed thoracenteses. J Clin Ultrasound 1994; 22:419–426.
11. Brandt WE. The thorax. In: Rumack MC, Wilson SR, Charboneau JW, eds. Diagnostic Ultrasound, 2nd ed. St. Louis, U.S.A.: Mosby, 1998:575–597.
12. O'Moore PV, Mueller PR, Simeone JF, et al. Sonographic guidance in diagnostic and therapeutic interventions in the pleural space. AJR Am J Roentgenol 1987; 149:1–5.
13. Grogan DR, Irwin RS, Channick R, et al. Complications associated with thoracentesis. A prospective, randomized study comparing three different methods. Arch Intern Med 1990; 150:873–877.
14. Kohan JM, Poe RH, Israel RH, et al. Value of chest ultrasonography versus decubitus roentgenography for thoracentesis. Am Rev Respir Dis 1986; 133:1124–1126.
15. Lipscomb DJ, Flower CD, Hadfield JW. Ultrasound of the pleura: An assessment of its clinical value. Clin Radiol 1981; 32:289–290.
16. Raptopoulos V, Davis LM, Lee G, et al. Factors affecting the development of pneumothorax associated with thoracentesis. AJR Am J Roentgenol 1991; 156:917–920.
17. Feller-Kopman D. Ultrasound-guided thoracentesis. Chest 2006; 129:1709–1714.
18. Diacon AH, Theron J, Bolliger CT. Transthoracic ultrasound for the pulmonologist. Curr Opin Pulm Med 2005; 11:307–312.
19. Mayo PH, Doelken P. Pleural ultrasonography. Clin Chest Med 2006; 27:215–227.
20. Diacon A, Brutsche M, Strobel W, et al. Where to puncture a pleural effusion: Tradition vs ultrasound. Schweiz Med Wochenschr 2000; 130(Suppl. 118):34S.
21. Colt HG, Brewer N, Barbur E. Evaluation of patient-related and procedure-related factors contributing to pneumothorax following thoracentesis. Chest 1999; 116:134–138.
22. Levine H, Szanto PB, Cugell DW. Tuberculous pleurisy. An acute illness. Arch Intern Med 1968; 122:329–332.
23. Abrams LD. A pleural-biopsy punch. Lancet 1958; 1:30–31.
24. Cope C. New pleural biopsy needle. JAMA 1958; 167:1107–1108.
25. Ogirala RG, Agarwal V, Aldrich TK. Raja pleural biopsy needle. A comparison with the Abrams needle in experimental pleural effusion. Am Rev Respir Dis 1989; 139:984–987.
26. O'Connor S, Yung T. A comparison of Abrams and Raja pleural biopsy needles. Aust N Z J Med 1992; 22:237–239.
27. Ogirala RG, Agarwal V, Vizioli LD, et al. Comparison of the Raja and the Abrams pleural biopsy needles in patients with pleural effusion. Am Rev Respir Dis 1993; 147: 1291–1294.
28. Morrone N, Algranti E, Barreto E. Pleural biopsy with Cope and Abrams needles. Chest 1987; 92:1050–1052.
29. Mungall IP, Cowen PN, Cooke NT, et al. Multiple pleural biopsy with the Abrams needle. Thorax 1980; 35:600–602.
30. Kirsch CM, Kroe DM, Azzi RL, et al. The optimal number of pleural biopsy specimens for a diagnosis of tuberculous pleurisy. Chest 1997; 112:702–706.
31. Seneff MG, Corwin RW, Gold LH, et al. Complications associated with thoracocentesis. Chest 1986; 90:97–100.

32. Poe RH, Israel RH, Utell MJ, et al. Sensitivity, specificity, and predictive values of closed pleural biopsy. Arch Intern Med 1984; 144:325–328.
33. Brandstetter RD, Karetzky M, Rastogi R, et al. Pneumothorax after thoracentesis in chronic obstructive pulmonary disease. Heart Lung 1994; 23:67–70.
34. Bartter T, Mayo PD, Pratter MR, et al. Lower risk and higher yield for thoracentesis when performed by experienced operators. Chest 1993; 103:1873–1876.
35. Aleman C, Alegre J, Armadans L, et al. The value of chest roentgenography in the diagnosis of pneumothorax after thoracentesis. Am J Med 1999; 107:340–343.
36. Doyle JJ, Hnatiuk OW, Torrington KG, et al. Necessity of routine chest roentgenography after thoracentesis. Ann Intern Med 1996; 124:816–820.
37. Petersen WG, Zimmerman R. Limited utility of chest radiograph after thoracentesis. Chest 2000; 117:1038–1042.
38. Carney M, Ravin CE. Intercostal artery laceration during thoracocentesis: Increased risk in elderly patients. Chest 1979; 75:520–522.
39. Lai JH, Yan HC, Kao SJ, et al. Intercostal arteriovenous fistula due to pleural biopsy. Thorax 1990; 45:976–978.
40. Ali J, Summer WR. Hemothorax and hyperkalemia after pleural biopsy in a 43-year-old woman on hemodialysis. Chest 1994; 106:1235–1236.
41. O'Rourke N, Garcia JC, Paul J, et al. A randomised controlled trial of intervention site radiotherapy in malignant pleural mesothelioma. Radiother Oncol 2007; 84:18–22.
42. Boutin C, Rey F, Viallat JR. Prevention of malignant seeding after invasive diagnostic procedures in patients with pleural mesothelioma. A randomized trial of local radiotherapy. Chest 1995; 108:754–758.
43. Sahn SA. State of the art. The pleura. Am Rev Respir Dis 1988; 138:184–234.
44. Patila J. Initial tuberculous pleuritis in the Finnish Armed Forces in 1939–1945 with special reference to eventual post pleuritits tuberculosis. Acta Tuberc Scand 1954; 36(Suppl.): 1–57.
45. Roper WH, Waring JJ. Primary serofibrinous pleural effusion in military personnel. Am Rev Respir Dis 1955; 71:616–634.
46. Berger HW, Mejia E. Tuberculous pleurisy. Chest 1973; 63:88–92.
47. Escudero Bueno C, Garcia Clemente M, Cuesta Castro B, et al. Cytologic and bacteriologic analysis of fluid and pleural biopsy specimens with Cope's needle. Study of 414 patients. Arch Intern Med 1990; 150:1190–1194.
48. Valdes L, Alvarez D, San Jose E, et al. Tuberculous pleurisy: A study of 254 patients. Arch Intern Med 1998; 158:2017–2021.
49. Heyderman RS, Makunike R, Muza T, et al. Pleural tuberculosis in Harare, Zimbabwe: The relationship between human immunodeficiency virus, CD4 lymphocyte count, granuloma formation and disseminated disease. Trop Med Int Health 1998; 3:14–20.
50. Villena V, Rebollo MJ, Aguado JM, et al. Polymerase chain reaction for the diagnosis of pleural tuberculosis in immunocompromised and immunocompetent patients. Clin Infect Dis 1998; 26:212–214.
51. Querol JM, Minguez J, Garcia-Sanchez E, et al. Rapid diagnosis of pleural tuberculosis by polymerase chain reaction. Am J Respir Crit Care Med 1995; 152(6 Pt 1):1977–1981.
52. Valdes L, San Jose E, Alvarez D, et al. Adenosine deaminase (ADA) isoenzyme analysis in pleural effusions: Diagnostic role, and relevance to the origin of increased ADA in tuberculous pleurisy. Eur Respir J 1996; 9:747–751.
53. Ferrer JS, Munoz XG, Orriols RM, et al. Evolution of idiopathic pleural effusion: A prospective, long-term follow-up study. Chest 1996; 109:1508–1513.
54. Burgess LJ, Maritz FJ, Le Roux I, et al. Combined use of pleural adenosine deaminase with lymphocyte/neutrophil ratio. Increased specificity for the diagnosis of tuberculous pleuritis. Chest 1996; 109:414–419.

55. Riantawan P, Chaowalit P, Wongsangiem M, et al. Diagnostic value of pleural fluid adenosine deaminase in tuberculous pleuritis with reference to HIV coinfection and a Bayesian analysis. Chest 1999; 116:97–103.

56. Burgess LJ, Maritz FJ, Le Roux I, et al. Use of adenosine deaminase as a diagnostic tool for tuberculous pleurisy. Thorax 1995; 50:672–674.

57. Valdes L, Alvarez D, San Jose E, et al. Value of adenosine deaminase in the diagnosis of tuberculous pleural effusions in young patients in a region of high prevalence of tuberculosis. Thorax 1995; 50:600–603.

58. Perez-Rodriguez E, Jimenez Castro D. The use of adenosine deaminase and adenosine deaminase isoenzymes in the diagnosis of tuberculous pleuritis. Curr Opin Pulm Med 2000; 6: 259–266.

59. Villena V, Lopez-Encuentra A, Echave-Sustaeta J, et al. Interferon-gamma in 388 immunocompromised and immunocompetent patients for diagnosing pleural tuberculosis. Eur Respir J 1996; 9:2635–2639.

60. Valdes L, San Jose E, Alvarez D, et al. Diagnosis of tuberculous pleurisy using the biologic parameters adenosine deaminase, lysozyme, and interferon gamma. Chest 1993; 103:458–465.

61. Light RW. Tuberculous pleural effusions. In: Light RW, ed. Pleural Diseases. Baltimore, U.S.A.: Lippincott Williams & Wilkins, 2001:182–195.

62. Loddenkemper R, Mai J, Scheffler N, et al. Prospective individual comparison of blind needle biopsy and of thoracoscopy in the diagnosis and differential diagnosis of tuberculous pleurisy. Scand J Respir Dis Suppl 1978; 102:196–198.

63. Gopi A, Madhavan SM, Sharma SK, et al. Diagnosis and treatment of tuberculous pleural effusion in 2006. Chest 2007; 131:880–889.

64. Prakash UB, Reiman HM. Comparison of needle biopsy with cytologic analysis for the evaluation of pleural effusion: Analysis of 414 cases. Mayo Clin Proc 1985; 60:158–164.

65. Dekker A, Bupp PA. Cytology of serous effusions. An investigation into the usefulness of cell blocks versus smears. Am J Clin Pathol 1978; 70:855–860.

66. Jarvi OH, Kunnas RJ, Laitio MT, et al. The accuracy and significance of cytologic cancer diagnosis of pleural effusions. (A followup study of 338 patients). Acta Cytol 1972; 16: 152–158.

67. Light RW. Pleural effusions related to metastatic malignancies. In: Light RW, ed. Pleural Diseases. Baltimore, U.S.A.: Lippincott Williams & Wilkins, 2001:108–134.

68. Rodriguez-Panadero F, Borderas Naranjo F, Lopez Mejias J. Pleural metastatic tumours and effusions. Frequency and pathogenic mechanisms in a post-mortem series. Eur Respir J 1989; 2:366–369.

69. Canto A, Rivas J, Saumench J, et al. Points to consider when choosing a biopsy method in cases of pleurisy of unknown origin. Chest 1983; 84:176–179.

70. Hucker J, Bhatnagar NK, al-Jilaihawi AN,et al. Thoracoscopy in the diagnosis and management of recurrent pleural effusions. Ann Thorac Surg 1991; 52:1145–1147.

71. Menzies R, Charbonneau M. Thoracoscopy for the diagnosis of pleural disease. Ann Intern Med 1991; 114:271–276.

72. Diacon AH, Wyser C, Bolliger CT, et al. Prospective randomized comparison of thoracoscopic talc poudrage under local anesthesia versus bleomycin instillation for pleurodesis in malignant pleural effusions. Am J Respir Crit Care Med 2000; 162:1445–1449.

73. Law MR, Hodson ME, Turner-Warwick M. Malignant mesothelioma of the pleura: Clinical aspects and symptomatic treatment. Eur J Respir Dis 1984; 65:162–168.

74. Stevens MW, Leong AS, Fazzalari NL, et al. Cytopathology of malignant mesothelioma: A stepwise logistic regression analysis. Diagn Cytopathol 1992; 8:333–341.

75. Wirth PR, Legier J, Wright GL Jr. Immunohistochemical evaluation of seven monoclonal antibodies for differentiation of pleural mesothelioma from lung adenocarcinoma. Cancer 1991; 67:655–662.

76. Frisman DM, McCarthy WF, Schleiff P, et al. Immunocytochemistry in the differential diagnosis of effusions: Use of logistic regression to select a panel of antibodies to distinguish adenocarcinomas from mesothelial proliferations. Mod Pathol 1993; 6:179–184.
77. Carella R, Deleonardi G, D'Errico A, et al. Immunohistochemical panels for differentiating epithelial malignant mesothelioma from lung adenocarcinoma: A study with logistic regression analysis. Am J Surg Pathol 2001; 25:43–50.
78. Brown RW, Clark GM, Tandon AK, et al. Multiple-marker immunohistochemical phenotypes distinguishing malignant pleural mesothelioma from pulmonary adenocarcinoma. Hum Pathol 1993; 24:347–354.
79. Diacon AH, Schuurmans MM, Theron J, et al. Safety and yield of ultrasound-assisted transthoracic biopsy performed by pulmonologists. Respiration 2004; 71:519–522.
80. Maskell NA, Gleeson FV, Davies RJ. Standard pleural biopsy versus CT-guided cutting-needle biopsy for diagnosis of malignant disease in pleural effusions: A randomised controlled trial. Lancet 2003; 361:1326–1330.
81. Lee P, Colt HG. Rigid and semirigid pleuroscopy: The future is bright. Respirology 2005; 10:418–425.
82. Lee P, Colt HG. State of the art: Pleuroscopy. J Thorac Oncol 2007; 2:663–670.
83. Boutin C, Rey F, Gouvernet J, et al. Thoracoscopy in pleural malignant mesothelioma: A prospective study of 188 consecutive patients. Part 2: Prognosis and staging. Cancer 1993; 72:394–404.

7
Chest Tubes

DEMONDES HAYNES and MICHAEL H. BAUMANN
Division of Pulmonary and Critical Care Medicine, University of Mississippi Medical Center,
Jackson, Mississippi, U.S.A.

I. Introduction

A. History

Reportedly, Hippocrates was the first to describe tube drainage of an infected pleural space (1). Continuous chest tube drainage of the pleural space incorporating an underwater seal device appears to have occurred first in the 1870s in a patient suffering empyema unresponsive to repeated aspiration (2). Extensive interest in effective methods of pleural drainage and experimentation investigating the appropriate role of these pleural drainage measures, including chest tube drainage, occurred after the 1917 postinfluenza epidemic of empyema (3). Postoperative use of chest tube drainage in thoracic surgery, including after lobectomy for suppurative lung disease, was reported in 1922 (4). However, not until the Korean War was postoperative chest tube placement standard after major thoracic surgical procedures (5).

B. Indications

Indications for chest tube (tube thoracostomy) placement are noted in Table 1 (1). Absolute contraindications do not exist, but careful consideration of the risks and benefits of chest tube placement should occur before placing a chest tube in a patient with a coagulopathy; consideration to correction of the disorder should be given if patient's stability permits (1,6). Chest tube insertion in an area of a dermatologic disorder should be avoided, if possible (6).

II. Chest Tube Placement Technique and Complications

Traditionally, the site of chest tube insertion has been determined by the material to be removed from the pleural space. Given that air rises to the least gravity-dependent portion of the chest, chest tube placement in the third to fifth intercostal space in the midaxillary line with the tube directed apically and anteriorly is suggested for pneumothorax. Alternately, the tube may be placed in the midclavicular line in the second intercostal space. Free flowing fluid, of any type, is best drained by placing the tube in the sixth intercostal space in the midaxillary line with the tube directed inferiorly and posteriorly (1). Image-directed tube placement by computed tomography or ultrasound is often used for the drainage of loculated pleural fluid.

Table 1   Indications for Chest Tube Placement

1. Pneumothorax
2. Empyema and parapneumonic effusion
3. Recurrent symptomatic effusion
4. Hemothorax
5. Chylothorax
6. Postoperatively in thoracic surgery
7. Bronchopleural fistula

Chest tubes traditionally have been placed by two major approaches, blunt dissection (incisional) and trocar insertion (1,6). Given concerns for damage to the underlying lung by utilizing a rigid, sharp trocar (1), many physicians prefer the blunt dissection approach. The development of chest tubes that may be placed by the Seldinger technique (guide wire placement) offers an additional alternative (7), which is described below. The reader is referred to two pictorial references outlining both the techniques (6,7).

Regardless of the insertion technique, the site chosen should be thoroughly cleaned with an antiseptic solution covering an adequate area allowing alternate insertion sites if needed. Generous use of local anesthesia with infiltration of the adjacent tissue and tissue superior to the rib is recommended. Limiting the anesthesia and insertion area to the tissues just above the superior surface of the rib is recommended to avoid damage to the neurovascular bundle located inferior to the rib above. If blunt dissection is planned, adequate anesthesia along the length of the incision site is required. Aspiration of air or fluid into the anesthetic syringe indicates entrance in the pleural space. Subsequent withdrawal of the needle to the point of absence of aspiration of either air or fluid indicates proximity to the visceral pleural surface. Liberal application of anesthetic to the visceral pleural surface is recommended.

After allowing several minutes for the development of adequate local anesthesia effects, make a small skin incision parallel to the superior surface of the rib with the length determined by the size of the tube being inserted. Usually, a 3- to 4-cm incision will suffice. Then, careful blunt dissection just above the rib's superior surface is accomplished using a Kelly clamp. Entrance to the pleural space is often heralded by the appearance of pleural fluid or the sound of air entering and leaving the chest through the insertion site due to respiratory fluctuation. The Kelly clamp is then used to widen the tract from the skin to pleural space. The Kelly is slowly withdrawn while simultaneously inserting a finger in the tract to maintain the tract and to allow digital sweeping of the immediate visceral pleural surface to clear any adjacent adhesions. The distal end of the chest tube (end inserted into the chest) is then clamped with forceps and inserted through the tract and into the pleural space. Rotation of the forceps with the distal tip of the chest tube clamped in the forceps will facilitate placement of the tube superiorly (apically) or inferiorly. A subsequent chest radiograph is obtained to confirm placement.

The chest tube placed by blunt dissection should be sewn in place using heavy suture material mounted on a curved cutting needle; we prefer 0 silk suture. A purse sting suture around the tube is suggested with a half square (surgeon's) knot left in place. The half-knot maintains tension in the purse string, thus sealing the chest tube within the pleural space. This also allows prompt closure of the wound upon tube removal and easy completion of the square knot. We keep the excess suture material in place and wrap it around the tube and tie it off allowing additional security against tube removal. This excess suture material also allows easy completion of a square knot upon tube removal. The site may be dressed using sealing antiseptic gauze (Adaptic X xeroform gauze nonadherent dressing, Johnson and Johnson, Arlington, TX, U.S.A.) serving to help seal the site against air leaks. Next, cut 4 × 4 gauze squares, (cut half way through creating a slit within which to place the chest tube), which are placed around the chest tube. Finally, after skin preparation with an adhesive substance (Benzoin Compound, tincture USP, Paddock Laboratories, Minneapolis, MN, U.S.A.), the site is taped. The most successful tape, in our practice, has been Microfoam (3M Medical, Surgical Division, St. Paul, MN, U.S.A.). Tape applied around the chest tube near the connection with the pleural drainage device (if used) in an umbilical/omental configuration adds security against tube removal.

Chest tubes may also be inserted using a Seldinger technique wherein a guide wire plays a central role in tube placement. This technique is core to many commercially available kits such as those made by the companies Arrow™ and Cook™. Both large and small bore chest tubes may be inserted by this approach. After adequate sterile cleansing of the site and local anesthesia, the pleural space is located with a sterile needle. Subsequently, a guide wire is placed through the needle into the space with the wire directed apically (for air) or inferiorly (for fluid) depending upon the material to be drained. Subsequently, a tract dilator (several graduated dilator sizes may be used for larger tubes) is passed. The actual chest tube is then placed over the guide wire and the wire removed. The tube may then be dressed similarly to tubes placed by blunt dissection. Commercially available kits often have tube-securing devices included.

Perhaps the most frequent complication of chest tube placement is patient discomfort during tube placement, tube residence, or tube removal (6). Harvey and Prescott noted that pain may be particularly problematic with larger tubes as compared to smaller tubes while in place; paradoxically no difference was noted between large and small tubes during tube insertion (8). Other common complications directly related to the tube itself include misplacement of the tube during insertion, disconnection of the tube while in place, and leakage around the tube possibly resulting in subcutaneous emphysema (6). Pneumothorax recurrence in mechanically ventilated patients may occur due to initial tube malposition. Radiographic demonstration of interlobar chest tube placement has a positive predictive value of 86% for pneumothorax recurrence. Optimally, the chest tube should parallel the chest wall and be in the anterior hemithorax in patients with a pneumothorax (9).

Few studies are available specifically addressing complications directly attributable to chest tubes. Millikan and colleagues prospectively assessed chest tube–related complications in the acute thoracic trauma setting (10). Out of 447 patients, four suffered a technical complication of chest tube placement by blunt dissection. These included diaphragm laceration (two patients), lung laceration (one patient), and one patient with avulsion injury to the lesser curve of the stomach, laceration to the left lobe of the liver, and left diaphragm defect. Of 1249 patients (trocar and blunt dissection chest tube placements), 30 cases of empyema occurred. No deaths were directly attributed to chest tube placement.

III. Specific Chest Tube–Related Questions

In general, this section addresses common questions related to chest tube placement. Specific answers to these questions related to common indications for chest tube placement will be explored further in section V (Selected Indications).

A. What Size Chest Tube Should Be Used?

Various sizes of chest tubes are now available increasing the options for treatment of various pleural conditions but potentially leading to selection of tube sizes inappropriate to the condition. Flow of a humid gas through a chest tube is governed by the Fanning equation ($v = \pi^2 r^5 P/fl$; where v is the flow, r is radius, l is length, P is pressure, and f is friction factor) (11–13). Flow is further complicated by the presence of liquids of various viscosities. Obviously, the critical factor in chest tube selection is the bore (internal diameter) of the tube and less so, the tube length. Hence, selection of a chest tube must take into account what is being drained and the rate at which the material is being formed. Patients with a large bronchopleural fistula on mechanical ventilation or patients with a briskly bleeding chest lesion require a larger tube than those patients with small air leaks or static pleural fluid collections.

Similarly, Poiseulle's law states that the flow of a liquid through a tube depends on the internal diameter (D), the length (L) of the tube, the viscosity of the liquid (η), and the pressure difference between its ends (ΔP):

$$\text{Flow rate} = \frac{\pi}{128} \frac{D^4 \Delta P}{\eta L}.$$

Therefore, if the diameter of a tube is doubled, flow will increase by a factor of 16, implying that small increases in the size of drainage tubes will result in substantial improvement in flow rates (14). Different fluids have different viscosities and should be taken into consideration when determining appropriate tube size for fluid drainage (15).

Knowledge of flow rates through various commercially available small-bore chest tubes (catheters) is key when considering their use. Generally, use of a small bore tube for fluid collection needs careful consideration, particularly if fluid production is brisk, given flow rates will be more limited for fluid than that for air. Additionally, not all small-bore catheters are of equal efficacy in their ability to handle air flow (16). This problem is compounded by the use of commercial thoracocentesis kits that contain drainage catheters as a source for indwelling catheters. As expected from the Fanning equation, smaller bore catheters handle lower flow rates with 8 Fr catheter rates ranging from 2.6 to 5.5 L of air per minute. Eight French thoracocentesis catheters handle significantly lower flow rates than the 8 Fr pneumothorax catheters made by the same manufacturer. Lower flow rates with the thoracocentesis catheter appear due to different proximal catheter hardware (16).

B. Should Suction Be Applied?

After placement of the chest tube, the tube may be connected to a pleural drainage unit (PDU). The option then exists to utilize suction regulated through the PDU to the pleural space. Limited information is available to provide clear guidance as to the role of suction in the various indications for chest tube placement. Notably air and free flowing fluid will generally drain from the chest without the need for suction. Suction becomes necessary when a compromising accumulation of air or fluid occurs due to their rate of development or due to the viscosity of fluid hampering efficient gravity drainage. See section III E (How should a chest tube be removed?) which discusses the role of suction in chest tube removal.

C.   How Can Re-expansion Pulmonary Edema Be Avoided?

Re-expansion pulmonary edema may occur after the drainage of pleural air or fluid (17). The etiology and risk factors leading to the development of re-expansion pulmonary are likely multifactorial (12). Increased vascular permeability, oxygen-free radical generation, and mechanical injury have been implicated as possible causes (18–20). Risk factors for re-expansion pulmonary edema appear to be young age, extent of lung collapse, and duration of collapse (17,21–23). Re-expansion pulmonary edema has also been shown to occur in the absence of suction and may occur in the contralateral lung (24). A related question regarding issues prompting concern for re-expansion pulmonary edema is how much pleural fluid should initially be removed during a diagnostic or therapeutic thoracocentesis or when placing a chest tube. The development of excess negative pleural pressures should be avoided and may herald the presence of a trapped lung (25,26) and reduced success of pleural sclerosis (25). Safe pleural fluid removal may continue as long as pleural pressures do not fall below −20 cm of water pressure (26).

However, the tools to measure pleural pressure during fluid removal are cumbersome and most clinicians do not measure pressures. The American Thoracic Society (ATS) recommends the removal of only one to one and a half liters of fluid at any one sitting provided the patient does not develop dyspnea, chest pain, or severe cough (27). Additionally, we perform all chest tube placements and thoracocenteses with an oxygen saturation monitor in place and discontinue drainage for a drop in saturation of more than 3% to 5% that does not resolve promptly with a short halt in fluid drainage. However, removal of several liters of fluid is likely safe in the patient with contralateral shift of the mediastinum (shift away from the fluid) who does not develop chest tightness, cough or dyspnea during fluid removal. The patient without mediastinal shift or with ipsilateral mediastinal shift (shift toward the fluid) likely has a fixed mediastinum, trapped lung, or endobronchial obstruction. In those patients, the chance of a marked fall in pleural pressure is increased and pleural pressure monitoring should be used or only a small volume of fluid (<300 mL) should be removed (27).

D.   Should Talc Be Used as a Pleural Sclerosant?

Talc is a successful (up to 91%) pleural sclerosant whether applied by chest tube (slurry) or poudrage (by thoracoscopy) for both pneumothorax and pleural effusion (28). However, controversy and debate regarding its use and possible side effects (including acute respiratory distress syndrome, ARDS) continues (29,30). The etiology of talc-associated respiratory failure is unclear. Small talc particle size may contribute to its distribution throughout the body and in turn be related to geographic origin of the talc (31). A trial from the United Kingdom revealed that smaller talc size (<10 μm) induced more local and systemic inflammation (32). Recent pleural disruption by pleural biopsy or other invasive procedures may promote systemic talc distribution (33). Given these findings and concerns, the patient should be informed of their options and associated risks before proceeding with talc pleural sclerosis. If talc is chosen, the dose is not clearly established. Doses of as little as 2 g by poudrage have been reported to be associated with ARDS (29).

Alternately, a large review notes a dose by poudrage or slurry of 5 g as successful and comparatively safe (28).

E. How Should a Chest Tube Be Removed?

Once the primary purpose for placement of a chest tube has passed, tube removal should be considered promptly. One of the most important issues to consider before tube removal is whether an air leak is present. Tube removal prior to cessation of an air leak, even a small leak, can lead to the development of a tension pneumothorax.

A commonly asked question is whether to remove a chest tube at the end of inspiration or the end of expiration (34). A randomized trial by Bell and colleagues assessing 102 chest tube placements in 69 patients suffering blunt or penetrating thoracic trauma requiring tube placement found no difference in the occurrence of post–chest tube removal pneumothoraces by either method (34). These findings occurred regardless of the mechanism of injury prompting tube placement, presence of hemothorax, history of thoracotomy or thoracoscopy, previous lung disease, or chest tube duration. Hence, patients having resolution of pneumothorax or a small stable pneumothorax by chest radiograph, lack of an air leak while the chest tube is applied to water seal, and as demonstrated in the current study, chest tube output less than 200 mL/day, may have their chest tube removed safely by either approach (34).

Whether to place a chest tube to suction or to water seal, both utilizing a PDU, prior to removal is not clear. A series of studies exploring this issue yield conflicting results and provide no definitive answer (35–37). Overall, continued chest tube suction after lung re-expansion and air leak cessation for several hours may be advisable before chest tube removal to reduce chest tube residence time and subsequent lung recollapse. Suction may also assist in the detection of small air leaks. Many recent studies advocate the use of suction with a subsequent switch to early underwater seal (38,39).

The optimal duration of suction after air-leak resolution has yet to be determined. Alternate approaches to the removal of a chest tube, including suction discontinuation and chest tube clamping to detect occult air leaks, are addressed by the American College of Chest Physicians (ACCP) consensus statement on the management of spontaneous pneumothorax (see section, spontaneous pneumothorax) (40). Additional randomized controlled trials are needed to determine the optimal approach to chest tube removal.

IV. The Pleural Drainage Unit (PDU)

Depending upon the clinical indication, once a chest tube is placed, a PDU may be attached to provide suction and/or water seal to prevent back flow of air into the pleural space. The same resistance considerations in choosing a chest tube need to be assessed for the connecting tubing and the multichambered drainage device comprising a PDU (12,16,41–43). Commercially available PDUs differ considerably in their flow rates and the accuracy of delivered negative pressures (16). An assessment of commercial PDUs available in the United States notes air-flow rate capabilities at -20 cm of water pressure vary with ranging from 10.8 to 42.1 L/min. The accuracy of the measured level of suction delivered varies significantly but may be of a magnitude that is not clinically significant (16).

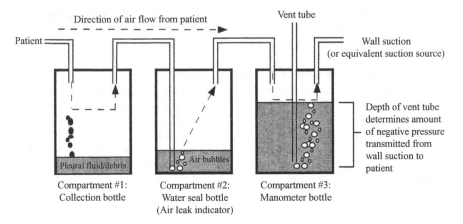

Figure 1   Three-compartment pleural drainage unit (PDU).

The assessed commercially available PDUs are all based upon the traditional three-chamber device (16). This three-chamber device (Fig. 1) is now commercially packaged into compartmentalized, durable, convenient single units providing easy mobility and specimen collection. The three compartments, sequentially, include the collection compartment (frequently with sampling ports) to trap liquid material and suspended debris from the patient's pleural space, while allowing any pleural air to pass through the next two compartments; the water-seal compartment to prevent air flow back to the patient's pleural space and to allow detection of an air leak (bronchopleural fistula); and the manometer compartment to regulate the amount of negative pressure transmitted back to the patient from the wall-suction device (or equivalent suction source). Commercial PDUs are available as "wet" or "dry" devices depending upon whether they have a traditional water-based manometer compartment or a system based upon a spring-loaded valve system (dry system) (16).

Simple one-way valve systems are available and commonly contained within commercial pneumothorax kits (16). Such a device may be attached to a chest tube in lieu of the more elaborate PDU devices described above. A Heimlich valve is such a device. Caution is urged when incorporating a Heimlich valve, or similar device, particularly when a patient is sent home with the device attached to a chest tube because of possible complications such as tension pneumothorax or brochopleural fistula (44–46). The presence of viscous material such as blood should be a relative contraindication to the use of any of these alternative PDU devices for the above-mentioned possible complications.

V.   Selected Indications

A.   Pneumothorax
Pulmonary medicine textbook and journal reviews subdivide pneumothoraces into spontaneous pneumothoraces (SP) and traumatic pneumothoraces (47,48). Spontaneous pneumothoraces occur without preceding trauma or an obvious underlying cause (12,47,48).

Spontaneous pneumothoraces are subdivided into primary and secondary. Primary spontaneous pneumothoraces (PSP) arise in patients without clinically obvious lung disease. Secondary spontaneous pneumothoraces (SSP) occur in patients with underlying lung disease, often chronic obstructive lung disease (12,47,48). Traumatic pneumothoraces result from direct or indirect trauma to the chest including those from diagnostic or therapeutic interventions. Traumatic pneumothoraces resulting from medical interventions are termed iatrogenic pneumothoraces (47).

Spontaneous Pneumothorax

Management of SP has been quite heterogeneous (49). The ACCP guidelines provide some management direction (40). Patient observation, simple aspiration, chest tube placement, surgical interventions including thoracoscopy and thoracotomy for management of SP patients are outlined. Observational management is the preferred ACCP guideline approach for stable PSP patients with a small pneumothorax (<3 cm lung collapse); some form of lung re-expansion procedure, such as chest tube placement, is recommended for a large (≥3-cm lung collapse) pneumothorax.

Chest tube placement plays a central role in the management of other SP patients in these ACCP guidelines, while simple aspiration has a limited place. Initial placement of a chest tube and hospital admission is preferred management of an unstable patient with a large (≥3-cm lung collapse) PSP or any SSP patient with a large pneumothorax or with clinical instability. Patients with a PSP (unlikely at risk for a large air leak) suitable for chest tube placement should have their lung re-expanded using a small bore catheter (≤14 Fr) or placement of a 16 to 22 Fr chest tube. Patients with a SSP, by the nature of their underlying lung disease, may be at greater risk of a large air leak or may require mechanical ventilation (40). Stable SSP patients not at great risk for a large air leak (not mechanically ventilated) who are chest tube candidates should have a 16 to 22 Fr chest tube placed; smaller tubes (≤14 Fr) may be acceptable in selected patients. Unstable SSP patients and SSP patients on mechanical ventilation should have a 24 to 28 Fr chest tube placed because of the risk for large air leaks (40). The British Thoracic Society (BTS) guidelines recommend simple aspiration for all PSP requiring intervention and in select SSP [small (<2 cm) pneumothoraces in minimally breathless patients under the age of 50 years] (50). This aspiration recommendation is based largely on a randomized prospective multicenter trial by Noppen and coworkers demonstrating that simple aspiration was as successful in treating first primary pnuemothoraces as immediate chest tube drainage (51).

Once placed, the initial management of the chest tube is quite variable (49). Limited information regarding the value of suction is available. So and Yu (52) and Minami and colleagues (53) found no clear advantage to the use of suction. The ACCP guidelines suggest attaching a chest tube to a water-seal device with or without suction as acceptable in most SP patients (40). If the lung does not re-expand promptly, suction should then be applied. A Heimlich valve may be incorporated in selected stable SP patients in lieu of a water-seal device, although the consensus of the ACCP expert group was a water-seal device is a better option in most SSP patients (40). Alternatively, the BTS guidelines only recommend adding suction after 48 hours for persistent air leak or failure of a pneumothorax to re-expand. They advocate that the addition of suction too early after the insertion of a chest tube, particularly in the case of spontaneous pneumothorax, may precipitate re-expansion pulmonary edema (50).

Once a chest tube is in place, tube directed pleural sclerosis for pneumothorax recurrence prevention is an available option. However, in PSP patients, thoracoscopy is the preferred recurrence prevention intervention, after the second pneumothorax event. Chest tube–directed pleural sclerosis is acceptable in patients with a PSP refusing surgery and for those with increased surgical risks (e.g., bleeding diathesis). Recurrence prevention by thoracoscopy, after the first pneumothorax episode, is preferred in patients with a SSP. Chest tube–directed pleural sclerosis my be used in certain circumstances based on patient contraindications to surgery, management preferences, and poor prognosis of underlying disease. As with PSP, doxycycline or talc slurry is the preferred sclerosant in SSP patients (40).

Once a pneumothorax air leak has resolved and recurrence prevention issues are addressed, removal of the chest tube is considered. Tubes should be removed in a staged sequence to ensure that any air leak has resolved before tube removal. A radiograph demonstrating lung re-expansion and no clinical evidence of an air leak is necessary. Any applied suction should be discontinued as part of this assessment (40). The role of chest tube clamping to ensure the absence of small air leaks not readily detected by monitoring the pleural drainage device water-seal chamber for bubbling remains controversial. The ACCP consensus group was divided regarding the utility of clamping with 47% and 59% of the group incorporating clamping as part of chest tube removal in PSP and SSP, respectively (40). Opponents of tube clamping raise concerns for the development of unnoticed lung collapse (54); supporters of clamping note that air leaks may not be obvious in the air-leak–indicator chamber and carefully monitored tube clamping may detect small air leaks and circumvent chest tube replacement due to an overlooked air leak (55). If clamping is incorporated, the tube should be clamped for approximately 4 hours in PSP and 5 to 12 hours in SSP with a subsequent chest radiograph obtained to assess for pneumothorax recurrence (40).

Traumatic Pneumothorax

Pneumothorax ranks second to rib fractures as the most common manifestation of traumatic chest injury and is noted in 40% to 50% of patients with chest trauma (56–58). Many of these pneumothoraces are occult (not seen on an initial chest radiograph but found by additional imaging) and may occur in up to 51% of trauma patients (58). Up to 20% of patients with chest trauma or multitrauma have an accompanying hemothorax not appreciated on the initial chest radiograph but revealed by chest computed tomography (59). Traumatic pneumothoraces should generally be treated with placement of a chest tube (57). Chest tube placement then serves the dual purpose evacuating both air and blood, affording the surgical team the opportunity to monitor the tempo of blood loss as a potential marker of the need for urgent operative intervention. Given the potential for the presence of both air and blood, a large bore tube (28–36 Fr) is recommended. Conservative management (close observation without chest tube placement) may be successful in carefully selected patients suffering a traumatic pneumothorax, particularly those not subjected to positive pressure mechanical ventilation (60).

Iatrogenic Pneumothorax

The incidence and causes of iatrogenic pneumothorax vary considerably. The most common causes of iatrogenic pneumothorax in the Veterans Administration patient population are transthoracic needle aspiration, subclavian vein catheterization, and thoracocentesis

(61,62). Treatment of a patient with an iatrogenic pneumothorax is quite variable. One text recommends observation and oxygen supplementation for patients not mechanically ventilated with minimal symptoms and a limited (<15%) pneumothorax (47). If a patient has more than minimal symptoms or a larger pneumothorax (>15%), simple aspiration is recommended (47). Patients with computed tomographic evidence of emphysema sustaining a pneumothorax during needle lung biopsy more often require chest tube placement than patients without evidence of emphysema (63). Given this information, initial placement of a small-bore chest tube and forgoing observation is recommended in such patients. Iatrogenic pneumothoraces secondary to positive pressure mechanical ventilation may develop tension pneumothorax and are likely to develop bronchopleural fistula (41). Such patients require placement of a larger bore chest tube and observation is not recommended.

B. Parapneumonic Pleural Effusions and Empyema

The most appropriate therapeutic approach to a parapneumonic effusion and empyema continues to be debated. The ACCP guidelines provide evidence-based direction while emphasizing the limited information available to base the suggested recommendations (64). The ACCP guidelines divide patients into four categories (64); however, the more recent BTS guidelines do not (65). The BTS guidelines recommend chest tube drainage in patients with the following: pH <7.2, LDH >1000 IU/L, low glucose (<2.2 mmol/L), or positive gram stain or culture (65). Both guidelines (64,65) recommend intrapleural fibrinolytics in some instances; however, these guidelines were published prior to the release of the Multicenter Intrapleural Sepsis Trial 1 (MIST 1) (66). The MIST 1 trial revealed that there were no significant differences between the groups treated with streptokinase versus the group not treated with streptokinase. Specifically, there was no benefit to streptokinase in terms of mortality, rate of surgery, radiographic outcomes, or length of hospital stay. However, there may still be a role for fibrinolytics in treating a small subgroup of patients who have an exceptionally large, chest tube–resistant collection of pleural fluid that causes substantial dyspnea, hypoxemia, or hypercapnia by the mechanical impairment of lung function (66).

C. Recurrent Symptomatic Pleural Effusions

Chest tube placement with subsequent introduction of pleural sclerosing agent offers the potential opportunity to prevent the re-accumulation of a recurrent symptomatic effusion. Although more commonly considered in recurrent symptomatic malignant effusions, this therapeutic maneuver may be useful in selected benign effusions as well.

Benign Pleural Effusions

A physician may consider preventing future recurrence of a benign effusion if it recurs with significant symptoms, if the physician is comfortable with the etiologic diagnosis, and no further invasive pleural diagnostic studies are planned. Generally, the patient should also be unresponsive to medical treatment of the underlying cause of the effusion. A diagnostic and therapeutic (talc poudrage) thoracoscopic approach may be taken or a chest tube may be placed with subsequent instillation of a pleural sclerosing agent.

Chest tube–directed pleurodesis successfully prevents effusion recurrence in nonmalignant exudative and transudative effusions (67,68). Talc pleurodesis demonstrates greater success (97%) than the overall success of other unspecified sclerosing agents combined (60%) in benign effusion cases (67). Underlying diagnoses and reported success with chest tube–directed talc pleurodesis include congestive heart failure (100%), liver cirrhosis (89%), systemic lupus erythematosus (100%), chylothorax (benign causes including lymphangioleiomyomatosis) (95%), yellow nail syndrome (100%), nephrotic syndrome (100%), peritoneal dialysis (100%), and unknown underlying causes (100%) (67).

Malignant Pleural Effusions

The American Thoracic Society (ATS) statement on the management of malignant pleural effusions (MPE) provides guidance on the role of chest tubes in malignant effusions (27). This statement notes that nearly all neoplasms have been reported to involve the pleural space with lung cancer frequently reported as the most common, accounting for approximately one-third of all malignant pleural effusions. Patients presenting with dyspnea potentially due to their malignant pleural effusion may be candidates for palliative intervention. If a therapeutic thoracocentesis provides marked symptom relief and the lung re-expands (no trapped lung or occluding endobronchial lesion), and the effusion rapidly re-accumulates with accompanying dyspnea, palliative treatment is warranted. However, if dyspnea is not relieved or the lung does not re-expand, a trapped lung or endobronchial lesion may be present and chest tube–directed sclerosis will likely fail (27). Traditionally, trapped lung has been a contraindication to chemical pleurodesis since there is not complete apposition of the parietal and visceral pleurae. One possible alternative in the patient with trapped lung and MPE is a chronic indwelling pleural catheter (Pleurx[TM]; Cardinal Health, Dublin, OH) as demonstrated in a small study where these catheters were placed in this patient population (69). All but one patient received symptomatic benefit (69). More study is needed in this area, however, this approach seems a viable option in this group of patients who have few other nonsurgical options.

Therapeutic options for symptomatic recurrent malignant effusions include therapeutic thoracocentesis (27) that may be repeated in selected patients expected to succumb to their disease shortly. Chemical pleurodesis directed by chest tube or thoracoscopy are additional options with the choice often dependent upon local expertise and availability of thoracoscopy. Talc slurry delivered by chest tube versus talc poudrage by thoracoscopy has similar success in malignant effusions (27,28).

Commonly, chest tube–directed pleurodesis is performed by a large-bore tube, however, similar success rates have been reported with smaller bore tubes (8– Fr) (70,71), and this success is noted in the ATS malignant effusion statement (27). The BTS guidelines also recommend using small-bore catheters (10–14 Fr) as the initial choice for effusion drainage and chemical pleurodesis (72). Once confirmation of lung re-expansion and fluid removal has been obtained radiographically, presclerosis narcotics and/or sedation are suggested given the pain frequently associated with sclerosis. The sclerosant diluted in 50 to 100 mL of sterile saline is introduced and the tube is clamped for one hour (27). The ATS statement does not suggest patient rotation (27). We also do not rotate patients administered agents in *solution* such as doxycycline based on a study demonstrating no difference in pleurodesis success for patients rotated and not rotated (73). Similarly, rotation adds no benefit for talc suspensions (slurry) (74). After clamping the tube for one hour after instillation of the sclerosant, the chest tube is then connected to a PDU with 20 cm of water suction until the 24-hour chest tube output is less than 150 mL (27).

Neither the ATS malignant effusion statement (27), a text (75), nor the BTS guidelines (72) suggest waiting to proceed with sclerosis until daily chest tube output of pleural fluid reaches an arbitrary minimum. The focus on when to introduce the sclerosing agent is upon the presence of successful lung re-expansion (27,75). Success appears similar whether waiting for a minimal amount of daily fluid production or with immediate application of the sclerosing agent after lung re-expansion (75). Similarly, intrapleural application of an anesthetic is not recommended for pain control, given no controlled studies support such a practice (75).

In addition to palliation that may be afforded by chest tube fluid drainage and pleural sclerosis, systemic therapy should be pursued particularly in malignant effusions likely to respond to chemotherapy and may be complimented by therapeutic thoracocentesis or pleurodesis. Breast cancer, small cell lung cancer, and lymphoma tend to be chemotherapy responsive (27).

As with a malignant pleural effusion associated with a trapped lung (above), a treatment alternative for any malignant pleural effusions is the placement of an indwelling pleural catheter (Pleurx™ catheter) (76). The Pleurx™ catheter is a 15.5 Fr catheter with fenestrations at the pleural end and a valve on the opposing end. External vacuum bottles can be used by the symptomatic patient at home to drain pleural fluid by appropriate attachment to the valve end of the catheter. A randomized study comparing the Pleurx™ catheter to doxycycline pleurodesis revealed improvement in dyspnea and quality of life was comparable in the two groups. It was also noted that 46% of the indwelling catheter patients had spontaneous pleurodesis (76). The BTS guidelines recommend the use of this catheter in select patients as well (72).

D. Hemothorax

Hemothoraces may be classified as traumatic, iatrogenic and, rarely, nontraumatic. A hemothorax is present when the pleural fluid hematocrit is $\geq 50\%$ of the peripheral blood. Given that a small amount of blood in the pleural space may visually appear significant, the hematocrit should be measured to clarify the issue in any bloody effusion (47). Drainage of a hemothorax is advisable to limit future potential complications including pleural infection (empyema) (1–5%) (77–79), retention of clotted blood in the pleural space (3%) (77), pleural effusion after chest tube removal (13%) (79), and fibrothorax (<1%) (77). As noted in relation to traumatic pneumothorax (above), 20% of hemothoraces in patients suffering chest trauma in a series by Trupka and colleagues may not be noted on routine chest radiograph but may be detected by chest computed tomography (59).

Chest tube placement should be considered in all of these hemothorax settings. The tube allows removal of the blood from the pleural space while permitting monitoring of the tempo of blood loss that may prompt a surgical intervention. Coincidental pneumothorax in the setting of trauma may also be removed. Drainage may also help mitigate the development of subsequent pleural infection and fibrothorax (79,80).

VI. Summary

Chest tube placement is a valuable therapeutic and, at times, diagnostic tool. A myriad of chest tube devices and support equipment including PDUs are available today. Knowledge of the appropriate use, placement, and limitations of these devices is key to the practice of chest medicine today. The few available randomized controlled trials regarding chest tube–related issues inadequately address the many aspects of chest tube management highlighting the need for additional studies. Such studies are necessary to assist clinicians to better utilize these important tools.

References

1. Miller KS, Sahn SA. Chest tubes. Indications, technique, management and complications. Chest 1987; 91:258–264.
2. Playfair GE. Case of empyema treated by aspiration and subsequently by drainage: Recovery. Br Med J 1875; 1:45.
3. Graham EA, Bell RD. Open pneumothorax: Its relation to the treatment of empyema. Am J Med Sci 1918; 156:839–871.
4. Lilienthal H. Resection of the lung for supportive infections with a report based on 31 consecutive operative cases in which resection was done or intended. Ann Surg 1922; 75:257–320.
5. Lawrence G. Closed chest tube drainage for pleural space problems. The primary therapeutic modality. In: Problems of the Pleural Space. Philadelphia, PA: W. B. Saunders Company, 1983:13–24.
6. Silver M, Bone RC. Techniques for chest tube insertion and pleurodesis. J Crit Illness 1993; 8:631–637.
7. Bone RC. The technique of small-catheter pleural aspiration. J Crit Illness 1993; 8:827–833.
8. Harvey J, Prescott RJ. Simple aspiration versus intercostal tube drainage for spontaneous pneumothorax in patients with normal lungs. BMJ 1994; 309:1338–1339.
9. Heffner JE, McDonald J, Barbieri C. Recurrent pneumothoraces in ventilated patients despite ipsilateral chest tubes. Chest 1995; 108:1053–1058.
10. Millikan J, Moore E, Steiner E, et al. Complications of tube thoracostomy for acute trauma. Am J Surg 1980; 140:738–741.
11. Batchelder TL, Morris KA. Critical factors in determining adequate pleural drainage in both the operated and nonoperated chest. Am Surg 1962; 28:296–302.
12. Baumann MH, Strange C. Treatment of spontaneous pneumothorax. A more aggressive approach? Chest 1997; 112:789–804.
13. Swenson EW, Birath G, Ahbeck A. Resistance to air flow in bronchospirometric catheters. J Thorac Surg 1957; 33:275–281.
14. Tattersall D, Traill Z, Gleeson F. Chest drains. Does size matter? Clin Radiol 2000; 55:415–421.
15. Park J, Kraus F, Haaga J. Fluid flow during percutaneous drainage procedures: An in vitro study of the effects of fluid viscosity, catheter size, and adjunctive urokinase. AJR 1993; 160:165–169.
16. Baumann M, Patel P, Roney C, et al. Comparison of function of commercially available pleural drainage units and catheters. Chest 2003; 123:1878–1886.
17. Trapnell DH, Thurston JGB. Unilateral pulmonary oedema after pleural aspiration. Lancet 1970; 1:1367–1369.
18. Jackson RM, Veal CF, Alexander CB, et al. Re-expansion pulmonary edema: A potential role for free radicals in its pathogenesis. Am Rev Respir Dis 1988; 137:1165–1171.
19. Pavlin DJ, Nessly ML, Cheney FW. Increased pulmonary vascular permeability as a cause of re-expansion pulmonary edema. Am Rev Respir Dis 1981; 124:422–427.
20. Sprung CL, Loewenherz JW, Baier H, et al. Evidence for increased permeability in reexpansion pulmonary edema. Am J Med 1981; 71:497–500.
21. Matsuura Y, Nomimura T, Murakami H, et al. Clinical analysis of reexpansion pulmonary edema. Chest 1991; 100:1562–1566.
22. Sautter RD, Dreher WH, MacIndoe JH, et al. Fatal pulmonary edema and pneumonitis after reexpansion of chronic pneumothorax. Chest 1971; 60:399–401.

23. Waqaruddin M, Bernstein A. Re-expansion pulmonary edema. Thorax 1975; 30:54–60.
24. Mahfood S, Hix WR, Aaron BL, et al. Reexpansion pulmonary edema. Ann Thorac Surg 1988; 45:340–345.
25. Lan R, Lo S, Chuang M, et al. Elastance of the pleural space: A predictor for the outcome of pleurodesis in patients with malignant pleural effusions. Ann Intern Med 1997; 126:768–774.
26. Light R, Jenkinson S, Minh V, et al. Observations on pleural fluid pressures as fluid is with drawn during thoracentesis. Am Rev Respir Dis 1980; 121:799–804.
27. Antony VB, Loddenkemper R, Astoul P, et al. Management of malignant pleural effusions. Am J Respir Crit Care Med 2000; 162:1987–2001.
28. Kennedy L, Sahn SA. Talc pleurodesis for the treatment of pneumothorax and pleural effusion. Chest 1994; 106:1215–1222.
29. Light RW. Talc should not be used for pleurodesis. Am J Respir Crit Care Med 2000; 162:2024–2026.
30. Sahn SA. Talc should be used for pleurodesis. Am J Respir Crit Care 2000; 162:2023–2024.
31. Ferrer J, Villarino MA, Tura JM, et al. Talc preparations used for pleurodesis vary markedly from one preparation to another. Chest 2001; 119:1901–1905
32. Maskell N, Lee Y, Gleeson F, et al. Randomized trials describing lung inflammation after pleurodesis with talc of varying particle size. Am J Respir Crit Care Med 2004; 170:377–382.
33. de Campos JRM, Vargas FS, Werebe EdC, et al. Thoracoscopy talc poudrage. A 15-year experience. Chest 2001; 119:801–806.
34. Bell RL, Ovadia P, Abdullah F, et al. Chest tube removal: End-inspiration or end-expiration? J Trauma 2001; 50:674–677.
35. Davis JW, Mackersie RC, Hoyt DB, et al. Randomized study of algorithms for discontinuing tube thoracostomy drainage. J Am Coll Surg 1994; 179:553–557.
36. Martino K, Merrit S, Boyakye K, et al. Prospective randomized trial of thoracostomy removal algorithms. J Trauma 1999; 46:369–373.
37. Sharma TN, Agnihotri S, Jain N, et al. Intercostal tube thoracostomy in pneumothorax. Factors influencing re-expansion of the lung. Indian J Chest Dis and All Sci 1988; 30:32–35.
38. Cerfolio R, Bass C, Katholi C. Prospective randomized trial compares suction versus water seal for air leaks. Ann Thorac Surg 2001; 71:1613–1617.
39. Reed M, Lyons J, Luchette F, et al. Preliminary report of a prospective, randomized trial of underwater seal for spontaneous and iatrogenic pneumothorax. J Am Coll Surg 2007; 204:84–90.
40. Baumann MH, Strange C, Heffner JE, et al. Management of spontaneous pneumothorax. An American College of Chest Physicians Delphi consensus statement. Chest 2001; 119:590–602.
41. Baumann MH, Sahn SA. Medical management and therapy of bronchopleural fistulas in the mechanically ventilated patient. Chest 1990; 97:721–728.
42. Capps JS, Tyler M, Rusch VW, et al. Potential of chest drainage units to evacuate broncho-pleural air leaks. Chest 1985; 88:57S.
43. Rusch VW, Capps JS, Tyler ML, et al. The performance of four pleural drainage systems in an animal model of bronchopleural fistula. Chest 1988; 93:859–863.
44. Crocker HL, Ruffin RE. Patient-induced complications of a Heimlich flutter valve. Chest 1998; 113:838–839.
45. Jones AE, Knoepp LF, Oxley DD. Bronchopleural fistula resulting from the use of a thoracic vent. A case report and review. Chest 1998; 114:1781–1784.
46. Mainini SE, Johnson FE. Tension pneumothorax complicating small-caliber chest tube insertion. Chest 1990; 97:759–760.
47. Light RW, Lee YCG. Pneumothorax, chylothorax, hemothorax, and fibrothorax. In: Mason RJ, Broaddus VC, Murray JF, Nadel JA, eds. Textbook of Respiratory Medicine, 4th ed. Philadelphia, PA: W. B. Saunders Company, 2005:1961–1988.
48. Sahn SA, Heffner JE. Spontaneous pneumothorax. N Engl J Med 2000; 342:868–874.

49. Baumann MH, Strange C. The clinician's perspective on pneumothorax management. Chest 1997; 112:822–828.
50. Henry M, Arnold T, Harvey J. BTS guidelines for the management of spontaneous pneumothorax. Thorax 2003; 58:39–52.
51. Noppen M, Alexander P, Driesen H, et al. Manual aspiration versus chest tube drainage in first episodes of primary spontaneous pneumothorax. A multicenter, prospective, randomized pilot study. Am J Respir Crit Care Med 2002; 165:1240–1244.
52. So S, Yu D. Catheter drainage of spontaneous pneumothorax: Suction or no suction, early or late removal? Thorax 1982; 37:46–48.
53. Minami H, Saka H, Senda K, et al. Small caliber catheter drainage for spontaneous pneumothorax. Am J Med Sci 1992; 304:345–347.
54. Miller AC. Treatment of spontaneous pneumothorax. The clinician's perspective on pneumothorax management. Chest 1998; 113:1423–1424.
55. Baumann MH, Strange C. Treatment of spontaneous pneumothorax. The clinicians' perspective on pneumothorax management. Chest 1998; 113:1424–1425.
56. Bridges KG, Welch G, Silver M, et al. CT detection of occult pneumothorax in multiple trauma patients. J Emerg Med 1993; 11:179–186.
57. Enderson BL, Abdalla R, Frame SB, et al. Tube thoracostomy for occult pneumothorax: A prospective randomized study of its use. J Trauma 1993; 35:726–730.
58. Wolfman NT, Myers WS, Glauser SJ, et al. Validity of CT classification on management of occult pneumothorax: A prospective study. AJR 1998; 171:1317–1320.
59. Trupka A, Waydhas C, Hallfeldt K, et al. Value of thoracic computed tomography in the first assessment of severely injured patients with blunt chest trauma: Results of a prospective study. J Trauma 1997; 43:405–411.
60. Johnson G. Traumatic pneumothorax: Is a chest drain always necessary? J Accid Emerg Med 1996; 13:173–174.
61. Despars JA, Sassoon CSH, Light RW. Significance of iatrogenic pneumothoraces. Chest 1994; 105:1147–1150.
62. Sassoon CSH, Light RW, O'Hara VS, et al. Iatrogenic pneumothorax: Etiology and morbidity. Respiration 1992; 59:215–220.
63. Cox JE, Chiles C, McManus CM, et al. Transthoracic needle aspiration biopsy: Variables that affect risk of pneumothorax. Radiology 1999; 212:165–168.
64. Colice GL, Curtis A, Deslaurierb, et al. Medical and surgical treatment of parapneumonic effusions. An evidence-based guideline. Chest 2000; 118:1158–1171.
65. Davies C, Gleeson F, Davies R. BTS guidelines for the management of pleural infection. Thorax 2003; 58:18–28.
66. Maskell N, Davies C, Nunn A, et al. U.K. Controlled trial of intrapleural steptokinase for pleural infection. N Engl J Med 2005; 352:865–874.
67. Glazer M, Berkman N, Lafair JS, et al. Successful talc slurry pleurodesis in patients with nonmalignant effusions. Report of 16 cases and review of the literature. Chest 2000; 117:1404–1409.
68. Sudduth CD, Sahn SA. Pleurodesis for nonmalignant pleural effusions. Recommendations. Chest 1992; 102:1855–1860.
69. Pien G, Gant M, Washam C, et al. Use of an implantable pleural catheter for trapped lung syndrome in patients with malignant pleural effusion. Chest 2001; 119:1641–1646.
70. Parker LA, Charnock GC, Delany DJ. Small bore catheter drainage and sclerotherapy for malignant pleural effusions. Cancer 1989; 64:1218–1221.
71. Seaton KG, Patz EF, Goodman PC. Palliative treatment of malignant pleural effusions: Value of small-bore catheter thoracostomy and doxycyline sclerotherapy. AJR 1995; 164:589–591.
72. Antunes G, Neville E, Duffy J, et al. BTS guidelines for the management of malignant pleural effusions. Thorax 2003; 58:29–38.

73. Dryzer S, Allen M, Strange C, et al. A comparison of rotation and nonrotation in tetracylcine pleurodesis. Chest 1993; 104:1763–1766.
74. Mager H, Maesen B, Verzijbergen F, et al. Distribution of talc suspension during treatment of malignant pleural effusion with talc pleurodesis. Lung Cancer 2002; 36:77–81.
75. Light R. Pleural effusions related to metastatic malignancies. In: Light R, ed. Pleural Diseases, 5th ed. Philadelphia, PA: Lippincott Williams and Wilkins, 2007:133–161.
76. Putnam JB, Light RW, Rodriguez RM, et al. A randomized comparison of indwelling pleural catheter and doxycycline pleurodesis in the management of malignant pleural effusions. Cancer 1999; 86:1992–1999.
77. Beall AC, Crawford HW, DeBakey ME. Considerations in the management of acute traumatic hemothorax. J Thorac Cardiovasc Surg 1976; 52:351–360.
78. Griffith GL, Todd EP, McMillin RD, et al. Acute traumatic hemothorax. Ann Thorac Surg 1978; 26:204–207.
79. Wilson JM, Boren CH, Peterson SR, et al. Traumatic hemothorax: Is decortication necessary? J Thorac Cardiovasc Surg 1979; 77:489–495.
80. Drummond DS, Craig RH. Traumatic hemothorax: Complications and management. Am Surg 1967; 33:403–408.

8

Interventional Radiology of Pleural Disease

JOHNY A. VERSCHAKELEN
University Hospitals, Gasthuisberg, Leuven, Belgium

I. Introduction

Percutaneous nonoperative procedures were first reported in the late 1800s. Leyden (1) was probably the first to perform a transthoracic needle biopsy to confirm the presence of a pulmonary infection. The lack of small-caliber needles, causing a high rate of complications, and the difficulties pathologists had in making a diagnosis from small samples or smears were responsible for the fact that these percutaneous diagnostic procedures did not experience widespread use until the 1960s. At that time, Dahlgren and Nordenström (2) introduced small-gauge needles, reducing the rate of pneumothorax, popularizing the technique of transthoracic fine needle sampling of the chest. At the same time, the first report on the use of fluoroscopy during transthoracic needle biopsy was published (3). Not until the late 1970s, however, did imaging-guided percutaneous insertion of drainage catheters in fluid collections of the lung and pleura become a routine procedure (4). Initially, fluoroscopy was the method of choice, but now many imaging techniques, including ultrasound (US), computed tomography (CT), and magnetic resonance (MR), are used to guide interventional procedures.

II. Imaging Guidance Modalities

A. Fluoroscopy

Uni- or biplanar fluoroscopy was the first imaging technique used to guide percutaneous pleural interventions. The technique is widely available, allows realtime control of the procedure, and gives an overview of the thorax (5). However, fluoroscopy is not suitable for every lesion. Small lesions may be difficult or impossible to identify. Some lesions may be superimposed on or not separable from normal thoracic structures. Another important limitation is that biopsy or drainage using fluoroscopic guidance may not be advisable if the lesion is adjacent to major cardiovascular structures, such as the aorta (6,7).

B. Ultrasonography

Ultrasound is well suited for interventional procedures in the pleura (8,9). Because of the development of high-resolution, high-frequency probes with special biopsy ports, ultrasonographically guided biopsy of small pleural lesions has become possible (10–13). Ultrasonography is particularly indicated to guide percutaneous aspiration and catheter drainage of a pleural fluid or air collection, even in small amounts (14–23) (Fig. 1). Advantages of this technique include real-time visualization during needle placement,

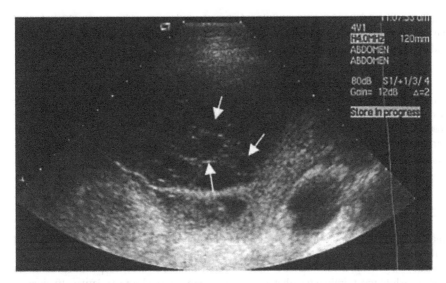

Figure 1 Ultrasonography is particularly indicated to guide percutaneous aspiration and catheter drainage of a pleural fluid collection. This technique is especially helpful to ensure accurate placement of the tube in the presence of septations (arrows).

decreasing the risk of injury to neighboring structures (vessels and nerves) and allowing real-time confirmation of procedure success (injection, drainage, biopsy), absence of ionizing radiation, and, in the case of biopsy of a mass, the ability to target nonnecrotic portions for sampling (11,24,25). In addition, US is a safe and convenient method of guiding interventional procedures at the bedside of the patient and obviates the need to transport patients on life-support devices to the radiology department (26,27). Tu et al. have shown in a prospective study of 94 medical care unit (MCU) patients having fever and evidence of pleural effusion that portable chest US and US-guided thoracocentesis are safe, feasible, and useful methods for diagnosing thoracic empyema (28). A disadvantage is that sonography is limited by attenuation of the beam as it transverses air-filled lung or pleura.

C. Computed Tomography
A major advantage of CT over fluoroscopy is its axial format and its exquisite anatomical detail (6,14,17,18,29). It is particularly useful for sampling lesions visible in only a single radiographic projection or when great imaging detail is required for the interventional procedure. The administration of intravenous contrast can be mandatory for the identification of tissue necrosis, fluid content, and identification of normal and abnormal vascular structures. CT allows for determination of an optimal cutaneous entry point for the biopsy needle or for tube placement. In addition, the introduction of CT continuous imaging, also called real-time CT and CT fluoroscopy, has improved the ease of performing interventional thoracic procedures because it allows real-time visualization of the lesion and of the progression of the needle or tube. In this way, the diagnostic accuracy can be improved and the duration of the procedure can be shortened (30–34). Compared with conventional spiral CT, there is also a markedly decreased patient radiation dose (35). A

disadvantage of CT-guided interventional procedures in comparison with US is indeed the need of ionizing radiation. Greater discomfort for the patient lying on the CT table and higher expenses may also be some of the disadvantages.

D. Magnetic Resonance

Although MR is often used for guidance of interventional procedures, little experience has been gained in thoracic or pleural interventions (36–38). This technique combines the absence of ionizing radiation with good anatomical detail and has become possible with the introduction of nonferromagnetic MR-compatible biopsy needles (39,40). Major disadvantages include, however, high cost, limited availability, and the length of the procedure.

III. Percutaneous Drainage of Thoracic Fluid and Air Collections

A. Parapneumonic Effusion and Empyema

Imaging plays an important part in the investigation and management of pleural fluid collection. The choice of treatment depends on the fluid characteristics (i.e., transudate vs. exudate). In general, a transudate or simple parapneumonic effusion responds to antibiotic therapy, while most drainage catheter placements are reserved for exudative effusions— either infectious, inflammatory, or neoplastic (41). In general, success of image-guided catheters depends on proper patient selection, the skills of the operator, and the ability to monitor daily chest tube function (42). Chest radiographs are the first-line investigation, and most pleural effusions are clearly visible. In large pleural collections, needle aspiration and drainage are often possible without imaging control.

Although chest radiographs and fluoroscopy (43) are used successfully to guide percutaneous catheter drainage of pleural effusion, both US and CT are more sensitive than chest radiographs for the detection and localization of pleural fluid, and both can be used to differentiate between transudates and exudates (44–46). Anechoic collections may be either exudates or transudates, but the presence of homogeneous internal echos and/or septations indicates an exudate. Multiple septa not only indicate exudates, but also predict difficulties with aspiration. Ultrasound guidance can in these cases ensure accurate placement of the drain (Fig. 1). Septa are seldom detectable on CT (16,43,45,47).

However, this latter technique is valuable to assess the underlying lung, mediastinum, chest wall, and subdiaphragmatic regions. It is especially useful in characterizing complex pleural and parenchymal disease and is used to guide drainage of collections that are difficult to access by way of an intercostal approach (e.g., paramediastinal collections). The presence of fibrin strand septations and loculations is an indication for the installation of fibrinolytic agents like streptokinase and urokinase, and again tube placement is facilitated when US is used to guide the procedure (48–51).

Drainage via thoracostomy, thoracocentesis, and antibiotics is standard therapeutic procedure for empyema (52–54). When these fail, excision of a rib for open drainage and open thoracostomy are more invasive alternatives (55). The success rate of closed drainage depends very much on the stage of the pleural effusion. A very high rate of clinical success may be expected when used in fubrinopurulent effusions. However, if drainage is delayed until a pleural peel has been formed, closed drainage will very likely fail and thoracotomy and decortication will be necessary (56). It has been shown that effusions up to four to six weeks in duration may be drained successfully, but those older than six weeks are likely to have an associated pleural peel (56,57). In addition, noninfected pleural collections are more adequately treated than empyemas. Keeling et al. have shown a failure rate of 19% in cases where empyemas were treated with small-bore catheter drainage (58), while in a study by Maier et al., CT- or US-guided pigtail catheter drainage failed in all of the 14 patients with fibropulrulent empyema and symptoms of sepsis (59). Shankar et al. have examined whether US appearance of thoracic empyema can predict outcome. They found that image-guided percutaneous catheter drainage was successful in 12 of 13 (92.3%) patients with anechoic empyemas; 53 of 65 (81.5%) with complex nonseptated empyemas, and in 15 of 24 (62.5%) patients with complex septated empyemas (60).

Failure of the thoracostomy tube can also be the result of a poorly positioned or non-functioning tube (61–63). Incorrect tube placement is not only responsible for inadequate drainage but can also produce complications such as pain, hypotension, subcutaneous emphysema, leakage, chylothorax, and bleeding (62,63). Large surgical studies have demonstrated the limitations of nonguided thoracostomy drainage of empyema (52,54) (Fig. 2). One report shows a 10% cure rate (52), while another shows a mortality rate of

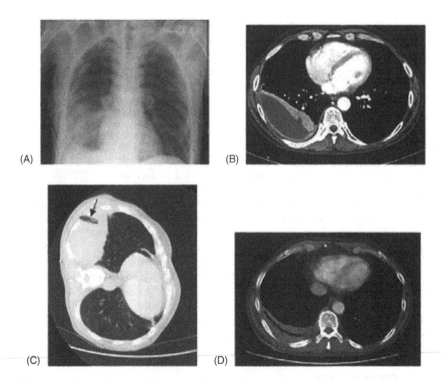

(A)	(B)	(C)	(D)

Figure 2	Chest X-ray and CT are valuable imaging modalities to locate the drain after a nonguided drainage of empyema. In this patient, chest X-ray (**A**) suggested and CT (**B**) confirmed incorrect placement of the thoracostomy tube. Under CT guidance, a new tube was placed (**C**) and treatment was successful. A follow-up CT (**D**) not only shows an important reduction in the amount of pleural fluid but also demonstrates the presence of extensive pleural thickening.

5% (54). Van Sonnenberg et al. (18) used CT and US to locate and drain empyemas in 17 patients, most of whom had failed to improve with conventional chest tube drainage due to a poorly positioned tube. Fifteen patients (88.2%) were treated successfully, averting surgery or further drainage. In four patients, the radiological procedure provided additional diagnostic information: two were found to have a bronchopleural fistula, in one patient a communication between the empyema and the esophagus was seen, and in one patient the empyema was communicating with a subphrenic abscess.

CT has also been used successfully to follow patients who underwent percutaneous catheter drainage for empyema (29) (Fig. 2). Up to four weeks after the removal of the catheter(s), CT scan demonstrated extensive pleural thickening in all of the 10 patients who entered the study. This pleural peel had decreased at 8 and 12 weeks; the pleura was essentially normal in four patients, demonstrated only a small area of plaque-like thickening in four patients, and was mildly thickened in two patients. Serial CT can be helpful in determining the necessity of decortication. Frequent cross-sectional imaging may also be needed to detect undrained loculations, so that additional drainage catheters can be placed if needed (56).

B. Malignant Pleural Disease and Pleural Effusions

Lung and breast carcinomas together with lymphoma are the most common causes of malignant pleural effusion (64). The majority of these pleural effusions require tube drainage with sclerosis to prevent recurrence. Imaging-guided drainage and chemical pleurodesis have become a well-accepted procedure for the management of malignant effusions (65,66). In addition, Davies et al. suggested that intrapleural streptokinase might be useful in the drainage of malignant multiloculated pleural effusions in patients who fail to drain adequately with a standard chest tube (67). In most cases, ultrasonography is used to guide catheter placement (68). This technique can also be used to guide transthoracic needle biopsy of pleural masses (8,13,69). Real-time ultrasound visualization allows accurate needle placement, shorter procedure time, and performance in debilitated and less cooperative patients (70). CT, on the other hand, is the method of choice for guiding biopsy of small pleural masses or for biopsy in those parts of the pleura that are hidden behind bone or aerated lung tissue (Fig. 3). In a series of 33 patients with diffuse or focal pleural thickening, pleural effusion, and suspected pleural malignancy, percutaneous CT- or US-guided cutting-needle biopsy revealed a sensitivity of 88%, a specificity of 100%, and an accuracy of 91% for the correct diagnosis of malignant disease including mesothelioma (71). In a larger series of 82 patients undergoing 85 image-guided pleural biopsies, a sensitivity of 76% and a specificity of 100% were found (27). This is much better than pleural biopsies performed without imaging guidance, where sensitivity varies from 48% to 56% for the detection of malignant pleural disease (72–74) and from 21% to 43% for the detection of malignant mesothelioma (75,76).

C. Pneumothorax

Pneumothorax can be either spontaneous or posttraumatic in origin. Common causes of traumatic pneumothorax include chest trauma, central venous catheter placement, transbronchial biopsy and transthoracic biopsy, or drainage procedures (77–79). Small

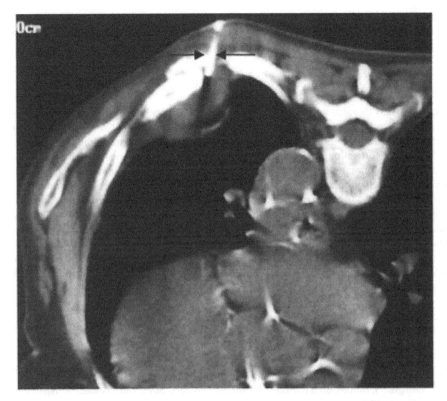

Figure 3 CT is the method of choice for guiding biopsy (arrows) of pleural masses that are hidden behind bone or aerated lung tissue.

or stable pneumothoraces in asymptomatic patients are usually observed. Drainage is performed for large or symptomatic air collections. Large air collections can be treated without imaging guidance. Fluoroscopy can be used to guide catheter placement, although CT is more often used when the pneumothorax occurred during a CT-guided interventional procedure. CT is also helpful in accessing loculated air collections (80).

IV. Imaging of Complications

The most common complications of transthoracic needle biopsy of lung lesions are pneumothorax and pulmonary hemorrhage ranging from 5% to 30% (10,81,82). These numbers are much smaller for pleural interventions since lung tissue is normally not punctured. Factors associated with higher incidence of pneumothorax include small pleural lesions, the presence of obstructive airways disease and emphysema, intractable coughing, increased duration of the procedure, and cavitary lesions.

Pulmonary hemorrhage is rare, but bleeding in the chest wall can occur when a vein or artery is damaged during the procedure. Special care should be taken to avoid intercostal and internal mammary vessels. The administration of intravenous contrast can be necessary to locate the internal mammary vessels on CT prior to the interventional procedure.

V. Video-Assisted Thoracic Surgery

Video-assisted thoracic surgery (VATS) has become a very useful diagnostic and therapeutic tool in the management of lung, pleural, and mediastinal disease (83,84). In the pleura, it has become the preferred surgical technique for pleural drainage, lyses of adhesions, decortication, and directed pleurodesis (83,85). Thoracoscopic biopsy has a sensitivity of approximately 91% to 98% in the detection of malignant pleural disease, including mesothelioma (86,87). Preoperative imaging, especially CT, is very important to assess location and extent of disease and to have an idea about the nature of the lesion(s). Since the anatomical relationships of the pleura and the pleural lesions remain relatively undisturbed during the procedure, imaging guidance or imaging-guided location of the lesion is rarely necessary. This is different for lung lesions that are often not visible during the VATS procedure. Three methods of preoperative image-guided location for VATS using CT guidance have been described: skin marking, transpleural staining, and wire placement (88–93). These procedures can help the surgeon to locate the pulmonary lesion but are performed less and less frequently as the experience with thoracoscopy increases (85).

References

1. Leyden OO. Über infectiöse Pneumonie. Dtsch Med Wochenschr 1883; 9:52–55.
2. Dahlgren S, Nordenström B. Needle Transthoracic Biopsy. Stockholm, Sweden: Almquist and Wiksell, 1966.
3. Hattori S, Matsuda M, Sugiyama T. Cytologic diagnosis of early lung cancer: Brushing methods under X-ray television fluoroscopy. Dis Chest 1964; 45:129–135.
4. Vainrub D, Husher DM, Guinn GA, et al. Percutaneous drainage of lung abscess. Am Rev Respir Dis 1978; 117:153–157.
5. Klein JS, Zarka M. Transthoracic needle biopsy: An overview. J Thorac Imaging 1997; 12:232–249.
6. van Sonnenberg E, Casola G, Ho M, et al. Difficult thoracic lesions: CT-guided biopsy experience in 150 cases. Radiology 1988; 167:457–461.
7. van Sonnenberg E, Wittich GR, Goodacre BW, et al. Percutaneous drainage of thoracic collections. J Thorac Imaging 1998; 13(2):74–82.
8. Heilo A, Stenwig AE, Solheim OP. Malignant pleural mesothelioma: US-guided histologic core-needle biopsy. Radiology 1999; 211:657–659.
9. Heilo A. Tumors in the mediastinum: US-guided histologic core-needle biopsy. Radiology 1993; 189:143–146.
10. Ikezoe J, Morimoto S, Kozuka T. Sonographically guided needle biopsy of thoracic lesions. Semin Intervent Radiol 1991; 8:15–22.
11. Pan JF, Yang PC, Chang DB, et al. Needle aspiration biopsy of malignant lung masses with necrotic centers. Improved sensitivity with ultrasound guidance. Chest 1993; 103: 1452–1456.
12. Yang PC, Chang DB, Yu CJ, et al. Ultrasoundguided core biopsy of thoracic tumors. Am Rev Respir Dis 1992; 146:763–767.

13. Yang PC. Ultrasound-guided transthoracic biopsy of peripheral lung, pleural, and chest-wall lesions. J Thorac Imaging 1997; 12:272–284.
14. Casola G, van Sonnenberg E, Keightley A, et al. Pneumothorax: Radiologic treatment with small catheters. Radiology 1988; 166:89–91.
15. Hunnam GR, Flower CDR. Radiologically-guided percutaneous catheter drainage of empyemas. Clin Radiol 1988; 39:121–126.
16. Merriam MA, Cronan JJ, Dorfman GDS, et al. Radiographically guided percutaneous catheter drainage of pleural fluid collections. AJR 1988; 151:1113–1116.
17. Silverman SG, Mueller PR, Saini S, et al. Thoracic empyema: Management with image-guided catheter drainage. Radiology 1988; 169:5–9.
18. van Sonnenberg E, Nakamoto SK, Mueller PR, et al. CT- and ultrasound-guided catheter drainage of empyemas after chest-tube failure. Radiology 1984; 151:349–353.
19. Parker LA, Melton JW, Delany DJ, et al. Percutaneous small-bore catheter drainage in the management of lung abscesses. Chest 1987; 92:213–218.
20. O'Moore PV, Mueller PR, Simeone JF, et al. Sonographic guidance in diagnostic and therapeutic interventions in the pleural space. AJR 1987; 149:1–5.
21. Cummin ARC, Wright NL, Joseph AE. Suction drainage: A new approach to the treatment of empyema. Thorax 1991; 46:259–260.
22. Morrison MC, Mueller PR, Lee MJ, et al. Sclerotherapy of malignant pleural effusion through sonographically placed small-bore catheters. AJR 1992; 158:41–43.
23. Sartori S, Tombesi P, Tassinari D, et al. Sonographically guided small-bore chest tubes and sonographic monitoring for rapid sclerotherapy of recurrent malignant pleural effusions. J Ultrasound Med 2004; 23(9):1171–1176.
24. Klein JS, Zarka MA. Transthoracic needle biopsy. Radiol Clin North Am 2000; 38:235–266.
25. Cohen M, Jacob D. Ultrasound guided interventional radiology. J Radiol 2007; 88(9 Pt 2):1223–1229.
26. Yu CJ, Yang PC, Chang DB, et al. Diagnostic and therapeutic use of chest sonography: Value in critically ill patients. AJR 1992; 159:695–701.
27. Benamore RE, Scott K, Richards CJ, et al. Image-guided pleural biopsy: Diagnostic yield and complications. Clin Radiol 2006; 61(8):700–705.
28. Tu CY, Hsu WH, Hsia TC, et al. Pleural effusions in febrile medical ICU patients: Chest ultrasound study. Chest 2004; 126(4):1274–1280.
29. Neff CC, vanSonnenberg E, Lawson DW, et al. CT follow-up of empyemas: Pleural peels resolve after percutaneous catheter drainage. Radiology 1990; 176:195–197.
30. White CS, Meyer CA, Templeton PA. CT fluoroscopy for thoracic interventional procedures. Radiol Clin North Am 2000; 38:303–322.
31. Sheafor DH, Paulson EK, Kliewer MA, et al. Comparison of sonographic and CT guidance techniques: Does CT fluoroscopy decrease procedure time? AJR 2000; 174: 939–942.
32. Ernst RD, Kim HS, Kawashima A, et al. Near realtime CT fluoroscopy using computer automated scan technology in nonvascular interventional procedures. AJR 2000; 174:319–321.
33. Daly B, Templeton PA. Real-time CT fluoroscopy: Evolution of an interventional tool. Radiology 1999; 211:309–315.
34. Meyer CA, White CS, Wu J, et al. Real-time CT fluoroscopy: Usefulness in thoracic drainage. AJR Am J Roentgenol 1998; 171(4):1097–1101.
35. Carlson SK, Bender CE, Classic KL, et al. Benefits and safety of CT fluoroscopy in interventional radiologic procedures. Radiology 2001; 219:515–520.
36. Adam G, Neuerburg J, Bucker A, et al. Interventional magnetic resonance. Initial clinical experience with a 1.5-tesla magnetic resonance system combined with c-arm fluoroscopy. Invest Radiol 1997; 32:191–197.

37. Buecker A, Adam G, Neuerburg JM, et al. MR-guided biopsy using a T2-weighted single-shot zoom imaging sequence (local look technique). J Magn Reson Imaging 1998; 8:955–959.
38. McLoud TC. CT and MR in pleural disease. Clin Chest Med 1998; 19(2):261–276.
39. Langen H-J, Kugel H, Grewe S, et al. MR guided biopsy using respiratory-triggered high-resolution T2-weighted sequences. AJR 2000; 174:834–836.
40. Lufkin R, Teresi L, Hanafee W. New needle for MR-guided aspiration cytology of the head and neck. AJR 1987; 149:380–382.
41. Light RW. Parapneumonic effusions and empyema. Clin Chest Med 1985; 6:55–62.
42. Moulton JS. Image-guided drainage techniques. Semin Respir Infect 1999; 14(1):59–72.
43. Westcott JL. Percutaneous catheter drainage of pleural effusion and empyema. AJR 1985; 144:1189–1193.
44. Yang PC, Luh KT, Chang DB, et al. Value of sonography in determining the nature of pleural effusion: Analysis of 320 cases. AJR 1992; 159:29–33.
45. Aquino SL, Webb WR, Gushiken BJ. Pleural exudates and transudates diagnosis with contrast enhanced CT. Radiology 1994; 192:803–808.
46. Tan Kendrick AP, Ling H, Subramaniam R, et al. The value of early CT in complicated childhood pneumonia. Pediatr Radiol 2002; 32(1):16–21 [Epub Nov. 15, 2001].
47. Light RW. Management of parapneumonic effusions (editorial; comment). Chest 1991; 100:892–893.
48. Ekingen G, Güvenç BH, Sözübir S, et al. Fibrinolytic treatment of complicated pediatric thoracic empyemas with intrapleural streptokinase. Eur J Cardiothorac Surg 2004; 263:503–507.
49. Moulton JS, Benkert RE, Weisiger KH, et al. Treatment of complicated pleural fluid collections with image-guided drainage and intracavitary urokinase. Chest 1995; 108:1252–1259.
50. Taylor RF, Rubens MB, Pearson MC, et al. Intrapleural streptokinase in the management of empyema. Thorax 1994; 49:856–859.
51. Chin NK, Lim TK. Controlled trial of intrapleural streptokinase in the treatment of pleural empyema and complicated parapneumonic effusions. Chest 1997; 111:275–279.
52. Davis WC, Johnson LF. Adult thoracic empyema revisited. Am Surg 1978; 44:362–368.
53. Ibarra-Pérez C, Selman-Lama M. Diagnosis and treatment of amebic "empyema". Report of eighty-eight cases. Am J Surg 1977; 134:283–287.
54. Sherman MM, Subramanian V, Berger RL. Management of thoracic empyema. Am J Surg 1977; 133:474–478.
55. Sahn SA. Diagnosis and management of parapneumonic effusions and empyema. Clin Infect Dis 2007; 45(11):1480–1486 [Epub Oct. 24, 2007].
56. Moulton JS. Image-guided management of complicated pleural fluid collections. Radiol Clin North Am 2000; 38(2):345–374.
57. Akhan O, Ozkan O, Akinci D, et al. Image-guided catheter drainage of infected pleural effusions. Diagn Interv Radiol 2007; 13(4):204–209.
58. Keeling AN, Leong S, Logan PM, et al. Empyema and effusion: Outcome of image-guided small-bore catheter drainage. Cardiovasc Intervent Radiol 2008; 31(1):135–141 [Epub Oct. 18, 2007].
59. Maier A, Domej W, Anegg U, et al. Computed tomography or ultrasonically guided pigtail catheter drainage in multiloculated pleural empyema: A recommended procedure? Respirology 2000; 5(2):119–124.
60. Shankar S, Gulati M, Kang M, et al. Image-guided percutaneous drainage of thoracic empyema: Can sonography predict the outcome? Eur Radiol 2000; 10(3):495–499.
61. Milfeld DJ, Mattox KL, Beall AC Jr. Early evacuation of clotted hemothorax. Am J Surg 1978; 136:686–692.
62. Maurer JR, Friedman PJ, Wing VW. Thoracostomy tube in an interlobar fissure: Radiologic recognition of a potential problem. AJR 1982; 139:1155–1161.

63. Webb WR, LaBerge J. Major fissure tube placement. Letter to the editor. AJR 1983; 140:1039.
64. Anderson CB, Philpott GW, Ferguson TB. The treatment of malignant pleural effusions. Cancer 1974; 33:916–922.
65. Marom EM, Patz EF Jr, Erasmus JJ, et al. Malignant pleural effusions: Treatment with small-bore-catheter thoracostomy and talc pleurodesis. Radiology 1999; 210:277–281.
66. Chen YM, Shih JF, Yang KY, et al. Usefulness of pig-tail catheter for palliative drainage of malignant pleural effusions in cancer patients. Support Care Cancer 2000; 8(5):423–426
67. Davies CWH, Traill ZC, Gleeson FV, et al. Intrapleural streptokinase in the management of malignant multiloculated pleural effusions. Chest 1999; 115:729–733.
68. Goff BA, Mueller PR, Muntz HG, et al .Small chest-tube drainage followed by bleomycin sclerosis for malignant pleural effusions. Obstet Gynecol 1993; 81:993–996.
69. Gleeson F, Lomas DJ, Flower CDR, et al. Powered cutting needle biopsy of the pleura and chest wall. Clin Radiol 1990; 41:199–200.
70. Sheth S, Hamper UM, Stanley DB, et al. US guidance for thoracic biopsy: A valuable alternative to CT. Radiology 1999; 210:721–726.
71. Adams RF, Gleeson FV. Percutaneous image-guided cutting-needle biopsy of the pleura in the presence of a suspected malignant effusion. Radiology 2001; 219:510–514.
72. von Hoff DD, Li Volsi V. Diagnostic reliability of needle biopsy of the parietal pleura: A review of 272 biopsies. Am J Clin Pathol 1975; 64:200–203.
73. Poe RH, Israel RH, Utell MJ, et al. Sensitivity, specificity, and predictive values of closed pleural biopsy. Arch Intern Med 1984; 144:325–328.
74. Dalyer WR, Eggleston JC, Erozan YS. Efficacy of pleural needle biopsy and pleural fluid cytopathology in the diagnosis of malignant neoplasm involving the pleura. Chest 1975; 67:536–539.
75. Ruffie P, Feld R, Minkin S, et al. Diffuse malignant mesothelioma of the pleura in Ontario and Quebec: A retrospective study of 332 patients. J Clin Oncol 1989; 7:1157–1168.
76. Achatzy R, Beba W, Ritschler R, et al. The diagnosis, therapy and prognosis of diffuse malignant mesothelioma. Eur J Cardiothorac Surg 1989; 3:445–448.
77. Conces DJ Jr, Tarver RD, Gray WC, et al. Treatment of pneumothoraces utilizing small caliber chest tubes. Chest 1988; 94:55–57.
78. Martin T, Fontana G, Olak J, et al. Use of a pleural catheter for the management of simple pneumothorax. Chest 1996; 110:1169–1172.
79. Minami H, Saka H, Senda K, et al. Small caliber catheter drainage for spontaneous pneumothorax. Am J Med Sci 1992; 304:345–347.
80. Klein JS. Interventional techniques in the thorax. Clin Chest Med 1999; 20:805–826.
81. Protopapas Z, White CS, Miller BH. Transthoracic needle biopsy practices: Results of a nationwide survey. Radiology 1996; 201(P):270.
82. Westcott JL. Direct percutaneous needle aspiration of localized pulmonary lesions: Results in 422 patients. Radiology 1980; 137:31–35.
83. Spirn PW, Shah RM, Steiner RM, et al. Image guided localization for video-assisted thoracic surgery. J Thorac Imaging 1997; 12:285–292.
84. Alrawi SJ, Raju R, Acinapura AJ, et al. Primary thoracoscopic evaluation of pleural effusion with local anesthesia: An alternative approach. JSLS 2002; 6(2):143–147.
85. Kaiser LR, Shrager JB. Video-assisted thoracic surgery: The current state of the art. AJR 1995; 165:1111–1117.
86. Boutin C, Rey F. Thoracoscopy in malignant mesothelioma: A prospective study of 188 consecutive patients. I. Diagnosis. Cancer 1993; 72:389–404.
87. Menzies R, Charbonneau M. Thoracoscopy for the diagnosis of pleural disease. Ann Intern Med 1991; 114:271–276.
88. Shah RM, Spirn PW, Salazar AM. Localization of peripheral pulmonary nodules for thorascopic excision: Value of CT-guided wire placement. AJR 1993; 161:279–283.

89. Mack MJ, Gordon MJ, Postma TW. Percutaneous localization of pulmonary nodules for thoracoscopic lung resection. Ann Thorac Surg 1992; 53:1123–1124.
90. Lenglinger FX, Schwarz CD, Artman W. Localization of pulmonary nodules before thoracoscopic surgery: Value of percutaneous staining with methylene blue. AJR 1994; 163:297–300.
91. Plumkett MB, Peterson MS, Landrenau RJ, et al. Peripheral pulmonary nodules: Preoperative percutaneous needle localization with CT guidance. Radiology 1992; 185:274–276.
92. Templeton PA, Krasna M. Localization of pulmonary nodules for thoracoscopic resection: Use of needle/wire breast-biopsy system. AJR 1993; 160:761–762.
93. Gossot D, Miaux Y, Guermazi A. The hook-wire technique for localization of pulmonary nodules during thoracoscopic resection. Chest 1994; 105:1467–1469.

9
Medical Thoracoscopy

PHILIPPE ASTOUL
Département des Maladies Respiratoires, Unité d'Oncologie Thoracique—Hôpital
Sainte-Marguerite, Marseille, France

I. Introduction

For a long time thoracoscopy was performed to achieve pneumonolysis in patients with tuberculosis. More recently many physicians in Europe have documented the usefulness of thoracoscopy for pneumonological indications other than tuberculosis. Taking into account that the evolution of medical technologies incited physicians to seek new and potentially less-invasive ways of performing diagnostic and therapeutic chest procedures, a distinction must be made between medical thoracoscopy, which may be video-assisted, and surgical thoracoscopy or video-assisted thoracoscopic surgery (VATS) (1,2).

Medical thoracoscopy is generally characterized as thoracoscopy performed under local anesthesia in the endoscopy suite with the use of nondisposable instruments, in general for diagnostic purposes. On the other hand, VATS is described as a keyhole surgical procedure in the operating room, under general anesthesia with one-lung ventilation using disposable instruments, in general for therapeutic purposes.

Thoracoscopy is only slightly more invasive than a simple percutaneous pleural needle biopsy but provides infinitely more information. In all cases where a chest tube is required, it should take a pneumonologist only a few minutes to introduce an endoscope via the same incision to inspect the pleura, to locate the adhesions, to take pleural samples, and to verify that the tube will be well positioned. In patients with primary pleural cancer, thoracoscopy is the only procedure that is able to give a diagnosis at the early stage of the disease, and for other pleural effusions, biopsies are made under visual control with a diagnostic rate of more than 95% of patients (3).

The use of thoracoscopy has been resumed as a result of considerable progress in modern techniques:

> Endoscopic telescopes have been greatly improved with extremely high optical quality despite their very small diameter (4).
>
> Adequate instrumentation, including video camera, forceps, endoscopic scalpel, and stapler, enables the physician or surgeon to carry out interventional thoracoscopy (5).
>
> Progress in anesthetics allows for a wide choice that ranges from local anesthesia in outpatients to general anesthesia (6,7).

Thoracoscopy can be performed for diagnostic as well as therapeutic purposes. The most frequent indication for diagnostic thoracoscopy is pleural effusion. Thoracoscopy in spontaneous pneumothorax may identify the cause of the pneumothorax. The most frequent indication for therapeutic thoracoscopy is pleurodesis (mostly chemical) to prevent recurrence of pleural effusion.

Thoracoscopy, while allowing full exploration of the pleural cavity, is much less invasive and incapacitating than thoracotomy (8). Complications are uncommon and rarely occur when the procedure is performed according to appropriate recommendations.

Diagnostic or therapeutic medical thoracoscopy is performed using one or several points of entry. In addition to visual inspection of the thoracic cavity, a number of procedures can be performed. Biopsies can be collected from the pleura and, more rarely, the lung. Adherences preventing exploration can be cut. Coagulation can be performed to stop bleeding or remove small blebs or superficial bullae in patients with spontaneous pneumothorax. A pleural drain is placed at the end of the examination to ensure prompt expansion of the lung against the chest wall. If lung biopsy or pleurodesis is performed, the mean duration of drainage is three to four days. In simple cases involving pleurisy, the examination can be performed as an ambulatory procedure (9).

To practice thoracoscopy, a chest physician needs specific training to learn thoracic anatomy, use of instrumentation (biopsy forceps, coagulation systems, video-endoscopic equipment), and surveillance of drainage during the recovery period.

II. Equipment and Technique

A. Equipment

Thoracoscopy can be performed either in a properly equipped operating room or in an endoscopy suite. The procedure room must be equipped with a procedure table, anesthesia equipment, Mayo stands, a roller tray for instruments, diathermo-coagulation, and patient-monitoring devices.

Thoracoscopic instruments have been designed to facilitate operative procedures. Forceps, graspers, lung manipulators, cautery and cutting devices, suction/irrigation instruments, and a variety of disposable and reusable pleural trocars and cannulas are currently available (10).

A rigid thoracoscope with a cold light source is used in most of the cases. Optics has been considerably improved, and telescopes have greater depth of field, magnification, and arc of vision. The major equipment requirements for medical thoracoscopy are trocars, telescopes, and forceps (Fig. 1). Trocars consist of an obturator and a cannula. To facilitate examination, trocars should not be too large; with a 7-mm trocar, insertion is easy, and painful, procedure-limiting pressure against the ribs is minimal. Telescopes are available with various angles of vision, including 180° (straightforward) and 50° or 90° (oblique). Illuminated forceps are ideal for biopsy of the parietal pleura under direct vision using a single point of entry. For biopsy of the diaphragmatic pleura or fibrous pleural lesions and for sampling the visceral pleura and the lung, 5-mm coagulating forceps via a 5-mm insulated trocar in a second point of entry is a more suitable device (1).

Visualization of the contents of the pleural cavity is facilitated by a video camera that is attached to the eyepiece of the rigid telescope. The size and quality of these cameras has considerably improved in recent years, and the addition of video makes viewing, documentation, and assistance during the procedures far easier than that present in the days of direct visualization. Newer telescopes magnify the subject being visualized

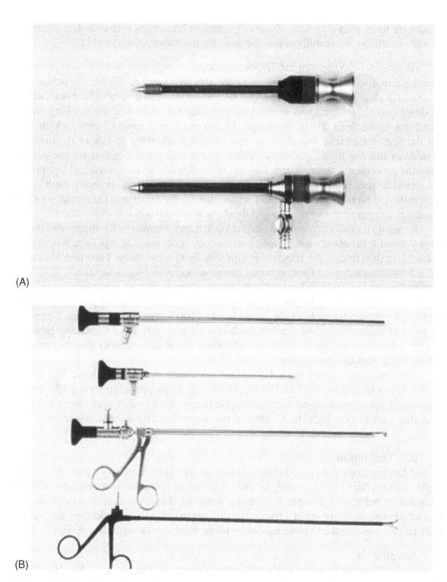

Figure 1 Major equipment for medical thoracoscopy: (**A**) trocars (5 and 7 mm) and (**B**) from top to bottom—7-mm telescope (0° angle), 4-mm telescope, illuminated forceps, and coagulating forceps.

(usually about 4× for a 7-mm rigid telescope), and the increased availability of the couplers of varying sizes allows greater depth of the field and increased field of vision without distortion to enhance visibility.

For routine patient care purposes, a single-chip video camera, a basic single standard medical-grade monitor or other video display, and simple video home system video recorder are more than sufficient. Eventually, smaller telescopes with excellent illumination and visualization capabilities may be used for microthoracoscopy (11).

Alternative Equipment for Thoracoscopy

Several alternative instruments were used for thoracoscopy. A flexible bronchoscopy was used for thoracoscopy (12,13). More recently, a dedicated semirigid thoracoscope was developed (12). Compared to rigid instruments, the control of the working end is limited due to the flexibility of the scope. The biopsy size is small (2 mm), which may limit the diagnostic yield, especially in case of mesothelioma. The size of the trocar is the same as that for rigid equipment, which means that the discomfort for the patient during the procedure is not reduced. The use of the flexible and the semirigid equipment have disadvantages of flexible instruments, that is, reduced maneuverability, high costs, vulnerability, difficult to sterilize, and small size of the biopsies. There are no clear advantages compared to that of the rigid thoracoscopy equipment.

Recently, minithoracoscopy was developed as an alternative for diagnostic thoracoscopy under local anesthesia. A minithoracoscopy set consists of rigid equipment with smaller sizes than that of the standard equipment. In a recent study, Tassi and Marchetti used a 3-mm thoracoscope for diagnostic thoracoscopy under local anesthesia (14). The diagnostic yield was 93% in his study. Rodriguez-Panadero et al. compared minithoracoscopy by using the 3-mm set and the 2-mm set to standard thoracoscopy using the 7-mm set (15). The diagnostic yield of the 3-mm set was 100%, the same as for the 7-mm set. The yield of diagnostic biopsies using the 2-mm set was only 40%. For taking biopsies with the minithoracoscope, it is always necessary to create a second port of entry, in contrast to the standard equipment.

Medical thoracoscopy must be carried out under sterile conditions. The thoracoscopy room should be sterilized in the same way as an operating room. The trocar, telescopes, forceps, connecting wire, fiberoptic fibers, and all other accessories are sterilized after careful cleaning (16). Calibrated talc is sterilized by autoclaving at 160°C.

B. Technique

Medical thoracoscopy is an invasive procedure that should be used only when other, more simple methods fail (17). Moreover, as with all technical procedures, appropriate training is mandatory before full competence can be achieved. The technique is very similar to chest tube insertion by means of a trocar, the difference being that, in addition, the pleural cavity can be visualized and biopsies can be taken from several intrapleural sites.

Anesthesia

Several modalities can be described based on the experience of the team, the local facilities, and the indications of the procedure (6,18). The preoperative evaluation of the patient includes spirometry, ECG, blood-gas analysis, and routine blood chemistry analysis.

Preoperative preparation may involve chest physiotherapy, bronchodilators, antibiotics, and corticosteroids to optimize pulmonary function in patients with obstructive lung disease. Current medications should generally be continued. Benzodiazepines are commonly used to produce anxiolysis and sedation. The role of preoperative medication has not been subjected to randomized study. Some authors routinely administer 0.4 to 0.8 mg of atropine s.c. prior to the procedure to prevent vasovagal reactions, with or without midazolam 5 mg (9). Sedation during the procedure is performed using incremental dosages of a narcotic (morphine or fentanyl) and a benzodiazepine. Agents to antagonize both morphine and benzodiazepine should be available (6).

Patients should have an intravenous cannula. Basic monitoring includes ECG and pulse oximetry. Supplementary oxygen should be provided to the patient to maintain oxygen saturation above 90%.

For taking a safe biopsy in patients using anticoagulant medication, International normalized ratio should be <2.0. Use of aspirin may prolong the bleeding time, but is not an absolute contraindication for taking biopsies.

Local Anesthesia

This is always recommended if the thoracoscopy procedure is to be briefed in a low-risk patient whose pleural cavity is free of adhesions. Local anesthesia is also preferable to general anesthesia in high-risk patients exhibiting poor general health, compromised respiratory function, or cardiac insufficiency.

General Anesthesia

General anesthesia may be necessary in some cases. It is the technique of choice for procedures requiring intubation. General anesthesia may be delivered and not preclude spontaneous ventilation, which is usually recommended. This method is a relief for patient and physician alike, since it allows time for multiple biopsies, section of extensive adhesions, and electrocautery (7).

There is no consensus in the literature on the appropriateness of performing thoracoscopy under local anesthesia (19,20).

Considerations which may help in choosing the most suitable anesthesiologic technique for thoracoscopy include:

(1) The mental status of the patient (patients afraid of any medical procedure should be offered general anesthesia. Children and mentally retarded patients should be treated under general anesthesia in all circumstances).
(2) The suspected duration and type of thoracoscopy: When a procedure is suspected to be long or painful, general anesthesia is preferred (e.g., multiloculated empyema). Potentially painful procedures are procedures with more than two ports of entry, or procedures followed by chemical pleurodesis. Although very effective, talc poudrage is known to be painful, especially in younger patients. Painless talc poudrage can be performed with intravenous propofol and morphine in a spontaneously breathing patient.

Endoscopy Procedure

The examination is performed with the patient lying on the healthy side. The entry site is generally made on the axilla midline in the third to seventh intercostal space. An absolute prerequisite for thoracoscopy is the presence of an adequate pleural space, which should be at least 6 to 10 cm in diameter. If not present, a pneumothorax is induced immediately on the operating table or the day before the procedure. If extensive pleuropulmonary adhesions are present, "extended thoracoscopy" without creating a pneumothorax can be carried out, but this requires special skills and should not be undertaken without any special training.

Induced Pneumothorax

A pleural trocar for making punctures, measuring 2 or 3 mm in diameter and 100 mm in length, is ideal for inducing pneumothorax. It is inserted into the pleural cavity, and by opening the trocar tap, the air is allowed to enter. The characteristic whistle of air can be heard as it passes through the trocar. As soon as the lung is in a state of equilibrium—an equal amount of air is heard entering the pleura during inhalation as leaving it during exhalation—the pleural trocar is removed and the thoracoscopy trocar is inserted (1,3).

Point of Entry (Single Vs. Multiple Points of Entry)

The puncture site is usually in the midaxillary zone between the third and sixth intercostal spaces because pleural adhesions are uncommon in this area. Choice of the point of entry can vary depending on the indication of the procedure. In patients with spontaneous pneumothorax, the offending leak is usually in the upper lobe so that the best location is between the third and fourth intercostal spaces. In patients with pleural effusion, the fifth, sixth, or seventh intercostal space is the best site of entry. Pulmonary biopsies are facilitated by entry through the fourth/fifth intercostal space. From the patient's viewpoint, the single-entry technique for thoracoscopy is preferred, especially under local anesthesia. Discomfort due to pain and stitches is limited to a single incision of 1 cm, similar to that for the chest tube insertion. Most of the cases of diagnostic thoracoscopy can be performed with a single port of entry. In the two point of entry technique, the optical telescope is not removed, but a second port of entry is created under visual control. A biopsy forceps is introduced through a second (smaller) trocar. The advantage of the two point of entry technique is a better view when biopsies are taken, and the possibility to obtain biopsies with electrocautery sealing, which is of advantage when biopsies are taken of the visceral pleura.

Examination

A procedure includes the following phases:

Careful aspiration of secretions.
Insufflation of air into the cavity, if necessary.
Section of adhesions preventing inspection.
Inspection using a lateral-viewing or a direct-viewing telescope. Perfect knowledge of normal and pathological endoscopic anatomy is mandatory. Biopsy can be performed with illuminated forceps through a single point of entry. When the parietal pleura is thin, specimens should be taken against the rib to avoid injuring the intercostal neurovascular bundle (1). In this regard, it is noteworthy that the main danger is hemorrhage from an intercostal vessel (21). A well-trained endoscopist can quickly create a second point of entry if he or she needs additional instrumentation to sever adhesions, take lung biopsies, and coagulate bleeding vessels.
Collection of multiple biopsy samples (wall, diaphragm, lung) for light microscopy, electronic microscopy, hormone receptor assay, mineral detection, bacteriology, and tumor culture.
Aspiration for fluid cytology.
Talc pleurodesis, if necessary.

At the end of the procedure, a chest tube is inserted and air aspirated. The surveillance of the patient is done in the recovering room, and a control chest X-ray is required. After a diagnostic thoracoscopy for pleural effusion, the tube can be removed as soon as the lung is clinically or radiologically re-expanded against the chest wall (22,23). Sometimes the patient can be discharged on the same day. After lung biopsy, tubing must be prolonged for 24 to 48 hours. After a therapeutic procedure, especially after talc pleurodesis, pleural drainage should be maintained until the lung is re-expanded, bubbling has stopped, and the volume of the fluid collected is less than 100 mL/day. This can take up to two to five days.

III. Complications and Contraindications

A. Complications

Thoracoscopy is one of the safest pneumonological examinations. In a review of 8000 cases, Viskum and Enk noted only one death (24). In this review, no mention of wound infection was found in any study, empyema occurred in only 12 out of 652 cases in three studies, and hemorrhage occurred in 6 out of 356 cases described in three other studies. O_2 desaturation during thoracoscopy under local anesthesia is reportedly less than 2%. Boutin and colleagues reported the mortality rate of 0.09% in a series of 4300 procedures (1). In an experience of more than 6000 thoracoscopies, Brandt and colleagues do not report the requirement for surgical intervention to stop bleeding caused by thoracoscopy (25). Reported mortality rates (<0.01%) are very low. Even several liters of fluid can be completely removed during thoracoscopy with little risk of pulmonary edema, becauseequilibration of pressures is provided by direct entrance of air through the cannula into the pleural space (2). If the re-expansion potential of the lung appears to be diminished, low-pressure suction should be applied. Such complication can be prevented by assessing the intrapleural pressure before the procedure (26). The most serious complication of thoracoscopy is air or gas embolism after air insufflation for artificial pneumothorax, which occurs very rarely (<0.1%), as long as necessary precautionary measures are observed. One of these recommendations is to use a double-balloon air insufflator to induce or to increase an artificial pneumothorax (1).

Although comparative studies have not been performed, it is possible that complication rates may be increased in this setting because of the increased morbidity of patients undergoing these procedures, the use of general anesthesia, and the invasive scope of procedures being performed (27).

B. Contraindications

Most complications can be avoided by proper selection of patients for thoracoscopy. Patients with severe chronic obstructive pulmonary disease and consequent respiratory insufficiency, with hypoxemia (PO_2 < 50 mm Hg) and hypercapnia, will not tolerate induction of a pneumothorax without further deterioration of the gas exchange, and are therefore not suitable candidates for thoracoscopy. When there is a contralateral lung or pleural involvement, thoracoscopy is not advisable unless general anesthesia and tracheal intubation is used. Patients with unstable cardiovascular status should not undergo thoracoscopy. Any patient with a history of cardiovascular disease should be evaluated by the cardiologist before thoracoscopy.

Cough, fever, and infection are relative contraindications for thoracoscopy. Treatment should be considered before a procedure is scheduled. Coagulation defects should be corrected before thoracoscopy.

Thoracoscopy will not be possible in case of complete symphysis of the visceral and parietal pleurae. In case of pleural adhesions, it is possible to create a pleural space by extended thoracoscopy (28). However, this technique should only be performed by experienced thoracoscopists.

Thoracoscopy is not attractive in severe pulmonary fibrosis; after induction of a pneumothorax, it can be difficult to re-expand the lung due to the loss of elasticity of the pulmonary tissue. Pulmonary biopsy in case of honeycombing may result in prolonged leakage and impaired re-expansion of the lung.

Pulmonary biopsy should be avoided in hydatid cysts, arteriovenous malformations, and other highly vascularized lesions.

IV. Clinical Applications

Taday, medical thoracoscopy is primarily a diagnostic procedure, but it can also be applied for therapeutic purposes (9,10,15).

A. Basic Indications for Medical Thoracoscopy

Pleural Effusion

Even algorithms for investigating pleural effusion of unknown etiology typically begin with thoracocentesis, diagnosis of pleural effusions is the prime indication for medical thoracoscopy (15,29–31). Because cytological examination is diagnostic in only 60% to 80% of patients with metastatic pleural involvement and in <20% of patients with mesotheliomas, thoracoscopic parietal pleural examination and biopsy present an opportunity to achieve earlier diagnosis, which is an important prognostic factor for such diseases (32).

Although the possibility of tuberculosis should not be ruled out, malignancy has been found more frequently in recent decades, and most experts agree that when the initial evaluation of a pleural effusion is nondiagnostic, especially when neoplastic disease is suspected, thoracoscopic exploration and parietal pleural biopsy should be considered (33). The diagnostic accuracy of thoracoscopy is between 90% and 100%, compared with an approximate sensitivity of 44% for closed needle pleural biopsy and 62% for fluid cytology; false negatives occur most frequently in cases of early malignant mesothelioma (29). If the patient has a malignancy and negative cytology on thoracocentesis, thoracoscopy is preferred over closed needle pleural biopsy because it will establish the diagnosis in >90% of cases (30).

Metastatic Pleural Malignancies

Needle biopsies are successful in only 50% of metastatic pleural malignancies. Moreover, unlike thoracoscopy, closed pleural biopsies are of little value for localized tumors and are of absolutely no use for metastatic tumors confined to the diaphragmatic, visceral, or mediastinal pleura. In fact, the success of closed techniques depends on tumor extension. The greater the extent of invasion, the more likely the closed biopsy is successful and high yield is achieved only in advanced stages of diseases. This explains why centers dealing with more advanced cancer report higher success rates with needle biopsy. Similarly, pleural fluid cytology exhibits variable success. A yield of 50% to 60% from pleural fluid cytology is certainly a more representative figure (34).

The main advantage of thoracoscopy is its ability to achieve early diagnosis when pleural biopsy and pleural fluid cytology have failed (31,32,35). In 85% of patients with malignancy, thoracoscopy reveals features suggestive of malignancy, including nodules 1 to 5 mm in diameter, large polypoid lesions, localized tumoral masses, rough, pale, thickened pleural surface, and hard, poorly vascularized pachypleuritis (Fig. 2). However,

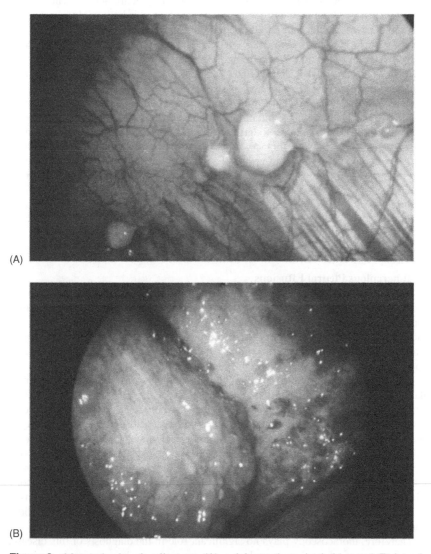

(A)

(B)

Figure 2 Metastatic pleural malignancy: (**A**) nodules on the parietal pleura and (**B**) intrapleural disseminated nodules.

since appearances can be misleading, macroscopic diagnosis must always be confirmed by histology. In this regard, it is important to note that some malignancies mimic non-specific inflammation and some inflammatory lesions can look like tumors (33). Even mesotheliomas have the appearance of ordinary inflammation rather than its fairly characteristic grape-like nodular form. Histopathological findings are the only criteria for certain diagnoses.

The major stumbling block for thoracoscopy in cancer patients is cases of adherent pleura (28,36). The ability to obtain a biopsy depends on the practitioner's skill at dividing and cutting adhesions, and there are some cases where biopsy is impossible.

Therapeutically, fluid can be completely and immediately removed during thoracoscopy with little risk of pulmonary edema. The re-expansion of the lung can be evaluated by visual inspection. Furthermore, the extent of intrapleural tumor spread can be described. The main advantage is certainly that talc poudrage can be performed during medical thoracoscopy.

Complete evacuation of pleural fluid, maximization of lung expandability by removing adhesions, and pleurodesis by talc insufflation results in short- and long-term success rates of >90% (37). Distribution of sterile, calibrated, asbestos-free talc powder on all pleural surfaces is confirmed by thoracoscopic visualization. Following pleurodesis, low-grade fevers should be expected in up to 30% of patients, and hospitalization duration averages 4.8 days. To date, talc poudrage is considered the best conservative option for pleurodesis (38). However, survival of patients with advanced pleural carcinomatosis is often short, and the risks and benefits of thoracoscopic pleurodesis must be carefully weighed against those of repeat thoracocentesis, tube thoracostomy, or bedside pleurodesis through an indwelling chest tube (39). Careful comparative studies are mandatory between these pleurodesis techniques.

Tuberculous Pleural Effusions
Tuberculosis now accounts for less than 10% of all effusions seen in Europe and the United States and a still lower percentage of all chronic cases. In 70% to 90% of cases, diagnosis may be achieved using specimens obtained by percutaneous needle biopsy for histology and culture in conjunction with culture of gastric contents aspirated immediately after awakening. With a second needle biopsy, definite diagnosis can be made in 95% of the cases (5,15).

The endoscopic appearance of tuberculosis consists of grayish-white granulomata blanketing the whole parietal and diaphragmatic pleura and, in particular, the costovertebral gutter (Fig. 3). Lesions have often lost their specific appearance by the time of thoracoscopy and mimic a simple inflammatory process, with increased vascularity, a reddish color, an important and sometimes hemorrhagic fibrinous reaction, and numerous adhesions. Thoracoscopy is usually unnecessary, therefore, to establish the diagnosis of a tuberculous effusion. A combined yield of only 6% for thoracoscopy is preceded by negative thoracocentesis and closed needle pleural biopsy has been reported. Thoracoscopy may be beneficial in difficult diagnostic situations, however, when lysis of adhesions is necessary or when larger amounts of tissue are warranted to assure diagnosis when drug resistance is suspected.

Therefore, thoracoscopy plays no significant role in the diagnosis of this disease, and the discovery of tuberculous granulomata on thoracoscopic biopsy sample is usually fortuitous.

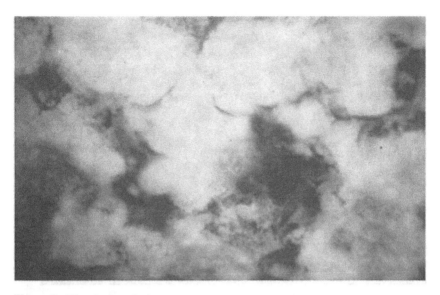

Figure 3   Pleural tuberculosis.

Malignant Mesothelioma

Diagnosis of malignant mesothelioma depends foremost on histological findings. In the past, histologists were reluctant to advance a diagnosis without an autopsy report to bolster their findings. With the increased incidence of this disease and the availability of immunohistochemical techniques, histologists are most forthcoming, although they still hide behind the cover of a group of experts ("panel"). Obtaining biopsy samples for diagnosis of mesothelioma is one of the best indications for thoracoscopy (40,41). However, the diagnosis of histological subtype of malignant pleural mesothelioma is difficult to assess and recent studies have shown the lack of correlation between thoracoscopic and surgical findings after extrapleural pneumonectomy (42,43).

Endoscopy is much less invasive than thoracotomy and allows equally good tissue sampling for pathological diagnosis. By allowing direct visualization of lesions, thoracoscopy facilitates the choice of biopsy sites and correlation of staging with survival. It also allows pulmonary biopsies to document prior exposure to asbestos.

Medical diagnostic thoracoscopy is indicated in any patient without precise histopathological diagnosis in whom clinical and laboratory findings raise suspicion of mesothelioma: cardinal characteristics are found in age between 55 and 60 years, previous exposure to asbestos, pleural effusion or radiological images showing irregular and nodular lesions of the parietal pleura, especially in the posterior and inferior part of the costovertebral gutter.

Macroscopically, the lesions range from 1–3 mm to 1 cm in diameter or even larger, depending on the stage (Fig. 4). In most patients, nodules and masses are associated with parietal pleural thickening up to several millimeters. In 20% of cases, nodules are small (1–5 mm in diameter). A typical aspect of mesothelioma is the "grape-like" aspect, which consists of a patch of closely spaced smooth, translucid, and poorly vascularized

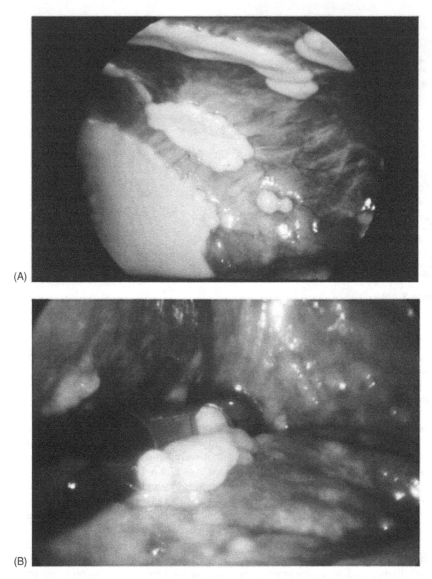

(A)

(B)

Figure 4 Malignant pleural mesothelioma (MPM): (**A**) early-stage disease (pleural plaques with neoplastic lymphangitis) and (**B**) advanced-stage disease.

nodules 5 to 10 mm in diameter with a clear or yellowish appearance. Upon biopsy, these lesions may be either friable and filled with sticky fluid or hard and difficult to remove. The "grape-like" aspect is typical than that of mesothelioma—generally, at the advanced stage—but it is not specific, since it is also encountered in patients with metastatic cancer of the pleura. Unlike benign inflammation, malignant thickness of the pleura associated with mesothelioma is hard and inelastic. When biopsy samples are taken, the cut edge is clear and there is little or no bleeding (44).

In 10% to 15% of all cases and in 50% of stage Ia cases, the lesions observed during thoracoscopy are macroscopically nonspecific: benign inflammation of the parietal or diaphragmatic pleura with lymphangitis in some of the cases. In these cases, a more discrete sign is irregular thickening located mainly in the posterior and inferior regions of the parietal pleura where lymphatic vessels are most numerous. The more nonspecific the lesions, the more biopsies should be taken (up to 15 or 20).

An important diagnostic finding is involvement of the visceral pleura and lung. These structures can be easily visualized during thoracoscopy. The visceral pleura is always less involved than the parietal pleura, with nodules being not only less numerous but also smaller. In many cases, the visceral pleura appears macroscopically normal, but routine biopsy should be performed to confirm or exclude the diagnosis (45).

In contrast with the high sensitivity of thoracoscopy, the combined sensitivity of fluid cytology and needle biopsy was only 38.2%. The overall sensitivity of these conventional methods is poor, and most investigators prefer open surgical biopsy, which is more painful, less safe, and less cost-effective than a surgical procedure.

Other Pleural Effusions

Pleural effusions associated with lung cancer result from direct carcinomatous involvement of the pleura or are paramalignant effusions (46). Even patients in whom cytological examination of pleural fluid is negative are often found on thoracotomy to have unresectable lesions. Thoracoscopy is preferable to thoracotomy for identifying this small group of patients who could potentially get benefit from a surgical resection (8). Thoracoscopy is also useful for staging both lung and esophageal cancer because it may complement cervical mediastinoscopy and allows staging of mediastinal lymphadenopathy. Ideally, diagnostic thoracoscopy and surgical resection can be performed sequentially during the same period of general anesthesia. Although curative resections can be performed thoracoscopically, it is unlikely that this technique will replace standard open surgical approaches for lobectomy and pneumonectomy.

Recurrent pleural effusions of benign etiology are frequently caused by heart failure, cardiac surgery, nephrotic syndrome, connective tissue diseases, and other inflammatory disorders (47) (Fig. 5). Thoracoscopy may be warranted when recurrent effusions cause symptoms and are not controlled by repeated large-volume thoracocentesis. Usually, pleural biopsy specimens are obtained to exclude infectious or neoplastic etiologies, and pleurodesis is performed. Results are usually excellent when talc is used, with success rates varying from 65% to >90%.

In some selected case of recurrent pleural effusions of nonmalignant etiology, including chylothorax, pleurodesis may be induced by applying talc poudrage during medical thoracoscopy (48).

Management of Recurrent Malignant Effusions by Thoracoscopic Talc Poudrage

Talc is superior to other agents, with more than 90% success rate for talc pleurodesis in the treatment of recurrent pleural effusions (49). Talc is an inexpensive and highly effective sclerosing agent when administered intrapleurally for symphysis. However, a controversy arose about the possible role of asbestos-free talc in inducing respiratory failure due to

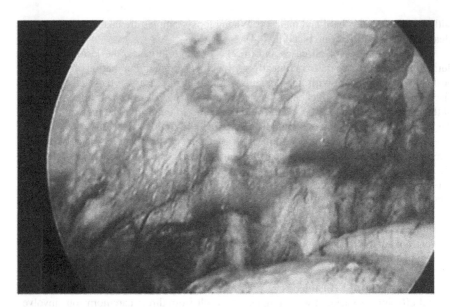

Figure 5 Endopleural sarcoidosis.

systemic distribution of particles after intrapleural injection (50,51). It is not clear so far whether the method of administration (slurry vs. poudrage) plays a major role in the development of respiratory failure; further experimental studies are needed to answer this question. However, recent publications have pointed out the importance of the quality of talc and the size of talc particles in the safety of pleural symphysis (52–55).

Talc poudrage pleurodesis can be performed by thoracoscopy under local anesthesia with conscious sedation or general anesthesia. Usually, the procedure is performed in patients with spontaneous breathing (56). Several technical details should be taken into account in order to achieve good pleurodesis and to avoid complications. All pleural fluid should be removed before insufflating talc. Fluid removal is easily done under visual control during thoracoscopy, as air is entering the pleural cavity without insufflation. This creates equilibrium in pressures. Complete collapse of the lung allows a good view of the pleural cavity and a careful analysis of visceral and parietal pleurae, as well as the opportunity to biopsy suspicious lesions and, at the end of the procedure, permits a wide distribution of the talc on dry tissue. Usually, less than 5 g of sterile, asbestos-free, calibrated talc is recommended to obtain symphysis in patients with MPE. Thoracoscopy allows repeated pleural inspection at the end of the procedure after talc insufflation to make sure that the powder is distributed over the pleural surface. Immediate talc poudrage can be done in cases of macroscopic or histologic evidence of malignancy and ineligibility of the patient for trials of intrapleural treatment. The safety and quality of such talc pleurodesis depends on the type of talc used (54,55), as well as the drainage technique and the time when pleurodesis is performed (56). The chest tube must be inserted as low as possible in the thorax, directed posteriorly toward the costovertebral gutter, and as close to the apex as possible for optimal drainage of residual fluid. This observation, however, has not been subject to a controlled study, and is not supported by all the authors of this manuscript, who think that positioning the drain caudally oriented would be more effective in removing all the new-forming pleural fluid.

Waiting for pleurodesis is detrimental to the patient because parietal nodules and/or cancerous thickening of the visceral pleura, which increase with time, can prevent adhesion of the lung to the chest wall, this being a prerequisite for successful pleurodesis. Therefore, patients with MPE are good candidates for thoracoscopy and talc pleurodesis if they meet the following criteria: (*i*) failure or unavailability of specific treatment, (*ii*) dyspnea that improves after large-volume thoracocentesis with subsequent and rapid recurrence of the pleural effusion, and (*iii*) absence of trapped lung as evidenced by previous thoracocenteses, contrast computed tomography (CT) or measurement of intrapleural pressures.

Thoracoscopic talc poudrage is a safe and efficient procedure for the management of patients with recurrent MPE (57). The cost of the procedure can be reduced by performing medical thoracoscopy in an endoscopy suite instead of an operating room. Despite the costs incurred by the technical procedure, it must be the treatment of choice for patients suffering this disabling disease (58).

Spontaneous Pneumothorax

If a chest tube is introduced by trocar technique, it is easy to use an optic for visual inspection of the lung and the pleural cavity. Then, thoracoscopy provides an excellent alternative to repeated chest tube drainage in patients with recurrent or prolonged (usually >5 days) pneumothorax for diagnostic and therapeutic purposes (59–61). Thoracoscopic findings in patients with spontaneous pneumothorax include, as described by Vanderschueren, normal appearance (type 1), pleural adhesions (type 2), small blebs (<2 cm) on the visceral pleural surface (type 3), and large bullae (>2 cm) (type 4) (62,63) [Figs. 6(A) and 6(B)]. Usually, these lesions are too fine to be seen on CT scans. The visibility of bullae and blebs can be enhanced if the patient performs a Valsalva maneuver or by creating positive airway pressure with the anesthesia mask during the procedure.

Lesions can be removed using electrocautery [Figs. 6(C) and 6(D)], argon plasma coagulation, or stapled lung resection if the skills and facilities for this technique are available, with results similar to those obtained after open thoracotomy (although the resultant pleurodesis may be somewhat less effective: recurrence rates are reportedly 5–10% vs. 1–3% after open thoracotomy). However, there is no proof to date that the endoscopic treatment of minimal lesions on the surface of the lung is required (61,64).

In case of recurrent pneumothorax, talc insufflation for pleurodesis may also be effective and is recommended by several teams. Talc poudrage achieves the best conservative treatment results, with a recurrence rate of <10% (65). However, it still remains a controversial issue due to severe secondary side effects. It seems that these complications are due to the quality of talc preparation, which must be carefully assessed (see section, management of recurrent malignant effusions by thoracoscopic talc poudrage).

Medical thoracoscopy is justified in all patients with spontaneous pneumothorax where tube drainage is indicated. This procedure offers several advantages: cost effectiveness (66,67), assessment of the underlying lesion under visual control, choice of the best treatment measures, and by severing of adhesions, if necessary, selecting the best location for chest tube placement (68,69).

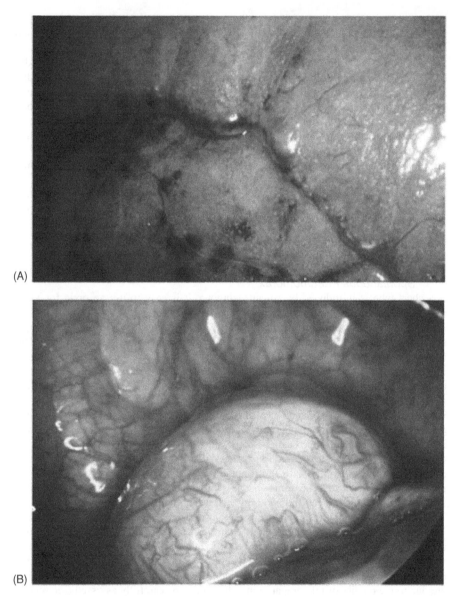

Figure 6   Pneumothorax: (**A**) blebs on the fissure (type III), (**B**) bullae (type IV), (**C**) coagulation of a bullae, and (**D**) adhesiolysis with electrocautery (type II).

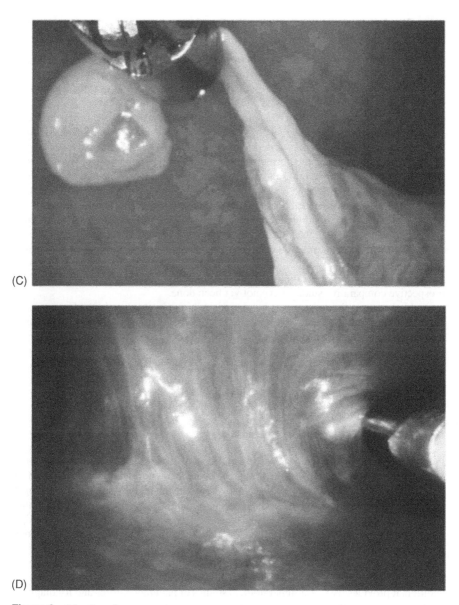

(C)

(D)

Figure 6 (*Continued*)

B. Advanced Indications for Medical Thoracoscopy

Empyema

Comprehensive reviews and evidence-based guidelines for the management of compli-cated parapneumonic effusion and empyema are available, but they do not deal compre-hensively with the role of thoracoscopy, apart from considering it an acceptable approach through surgery (70–73).

Medical thoracoscopy can be useful in the management of early empyema (74,75). During the exudative and organizing phase of empyema, in cases with multiple loculations, thoracoscopic visualization allows debridement of fibrinous adhesions and evacuation of loculated fluid in removing the fibrinopurulent membranes by forceps to create one single pleural cavity (Fig. 7). In draining and irrigating the pleural cavity much more successfully, this procedure may shorten the length of hospital stay and avoid thoracotomy. However, this treatment should be carried out early in the course of empyema, before the adhesions become too fibrous and adherent (75). The timing of thoracoscopic intervention is critical and should be considered if the indication for a placement of a chest tube is present (76,77). This procedure is similar to chest tube placement that allows the creation of a single pleural cavity. The precise role for thoracoscopy instead of chest tube drainage, instillation of fibrinolytic agents, rib resection, or thoracotomy-decortication is still controversial, and prospective comparative studies have not yet been done.

In summary, the presence of loculations, which are characteristic of complicated parapneumonic effusion and fibrinopurulent empyema, frequently makes the effusion resistant to drainage with a single chest tube. In these situations, either intrapleural fibrinolytics (78–81), medical thoracoscopy, VATS or, in advanced cases of chronic fibrotic empyema, open surgical decortication is used. There are considerable differences in using these approaches between different hospitals, regions, and countries, based more on individual clinical choice than on scientific data.

Diffuse Pulmonary Diseases

Forceps lung biopsy during thoracoscopy under local anesthesia has been used for many years by pneumonologists but its employment has been considerably reduced with the advent of VATS, particularly in diffuse lung disease (5), although a study demonstrating its utility was published in 1999 (82). Thus, it is important that interventional pneumonolo-gists remain familiar with a technique that can be still relevant. Thoracoscopic lung biopsy helps to establish the diagnosis of diffuse or focal interstitial lung disease and pulmonary infection, in particular when transbronchial biopsy (TBB) or bronchoalveolar lavage has failed to provide a diagnosis (83). The possibility of taking several biopsies from different sites under visual control and the lower morbidity are the most important advantages. In addition, it provides tissue for mineralogical studies of pneumoconioses and for diagnosis of pulmonary infiltrates or peripheral nodular lesions of unknown etiology.

Specimens are usually obtained using a cup biopsy forceps, which is dipped in the lung parenchyma. After lung palpation with the forceps in the closed position, the forceps is opened, the lung is grasped, and the forceps is closed while applying short pulses of diathermy coagulation (Fig. 8). In many cases, patients can be discharged from the hospital in fewer than three days with little morbidity. Postoperative stay in an ICU is rarely necessary (84).

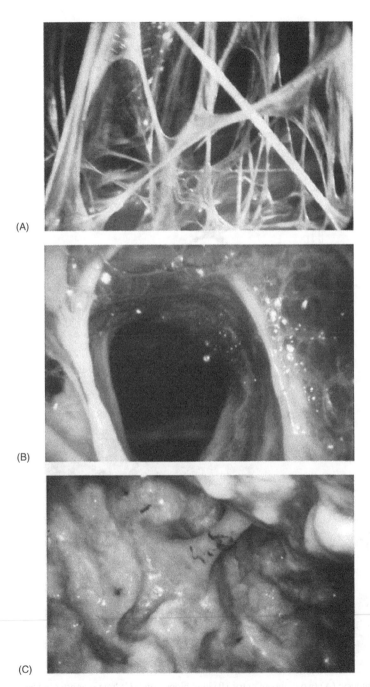

Figure 7 Empyema: (**A**) early-stage parapneumonic effusion, (**B**) endopleural purulent adhesions, and (**C**) empyema.

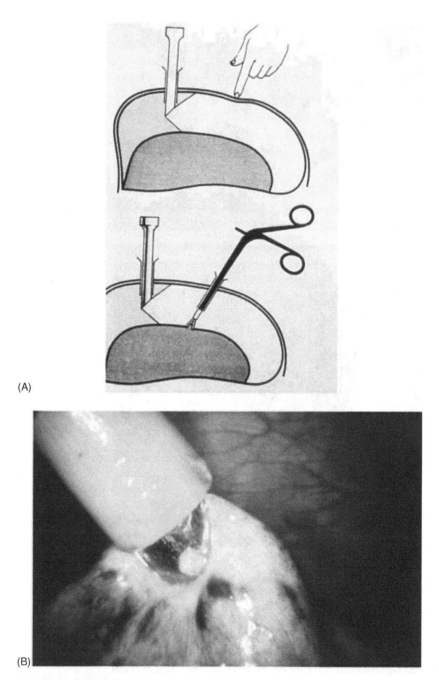

(A)

(B)

Figure 8   Lung biopsy: (**A**) two points of entry, (**B**) lung biopsy, and (**C**) lung scar after biopsy.

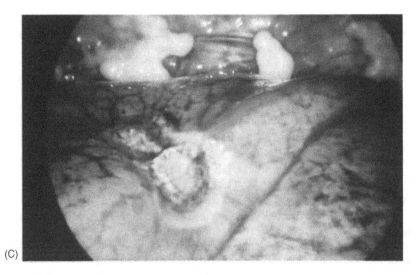

(C)

Figure 8 (*Continued*)

The diagnostic rate of diseases such as pneumoconiosis, sarcoidosis, or carcinomatous lymphangitis is very high. Frequently, more than 90% of samples taken are useful for analysis. The diameter of the biopsies varies from 2.1 to 6.6 mm—much larger than TBB. Coagulation artefacts are not a major problem if coagulation time is kept to <2 seconds. The diagnostic accuracy of the technique depends on the distribution pattern of the interstitial disease, the lobular compartment involved, and the histological specificity of the disease.

Diagnoses of idiopathic interstitial pneumonitis could be made with confidence. Although the diagnosis of suspected pulmonary vasculitis or other pulmonary vascular disorders is more difficult and the technique of medical thoracoscopy is less powerful in such cases, it remains useful in suspected vascular pathology, especially if there are lesions in the smaller pulmonary arterioles (82).

No major complications such as important bleeding or persistent fistula usually occur after the procedure. However, prolonged air leak is the most troublesome problem, which is not correlated with the number or size of biopsies but to the preexisting total lung capacity and static compliance. Such a complication is to be anticipated in patients with very stiff or honeycombing lungs where the use of a stapler or open lung biopsy with a suture may be a reasonable alternative. Medical thoracoscopic lung biopsy must be avoided in case of suspected major pleural adhesions, in severe pulmonary hypertension, and in a very sick ventilated patients, in whom open lung biopsy carries less risk.

Thoracoscopy has prompted many practitioners to consider lung biopsy earlier in the management algorithm of patients with parenchymal disease of unclear origin, especially when bronchoscopic lung biopsies have been nondiagnostic.

Vaso-Motor Syndrome of the Upper Limb

Interruption of the upper dorsal sympathetic chain at the D2 and D3 level represents a permanent cure in patients with Raynaud's syndrome, causalgia, or essential hyperhidrosis (85). Thoracoscopic sympathectomies are performed by using either electrocautery, dissection, or excision (86). Sympathectomy by medical thoracoscopy route is feasible, and this technique has been proven simple and safe with skill practitioners, with excellent short-term clinical results (87,88). Side effects and complications are minor (compensatory hyperhidrosis) or self-limiting (pain). The key problem is to prevent Horner's syndrome in avoiding the stellate ganglion with careful examination of the upper posterior part of the pleural cavity.

Exposure is usually through the anterior chest wall, and procedures can be performed bilaterally at a single setting (89,90).

Intrapleural Treatment

Intrapleural immunotherapy or chemotherapy can be administered after thoracoscopic placement of intrapleural implantable access system to treat cancer (91). Proper placement of the catheter under thoracoscopic guidance ensures that the drug is applied directly to the lesions (92,93). The subcutaneous location of the site reduces the risk of infection (94). The main indications for intrapleural therapy are malignant pleural mesothelioma as single treatment or in multimodal strategy as neoadjuvant treatment.

V. Conclusion

Potential advantages of thoracoscopy over more conventional techniques include certainty of representative tissue for diagnosis, reduced requirements for postoperative analgesia, shorter hospital stays, and a shorter duration of chest tube drainage compared with thoracotomy. The thoracoscopic approach to pleural and lung diseases has to demonstrate safety and cost-effectiveness compared with more conventional approaches. Potential adverse events including bleeding, persistent pneumothorax, intercostal nerve and vessel injury, cardiac disturbances, complications related to anesthesia, respiratory failure, wound infections, and malignant seeding of the chest wall have been reported; procedure-related mortality is rare (0.24%, comparable to that of bronchoscopic biopsy) in experienced hands.

Future directions in the field of medical thoracoscopy include developing "mini-invasive" procedures (95). One of the most exciting tasks in this field is to develop physician training and to provide education, allowing chest physicians to analyze the pleural cavity and enhance their understanding of anatomical relationships and pleuropulmonary physiology (96).

References

1. Boutin C, Viallat JR, Aelony Y. Practical Thoracoscopy. Heidelberg: Springer Verlag, 1991.
2. Loddenkemper R. Thoracoscopy—State of the art. Eur Respir J 1998; 11:213–221.
3. Boutin C, Astoul P. Diagnostic thoracoscopy. Clin Chest Med 1998; 19:295–309.
4. Colt HG. Thoracoscopy: Window to the pleural space. Chest 1999; 116:1409–1415.
5. Loddenkemper R, Schonfeld N. Medical thoracoscopy. Curr Opin Pulm Med 1998; 4:235–238.
6. Migliore M, Guiliano R, Aziz T, et al. Four-step local anesthesia and sedation for thoracoscopic diagnosis and management of pleural diseases. Chest 2002; 121:2032–2035.

7. Plummer S, Hartley M, Vaughan RS. Anaesthesia for telescopic procedures in the thorax. Br J Anaesth 1998; 80:223–234.

8. Landreneau RJ, Mack MJ, Dowling RD, et al. The role of thoracoscopy in lung cancer management. Chest 1998; 113(Suppl. 1):6S–12S.

9. Mathur PN, Astoul P, Boutin C. Medical thoracoscopy: Technical details. Clin Chest Med 1995; 16:479–486.

10. Little AG. Thoracoscopy: Current status. Curr Opin Pulm Med 1996; 2:315–319.

11. Yamada S, Kosaka A, Masuda M, et al. Minimally invasive lung and pleural biopsies using 2-mm and standard thoracoscopic equipment. Jpn J Thorac Cardiovasc Surg 2000; 48:700–702.

12. Davidson AC, George RJ, Sheldon CD, et al. Thoracoscopy: Assessment of a physician service and comparison of a flexible bronchoscope used as a thoracoscope with a rigid thoracoscope. Thorax 1988; 43:327–332.

13. Ernst A, Hersh CP, Herth F, et al. A novel instrument for the evaluation of the pleural space. Chest 2002; 122:1530–1534.

14. Tassi G, Marchetti G. Minithoracoscopy. A less invasive approach to thoracoscopy. Chest 2003; 124:1975–1977.

15. Rodriguez-Panadero F, Janssen J, Astoul P. Thoracoscopy: General overview and management of pleural effusion. Eur Respir J 2006; 28;409–422. Review.

16. Mathur P, Martin WJ. Clinical utility of thoracoscopy. Chest 1992; 4:1–4.

17. Light RW. Diagnostic principles in pleural disease. Eur Respir J 1997; 10:476–481.

18. Danby CA, Adebonojo SA, Moritz DM. Video-assisted talc pleurodesis for malignant pleural effusions utilizing local anesthesia and IV sedation. Chest 1998; 113:739–742.

19. Harris RJ, Kavuru S, Rice TW, et al. The diagnostic and therapeutic utility of thoracoscopy. Chest 1995; 108:828–841.

20. Aelony Y, Boutin C. Local anesthesia with thoracoscopic talc poudrage pleurodesis. Chest 1996; 110:1126.

21. DeCamp MM Jr, Jaklitsch MT, Mentzer SJ, et al. The safety and versatility of video-thoracoscopy: A prospective analysis of 895 consecutive cases. J Am Coll Surg 1995; 18: 113–120.

22. Russo L, Wiechmann RJ, Magovern JA, et al. Early chest tube removal after video-assisted thoracoscopic wedge resection of the lung. Ann Thorac Surg 1998; 66:1751–1754.

23. Astoul Ph, Boutin C, Seitz B, et al. Diagnostic thoracoscopy in short term hospitalization. Acta Endo 1990; 20:79–83.

24. Viskum K, Enk B. Complications of thoracoscopy. Poumon Coeur 1981; 37:25–28.

25. Brandt HJ, Loddenkemper R, Mai J. Atlas of Diagnostic Thoracoscopy. New York: Thieme Stuttgart, 1985.

26. Lan RS, Lo SK, Chuang ML, et al. Elastance of the pleural space: A predictor for the outcome of pleurodesis in patients with malignant pleural effusion. Ann Intern Med 1997; 126:768–774.

27. Hansen M, Faurschou P, Clementsen P. Medical thoracoscopy, results and complications in 146 patients: A retrospective study. Respir Med 1998; 9:228–232.

28. Janssen JP, Boutin C. Extended thoracoscopy: A biopsy method to be used in case of pleural adhesions. Eur Resp J 1992; 5:763–766.

29. Colt HG. Thoracoscopic management of malignant pleural effusions. Clin Chest Med 1995; 16:505–518.

30. Colt HG. Thoracoscopy: A prospective study of safety and outcome. Chest 1995; 108:324–329.

31. Rodriguez-Panadero F. Malignant pleural diseases. Monaldi Arch Chest Dis 2000; 55:17–19.

32. Wilsher ML, Veale AG. Medical thoracoscopy in the diagnosis of unexplained pleural effusion. Respirology 1998; 3:77–80.

33. de Groot M, Walther G. Thoracoscopy in undiagnosed pleural effusions. S Afr Med J 1998; 88:706–711.

34. Renshaw AA, Dean BR, Antman KH, et al. The role of cytologic evaluation of pleural fluid in the diagnosis of malignant mesothelioma. Chest 1997; 111:106–109.
35. McLean AN, Bicknell SR, McAlpine LG, et al. Investigation of pleural effusion: An evaluation of the new Olympus LTF semiflexible thoracofiberscope and comparison with Abram's needle biopsy. Chest 1998; 114:150–153.
36. Mason AC, Miller BH, Krasna MJ, et al. Accuracy of CT for the detection of pleural adhesions: Correlation with video-assisted thoracoscopic surgery. Chest 1999; 115:423–427.
37. Aelony Y, King R, Boutin C. Thoracoscopic talc poudrage pleurodesis for chronic reccurent pleural effusions. Ann Intern Med 1991; 115:778–782.
38. Aelony Y, King RR, Boutin C. Thoracoscopic talc poudrage in malignant pleural effusions: Effective pleurodesis despite low pleural pH. Chest 1998; 113:1007–1012.
39. Light RW. Diseases of the pleura: The use of talc for pleurodesis. Curr Opin Pulm Med 2000; 6:255–258.
40. Boutin C, Rey F. Thoracoscopy in pleural mesothelioma. A prospective study of 188 consecutive patients. Part I: Diagnosis. Cancer 1993; 72:389–393.
41. Canto A, Guijarro R, Arnau A, et al. Videothoracoscopy in the diagnosis and treatment of malignant pleural mesothelioma with associated pleural effusions. J Thorac Cardiovasc Surg 1997; 45:16–19.
42. Bueno R, Reblando J, Glickman J, et al. Pleural biopsy: A reliable method for determining the diagnosis but not subtype in mesothelioma. Ann Thorac Surg 2004; 78:1774–1776. Review.
43. Greillier L, Cavailles A, Fraticelli A, et al. Accuracy of pleural biopsy using thoracoscopy for the diagnosis of histologic subtype in patients with malignant pleural mesothelioma. Cancer 2007; 110;2248–2252.
44. Boutin C, Frenay C, Astoul P. Endoscopic diagnosis of mesothelioma. Rev Mal Respir 1999; 16:1257–1262.
45. Boutin C, Rey F, Gouvernet J, et al. Thoracoscopy in pleural malignant mesothelioma: A prospective study of 188 patients. Part 2: Prognosis and staging. Cancer 1993; 72:394–404.
46. Sahn SA. Pleural diseases related to metastatic malignancies. Eur Respir J 1997; 10:1907–1913.
47. Mouroux J, Perrin C, Venissac N, et al. Management of pleural effusion of cirrhotic origin. Chest 1996; 109:1093–1096.
48. Mares DC, Mathur PN. Medical thoracoscopic talc pleurodesis for chylothorax due to lymphoma: A case series. Chest 1998; 114:731–735.
49. Walker-Renard P, Vaughan LM, Sahn SA. Chemical pleurodesis for malignant pleural effusions. Ann Intern Med 1994; 120:56–64.
50. Light RW. Talc for pleurodesis? Chest 2002; 122:1506–1508.
51. Werebe EC, Cazetti R, Milanez de Campos JR, et al. Systemic distribution of talc after intrapleural administration in rats. Chest 1999; 115:190–193.
52. Fraticelli A, Robaglia-Schlupp A, Helene Riera H, et al. Distribution of calibrated talc after intrapleural administration: An experimental study in rats. Chest 2002; 122:1737–1741.
53. Ferrer J, Villarino MA, Tura JM, et al. Talc preparation used for pleurodesis vary markedly from one preparation to another. Chest 2001; 119:1901–1905.
54. Ferrer J, Montes JF, Villarino MA, et al. Influence of particle size on extrapleural talc dissemination after talc slurry pleurodesis. Chest 2002; 122:1018–1027.
55. Maskell NA, Lee YC, Gleeson FV, et al. Randomized trials describing lung inflammation after pleurodesis with talc of varying particle size. Am J Respir Crit Care Med 2004; 170: 377–382.
56. Viallat JR, Rey F, Astoul P, et al. Thoracoscopic talc poudrage pleurodesis for malignant effusions. A review of 360 cases. Chest 1996; 110:1387–1393.
57. Janssen JP, Collier G, Astoul P, et al. Safety of pleurodesis with talc poudrage in malignant pleural effusion: A prospective cohort study. Lancet 2007; 369:1535–1539.

58. Cardillo G, Faciolo F, Carbone L, et al. Long-term follow-up of video-assisted talc pleurodesis in malignant recurrent effusions. Eur J Cardiothorac Surg 2002; 21:302–305.
59. Janssen JP, Schramel FM, Sutedja TG, et al. Videothoracoscopic appearance of first and recurrent pneumothorax. Chest 1995; 108:330–334.
60. Delaunois L, El Khawand C. Medical thoracoscopy in the management of pneumothorax. Monaldi Arch Chest Dis 1998; 53:148–150.
61. Tschopp JM, Rami-Porta R, Noppen M, et al. Management of spontaneous pneumothorax: State of the art. Eur Respir J 2006; 28:1–14.
62. Schramel FMNH. Current aspects of spontaneous pneumothorax. Eur Respir J 1997; 10: 1372–1379.
63. Sahn SA, Heffner JE. Spontaneous pneumothorax. N Engl J Med 2000; 342:868–874.
64. Milanez JRC, Vargas FS, Filomeno LTB, et al. Intrapleural talc for the prevention of recurrent pneumothorax. Chest 1994; 106:1162–1165.
65. Tschopp JM, Brutsche M, Frey JG. Treatment of complicated spontaneous pneumothorax by simple talc pleurodesis under thoracoscopy and local anaesthesia. Thorax 1997; 52:329–332.
66. Schramel FM, Sutedja TG, Braber JC, et al. Costeffectiveness of video-assisted thoracoscopic surgery versus conservative treatment for first time or recurrent spontaneous pneumothorax. Eur Respir J 1996; 9:1821–1825.
67. Tschopp JM, Boutin C, Astoul P, et al. talcage by medical thoracoscopy for primary spontaneous pneumothorax is more cost-effective than drainage: a randomised study. Eur Respir J 2002; 20:1003–1009.
68. Miller AC, Harvey JE. Guidelines for the management of spontaneous pneumothorax. Standards of Care Committee—British Thoracic Society. BMJ 1993; 307:114–116.
69. Baumann MH, Strange C, Heffner JE, et al. Management of spontaneous pneumothorax. An American College of Chest Physicians Delphi Consensus statement. Chest 2001; 119:590–602.
70. Sahn SA. Management of complicated parapneumonic effusions. Am Rev Respir Dis 1993; 148:813–817.
71. Davies CW, Gleeson FV, Davies RJ. On behalf of the Pleural Disease Group. Standards of Care Committee. British Thoracic Society. BTS guidelines for the management of pleural infection. Thorax 2003; 58(Suppl. 2):ii18–ii28.
72. Alfageme I, Munoz F, Pena N, et al. Empyema of the thorax in adults. Etiology, microbiologic findings, and management. Chest 1993; 103:839–843.
73. Colice GL, Curtis A, Deslauriers J, et al. Medical and surgical treatment of parapneumonic effusions. An evidence-based guideline. Chest 2000; 18:1158–1171.
74. Striffeler H, Gugger M, Im Hof V, et al. Video-assisted thoracoscopic surgery for fibrinopurulent pleural empyema in 67 patients. Ann Thorac Surg 1998; 65:319–323.
75. Karmy-Jones R, Sorenson V, Horst HM, et al. Rigid thorascopic debridement and continuous pleural irrigation in the management of empyema. Chest 1997; 111:272–274.
76. Silen ML, Naunheim KS. Thoracoscopic approach to the management of empyema thoracis: Indications and results. Chest Surg Clin N Am 1996; 6:491–499.
77. Cassina PC, Hauser M, Hillejan L, et al. Video-assisted thoracoscopy in the treatment of pleural empyema: Stage-based management and outcome. J Thorac Cardiovasc Surg 1999; 117:234–238.
78. Maskell NA, Davies CW, Nunn AJ, et al. UK controlled trial of intrapleural streptokinase for pleural infection. N Engl J Med 2005; 352:865–874.
79. Davies RJO, Traill ZC, Gleeson FV. Randomized controlled trial of intrapleural streptokinase in community acquired pleural infection. Thorax 1997; 52:416–421.
80. Bouros D, Schiza S, Tzanakis N, et al. Intrapleural urokinase *versus* normal saline in the treatment of complicated parapneumonic effusions and empyema. Am J Respir Crit Care Med 1999; 159:37–42.

81. Thomson AH, Hull J, Kumar MR, et al. A randomized trial of intrapleural urokinase in the treatment of childhood empyema. Thorax 2002; 57:343–347.
82. Vansteenkiste J, Verbeken E, Thomeer M, et al. Medical thoracoscopic lung biopsy in interstitial lung disease: A prospective study of biopsy quality. Eur Respir J 1999; 14:585–590.
83. Krasna MJ, White CS, Aisner SC, et al. The role of thoracoscopy in the diagnosis of interstitial lung disease. Ann Thorac Surg 1995; 59:348–351.
84. Ravini M, Ferraro G, Barbieri B, et al. Changing strategies of lung biopsies in diffuse lung diseases: The impact of video-assisted thoracoscopy. Eur Respir J 1998; 11:99–103.
85. Di Lorenzo N, Sica GS, Sileri P, et al. Thoracoscopic sympathectomy for vasospastic diseases. J Soc Laparoendosc Surg 1998; 2:249–253.
86. Noppen M, Herregodts P, D'haese J, et al. A simplified T2–T3 thoracoscopic sympatholysis technique for the treatment of essential hyperhidrosis: Short-term results in 100 patients. J Laparoendosc Surg 1996; 6:151–159.
87. Noppen M, Vincken W. Thoracoscopic sympathicolysis for essential hyperhidrosis: Effects on pulmonary function. Eur Respir J 1996; 9:1660–1664.
88. Noppen M, Dendale P, Hagers Y, et al. Changes in cardiocirculatory autonomic function after thoracoscopic upper dorsal sympathicolysis for essential hyperhidrosis. J Auton Nerv Syst 1996; 60:115–120.
89. Noppen M, Dab I, D'Haese J, et al. Thoracoscopic T2–T3 sympathicolysis for essential hyperhidrosis in childhood: Effects on pulmonary function. Pediatr Pulmonol 1998; 26: 264–264.
90. Noppen M, Sevens C, Gerlo E, et al. Plasma catecholamine concentrations in essential hyperhidrosis and effects of thoracoscopic D2–D3 sympathicolysis. Eur J Clin Invest 1997; 27: 202–205.
91. Driesen P, Boutin C, Viallat JR, et al. Implantable access system for prolonged intrapleural immunotherapy. Eur Respir J 1994; 7:1889–1892.
92. Astoul Ph, Bertault-Peres P, Durand A, et al. Pharmacokinetics of intrapleural recombinant interleukin-2 in immunotherapy for malignant pleural effusion. Cancer 1994; 73:308–313.
93. Monjanel-Mouterde S, Frenay C, Catalin J, et al. Pharmacokinetics of intrapleural cisplatin for the treatment of malignant pleural effusions. Oncol Rep 2000; 7:171–175.
94. Astoul Ph, Picat-Joossen D, Viallat JR, et al. Intrapleural administration of interleukin-2 for the treatment of patients with malignant pleural mesothelioma. Cancer 1998; 83:2099–2104.
95. d'Alessandro AA. Microthoracoscopy at the cutting edge of thoracic surgery. J Laparoendosc Adv Surg Tech A 1997; 7:313–318.
96. Yim AP. Training in thoracoscopy in the Asia-Pacific. Int Surg 1997; 82:22–23.

10
Therapeutic Use of Thoracoscopy for Pleural Diseases

PIERRE-EMMANUEL FALCOZ
Université Louis Pasteur and Hôpitaux Universitaires de Strasbourg, Strasbourg, France
PASCAL THOMAS
Université de Marseille, Hôpital Sainte Marguerite, Marseille, France
GILBERT MASSARD
Université Louis Pasteur and Hôpitaux Universitaires de Strasbourg, Strasbourg, France

I. Introduction

The therapeutic use of thoracoscopy is not a recent addition to our armamentarium (1). Illustrations in physiology textbooks from the 1950s show ports, forceps, and hooks similar to those still in use; optical interface with video transmission and the creation of endoscopic staplers and disposable instruments are the extent of new technology. For half a century, thoracoscopy has been an important adjunct to collapse therapy for tuberculosis, which was the mainstay of treatment prior to the advent of major antituberculous drugs. Thoracoscopy was used to separate pleural adhesions in order to create pneumothorax. It is therefore paradoxical that now one of the main indications for thoracoscopy is treatment of pneumothorax!

For approximately 15 years, surgeons, physicians, and patients have been subjected to a campaign in favor of minimally invasive techniques. The exponential development of these techniques has reinvigorated the biomedical industry. This chapter will critically review the therapeutic use of videothoracoscopy in pleural diseases to define the optimal indications and compare it to classic alternatives where available.

II. Potential Indications for Therapeutic Thoracoscopy

Use of thoracoscopy for diagnostic purposes in pleural diseases is described elsewhere in this book. We therefore concentrate here on the treatment of pleural diseases and more particularly on the management of empyema and spontaneous pneumothorax.

Traditional indications also included pleurodesis for recurrent pleural effusions (in particular metastatic effusions) with talc poudrage or various other irritative substances. The sine qua non condition for a successful pleurodesis in this setting is that the lung is able to re-expand and completely seal the pleural space. Therefore, it is mandatory to perform this pleurodesis at an early stage, before metastatic deposits on the visceral pleura encase the lung. It is well known that talc is both the most efficient and the least expensive material; we therefore consider that this indication does not need any further development (2).

Several single-case reports describe successful management of chylothorax with thoracoscopic ligation of the thoracic duct. However, chylothorax remains a rare event, and it is impossible to estimate the proportion of patients amenable to safe thoracoscopic management, as the proportion of those managed by formal thoracotomy remains unknown. We consider this indication as—hopefully—anecdotal and will not further develop this issue (3,4).

In stable patients with traumatic hemothorax, early thoracoscopy may allow for adequate cleaning of the pleural space and thus avoid clotting; early recognition of various underlying traumatic lesions such as rupture of the diaphragm, rupture of the pericardium, and parenchymal tears will lead to adequate early management (5,6). However, many patients are either unstable or cannot be brought to immediate thoracoscopy because of associated extrathoracic injuries; classic treatment with chest tube placement followed by thoracotomy, if required, by persistent bleeding still has its place.

III. Preliminary Remarks

We consider all procedures described below as surgical procedures to be undertaken only by certified thoracic surgeons. In Europe, we recommend certification by the National Colleges of Thoracic Surgeons. This certification should progressively be replaced by the recently awarded European Board of Cardiothoracic Surgery, which is promoted by the European Association for Cardiothoracic Surgery and by the European Society of Thoracic Surgeons. Any of these procedures (that are mentioned below) may result in life-threatening intraoperative complications with disastrous consequences, unless a skilled thoracic surgeon may immediately convert them to thoracotomy and proceeds with a classic open operation. According on intraoperative findings, extensive surgical background is required to guarantee adequate surgical decision making.

Although such procedures have been conducted under local anesthesia since their inception, it seems preferable for both the patient and the surgeon to use general anesthesia. Anesthesia should be administered with double lumen intubation, or at least one should use bronchial blockers to achieve safe single lung ventilation—the only way to allow a thorough inspection of the pleural cavity is to take the lung down by stopping its ventilation. Administration of general anesthesia will also avoid loss of precious time should a serious complication occur.

IV. Video-Assisted Thoracic Surgery Management of Empyema

At first look, treatment modalities for empyema are confusing. When comparing different publications, it appears that patient populations and diagnostic criteria differ, that classifications have not been homogenized, and that guidelines for treatment depend on the type of unit (surgery, pulmonology, internal medicine, or intensive care) the patient has been admitted to. Finally, endpoints of such studies also fail to converge.

We should also clearly separate two very different entities: parapneumonic empyema and secondary empyema (Table 1). In the event of parapneumonic empyema, early surgical intervention is a valuable option. When facing secondary empyema, the individual prognosis depends on the precise cause; most often complex surgery is required in such patients. The most common cause of secondary empyema is postoperative, as happens following pneumonectomy, lobectomy, or esophageal resection. Empyema may also be associated with mediastinitis in patient with spontaneous or instrumental esophageal

Table 1 Causes of Empyema

Primary lung infection
  Parapneumonic
  Tuberculosis
Postoperative complications
  Lobectomy
  Pneumonectomy
  Esophageal resection
Diffusion of neighboring infection
  Mediastinitis (esophageal disruption)
  Descending necrotizing mediastinitis
  Spinal abscess
  Subphrenic abscess

---

disruption or with necrotizing descending mediastinitis originating from a dental or tonsillar abscess. These days is rare that a subphrenic abscess is not diagnosed prior to its spreading to the pleural cavity. Finally, spinal abscesses may also drain to the pleura.

A. Principles of Treatment for Empyema

From a theoretical point of view, cure of empyema requires evacuation and cleaning of the pleural space and complete re-expansion of the lung. Expansion of the lung will seal the pleural space, which eventually marks healing of empyema. In modern medicine, this double goal should be reached as quickly as possible in order to reduce duration of treatment and hospital stay and duration of physical disability. The slight increase in the cost of treatment because of using modern tools should be counterbalanced favorably by the reduction of the global cost.

The process of parapneumonic empyema is well documented (7). The first stage is the exudative phase, when plasma with high protein content escapes towards a free pleural space. This stage is usually very short—no longer than 48 hours. The second stage is the fibrinopurulent stage, in which fibrin deposits on the visceral pleura become thicker, septa develop between the parietal and visceral pleurae, and loculations appear. The duration of this stage is about 14 days. The third stage is the organizing phase. The pleural peel is well defined, and ingrowth of fibroblasts transforms the initially soft, jelly-like material into a firm envelope. We now observe progressive encasement of the lung, inhibiting spontaneous re-expansion.

B. Stage 1 Empyema: Minimally Invasive Treatment Not Required

Patients with stage 1 empyema can be successfully managed without the use of minimally invasive surgical techniques. Simple thoracocentesis or, even better, tube thoracostomy may evacuate the pleural effusion and hence re-expand the lung (8). Antibiotics and physiotherapy will definitely cure the patient. Unfortunately, patients are seldom caught at this stage.

C. Stage 3 Empyema: Minimally Invasive Treatment No Longer Possible?

In patients with stage 3 empyema, external drainage cannot succeed because spontaneous re-expansion of the lung is no longer possible; in such patients, a formal decortication needs to be performed to free the surface of the lung. Most surgeons will advocate an open approach to guarantee a safe procedure (9–11). Such aggressive surgery ensures rapid relief from sepsis at a low mortality even in very ill patients: (9) despite high sepsis or low-performance status, mortality was limited to 3.9%.

However, some very skilled surgeons have reported successful decortication using video-assisted thoracic surgery (VATS). One of the teams promoting its use is the group from Krasnodar, Russia (12). Similarly, Chan and coworkers recently published their experience over a five-year period (13). VATS decortication was successfully used in 41 patients—no patients required conversion to thoracotomy; exclusive use of VATS gave less pain and greater patient acceptance. The authors concluded that VATS allows equally effective decortication for empyema as thoracotomy, in experienced hands.

D. Stage 2 Empyema: Minimally Invasive Treatment Optional

In patients with fibrilopurulent empyema, there are four options:

1. Repeated thoracocentesis
2. External drainage
3. Intrapleural fibrinolysis
4. Minimally invasive debridement

Each of these options requires backup with antibiotic treatment and aggressive chest physiotherapy. It is now well accepted that repeated thoracocentesis has a high failure rate and that early placement of a chest tube may be beneficial. The chest tube offers the possibility to proceed with intrapleural fibrinolysis if required. Most authors also agree that biochemistry is of limited use to define treatment and that computed tomography (CT) scan offers the optimal information needed to choose the suitable option (8,14,15).

Classic treatment was made with external drainage, followed by daily pleural lavages through the chest tube for two to three weeks. With modern health care economics and social evolution, quicker treatment options must be promoted. Fibrinolytic therapy has been used since the 1960s to accelerate detersion of fibrinous material, and its benefit has been stressed by recent scientific studies (16,17). Diacon et al. reported a primary success rate of 82%, with a mean duration of treatment of 4.2 days (16). With a slightly longer treatment time of seven days, Misthos et al. were able to increase the primary success rate to 88% (17). However, in a recent review, Bouros and coworkers (18) advocated the use of intrapleural fibrinolytic therapy for patients who fail chest tube drainage or who require a period of medical stabilization before surgery is performed.

Some authors question the precise mechanism of such treatments: Is success due to effective fibrinolysis, or does increase of exudate by stimulation of the pleura help to wash out the pleural deposits (19,20)?

With the explosive development of videothoracoscopic surgery, minimally invasive debridement of empyema has been advanced. It is of note that the approach is not new, because early pleural debridement with thoracotomy was recommended during the 1980s. At that time, such an approach was not easily accepted by pulmonologists or by patients

(21,22). Weissberg and Refaely used classic "optical" thoracoscopy for many years, which has been replaced by video equipment (23).

Angelillo Mackinlay reported the first study showing favorable results with VATS. They reported a 100% success rate, with a median duration of treatment of 4.3 days (24). These optimistic data were recently confirmed by Solaini et al., who reported a primary success rate of 91.8% and median duration of hospital stay of 7.1 days (25).

Further comparison of treatments requires controlled trials. To date, Medline research identified a single randomized study comparing fibrinolysis to VATS debridement (26), included in a Cochrane Systematic Review (27). Unfortunately, it was a relatively low cohort of patients. Nevertheless, the results strongly support early operative management. Chest tube time was 5.8 days in the surgical group and 9.8 days in the streptokinase group; total hospital stay was 8.7 days in the surgical group and 12.8 days in the strep-tokinase group. Primary success rate was 91% after surgical debridement and 44% after fibrinolysis. Total estimated cost was $16,642 in surgical patients and $24,052 in medical patients. These data suggest that early operative management may considerably reduce the duration of treatment and favor an earlier return to occupational habits. Another advantage of surgery is that the stage of empyema may be assessed adequately and that conversion to classic decortication is feasible at once, if required.

Chest physicians' opinions about these different treatment options were elicited by questionnaire at an interactive symposium of the American College of Chest Physicians (Table 2). For example, more than two-thirds physicians were in favor of immediate surgery for multiloculated empyema (28).

E. Tuberculous Empyema

At an early stage, before encasement of the lung, tuberculous empyema may be determined by simple pleural biopsy, and its treatment based on drainage and specific antituberculous therapy is most often effective. The problem is different when the diagnosis is made at the stage of pulmonary encasement. Antibiotic therapy may well halt the infectious process, but re-expansion of the lung requires formal decortication. This is usually performed by a conventional thoracotomy approach. However, Porkhanov and colleagues have used a technique of video-assisted decortication where the pleural pocket is entered and the visceral peel is dissected off the surface of the lung from the pleural reflexions toward the

Table 2 Physician Opinions of Optimal Treatment of Multiloculated Empyema

Type of treatment	% Of physicians in favor of treatment	Total % in favor of treatment
Medical treatment		
Bedside chest tube	8	ns
Multiple CT-guided catheters	7	ns
Chest tube + fibrinolysis	14	29
Surgical treatment		
Thoracotomy + chest tubes	22	ns
Formal decortication	49	71

ns: not stated.
Source: Adapted from Ref. 28.

center (12). Such operations require great experience. It is quite understandable that in countries with a high prevalence of pleural tuberculosis and little money allotted to health care, a reduction in hospital stay is sought. This applies especially to the countries of the former Soviet Union. In addition, Yim et al. (29) have also proposed VATS for treatment of pulmonary tuberculosis—8 decortications, 17 wedge lung resections, 8 drainages of empyema, and 9 lobectomies in their cohort of 62 patients—concluding that it is an effective therapeutic modality in selected patients.

F. Postpneumonectomy Empyema: A Potential Indication for VATS?

Empyema is observed as a complication of pneumonectomy, with a reported prevalence varying from 2% to 10% in most series; risk factors for empyema are pneumonectomy for benign disease, completion pneumonectomy, intraoperative spillage from infected parenchymal cavities, and postoperative hemothorax (30,31). Classic management has consisted of either tube thoracostomy with repeated lavage or open window thoracostomy with iterative gauze packing.

Recent publications underline the contribution of VATS in the management of this complication (32–34). Thoracoscopy allows for complete debridement and removal of fibrinous deposits and septations, and is generally followed by pleural irrigation for several days until pleural fluid cultures become sterile. Hollaus et al. reported successful management without long-term recurrence in patients followed for 204 to 1163 days (32). Bagan et al. advocated the interest of combining antibiotic irrigation and VATS debridement (34).

V. Vats Management for Spontaneous Pneumothorax

Recurrent spontaneous pneumothorax is a disabling disorder, which may present either in young and otherwise healthy patients (primary pneumothorax) or as a complication of an underlying lung disease (secondary pneumothorax). Minimally invasive management has two advantages: earlier return to occupational habits for younger patients and less physiological harm due to less-operative trauma in older ones. It is possible to distinguish two different philosophies of approach: the medical approach, based on chemical pleurodesis, which may be undertaken by blinded instillation or thoracoscopy (35,36); and the minimally invasive surgical approach, which merely reproduce the classic surgical techniques formerly performed by open surgery.

A. Indications

Indication of chemical pleurodesis or surgical management should refer to the potential risk of recurrence. Recurrence rates after chest tube drainage of a first episode range from 10% to 21%; recurrence after a second episode is estimated close to 50% and may reach 80% following a third episode (37,38). Therefore, "classic" indications are defined as follows:

- Second ipsilateral recurrence
- First contralateral recurrence
- Bilateral simultaneous pneumothorax
- Persisting pneumothorax (air leaks beyond day 7 of tube drainage)
- Spontaneous hemopneumothorax
- At-risk professions (pilots, scuba divers, etc.)

B. Classic Surgical Treatment

The principles of surgical management for primary spontaneous pneumothorax include (1) treatment of the apex and (2) pleurodesis. Treatment of the apex means resection of visible blebs, suture of perforations, and even blind apical resection when no obvious lesion has been identified. Pleurodesis may be performed either by pleural abrasion or by parietal pleurectomy (39,40). Pleural abrasion theoretically preserves the extrapleural space, which should be helpful in the hypothesis of a subsequent ipsilateral thoracotomy. Most authors cited a chemical abrasion of the visceral pleura by iodine or silver nitrate (41,42). These operations performed through a classic or muscle-sparing thoracotomy provided excellent results, with less than 1% recurrence (Table 3) (42–44). Pleurectomy has been credited with a slight advantage over abrasion: recurrence rate was 0.4% following pleurectomy ($n = 752$) and 2.3% after abrasion ($n = 301$) (44). Although the primum movens of spontaneous pneumothorax is a lung disorder, pleurodesis appears to be mandatory; Körner and colleagues have performed apical wedge resections without pleurodesis through thoracotomy, resulting in a recurrence rate of 5% (45). Incidence of postoperative complications has been close to 15% (Table 3), with most complications related to the patients' status (e.g., COPD) rather than to the thoracotomy itself. When separating primary and secondary pneumothorax, it appeared that significantly more complications occurred in patients with underlying lung disease—the respective rates were 26.3% for secondary pneumothorax versus 7.2% for primary pneumothorax ($p < 0.01$) (42). The main complications were hemothorax and prolonged air leaks. Postoperative hemothorax is seen more particularly following pleurectomy and occurred in 0% to 4% of cases. Total pleurectomy led to an increased complication rate when compared to apical pleurectomy (44). Prolonged air leaks have been observed in 5% to 10% of patients and were more frequent in patients with COPD (41).

Most classic series reported by European centers relate a prolonged postoperative hospital stay close to 14 days, which may be due to "cultural" reasons—chest tubes were left in place for four to six days as a rule, and both patients and doctors believed that thoracotomy required a hospitalization of at least two weeks for adequate recovery. Nonetheless, hospital stay was prolonged by four days in patients with secondary pneumothorax (42).

We should also mention a classic approach that can be considered as the precursor of minimally invasive surgery: the transaxillary minithoracotomy was popularized by Becker and Munro in 1976 (46). The operation is made through an incision placed just below the axillary hairline and extended over 5 to 6 cm at the most; the chest is entered through the third intercostal space. Apical pleurectomy or abrasion is performed, and the apexes of the upper and lower lobe are carefully inspected. Blebs or bullae can be drawn

Table 3 Outcome Following Open Surgery for Spontaneous Pneumothorax

N	Pleurodesis	Complications (%)	Recurrence (%)	Follow-up (mo)	References
400	Abrasion	15	0.25	ns	(41)
107	Abrasion	14	0	27	(42)
278	Pleurectomy	6.5	1	84	(43)
233	Pleurectomy	17	0.4	56	(44)
120	None	ns	5	ns	(45)

ns: not stated.

to the level of the skin and stapled outside the chest. A single tube is left for 24 hours. In 1980, Deslauriers and colleagues published their experience with 362 consecutive patients (47). Four patients required reoperation for bleeding ($n = 3$) or air leak ($n = 1$), and a further 30 experienced minor complications (9.4%). Mean hospital stay was six days. Only 2 (0.4%) patients were presented with recurrent pneumothorax.

C. Chemical Pleurodesis

Chemical pleurodesis has been promoted by chest physicians comfortable with thoracoscopy, thus prolonging the traditions of physiology. The basic principle is to create a "chemical pleuritis," scarring from which will cause dense adhesions. The most popular agents, silver nitrate, tetracycline, minocycline, and talc share the substantial advantage of low cost. Although a recent publication has shown rather encouraging results (48), silver nitrate has lost favor over the years because its application is particularly painful and induces a major exudative reaction (35). Injectable tetracycline is no longer commercially available; besides, results with it were not satisfactory, since the recurrence rate was estimated at 16% in a series of 390 consecutive patients (49). Additional minocycline pleurodesis seems to have better results—less than 2% recurrence at a mean follow-up of 29 months (50). However, talc poudrage has the lowest recurrence rate of all chemical agents (2). In a comparative trial including 96 patients, recurrence rate was 36% after simple drainage, 13% following tetracycline pleurodesis, and 8% after talc poudrage (51). The reported failure rates after talc poudrage range from 3% to 15% (36,52–54) (Table 4). Half of the failures are immediate failures, prompting repeated thoracoscopy or subsequent thoracotomy (36). Concerns about talc poudrage also include asbestos contamination and restrictive changes of lung function. Fear of asbestos contamination can be excluded; no single case of mesothelioma occurred in a cohort of 210 patients followed for 14 to 40 years (55). Further, the threat of restrictive respiratory impairment is equally unfounded: in a series of 50 patients evaluated five years after videothoracoscopic talc poudrage, lung function was not impaired (56); spirometry showed normal values in 42 patients reviewed by Guérin et al. (36).

However, most surgeons favor pleural abrasion or pleurectomy because granuloma formation is considered excessive and might offer a challenging barrier in the event of a subsequent ipsilateral thoracotomy. In contrast, patchy distribution of talc will lead to incomplete pleurodesis and require a subsequent thoracotomy to complete pleurodesis in technically critical conditions. The more recently developed fibrin glue is not an option because the recurrence rate of 25% is unacceptable (57). In addition, this type of material has a relatively high cost and entails biological risks.

Table 4 Success Rates with Talc Poudrage for Spontaneous Pneumothorax

No. of patients	Success rate (%)	References
109	87	(36)
200	92.7	(52)
356	88	(53)
861	>97	(54)

In conclusion, results of chemical pleurodesis are not satisfactory; therefore, talc poudrage should be restricted to otherwise inoperable patients with secondary pneumothorax.

D. Global Results with VATS

As expected, the use of a modern approach to the pleural cavity has not yet ended the debate on pleurodesis. Most authors have merely transferred their usual technique to minimally invasive procedures, and the majority seems to favor abrasion (58–60). As previously recommended, isolated resection of blebs without pleurodesis is seldom performed (61). Other publications show that technique has evolved with growing experience; Inderbitzi and colleagues performed isolated ligation or wedge excision without pleurodesis for half of their patients and subsequently added apical pleurectomy to the procedure (37). We will discuss the results with reference to open surgery, in particular for postoperative complications and quality of long-term prevention of recurrence.

Complications

Complication rates are quite similar to those for open thoracotomy (62,63). In a decision analysis study by Falcoz and colleagues, the total complication rate was 10% (63): 7.5% were considered as imperfect results (minor air leak, pleural effusion, incomplete re-expansion, short-term ipsilateral recurrent pneumothorax), whereas 2.5% were identified as major complications (hemothorax, pleural infection, prolonged air leak, long-term ipsilateral recurrent pneumothorax). In addition, when considering the cause of pneumothorax, the complication rate was 6.75% for primary pneumothorax versus 27.7% for secondary pneumothorax (59). The most frequent complication is prolonged air leak (>5 days), observed in approximately 8% of patients (37,60,64). Initial failure of pleurodesis and hemothorax requires reoperation; the incidence of reoperation has been close to 5% (58).

Recurrence After Surgery

Most series suggest that at medium term (less than three years of follow-up), the recurrence rate ranges from 5% to 10% (Table 5). In addition, "failure during hospitalization treated by thoracotomy" (62) should be considered as an early recurrence. Recurrences are certainly

Table 5 Recurrence Rates Following VATS for Spontaneous Pneumothorax

No. of patients	Follow-up (mo)	% Recurrence	% Lost for follow-up	References
79	19.6	8.3	6.3	(37)
163	24.5	3.6[a]	8.5	(58)
100	30	3	ns	(59)
113	13.1	4.1	10	(60)
100	17	4	ns	(64)
109	53.2	4.6	0	(65)
99	29	4.8	0	(66)
94	48	3.1	0	(67)

ns: not stated.
[a]3.6% long-term recurrence, but 4 early failures requiring reoperation by thoracotomy, which equals a total of 6% of failures.

increased when compared to thoracotomy: in a comparison study, recurrence rate was significantly different after thoracotomy than after VATS (0.4% vs. 6%, respectively) (62). A multicenter study by Naunheim and colleagues (60) reported a heterogeneous series of 113 patients, since pleurodesis differed: abrasion, 45%; sclerotic agents, 24%; laser, 13%; pleurectomy, 10%; and none, 10%. The overall recurrence rate was 4.1%, and actuarial freedom of recurrence was estimated at 95% at 6 months. Similarly, Bertrand and colleagues (58) reported a freedom of recurrence of 95% at 42 months in a review of 163 patients. In the latter series, three patients had a complete recurrence requiring a second operation, and three had partial recurrence managed conservatively, which accounts for a recurrence rate of 3.6%.

However, four patients were reoperated via thoracotomy for immediate failure during the initial postoperative hospital stay; when including these patients, the total rate of recurrence was 6%. A national survey in the United States reported a 7% failure rate in 1993 (68). Be that as it may, no definitive conclusion as to recurrence rates can be drawn without a controlled trial, or a systematic review (see section, controlled studies). Also, published series probably underestimate the real recurrence rate: follow-up is short and 8.5% to 10% of patients are lost to follow-up (58,60). This proportion of patients lost to follow-up seems far too high for a benign disease and short-term surveillance; it is likely that patients with postoperative recurrence choose a different surgeon, as they would for failed hernia repair or recurring varicose veins.

Recurrence depends on surgical technique; compared to open surgery, it is the lowest when both apical resection and pleurodesis have been performed. The importance of apical stapling has been particularly stressed by Naunheim and colleagues (60). In a univariate analysis, two factors predicted recurrence. When no bleb had been identified, the recurrence rate was 27.3% versus 0% and 2.7% when 1 or multiple blebs were seen. Apical stapling reduced recurrence rate to 1.8% versus 23% when no excision was made (60). Mouroux and colleagues (59) confirmed these data in a series of 100 consecutive patients. Overall recurrence rate was 3%; 2 out of 10 patients without apical stapling recurred (20%) versus 1 out of 87 in whom an apical lesion had been wedged (1.5%).

The importance of pleurodesis is nicely demonstrated by Inderbitzi and colleagues (37), who observed a total of 6 recurrences in 72 patients (8.3%). The results varied considerably, and appeared that combined resection of blebs and pleurodesis is the safest treatment (Table 6). In contrast, isolated ligation of bullae had a failure rate of 19.2% when including prolonged air leaks; therefore, the results did not differ from those for simple chest tube drainage. Chemical pleurodesis instead of abrasion or pleurectomy is also less successful: combination of thoracoscopic bullectomy and tetracycline pleurodesis resulted in an early failure rate of 9% (69).

Table 6 Recurrence with Respect to Operative Technique

Technique	Recurrence rate	% Recurrence
Isolated ligation of bulla	3/26	11.5
Isolated wedge resection	1/14	7.1
Isolated pleurectomy	1/16	6.3
Pleurectomy + wedge	1/18	5.6

Source: Adapted from Ref. 37.

Causes of Recurrence

It is not likely that learning curve alone can explain the less than optimal results of VATS. Bertrand and colleagues (58) failed to show any difference between two subsequent time periods.

Why should there be less success when the technique allows for improved visibility in comparison to a minithoracotomy? Presumably, fewer blebs are recognized and treated during VATS (58). Open surgery is usually performed with single-lumen intubation, while VATS requires double-lumen intubation and one lung ventilation. Single-lung ventilation will deflate blebs as well as the lung, so that blebs may be missed despite careful inspection of the apex. Remaining blebs or bullae are commonly identified during reoperation after failed VATS. A second reason might be a certain disinclination to use abrasion. With magnification, the perception of hemorrhage is exaggerated and a less than optimal abrasion may be performed. Finally, the area between the trocars remains out of view and may not be abraded adequately.

The lower degree of tissue trauma and the less-intense biological reaction observed with VATS might result in less-efficient pleurodesis: release of inflammatory and vasoactive mediators (C-reactive protein, prostacyclin, and thromboxane A_2) was significantly lower in VATS patients as compared to a similar sample of thoracotomy patients (70).

E. Potential Advantages of VATS

Improved Intraoperative Visibility

From a theoretical point of view, thoracoscopy offers a complete panoramic view of the pleural cavity and underlying lung, which cannot be achieved by a small-sized thoracotomy. This improved visualization is certainly a major advantage to the teaching surgeon, who can easily follow his trainee at each step of the operation.

Catamenial pneumothorax is a situation in which VATS should be advantageous. This variant is related either to pleural endometriosis or to diaphragmatic perforations. In the latter case, permanent cure is achieved after adequate repair of the diaphragm. VATS certainly offers an improved view of the diaphragm in comparison to a minithoracotomy (71).

Duration of Postoperative Hospital Stay and Disability

Although there have not been many randomized studies, we may anticipate that VATS allows a reduction in hospital stay of about four days (Table 7). However, this reduction in hospital stay is not solely explained by the new technology. In Western Europe, economic considerations and administrative pressure have had a major impact on discharge policy (72,73). Psychologically, VATS is considered as "less than surgery" by both patients and physicians, leading to earlier discharge. In former series, even axillary thoracotomy was often regarded as a reason for routine hospitalization for at least 10 days, although patients might have been fit for an earlier discharge. Further, hospital stay obviously depends on drainage time; minimally invasive techniques certainly have led to revised policies and promotion of early removal of chest tubes (74,75).

Postoperative Pain

VATS avoids large trans-sections of chest wall muscles and the particularly painful spreading of ribs. Reduced surgical trauma should result in a considerable reduction of

Table 7 Comparative Duration of Postoperative Hospital Stay

| Country | Hospital length of stay (days) | | References |
	VATS	Thoracotomy	
France	6.9	10.3	(58)
France	8	ns	(59)
France	9.5	14	(62)
France	7	11.5	(72)
France	5.4	10.5	(63)
Switzerland	4.2	ns	(37)
United States	4.3	ns	(60)
Hong Kong	4	ns	(64)
Italy	3.8	ns	(73)

ns: not stated.

postoperative pain. Subjectively, most patients having undergone bilateral operations state that VATS is less painful. Dumont and colleagues demonstrated a significantly lower level of pain after VATS when compared to a control group operated through lateral thoracotomy: 42% of VATS patients required level 3 analgesics versus 95% in the case of formal thoracotomy (62). With a similar methodology, Hazelrigg and colleagues compared 20 and 26 patients gathered in a multicenter trial; 7.7% of VATS patients and 70% of thoracotomy patients required parenteral narcotics after 48 hours (76).

Another distressing problem in thoracic surgery is persistent pain for long term. Such pain is usually explained by intercostal nerve injury and intraoperative tension on the costo-vertebral joints due to the use of rib spreaders. Bertrand and colleagues estimated that 63% of patients experienced residual chest pain following VATS for pneumothorax, which was considered minimal in 58%, moderate in 38%, and severe in 4%. Comparatively, 61% had persistent pain following lateral thoracotomy for pneumothorax, considered minimal in 65%, moderate in 33%, and severe in 2% (58). Mouroux reported a similar incidence of severe chest pain of 3% (59). Passlick and colleagues (77) reported that with a mean follow-up of 59 months, 31.7% of patients complained of chronic pain and 3.3% required daily pain medications. The incidence of chronic pain was increased following pleurectomy (47.1%) when compared to abrasion (25.6%). In addition, Sihoe and coworkers reported that with a median follow-up of 19 months, 52.9% of patients experienced paresthesia as a postoperative complication distinct from their wound pain (78). These studies show that chronic pain has not been reduced by VATS. In fact, use of relatively large instruments in narrow intercostal spaces causes significant crushing injury to the intercostal nerves. Because of this, Jutley and colleagues (79) along with Salati and coworkers (73) promoted the use of uniportal VATS technique, arguing that postoperative pain and paresthesia incidence was lower than with "standard" three-port VATS.

Return to Activity

Return to occupational activity has been evaluated in two series with reference to historic control groups. A first series demonstrated a return to activity within a mean of 42 days after VATS and 74 days after thoracotomy (58). In a second series comparing two groups of 16 patients, return to work was possible 1 month after VATS and 2.6 months after thoracotomy ($p < 0.002$); leisure activities were resumed at 2 months after VATS and 4 months after thoracotomy ($p < 0.0005$) (72). One should not neglect a changing philosophy towards postoperative recovery between these two comparisons. A prospective randomized study, published in 2004, concluded that there were no differences in the patients tacking up their normal activities again when comparing axillary thoracotomy and VATS: 33.9 ± 12.8 days for VATS versus 34.4 ± 14.4 days for axillary thoracotomy (80). Finally, when comparing VATS and minithoracotomy postoperative quality-of-life evolution, significant differences were seen in favor of VATS in the framework of thoracic pain evaluation at 6 months (81).

Cost-efficiency

Cost of treatment must be taken into account because pneumothorax is a rather common problem. At first look, VATS might be less expensive owing to a shorter hospital stay. Falcoz and coworkers showed a reduction of four days of length of stay when comparing VATS to a conservative approach, corresponding to a reduction in cost of €3189 per patient (63). In addition, Dumont and colleagues demonstrated that hospital stay was reduced by 4.5 days when comparing VATS patients to a control group (62). The reduction in cost was estimated at $2300, whereas the increase in cost due to stapling material was estimated at $245. The shorter hospital stay should counterbalance the enhanced cost for disposable surgical materials. However, the conclusions of these two studies are biased, because shortening of hospital stay is not the result only of a changing operative approach. Hence, accurate cost analysis should not focus only on hospital stay, which might be the same for VATS and for open surgery with a limited thoracotomy (46,47). An objective cost analysis should also take into account hidden costs (prolonged OR time, video equipment, and disposable materials), as well as the increased cost of double-lumen catheter intubation, which is mandatory for VATS. Besides, many colleagues perform routine CT scans preoperatively to decrease the risk of missing blebs (82). Cost of recurrence should also be considered; also, the psychological impact of recurrence in operated patients is inestimable (83).

Van Schil presented, in 2003, a critical review of cost analysis of VATS versus thoracotomy (84). Only three studies specifically addressed cost analysis in the framework of pneumothorax. In a comparative retrospective study of 60 patients, Crisci and Coloni used a variety of surgical procedures ranging from bullectomy and pleurectomy to abrasion only (85). Compared with limited thoracotomy, operating time, length of hospitalization, and day of chest tube removal were shorter in the VATS group. The total cost of VATS was 22.7% lower than in the thoracotomy group. However, in the VATS group the cost of the video equipment was not calculated. Moreover, a secondary pneumothorax was present in 40% of patients in the thoracotomy group compared with 26.7% in the VATS group. Bullectomy and pleurectomy were more often performed in the thoracotomy group suggesting more extensive bullous disease, which could already induce a longer hospital stay. In a prospective but nonrandomized study of 66 patients with a persisting or recurrent pneumothorax, 36 had a VATS procedure and 30 were operated on by way of a transaxillary minithoracotomy (86). The choice of the specific procedure was made by the patients themselves. No advantage of VATS was shown in operating time, analgesic consumption, duration of chest-tube drainage, or postoperative recurrences. Due to the use of disposable instruments, the cost was higher for a VATS approach. In a retrospective case series, cost was analyzed in 0 patients with spontaneous pneumothorax: 22 treated by VATS and 28 by a limited axillary thoracotomy (87). There was no difference in operating time, but the length of stay was shorter in the VATS group. However, the overall cost of VATS was not different than that of a limited thoracotomy. This study also looked at socioeconomic cost, which was lower in the VATS group since the latter missed significantly less time from work postoperatively. This study concluded that VATS was a cost-effective and better-tolerated procedure for the treatment of spontaneous pneumothorax compared with an open technique.

Knowing that some authors recommend VATS at the first episode (88,89), we need to further evaluate the increased cost due to expanded indications. Morimoto and colleagues concluded that even if thoracoscopic surgery at the first episode significantly increased costs, it remains acceptable from a cost-effectiveness perspective (89).

F. Controlled Studies

Nonrandomized reports emanating from single institution provide weak evidence for comparisons of effectiveness. Even randomized studies are frequently underpowered to detect meaningful difference, and surrogates are often used. The need for a systematic review and meta-analysis of the evidence from the literature, concerning this relatively frequent disease, is real. Effectively, without this evidence it is not possible to make recommendations for best practice or to provide guidance for its wider application.

To date, two systematic reviews have been published. Sedrakayan and colleagues made a systematic review of randomized trials only (90). They sought to determine if VATS was associated with better clinical outcomes than that of thoracotomy for three common thoracic surgery procedures, among which there was surgery for pneumothorax. Four trials compared VATS with conventional method in 179 patients. In the trials that reported this information, the average age of participant was 34 years and 27% were women. The authors concluded that VATS was associated with better clinical outcome (shorter length of hospital stay, less pain or use of pain medication) and seemed to have a complication profile (no significant difference in early outcome, failure or recurrence) comparable to that of open surgery with limited incisions for the treatment of pneumothorax. Obviously, no definitive conclusion can be drawn from this study, even if methodologically irreproachable. Indeed, evidence supporting similar recurrence rates between VATS and open surgery for the treatment of recurrent pneumothorax is questionable. Hence, Barker and coworkers did a systematic review of randomized and nonrandomized trials to compare the recurrence rates between the two forms of surgical access (91). A total of 29 studies (4 randomized and 25 nonrandomized) were eligible for inclusion. In studies that did the same pleurodesis through two different forms of access, the relative risk of recurrence in patients undergoing VATS compared with open surgery was similar between randomized and nonrandomized studies, yielding an overall relative risk of 4.731. Whatever be the choice of the type of comparison included in the model (all comparative studies, high-quality studies, simulation), the relative risk of recurrence remained stable. The authors concluded that both randomized and nonrandomized trials are consistent in recurrence of pneumothoraces and show a four-fold increase when a similar pleurodesis procedure is done with a VATS approach compared with an open approach.

G. Should VATS Be Recommended for an Initial Episode of Pneumothorax?

The advent of VATS has certainly promoted an earlier and more aggressive approach. Obviously, most colleagues will perform an operation at the first recurrence based on the fact that spontaneous recurrence rate is certainly in excess of 50%. Besides, advantages of such a "clinical" intuitive attitude have been demonstrated in a recent study (63). The definition of persistent pneumothorax has also been remastered, knowing that an air leak persisting beyond 48 hours is unlikely to seal.

However, we consider excessive the recommendation to operate as soon as the first episode (88,92). Some colleagues argue that immediate thoracoscopy under local anesthesia—awake VATS surgery—will select the patients at risk for recurrence when disclosing apical blebs. But there is no proven correlation between thoracoscopic findings and patterns of recurrence (51). Outside of large teaching hospitals, such a strategy is further limited by the lack of availability of experienced and skilled physicians (53). Pompeo and coworkers highlight the fact that the high level of recurrence rate (20–60%) observed after conservative management compares unfavorably with that reported after immediate surgery; cost analysis showed a reduction in overall hospital charges in the awake arm, a finding—according to the authors—that supports immediate surgical treatment for these patients (92). Schramel and colleagues concluded that VATS should be performed for first episodes by comparing total cost of conservative management and thoracoscopic management over two time periods (88). However, this study is biased because surgical patients of the control group underwent formal thoracotomy; when total hospitalization is taken into account, including waiting time before VATS, cost-efficiency does not result.

H. Management of Recurrent Pneumothorax Following VATS Treatment

This situation is encountered in 5% to 10% of patients having undergone VATS pleurodesis, and it is therefore surprising that only two studies have been dedicated to this question (93,94). Most surgeons would assume that if VATS has failed at the first attempt, it would be insufficient at the second attempt as well, and they would recommend an open approach. Also, almost 50% of patients show bullae during reoperation that obviously were not identified during VATS.

Ingolfsson and coworkers performed 15 redo operations for failure after VATS treatment for spontaneous pneumothorax. Seven of the reoperations were thoracotomies and eight were VATS, all successful at follow-up. Pleurodesis was mainly achieved with partial pleurectomy, in an average of 17 months after the primary operation (93). The authors identified three risk factors of having redo surgery: younger patients, patients operated on for recurrent or secondary pneumothorax with emphysema, and patients that were not operated on with a wedge resection during the primary surgical procedure. Cardillo and colleagues performed 19 reoperations with VATS techniques. The conversion rate was 5.2% (1 patient). Pleurodesis was achieved with talc poudrage, and apical resection was added in 10 patients because of bullae or leak. There has been no recurrence with a mean follow-up of 32 months (94). On the basis of these experiences, we conclude that an attempt at repeated VATS is justified, provided that the operating surgeon has sufficient experience.

VI. Conclusion

Minimally invasive surgery has become a major tool for the treatment of pleural diseases such as spontaneous pneumothorax and parapneumonic empyema. Shortened duration of recovery and excellent medium-term results justify an early and aggressive approach to empyema, which, like many diseases, profits from early diagnosis and treatment.

The final judgment regarding the use of VATS for spontaneous pneumothorax requires some deliberation. Chemical pleurodesis should be limited to otherwise inoperable patients. VATS pleurectomy or pleural abrasion probably allows for less postoperative pain and a shorter hospital stay when compared to an open approach; however, long-term prevention of recurrent pneumothorax remains less than optimal with VATS techniques. Economic considerations might reawaken the interest of the surgical community in transaxillary minithoracotomy.

References

1. Dumarest F. La pratique du Pneumothorax Thérapeutique. Paris, France: Masson Edit, 1945.
2. Walker-Renard PB, Vaughan ML, Sahn SA. Chemical pleurodesis for malignant pleural effusion. Ann Intern Med 1994; 120:56–64.
3. Wurnig PN, Hollaus PH, Ohtsuka T, et al. Thoracoscopic direct clipping of the thoracic duct for chylopericardium and chylothorax. Ann Thorac Surg 2000; 70:1662–1665.
4. Buchan KG, Hosseinpour AR, Ritchie AJ. Thoracoscopic thoracic duct ligation for traumatic chylothorax. Ann Thorac Surg 2001; 72:1366–1367.
5. Thomas P, Moutardier V, Ragni J, et al. Video-assisted repair of a ruptured right hemidiaphragm. Eur J Cardiothorac Surg 1994; 8:157–159.
6. Lang-Lazdunski L, Mouroux J, Pons F, et al. Role of videothoracoscopy in chest trauma. Ann Thorac Surg 1997; 63:327–331.
7. De Hoyos A, Sundaresan S. Thoracic empyema. Surg Clin N Am 2002; 82:643–671.
8. Sasse S, Nguyen TK, Mulligan M, et al. The effects of early chest tube placement on empyema resolution. Chest 1997; 111:1679–1683.
9. Molnar TF. Current surgical treatment of thoracic empyema in adults. Eur J Cardiothorac Surg 2007; 32:422–430.
10. Le Mense GP, Strange C, Sahn SA. Empyema thoracis. Therapeutic management and outcome. Chest 1995; 107:1532–1537.
11. Cassina PC, Hauser M, Hillejan L, et al. Video-assisted thoracoscopy in the treatment of pleural empyema: Stage based management and outcome. J Thorac Cardiovasc Surg 1999; 117:234–238.
12. Porkhanov VA, Bodnia VN, Kononenko VB, et al. Videoassisted thoracoscopy in treatment of pleural empyema. Khirurgia (Mosk) 1999; 11:40–43.
13. Chan DT, Sihoe AD, Chan S, et al. Surgical treatment for empyema thoracis: Is video-assisted thoracic surgery "better" than thoracotomy? Ann Thorac Surg 2007; 84:225–231.
14. Heffner JE, McDonald J, Barbieri C, et al. Management of parapneumonic effusions. An analysis of physicians practice patterns. Arch Surg 1995; 130:433–438.
15. Levinson GM, Pennington DW. Intrapleural fibrinolitics combined with image guided chest tube drainage for pleural infection. Mayo Clin Proc 2007; 82(4):407–413.
16. Diacon AH, Theron J, Schuurmans MM, et al. Intrapleural streptokinase for empyema and complicated parapneumonic effusions. Am J Respir Crit Care Med 2004; 170:49–53.
17. Misthos P, Sepsas E, Konstantinou M, et al. Early use of intraplaural fibrinolitics in the management of postpneumonic empyema. A prospective study. Eur J Cardiothorac Surg 2005; 28:599–603.

18. Bouros D, Tzouvelekis A, Antoniou KM, et al. Intrapleural fibrinolitic therapy for pleural infection. Pulm Pharmacol Ther 2007; 20:616–626.
19. Chin NK, Lim TK. Controlled trial of intrapleural streptokinase in the treatment of pleural empyema and complicated parapneumonic effusions. Chest 1997; 111:275–279.
20. Sahn SA. Diagnosis and management of parapneumonic effusions and empyema. Clin Infect Dis 2007; 45:1480–1486.
21. Van Way C, Narrod J, Hopeman A. The role of early limited thoracotomy in the treatment of empyema. J Thorac Cardiovasc Surg 1988; 96:436–439.
22. Hutter JA, Harari D, Braimbridge MV. The management of empyema thoracis by thoracoscopy and irrigation. Ann Thorac Surg 1985; 39:517–520.
23. Weissberg D, Refaely Y. Pleural empyema: 24-year experience. Ann Thorac Surg 1996; 62:1026–1029.
24. Angelillo Mackinlay TA, Lyons GA, Chimondeguy DJ, et al. VATS debridement versus thoracotomy in the treatment of loculated postpneumonia empyema. Ann Thorac Surg 1996; 61:1626–1630.
25. Solaini L, Prusciano F, Bagioni P. Video-assisted thoracic surgery in the treatment of pleural empyema. Surg Endosc 2007; 21:280–284.
26. Wait MA, Sharma S, Hohn J, et al. A randomized trial of empyema therapy. Chest 1997; 111:1548–1551.
27. Coote N, Kay E. Surgical versus non-surgical management of pleural empyema. Cochrane Database Syst Rev 2005; 4:Art No. CD001956.
28. Strange C, Sahn SA. The clinician's perspective on parapneumonic effusions and empyema. Chest 1993; 103:259–261.
29. Yim AP, Izzat MB, Lee TW. Thoracoscopic surgery for pulmonary tuberculosis. World J Surg 1999; 23(11):114–117.
30. Massard G, Lyons G, Wihlm JM, et al. Early and long-term results after completion pneumonectomy. Ann Thorac Surg 1995; 59:196–200.
31. Massard G, Dabbagh A, Wihlm JM, et al. Pneumonectomy for chronic infection is a high-risk procedure. Ann Thorac Surg 1996; 62:1033–1037.
32. Hollaus PH, Lax F, Wurnig PN, et al. Videothoracoscopic debridement of the postpneumonectomy space in empyema. Eur J Cardiothorac Surg 1999; 16:283–286.
33. Gossot D, Sterne JB, Galetta D, et al. Thoracoscopic management of postpneumonectomy empyema. Ann Thorac Surg 2004; 78:273–276.
34. Bagan P, Boissier F, Berna P, et al. Postpneumonectomy empyema treated with a combination of antibiotic irrigation followed by videothoracoscopic debridement. J Thorac Cardiovasc Surg 2006; 132:708–710.
35. Wied U, Halkier E, Hoeier-madsen K, et al. Tetracycline versus silver nitrate pleurodesis in spontaneous pneumothorax. J Thorac Cardiovasc Surg 1983; 86:591.
36. Guérin JC, Champel F, Biron E, et al. Talcage pleural par thoracoscopie dans le traitement du pneumothorax. Rev Mal Resp 1985; 2:25–29.
37. Inderbitzi RGC, Leiser A, Furrer M, et al. Three years experience in videoassisted thoracic surgery (VATS) for spontaneous pneumothorax. J Thorac Cardiovasc Surg 1994; 107: 1410–1415.
38. Cran IR, Rumball CA. Survey of spontaneous pneumothorax in the Royal Air Force. Thorax 1967; 22:462–465.
39. Gaensler EA. Parietal pleurectomy for recurrent spontaneous pneumothorax. Surg Gynecol Obstet 1956; 102:293–308.
40. Clagett OT. The management of spontaneous pneumothorax. J Thorac Cardiovasc Surg 1968; 55:761–762.
41. Dumont P, Nebia A, Roeslin N, et al. Traitement chirurgical du pneumothorax. Etude d'une série de 400 cas. Ann Chir Chir Thorac Cardio-vasc 1995; 49:235–240.

42. Thomas P, Le Mee F, Le Hors H, et al. Résultats du traitement chirurgical des pneumothorax persistants ou récidivants. Ann Chir Chir Thorac Cardio-vasc 1993; 47:136–140.

43. Thévenet F, Gamondès JP, Bodzongo D, et al. Pneumothorax spontané et rcidivant. Traitement chirurgical. A propos de 278 observations. Ann Chir Chir Thorac Cardio-vasc 1992; 46: 165–169.

44. Weeden D, Smith GH. Surgical experience in the management of spontaneous pneumothorax, 1972–82. Thorax 1983; 38:737–743.

45. Körner H, Andersen KS, Stangeland L, et al. Surgical treatment of spontaneous pneumothorax by wedge resection without pleurodesis or pleurectomy. Eur J Cardiothorac Surg 1996; 10: 656–659.

46. Becker RM, Munro DD. Transaxillary minithoracotomy: The optimal approach for certain pulmonary and mediastinal lesions. Ann Thorac Surg 1976; 22:254–259.

47. Deslauriers J, Beaulieu M, Després JP, et al. Transaxillary pleurectomy for treatment of spontaneous pneumothorax. Ann Thorac Surg 1980; 30:569–574.

48. Marcheix B, Brouchet L, Renaud C, et al. Videothoracoscopic silver nitrate pleurodesis for primary spontaneous pneumothorax: An alternative to pleurectomy and pleural abrasion? Eur J Cardiothorac Surg 2007; 31:1106–1109.

49. Olsen PS, Andersen HO. Long-term results after tetracycline pleurodesis in spontaneous pneumothorax. Ann Thorac Surg 1992; 53:1015–1017.

50. Chen JS, Hsu HH, Chen RJ, et al. Additional minocycline pleurodesis after thoracoscopic surgery for primary spontaneous pneumothorax. Am J Respir Crit Care Med 2006; 173: 548–554.

51. Almind M, Lange P, Viskum K. Spontaneous pneumothorax: Comparison of simple drainage, talc pleurodesis, and tetracycline pleurodesis. Thorax 1989; 44:623–627.

52. El Khawand C, Marchandise FX, Mayne A, et al. Pneumothorax spontané. Résultats du talcage sous thoracoscopie. Rev Mal Resp 1995; 12:275–281.

53. Van de Brekel JA, Duurkens VA, Vanderschueren RG. Pneumothorax. Results of thoracoscopy and pleurodesis with talc poudrage and thoracotomy. Chest 1993; 103:345–347.

54. Cardillo G, Carleo F, Giunti R, et al. Videothoracoscopic talc poudrage in primary spontaneous pneumothorax: A single institution experience in 861 cases. J Thorac Cardiovasc Surg 2006; 131:322–328.

55. Chappel AG, Johnson A, Charles J, et al. A survey of the long term effects of talc and kaolin pleurodesis. Br J Dis Chest 1979; 73:285–288.

56. Cardillo G, Carleo F, Carbone L, et al. Long-term lung function following videothoracoscopic talc poudrage for primary spontaneous recurrent pneumothorax. Eur J Cardiothorac Surg 2007; 31:802–807.

57. Guérin JC, Van Der Schueren RG. Traitement des pneumothorax récidivants par application de colle de fibrine sous endoscopie. Rev Mal Resp 1989; 6:443–445.

58. Bertrand PC, Regnard JF, Spaggiari L, et al. Immediate and long-term results after surgical treatment of primary spontaneous pneumothorax by VATS. Ann Thorac Surg 1996; 61: 1641–1645.

59. Mouroux J, Elkaïm D, Padovani B, et al. Video-assisted thoracoscopic treatment of spontaneous pneumothorax: Technique and results of one hundred cases. J Thorac Cardiovasc Surg 1996; 112:385–391.

60. Naunheim KS, Mack MJ, Hazelrigg SR, et al. Safety and efficacy of video-assisted thoracic surgical techniques for the treatment of spontaneous pneumothorax. J Thorac Cardiovasc Surg 1995; 109:1198–1204.

61. Nezu K, Kushibe K, Tojo T, et al. Thoracoscopic wedge resection of blebs under local anesthesia with a sedation for treatment of a spontaneous pneumothorax. Chest 1997; 111:230–235.

62. Dumont P, Diemont F, Massard G, et al. Does a thoracoscopic approach for surgical treatment of spontaneous pneumothorax represent progress? Eur J Cardiothorac Surg 1997; 11:27–31.

63. Falcoz PE, Binquet C, Clement F, et al. Management of the second episode of spontaneous pneumothorax: A decision analysis. Ann Thorac Surg 2003; 76:1843–1848.
64. Yim AP, Ho JK. One hundred consecutive cases of video-assisted thoracoscopic surgery for primary spontaneous pneumothorax. Surg Endosc 1995; 9:332–336.
65. Hatz RA, Kaps MF, Meimarakis G, et al. Long-term results after video-assisted thoracoscopic surgery for first-time and recurrent spontaneous pneumothorax. Ann Thorac Surg 2000; 70:253–257.
66. Passlick B, Born C, Haussinger K, et al. Efficiency of video-assisted thoracic surgery for primary and secondary spontaneous pneumothorax. Ann Thorac Surg 1998; 65:324–327.
67. Ayed AK, Chandrasekaran C, Sukumar M. Video-assisted thoracoscopic surgery for primary spontaneous pneumothorax: Clinicopathological correlation. Eur J Cardiothorac Surg 2006; 29:221–225.
68. Cole FH Jr, Cole FH, Khandekar A, et al. Videoassisted thoracic surgery: Primary treatment for spontaneous pneumothorax? Ann Thorac Surg 1995; 60:931–935.
69. Waterworth PD, Kallis P, Townsend ER, et al. Thoracoscopic bullectomy and tetracycline pleurodesis for the treatment of spontaneous pneumothorax. Respir Med 1995; 89:563–566.
70. Gebhard FT, Becher HP, Gerngross H, et al. Reduced inflammatory response in minimal invasive surgery of pneumothorax. Arch Surg 1996; 131:1079–1082.
71. Alifano M, Jablonski C, Falcoz PE et al. Catamenial and noncatamenial, endometriosis related and nonendometriosis related pneumothorax referred for surgery. Am J Respir Crit Care Med 2007; 176:1048–1053.
72. Bernard A, Bélichard C, Goudet P, et al. Pneumothorax spontané. Comparaison de la thoracoscopie et de la thoracotomie. Rev Mal Respir 1993; 10:433–436.
73. Salati M, Brunelli A, Xiume F, et al. Uniportal video-assisted thoracic surgery for primary spontaneous pneumothorax: Clinical and economic analysis in comparison to the traditional approach. Interact CardioVasc Thorac Surg 2008; 7:63–66.
74. Henry M, Arnold T, Harvey J. BTS guidelines for the management of spontaneous pneumothorax. Thorax 2003; 58(Suppl. II):ii39–ii52.
75. Kuester JR, Frese S, Stein RM, et al. Treatment of primary spontaneous pneumothorax in Switzerland: Results of a survey. Interact Cardiovasc Thorac Surg 2006; 5:139–144.
76. Hazelrigg SR, Landreneau RJ, Mack M, et al. Thoracoscopic stapled resection for spontaneous pneumothorax. J Thorax Cardiovasc Surg 1993; 105:389–393.
77. Passlick B, Born C, Sienel W, et al. Incidence of chronic pain after minimally invasive surgery for spontaneous pneumothorax. Eur J Cardiothorac Surg 2001; 19:355–359.
78. Sihoe AL, Au SW, Cheung ML, et al. Incidence of chest wall paresthesia after video-assisted thoracic surgery for primary spontaneous pneumothorax. Eur J Cardiothorac Surg 2004; 25:1054–1058.
79. Jutley RS, Khalil MW, Rocco G. Uniportal vs standard three-port VATS technique for spontaneous pneumothorax: Comparison of postoperative pain and residual paraesthesia. Eur J Cardiothorac Surg 2005; 28:43–46.
80. Freixinet JL, Canalis E, Julia G, et al. Axillary thoracotomy versus videothoracoscopy for the treatment of primary spontaneous pneumothorax. Ann Thorac Surg 2004; 78:417–420.
81. Balduyck B, Hendricks J, Lauwers P, et al. Quality of life evolution after surgery for primary or secondary spontaneous pneumothorax: A prospective study comparing different surgical techniques. Interact Cardiovasc Thorac Surg 2008; 7:45–49.
82. Warner BW, Bailey WW, Shipley RT. Value of computed tomography of the lung in the management of primary spontaneous pneumothorax. Am J Surg 1991; 162:39–42.
83. Nazari S. Psychological implications in the surgical treatment of pneumothorax. Ann Thorac Surg 1997; 63:1830.
84. Van Schil P. Cost analysis of video-assisted thoracic surgery versus thoracotomy: Critical review. Eur Resp J 2003; 22:735–738.

85. Crisci R, Coloni GF. Video-assisted thoracoscopic surgery versus thoracotomy for recurrent spontaneous pneumothorax. A comparison of results and costs. Eur J Cardiothorac Surg 1996; 10:556–560.
86. Kim KH, Kim HK, Han JY, et al. Transaxillary minithoracotomy versus video-assisted thoracic surgery for spontaneous pneumothorax. Ann Thorac Surg 1996; 61:1510–1512.
87. Hyland MJ, Ashrafi AS, Crepeau A, et al. Is video-assisted thoracoscopic surgery superior to limited axillary thoracotomy in the management of spontaneous pneumothorax? Can Respir J 2001; 8:339–343.
88. Schramel FM, Sutedja TG, Braber JC, et al. Costeffectiveness of video-assisted thoracoscopic surgery versus conservative treatment for first time or recurrent spontaneous pneumothorax. Eur Respir J 1996; 9:1821–1825.
89. Morimoto T, Shimbo T, Noguchi Y, et al. Effects of timing of thoracoscopic surgery for primary spontaneous pneumothorax on prognosis and costs. Am J Surg 2004; 187:767–774.
90. Sedrakayan A, Van der Meulen J, Lewsey J, et al. Video assisted thoracic surgery for treatment of pneumothorax and lung resections: Systematic review of randomized clinical trials. BMJ 2004; 329:1008–1011.
91. Barker A, Maratos EC, Edmonds L, et al. Recurrence rates of video-assisted thoracoscopic versus open surgery in the prevention of recurrent pneumothoraces: A systematic review of randomized and non-randomized trials. Lancet 2007; 370:329–335.
92. Pompeo E, Tacconi F, Mineo D, et al. The role of awake video-assisted thoracoscopic surgery in spontaneous pneumothorax. J Thorac Cardiovasc Surg 2007; 133:786–790.
93. Ingolfsson I, Gyllstedt E, Lillo-Gil R, et al. Reoperations are common following VATS for spontaneous pneumothorax: Study of risk factors. Interact CardioVasc Thorac Surg 2006; 5:602–607.
94. Cardillo G, Facciolo F, Regal M, et al. Recurrences following videothoracoscopic treatment of primary spontaneous pneumothorax: The role of redo-videothoracoscopy. Eur J Cardiothorac Surg 2001; 19:396–399.

11
Pleurodesis

FRANCISCO RODRIGUEZ-PANADERO
Unidad Médico-Quirúrgica de Enfermedades Respiratorias, Hospital Universitario
Virgen del Rocío, Sevilla, Spain

Pleurodesis is defined as the symphysis between the visceral and parietal pleural surfaces that prevents accumulation of either air or fluid in the pleural space. Its main indications are malignant pleural effusions (MPE) and pneumothorax, although some benign effusions may occasionally require this treatment also.

I. Pleurodesis in MPE

Most of the patients undergoing a pleurodesis procedure have a symptomatic MPE. When this condition is diagnosed, palliative therapy should be considered with special evaluation of the patient's symptoms, general health and functional status, and expected survival. The main indication for treatment in such cases is relief of dyspnea, which is dependent on both the volume of the effusion and the underlying condition of the lungs and pleura. Therapeutic thoracocentesis should be performed in virtually all dyspneic patients with MPE to determine its effect on breathlessness, and rate and degree of recurrence. This is especially important in patients who are present with a massive pleural effusion and contralateral mediastinal shift (Fig. 1), and those patients are also the obvious candidates for a pleurodesis procedure. Also, rapid recurrence of the effusion dictates the need for immediate treatment, while stability and absence of symptoms may warrant observation. If dyspnea is not relieved by thoracocentesis, other causes should be investigated such as lymphangitic carcinomatosis, atelectasis, thromboembolism, and tumor embolism.

If the effusion is small (less than one-third of the hemithorax) and cytology is positive, the best choice would be to apply chemotherapy if the primary is known and it is sensitive to that treatment (breast, ovary, small-cell lung cancer, lymphoma, etc.) and to observe the evolution of the pleural effusion. When cytology is negative and/or the primary is unknown, thoracoscopy would be recommended; because the diagnosis yield is high, large specimens can be taken under visual control for special studies (immunohistochemistry and others), and talc poudrage for pleurodesis can also be performed at the same time. According to our experience, pleurodesis would be required in about two-thirds of patients with malignant effusion sooner or later (1). In the presence of a large and recurrent effusion, the choice is clearly defined in favor of pleurodesis, preferably using talc. This should be done as early as possible (2) in order to prevent development of a trapped lung, which could provoke a failure in lung re-expansion and pleurodesis. When the effusion is relatively small (less than one-third of the hemithorax), one wonders if this particular patient is ever going to need any pleurodesis procedure. The answer would be

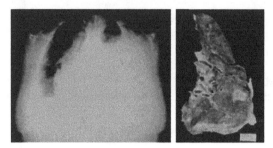

Figure 1   Contralateral mediastinal shift in a patient with lymphoma. Talc pleurodesis was successfully achieved, as shown in the autopsy specimen (*on the right*).

obvious if the effusion remains stable and is well tolerated, but in an undefined proportion of cases, it would progress to a larger effusion, with the subsequent deterioration of the patient's condition and advancement of the disease. This could lead to a trapped lung, thus making any pleurodesis attempt risky and unlikely to be successful. According to a prospective study from our group, serial determinations of pH and D-dimer in pleural fluid would be of help in predicting which patients are more likely to need pleurodesis (3): patients requiring pleurodesis over the follow-up period showed a declining pH on serial determinations, and the pleural fluid D-dimer median levels were growing higher in the pleurodesis group than in those who never required a pleurodesis procedure.

Before attempting pleurodesis, the ability for the lung to re-expand should be demonstrated. Failure of complete lung expansion occurs when main-stem bronchial occlusion by tumor or trapped lung due to extensive pleural tumor infiltration is present. If the mediastinum is centered in the presence of a large pleural effusion or the lung does not expand completely after pleural drainage, an endobronchial obstruction or trapped lung should be suspected. Bronchoscopy is mandatory if the bronchial obstruction is suspected (Fig. 2), but management of trapped lung can be much more complex. It can be detected on contrast computed tomography (CT) scans [Figs. 3(A) to 3(C)], and pleural pressure

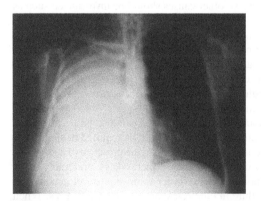

Figure 2   Pleural effusion with ipsilateral mediastinal shift and loss of volume of the right hemithorax in a patient with past history of contralateral breast cancer. Endobronchial metastatic involvement was found at bronchoscopy.

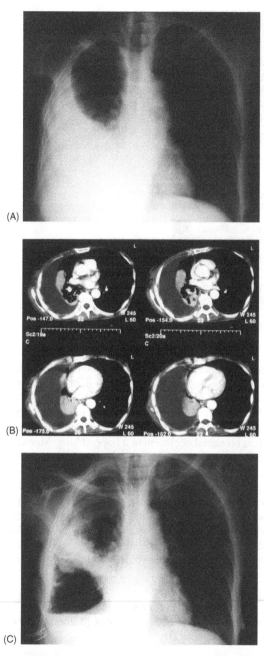

Figure 3 (**A**) Metastatic pleural effusion of cholangiocarcinoma. The effusion was present for more than six months before drainage was attempted. (**B**) CT findings on the same patient. The visceral pleura is markedly thickened, especially on the right lower lobe. (**C**) Same patient of parts (A) and (B). The middle and lower lobe did not re-expand after chest tube placement.

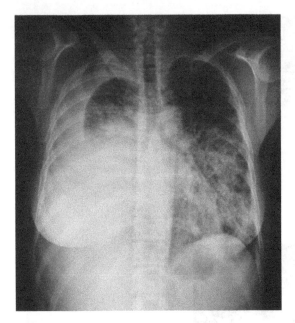

Figure 4 Extensive bilateral involvement is a formal contraindication to talc poudrage in this patient with lung cancer.

measurement during thoracocentesis might also be useful. In patients with mediastinum centered or with ipsilateral shift, the likelihood of a precipitous drop in pleural pressure is increased, and either pleural pressure should be monitored during thoracocentesis or only a small volume of fluid should be removed. In the patient with ipsilateral mediastinal shift, it is unlikely that removal of pleural fluid will result in significant relief of dyspnea (Fig. 4), since there is either main-stem bronchial occlusion or a trapped lung. Moreover, pleurodesis is hardly indicated in this case, and other alternative measures should be considered (see below).

An initial pleural pressure of -10 cm H_2O at thoracocentesis makes trapped lung likely (4). According to Lan and coworkers, pleural elastance seems to be the best predictor for trapped lung and outcome of pleurodesis (5). In the absence of endobronchial obstruction, cut points of -19 cm H_2O with the removal of 500 mL of pleural fluid are predictive of trapped lung. Measurement of the pleural pressure during thoracocentesis may, however, be cumbersome, and the pressure curve profile can differ significantly between patients (6).

A. Definition of Success or Failure of Pleurodesis in MPE

According to the ATS/ERS consensus statement on Management of Malignant Pleural Effusions, the following definitions were proposed (7):

Successful pleurodesis
    (i) Complete success: Long-term relief of symptoms related to the effusion, with absence of fluid reaccumulation on chest radiographs until death.

(ii) Partial success: Diminution of dyspnea related to the effusion, with only partial reaccumulation of fluid (less than 50% of the initial radiographic evidence of fluid), with no further therapeutic thoracocenteses required for the remainder of the patient's life.

Failed pleurodesis: Lack of success as defined above. Comparative studies of different pleurodesis techniques should evaluate outcomes using time-to-event analyses, censoring patients who are lost to follow-up. Data should be reported with and without inclusion of patients who die within one month of pleurodesis.

B. Pleural pH and Outcome of Pleurodesis in MPE

Pleural fluid pH and glucose can be of help as a first approach to a patient in whom pleurodesis is being considered, as a low glucose/pH has been associated with short survival and poor results of pleurodesis (8,9). In our thoracoscopy series, we found a complete successful pleurodesis in 79% of the patients with pH $\geq$ 7.30, whereas it was successful in only 40% of those with pH lower than 7.20, and in none of the patients with pH $<$ 7.15. The association between pH and outcome of pleurodesis was also reported by others (10,11), and we found that a low pH correlates with the presence of a trapped lung. However, Heffner and coworkers reported in a meta-analysis study that, although pH was by itself an independent predictor of survival, it had insufficient predictive accuracy for selecting patients for pleurodesis (12). Nevertheless, the impact of mesothelioma cases may have been underestimated in that study, since patients with mesothelioma tend to survive longer than those with metastatic pleural carcinoma (13), and they have also a tendency to present with a lower pH, due to the marked pleural thickening caused by mesothelioma. Therefore, it is likely that the inclusion of those mesothelioma patients provoked a double-way bias on the pH-survival relationship in the Heffner studies (they survive longer and—on the other hand—have an average lower pH than metastatic carcinomas).

C. Contraindications to Pleurodesis in MPE

Like any other invasive procedure, pleurodesis, especially thoracoscopic talc poudrage, is contraindicated in cases of intractable coagulation disorders, and severe respiratory insufficiency is also a contraindication ($Pco_2 > 55$ mm Hg). Moreover, pleurodesis should not be attempted in patients with a significant contralateral involvement of the lung, since they are likely to develop acute respiratory failure (Fig. 4). The presence of a bilateral pleural effusion might also be problematic, unless all the effusion is removed from the contralateral side before attempting pleurodesis on one side. Simultaneous pleurodesis should not be attempted in any case, because the likelihood of developing complications is high.

II. Pleurodesis in Pneumothorax

The main problem in managing pneumothorax—either primary or secondary—lies in the rate of recurrence, which is unacceptably high when drainage alone is used. Therefore, a pleurodesis technique is frequently required to be on the safer side and achieve a pleural symphysis. In a prospective randomized study, Almind and coworkers compared the recurrence of pneumothorax using drainage alone, and drainage plus tetracycline or talc and found a rate of 36%, 13%, and 8%, respectively, after an average follow-up of 4.6 years (14). Alfageme and coworkers found a 9% recurrence rate with tetracycline pleurodesis as compared to 35% in patients with drainage alone (15). In another multicenter, prospective, randomized study including 108 patients, Tschopp and coworkers found a 5% recurrence rate at five-year follow-up after thoracoscopic talc poudrage, as compared to 34% with pleural drainage alone (16).

Thoracotomy has been performed frequently in the past to prevent recurrence in high-risk patients with pneumothorax (aviators, patients with diving duties, etc.), but there is a growing trend to use video-assisted thoracoscopic surgery (VATS), which allows for the endoscopic resection of the bullae or blebs, as well as for pleurodesis, either through mechanical abrasion of the parietal pleura or application of localized apical talc pleurodesis (17,18). Some controversy exists as to what would be the choice for patients with *secondary* spontaneous pneumothorax (i.e., with known underlying lung disease), especially those who have evidence of bullae on CT scans. In a survey conducted by the German Society for Thoracic Surgery, Hurtgen and coworkers reported the results of 1365 VATS procedures (19) and found an overall 10.2% rate of recurrence when only bleb resection was done (with no pleurodesis procedure added). Thoracoscopic pleural abrasion had also a rather high recurrence rate in their series (7.9%, but it depended on the extension of the abrasion performed). The VATS procedure is, however, expensive and requires general anesthesia with double-lumen tracheal intubation. According to Naunheim and coworkers (20), the rate of recurrence with VATS varies widely depending on identification and subsequent ablation of blebs. On the other hand, there is some controversy on the actual site of air leakage in pneumothorax, even when emphysematous-like changes are found (21). Therefore, talc pleurodesis should be considered as a supplement to bleb resection in patients with high risk of recurrence of the pneumothorax.

Iatrogenic pneumothorax—which occurs mostly as a complication of transthoracic needle aspiration—may be managed by observation or small-bore–chest tube placement, depending upon patient stability and the size of the pneumothorax (22).

Although long-term effects of talc application has been shown to cause little impairment to lung function (23–25), there is some concern about its generous use for pleurodesis in pneumothorax, especially in young patients, who might require a thoracotomy for lung cancer or some other cause (i.e., lung transplantation in cystic fibrosis) in the future (26).

In view of the above arguments, the approach to the patient with pneumothorax remains controversial (27). There is a wide agreement in treating a first episode of pneumothorax in young patients with a small-bore pleural catheter alone. It a prolonged air-leak or recurrence of pneumothorax is observed, VATS would be the technique of choice, whereas a thoracoscopic talc poudrage would be the preferred procedure in elderly patients with spontaneous pneumothorax (28). These patients might not tolerate VATS because the need for general anesthesia and single-lung ventilation. On the other hand, Noppen and coworkers have demonstrated that thoracoscopic talc poudrage is as efficient and safe in persistent secondary pneumothorax than in recurrent primary spontaneous pneumothorax (29). In patients with advanced COPD and pneumothorax, talc-slurry application through the chest tube might be the only available choice.

Pleurodesis using autologous blood "patch" appears to be effective in some difficult cases (30), and it has been used successfully in postoperatory persistent air leak

(31). However, to prevent severe complications, it is recommended that "blood patch" pleurodesis be performed only through large-bore intercostal catheters, that blood is rapidly transferred into the catheter tubing, a sterile saline flush, and full resuscitation equipment is available, and the operator is skilled in the management of tension pneumothorax (32).

Cystic fibrosis patients have a marked tendency to develop repeated and bilateral pneumothoraces, but they can be candidates for lung transplantation as well, and they therefore need a treatment that will be efficient and yet allow for an eventual thoracotomy. Chest drainage with underwater sealing would be the choice for a few days, with subsequent VATS, bullectomy, and apical pleurodesis if the air leak persists (33,34).

III. Pleurodesis in Benign Effusions

Although this is a rather uncommon indication for pleurodesis, there are a few occasions where patients with benign effusions, such as those with persistent effusion from cardiac, renal, or cirrhotic origin that are not responsive to standard treatment, require a pleurodesis procedure. According to Sudduth and Sahn, the following three criteria should be met (35):

The effusion must be symptomatic.

The presence of a trapped lung should be excluded.

Pleurodesis should be reserved for those cases where there is no other therapeutic alternative or when other measures have failed.

Vargas and coworkers reported their experience with a low dose (2 g) of talc in those conditions with a very good success rate (36). According to my own experience, I would add some supplementary recommendations to those mentioned above.

Talc pleurodesis in effusions of cardiac origin is usually successful, but a combined standard medical treatment should also be applied.

Management of pleural effusions associated to cirrhosis of the liver is very difficult (especially when ascites is present) because some communications between the abdominal and pleural cavity exist frequently. Those peritoneal-pleural fistulas can occasionally be seen at thoracoscopy and make pleurodesis rarely successful (37). Octreotide, a somatostatin synthetic analog, has been shown to be useful in controlling those problematic effusions (38).

Patients in peritoneal dialysis can also develop pleural effusions, due to transdiaphragmatic communications, and they can be managed with temporal change from peritoneal to hemodialysis and then inducing pleurodesis with intrapleural instillation of talc or doxycycline.

Chylothorax is also occasionally difficult to manage, as it is absolutely necessary that chyle flux through the thoracic duct be reduced to a minimum. This can be achieved by using a special diet or, more importantly, suspending gastrointestinal feeding and giving intravenous hyper alimentation instead. Management of patients with chylothorax is especially difficult when it is associated to malignancy (particularly lymphoma), but intravenous feeding and eventual pleurodesis can be also necessary in benign conditions when there is a recurrent chylothorax.

IV. Choice of Sclerosing Agent

According to the ERS/ATS consensus statement on Management of Malignant Pleural Effusions (7), which included a comprehensive review of the success with the most relevant agents, talc was found to be the best sclerosant regarding rate of success. In a multicenter study, Dresler et al. obtained a similar overall efficacy for talc poudrage and "slurry" forms of administration; however, they found that poudrage was better in metastatic lung and breast carcinomas (39). In a randomized series including 57 patients, Yim et al. found no significant difference in results when comparing talc poudrage and slurry (40). However, in another randomized study comparing talc poudrage and slurry in 55 patients with MPE, Mañes and coworkers in our Group found a significantly higher rate of recurrences with talc slurry than with poudrage (41). Therefore, this issue is not definitely solved, and our Group is currently working in broadening our previous randomized series. Potential disadvantages of slurry include lack of uniform distribution and accumulation in dependent areas of the pleural cavity, with subsequent incomplete pleurodesis and multiple loculations. Also, we have found that most of the talc administered in the slurry form might be eventually eliminated through the chest tube with the saline solution after the drain is unclamped. The use of some iodide compounds (thymol or povidone) has been proposed as an alternative to talc for pleurodesis, although they are not free of complications (42). Moreover, iodide might provoke severe adverse effects when instilled into the pleural space, especially in allergic patients (43).

For interested readers, I would recommend several reviews on choice of sclerosants for pleurodesis (7,41,44–46). However, I think that a few agents deserve a dedicated comment.

A. Tetracycline Derivatives for Pleurodesis

Doxycycline

According to one experimental study done in rabbits, doxycycline is as effective as tetracycline for pleurodesis; its effect is independent of the acidity of the doxycycline solution, and moderate concentrations of the substance (10 mg/kg) can produce excellent results (47). Although it requires repeated instillations in some cases, its effectiveness has been demonstrated clinically in several studies and it can be applied through a small-bore pleural catheter (48–50). Pain with doxycycline is an important issue, and heavy analgesia is therefore recommended.

Minocycline

Minocycline has also been proposed as a substitute for tetracycline in some studies, including treatment of pneumothorax and also refractory hepatic hydrothorax (51,52). However, minocycline has been reported to cause serious, albeit rare, adverse effects including serum sickness–like and hypersensitivity syndrome reactions and drug-induced lupus (53). Also, it can provoke vestibular symptoms when the doses usually required for pleurodesis are given, and a high rate of hemothorax after intrapleural application of those high doses has been reported in experimental studies (54).

B. Other Sclerosing Agents

Bleomycin: This agent does not appear to be effective in experimental animal studies (55), and it has been shown to be inferior to talc in clinical practice (56). In addition, it is expensive and also has the risk of significant systemic toxicity.

Sodium hydroxide: It has been used mostly in South America, with acceptable effectiveness reported (57). As with many other sclerosants, pain is an important issue. However, according to Teixeira and coworkers (58), control of pain should not include intrapleural administration of lidocaine, since it reacts with NaOH, with subsequent partial deactivation and reduction of the sclerosing effect.

Silver nitrate: Silver nitrate was the first reported agent injected into the pleural space to provoke pleurodesis (in pneumothorax) by Spengler in 1906 (59), and it has been proposed as a valid alternative to talc by some authors (60). In an experimental study, Vargas and coworkers showed a superiority of silver nitrate over talc slurry in producing pleurodesis in rabbits (61). However, a striking finding in their study was that the mean degree of alveolar inflammation in the silver nitrate group was significantly higher than in the talc group. If this can be extrapolated to humans, it would mean that patients submitted to silver nitrate pleurodesis would be in a greater risk of developing early pulmonary complications after its application.

TGF-β2: A few reports have reported on the effectiveness of TGF-β2 in experimental pleurodesis (62,63). Although these results look promising, the cost of this treatment would likely be extremely high, and—up to my knowledge—it has not been yet applied in humans.

V. Technical Aspects of Pleurodesis

Size of chest tube: A small-bore catheter has been sometimes proposed for pleurodesis (64–66), but I believe that a 20 to 28 F chest tube should always be recommended whenever talc is applied in order to prevent obstruction of the drainage by clots.

Time of drainage prior to pleurodesis: Although it is frequently quoted in the literature that the amount of pleural fluid drained per day should be reduced to less than 100 to 150 mL before proceeding to pleurodesis, there is sufficient evidence that the only condition really needed is the ability of the lung to re-expand. Therefore, I would recommend applying the sclerosant as soon as possible after chest tube insertion, once the lung expandability has been demonstrated, since a prolonged drainage might provoke adhesions and multiloculations before the sclerosing procedure, thus impairing the symphysis process itself.

Rate of suction: To prevent re-expansion pulmonary edema, carefully graded and progressive suction should be applied and maintained until the amount of fluid aspirated per day is less than 100 mL. We usually put the drainage in water seal without suction for about 3 hours following talc poudrage, and then begin to apply gentle suction (2–5 cm H_2O). That suction rate can be then doubled every 3 hours until about -20 cm H_2O are reached.

Air leak can occur during lung re-expansion (67), especially in patients who have necrotic tumor nodules in the visceral pleura. In our experience, this is more likely to occur in patients who had undergone chemotherapy previously, even if no biopsies of the lung or visceral pleura were taken during the thoracoscopy procedure.

VI. Mechanisms of Pleurodesis

The underlying, common response in the pleural space to the instillation of a pleurodesis agent is *inflammation*, and inflammation resolves with the subsequent development of fibrosis. Pleurodesis can also be achieved by abrading the pleural surface as is often done for patients with pneumothoraces following surgical removal of blebs on the surface of the lung. This implies that perturbation of normal pleural mesothelial cells allows for the initiation of an inflammatory process that eventually results in the development of symphysis between the visceral and parietal pleural surfaces. Following instillation of talc, there is a rapid neutrophil influx in the pleural space, reaching a peak about 24 hours. The chemokine interleukin-8 (IL-8) correlates with the level of neutrophils seen in the pleural space, indicating that the sclerotic agent, in this instance talc, has initiated the release of neutrophil chemokines in the pleural space (68). Once neutrophils are recruited to the pleural space, they themselves can be sources of further cytokine release, which then perpetuates the inflammatory cascade.

The inflammatory response to the sclerosant can be significantly inhibited by corti-costeroids (69), and—according to our own experience—simultaneous steroid treatment is associated with an increased rate of failed pleurodesis in clinical practice.

A second critical response to a sclerosing agent is the initiation of the *coagulation cascade* and a decrease in the pleural fibrinolytic activity. This is necessary for the early formation of fibrin links between the visceral and parietal pleurae, in order to make the symphysis of the two layers possible. Fibrinolytic activity—as expressed by D-dimer levels—shows a decline 24 hours after talc poudrage in patients who have successful pleurodesis. On the other hand, D-dimer activity is not decreased after talc poudrage in patients with unsuccessful pleurodesis (70). Since there are some commercial kits available to perform rapid neutrophils count and D-dimer determination, we currently use them in combination in order to monitor the ongoing biologic process after intrapleural talc instillation. Thus, patients who are developing a good inflammatory response show a typical pattern with rapidly increasing neutrophils and declining D-dimer in serial samples of pleural fluid after talc poudrage (71). If this does not occur, or the response to talc is poor, we attempt to enhance the pleurodesis process by increasing the suction rate and prolonging the time of drainage in order to provoke a better pleural symphysis through mechanical irritation and tight apposition of the visceral and parietal pleura layers. The formation of a fine latticework of fibrin (the end product of the coagulation cascade) between the visceral and parietal pleurae then allows the third step of the inflammatory cascade to be initiated. This process leads to *proliferation of fibroblasts*, which form strong adhesive links between the visceral and parietal pleural surfaces, obliterating the pleural space. Several fibroblast growth factors have been found to be present in the pleural fluid of patients given sclerosing agents. These include platelet-derived growth factor (PDGF), basic fibroblast growth factor (bFGF), and transforming growth factor-β (TGF-β). Patients with successful pleurodesis have a marked increase in the amount of bFGF in their pleural fluids, and those with unsuccessful pleurodesis had significantly lower amounts of bFGF (72). There appears to be a significant inverse correlation between the release of bFGF into the pleural fluids of patients who have MPE and the tumor size, as evaluated by objective grading during thoracoscopy. Thus, patients with extensive pleural involvement by tumor do not have a high bFGF production by the mesothelial cells. However, when talc was instilled early into patients in the course of their malignant pleural disease while there still remained significant surface area of pleural mesothelial cells exposed to the sclerosing agent, there was a much higher level of bFGF, and pleurodesis was successful. This is consistent with clinical experience, where achieving sclerosis in patients with a far advanced malignant pleural involvement is difficult when compared to those early in the course of their disease. Thus, an exuberant and vigorous response by pleural mesothelial cells appears to be critical for achieving pleurodesis.

In summary, initiation of pleurodesis by instillation of a sclerotic agent into the pleural space is associated with a sequence of inflammatory events leading to pleural fibrosis. These steps involve an inflammatory cascade of increased phagocytic cellular trafficking in the pleural space, the laying down of a lattice fibrin network between the visceral and parietal pleurae, and finally, the exuberant growth and proliferation of pleural fibroblasts leading to loss of tissue margins between the two surfaces.

VII. Side Effects and Complications of Pleurodesis
Pain and transient fever, due to release of proinflammatory mediators, are common side effects associated with pleurodesis performed with practically any sclerosant. However, other worrying complications that have been reported with the procedure are as follows:

A. Re-expansion Edema
In order to prevent re-expansion lung edema, careful and graded suction should be applied. We usually leave the drain connected to water-seal without suction for at least 3 hours following the pleurodesis procedure, and then apply increasing suction gradually. Pulmonary edema can occur when re-expanding the lung in pneumothorax and malignant effusions, even without application of any sclerosant. Although the edema usually appears on the ipsilateral hemithorax, Mahfood and coworkers reported three cases in which it was contralateral, with fatal outcome in two cases (73). The mechanism for this complication is not fully understood; however, a too rapid re-expansion, especially if the lung was collapsed for several weeks, may play an important role, as pointed out by several authors (74) and also confirmed by our experience.

B. Persistent Air Leak
It can occur during lung re-expansion, especially in patients with necrotic tumor nodules in the visceral pleura. In our experience, this especially occurs in patients that have been submitted to previous chemotherapy, even if no biopsies of the visceral pleural were taken.

C. Acute Respiratory Distress or Pneumonitis
Acute respiratory distress or pneumonitis has been described in some cases of talc pleurodesis (75–77). The precise pathophysiologic mechanism responsible for this severe complication is still unclear, but it appears that a high dose of talc used might have played a significant role in some cases. Also, the *size of talc particles* used for pleurodesis appears to be critical (78). In a study on experimental talc-slurry pleurodesis, Kennedy and coworkers found prominent perivascular infiltrates with mononuclear inflammation in the underlying lung, and they speculated that some mediators might spread through the

pulmonary circulation (79). There is some concern about the systemic absorption of the sclerosing agents, and this is suspected to be the rule for almost all of the soluble agents that are instilled into the pleural space. In contrast, talc is thought to persist in the pleura for a long time, thus accounting—at least in part—for its better results in pleurodesis. However, there are some disturbing reports on the finding of talc particles in distant organs after talc pleurodesis, both in animals (80) and humans (81). Our experience with four autopsies in patients that had undergone thoracoscopic talc poudrage is, however, completely different, since no talc was found beyond the pleura in any case. It seems that size of particles might play an important role in the whole process (82,83), and a recent European multicenter study on safety of talc poudrage using large-size–particle talc (with 25.6 μm median diameter) found no cases of acute respiratory distress in a series including 558 patients (84).

D. Possible Activation of the Systemic Coagulation

One special aspect to be considered is the possible activation of the systemic coagulation following pleurodesis. Agrenius and coworkers reported an increase in coagulation and inhibition of fibrinolytic activity in the pleural space after instillation of quinacrine as a sclerosing agent (85,86). We also demonstrated similar effects after talc pleurodesis in our patients (70) and were subsequently concerned about the possible systemic implications of the pleural coagulation/fibrinolysis imbalance that is involved in the pleurodesis process itself. Prompted by this concern and by our finding of two cases of massive pulmonary embolism after talc pleurodesis, we performed a preliminary study on simultaneous pleural/plasma determination of markers for coagulation and fibrinolysis, and found that an activation of the systemic coagulation is frequently observed after talc poudrage (87) and that this side effect can be partially controlled with prophylactic heparin (88). The relevance of this finding in clinical practice is still unclear, but some early deaths (less than 30 days) following pleurodesis procedures (up to 43% in the series of Seaton and coworkers) (48) may be in part related to an undetected pulmonary embolism, and not to advanced neoplastic disease, as it is commonly believed.

VIII. Other Alternatives to Pleurodesis

When pleurodesis fails or is contraindicated, several options are available.

Repeat pleurodesis: It is especially appropriate in patients that have a good performance status and with a high recurrence rate. According to our experience, a second talc poudrage procedure, with increased dosage of talc, can be helpful in selected cases.

Pleuroperitoneal shunt: It can be useful in patients that have a trapped lung and that are in a generally good condition, provided that they have no significant ascites (89).

Parietal pleurectomy: Parietal pleurectomy by thoracotomy is very effective in controlling the effusion, but it is associated with significant morbidity. Instead, thoracoscopic parietal pleural abrasion or partial pleurectomy can be effectively performed through video-assisted thoracoscopic surgery (VATS).

Indwelling pleural catheter: In patients with an expected short survival (poor performance status, and usually presenting with very low pleural pH), placement of an indwelling pleural catheter connected to a vacuum bottle or a disposable bag can be an acceptable choice. Tremblay and Michaud have reported very good results in a series of 250 cases treated with a tunnelled pleural catheter for MPEs (90).

Repeated thoracocentesis: In cases with very poor general condition, repeated thoracocentesis may be the only choice available. However, this option should be kept in very last place since discomfort, risks of infection, and protein depletion can significantly adversely affect the already poor quality of life of those patients.

Acknowledgments

Part of the research mentioned by our group was funded by grants FIS 96/0449, FIS 98/0419, and FIS 05/0289.

References

1. Rodriguez-Panadero F, Antony VB. Pleurodesis: State of the art. Eur Respir J 1997; 10:1648–1654.
2. Steger V, Mika U, Toomes H, et al. Who gains most? A 10-year experience with 611 thoracoscopic talc pleurodeses. Ann Thorac Surg 2007; 83(6):1940–1945.
3. Romero Romero B, Diaz-Cañaveral L, Laserna E, et al. The need for chemical pleurodesis in patients with malignant pleural effusion is associated to decline of pH and high levels of D-dimer in serial pleural fluid samples. Am J Respir Crit Care Med 2001; 163(5):A903.
4. Light RW, Jenkinson SG, Minh V, et al. Observations on pleural pressure as fluid is withdrawn during thoracentesis. Am Rev Respir Dis 1980; 121:799–804.
5. Lan RS, Lo SK, Chuang ML, et al. Elastance of the pleural space: A predictor for the outcome of pleurodesis in patients with malignant pleural effusion. Ann Intern Med 1997; 126:768–774.
6. Villena V, Lopez-Encuentra A, Pozo F, et al. Measurement of pleural pressure during therapeutic thoracentesis. Am J Respir Crit Care Med 2000; 162:1534–1538.
7. Antony VB, Loddenkemper R, Astoul P, et al. Management of malignant pleural effusions. Am J Respir Crit Care Med 2000; 162:1987–2001.
8. Rodriguez-Panadero F, Lopez-Mejias J. Low glucose and pH levels in malignant pleural effusions: Diagnostic significance and prognostic value in respect to pleurodesis. Am Rev Respir Dis 1989; 139:663–667.
9. Sanchez-Armengol A, Rodriguez-Panadero F. Survival and talc pleurodesis in metastatic carcinoma revisited. Report on 125 cases. Chest 1993; 104:1482–1485.
10. Sahn SA, Good JT Jr. Pleural fluid pH in malignant effusions: Diagnostic, prognostic and therapeutic implications. Ann Intern Med 1988; 108:345–349.
11. Martínez-Moragón E, Aparicio J, Sanchis J, et al. Malignant pleural effusion: Prognostic factors for survival and response to chemical pleurodesis in a series of 120 cases. Respiration 1998; 65:108–113.
12. Heffner JE, Nietert PJ, Barbieri C. Pleural fluid pH as a predictor of survival for patients with malignant pleural effusions. Chest 2000; 117:79–86.
13. Rodriguez-Panadero F, Del Rey Pérez JJ. Survival of malignant pleural mesotheliomas as compared to metastatic carcinomas. Eur Respir Rev 1993; 3(11):208–210.
14. Almind M, Lange P, Viskum K. Spontaneous pneumothorax: Comparison of simple drainage, talc pleurodesis, and tetracycline pleurodesis. Thorax 1989; 44:627–630.
15. Alfageme I, Moreno L, Huertas C, et al. Spontaneous pneumothorax. Long-term results with tetracycline pleurodesis. Chest 1994; 106:347–350.

16. Tschopp JM, Boutin C, Astoul P, et al. Talcage by medical thoracoscopy for primary sponta-
     neous pneumothorax is more cost-effective than drainage: A randomised study. Eur Respir J
     2002; 20(4):1003–1009.
17. Jannsen JP, van Mourik J, Cuesta Valentin M, et al. Treatment of patients with spontaneous
     pneumothorax during videothoracoscopy. Eur Respir J 1994; 7:1281–1284.
18. Cardillo G, Carleo F, Giunti R, et al. Videothoracoscopic talc poudrage in primary spontaneous
     pneumothorax: A single-institution experience in 861 cases. J Thorac Cardiovasc Surg 2006;
     131(2):322–328.
19. Hurtgen M, Linder A, Friedel G, et al. Video-assisted thoracoscopic pleurodesis. A survey
     conducted by the German Society for Thoracic Surgery. Thorac Cardiovasc Surg 1996; 44:199–
     203.
20. Naunheim KS, Mack MJ, Hazelrigg SR, et al. Safety and efficacy of video-assisted thoracic
     surgical techniques for the treatment of spontaneous pneumothorax. J Thorac Cardiovasc Surg
     1995; 109(6):1198–1204.
21. Noppen M, Baumann MH. Pathogenesis and treatment of primary spontaneous pneumothorax:
     An overview. Respiration 2003; 70(4):431–438.
22. Baumann MH, Noppen M. Pneumothorax. Respirology 2004; 9(2):157–164.
23. Viskum K, Lange P, Mortensen J. Long term sequelae after talc pleurodesis for spontaneous
     pneumothorax. Pneumologie 1989; 43(2):105–106.
24. Gyorik S, Erni S, Studler U, et al. Long-term follow-up of thoracoscopic talc pleurodesis for
     primary spontaneous pneumothorax. Eur Respir J 2007; 29(4):757–760.
25. Hunt I, Barber B, Southon R, et al. Is talc pleurodesis safe for young patients following primary
     spontaneous pneumothorax? Interact Cardiovasc Thorac Surg 2007; 6(1):117–120.
26. Steger V, Walles T, Walker T, et al. Long-term follow-up of thoracoscopic talc pleurodesis for
     primary spontaneous pneumothorax. Eur Respir J 2007; 30(3):598–599.
27. Berger R. Pleurodesis for spontaneous pneumothorax. Will the procedure of choice please
     stand up? Chest 1994; 106:992–994.
28. Tschopp JM, Brutsche M, Frey JG. Treatment of complicated spontaneous pneumothorax
     by simple talc pleurodesis under thoracoscopy and local anaesthesia. Thorax 1997; 52:329–
     332.
29. Noppen M, Meysman M, d'Haese J, et al. Comparison of video-assisted thoracoscopic talcage
     for recurrent primary versus persistent secondary spontaneous pneumothorax. Eur Respir J
     1997; 10(2):412–426.
30. Cagirici U, Sahin B, Cakan A, et al. Autologous blood patch pleurodesis in spontaneous
     pneumothorax with persistent air leak. Scand Cardiovasc J 1998; 32:75–78.
31. Rivas de Andres JJ, Blanco S, De la Torre M. Postsurgical pleurodesis with autologous blood
     in patients with persistent air leak. Ann Thorac Surg 2000; 70(1):270–272.
32. Williams P, Laing R. Tension pneumothorax complicating autologous "blood patch" pleurode-
     sis. Thorax 205; 60(12):1066–1067.
33. Noppen M, Dhondt E, Mahler T, et al. Successful management of recurrent pneumothorax in
     cystic fibrosis by localized apical thoracoscopic talc poudrage. Chest 1994; 106:262–264.
34. Stringel G, Amin NS, Dozor AJ. Video-assisted thoracoscopy in the management of recurrent
     spontaneous pneumothorax in the pediatric population. JSLS 1999; 3:113–116.
35. Sudduth C, Sahn SA. Pleurodesis for nonmalignant pleural effusions. Recommendations.
     Chest 1992; 102:1855–1860.
36. Vargas FS, Milanez JRC, Filomeno LTB, et al. Intrapleural talc for the prevention of recurrence
     in benign or undiagnosed pleural effusions. Chest 1994; 106:1771–1775.
37. Nakamura A, Kojima Y, Ohmi H, et al. Peritoneal-pleural communications in hepatic hydrotho-
     rax demonstrated by thoracoscopy. Chest 1996; 109:579–581.
38. Barreales M, Saenz-Lopez S, Igarzabal A, et al. Refractory hepatic hydrothorax: Successful
     treatment with octreotide 2005; 97(11):830–835.

39. Dresler CM, Olak J, Herndon JE, et al. Phase III intergroup study of talc poudrage vs talc slurry sclerosis for malignant pleural effusion. Chest 2005; 127:909–915.
40. Yim AP, Chan AT, Lee TW, et al. Thoracoscopic talc insufflation versus talc slurry for symptomatic malignant pleural effusion. Ann Thorac Surg 1996; 62(6):1655–1658.
41. Rodriguez-Panadero F, Jannsen JP, Astoul P. Thoracoscopy: General overview and place in the diagnosis and management of pleural effusion. Eur Respir J 2006; 28:409–421.
42. Xie C, McGovern JP, Wu W, et al. Comparisons of pleurodesis induced by talc with or without thymol iodide in rabbits. Chest 1998; 113:795–799.
43. Agarwal R, Aggarwal AN, Gupta D, et al. Efficacy and safety of iodopovidone in chemical pleurodesis: A meta-analysis of observational studies. Respir Med 2006; 100(11): 2043–2047.
44. Walker-Renard PB, Vaughan LM, Sahn SA. Chemical pleurodesis for malignant pleural effusions. Ann Intern Med 1994; 120:56–64.
45. Rodriguez-Panadero F. Current trends in pleurodesis. Curr Opin Pulm Med 1997; 3:319–325.
46. Dikensoy O, Light RW. Alternative widely available, inexpensive agents for pleurodesis. Curr Opin Pulm Med 2005; 11(4):340–344.
47. Hurewitz AN, Lidonicci K, Wu CL, et al. Histologic changes of doxycycline pleurodesis in rabbits: Effect of concentration and pH. Chest 1994; 106:1241–1245.
48. Seaton KG, Patz EF Jr, Goodman PC. Palliative treatment of malignant pleural effusions: Value of small-bore catheter thoracostomy and doxycycline sclerotherapy. Am J Roentgenol 1995; 164:589–591.
49. Pulsiripunya C, Youngchaiyud P, Pushpakom R, et al. The efficacy of doxycycline as a pleural sclerosing agent in malignant pleural effusion: A prospective study. Respirology 1996; 1: 69–72.
50. Porcel JM, Salud A, Nabal M, et al. Rapid pleurodesis with doxycycline through a small-bore catheter for the treatment of metastatic malignant effusions. Support Care Cancer 2006; 14(5):475–478.
51. Chen JS, Hsu HH, Kuo SW, et al. Effects of additional minocycline pleurodesis after thoracoscopic procedures for primary spontaneous pneumothorax. Chest 2004; 125(1):50–55.
52. Lin CC, Wu JC, Chang SC, et al. Resolution of refractory hepatic hydrothorax after chemical pleurodesis with minocycline. Zhonghua Yi Xue Za Zhi (Taipei) 2000; 63(9):704–709.
53. Knowles SR, Shapiro L, Shear NH. Serious adverse reactions induced by minocycline. Report of 13 patients and review of the literature. Arch Dermatol 1996; 132:934–939.
54. Light RW, Wang NS, Sassoon CSH, et al. Comparison of the effectiveness of tetracycline and minocycline as pleural sclerosing agent in rabbits. Chest 1994; 106:577–582.
55. Vargas FS, Wang N-S, Lee HM, et al. Effectiveness of bleomycin in comparison to tetracycline as pleural sclerosing agent in rabbits. Chest 1993; 104:1582–1584.
56. Hartman DL, Gaither JM, Kesler KA, et al. Comparison of insufflated talc under thoracoscopic guidance with standard tetracycline and bleomycin pleurodesis for control of malignant pleural effusions. J Thorac Cardiovasc Surg 1993; 105(4):743–747.
57. Vargas FS, Carmo AO, Teixeira LR. A new look at old agents for pleurodesis: Nitrogen mustard, sodium hydroxide, and silver nitrate. Curr Opin Pulm Med 2000; 6:281–286.
58. Teixeira LR, Vargas FS, Carmo AO, et al. Effectiveness of sodium hydroxide as a pleural sclerosing agent in rabbits: Influence of concomitant intrapleural lidocaine. Lung 1996; 174:325–332.
59. Spengler L. Zur chirurgie des pneumothorax: Mitteilung über 10 eigene fálle von geheilten tuberkulosen pneumothorax, verbunden in 6 fallen mit gleichzeitiger heilung der lungentuberkulose. Beitr Z Klin Chir 1906; 49:68–89.
60. Paschoalini Mda S, Vargas FS, Marchi E, et al. Prospective randomized trial of silver nitrate vs talc slurry in pleurodesis for symptomatic malignant pleural effusions. Chest 2005; 128(2):684–689.

61. Vargas FS, Teixeira LR, Vaz MA, et al. Silver nitrate is superior to talc slurry in producing pleurodesis in rabbits. Chest 2000; 118:808–813.

62. Light RW, Cheng DS, Lee YC, et al. A single intrapleural injection of transforming growth factor-beta2 produces excellent pleurodesis in rabbits. Am J Respir Crit Care Med 2000; 162:98–104.

63. Lee YC, Lane KB, Parker RE, et al. Transforming growth factor beta2 (TGF-beta2) produces effective pleurodesis in sheep with no systemic complications. Thorax 2000; 55:1058–1062.

64. Clementsen P, Evald T, Grode G, et al. Treatment of malignant pleural effusion: Pleurodesis using a small percutaneous catheter. A prospective randomized study. Respir Med 1998; 92:593–596.

65. Marom EM, Patz EF Jr, Erasmus JJ, et al. Malignant pleural effusions: Treatment with small-bore catheter thoracostomy and talc pleurodesis. Radiology 1999; 210(1):277–281.

66. Villanueva AG, Gray AW Jr, Shahian DM, et al. Efficacy of short term versus long term tube thoracostomy drainage before tetracycline pleurodesis in the treatment of malignant pleural effusions. Thorax 1994; 49:23–25.

67. Chang YC, Patz EF Jr, Goodman PC. Pneumothorax after small-bore catheter placement for malignant pleural effusions. Am J Roentgenol 1996; 166(5):1049–1051.

68. Hartman DL, Antony VB, Hott JW, et al. Thoracoscopic talc insufflation increases pleural fluid IL-8 levels in patients with malignant pleural effusions. Am J Respir Crit Care Med 1994; 149(Suppl. 2, 2):A974.

69. Xie C, Teixeira LR, McGovern JP, et al. Systemic corticosteroids decrease the effectiveness of talc pleurodesis. Am J Crit Care Med 1998; 157:1441–1444.

70. Rodriguez-Panadero F, Segado A, Martin Juan J, et al. Failure of talc pleurodesis is associated with increased pleural fibrinolysis. Am J Respir Crit Care Med 1995; 785–790.

71. Psathakis K, Calderon-Osuna E, Romero-Romero B, et al. The neutrophilic and fibrinolytic response to talc can predict the outcome of pleurodesis. Eur Respir J 2006; 27(4):817–821.

72. Antony VB, Nasreen N, Mohammed KA, et al. Talc pleurodesis: Basic fibroblast growth factor mediates pleural fibrosis. Chest 2004; 126(5):1522–1528.

73. Mahfood S, Hix WR, Aaron BL, et al. Reexpansion pulmonary edema. Ann Thorac Surg 1988; 45:340–345.

74. Nakamura H, Ishizaka A, Sawafuji M, et al. Elevated levels of interleukin-8 and leukotriene B4 in pulmonary edema fluid of a patient with reexpansion pulmonary edema. Am J Respir Crit Care Med 1994; 149:1037–1040.

75. Rinaldo JE, Owens GR, Rogers RM. Adult respiratory distress syndrome following intrapleural instillation of talc. J Thorac Cardiovasc Surg 1983; 85:523–526.

76. Bouchama A, Chastre J, Gaudichet A, et al. Acute pneumonitis with bilateral pleural effusion after talc pleurodesis. Chest 1984; 86:795–797.

77. Rehse DH, Aye RW, Florence MG. Respiratory failure following talc pleurodesis. Am J Surg 1999; 177:437–440.

78. Maskell NA, Lee YC, Gleeson FV, et al. Randomized trials describing lung inflammation after pleurodesis with talc of varying particle size. Am J Respir Crit Care Med 2004; 170:377–382.

79. Kennedy L, Harley RA, Sahn SA, et al. Talc slurry pleurodesis: Pleural fluid and histologic analysis. Chest 1995; 107:1707–1712.

80. Campos Werebe E, Pazetti R, Milanez de Campos JR, et al. Systemic distribution of talc after intrapleural administration in rats. Chest 1999; 115:190–193.

81. Milanez de Campos JR, Campos Werebe E, Vargas FS, et al. Respiratory failure due to insufflated talc. Lancet 1997; 349:251–252.

82. Ferrer J, Villarino MA, Tura JM, et al. Talc preparations used for pleurodesis vary markedly from one preparation to another. Chest 2001; 119:1901–1905.

83. Navarro Jiménez C, Gómez Izquierdo L, Sánchez Gutiérrez C, et al. Análisis morfométrico y mineralógico de 14 muestras de talco usado para pleurodesis en distintos países de Europa y América. Neumosur 2005; 17(3):197–202.

84. Jannsen JP, Collier G, Astoul P, et al. Safety of talc poudrage in malignant pleural effusion. Lancet 2007; 369:1535–1539.
85. Agrenius V, Chmielewska J, Widström O, et al. Increased coagulation activity of the pleura after tube drainage and quinacrine instillation in malignant pleural effusion. Eur Respir J 1991; 4:1135–1139.
86. Agrenius V, Chmielewska J, Widström O, et al. Pleural fibrinolytic activity is decreased in inflammation as demonstrated in quinacrine pleurodesis treatment of malignant pleural effusion. Am Rev Respir Dis 1989; 140:1381–1385.
87. Rodriguez-Panadero F, Segado A, Torres I, et al. Thoracoscopy and talc poudrage induce an activation of the systemic coagulation system. Am J Respir Crit Care Med 1995; 151:A357.
88. Rodriguez-Panadero F, Segado A, Martin Juan J, et al. Activation of systemic coagulation in talc poudrage can be (partially) controlled with prophylactic heparin. Am J Respir Crit Care Med 1996; 153:A458.
89. Petrou M, Kaplan D, Goldstraw P. The management of recurrent malignant pleural effusions: The complementary role of talc pleurodesis and pleuro-peritoneal shunting. Cancer 1995; 75:801–805.
90. Tremblay A, Michaud G. Single-center experience with 250 tunnelled pleural catheter insertions for malignant pleural effusion. Chest 2006; 129:362–368.

12

Translational Research in Pleural Diseases

GEORGIOS T. STATHOPOULOS
Department of Critical Care and Pulmonary Services, General Hospital "Evangelismos",
School of Medicine, University of Athens, Athens, Greece

JOOST P. J. J. HEGMANS
Department of Pulmonary Medicine, Erasmus MC, Rotterdam, The Netherlands

Y. C. GARY LEE
Department of Medicine & Lung Institute of Western Australia, University of Western Australia
and Sir Charles Gairdner Hospital, Perth, Australia

I. Introduction

Pleural diseases affect over 3000 patients per million population and can arise from more than 50 lung and extra-pulmonary disorders (1). The causes of pleural diseases, their molecular mechanisms, diagnosis, and their best treatments are often complex—and require consideration of both local (pleural) and systemic factors. Our knowledge on the pathogenesis of pleural diseases remains limited, and in part accounts for relatively lack of novel therapies in pleural diseases in the last few decades.

In addition, clinical treatments in pleural diseases are often based on "conventional wisdom" rather than on vigorously scrutinized scientific validation. The efficacy and safety of many of the clinically employed treatments have not been robustly proven in preclinical settings before being used in humans. Examples include many compounds used in humans for pleurodesis, such as povidone iodine which has recently been linked to serious adverse events (2). Even talc, first used in the 1930s and currently the most commonly used agent, has not undergone thorough modern drug-safety testing (3) and an association of pleurodesis with small-particle–size talc and subsequent systemic inflammation and ARDS with a 2.3% mortality, has only been revealed recently (4–6).

Translational research in pleural disease is desperately needed to further our understanding of the mechanisms of common pleural diseases and in evaluating and establishing novel therapies. Exciting progresses have been made in recent years. Animal model work, in vitro cellular experiments, and latest molecular technologies, for example, microarray global gene profiling and proteomics, have all been employed and serve separate and important roles in translational pleural research (7). It is likely that other advanced technologies, for example, metabolomics, will soon be applied as well.

The pleural cavity is lined by a monolayer of multipotent mesothelial cells on the parietal, visceral, and diaphragmatic pleurae. In healthy state, the mesothelial cells significantly outnumber infiltrating cells (e.g., leukocytes) in the pleural cavity. The close relationship between the pleural cavity and the blood supply in the pleura allows easy exchange of important mediators (e.g., cytokines) and rapid influx of inflammatory cells in disease states (8). Pathogenesis of pleural diseases therefore involves complicated interactions among mesothelial cells, infiltrating inflammatory (and/or malignant) cells, and their cellular products as well as numerous mediators from plasma extravasation. These complex situations cannot be studied adequately in vitro, and necessitates the use of animal models or examination of ex vivo clinical specimens. Conversely, in vitro work is important in establishing the cellular source(s) and responses driving the biologic observations.

II. Laboratory Analyses of Pleural Fluid and Tissue Samples

A large number of published pleural research papers examined proteins in pleural fluid and/or tissues, often by enzyme-linked immunosorbent assays and immunohistochemistry. These studies have revealed mediators differentially expressed in pleural effusions of different etiologies, which may provide valuable diagnostic tools or unveil novel knowledge on disease pathology. For example, numerous studies have found increased levels of adenosine deaminase (ADA) and interferon (IFN)-γ in tuberculous pleural effusions (9–12). These findings have been rapidly translated into diagnostic tests for tuberculosis (TB), now used clinically worldwide (13–18).

The biologic roles of the identified candidate proteins in pleural disease can be explored using in vitro and in vivo studies. For example, comparative studies of human pleural fluid samples have identified increased expressions of vascular endothelial growth factor (VEGF) and its receptors in pleural malignancies (19–22), which was corroborated by laboratory studies showing that VEGF is a major therapeutic target in malignant effusion formation (23,24). This knowledge has led to the trials of VEGF antagonists, for example, bevacizumab, in both malignant and benign pleural effusions with promising results (25,26).

This type of studies have shortcomings: they can only investigate one protein in isolation each time, and are likely to be surpassed by technologies of mass screening for candidate genes or proteins. Researchers must also be aware that exudative effusions, by definition, contain high levels of protein. Hence, finding elevated levels of a protein in effusions does not necessarily mean that it carries a diagnostic or pathogenic role. Furthermore, the conventional assumption that protein levels in the pleural fluid represent those in the pleural tissues/tumors has recently been challenged (27). Experimental studies are thus important to determine whether proteins found over- or under-expressed in pleural tissues and fluids actually bear a significant pathogenic role.

III. In Vitro Research With Mesothelial Cells

Mesothelial cells are capable of producing a wide array of mediators that are involved in key biologic processes in the pleural space, such as inflammation, fibrosis, vascular permeability, angiogenesis, etc. (28). In addition, they possess potent phagocytic activity and can transform into fibroblast-like cells upon stimulation (a process referred to as epithelial-to-mesenchymal transition). Mesothelial cell experiments are performed using either immortalized (usually virally transformed) cell lines or primary cells harvested from the pleura, peritoneum or occasionally pericardium. While mesothelial cells from different serosal cavities are postulated to have similar biologic behaviors, this has not been corroborated. Normal human pleural mesothelial cells are difficult to isolate, and have most commonly been isolated from pleural effusions due to heart failure (29,30).

Concerns have been expressed that mesothelial cells obtained from human transudative effusions may not truly represent "normal" mesothelial cells, as they have likely been exposed to mediators. Primary culture of pleural mesothelial cells from animals, for example, rabbits or mice (31,32), has been used as alternatives.

IV. In Vivo Models of Pleural Diseases

A. Introduction

In vivo studies are essential in translational research as pleural pathologies are inevitably a result of complicated interactions that can only be adequately studied in vivo. Animal studies are also essential in evaluating the efficacy, safety, and pharmacokinetics of novel therapeutic modalities.

A good understanding of the advantages and limitations of the available models is essential to design meaningful in vivo experiments. Rabbits, mice, rats, and sheep are the commonest animal species used in pleural research. Smaller animals (e.g., mice) cost less and are easier to handle but make intrapleural injections difficult and provide limited amount of biologic samples.

Important anatomical variations of the pleura exist among species. First, many animals (e.g., mice, dogs) have incomplete mediastina, and the two pleural cavities communicate freely, prohibiting the use of the contralateral pleura as a control. Second, larger animals (e.g., sheep) have a thick visceral pleura resembling that of humans, but smaller animals (e.g., mice) have a thin visceral membrane. This difference bears implications on fluid and particulate transport across the pleura.

The pleural cavity can be assessed in many ways. Direct intrapleural injection with a fine needle is the least invasive. Small injection volume is adequate, as the injectate will be distributed throughout the whole pleural surface by respiratory motions. Alternatively, placement of small plastic "chest tubes" allows repeated intrapleural treatment and/or sampling (e.g., lavage). This provides longitudinal data on the biologic changes within the pleural space, helping to reduce the number of animals required in time-course studies (7).

Commonly used end-points in animal pleural studies include lethality (e.g., in malignant effusion models), adhesions/pleurodesis scores (e.g., in empyema or pleurodesis studies), and pleural fluid volume (e.g., in empyema or malignant effusion studies). Different biologic samples can be collected to provide additional information. Pleural tissues allow histologic assessment, for example, for inflammatory or fibrotic changes. Pleural fluid and blood can be assayed for cellular and protein contents and drug levels in pharmacokinetic studies. Pleural vascular permeability can be tested, for example, with Miles assay. Increasingly, animal-imaging techniques, for example, MRI or ultrasonography, are employed which can provide longitudinal data in a noninvasive fashion.

No animal model is ideal. A thorough understanding of the advantages and limitations of various animal species and models is essential in order to design the most suitable in vivo model or in vitro experiment that provides the best chance of answering the scientific question(s) raised.

B. Specific Translational Use of Animal Models in Various Pleural Diseases

Animal models have been developed for the study of a variety of pleural pathologies. Employment of the suitable model can provide significant insights and answers specific

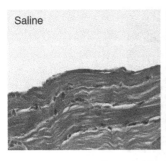
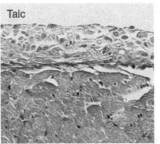

Figure 1   Collagen deposition in the mouse mesothelial layer after intraperitoneal delivery of talc. Trichrome stain (black) illustrates collagen deposits.

clinical questions or explores new findings from bench research, as illustrated by examples below. Detailed description of various animal models employed in pleural research is outside the scope of this chapter and can be found elsewhere (7).

Pleural Fibrosis/Pleurodesis Model

Animal studies of pleurodesis represent one of the most common types of in vivo pleural research (33–37). The efficacy and safety of conventional agents, for example, talc, doxy-cycline, bleomycin, and silver nitrate have been extensively assessed in animal models (Fig. 1). The importance of using animal studies of pleural fibrosis in the translational crosstalk between laboratory investigations and clinical practice is highlighted by two recent examples.

First, clinical observations of acute respiratory failure after talc pleurodesis have raised significant concerns in the past few years. It was postulated that extrapleural migration of small-particle–size talc induces systemic and pulmonary inflammation. Research using a rabbit model of pleurodesis was used to test and helped unveil relations between talc preparations with different particle sizes and their toxicity (38,39). The results of these studies and other clinical observations led to a recent observational series confirming that large-particle–size talc has a better safety profile (40).

The usefulness of animal models in drug development can be seen in a series of experimental work on transforming growth factor (TGF)-β as a pleurodesing agent. Based on the profibrotic role of TGF-β shown in other organ systems, pilot studies were performed with intrapleural instillation of this cytokine and demonstrated potent induction of pleurodesis without eliciting local inflammation or systemic complications (34,35). Clinical trials are under planning to evaluate TGF-β as a pleurodesing agent in patients with malignant pleural effusions.

Malignant Pleural Effusion Models

Animal studies can shed light on the pathophysiology of pleural diseases in which the disease mechanisms are unclear. The insights gained from this type of experimental studies can lead to new therapeutic targets, as seen in recent studies on VEGF, and of tumor necrosis factor (TNF)-α/nuclear factor (NF)-κB (23,24,41–43). Most animal studies on malignant pleural effusions have been performed using mice-rendered immunodeficient (e.g., severe combined immunodeficient mice) (44,45), which precludes the evaluation of the host defense mechanism in malignant pleural diseases and of novel therapies.

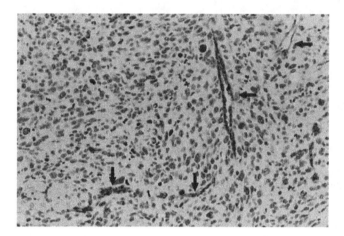

Figure 2 Histologic section through pleural tumor resulting from direct intrapleural injection of Lewis lung carcinoma in C57BL/6 mouse, stained with antifactor VIII–related antigen antibody. Arrows indicate new blood vessels.

A recently established murine model of pleural adenocarcinoma using immunocompetent mice represents a significant step toward translational pleural research. Carcinoma cells are implanted intrapleurally or systemically—the latter often results in pleural metastases, especially from lung deposits of the tumor. The resultant malignant effusions are rich in inflammatory cells and cytokines, and the pleural tumor deposits exhibit abundant angiogenesis (Fig. 2). Lethality usually results from either local effects (e.g., respiratory compromise from the effusions) or systemic effects (e.g., cachexia and distant metastases). Using these models, the role of important mediators and biologic pathways (e.g., VEGF/VEGFR, IL-6/Stat3, and TNF-α/NF-κB) in effusion formation has been uncovered (23,24,27,41–43). Other studies have assessed the efficacy of novel therapies, such as IL-12 and IL-15 (46), inhibitors of topoisomerase II (47) and of VEGF-receptor tyrosine kinase (23), and zoledronic acid (27). The intrapleural injection model has also been successfully applied to transgenic mice, such as nitric oxide synthase and TNF-α knockouts (43,48).

Other Models

Preclinical models of pleural diseases have also been widely used as surrogate systems for the study of inflammation [especially using the carrageenan pleurisy model in mice, rats or rabbits (49–51)] and the mechanisms of allergic responses. In the latter, ovalbumin-sensitized rats or mice, upon challenges by intrapleural injection of ovalbumin, develop mast cell degranulation, IgE accumulation, and eosinophil chemotaxis (52,53). The role of novel mediators in inflammatory pathways and the efficacy of new therapies can be evaluated with these models (52–55).

Animal models of empyema have also facilitated the study of the pathogenesis of the disease. Availability of knockout mice, for example, has revealed the important role of CD4+ lymphocytes in empyema-associated inflammation and bacterial clearance (56). Animal studies have been used to examine interventional therapies for empyema, for example, repeated early thoracocentesis (57), early chest tube insertion (58), and intrapleural delivery of fibrinolytics for empyema (59). These models have also allowed pharmacokinetic studies of antibiotics into the pleural space (60–62).

Findings from experimental models of asbestos exposure and mesothelioma have yielded significant insight on mesothelioma pathobiology, diagnosis, and therapy. For instance, a study of the sequential changes in gene expression observed in asbestos-exposed rats identified several candidate markers of asbestos-induced carcinogenesis, including osteopontin (63). The findings were recapitulated in clinical studies—serum osteopontin reflects tumor progression and has supportive diagnostic value in mesothelioma (64). The observation of malignant mesothelioma development in hamsters after pleural, pericardial, or peritoneal injection of simian virus 40 (SV40) led to an extensive list of laboratory and clinical studies on this virus, especially as a cofactor of mesothelioma development (65). In vivo animal research has aided in unveiling biologic pathways of mesothelioma formation and progression (66–69). Animal models have also been extensively applied to evaluate therapies for malignant mesothelioma (70,71).

Similarly, animal models have provided major value in translational research of TB pleuritis (72,73), and have also provided opportunities to study less-common conditions such as pleural effusions from esophageal rupture, rheumatoid arthritis, benign asbestos pleuritis, etc. Preclinical models have also played an important role in our understanding of the physiologic changes with pleural fluid accumulation or pneumothoraces.

V. New Technologies for Translational Pleural Research

A wide range of powerful new technologies are now available for translational research and some have already been employed in pleural research. These modalities can screen the expression of a huge number of genes [e.g., cDNA microarrays (74)] or proteins [e.g., mass spectrometry (75)], and reveal a massive amount of novel information from a single experiment that previously would not have been feasible. Transcriptome sequencing to detect mutations from mesothelioma samples have been recently attempted (76), as had comparative genomic hybridization to assess gene copy numbers (77). As these technologies become more readily available and affordable, it is anticipated that they would be employed more often in pleural research in the very near future.

Genomic and proteomic techniques are able to uncover genes or proteins that are over- or under-expressed in disease states. The data may offer significant insight on disease pathogenesis, and identify genes or proteins (or clusters of them) that can act as novel biomarkers for disease diagnosis, monitoring and/or predicting prognosis, or response to treatment. Whichever of these technologies be used, careful definition of patient phenotypes is crucial. Discordant results from similar studies can often be explained by the differences in patient populations recruited. Data are also influenced by variations in sample collection methods, technology platforms used, and the bioinformatics used for data analyses (78). The technologies are advancing at a lightning speed and often outpaced the recognition of its limitations. Researchers must understand the principles and practicalities of the techniques to recognize the limitations of the data generated.

A. Microarray

In the past decade, global gene profiling using DNA microarray technology has been successfully applied to researches of many disciplines, especially mesothelioma research.

This technology can screen the RNA expression of tens of thousands of genes simultaneously, providing information that previously would take decades to achieve.

DNA microarray requires collection of samples promptly after being obtained to minimize RNA degradation. To date the most common source of samples are pleural tissues excised during resection of mesothelioma. One potential shortcoming is that the samples may contain a combination of tumor and neighboring benign pleura and varying amount of connective tissues. RNA is then extracted from the samples and its quality and quantity are assessed (74,78,79). Complementary DNA is synthesized, labeled, and hybridized with gene-specific (single-stranded DNA) probes on the array chips. The most commonly used method is a single-color array, for example, Affymetrix GeneChips. A two-color approach is sometimes used in which the sample and a control are labeled with different dyes and hybridized to the same array. The amount of DNA hybridized to the probes is quantified by measuring the fluorescence intensity, and compared with that of housekeeping genes (74).

As many as over 54,000 genes can be studied simultaneously in a single gene chip. The vast amount of data generated requires specialized bioinformatics for analyses. First, the data need to be normalized to allow comparisons within and between samples. This is followed by "filtering", which screens and identifies candidate genes according to the pre-set criteria. Data can often be filtered in many different ways, with different results, as according to the objective of the experiment. For example, if the purpose is to identify the key candidate genes of high reproducibility, the cutoff of fold increase may be set high to filter away marginally over- or under-expressed genes. On the other hand, grouping of the gene expression into common "pathways" (e.g., metabolic, inflammatory, angiogenesis, etc.) may be helpful to gain insight on overall disease pathology, and may require different filtering strategies. It is well known that the end product of the analyses is critically dependent on the bioinformatics platform and the filtering conditions used (74,79).

Although the microarray technique is extremely powerful, limitations exist. Gene chips are expensive, and most studies have included small number of samples (as few as two in one publication on mesothelioma; see Ref. 80). This is clearly inadequate to cover the variations in phenotypes encountered in clinical settings. A recent study on transcriptome sequencing of mesothelioma further confirmed that mesotheliomas are often heterogenous: each sample in that study contained a different mutation profile (76). It is likely that expression patterns are different during different stages of mesothelioma development even within the same patient. Most studies published are cross-sectional in nature, and the reproducibility within individuals is unclear. Little is known about whether the expression patterns of different parts of the pleura of the same patient are concordant.

Differential gene expressions identified by DNA microarrays, do not necessarily translate into differences in protein production. In our experience, DNA microarrays are more sensitive in detecting genes over-expressed in disease states than genes whose expressions are suppressed. In these regards, proteomics (see below) have at least a complimentary (if not superior) role.

Microarray Studies in Pleural Diseases

Many studies have profiled the gene expression of mesothelioma cells or tissues against controls (usually benign pleura or other tumors, especially adenocarcinomas) (Fig. 3). The results are discordant among studies, though a reasonable amount of overlap does exist.

Data from microarray profiling of cell lines are generally different from studies using excised human tumors. This is perhaps not surprising as global gene expressions are

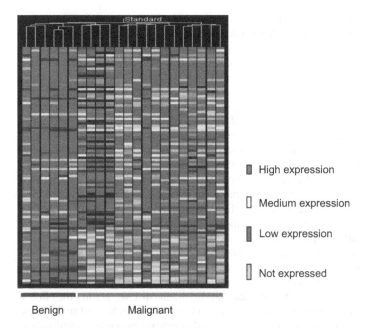

High expression

Medium expression

Low expression

Not expressed

Benign   Malignant

Figure 3 Global gene profiling was performed on human pleural tissues of malignant (mesothe-lioma or adenocarcinoma) and benign etiologies using Affymetrix GeneChips. This figure is a clustering tree showing genes with significant difference in expression among groups. In the clus-tering process, samples are aligned such that those with the most similar overall expression profiles are put adjacent to each other. Each column represents the gene expression of one sample; each horizontal line represents the expression of a gene. The level of expression is reflected by the color.

likely to be significantly influenced by surrounding environment in vivo, thus accounting for the differences observed from in vitro experiments. Recent studies have also shown that mesothelioma cells acquired further chromosomal copy-number changes with passages, which cast a further variable to profiling studies using cell lines (80).

Laser capture microdissection is a technique that allows selection of cells of interest from histologic specimens so that the gene expression profile of cells in their "natural" environment can be assessed. The amount of RNA from cells captured by this method is often limited, and amplification is necessary to obtain enough RNA for microarray profiling. This method potentially allows accurate comparison of gene expression of disease and normal tissues within the same individual, thereby eliminating differential gene expressions arising from interindividual differences unrelated to the disease process. This has been applied in mesothelioma research and has shown, using a microarray chip of 10,000 genes, differential expression of 14 genes between mesothelioma and controls (81). Overexpression of ferritin light peptide was further confirmed by real-time polymerase chain reaction (RT-PCR) (81).

Various microarray studies have revealed novel molecules that may play important roles in the biology of mesothelioma. Gordon et al. found that NME2, CRI1, PDGF-C and GSN were differentially expressed in mesothelioma over benign controls at RNA and protein levels (82). Using a mixture of human tissue samples and cell lines, Hoang et al.

discovered an overexpression of matriptase in epithelioid mesothelioma (83). Microarray studies with mesothelioma cell lines have unveiled different candidate genes, for example, gp96 (84), galectin-3–binding protein (84), laminin receptor (84), fra-1 (85), JAGGED1 (86), cyclin D2 (86), etc. It is important to note that genes identified in some of these studies had not been verified in separate cohorts.

Diagnosis of mesothelioma is not always straightforward, and differentiation from adenocarcinoma can be difficult. Microarray has been performed to identify "signature patterns" of clusters of genes, which can aid the diagnosis of malignant mesothelioma. There is no single molecule that is pathognomonic for mesothelioma in all the studies published. A gene profiling study of 33 mesotheliomas and 190 lung adenocarcinomas identified a panel of 17 genes that may aid differentiation of these two malignancies (87). Using an array of over 54,000 genes, Davidson et al. showed a different gene expression signature pattern for peritoneal mesotheliomas compared with ovarian carcinomas (88). Microarray has also revealed significantly different gene expression profiles of epithelioid and biphasic mesotheliomas (89)—the two most common subtypes of mesothelioma and are known to have different prognosis.

Traditionally, microarray data are analyzed by comparing the expression of the same gene between disease (e.g., mesothelioma) and control groups. An alternative approach using the ratios of the expression of different gene pairs within the same sample has been tested in mesothelioma. Such approach may aid diagnosis (90), predict the clinical outcome in mesothelioma patients (91), and treatment response (92). Several studies have also revealed other combination of genes that predict disease progression and patient survival. One set of such "gene classifier" has been derived from one cohort and validated (with 76% accuracy) in another (93), though the number of patients in each of the cohorts was small.

B. Proteomics

Proteomics involves the comprehensive study of all proteins in body fluids, tissues or cell types under given conditions. It consists of the identification and quantification of proteins as well as the comprehensive study of their structure, localization, modification, interactions, activities, and functions (94). Proteomic technologies can help to characterize the disease mechanism, and identify biomarkers and novel therapeutic targets. The proteomic field is rapidly changing, constantly reshaped by the advent of new technologies and scientific breakthroughs. Proteomics have recently been applied to the study of pleural diseases, and can potentially bring about important medical advances in pleural research.

Principles of Proteomic Analyses

Individual cells produce thousands of proteins, each with specific functions. The collection of proteins in a cell is known as the proteome, and, unlike the genome which is constant irrespective of cell type, it differs from cell to cell and is constantly changing through its biochemical interactions with the genome and the environment. It changes from moment to moment in response to tens of thousands of intra- and extra-cellular environmental signals such as other proteins, pH, hypoxia, and drug administration, and changes continuously with processes such as ageing, stress, or disease. The level of expression of the proteins varies from very low, for example, a few copies per cell, to extremely abundant. Some proteins are expressed for short time periods in life, for example, during embryonic development, while others may be continually expressed.

A number of options are available to profile and identify proteins. It relies mainly on the separation of a protein sample by two-dimensional (2D) electrophoresis, which separates proteins first by isoelectric point and then by molecular weight (95). Protein spots in a gel can be visualized using a variety of chemical stains or fluorescent markers. Once proteins are separated and stained, they have to be characterized by mass spectrometry (MS) (96). Basic types of mass analyzers are the matrix-assisted laser desorption–ionization time of flight (MALDI-TOF), quadrupole (Q), quadrupole "ion trap" (IT), and Fourier transform ion cyclotron (FT-ICR-MS or FTMS).

In short, spots of interest are excised from the gel, destained, and subsequently digested with proteolytic enzymes and/or chemicals. On average, the resulting peptides have the right size to be detected by MS and are first mixed with a UV-absorbing organic acid, also known as matrix solution (e.g., α-cyano-4-hydroxy-*trans*-cinnamic acid) which causes the peptide to form crystals. When irradiated with UV-laser pulses, the peptide/matrix crystals become detached (desorption), and gaseous ions are liberated (ionization). The charged molecules are accelerated through a strong electric field within a high vacuum, and a recording is taken of how long the peptides take to travel a specified distance and strike a detector. Ionized peptides are thus separated on the basis of their mass-to-charge (m/z) ratio—the higher the mass of the particle relative to its charge, the longer its flight time.

Detected peptides/ions are displayed as a unique series of peaks that are referred to as the peptide mass fingerprint (PMF). This mass-mapping spectrum of peptide peaks is then compared with the virtual peptide masses predicted from theoretical digestion of protein sequences currently contained within databases (e.g., UniProt, Swiss-Prot, NCBI) and the protein can be identified. This approach was used to study the proteome of human malignant pleural effusions (97–100). Although many protein spots were present in a 2D gel map and could subsequently be identified by MS, the value for clinical medicine was limited (101). Most proteins detected were previously reported in the literature to be present in serum and did not originate from diseased cells or contain disease-specific information. Better results can be obtained by reducing the sample complexity by capturing proteins to specific matrices before MS to allow a better detection of low-abundance proteins (102,103).

Proteomic studies have shown that specific proteins are expressed at different anatomic sites in primary tumors, effusions, and solid metastases, and might have different prognostic value (104–106). MALDI-TOF technology was also used to characterize the proteins present in exosomes isolated from malignant pleural effusions from different cancerous origins (107). Exosomes are small natural membrane vesicles released by a wide variety of cell types. The biologic functions of exosomes are only slowly unveiled, but it is clear that they serve to remove unnecessary cellular proteins and act as intercellular messengers. Proteomic studies are being performed to gather information on their potential biologic functions (108,109).

Other proteomic platforms that are used to characterize pleural effusions are protein (micro) arrays (110,111). These arrays are prepared by printing the captured proteins on filters or coated microscope slides using purified or recombinant proteins, crude mixtures, or antibodies.

Before starting a proteomic study, the advantages and disadvantages of various methods must be assessed in order to choose the best suitable approach. The choice of an appropriate methodology will depend on the goals of the specific study, amount and number of samples, availability of resources, etc. (112). Ongoing rapid developments in separation techniques, automation, sample throughput, and bioinformatics will further stimulate the investigation of pleural effusions and will ultimately lead to new insights into the causative mechanisms of diseases. The application of this technology to pleural research is still in its early stage. Due to the aforementioned current limitations, proteomics at present cannot replace standard diagnostic procedures (e.g., pleural tissue biopsy), but holds great promise for identifying novel diagnostic and therapeutic targets to revolutionize the clinical approach to pleural diseases.

VI. Conclusions

In contrast to empiric approaches of the past, contemporary evidence-based medicine requires rational and in-depth investigations of disease pathogenesis and therapy. In this regard, crosstalk between in vitro and in vivo studies of animals and human has proven invaluable in furthering knowledge on disease pathobiology and in advancing therapeutics. In recent years, pleural disease research has adopted this new paradigm of translational research. The development of novel animal models of virtually any pleural disease and the introduction of modern molecular biology tools have facilitated unprecedented amount of functional studies attempting to decipher pathogenesis of pleural diseases. These, coupled with new high-throughput methods of mass-examination of genes and proteins, will hopefully lead to the design of novel therapies against various pleural diseases in the very near future.

References

1. Light RW, Lee YCG. Textbook of Pleural Diseases, 2nd ed. London, U.K.: Arnold Press, 2008.
2. Wagenfeld L, Zeitz O, Richard G. Visual loss after povidone-iodine pleurodesis. New Engl J Med 2007; 357:1264–1265.
3. Davies HE, Lee YC, Davies RJ. Pleurodesis for malignant pleural effusion: talc, toxicity and where next? Thorax 2008; 63:572–574.
4. West SD, Davies RJO, Lee YCG. Pleurodeses for malignant pleural effusions: Current controversies and variations in practices. Curr Opin Pulm Med 2004; 10:305–310.
5. West SD, Lee YCG. Current management of malignant pleural mesothelioma. Clin Chest Med 2006; 27:335–354.
6. Dresler CM, Olak J, Herndon II JE, et al. Phase III intergroup study of talc poudrage vs talc slurry sclerosis for malignant pleural effusion. Chest 2005; 127:909–915.
7. Stathopoulos GT, Lee YCG. Experimental Models: Pleural diseases other than mesothelioma. In: Light RW, Lee YC (eds.), Textbook of Pleural Diseases (2nd ed.). London, UK: Hodder-Arnold, 2007:169–186.
8. Lee YCG. Mesothelial cell in pleural disease: An active player or innocent bystander. In: Luh K-T, ed. 7th Congress of the Asian Pacific Society of Respirology. Taipei, Taiwan: Monduzzi Editore—MEDIMOND Inc., 2002:101–105.
9. Ribera E, Ocaña I, Martinez-Vazquez JM, et al. High level of interferon gamma in tuberculous pleural effusion. Chest 1988; 93:308–311.
10. Shimokata K, Kishimoto H, Takagi E, et al. Determination of the T-cell subset producing gamma-interferon in tuberculous pleural effusion. Microbiol Immunol 1986; 30:353–361.
11. Ribera E, Ocaña I, Martinez-Vazquez JM, et al. High level of interferon gamma in tuberculous pleural effusion. Chest 1988; 93:308–311.
12. Lee YC, Rogers JT, Rodriguez RM, et al. Adenosine deaminase levels in nontuberculous lymphocytic pleural effusions. Chest 2001; 120:356–361.

13. Mazurek GH, Jereb J, Lobue P, et al. Division of Tuberculosis Elimination, National Center for HIV, STD, and TB Prevention, Centers for Disease Control and Prevention (CDC). Guidelines for using the QuantiFERON-TB Gold test for detecting mycobacterium tuberculosis infection, United States. MMWR Recomm Rep 2005; 54:49–55.

14. Hotta K, Ogura T, Nishii K, et al. Whole blood interferon-gamma assay for baseline tuberculosis screening among Japanese healthcare students. PLoS ONE 2007; 2:e803.

15. Villena V, López-Encuentra A, Pozo F, et al. Interferon gamma levels in pleural fluid for the diagnosis of tuberculosis. Am J Med 2003; 115:365–370.

16. Valdés L, San José E, Alvarez D, et al. Diagnosis of tuberculous pleurisy using the biologic parameters adenosine deaminase, lysozyme, and interferon gamma. Chest 1993; 103:458–465.

17. Ocaña I, Martinez-Vazquez JM, Segura RM, et al. Adenosine deaminase in pleural fluids. Test for diagnosis of tuberculous pleural effusion. Chest 1983; 84:51–53.

18. Daniil ZD, Zintzaras E, Kiropoulos T, et al. Discrimination of exudative pleural effusions based on multiple biological parameters. Eur Respir J 2007; 30:957–964.

19. Kraft A, Weindel K, Ochs A, et al. Vascular endothelial growth factor in the sera and effusions of patients with malignant and nonmalignant disease. Cancer 1999; 85:178–187.

20. Thickett DR, Armstrong L, Millar AB. Vascular endothelial growth factor (VEGF) in inflammatory and malignant pleural effusions. Thorax 1999; 54:707–710.

21. Cheng D, Rodriguez RM, Perkett EA, et al. Vascular endothelial growth factor in pleural fluid. Chest 1999; 116:760–765.

22. Sack U, Hoffmann M, Zhao XJ, et al. Vascular endothelial growth factor in pleural effusions of different origin. Eur Respir J 2005; 25:600–604.

23. Yano S, Herbst RS, Shinohara H, et al. Treatment for malignant pleural effusion of human lung adenocarcinoma by inhibition of vascular endothelial growth factor receptor tyrosine kinase phosphorylation. Clin Cancer Res 2000; 6:957–965.

24. Yano S, Shinohara H, Herbst RS, et al. Production of experimental malignant pleural effusions is dependent on invasion of the pleura and expression of vascular endothelial growth factor/vascular permeability factor by human lung cancer cells. Am J Pathol 2000; 157:1893–1903.

25. Pichelmayer O, Zielinski C, Raderer M. Response of a nonmalignant pleural effusion to bevacizumab. N Engl J Med 2005; 353:740–741.

26. Pichelmayer O, Gruenberger B, Zielinski C, et al. Bevacizumab is active in malignant effusion. Ann Oncol 2006; 17:1853.

27. Stathopoulos GT, Moschos C, Loutrari H, et al. Zoledronic acid is effective against experimental malignant pleural effusion. Am J Respir Crit Care Med 2008; 178:50–59 [Epub ahead of print] doi:10.1164/rccm.200710-1513OC.

28. Lee YCG, Lane KB. Cytokines in pleural diseases. In: Light RW, Lee YCG, eds. Textbook of Pleural Diseases. London, U.K.: Arnold Press, 2003:63–89.

29. Marchi E, Liu W, Broaddus VC. Mesothelial cell apoptosis is confirmed in vivo by morphological change in cytokeratin distribution. Am J Physiol Lung Cell Mol Physiol 2000; 278:L528–L535.

30. Antony VB, Owen CL, Hadley KJ. Pleural mesothelial cells stimulated by asbestos release chemotactic activity for neutrophils in vitro. Am Rev Respir Dis 1989; 139(1):199–206.

31. Lee YCG, Knight DA, Lane KB, et al. Activation of proteinase activated receptor-2 in mesothelial cells induces pleural inflammation. Am J Physiol Lung Cell Mol Physiol 2005; 288:L734–L740.

32. Lee YCG, Malkerneker D, Thompson PJ, et al. Transforming growth factor-β induces vascular endothelial growth factor elaboration from pleural mesothelial cells in vivo and in vitro. Am J Respir Crit Care Med 2002; 165:88–94.

33. Marchi E, Vargas FS, Acencio MMP, et al. Pleurodesis: A novel experimental model. Respirology 2007; 12:500–504.

34. Light RW, Cheng DS, Lee YCG, et al. A single intrapleural injection of transforming growth factor beta-2 produces an excellent pleurodesis in rabbits. Am J Respir Crit Care Med 2000; 162:98–104.

35. Lee YCG, Lane KB, Parker RE, et al. Transforming growth factor beta-2 (TGFb2) produces effective pleurodesis in sheep with no systemic complications. Thorax 2000; 55: 1058–1062.

36. Werebe EC, Pazetti R, Milanez de Campos JR, et al. Systemic distribution of talc after intrapleural administration in rats. Chest 1999; 115:190–193.

37. Cohen RG, Shely WW, Thompson SE, et al. Talc pleurodesis: Talc slurry versus thoracoscopic talc insufflation in porcine model. Ann Thorac Surg 1996; 62:1000–1002.

38. Ferrer J, Montes JF, Villarino MA, et al. Influence of particle size on extrapleural talc dissemination after talc slurry pleurodesis. Chest 2002; 122:1018–1027.

39. Maskell NA, Lee YC, Gleeson FV, et al. Randomized trials describing lung inflammation after pleurodesis with talc of varying particle size. Am J Respir Crit Care Med 2004; 170: 377–382.

40. Janssen JP, Collier G, Astoul P, et al. Safety of pleurodesis with talc poudrage in malignant pleural effusion: A prospective cohort study. Lancet 2007; 369:1535–1539.

41. Yeh HH, Lai WW, Chen HH, et al. Autocrine IL-6-induced Stat3 activation contributes to the pathogenesis of lung adenocarcinoma and malignant pleural effusion. Oncogene 2006; 25:4300–4309.

42. Stathopoulos GT, Zhu Z, Everhart MB, et al. Nuclear factor-kappa B affects tumor progression in a mouse model of malignant pleural effusion. Am J Respir Cell Mol Biol 2006; 34:142–150.

43. Stathopoulos GT, Kollintza A, Moschos C, et al. Tumor necrosis factor-alpha promotes malignant pleural effusion. Cancer Res 2007; 67:9825–9834.

44. Kraus-Berthier L, Jan M, Guilbaud N, et al. Histology and sensitivity to anticancer drugs of two human non-small cell lung carcinomas implanted in the pleural cavity of nude mice. Clin Cancer Res 2000; 6:297–304.

45. Astoul P, Colt HG, Wang X, et al. Metastatic human pleura ovarian cancer model constructed by orthotopic implantation of fresh histologically-intact patient carcinoma in nude mice. Anticancer Res 1993; 13:1999–2002.

46. Kimura K, Nishimura H, Matsuzaki T, et al. Synergistic effect of interleukin-15 and interleukin-12 on antitumor activity in a murine malignant pleurisy model. Cancer Immunol Immunother 2000; 49:71–77.

47. Kraus-Berthier L, Jan M, Guilbaud N, et al. Histology and sensitivity to anticancer drugs of two human non-small cell lung carcinomas implanted in the pleural cavity of nude mice. Clin Cancer Res 2000; 6:297–304.

48. Wang B, Xiong Q, Shi Q, et al. Genetic disruption of host nitric oxide synthase II gene impairs melanoma-induced angiogenesis and suppresses pleural effusion. Int J Cancer 2001; 91:607–611.

49. Bliven ML, Otterness IG. Carrageenan pleurisy. Methods Enzymol 1988; 162:334–339.

50. Vinegar R, Truax JF, Selph JL, et al. Pathway of onset, development and decay of carrageenan pleurisy in the rat. Fed Proc 1982; 41:2588–2595.

51. Strange C, Tomlinson JR, Wilson C, et al. The histology of experimental pleural injury with tetracycline, empyema and carrageenan. Exp Mol Pathol 1989; 51:205–219.

52. Klein A, Talvani A, Cara DC, et al. Stem cell factor plays a major role in the recruitment of eosinophils in allergic pleurisy in mice via the production of leukotriene B4. J Immunol 2000; 164:4271–4276.

53. Pasquale CP, E-Silva PM, Lima MC, et al. Suppression by cetirizine of pleurisy triggered by antigen in actively sensitized rats. Eur J Pharmacol 1992; 223:9–14.

54. Martins MA, Castro-Faria-Neto HC, Bozza PT, et al. Role of PAF in the allergic pleurisy caused by ovalbumin in actively sensitized rats. J Leukoc Biol 1993; 53:104–111.

55. Martins MA, Pasquale CP, E-Silva PM, et al. Eosinophil accumulation in the rat pleural cavity after mast cell stimulation with compound 48/80 involves protein synthesis and is selectively suppressed by dexamethasone. Int Arch Allergy Appl Immunol 1990; 92:416–424.
56. Mohammed KA, Nasreen N, Ward MJ, et al. Induction of acute pleural inflammation by *Staphylococcus aureus*. I. CD4+ T cells play a critical role in experimental empyema. J Infect Dis 2000; 181:1693–1699.
57. Sasse S, Nguyen T, Texeira LR, et al. The utility of daily therapeutic thoracentecis for the treatment of early empyema. Chest 1999; 116:1703–1708.
58. Sasse S, Nguyen TK, Mulligan M, et al. The effects of early chest tube placement on empyema resolution. Chest 1997; 111:1679–1683.
59. Zhu Z, Hawthorne ML, Guo Y, et al. Tissue plasminogen activator combined with human recombinant deoxyribonuclease is effective therapy for empyema in a rabbit model. Chest 2006; 129:1577–1583.
60. Strahilevitz J, Lev A, Levi I, et al. Experimental pneumococcal pleural empyema model: The effect of moxifloxacin. J Antimicrob Chemother 2003; 51:665–669.
61. Teixeira LR, Sasse SA, Villarino MA, et al. Antibiotic levels in empyemic pleural fluid. Chest 2000; 117:1734–1739.
62. Liapakis IE, Light RW, Pitiakoudis MS, et al. Penetration of clarithromycin in experimental pleural empyema model fluid. Respiration 2005; 72:296–300.
63. Sandhu H, Dehnen W, Roller M, et al. mRNA expression patterns in different stages of asbestos-induced carcinogenesis in rats. Carcinogenesis 2000; 21:1023–1029.
64. Pass HI, Lott D, Lonardo F, et al. Asbestos exposure, pleural mesothelioma, and serum osteopontin levels. N Engl J Med 2005; 353:1564–1573.
65. Cicala C, Pompetti F, Carbone M. SV40 induces mesotheliomas in hamsters. Am J Pathol 1993; 142:1524–1533.
66. Marzo AL, Fitzpatrick DR, Robinson BWS, et al. Antisense oligonucleotides specific for transforming growth factor beta2 inhibit the growth of malignant mesothelioma both in vitro and in vivo. Cancer Res 1997; 57:3200–3207.
67. Janne PA, Taffaro ML, Salgia R, et al. Inhibition of epidermal growth factor receptor signaling in malignant pleural mesothelioma. Cancer Res 2002; 62:5242–5247.
68. Mazieres J, You L, He B, et al. Wnt2 as a new therapeutic target in malignant pleural mesothelioma. Int J Cancer 2005; 117:326–332.
69. Frizelle SP, Grim J, Zhou J, et al. Re-expression of p16INK4a in mesothelioma cells results in cell cycle arrest, cell death, tumor suppression and tumor regression. Oncogene 1998; 16:3087–3095.
70. Scagliotti GV, Novello S. State of the art in mesothelioma. Ann Oncol 2005; 16:ii240–ii245.
71. Khokhar NZ, She Y, Rusch VW, et al. Experimental therapeutics with a new 10-deazaaminopterin in human mesothelioma: Further improving efficacy through structural design, pharmacologic modulation at the level of MRP ATPases, and combined therapy with platinums. Clin Cancer Res 2001; 7(10):3199–3205.
72. Allen SS, McMurray DN. Coordinate cytokine gene expression in vivo following induction of tuberculous pleurisy in guinea pigs. Infect Immun 2003; 71:4271–4277.
73. Allen SS, Cassone L, Lasco TM, et al. Effect of neutralizing transforming growth factor β1 on the immune response against mycobacterium tuberculosis in guinea pigs. Infect Immun 2004; 72:1358–1363.
74. Quachenbush J. Microarray analysis and tumor classification. New Engl J Med 2006; 354:2463–2472.
75. Hegmans J, Lambrecht B. Proteomics in pleural disease. In: Light RW, Lee YCG, eds. Textbook of Pleural Diseases, 2nd ed. London, U.K.: Arnold Press, 2008.
76. Sugarbaker DJ, Richards WG, Gordon GJ, et al. Transcriptome sequencing of malignant pleural mesothelioma tumors. Proc Natl Acad Sci U S A 2008; 105(9):3521–3526.

77. Lindholm PM, Salmenkivi K, Vauhkonen H, et al. Gene copy number analysis in malignant pleural mesothelioma using oligonucleotide array CGH. Cytogenet Genome Res 2007; 119(1–2):46–52.

78. Pusztai L. Chips to bedside: Incorporation of microarray data into clinical practice. Clin Cancer Res 2006; 12:7209–7214.

79. Wiltgen M, Tilz GP. DNA microarray analysis: Principles and clinical impact. Hematology 2007; 12:271–287.

80. Zanazzi C, Hersmus R, Veltman IM, et al. Gene expression profiling and gene copy-number changes in malignant mesothelioma cell lines. Genes Chromosomes Cancer 2007; 46(10):895–908.

81. Mohr S, Bottin MC, Lannes B, et al. Microdissection, mRNA amplification and microarray: A study of pleural mesothelial and malignant mesothelioma cells. Biochimie 2004; 86(1): 13–19.

82. Gordon GJ, Rockwell GN, Jensen RV, et al. Identification of novel candidate oncogenes and tumor suppressors in malignant pleural mesothelioma using large-scale transcriptional profiling. Am J Pathol 2005; 166:1827–1840.

83. Hoang CD, D'Cunha J, Kratzke MG, et al. Gene expression profiling identifies matriptase overexpression in malignant mesothelioma. Chest 2004; 125:1843–1852.

84. Singhal S, Wiewrodt R, Malden LD, et al. Gene expression profiling of malignant mesothelioma. Clin Cancer Res 2003; 9:3080–3097.

85. Ramos-Nino ME, Scapoli L, Martinelli M, et al. Microarray analysis and RNA silencing link fra-1 to cd44 and c-met expression in mesothelioma. Cancer Res 2003; 63:3539–3545.

86. Kettunen E, Nissen AM, Ollikainen T, et al. Gene expression profiling of malignant mesothelioma cell lines: cDNA array study. Int J Cancer 2001; 91(4):492–496.

87. Holloway AJ, Diyagama DS, Opeskin K, et al. A molecular diagnostic test for distinguishing lung adenocarcinoma from malignant mesothelioma using cells collected from pleural effusions. Clin Cancer Res 2006; 12:5129–5135.

88. Davidson B, Espina V, Steinberg SM, et al. Proteomic analysis of malignant ovarian cancer effusions as a tool for biologic and prognostic profiling. Clin Cancer Res 2006; 12: 791–799.

89. Sun X, Wei L, Liden J, et al. Molecular characterization of tumour heterogeneity and malignant mesothelioma cell differentiation by gene profiling. J Pathol 2005; 207(1):91–101.

90. Gordon GJ, Jensen RV, Hsiao LL, et al. Translation of microarray data into clinically relevant cancer diagnostic tests using gene expression ratios in lung cancer and mesothelioma. Cancer Res 2002; 62:4963–4967.

91. Gordon GJ, Rockwell GN, Godfrey PA, et al. Validation of genomics-based prognostic tests in malignant pleural mesothelioma. Clin Cancer Res 2005; 11:4406–4414.

92. Gordon GJ, Jensen RV, Hsiao LL, et al. Using gene expression ratios to predict outcome among patients with mesothelioma. J Natl Cancer Inst 2003; 95:598–605.

93. Pass HI, Liu Z, Wali A, et al. Gene expression profiles predict survival and progression of pleural mesothelioma. Clin Cancer Res 2004; 10:849–859.

94. Fields S. Proteomics in genomeland. Science 2001; 291:1221–1224.

95. Gorg A, Weiss W, Dunn MJ. Current two-dimensional electrophoresis technology for proteomics. Proteomics 2004; 4:3665–3685.

96. Aebersold R, Mann M. Mass spectrometry-based proteomics. Nature 2003; 422:198–207.

97. Davidson B, Espina V, Steinberg SM, et al. Proteomic analysis of malignant ovarian cancer effusions as a tool for biologic and prognostic profiling. Clin Cancer Res 2006; 12:791–799.

98. Hsieh WY, Chen MW, Ho HT, et al. Identification of differentially expressed proteins in human malignant pleural effusions. Eur Respir J 2006; 28:1178–1185.

99. Tyan YC, Wu HY, Su WC, et al. Proteomic analysis of human pleural effusion. Proteomics 2005; 5:1062–1074.

100. Tyan YC, Wu HY, Lai WW, et al. Proteomic profiling of human pleural effusion using two-dimensional nano liquid chromatography tandem mass spectrometry. J Proteome Res 2005; 4:1274–1286.
101. Adkins JN, Varnum SM, Auberry KJ, et al. Toward a human blood serum proteome: Analysis by multidimensional separation coupled with mass spectrometry. Mol Cell Proteomics 2002; 1:947–955.
102. Fetsch PA, Simone NL, Bryant-Greenwood PK, et al. Proteomic evaluation of archival cytologic material using SELDI affinity mass spectrometry: Potential for diagnostic applications. Am J Clin Pathol 2002; 118:870–876.
103. Soltermann A, Ossola R, Kilgus-Hawelski S, et al. N-Glycoprotein profiling of lung adenocarcinoma pleural effusions by shotgun proteomics. Cancer 2008; 114:124–133.
104. Yanagisawa Y, Sato Y, Asahi-Ozaki Y, et al. Effusion and solid lymphomas have distinctive gene and protein expression profiles in an animal model of primary effusion lymphoma. J Pathol 2006; 209:464–473.
105. Yanagisawa K, Shyr Y, Xu BJ, et al. Proteomic patterns of tumour subsets in non-small-cell lung cancer. Lancet 2003; 362:433–439.
106. Davidson B. Anatomic site-related expression of cancer-associated molecules in ovarian carcinoma. Curr Cancer Drug Targets 2007; 7:109–120.
107. Bard MP, Hegmans JP, Hemmes A, et al. Proteomic analysis of exosomes isolated from human malignant pleural effusions. Am J Respir Cell Mol Biol 2004; 31:114–121.
108. Thery C, Boussac M, Veron P, et al. Proteomic analysis of dendritic cell-derived exosomes: A secreted subcellular compartment distinct from apoptotic vesicles. J Immunol 2001; 166:7309–7318.
109. Hegmans JP, Bard MP, Hemmes A, et al. Proteomic analysis of exosomes secreted by human mesothelioma cells. Am J Pathol 2004; 164:1807–1815.
110. Kothmaier H, Quehenberger F, Halbwedl I, et al. EGFR and PDGFR differentially promote growth in malignant epithelioid mesothelioma of short and long term survivors. Thorax 2008; 63:345–351.
111. Hegmans JP, Hemmes A, Hammad H, et al. Mesothelioma environment comprises cytokines and T-regulatory cells that suppress immune responses. Eur Respir J 2006; 27:1086–1095.
112. Mischak H, Apweiler R, Banks RE, et al. Clinical proteomics: A need to define the field and to begin to set adequate standards. Proteomics Clin Appl 2007; 1:148–156.

13
Clinical Evaluation of the Patient with a Pleural Effusion

STEVEN A. SAHN
Division of Pulmonary, Critical Care, Allergy and Sleep Medicine, Medical University of South Carolina, Charleston, South Carolina, U.S.A.

I. Introduction

The clinical recognition of a pleural effusion, either on physical examination or radiologically, is a marker that an abnormal physiologic state has resulted in greater formation than removal of pleural fluid. Disease in virtually any organ can cause a pleural effusion (1). In the diagnostic approach to the patient with a pleural effusion, the clinician must be cognizant that not only disease in the thorax can be causative but disease in organs juxtaposed to the diaphragm, such as the liver or spleen, can as well. Furthermore, systemic diseases, such as systemic lupus erythematosus and rheumatoid arthritis, may involve the pleura, as can diseases of the lymphatic system, such as yellow nail syndrome. Therefore, the evaluation of a pleural effusion must begin with a complete history and physical examination and follow with pertinent laboratory tests to formulate a pre-thoracentesis diagnosis.

II. Value of Pleural Fluid Analysis

The clinician should be aware that pleural fluid analysis in isolation can establish a definitive (i.e., positive cytology, empyema) diagnosis in only a minority of patients, and the number of definitive diagnoses will vary with the population being evaluated. In a prospective study of 129 patients with pleural effusion, thoracenteses provided a definitive diagnosis in only 18% of patients and a presumptive diagnosis in 55% of patients (2). In the remaining 27% of patients, the pleural fluid findings were not helpful diagnostically, as the values were compatible with two or more clinical possibilities; however, in a number of these patients, the findings were useful in excluding other possible diagnoses, such as empyema. Therefore, history and physical examination, radiologic evaluation, and ancillary blood tests are crucial in generating a pre test diagnosis. Pleural fluid analysis is a valuable test that may not provide an initial definitive diagnosis but can allow a confident clinical diagnosis if there is a thoughtful pre-thoracentesis evaluation.

Diagnoses that can be established definitively by pleural fluid analysis with the appropriate diagnostic tests are shown in Table 1 (1,3).

III. Symptoms with Pleural Effusions

The patient may present with (lupus pleuritis) (4) or without (BAPE) (5) symptoms related to the pleural effusion. Patients without underlying cardiopulmonary disease who

Table 1 Diagnoses That Can be Established Definitively by Pleural Fluid Analysis

Diseases	Diagnostic pleural fluid tests
Chylothorax	Triglycerides ($>$110 mg/dL); presence of chylomicron
Duropleural fistula	Presence of B_2-transferrin
Empyema	Observation (pus, putrid odor)
Esophageal rupture	Presence of salivary amylase, pleural fluid acidosis (often as low as 6.00); presence of food particles
Extravascular migration of central venous catheter	Milky if lipids are infused; glucose pleural fluid/serum ratio substantially $>$ 1.0
Fungal pleurisy	Positive KOH stain, culture
Hemothorax	Hematocrit (pleural fluid/blood ratio $\geq$ 0.5)
Lupus pleuritis	Lupus erythematosus (LE) cells present
Malignancy	Positive cytology
Peritoneal dialysis	Total protein $<$ 1 g/dL and glucose 300–400 mg/dL
Rheumatoid pleurisy	Characteristic cytology
Tuberculous effusion	Positive acid-fast bacillus (AFB) stain, culture; adenosine deaminase (ADA) $>$ 40–60 U/L
Urinothorax	Creatinine (pleural fluid/serum ratio $>$ 1.0)

From Sahn SA. The diagnostic value of pleural fluid analysis. Sem Respir Crit Care Med 1995;16:269–78 (www.chestjournal.org), with permission.

develop a small effusion may be asymptomatic and the effusion discovered by routine chest radiograph. When patients with a pleural effusion are symptomatic, dyspnea and chest pain are the most common findings. Dyspnea may be caused by a large or massive pleural effusion in a patient with normal lungs, a moderate effusion with underlying lung disease, and a small effusion with severe lung disease. A large pleural effusion causes ipsilateral mediastinal shift, depression of the ipsilateral diaphragm, outward movement of the ipsilateral chest wall, and lung compression when there is absence of an endobronchial lesion or a fixed mediastinum. The breathlessness perceived by patients with a large to massive pleural effusion is due to its effect on the previously mentioned structures with input by neurogenic receptors from the lung and chest wall (6). Small-to-moderate effusions tend to cause lung displacement rather than lung compression and generally have minimal to no effect on pulmonary function (7). Chest pain with splinting and atelectasis or a primary parenchymal process from infection or malignancy may be the major cause of dyspnea in patients with a small-to-moderate pleural effusion.

Patients with a pleural effusion may present with pleuritic chest pain, which is associated with pleural inflammation; the pain will vary with the degree of pleural inflammation (8). Pleuritic chest pain has been described as having a stitch in the side, stabbing, or shooting. It may be exacerbated by deep inspiration, cough, or sneeze. Any maneuver that results in chest wall splinting, such as manual pressure over the chest wall, will minimize the pain. However, a splinting maneuver will not differentiate other causes of pleuritic-like chest pain, such as rib fractures, from inflammation of the pleura per se.

With inflammation of the costal pleura, pain is located directly over the site of pleural involvement, often with associated tenderness on pressure; cutaneous hypersensitivity and abdominal pain are absent. When the lateral anterior and parts of the posterior diaphragmatic pleura are inflamed, the perceived pain covers a more diffuse area including the lower thorax, back, and abdomen; this pain, typically accompanied by cutaneous hyperesthesia, is exacerbated by pressure and muscle rigidity. Inflammation of the central portion of the diaphragmatic pleura does not elicit pain in the immediate area but results in referred pain to the ipsilateral posterior neck, shoulder, and trapezius muscle; the pain is associated with tenderness, hyperesthesia, hyperalgesia, and muscle spasm. The referred pain from central diaphragmatic inflammation occurs because the majority of the sensory fibers of the phrenic nerve enter at the C4 level of the spinal cord, the usual entry point of sensation from the shoulder (8).

The primary symptoms of a pleural effusion, chest pain, and dyspnea, are nonspecific; therefore, further history is important in limiting the differential diagnosis prior to pleural fluid analysis. Features such as loss of consciousness in an alcoholic who presents with fever suggests that the effusion is an anaerobic empyema (9). The acute onset of dyspnea and ipsilateral chest pain in an individual who sustained a recent leg fracture that required a cast suggests that the effusion is caused by a pulmonary embolism (10). Pleural effusion from asbestos exposure, benign asbestos pleural effusion (BAPE), should be suspected in a man who was a shipyard worker for the past 20 years (5). A patient who sustained a myocardial infarction two weeks previously and presents with fever, dyspnea, and pleuritic chest pain may have the post cardiac injury syndrome (11). Barogenic esophageal rupture should be considered in the patient who provides a history of severe retching and upper abdominal or lower chest pain (12). A known diagnosis of systemic lupus erythematosus or a history of taking procainamide should raise the possibility of lupus pleuritis (13). A history of sarcoidosis (14), rheumatoid disease (15), or chronic dialysis (uremic pleural effusion, tuberculous effusion) (16,17) should alert the clinician to the possible cause of the pleural effusion. Although the number of drugs that are associated with pleural disease is substantially less than those reported to cause parenchymal disease, drug-induced pleural disease should always be considered in the patient who presents with an undiagnosed exudative effusion (18). Drugs associated with pleural fluid eosinophilia are shown in Table 2.

IV. Physical Examination

Pleural fluid separates the lung from the chest wall and interferes with sound transmission. The physical signs of a pleural effusion will vary depending upon the volume of pleural fluid and the degree of lung compression. The examination will also be affected by the status of the underlying lung and the patency of the bronchial tree.

A small amount of pleural fluid (approximately 250–300 mL) will be difficult to detect on physical examination (19). With about 500 mL of fluid, the following physical findings typically are present: *(i)* dullness to percussion; *(ii)* decreased fremitus; and *(iii)* normal vesicular breath sounds, possibly of lower intensity compared to the contralateral side. When the effusion volume exceeds 1000 mL, there usually is *(i)* mild bulging and an absence of inspiratory retraction of the lower intercostal spaces; *(ii)* decreased expansion of the ipsilateral chest wall; *(iii)* dullness to percussion to the level of the scapula and possibly to the axilla; *(iv)* decreased or absent fremitus at the posterior base and laterally; *(v)* decreased bronchovesicular breath sounds at the upper level of the effusion; and *(vi)* egophony at the upper level of the effusion. If there is greater lung compression, auscultation may reveal bronchial breath sounds (19).

Table 2   Drugs Associated with an
Eosinophilic Pleural Effusion

- Acyclovir*
- Antidepressants
  - Amitriptyline*
  - Desipramine**
  - Imipramine**
  - Tricyclic antidepressants
- Beta-blockers
  - Acebutolol**
  - Atenolol*
  - Betaxolol*
  - Celiprolol*
  - Metoprolol*
  - Nadolol*
  - Oxprenolol*
  - Pindolol*
  - Practolol***
  - Propranolol**
  - Sotalol*
- Bromocriptine*
- Clozapine**
- Dantrolene**
- Fenfluramine/dexfenfluramine**
- Fluoxentine*
- Gliclazide*
- Infliximab*
- Isotretinoin**
- Mesalamine**
- Nitrofurantoin****
- Propylthiouracil***
- Simvastin**
- Sulfasalazine***
- Tizanidine*
- Trimipramine**
- Valproic acid**

---

* 1 to 5 reports
** ~10
*** 20 to 100
**** >100
From Pneumotox.com

With a massive pleural effusion, physical examination will show: *(i)* bulging of the intercostal spaces; *(ii)* virtual absence of chest wall expansion; *(iii)* a dull percussion note over the entire hemithorax; *(iv)* absent breath sounds over the majority of the chest with possible bronchovesicular or bronchial breath sounds at the uppermost portion of the effusion; *(v)* egophony at the upper level of the effusion; and *(vi)* palpation of the liver or spleen due to significant diaphragmatic depression (19).

In the setting of a transudative pleural effusion, the pre-thoracentesis history and physical examination should increase the likelihood of a presumptive diagnosis. Patients with congestive heart failure typically relate symptoms of orthopnea and paroxysmal nocturnal dyspnea and have an S3 gallop and bibasilar, fine crackles usually associated with increased jugular venous pressure. Patients with hepatic hydrothorax show the stigmata of cirrhosis and typically have clinical ascites. Those with nephrotic syndrome and a pleural effusion usually have anasarca. Patients most likely to have atelectatic effusions are those who are post operative (20), in an intensive care unit (21), or have upper abdominal or lower chest pain.

V. Laboratory Tests

A. Peripheral Leukocyte Count

The finding of peripheral leukocytosis with a left shift with an associated pleural effusion suggests a bacterial infection, most commonly from pneumonia; however, other diagnoses to consider include subphrenic abscess, esophageal rupture, hepatic or splenic abscess, or severe inflammation as with pancreatitis. Leukopenia with a pleural effusion may be seen with systemic lupus erythematosus, viral pleurisy, severe pneumonia with sepsis, or pneumonia in an HIV positive patient.

B. Chest Radiograph

Finding an isolated pleural effusion or associated findings on chest radiograph may narrow the differential diagnosis prior to pleural fluid analysis (1). When the only abnormality on the chest radiograph is a pleural effusion, the clinician should consider infectious causes, such as tuberculosis or viral pleurisy, in addition to a focal bacterial pneumonia. Connective tissue diseases, such as rheumatoid pleurisy and lupus pleuritis, should be considered in the appropriate clinical setting. Metastatic carcinoma, non-Hodgkin lymphoma, body cavity lymphoma, and leukemia can also be present as a solitary pleural effusion. Other entities where a pleural effusion may be the only radiographic abnormality include benign asbestos pleural effusion (BAPE), pulmonary embolism, drug-induced pleural disease, yellow nail syndrome, hypothyroidism, uremic pleuritis, chylothorax, and constrictive pericarditis. When the effusion is massive and causes contralateral mediastinal shift, the most likely diagnosis is carcinoma, usually a non-lung primary (22). When there is no contralateral shift, lung cancer (23) and malignant mesothelioma (24) are most likely.

A pleural effusion as the only radiographic abnormality may also be associated with disease below the diaphragm. This radiographic finding is seen with transudates from hepatic hydrothorax, nephrotic syndrome, urinothorax, and peritoneal dialysis, and exudates from acute pancreatitis and pancreatic pseudocyst, Meigs' syndrome, chylous ascites, subphrenic abscess, hepatic abscess, and splenic abscess or infarction (1).

When a patient has bilateral effusions on chest radiograph, the effusion is most often a transudate caused by congestive heart failure; nephrotic syndrome, hypoalbuminemia, peritoneal dialysis, and constrictive pericarditis also need to be considered. Bilateral exudative effusions occur with malignancy, usually a non-lung primary or lymphoma, lupus pleuritis, and yellow nail syndrome (25).

In patients whose chest radiograph show a pleural effusion with interstitial lung disease, the differential diagnosis includes congestive heart failure, rheumatoid disease, asbestos-induced pleuropulmonary disease, lymphangitic carcinomatosis, lymphangi-oleiomyomatosis (LAM), viral and mycoplasma pneumonia, Waldenstrom macroglob-ulinemia, sarcoidosis, and *Pneumocystis carinii* pneumonia.

Pleural effusions associated with pulmonary nodules suggest metastatic cancer, Wegener granulomatosis, rheumatoid disease, septic pulmonary emboli, sarcoidosis, and tularemia.

C. Pleural Fluid Analysis

Virtually all patients with a newly discovered pleural effusion should have a thoracentesis performed to aid in diagnosis and management. Exceptions would be a secure clinical diagnosis, such as typical congestive heart failure, and a very small volume of pleural fluid, as with viral pleurisy. Observation may be warranted in the above situations; however, if the clinical situation worsens, a thoracentesis should be performed promptly. Only 30 to 50 mL of pleural fluid is needed for complete pleural fluid analysis. An effusion that layers on a lateral decubitus radiograph of at least 10 mm from the inside of the chest wall to the fluid line is generally safe to sample by thoracentesis if the physical examination is confirmatory. Thoracentesis with ultrasound guidance should be used to sample a very small or loculated effusion that is not clearly localized by examination. However, we recommend that pleural ultrasound should be used routinely for all thoracenteses to insure patient safety. Shortly, it will be mandated that pulmonary fellows are competent in pulmonary ultrasonography.

Observation of Pleural Fluid

Some diagnoses can be established immediately at the bedside by visual examination of the fluid (Table 3). For example, if pus is aspirated from the pleural space, the diagnosis of empyema is established, and if the pus has a putrid odor, anaerobic organisms are causative. A chylothorax can be suspected if there is milky fluid; however, this appearance could also be due to empyema or a cholesterol effusion. Centrifugation of the specimen will be helpful, for if the supernatant remains turbid, a lipid effusion (either chylothorax or cholesterol effusion) is likely; if the supernatant clears, the turbidity is caused by a large number of leukocytes. With a frankly bloody effusion, a diagnosis of hemothorax (pleural fluid hematocrit >40–50% of the blood hematocrit) must be excluded as it requires different management than a hemorrhagic effusion (usual PF hematocrit <5%). Brownish, anchovy-paste fluid is virtually diagnostic of an amebic liver abscess that has ruptured through the diaphragm into the right pleural space (26). If the pleural effusion is the color of the enteral feeding or central venous line infusate, the diagnosis that the feeding tube has entered the pleural space (27) and the vascular catheter has migrated out of the vessel (28), respectively, is confirmed. A fluid that appears to contain debris is characteristic of rheumatoid pleurisy (29), and a clear yellow fluid that has the smell of ammonia suggests a urinothorax (30).

Transudates and Exudates

The determination of whether an effusion is a transudate or an exudate is an important diagnostic step in pleural fluid analysis. Because the cause of a transudative effusion is relatively straightforward based on the clinical presentation, the patient typically does not require an extensive diagnostic evaluation (Table 4). In contrast, finding an exudative

Table 3 Observations of Pleural Fluid Helpful in Diagnosis

Color of Fluid	Suggested Diagnosis
Pale yellow (straw)	Transudate, some exudates
Red (bloody)	Malignancy, BAPE, PCIS, or pulmonary infarction in absence of trauma
White (milky)	Chylothorax, cholesterol effusion or empyema
Brown	Long-standing bloody effusion; amebic liver abscess rupture
Black	*Aspergillus niger* infection
Yellow-green	Rheumatoid pleurisy
Color of enteral tube feeding or central venous line infusate	Feeding tube has entered the pleural space; extravascular catheter migration

Character of Fluid	Suggested Diagnosis
Pus	Empyema
Viscous	Mesothelioma
Debris-like	Rheumatoid pleurisy
Turbid	Inflammatory exudate of lipid effusion
Anchovy paste	Amebic liver abscess rupture

Odor of Fluid	Suggested Diagnosis
Putrid	Anaerobic empyema
Ammonia	Urinothorax

BAPE = benign asbestos pleural effusion
PCIS = post cardiac injury syndrome

Table 4 Causes of Transudative Pleural Effusions

Diagnosis	Comment
Congestive heart failure	Acute diuresis can increase PF protein & LDH concentrations into exudative range
Cirrhosis	Can occur without clinical ascites
Nephrotic syndrome	Typically small & bilateral & subpulmonic; with a unilateral effusion consider pulmonary embolism
Peritoneal dialysis	Small right effusion most common one day to eight years after initiating dialysis; acute massive right effusion in women 1 day to two years after initiating dialysis
Hypoalbuminemia	Edema fluid rarely isolated to pleural space; small bilateral effusions
Urinothorax	Unilateral effusion caused by ipsilateral obstructive uropathy
Atelectasis	Small effusion caused by increased intrapleural negative pressure; common in ICU patients
Constrictive pericarditis	Bilateral effusions with normal heart size
Trapped lung	Unilateral effusion from remote inflammatory process
Duropleural fistula	Trauma and surgery most common causes; a subarachnoid-pleural fistula
Ventriculopleural fistula	Pleural fluid is cerebrospinal fluid in uncomplicated fistulas

Table 5 Causes of Exudative Pleural Effusions

Infectious	Malignancy	Connective Tissue Disease
Actinomyces	Carcinoma	Bechet Syndrome
Atypical pneumonias	Chylothorax	Churg-Strauss syndrome
Bacterial pneumonia	Leukemia	Familial Mediterranean Fever
Esophageal rupture, barogenic	Lymphoma	Lupus pleuritis
Fungal disease	Mesothelioma	Mixed connective tissue disease
Hepatic abscess		Rheumatoid pleurisy
Hepatitis	**Other Inflammatory**	Wegener granulomatosis
Nocardia	ARDS	
Parasites	BAPE	**Endocrine Dysfunction**
Subphrenic abscess	Post cardiac injury syndrome	Hypothyroidism
Splenic abscess	Pulmonary infarction	Ovarian hyperstimulation
Tuberculous effusion	Sarcoidosis	syndrome
	Uremic pleurisy	
Iatrogenic		**Lymphatic Abnormalities**
Central venous catheter	**Increased Negative**	Lymphangiectasis
misplacement/migration	**Intrapleural pressure**	Lymphangioleiomyomatosis
Drug-induced	Atelectasis	(chylothorax)
Enteral feeding tube entering	Cholesterol effusion	Yellow nail syndrome
pleural space	Trapped lung	
Esophageal perforation		**Transdiaphragmatic**
Esophageal sclerotherapy		**Movement of Fluid from**
Hemothorax		**Abdomen into Pleura Space**
Radiation pleuritis		Chylous ascites
		Meigs syndrome
Trauma		Pancreatitis, acute
Chylothorax		Pancreatitis, chronic
Hemothorax		Peritoneal carcinomatosis
		Peritoneal lymphomatosis
		Urinothorax

pleural effusion presents a much larger number of possibilities and may be diagnostically problematic, requiring a multiplicity of tests (Table 5).

Exudative effusions, caused predominantly by neoplasms, inflammation, infection, or inflammatory processes or impaired lymphatic pleural space drainage, are characterized by the presence of higher concentrations of large-molecular-weight proteins than transudative effusions, the by-product of hydrostatic and oncotic pressure imbalance. Although an early approach to detect exudates was the measurement of pleural fluid specific gravity, pleural fluid protein later replaced this measurement. However, pleural fluid protein concentration alone has insufficient sensitivity as a screening strategy. Light and colleagues (31) reported the use of pleural fluid protein and LDH values compared to serum values in a combination test. These criteria "established" the presence of an exudate if one or more of three criteria were satisfied. A modification of these three criteria are as follows: (i) a pleural fluid-to-serum protein ratio of >0.5; (ii) a pleural fluid-to-serum lactate dehydrogenase (LDH) ratio of >0.6; and (iii) a pleural fluid LDH concentration

>0.67 of the upper limits of normal for a laboratory's serum LDH value. Heffner and co workers (32), using pooled data from several primary investigations, reported that Light's criteria had a sensitivity of 98% and a specificity of 74% in identifying an exudative effusion. They also reported results from a meta-analysis of over 1400 patients that decision thresholds, determined by receiver operating characteristic (ROC) analysis for separation of transudates and exudates, had a similar cut point for pleural fluid-to-serum protein ratio of >0.5 but a different LDH cut point (>0.45, the upper limits of normal of serum) (21). In a ROC analysis of 200 consecutive patients, Joseph and colleagues (33) found that a PF LDH of >0.82 of the upper limits of normal of the serum LDH had excellent discriminative value. They also noted that, because pleural fluid LDH concentration is not influenced by the serum LDH concentration, there is no basis for using the pleural fluid-to-serum LDH ratio in the diagnostic separation of transudative or exudative pleural effusions. Other investigators have suggested the use of pleural fluid cholesterol as a discriminating test between transudates and exudates and that pleural fluid cholesterol has a lower sensitivity but higher specificity compared with Light's criteria (34–36). It has been suggested, therefore, that pleural fluid cholesterol can be used as a confirmatory test for patients who have a condition usually associated with a transudate, such as congestive heart failure with diuretic therapy, but have an exudate by Light's criteria. Clinicians should understand that pleural fluid values simply enhance or diminish their pretest probability that the fluid is an exudative effusion. The degree of clinical suspicion, whether high or low, should not be affected by a borderline test result.

Total Protein and LDH Concentrations
The total pleural fluid protein concentration may be clinically helpful. For example, a tuberculous pleural effusion rarely has a total protein concentration < 4.0 g/dL, while protein concentrations show a wide range in parapneumonic effusions and carcinomatous and lymphomatous pleural effusions (31). When a total protein concentration of 7.0 to 8.0 g/dL is detected, Waldenstrom macroglobulinemia (37) and multiple myeloma (38) should be considered.

Several features about the pleural fluid LDH may also help in the diagnostic evaluation of a pleural effusion. With a discordant exudate (an exudate by protein but not LDH criterion), the differential should include malignancy, resolving parapneumonic effusion, sarcoidosis, chylothorax, yellow nail syndrome, and a hypothyroid effusion. When an exudate is discordant by LDH only, malignancy (31), parapneumonic effusions (31), and *Pneumocystis carinii* pneumonia should be considered (39). With an upper limit of normal of the serum LDH of 200 IU/L, finding a pleural fluid LDH concentration of >1000 IU/L narrows the differential diagnosis to a complicated parapneumonic effusion or empyema (40,41), rheumatoid pleurisy (42), or pleural paragonimiasis (43); an LDH value >1000 IU/L is less often observed with malignancy and rarely with a tuberculous effusion (31).

Most transudates have nucleated cell counts <500/μL, while most exudates are have >1000 nucleated cells/μL (1,44). The total pleural fluid nucleated cell count is rarely diagnostic; however, counts >50,000/μL are usually seen only in complicated parapneumonic effusions and empyema but can occasionally occur in acute pancreatitis and with a large pulmonary infarction (1,44). Pleural fluid nucleated cell counts >10,000/μL are typically noted in uncomplicated parapneumonic effusions and may occasionally be found with pulmonary infarction, acute pancreatitis, malignancy, tuberculosis, postcardiac injury syndrome, and lupus pleuritis (1,45). Chronic exudates typified by tuberculous pleural effusion and malignancy usually have nucleated cell counts <5000/μL (46,47). When pus is aspirated from the pleural space, the nucleated cell count may be less than anticipated, even as low as a few hundred neutrophils, because the remainder of the neutrophils have undergone autolysis from the harsh environment of a low pH and low oxygen tension. Pus, a yellowish-white, creamy, thick, opaque fluid assumes its appearance because of cellular debris, fibrin, and coagulated pleural fluid.

The timing of thoracentesis in relation to acute pleural injury determines the predominant cellular population. The acute response to pleural injury attracts neutrophils to the pleural space (48). Interleukin-8 (IL-8) is one of the major chemotaxins that attracts neutrophils to the pleural space (49,50). It has been demonstrated that absolute neutrophil counts correlate directly with IL-8 levels, with the highest IL-8 levels being found in purulent effusions (50). With the cessation of acute injury, over the next few days, mononuclear cells move into the pleural space from the peripheral blood, and thus, macrophages become the predominant cell (51). In chronic exudative effusions, the lymphocyte predominates. Therefore, in diseases in which the patient presents shortly after the onset of symptoms, such as bacterial pneumonia, pulmonary embolism with infarction, and acute pancreatitis, neutrophils predominate. In diseases with a more insidious onset, such as malignancy and a tuberculous effusion, the predominant cell is the lymphocyte.

The finding of ≥80% lymphocytes limits the possibilities of the exudative pleural effusion (3) (Table 6). The most common of these diagnoses is a tuberculous pleural effusion (52). Other causes include lymphoma (52), yellow nail syndrome (53), chronic rheumatoid pleurisy (47,54), sarcoidosis (55), trapped lung (56), chylothorax (57), and acute lung rejection (58). All of the above-mentioned diagnoses can occur when the lymphocyte population is <80%; however, the lymphocyte percentage in these effusions is rarely <50%. In contrast to lymphoma, only about 60% of patients with a carcinomatous pleural effusion have lymphocyte populations of >50% to 70% (52). An undiagnosed lymphocytic-predominant exudative effusion is the most appropriate indication for percutaneous pleural biopsy and the most sensitive diagnostic procedure in a tuberculous pleural effusion (59,60). Non-Hodgkin lymphoma and carcinoma, and occasionally sarcoidosis and rheumatoid pleurisy, may be diagnosed by percutaneous pleural biopsy.

Table 6 Pleural Fluid Lymphocyte Predominant (≥80%) Exudates

Disease	Comment
Acute lung rejection	New or increased effusion 2–6 weeks following transplant
Chylothorax	2000–20,000 lymphocytes/μl; lymphoma most common cause
Lymphoma	Often 100% lymphocytes; diagnostic yield on cytology or pleural biopsy higher with non-Hodgkin lymphoma
Rheumatoid pleurisy (chronic)	<5% of patients with RA; males with rheumatoid nodules and low pleural fluid pH and glucose and LDH > 1000 IU/L
Sarcoidosis	Usually >90% lymphocytes; protein discordant exudate
Uremic pleurisy	Typically occurs in patients on dialysis for 1–2 years; tends to resolve in 4–6 weeks spontaneously
Yellow nail syndrome	A cause of a persistent pleural effusion

Table 7 Pleural Fluid Eosinophila (PFE)*

Disease	Comment
Pneumothorax	Tissue eosinophilia an early constant finding
Hemothorax	May take 1–2 weeks for PFE to develop
BAPE	30% incidence; up to 50% eosinophils
Pulmonary embolism	Associated with radiographic infarction and hemorrhagic effusion
Previous thoracentesis	Usually caused by pneumothorax or significant bleeding
Parasitic disease	Paragonimiasis, hydatid disease, amebiasis, ascariasis
Fungal disease	Histoplasmosis, coccidioidomycosis
Drug-induced	Dantrolene, bromocriptine, nitrofurantoin
Lymphoma	Hodgkin disease
Carcinoma	Prevalence of PFE the same in malignant and non-malignant effusions
Churg-Strauss syndrome	PFE is usual finding
Tuberculous effusion	Rare

*PFE = PF eosinophils/total nucleated PF cells ≥10%

Pleural fluid eosinophilia (PFE) is defined as a pleural fluid eosinophil count ≥10% of the total nucleated cell count (Table 7). IL-5 appears to be an important chemotactic factor attracting bone marrow–produced eosinophils into the pleural space (61). In patients who require early thoracotomy for treatment of a spontaneous pneumothorax, eosinophilic pleuritis is commonly encountered (62). While eosinophils appear to move rapidly (within hours) into the pleural space following pneumothorax, in contrast following hemothorax, eosinophils do not to appear in pleural fluid for 7 to 14 days (63). Interestingly, PFE is associated with peripheral blood eosinophilia following trauma that persists until all pleural fluid resolves (64). BAPE is a common cause of PFE, occurring in 30% to 50% of patients, with eosinophil percentages often peaking at 50% (65,66); frequently, these effusions are hemorrhagic. The most common cause of PFE is air or blood in the pleural space (63,67); therefore, pneumothorax, hemothorax, BAPE, pulmonary embolism with infarction, and carcinoma are known causes of pleural fluid eosinophilia. Two recent studies found that the prevalence of PFE was same in malignant and non malignant effusions (68,69). Other causes of PFE include parasitic disease, fungal disease, drug-induced pleurisy, Churg–Strauss syndrome, and Hodgkin lymphoma. A tuberculous effusion is a rare cause of pleural fluid eosinophilia.

Pleural fluid macrophages that originate from the blood monocyte (51) are not of diagnostic value. Mesothelial cells are exfoliated into normal pleural fluid in small numbers. Although mesothelial cells are common in transudative effusions and some exudates, they are rare in a tuberculous effusion probably because of the extensive pleural involvement by the intrapleural hypersensitivity reaction that inhibits mesothelial cells shedding into the pleural space (52,70). This same phenomenon is observed with inflammatory processes, such as empyema, chemical pleurodesis, rheumatoid pleurisy, and chronic malignant effusions.

A large number of plasma cells in pleural fluid suggests multiple myeloma with pleural involvement (38). A small number of plasma cells in serous fluid is non diagnostic and have been observed in a number of non malignant diseases.

Pleural Fluid Glucose and pH

A pleural fluid glucose or pH should be measured on all exudative pleural effusions because it can (i) narrow the differential diagnosis (71–73); (ii) provide management strategies for parapneumonic effusions (40,41,74–76); and (iii) in malignant pleural effusions, provide information relating to the extent of pleural involvement with tumor, ease of diagnosis, prognosis, and management (77–81). A low pleural fluid glucose is defined as a glucose concentration <60 mg/dL with a normal serum glucose or a pleural fluid-to-serum glucose ratio <0.5. A low pleural fluid pH is defined as a pH value <7.30 with a normal blood pH. Normal pleural fluid has a pH of approximately 7.60 (82), transudates have a pH ranging from 7.45 to 7.55, and most exudates have a pH ranging from 7.30 to 7.45 (1,71,73). Therefore, finding a pleural effusion with a pH <7.30 signifies a substantial accumulation of hydrogen ions in the pleural space. There is a direct relationship between pleural fluid pH and glucose; if the pleural fluid pH is low, the glucose is low, and when the pH is normal, the glucose is normal (71,72,76). This correlation suggests that the pathophysiologic processes responsible for this biochemical phenomena are interrelated. The mechanism of the low pH and glucose in a parapneumonic effusion/empyema and esophageal rupture is an increased rate of glucose utilization by neutrophil phagocytosis and bacteria metabolism with the accumulation of the end-products of glycolysis, CO_2, and lactic acid, causing the pH to decrease (83). In contrast, in malignant (84) and rheumatoid (85,86) pleural effusions, the mechanism of the low pH and glucose is related to an abnormal pleural membrane rather than increased metabolic activity in pleural fluid. The abnormally thickened pleura in rheumatoid pleurisy and malignancy creates a barrier to glucose entry into the pleural space and to the efflux of CO_2 and lactic acid causing the glucose and pH to fall. The mechanism in tuberculous and lupus pleuritis has not been extensively studied but probably represents a combination of the above-mentioned mechanisms.

Table 8 shows the usual pleural fluid pH and glucose, as well as the ranges and incidence, in the diagnoses associated with a low pleural fluid pH and glucose. The lowest pH tends to be found in parapneumonic empyema (40,41,73,76) and esophageal rupture (87), both of which can result in an anaerobic empyema. A glucose of zero is found virtually only in rheumatoid pleural effusions (72,85) and empyemas (72). In malignancy, a tuberculous effusion, and lupus pleuritis, the pH and glucose values tend to be higher than

Table 8 Diagnoses Associated with Pleural Fluid Acidosis (pH < 7.30) and Low Glucose Concentration (<60 mg/dL or PF/S < 0.5)

Diagnosis	pH Range (Incidence)	Glucose Range (mg/dL)
CPE/empyema	5.50–7.29 (~100%)	0–40
Esophageal rupture	5.50–7.00 (~100% by 48 hrs)	20–59
Rheumatoid pleurisy	6.80–7.10 (80%)	0–30
Malignancy	6.95–7.29 (33%)	30–59
Tuberculous effusions	7.00–7.29 (20%)	30–59
Lupus pleuritis	7.00–7.29 (20%)	30–59

PF/S = pleural fluid/serum
CPE = complicated parapneumonic effusion

with the aforementioned diagnoses (71–73). Pleural fluid pH should always be measured in a radiometer system.

Pleural Fluid Amylase

The finding of an amylase-rich pleural effusion, defined as a pleural fluid amylase in excess of the upper limits of normal for serum amylase or a pleural fluid/serum amylase >1.0, signifies that the exudative effusion is either due to pancreatic disease (88–91), malignancy (90,92,93), or esophageal rupture (94–96). A pleural fluid high in amylase can be observed with acute or chronic pancreatitis, the latter associated with pseudocyst formation and a fistulous tract into the mediastinum or pleural space. Rare causes of an amylase-rich effusion include pneumonia, ruptured ectopic pregnancy, hydronephrosis, and cirrhosis (90). Several mechanisms are responsible for the formation of a pancreatic pleural effusion and include direct contact of the pancreatic enzymes with the diaphragmatic pleura, movement of ascitic fluid into the pleural space transdiaphragmatically along a pressure gradient (97,98), and movement of fluid through a fistulous tract from the pseudocyst to the pleural space (91), and retroperitoneal movement into the mediastinum creating mediastinitis and eventual rupture into the pleural cavity (99,100). Pleural fluid amylase increases in concentration because of impaired lymphatic pleural space drainage; this mechanism in combination with more rapid clearance of amylase by the kidney is the explanation for the pleural fluid to serum amylase ratio being >1.0.

The pleural fluid amylase may be normal in the early phase of acute pancreatitis but increases over time (88). In chronic pancreatitis, the pleural fluid amylase is always elevated and may reach extremely high levels, often >100,000 IU/L (92). Serum amylase may be elevated due to back-effusion from the pleural space or may be normal (101).

Approximately 10% to 14% of patients with a malignant pleural effusion present with an increased pleural fluid amylase concentration (88,90,93,102). Isoenzyme analysis of these amylase-rich malignant pleural effusions demonstrate that most of the amylase is of the salivary type (88,90,93). The most common malignancy causing a salivary, amylase-rich pleural effusion is adenocarcinoma of the lung with adenocarcinoma of the ovary being the next most frequent (90,93). Other types of lung cancer, as well as lymphoma and leukemia, have also been associated with a salivary-like, amylase-rich pleural effusion (90,93). Clinically, the finding of a salivary isoamylase–rich effusion makes it highly likely that the effusion is due to malignancy in the absence of esophageal rupture. Statistically, the tumor is most likely to be an adenocarcinoma of the lung and not mesothelioma, as the latter tumor has not been reported to be associated with a high salivary amylase level.

Adenosine Deaminase

Adenosine deaminase (ADA), an enzyme important in the degradation of purines, is required for lymphoid cell differentiation and is involved in monocyte-macrophage maturation. Pleural fluid-to-serum ADA ratios >1 have been observed in a tuberculous effusion, rheumatoid pleurisy, and empyema, while other exudates have similar ADA levels in pleural fluid and serum (103). Furthermore, effusions from patients with a tuberculous effusion, rheumatoid pleurisy, and empyema have higher ADA activity than other exudates and congestive heart failure. Pleural fluid ADA levels above 70 U/L are highly suggestive of a tuberculous effusion, while levels below 40 U/L make the diagnosis unlikely (104,105). However, patients with rheumatoid pleuritis may have pleural fluid ADA levels exceeding 70 U/L (106), and high levels have also been found in empyema, lymphoma, and leukemia (107). Recent data suggests that the determination of ADA isoenzymes enhances the diagnostic utility of ADA activity. In tuberculous effusions, ADA2, probably reflecting monocyte/macrophage origin, is responsible for increased ADA content in contrast to ADA1, which originates from lymphocyte or neutrophil turnover, and causes the increased ADA in parapneumonic effusions (108).

Cytologic Examination

Pleural fluid cytologic examination has a positive diagnostic yield in 40% to 90% of patients with pleural malignancy (109,110). An important reason for the variability in diagnostic yield is that the effusion may be paramalignant (111). Paramalignant effusions are effusions associated with a known malignancy but pleural fluid cytology is negative. These effusions can be caused by local effects of the tumor (obstructive atelectasis or pneumonia and impaired lymphatic drainage of the pleural space), systemic effects (pulmonary embolism), and results of therapy (radiation). Other explanations for the variability in cytologic diagnosis include the tumor type, high positivity with adenocarcinoma and low with Hodgkin disease (112), the number of specimens submitted (yields tend to increase with additional specimens due to exfoliation of fresher cells), and the interest and expertise of the cytopathologist (113).

Many serous samples have the tendency to clot making cytologic examination problematic. Pleural fluid should be placed immediately into sterile containers with an anticoagulant; heparin (200 units) is a satisfactory anticoagulant for up to 20 mL of pleural fluid. Although it is preferable to examine the pleural fluid cells immediately, a delay of up to 24 hours generally is not deleterious provided there is no bacterial contamination. The cells in bloody fluid tend to show more rapid deterioration than serous fluids (114). The volume of pleural fluid submitted for cytologic evaluation is probably not critical, as a few milliliters will have a diagnostic value similar to 1000 mL.

References

1. Sahn SA. The pleura. Am Rev Respir Dis 1988; 138:184–234.
2. Collins TR, Sahn SA. Thoracentesis: Complications, patient experience and diagnostic value. Chest 1987; 91:817–811.
3. Sahn SA. Diagnostic value of pleural fluid analysis. Clin Chest Med 1995; 16:269–278.
4. Good JT Jr, King TE, Antony VB, et al. Lupus pleuritis: Clinical features in pleural fluid characteristics with special reference to pleural fluid anti-nuclear antibodies. Chest 1983; 84:714–718.
5. Epler GR, McLoud TC, Gaensler EA. Prevalence and incidence of benign asbestos pleural effusion in a working population. JAMA 1982; 247:617–622.
6. Estenne M, Yernault JC, De Troyer A. Mechanism of relief of dyspnea after thoracentesis in patients with large pleural effusions. Am J Med 1983; 74:813–819.
7. Anthonisen NR, Martin RR. Regional lung function in pleural effusion. Am Rev Respir Dis 1977; 116:201–207.
8. Sahn SA, Heffner JE. Approach to the patient with pleurisy. In: Kelley WN, ed. Textbook of Internal Medicine (2nd ed). Philadelphia, PA: JB Lippincott Co, 1991:1887–1890.
9. Bartlett JG, Finegold SM. Anaerobic infections of the lung and pleural space. Am Rev Respir Dis 1974; 110:56–77.
10. Bynum LJ, Wilson JE III. Radiographic features of pleural effusions in pulmonary embolism. Am Rev Respir Dis 1978; 117:829–834.

11. Stelzner TJ, King TE Jr, Antony VB, et al. Pleuropulmonary manifestations of the post cardiac injury syndrome. Chest 1983; 84:383–387.
12. Bladergroen M, Lowe J, Postlethwaite R. Diagnosis and recommended management of esophageal perforation and rupture. Ann Thorac Surg 1986; 42:235–239.
13. Goode JT Jr, Antony VB, King TE Jr, et al. Lupus pleuritis: Clinical features and pleural fluid characteristics with special reference to anti-nuclear antibody titers. Chest 1983; 84: 714–718.
14. Huggins JT, Doelken P, Sahn SA, et al. Pleural effusions in a series of 181 outpatients with sarcoidosis. Chest 2006; 129:1599–1604.
15. Walker WC, Wright V. Rheumatoid pleuritis. Ann Rheum Dis 1967; 26:464–474.
16. Berger HW, Rammohan G, Neff MS, et al. Uremic pleural effusion. A study in 14 patients on chronic dialysis. Ann Intern Med 1975; 82:362–364.
17. Gopi A, Madhvan H, Sharma S, et al. Diagnosis and treatment of tuberculous pleural effusion in 2006. Chest 2007; 131:880–889.
18. Sahn SA. Drug-induced pleural disease. In: Camus P, Rosenow E (eds.), Drug-Induced Iatrogenic Lung Disease. London: Hodder Arnold. 2009, in press.
19. Hopkins HU. Principles and methods of physical diagnosis (3rd ed). Philadelphia, PA: W.B. Saunders, 1965:202–230.
20. Heidecker J, Sahn SA. The spectrum of pleural effusion after coronary artery bypass grafting surgery. Clin Chest Med 2006; 27:267–283.
21. Mattison L, Coppage L, Alderman D, et al. Pleural effusion in the medical intensive care unit: Prevalence, causes, and clinical implications. Chest 1997; 111:1018–1023.
22. Maher GG, Berger HW. Massive pleural effusions: malignant and non-malignant causes in 46 patients. Am Rev Respir Dis 1972; 105:458–460.
23. Liberson M. Diagnostic significance of the mediastinal profile in massive unilateral pleural effusions. Am Rev Respir Dis 1963; 88:176–180.
24. Heller RM, Janower ML, Weber AL. The radiological manifestations of malignant pleural mesothelioma. Am J Roentgenol 1970; 108:53–59.
25. Rabin CB, Blackman NS. Bilateral pleural effusion. Its significance in association with a heart of normal size. J Mt Sinai Hosp 1957; 24:45–53.
26. Roberts PP. Parasitic infections of the pleural space. Semin Respir Infect 1988; 3:362–382.
27. Miller KS, Tomlinson JR, Sahn SA. Pleuropulmonary complications of enteral tube feedings. Two reports, review of the literature, and recommendations. Chest 1985; 88: 230–233.
28. Ellis LM, Vogel SB, Copeland EM. Central venous catheter vascular erosions. Diagnosis and clinical course. Ann Surg 1989; 209:475–478.
29. Nosanchuk JS, Naylor B. A unique cytologic picture in pleural fluid from patients with rheumatoid arthritis. Am J Clin Pathol 1968; 50:330–335.
30. Stark DD, Shanes JG, Baron RL, et al. Biochemical features of urinothorax. Arch Intern Med 1982; 42:1509–1511.
31. Light RW, MacGregor MI, Luchinger PC, et al. Pleural effusions: The diagnostic separation of transudates and exudates. Ann Intern Med 1972; 77:507–513.
32. Heffner JE, Brown LK, Barbieri C. Diagnostic value of tests that discriminate between exudative and transudative pleural effusions. Chest 1997; 111:970–979.
33. Joseph J, Badrinath P, Basran G, et al. Is the pleural fluid transudate or exudate? A revisit of the diagnostic criteria. Thorax 2001; 56:867–870.
34. Hamm H, Brohan U, Bohmer R, et al. Cholesterol in pleural effusions: A diagnostic aid. Chest 1987; 92:296–302.
35. Costa M, Quiroga T, Cruz E. Measurement of pleural fluid cholesterol and lactate dehydrogenase. A simple and accurate set of indicators for separating exudates from transudates. Chest 1995; 108:1260–1263.

36. Gil Suay V, Martinez Moragon E, Cases Viedma E, et al. Pleural cholesterol in differentiating transudates and exudates. A prospective study of 232 cases. Respiration 1995; 62:57–63.
37. Winterbauer RH, Riggins RCK, Griesman FA, et al. Pleuropulmonary manifestations of Waldenstrom's macroglobulinemia. Chest 1974; 66:368–375.
38. Rodriguez JN, Pereira A, Martinez JC, et al. Pleural effusion in multiple myeloma. Chest 1994; 105:622–624.
39. Horwitz ML, Schiff M, Samuels J, et al. *Pneumocystis carinii* pleural effusion. Pathogenesis and pleural fluid analysis. Am Rev Respir 1993; 148:232–234.
40. Light RW, Girard WM, Jenkinson SG, et al. Parapneumonic effusions. Am J Med 1980; 69:507–511.
41. Potts DE, Levin DC, Sahn SA. Pleural fluid pH in parapneumonic effusions. Chest 1976; 70:328–331.
42. Pettersson T, Klockars M, Helmstrom PE. Chemical and immunological features of pleural effusions: Comparison between rheumatoid arthritis and other diseases. Thorax 1982; 37: 354–361.
43. Johnson JR, Falk A, Iber C, et al. Paragonimiasis in the United States. A report of nine cases in Hmong immigrants. Chest 1982; 82:168–171.
44. Light RW, Erozan YS, Ball WC Jr. Cells in pleural fluid: Their value and differential diagnosis. Arch Intern Med 1973; 132:854–860.
45. Light RW, Pleural Diseases (3rd ed). Baltimore: Williams & Wilkins, 1995:36–74.
46. Berger HW, Mejia E. Tuberculous pleurisy. Chest 1973; 63:88–92.
47. Pettersson T, Riska H. Diagnostic value of total and differential leukocyte counts in pleural effusions. Acta Med Scand 1981; 210:129–135.
48. Antony VB, Repine JE, Sahn SA. Experimental models of inflammation in the pleural space. In: Chretein J, Bignon N, Hirsch A (eds.). The Pleura in Health and Disease. New York: Marcel Dekker, 1985.
49. Antony VB, Godbey SW, Kunkel SL, et al. Recruitment of inflammatory cells to the pleural space. Chemotactic cytokines, IL–8, and monocyte chemotactic peptide–1 in human pleural fluids. J Immunol 1993; 151:7216–7223.
50. Broaddus VC, Hebert CA, Vitangcol RV, et al. Interleukin-8 as a major neutrophil chemotactic factor in the pleural liquid of patients with empyema. Am Rev Respir Dis 1992; 146: 825–830.
51. Antony VB, Sahn SA, Antony AC, et al. Bacillus Calmette-Guerin-stimulated neutrophils release chemotaxins for monocytes in rabbit pleural spaces and in vitro. J Clin Invest 1985; 76:1514–1521.
52. Yam LT. Diagnostic significance of lymphocytes in pleural effusion. Ann Intern Med 1967; 66:972–982.
53. Nordkild P, Kromanr–Andersen H, Struve-Christiensen E. Yellow nail syndrome—the triad of yellow nails, lymphedema, and pleural effusion. Acta Med Scand 1986; 219:221–227.
54. Sahn SA, Kaplan RL, Maulitz RM, et al. Rheumatoid pleurisy. Observation on the development of low pleural fluid pH and glucose levels. Arch Intern Med 1980; 140: 1237–1238.
55. Nicholls AJ, Friend JAR, Legge JS. Sarcoid pleural effusions: Three cases and review of the literature. Thorax 1980; 35:277–281.
56. Doelken P, Sahn SA. Trapped lung. Sem Respir Crit Care Med 2001; 22:631–636.
57. Yoffey JM, Cortice FC. Lymphatics, Lymph, and Lymphoid Tissue. Cambridge: Harvard University Press, 1956; 323–390.
58. Judson MA, Handy JR, Sahn SA. Pleural effusion from acute lung rejection. Chest 1997; 111:1128–1130.
59. Scharer L, McClemant JH. Isolation of tubercle bacilli from needle biopsy specimens of parietal pleura. Am Rev Respir Dis 1968; 97:466–468.

60. Levine H, Metzger W, Lacera D, et al. Diagnosis of tuberculous pleurisy by culture of pleural biopsy specimen. Arch Intern Med 1970; 126:269–271.
61. Nakamura Y, Ozaki T, Yanagawa H, et al. Eosinophil colony-stimulating factor induced by administration of interleuken-2 into the pleural cavity of patients with malignant pleurisy. Am Rev Respir Cell Molecul Biol 1990; 3:291–300.
62. Askin FB, McCann BG, Kuhn C. Reactive eosinophilic pleuritis. Arch Pathol Lab Med 1997; 101:187–191.
63. Spriggs AI, Boddington MM. The Cytology of Effusions (2nd ed). In: New York: Grune & Stratton 1986.
64. Maltais F, Laberge F, Cormier Y. Blood hypereosinophilia in the course of posttraumatic pleural effusion. Chest 1990; 98:348–351.
65. Mattson SB. Monosymptomatic exudative pleurisy in persons exposed to asbestos dust. Scand J Respir Dis 1975; 56:263–272.
66. Hillerdal G, Ozesmi M. Benign asbestos pleural effusion: 73 exudates 160 patients. Eur J Respir Dis 1987; 71:113–121.
67. Adelman M, Albelda SM, Gottlieb J, et al. Diagnostic utility of pleural fluid eosinophilia. Am J Med 1984; 77:915–920.
68. Rubins JB, Rubins HB. Etiology and prognostic significance of eosinophilic pleural effusions. A prospective study. Chest 1996; 110:1271.
69. Martinez-García MA, Cases-Viedma E, Cordero-Rodriguez PJ, et al. Diagnostic utility of eosinophils in the pleural fluid. Eur Respir J 2000; 15:1666–1669.
70. Hurwitz S, Leiman G, Shapiro C. Mesothelial cells in pleural fluid: TB or not TB? So African Med J 1980; 57:937–939.
71. Sahn SA. Pleural fluid pH in the normal state and in diseases affecting the pleural space. In: Chretien J, Bignon N, Hirsch A (eds.). The Pleura in Health and Disease. New York: Marcel Dekker, 1985:253–266.
72. Sahn SA. Pathogenesis and clinical features of diseases associated with a low pleural fluid glucose. In: Chretien J, Bignon N, Hirsch A (eds.). The Pleura in Health and Disease. New York: Marcel Dekker, 1985:267–285.
73. Good JT Jr, Taryle DA, Maulitz RM, et al. The diagnostic value of pleural fluid pH. Chest 1980; 78:55–59.
74. Heffner JE, Brown LK, Barbieri C, et al. Pleural fluid chemical analysis in parapneumonic effusions. A meta-analysis. Am J Respir Crit Care Med 1995; 151:1700–1708.
75. Colice GL, Curtis A, Deslauriers J, et al. Medical and surgical treatment of parapneumonic effusions. Chest 2000; 118:1158–1171.
76. Potts DE, Taryle DA, Sahn SA. The glucose-pH relationship in parapneumonic effusions. Arch Intern Med 1978; 138:1378–1380.
77. Sahn SA, Good JT Jr. Pleural fluid pH in malignant effusions. Diagnostic, prognostic and therapeutic implications. Ann Intern Med 1988; 108:345–349.
78. Rodriguez-Panadero F, Lopez-Mejias J. Low glucose and pH levels in malignant pleural effusions. Diagnostic significance and prognostic value in respect to pleurodesis. Am Rev Respir Dis 1989; 139:663–667.
79. Rodriguez-Panadero F, Lopez-Mejias J. Survival time of patients with pleural metastatic carcinoma predicted by glucose and pH studies. Chest 1989; 95:320–324.
80. Heffner JE, Nietert PJ, Barbieri C. Pleural fluid pH as a predictor of survival for patients with malignant pleural effusions. Chest 2000; 117:79–86.
81. Heffuer JE, Nietert PJ, Barbieri C. Pleural fluid pH as a predictor of pleurodesis failure. Chest 2000; 117:87–95.
82. Sahn SA, Wilcox ML, Good JT Jr, et al. Characteristics of normal rabbit pleural fluid: Physiologic and biochemical implications. Lung 1979; 156:63–69.

83. Sahn SA, Reller LB, Taryle DA, et al. The contribution of leukocytes and bacteria to the low pH of empyema fluid. Am Rev Respir Dis 1983; 128:811–815.
84. Good JT Jr, Taryle DA, Sahn SA. The pathogenesis of low glucose, low pH malignant effusions. Am Rev Respir Dis 1985; 131:737–741.
85. Carr DT, McGuckin WF. Pleural fluid glucose. Am Rev Respir Dis 1968; 97:302–305.
86. Taryle DA, Good JT Jr, Sahn SA. Acid generation by pleural fluid: Possible role in the determination of pleural fluid pH. J Lab Clin Med 1979; 93:1041–1046.
87. Good JT Jr, Antony VB, Reller RB, et al. The pathogenesis of the low pleural fluid pH in esophageal rupture. Am Rev Respir Dis 1983; 127:702–704.
88. Light RW, Ball WC. Glucose and amylase in pleural effusions. JAMA 1973; 225:257–260.
89. Kaye MD. Pleuropulmonary complications of pancreatitis. Thorax 1968; 23:297–306.
90. Joseph J, Viney S, Beck P, et al. A prospective study of amylase-rich pleural effusion with special reference to amylase isoenzyme analysis. Chest 1992; 102:1455–1459.
91. Rockey DC, Cello JP. Pancreaticopleural fistula: a report of 7 cases and review of the literature. Medicine 1990; 69:332–344.
92. Ende N. Studies of amylase activity in pleural effusions and ascites. Cancer 1960; 13: 283–287.
93. Kramer MR, Sepero RJ, Pitchenik AE. High amylase in neoplasm-related pleural effusions. Ann Intern Med 1989; 110:567–569.
94. Abbott OA, Mansour KA, Logan WD Jr, et al. Atraumatic so-called "spontaneous" rupture of the esophagus. A review of 47 personal cases with comments on a new method of surgical therapy. J Thorac Cardiovasc Surg 1970; 59:67–83.
95. Sherr HP, Light RW, Merson MH, et al. Origin of pleural fluid amylase in esophageal rupture. Ann Intern Med 1972; 76:985–986.
96. Maulitz RM, Good JT Jr, Kaplan RL, et al. The pleuropulmonary consequence of esophageal rupture: An experimental model. Am Rev Respir Dis 1979; 120:363–367.
97. Perry TT. Role of lymphatic vessels in the transmission of lipase in disseminated pancreatic lymphatic necrosis. Arch Pathol 1947; 43:456–465.
98. Dumont AE, Doubilet H, Mulholand JH. Lymphatic pathways of pancreatic secretion in man. Ann Surg 1960; 153:403–409.
99. Camaro JL. Chronic pancreatic ascites in pancreatic pleural effusions. Gastroenterol 1978; 74:134–140.
100. Tombroff M, Loick A, Dekoster JP, et al. Pleural effusions with pancreatico-pleural fistula. Br Med J 1973; 1:330–331.
101. Lueng AKC. Pancreatic pleural effusion with normal serum amylase levels. J Royal Soc Med 1985; 78:698.
102. Buckler H, Honeybourne D. Raised pleural fluid amylase level as an aid in the diagnosis of adenocarcinoma of the lung. Br J Clin Pract 1984; 38:359–361, 371.
103. Pettersson T, Kaarina O, Weber TH. Adenosine deaminase in the diagnosis of pleural effusions. Acta Med Scand 1984; 215:299–304.
104. Ocana I, Martinez-Vazquez JM, Segura RM, et al. Adenosine deaminase in pleural fluids. Test for diagnosis of tuberculous pleural effusion. Chest 1983; 84:51–53.
105. Fontan Bueso J, Verea Hernando H, Garcia–Buela JP, et al. Diagnostic value of simultaneous determination of pleural adenosine deaminase and pleural lysozyme/serum lysozyme ratio pleural effusions. Chest 1988; 93:303–307.
106. Ocana I, Ribera E, Martinez-Vazquez JM, et al. Adenosine deaminase activity in rheumatoid pleural effusion. Ann Rheum Dis 1988; 47:394–397.
107. Ungerer JP, Grobler SM. Molecular forms of adenosine deaminase in pleural effusions. Enzyme 1988; 40:7–13.

108. Ungerer JP, Oosthuizen RM, Retief JH, et al. Significance of adenosine deaminase activity and its isoenzymes in tuberculous effusions. Chest 1994; 106:33–37.
109. Grunze H. The comparative diagnostic accuracy, efficacy, and specificity of cytologic techniques used in the diagnosis of malignant neoplasm and serous effusions of the pleuroperitoneal cavities. Acta Cytol 1964; 8:150–164.
110. Jarvi OH, Kunnas RJ, Laitio MT, et al. The accuracy and significance of cytologic cancer diagnosis of pleural effusions. Acta Cytol 1972; 16:152–157.
111. Sahn SA. Malignant pleural effusions. Semin Respir Med 1987; 9:43–53.
112. Naylor B, Schmidt RW. The case for exfoliate cytology of serous effusions. Lancet 1964; 1:711–712.
113. Melamed MR. The cytological presentation of malignant lymphomas and related diseases and effusions. Cancer 1963; 16:413–431.
114. Johnson WD. The cytological diagnosis of cancer in serous effusions. Acta Cytol 1966; 10: 161–172.

14

Discrimination Between Transudative and Exudative Pleural Effusions: Evaluating Diagnostic Tests in the Pleural Space

JOHN E. HEFFNER

Providence Portland Medical Center, Portland, Oregon, U.S.A.

I. Introduction

The initial step in evaluating pleural effusions is performance of a thorough history and physical examination with a review of available imaging and laboratory studies. This evaluation may allow a presumptive diagnosis and therapeutic plan if the patient fits a well-established clinical profile, such as congestive heart failure with an associated right-sided pleural effusion. Conversely, if the etiology of the effusion remains uncertain after initial evaluation or if the effusion fails to respond to a therapeutic trial for a presumed diagnosis, a thoracocentesis is indicated for pleural fluid analysis. Routine pleural fluid tests may diagnose the specific etiology of the effusion as occurs with a positive–pleural fluid Gram stain in patients with an empyema or positive–pleural fluid cytology with a malignant pleural effusion.

The etiologies of many effusions, however, remain uncertain after routine pleural fluid analysis. For such patients, classification of pleural fluid as an exudate or transudate allows clinicians to simplify their differential diagnoses and pursue the more likely diagnoses with further testing (1). An exudative effusion presents a differential diagnosis of various inflammatory and malignant conditions, which usually warrants additional diagnostic testing that may include pleural biopsy. Conversely, the presence of a transudative effusion may limit the need for further pleural evaluations because these effusions are often attributable to clinically apparent conditions, such as congestive heart failure, cirrhosis with ascites, or nephrosis. Accurate classification of effusions, therefore, is fundamentally important in managing patients with pleural disease.

It should be emphasized, however, that classification of an effusion as an exudate or transudate for any individual patient by existing techniques represents an inexact, probabilistic statement of what conditions are more likely than others as potential etiologies of an effusion. As is true for all laboratory tests, clinicians must combine other clinically relevant information about a patient with the results of pleural fluid classification to successfully construct an efficient algorithm for diagnostic evaluation (2). This chapter will review the value and limitations of available approaches for discriminating between exudative and transudative effusions and propose a Bayesian strategy for utilizing this information in patient care, which helps to keep the limitations of pleural fluid classification in mind.

II.   Approaches to Diagnosis and Available Tests

Exudative effusions are defined by the presence of high concentrations of relatively large molecular weight compounds in pleural fluid. Conditions associated with exudative effusions alter pleural membrane permeability and allow large molecules to diffuse from serum into the pleural space or slow the egress of these molecules by blocking pleural lymphatics. Most commonly used tests for classifying effusions measure the concentrations of these compounds in pleural fluid and often compare their results with concentrations measured in serum.

Pleural fluid protein (3) and lactate dehydrogenase (LDH) (4) are the two large molecular weight compounds that were noted nearly 50 years ago to exist in higher concentrations in exudates as compared with transudates. Various diagnostic rules have incorporated pleural fluid protein and LDH in the pursuit of a strategy to classify pleural effusions with the highest possible accuracy. Light's rule is the most commonly used strategy (1) and includes three criteria: (1) a pleural fluid LDH of more than 67% of the upper limits of normal for the laboratory's serum value, (2) a pleural fluid-to-serum LDH ratio >0.6, and (3) a pleural fluid-to-serum protein ratio >0.5 (1). These criteria are used in an "or" rule wherein a positive result for any one criterion defines an exudate.

Many clinical studies find that Light's rule has a sensitivity of 95% to 97%, a specificity of 65% to 80%, and an overall diagnostic accuracy of 88% to 93% for identifying exudates (1,5–7). Because of its high sensitivity, Light's rule performs well as a screening test for detecting nearly all of the exudates that exist in populations of patients undergoing pleural fluid analysis. Screening studies intentionally select cutoff points that promote a high sensitivity so as to avoid missing any patients with the "target condition," which is considered to have the greatest clinical implications for patients. In this instance, the target condition is an exudative effusion, which is considered more important to identify than that of a transudative effusion because of the association of infections and cancer with exudates. Despite the high sensitivity, the identification of a transudative effusion by Light's criteria does not exclude the possibility of a malignant etiology considering that 5% of malignant pleural effusions present with transudates by Light's rule (8).

Due to its only moderate specificity, however, Light's rule misclassifies as exudates 15% to 30% of transudative effusions (6,9,10). This misclassification exposes some patients with true transudates to potential risks of unnecessary diagnostic studies if clinicians over rely on the results of Light's rule without considering a patient's entire clinical picture.

This considerable misclassification of transudative effusions appears to conflict with the frequent promotion of Light's rule as an ideal classification strategy because of its high ~90% overall diagnostic accuracy (11). One should note, however, that this diagnostic accuracy derives at least partly from spectrum effect inherent in the patient populations enrolled in the studies that examined the rule's diagnostic performance. Most of these populations had large proportions of patients with extreme values for pleural fluid test results that were distant from the three criteria's cutoff points (Fig. 1). These extreme values suggest that large proportions of patients had conditions that were associated with clearly established exudates or transudates, which would predictably inflate the diagnostic performance of any laboratory test (12,13). When patients with pleural fluid results closer to the cutoff points of Light's rule are evaluated, the overall diagnostic accuracy of the rule degrades to 65% to 70% (14) (Table 1). Clinicians should not believe, therefore, that

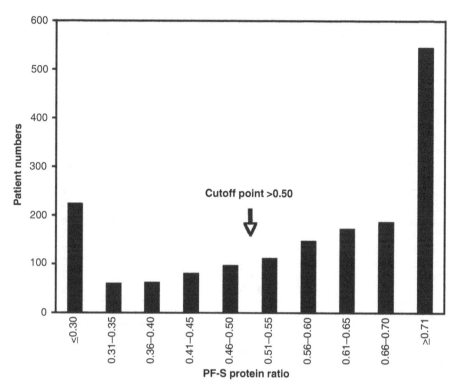

Figure 1 A meta-analysis of 1448 patients demonstrated that most patients evaluated for pleural fluid tests have test results far from cutoff points as shown by these data for the pleural fluid-to-serum (PF-S) protein ratio. Data extracted from Ref. 6.

a diagnostic rule that has a high overall diagnostic accuracy for populations of patients correctly classifies every individual patient with an equivalent degree of accuracy (12).

Another limitation of Light's rule relates to its inclusion of two criteria that are mathematically coupled and, consequently, do not function well when combined in a diagnostic rule due to multicollinearity effects (15). Both the criteria "pleural fluid LDH" and "pleural fluid-to-serum LDH ratio" contain the same term of "pleural fluid LDH." As a result, these two criteria have a high correlation coefficient of 0.84 and essentially analyze pleural fluid for the same biochemical feature, that is, LDH concentration. Heffner and coworkers (6) proposed an "Abbreviated Light's rule" that removes the LDH ratio criterion and thereby simplifies Light's rule that yet maintains a high overall diagnostic accuracy equivalent to the three-criteria rule (6). The high diagnostic accuracy of the Abbreviated Light's rule as compared with the full three-criteria rule was recently confirmed (16).

Elimination of mathematical coupling by using the Abbreviated Light's rule, however, changes the cutoff point for pleural fluid LDH from 67% of the upper limits of normal to 45% when each of Light's rule are examined individually by receiver operating characteristics (ROC) analysis (6). Light's group recently confirmed this lower cutoff

Table 1 A Meta-Analysis of Light's Rule Demonstrates That the Overall Diagnostic Accuracy of the Rule Degrades As Any One Criterion Returns Values Close to Its Cutoff Point

LDH-R ratio	*n*	Diagnostic accuracy (%)
≤0.30	164	94
0.31–0.35	60	95
0.36–0.40	65	92
0.41–0.45	46	83
0.46–0.50	48	65
0.51–0.55	37	73
0.56–0.60	37	76
0.61–0.65	42	76
0.66–0.70	42	71
0.71–0.75	52	79
0.76–0.80	38	76
0.81–0.85	39	85
0.86–0.90	36	89
0.91–0.95	24	92
0.96–1.00	35	97
>1.00	817	98
Total patients	1582	92

In this table, the diagnostic accuracy of Light's rule is shown across the values of pleural fluid-to-serum LDH with the overall accuracy for the entire sample being 92%. LDH-R denotes pleural fluid-to-serum lactate dehydrogenase ratio.
Source: Adapted from Ref. 14.

point using similar ROC techniques in a retrospective analysis of 1490 patients with pleural effusions (17).

The importance of accurate classification of pleural effusions and the moderate specificity of Light's rule have stimulated many investigators to evaluate other pleural fluid tests and diagnostic rules and compare their performance with Light's rule. The goals of these studies are twofold: to develop a test or testing rule that (1) retains the high sensitivity of Light's rule but improves its specificity and/or (2) to improve the rule's clinical utility by decreasing cost or eliminating the need for companion serum tests as required by Light's rule.

Examined tests include pleural fluid-to-serum albumin ratio (5,9), pleural fluid cholesterol (18–23), pleural fluid-to-serum cholesterol ratio (9,19–22), pleural fluid-to-serum bilirubin ratio (9,24), pleural fluid-to-serum cholinesterase ratios (25), cell-free DNA (26), and a host of other tests that include aspartate transaminase, interleukin-1β, uric acid, C-reactive protein, alanine transaminase, alkaline phosphatase, creatinine kinase, ferritin, interleukin-8, tumor necrosis factor-α, and γ-glutamyltransferase to name a few (2). The cutoff points established for the most commonly proposed tests are shown in Table 2. The cutoff points for tests utilizing pleural fluid cholesterol differ between reports because of the small sample sizes of the primary studies. Our group published a meta-analysis of these primary studies using patient-level data provided by the primary

Table 2 Cutoff Points Proposed for Various Pleural Fluid Tests

Test	Reported cutoff points	Meta-analysis cutoff points (6)
Pleural fluid protein (g/dL)	>3 (42)	>2.9
Pleural fluid-to-serum protein ratio	>0.5 (43)	>0.5
Pleural fluid LDH	>0.67 upper limits of normal (43) >0.47 upper limit of normal (17)	>0.45 of upper limits of normal
Pleural fluid-to-serum LDH ratio	>0.6 (43)	>0.6
Pleural fluid cholesterol (mg/dL)	>54 (21) >55 (22) >60 (19,20,23)	>45
Pleural fluid-to-serum cholesterol ratio	>0.3 (9,19)	>0.3
Albumin gradient (g/dL)	≤1.2 (5,9)	≤1.2
Pleural fluid-to-serum bilirubin ratio	>0.6 (9,24)	>0.6

Source: Adapted from Ref. 6.

investigators and reported cutoff points for the aggregate population of 1448 patients (6) (Table 2).

Our meta-analysis demonstrated that most of the evaluated pleural tests have similar diagnostic performance compared with the individual criteria of Light's rule, as demonstrated by overlapping 95% confidence intervals (Table 3) (6). A more recent series of 471 patients examined by ROC analysis demonstrated similar equivalency of pleural fluid tests (23). This result is expected considering the shared biologic rationale of these tests, which is the detection of large molecular weight compounds in exudative pleural fluid.

As investigators have proposed new diagnostic tests, such as pleural fluid cholesterol, commentators have often compared the diagnostic accuracy of each new test with the full three-criteria Light's rule and found Light's rule to have a higher sensitivity albeit the new test might have a higher specificity. This observation, however, is expected considering the reciprocal relationship of sensitivity with specificity and the impact of combining individual tests in "or" rules, which will be discussed later.

III. Measures of Diagnostic Accuracy

A. Sensitivity and Specificity

Sensitivity describes the proportion of patients with the target condition (exudate) who are correctly classified by a positive test result. Specificity is the proportion of patients without the target condition (a transudate) who have a negative test result. Although sensitivity and specificity are commonly reported to profile the performance of tests, these terms actually provide the clinician with limited information as to how a positive or negative

Table 3 Diagnostic Accuracy of Individual Pleural Fluid Tests

Pleural fluid test	Sensitivity (%) (95% CI)	Specificity (%) (95% CI)	+PV (%) (95% CI)	−PV (%) (95% CI)	AUC (95% CI)
P-PF, $n = 1187$	91.5 (89.3–93.7)	83.0 (77.6–88.4)	94.6 (93.8–97.1)	75.0 (69.1–80.9)	94.2 (92.6–95.9)
P-R, $n = 1393$	89.5 (87.4–91.6)	90.9 (87.4–94.5)	96.9 (95.6–98.1)	73.3 (68.4–78.1)	95.4 (94.3–96.7)
LDH-PF, $n = 1438$	88.0 (85.8–90.3)	81.8 (77.1–86.6)	93.9 (92.2–95.6)	68.3 (63.1–73.6)	93.3 (91.8–94.8)
LDH-R, $n = 1388$	91.4 (89.4–93.3)	85.0 (80.6–89.4)	95.1 (93.5–96.6)	75.7 (70.7–80.7)	94.7 (93.4–96.0)
C-PF, $n = 1348$	89.0 (86.8–91.2)	81.4 (76.6–86.2)	93.8 (92.1–95.5)	70.1 (64.8–75.3)	93.3 (91.7–94.8)
C-R, $n = 1123$	92.0 (90.1–93.9)	81.4 (76.6–86.2)	94.0 (92.3–95.7)	76.3 (71.2–81.4)	94.1 (92.5–95.7)
A-G, $n = 386$	86.8 (82.2–91.4)	91.8 (86.4–97.3)	95.8 (93.0–98.7)	76.3 (68.6–83.9)	94.0 (91.3–96.6)
BILI-R, $n = 303$	84.3 (79.3–89.3)	61.1 (51.2–70.9)	82.3 (77.1–87.5)	64.4 (54.6–74.3)	81.3 (76.3–86.4)

Abbreviations: AUC, area under the curve; P-PF, pleural fluid protein; P-R, pleural fluid-to-serum protein ratio; LDH-PF, pleural fluid LDH; LDH-R, pleural fluid-to-serum LDH ratio; C-PF, pleural fluid cholesterol; C-R, pleural fluid-to-serum cholesterol ratio; A-G, pleural fluid-to-serum albumin gradient; BILI-R, pleural fluid-to-serum bilirubin ratio; PV, predictive value; CI, 95% confidence interval.
Source: Adapted from Ref. 6.

test result increases or decreases the probability that a patient has an exudative effusion (27,28). If a test has 100% sensitivity, a *negative* test *rules out* the target condition. If a test has 100% specificity, a *positive* test *rules* in the target condition. Lower values for sensitivity and specificity leave clinicians in varying degrees of uncertainty about the clinical meaning of any test result.

Also, the actual values of sensitivity and specificity for any diagnostic test are reciprocally interrelated, which has created confusion in the literature regarding the relative merits of the three-criteria Light's rule as compared with competing single pleural fluid tests. As stated earlier, Light's rule has been described as having a higher sensitivity but lower specificity as compared with other pleural fluid tests (1,7). This observation, however, results from the reciprocal linkage of sensitivity with specificity rather than any unique attributes of Light's rule. When a combination of two or more tests are used with an "or" rule, as is done with Light's rule, the chance of identifying patients with the target condition (i.e., exudative effusion or "true positives") increases, which raises the test's sensitivity. The cost of raising sensitivity includes the increased probability that patients without the target condition will be misidentified as having the condition (i.e., patients with transudates misclassified as having exudates, "false positives"). Increasing the false-positive rate necessarily lowers the test's specificity. Light's rule, therefore, would be expected to have a lower specificity as compared with diagnostic approaches that use a single pleural fluid test even if the *single* test has the same diagnostic performance as each of the three tests that compose Light's rule. Indeed, the reason Light's rule combines three tests in an "or" rule is to increase sensitivity beyond the measured sensitivity of each of its individual criteria.

It follows, therefore, that efforts to identify a single pleural fluid test with an equivalent sensitivity but higher specificity than Light's rule will be challenging because of the inherent advantage of "or" combination rules in inflating sensitivity. A new single test, however, might appear to have a higher specificity than Light's rule only because combination "or" rules sacrifice specificity so as to increase sensitivity. This sacrifice of specificity by Light's rule to improve its function as a screening test explains why it misclassifies 15% to 30% of transudates as exudates, as previously mentioned.

One could wonder, however, if other combinations of pleural fluid tests combined in "or" rules could provide a higher or equivalent sensitivity with a higher specificity as compared with Light's rule. Our meta-analysis of 1448 patients compared the diagnostic performance of all permutations of the tests reported in Table 3 and found that many combinations had similar and, for some, higher performance as compared with Light's rule but none demonstrated major diagnostic improvements to a clinically important degree (6).

This result is expected, however, considering the similar diagnostic performance of most of the individual criteria (including those in Light's rule) reported. More of the recent studies have similarly demonstrated marginal improvements in diagnostic accuracy of various test combination rules as compared with Light's rule (23). It appears, therefore, that it will be difficult if not impossible to develop new tests combined in "or" rules that supercede Light's rule, as sought by the first goal of examining tests stated above.

But the second goal of this line of research is to identify test rules with greater clinical utility or ease of use as compared with Light's rule. Our meta-analysis (6) and another recent study (23) demonstrated that several combinations of tests, which did not require serum samples, combined in an "or" rule favorably compared to Light's rule (Table 4). It is possible, therefore, to simplify pleural fluid analysis with the use of these new rules without losing diagnostic performance.

Table 4 Relative Diagnostic Performance of Pleural Fluid Test Combinations Used in "Or" Rules for Identifying Exudative Pleural As Compared with Light's Rule

Pleural fluid test	Sensitivity (%)	Specificity (%)	+PV (%)	−PV (%)
P-PF or LDH-PF	94.0	75.1	92.3	79.8
P-PF or C-PF	94.9	78.7	93.4	82.9
LDH-PF or C-PF	97.5	71.9	91.7	90.1
P-PF or LDH-PF or C-PF	98.4	70.4	91.3	93.2
P-R or LDH-PF or LDH-R[a]	97.9	74.3	92.3	91.7

Although the alternative test rules do not require serum samples, they perform as well as Light's rule. Data extracted from Ref. 6.
[a]Denotes Light's rule. The cutoff point for exudates for pleural fluid cholesterol (C-PF) was >45 mg/dL.
Abbreviations: P-PF, pleural fluid protein; P-R, pleural fluid-to-serum protein ratio; LDH-PF, pleural fluid LDH; LDH-R, pleural fluid-to-serum LDH ratio; C PF, pleural fluid cholesterol; PV, predictive value.

B. Positive and Negative Predictive Values

Considering the limitations of sensitivity and specificity, many clinicians prefer to consider the positive and negative predictive values of tests as a more clinically useful measures of diagnostic performance. The positive predictive value describes the proportion of patients with a positive test who have the target condition (i.e., an exudative effusion). The negative predictive value describes the proportion of patients with a negative test who do not have the target condition (i.e., a transudative effusion). Knowledge of the positive and negative predictive values of a test allows clinicians to use the test result for estimating the probability that a patient has the target condition and represents an advancement over the information provided by knowledge of a test's sensitivity and specificity. As shown in Tables 3 and 4, the positive and negative predictive values of various pleural fluid tests and test combinations compare favorably with each other and Light's rule.

Predictive values present problems in clinical practice, however, because they are influenced by the prevalence of the target disorder in the tested population. Our meta-analysis of primary studies comprised a population wherein 75% of patients who undergo diagnostic thoracocentesis had exudates (6). The predictive values of pleural fluid tests listed in Table 3 are based on a 75% prevalence of exudative effusions in the tested population. If thoracocentesis is performed in populations of patients with a different prevalence of exudates as compared with transudates, clinicians cannot assume that positive and negative test results signify the positive and negative predictive values listed in Table 3.

A fundamental limitation of Light's rule and similar combination "or" rules relates to their dichotomization of test results into binary classifications of "exudates present" or "exudates absent" (i.e., the latter being equivalent to "transudate present") (29). Pleural fluid tests generate results along a continuous range of numeric values, which require cutoff points to dichotomize patients into two groups. Patients with extreme test results toward the exudative range and those with values just across the exudative cutoff point are all classified the same even though the probability of correct classification as an exudate is greater for patients with extreme values. Consequently, most of the rich diagnostic information contained in the continuous numeric test results is lost in the dichotomization process. Pleural experts are aware of the clinical importance of this lost information in their discussions of the varying differential diagnoses that exist with increasing pleural fluid concentrations of protein and LDH (30). Exudative effusions due to tuberculous pleurisy, for instance, rarely have pleural fluid values below 4 g/dL while congestive heart failure effusions misclassified by Light's rule as exudates have pleural fluid proteins just on the exudative side of the cutoff point (30). Some quantitative measure is needed to capture this information contained within continuous numeric pleural fluid test results to assist clinicians in estimating the likelihood that an exudative effusion exists and the differential diagnoses presented by the tests' results. This information can be gleaned by considering likelihood ratios.

C. Likelihood Ratios

Likelihood ratios measure test performance in a manner that captures all of the information contained in numeric test results and provide clinicians with the probability that a target condition (i.e., exudates) actually exists. Likelihood ratios quantify the likelihood of a given test result in patients with a condition compared with the likelihood of the same result in patients without the condition (29,31). In contrast to predictive values, likelihood ratios do not depend on the prevalence of the target condition in the test population.

Likelihood ratios can be calculated as binary likelihood ratios (above and below the cutoff point for exudates), as multilevel likelihood ratios (above or below multiple levels along a continuum of test results), or as continuous likelihood ratios (as a function of every possible test result along the numeric test result continuum) (Table 5). Multilevel and continuous likelihood ratios, in contrast to other measures of test performance, provide information about how much various test results along a continuum of results increase or decrease the probability that a patient has an exudative effusion (Fig. 2). Likelihood ratios above a value of 1 increase the likelihood that an exudate exists, and ratios below 1 decrease the probability of an exudate making a transudate more likely.

Table 5 Method for Calculating Likelihood Ratios

P-R result	Exudates, *n*	Transudates, *n*	Multilevel LR
≥0.71	544	2	93.03
0.66–0.70	186	2	31.80
0.61–0.65	161	13	4.24
0.56–0.60	136	13	3.58
0.51–0.55	92	21	1.50
0.46–0.50	57	41	0.48
0.41–0.45	36	46	0.27
0.36–0.40	19	44	0.15
0.31–0.35	10	51	0.07
≤0.30	25	200	0.04
Total	1266	433	

LRs are calculated by separating patients into multiple levels grouped by strata of test results and by target conditions (e.g., exudates and transudates). Likelihood ratios are then derived by the proportion of total exudates within a strata divided by the total transudates within the same strata. For instance, the LR for effusions with a pleural fluid-to-serum protein ratio >0.71 is (544/1266)/(2/433) = 93.03.
Abbreviations: P-R, pleural fluid-to-serum protein ratio; LR, likelihood ratio.
Source: Adapted from Ref. 14.

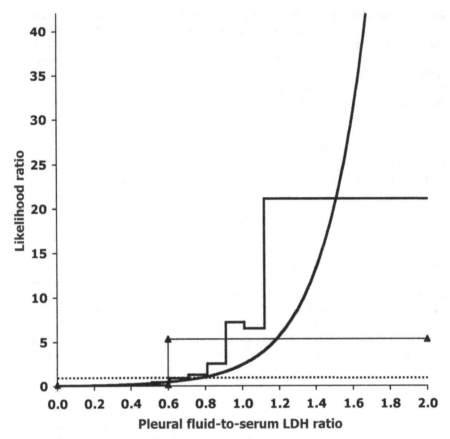

Figure 2 Binary (*bilevel straight lines*), multilevel (*staircase straight lines*), and continuous likelihood ratios (*exponential curve*) as functions of pleural fluid-to-serum (PF-S) LDH. Continuous likelihood ratios represent the most accurate values for discrete measures of pleural fluid tests. As shown, binary estimates of likelihoods, as contained in the dichotomous Light's rule overestimate near the cutoff point and underestimate at high values of the LDH ratio the actual likelihood ratio value. Multilevel likelihood ratios should progressively increase in value as PF-S LDH increases; the example shown dips in value at a PF-S LDH value of 1.0 because of vagaries of the dataset used. *Source*: Adapted from Ref. 14.

Clinicians use likelihood ratios to modulate the degree to which their pretest suspicion of an exudate is altered by a test result. To do so, physicians first estimate the pretest probability of an exudative effusion based on the patient's clinical presentation (32). For instance, a 50-year-old patient with congestive heart failure and a slowly resolving pleural effusion after diuretic therapy might be thought most likely to have a transudative effusion. Because the patient is also a heavy smoker, a clinician might also be concerned about an atypical presentation of a malignant effusion. The clinician's suspicion would probably remain low for an exudate, however, in this setting of heart failure, and the clinician might estimate the pretest probability of an exudate at only ~10%. This pretest probability can be transformed to pretest odds by the following equation: pretest odds = pretest probability/(1.00 − pretest probability), which, in this example, would be 0.11 [i.e., 0.10/(1.00 − 0.10)].

Posttest odds can be calculated by multiplying pretest odds by the likelihood ratio of the test result. For this example, the first pleural fluid test result obtained by the clinician was a pleural fluid-to-serum protein ratio of 0.6. By Light's rule, even without knowledge of the results of the other two Light's criteria, the effusion would be classified as an exudate. Because the clinician might remain convinced that heart failure undergoing diuresis was the cause of the effusion, the physician would be tempted to classify the effusion as an exudate and pursue additional diagnostic evaluations. Some experts would recommend follow up pleural fluid tests in this setting, such as measurement of the albumin gradient (1).

Multilevel or continuous likelihood ratios, however, provide a more accurate classification of the effusion than a binary approach. Referring to a source of multilevel likelihood ratios for different pleural fluid tests, the clinician would find that the likelihood ratio for a pleural fluid-to-serum protein ratio test result of 0.55 would be 1.50 (Table 5). This value indicates that a test result of 0.55 increases the pretest odds of an exudate by a factor of only 1.50. This low value for the likelihood ratio would be expected because the test result of 0.55 is only slightly higher than the cutoff point (0.5) for protein ratios, when these tests are used in the traditional dichotomous manner of Light's rule. The pretest odds of 0.11 is multiplied by 1.50 to give the posttest odds of 0.17. Because clinicians find probabilities more easily interpretable, the posttest probability can be calculated by the following equation: posttest probability = posttest odds/(posttest odds + 1.00). This equation computes a posttest probability of an exudative effusion of 0.15 or 15%. Since the probability of an exudate is only 15%, the clinician would conclude that the patient most likely (85% likelihood) has a transudate. Even though the test was "positive" for an exudate by the traditional Light's rule, the borderline positive result did not raise the clinician's pretest estimation of the probability of an exudate sufficiently to alter the diagnosis of a transudative effusion due to congestive heart failure and initiate additional diagnostic studies.

Likelihood ratios progressively increase or decrease the further a test result is above or below the cutoff point used to determine a "positive" or "negative" test result. Test results near the cutoff point result in likelihood ratios close to 1, which alter the pretest probability of the target condition to only marginal degrees. Extremely high or low results generated by test results far beyond the cutoff points produce extremely high or low likelihood ratios, which have a large effect in changing the pretest probability of disease. Likelihood ratios calculated at many points along test result values, therefore, provide the clinician with more information regarding the meaning of a test result as compared with strategies that bin both borderline and extreme test results into dichotomous categories of "condition present" (exudate) and "condition absent" (transudate) (31–33).

To demonstrate the value of this added information for the previous example, now consider that the pleural fluid-to-serum protein ratio was much higher than 0.55, such as 0.72, which is associated with a multilevel likelihood ratio of 93 (Table 5). Repeating the same calculations with this new likelihood ratio yields a posttest probability of an exudate of 94% (posttest odds = 0.17 × 93 = 15.8; posttest probability = 15.8/(1 + 15.8) = 0.94). With this second laboratory result, the clinician would more confidently diagnose an exudate and initiate further evaluation for a malignancy despite the presence

Table 6   Use of Likelihood Ratios to Calculate Posttest Probability Using Results of Three
Tests That Measure Protein and Lactate Dehydrogenase (LDH) in Serum and Pleural Fluid
Samples (Light's rule)

Pleural fluid results
  Pleural fluid-to-serum protein ratio = 0.46
  Pleural fluid LDH (fraction of lab normal) = 0.63
  Pleural fluid-to-serum LDH ratio = 0.72
Calculation of posttest probability
  Pretest probability of an exudate = 25%
  Pretest odds = pretest probability/(1.00−pretest probability) = 0.25/(1.00−0.25) = 0.33
  Pleural fluid protein ratio likelihood ratio (LR) = 0.48
  Posttest odds$_1$ = pretest odds × LR = 0.33 × 0.48 = 0.16
  Pleural fluid LDH likelihood ratio = 1.69
  Posttest odds$_2$ − 0.16 × 1.69 = 0.27
  Pleural fluid LDH ratio likelihood ratio = 1.27
  Posttest odds$_3$ = 0.27 × 1.27 = 0.34
  Posttest probability of an exudate = posttest probability/(1.00 + posttest probability) =
    0.34/(1.00 + 0.34) = 0.25 = 25%

Likelihood ratios were obtained from values reported in Ref. 14.

of heart failure. In both examples, the pleural fluid test was "positive" for an exudate by
Light's rule, but only the second example was established as exudative when evaluated
by likelihood ratios.

Likelihood ratios from different tests can be combined in a serial manner to increase
diagnostic certainty if each of the tests is independent of the others. In the instance of the
three-criteria Light's rule, a clinician may decide to use the likelihood ratios attached to
each of the three criteria's test results to calculate posttest odds in a serial manner (Table
6). The example in Table 6 presents a patient classified by Light's rule with an exudate.
Serial application of likelihood ratios in this example, however, shows that test results
do not change the clinician's low 25% pretest suspicion of an exudate. We should again
emphasize that tests must be independent of each other to be used serially. Because the two
criteria in Light's rule that use LDH are mathematically coupled, they should not be used
serially. The two criteria in the Abbreviated Light's rule, however, can be used serially.

The above discussion is not intended to encourage physicians to perform the necessary calculations to use Bayesian equations and likelihood ratios in everyday clinical
practice for evaluating pleural effusions. Although the availability of handheld and ward
computers make use of these simple arithmetic tools feasible, the major limitation of this
approach is the absence of quantitative scoring systems that assist clinicians in estimating pretest probabilities of exudative effusions from available clinical information. This
limitation, however, is not insurmountable considering advances made for other medical
conditions. For instance, the diagnosis of deep venous thrombosis has been greatly assisted
by validated scoring systems, such as the Wells score, that assist clinicians in constructing
quantitative pretest probabilities (34). Also, specialized techniques, such as classification
and regression tree (CART) analysis that incorporate clinical factors in addition to pleural
fluid results in sequential manners, have been shown to improve classification of pleural
effusions and will eventually become bedside informatics resources (35). The primary

purpose of understanding multilevel and continuous likelihood ratios is to gain insight into the marginal value of pleural fluid test results when they return values close to their cutoff points.

Other limitations to the use of likelihood ratios relate to the quality of the primary studies that examine the diagnostic accuracy of pleural fluid tests. Such studies are difficult to perform rigorously because no gold standard test exists to classify effusions as exudative and transudative. Consequently, various clinical studies (lung scans, echocardiographic examinations, pleural biopsies) are performed on subsets of study patients to establish the underlying disease (e.g., heart failure, lung cancer, pulmonary embolism). Once the underlying condition is diagnosed, effusions are categorized as the type (exudate or transudate) that is typically associated with the underlying condition. In almost all studies, different batteries of tests and imaging studies were applied to different patients based on their clinical presentation. This verification bias results in considerable uncertainties regarding study patients' underlying diagnoses and true pleural fluid classifications (36).

Other limitations of existing studies pertain to deficiencies in study design. Although standards for evaluating diagnostic tests are well described (37), these standards have been incompletely applied in most studies that examine the diagnostic accuracy of pleural fluid tests (6,12,38).

IV. Conclusions

Pleural tests and diagnostic rules do not establish the exudative or transudative nature of a pleural effusion with a high degree of certainty for an individual patient. Classification of an effusion is only a "point of departure" for evaluating an effusion and should be considered a probabilistic statement that helps to trim the differential diagnosis. Clinicians should consider their level of confidence in making such probabilistic statements to determine the need for additional testing and the appropriateness of therapeutic interventions. Most of the available pleural fluid tests and combination test rules have similar diagnostic performance. If the patient's clinical features do not match the test results, clinicians should pursue alternative diagnoses and recall that pleural fluid tests only alter the pretest probability of a diagnosis given the clinical information that the clinician already has at hand (29,39).

Although tradition supports the ongoing use of Light's rule, other rules have similar diagnostic value and some have greater clinical utility because they obviate the need for serum testing. If Light's rule is used, the "abbreviated" rule is preferred because of the multicollinearity of the two LDH-based Light's criteria. The cutoff for the pleural fluid LDH criterion in the abbreviated rule is 45% of the laboratory normal value. If clinicians choose to avoid serum testing, other combination rules, such as the two-criteria rule that combines pleural fluid protein and cholesterol or the three-criteria rule that combines pleural fluid protein, cholesterol, and LDH have high diagnostic accuracy (6). As occurs with all "or" rules, the addition of each new criterion likely increases sensitivity at the expense of decreasing specificity.

The use of multilevel likelihood ratios rather than binary classification rules will improve diagnostic accuracy in classifying pleural effusions, but their application in clinical practice awaits validation of clinical scoring systems that aid clinicians in estimating pretest probabilities of an exudate. Understanding their use, however, provides insight into the limitations of binary classification systems, such as Light's rule, that do not incorporate all of the information contained within numeric continuous test result data.

In the future, advances in pleural fluid testing will most likely obviate the utility of rules that classify pleural effusions as exudates or transudates. Polymerase chain reaction techniques, for instance, offer opportunities to identify pathogens in pleural fluid (40) and evidence of neoplastic cell changes associated with malignant pleural effusions (41). As techniques for making specific etiologic diagnoses for pleural effusions advance our reliance on simple classification schema will diminish. In the meantime, clinicians should have a clear understanding of the value and limitations of pleural fluid analysis.

References

1. Light RW. Pleural Disease, 5th ed. Philadelphia, PA: Lippincott Williams & Wilkins, 2007.
2. Heffner JE. Discriminating between transudates and exudates. Clin Chest Med 2006; 27:241–252.
3. Carr DT, Power MH. Clinical value of measurement of concentration of protein in pleural fluid. N Engl J Med 1958; 259:926–927.
4. Chandrasekhar AJ, Palatao A, Dubin A, et al. Pleural fluid lactic acid dehydrogenase activity and protein content. Arch Intern Med 1969; 123:48–50.
5. Roth BJ, O'Meara TF, Cragun WH. The serum-effusion albumin gradient in the evaluation of pleural effusions. Chest 1990; 98:546–549.
6. Heffner JE, Brown LK, Barbieri CA. Diagnostic value of tests that discriminate between exudative and transudative pleural effusions. Primary Study Investigators. Chest 1997; 111:970–980.
7. Romero S, Martinez A, Hernandez L, et al. Light's criteria revisited: Consistency and comparison with new proposed alternative criteria for separating pleural transudates from exudates. Respiration 2000; 67:18–23.
8. Ashchi M, Golish J, Eng P, et al. Transudative malignant pleural effusions: Prevalence and mechanisms. South Med J 1998; 91:23–26.
9. Burgess L, Maritz FJ, Taljaard JJF. Comparative analysis of the biochemical parameters used to distinguish between pleural transudates and exudates. Chest 1995; 107:1604–1609.
10. Vives M, Porcel JM, Vicente de Vera M, et al. A study of Light's criteria and possible modifications for distinguishing exudative from transudative pleural effusions. Chest 1996; 109:1503–1507.
11. Lee YC, Davies RJ, Light RW. Diagnosing pleural effusion: Moving beyond transudate–exudate separation. Chest 2007; 131:942–943.
12. Heffner JE. Evaluating diagnostic tests in the pleural space. Differentiating transudates from exudates as a model. Clin Chest Med 1998; 19:277–293.
13. Mulherin SA, Miller WC. Spectrum bias or spectrum effect? Subgroup variation in diagnostic test evaluation. Ann Intern Med 2002; 137:598–602.
14. Heffner JE, Highland K, Brown LK. A meta-analysis derivation of continuous likelihood ratios for diagnosing pleural fluid exudates. Am J Respir Crit Care Med 2003; 167:1591–1599.
15. Katz MH. Multivariable analysis. A practical guide for clinicians, 1st ed. Cambridge, MA: University Press, 1999.
16. Gonlugur U, Gonlugur TE. The distinction between transudates and exudates. J Biomed Sci 2005; 12:985–990.
17. Porcel JM, Pena JM, Vicente de Vera C, et al. Bayesian analysis using continuous likelihood ratios for identifying pleural exudates. Respir Med 2006; 100:1960–1965.
18. Costa M, Quiroga T, Cruz E. Measurement of pleural fluid cholesterol and lactate dehydrogenase. A simple and accurate set of indicators for separating exudates from transudates. Chest 1995; 108:1260–1263.
19. Hamm H, Brohan U, Bohmer R, et al. Cholesterol in pleural effusions. A diagnostic aid. Chest 1987; 92:296–302.

20. Romero S, Candela A, Martín C, et al. Evaluation of different criteria for the separation of pleural transudates from exudates. Chest 1993; 104:399–404.
21. Suay VG, Moragón EM, Viedma EC, et al. Pleural cholesterol in differentiating transudates and exudates. A prospective study of 232 cases. Respiration 1995; 62:57–63.
22. Valdés L, Pose A, Suàrez J, et al. Cholesterol: A useful parameter for distinguishing between pleural exudates and transudates. Chest 1991; 99:1097–1102.
23. Leers MP, Kleinveld HA, Scharnhorst V. Differentiating transudative from exudative pleural effusion: Should we measure effusion cholesterol dehydrogenase? Clin Chem Lab Med 2007; 45:1332–1338.
24. Meisel S, Shamiss A, Thaler M, et al. Pleural fluid to serum bilirubin concentration ratio for the separation of transudates and exudates. Chest 1990; 98:141–144.
25. Garcia Pachon E, Padilla Navas I, Molina Siles M, et al. Pleural fluid to serum cholinesterase ratio to discriminate between transudates and exudates: Reevaluation in 177 patients. Rev Clin Esp 1998; 198:129–132.
26. Chan MH, Chow KM, Chan AT, et al. Quantitative analysis of pleural fluid cell-free DNA as a tool for the classification of pleural effusions. Clin Chem 2003; 49:740–745.
27. Sheps SB, Schechter MT. The assessment of diagnostic tests: A survey of current medical research. JAMA 1984; 252:2418–2422.
28. Riegelman RK, Hirsch RP. Studying a Study and Testing a Test. How to Read the Medical Literature, 2 ed. Boston, MA: Little Brown and Co., 1989.
29. Sox HC, Blatt MA, Higgins MC, et al. Medical Decision Making. Philadelphia, PA: American College of Physicians, 2007.
30. Sahn SA, Heffner JE. Pleural fluid analysis. In: Light RW, Lee GYC, eds. Textbook of Pleural Diseases. London, U.K.: Arnold, 2003:191–209.
31. Jaeschke R, Guyatt G, Sackett D. Users' guides to the medical literature. III. How to use an article about a diagnostic test. JAMA 1994; 271:703–707.
32. Sackett DL, Straus SE, Richardson WS, et al. Evidence-based medicine. How to practice and teach EBM, 2nd ed. Edinburgh, U.K.: Churchill Livingstone, 2000.
33. Heffner JE, Sahn SA, Brown LK. Multilevel likelihood ratios for identifying exudative pleural effusions. Chest 2002; 121:1916–1920.
34. Goodacre S, Stevenson M, Wailoo A, et al. How should we diagnose suspected deep-vein thrombosis? QJM 2006; 99:377–388.
35. Esquerda A, Trujillano J, Lopez de Ullibarri I, et al. Classification tree analysis for the discrimination of pleural exudates and transudates. Clin Chem Lab Med 2007; 45:82–87.
36. Diamond GA. Off Bayes: Effect of verification bias on posterior probabilities calculated using Bayes' theorem. Medical Decision Making 1992; 12:22–31.
37. Bossuyt PM, Reitsma JB, Bruns DE, et al. The STARD statement for reporting studies of diagnostic accuracy: Explanation and elaboration. Ann Intern Med 2003; 138:W1–W12.
38. Heffner JE, Feinstein D, Barbieri C. Methodologic standards for diagnostic test research in pulmonary medicine. Chest 1998; 114:877–885.
39. Begg CB. Biases in the assessment of diagnostic tests. Stat Med 1987; 6:411–423.
40. Liu KT, Su WJ, Perng RP. Clinical utility of polymerase chain reaction for diagnosis of smear-negative pleural tuberculosis. J Chin Med Assoc 2007; 70:148–151.
41. Holloway AJ, Diyagama DS, Opeskin K, et al. A molecular diagnostic test for distinguishing lung adenocarcinoma from malignant mesothelioma using cells collected from pleural effusions. Clin Cancer Res 2006; 12:5129–5135.
42. Leuallen EC, Carr DT. Pleural effusion, a statistical study of 436 patients. N Engl J Med 1955; 1955:79–83.
43. Light RW, MacGregor I, Luchsinger PC, et al. Pleural effusion: The diagnostic separation of transudates and exudates. Ann Intern Med 1972; 77:507–513.

15

Transudative Pleural Effusions

UDAYA B. S. PRAKASH

Pulmonary and Critical Care, Mayo Clinic College of Medicine, Mayo Clinic, Rochester, Minnesota, U.S.A.

I. Introduction

A transudate can be defined as any fluid that has passed through a membrane or interstice, or exuded through a tissue. By definition, a transudate contains minimal quantities of protein and colloids, or cells. A transudate has protein concentration of ~1.0 g/dL and a low specific gravity (<1.016). A transudative pleural effusion denotes accumulation of an abnormal quantity of a transudate in the pleural space. The formation and the accumulation of a transudate in the pleural space occur when the systemic factors influencing the formation or absorption of pleural fluid are altered (1). This occurs when there is an increase in the hydrostatic pressure or a decrease in the oncotic pressure, or a combination of these two factors. The pleural fluid may originate in the lung, the pleura, or the peritoneal cavity. The permeability of the capillaries to proteins is normal in the area where the fluid forms (2,3). In patients with transudative pleural effusions, the pleural membranes themselves are normal and unaffected by pathologic process. The pleural surface is usually inflamed or involved by the underlying process in exudative pleural effusions. An exudative pleural effusion has high protein content, higher specific gravity, and tends to be cellular and turbid in appearance.

II. Definition

From a clinical perspective, a transudate implies that the pleural membranes are not themselves diseased and that a transudative effusion is a benign (nonmalignant) effusion caused by extrapleural disease (4,5). This clinically important knowledge warrants methods to separate a transudate from an exudate. A broad clinical classification of pleural effusions into transudates and exudates is based on the biochemical analysis of the pleural fluid. The criteria used to differentiate the transudate from the exudate are shown in Table 1. Of all the diagnostic criteria used to separate a transudate from an exudate, the criteria recommended by Light and colleagues have been used extensively by clinicians (6–9). These criteria include the following measurements: pleural fluid-to-serum protein ratio <0.5, pleural fluid-to-serum lactic dehydrogenase (LDH) ratio <0.6, or pleural fluid LDH <67% of the upper limits of normal for the serum LDH. However, these criteria have been shown to misclassify up to 30% of transudates into exudates (10–16). Further, these criteria are not completely reliable in patients who are on diuretic therapy (17). In order to better define a transudate, modifications in these criteria have been suggested (8,18–20). It is recommended that if a patient is thought to have a transudative effusion

Table 1 Biochemical Features of Transudative Pleural Effusions

Pleural fluid protein (g/dL)	≤3.0
Pleural fluid specific gravity	≤1.020
Pleural fluid protein/serum protein	≤0.5[a]
Pleural fluid LDH/serum LDH	≤0.6[a]
Pleural fluid LDH (IU/L)	≤200[a]
Pleural fluid LDH	<2/3 of upper limit of normal[b]
Pleural fluid cholesterol (mg/dL)	<45
Pleural fluid/serum cholesterol	<0.3
Albumin gradient (serum–pleural level) (g/dL)	≤1.2
Pleural fluid/serum bilirubin	≤0.6

LDH: lactic dehydrogenase.

[a] Light et al. (6,7) have concluded that any pleural effusion that meets these criteria is classified as a transudate. This criterion is commonly used in clinical practice.

[b] Pleural fluid level at upper limit of normal serum; this criterion can be applied when serum sample is not available.

by clinical criteria, but the fluid is identified as exudative by Light's criteria, an albumin gradient (difference between serum and pleural fluid albumin) be obtained. If this is above 1.2 g/dL, the exudative categorization by Light's criteria can be ignored and the effusion be considered a transudate (3). Numerous other biochemical tests of the pleural fluid have been studied in an effort to find the most helpful test to separate a transudative pleural effusion from an exudative pleural effusion. These include pleural levels of adenosine deaminase (21), cholesterol (22–24), bilirubin (25), cholinesterase (26), albumin gradient (7,11,27,28), pleural fluid viscosity (29), and protein gradient (30). The commonly used tests to differentiate a transudate from an exudate are summarized in Table 2 (31).

Ultrasound examination of the pleural space in patients with pleural effusion is very useful in evaluation of the location, loculation, and in the performance of thoracentesis

Table 2 Commonly Used Test Rules to Establish the Presence of a Transudative Pleural Effusion

Light's criteria
    Pleural fluid-to-serum LDH ratio <0.6 or
    Pleural fluid LDH <67% of the upper limits of normal for the serum LDH value or
    Pleural fluid-to-serum protein ratio <0.5
Abbreviated Light's criteria
    Pleural fluid LDH <67% of the upper limits of normal for the serum LDH value or
    Pleural fluid-to-serum protein ratio <0.5
Two-criteria pleural fluid rule without a blood test component
    Pleural fluid LDH <67% of the upper limits of normal for the serum LDH value or
    Pleural fluid cholesterol <45 mg/dL
Three-criteria pleural fluid rule without a blood test component
    Pleural fluid LDH <67% of the upper limits of normal for the serum LDH value or
    Pleural fluid cholesterol <45 mg/dL or
    Pleural fluid protein <3.0 g/dL

Source: Adapted from Ref. 31.

(32–34). This technique has been studied to determine its efficacy in differentiating a transudate from an exudate. Complex nonseptated echoic effusions tend to be exudates, whereas transudates may exhibit nonseptated and anechoic patterns (34,35). Importantly, ultrasound characteristics of the pleural effusion should not be the sole determinant of a transudate.

III. Pathogenesis

A small amount of transudate is present in the pleural space of all healthy individuals. This fluid has normal mechanical and physiological roles. The normal volume of pleural fluid is 0.1 to 0.3 mL/kg of body weight (36). Accumulation of abnormal quantities of pleural fluid denotes an underlying pathology or disease process, either in the pleura itself or in an extrapleural site or organ. In either situation, excess fluid accumulates in the pleural space when fluid collection exceeds normal removal mechanisms. The fluid dynamics in the pleural space are regulated by the hydrostatic, oncotic, and intrapleural pressures. Changes in capillary permeability (inflammation), increased hydrostatic pressure, decreased plasma oncotic pressure, impaired lymphatic drainage, increased negative intrapleural pressure, or movement of fluid (through diaphragmatic pores and lymphatic vessels) from the peritoneum can result in collection of abnormal quantities of fluid in the pleural space. In congestive cardiac failure, for example, an increase in transcapillary hydrostatic pressure leads to transudation of fluid across the capillary membrane into the pleural space. Even in this abnormal situation, when a transudative fluid accumulates in the pleural space, it is the result from the egress of fluid through a pleural membrane that is usually intact and not affected by the underlying pathology. The most common cause of a transudative pleural effusion is congestive cardiac failure, especially when the pulmonary artery wedge pressure exceeds 25 mm Hg. The most common cause of an exudative pleural effusion is pneumonia (parapneumonic effusion).

IV. Diagnosis

The initial step in the management of a pleural effusion is to determine if it is a transudate or an exudate. As discussed above, a variety of tests have been used to separate a transudate from an exudate. It is, however, important to recognize that not infrequently, the biochemical analysis may provide inconclusive results. This occurs if the fluid is collected and analyzed during the transitional phase, when the ongoing pathologic process adds additional protein and/or cells to the transudative fluid. Eventually, such effusions manifest biochemical features of an exudate. Because of this possibility, clinicians should be cautious of quickly adhering to a definitive diagnosis based purely on the biochemical features of pleural fluid. Another pitfall of wholly relying on the biochemical criteria is exemplified by the inadvertent addition of protein-rich blood to the pleural fluid during thoracentesis if the procedure results in trauma to the intercostal vasculature. Postural changes may also affect the biochemical analysis. Compared with thoracentesis performed in supine posture, fluid aspirated in sitting position may show tendency to be an exudate (37). From a clinical perspective, this is not a significant factor.

From a clinician's perspective, it is not necessary to perform all the tests to differentiate a transudate from an exudate. Even with extensive and repeated biochemical analysis of pleural fluid, classification of pleural fluid into transudates and exudates does not permit consideration of all causes. It is more useful to consider the cause of pleural effusion based on the potential cause or source of pleural effusion as determined by clinical features. Clinical suspicion of underlying disorder is important in considering the cause and nature of pleural effusion. It is important to recognize that pleural fluid caused by the same disease process, for example, congestive heart failure or malignancy, can be classified either as a transudate or an exudate based on biochemical analysis.

Determining whether an abnormal pleural collection is a transudate or exudate is an important initial step in evaluating pleural effusions of uncertain etiology. If an obvious etiology for the pleural effusion is clinically evident, then the biochemical analysis of the pleural fluid to determine if it is a transudate or exudate assumes secondary importance, or becomes unnecessary. From a clinical perspective, a transudative pleural effusion indicates limited diagnostic possibilities and this generally precludes further diagnostic testing. Continuing attempts to better define a transudate from an exudate may not provide more helpful information than that derived from the criteria of Light and colleagues. The efforts are better spent in identifying disease-specific diagnostic markers of pleural effusions (38).

V. Etiologies

A number of clinical conditions cause transudative pleural effusion. Exudative pleural effusions are much more commonly encountered in clinical practice. In a study of 1257 pleural effusions, transudates were observed in only 16% of patients (39). The common causes are listed in Table 3. Many of the entities listed can cause either a transudate or an exudate. The occurrence of transudative pleural effusion in various conditions does not imply that the main clinical condition alone is responsible for the pleural effusion. In many patients, the presence of pleural effusion may be caused by more than one disorder. The following paragraphs describe many of the entities known to cause transudative pleural effusions.

Table 3 Etiology of Transudative
Pleural Effusions

Congestive heart failure
Hepatic hydrothorax
Nephrotic syndrome
Peritoneal dialysis
Fontan operation
Urinothorax
Superior vena caval obstruction
Atelectasis
Misplaced central line
Pericardial disease[a]
Myxedema[a]
Pulmonary emboli[a]
Malignancy[a]
Sarcoid[a]
Amyloidosis[a]

[a]Effusion may be transudative or exudative.

A. Congestive Cardiac Failure

In congestive cardiac failure, an increase in pulmonary capillary hydrostatic pressure facilitates movement of the edema fluid through the visceral pleura into the pleural space. The pleural effusion is caused by the abnormal elevation in the left-sided pressure, and correlates with the capillary wedge pressure (40,41). The appearance of pleural effusion in congestive cardiac failure is usually preceded by alveolar and interstitial edema (41,42). In an animal lung model, volume loading led to an increase in transudation of fluid across the lung and into the pleural space. The protein concentration in the lung lymph and pleural effusion was identical, and the total volume of pleural fluid constituted 25% of all edema fluid in the lung (43). A study in an intact sheep model of high-pressure pulmonary edema showed that left atrial hypertension resulted in pleural fluid formation, but only after pulmonary edema had developed (44). These observations indicate that patients with congestive heart failure are more likely to develop pleural effusion if pulmonary edema is present (41). There is no association between pleural effusion and chronic pulmonary arterial and right atrial hypertension (45).

Congestive cardiac failure is the most common cause of the transudative pleural effusion and accounts for more than 85% of all transudates (46). An autopsy series in the 1950s noted a 72% incidence of pleural effusion with volumes exceeding 250 mL (47). In a study of 204 patients with transudative pleural effusions, 73% were secondary to congestive cardiac failure (39). In a meta-analysis of 377 patients with transudates, 72% were caused by congestive cardiac failure (8). A significant number of patients with decompensated congestive cardiac failure will exhibit pleural effusion. Pleural effusions are more frequent in middle-aged and older patients. In such patients, serial chest roentgenographs commonly show chronic small bilateral pleural effusions.

Pleural effusions associated with congestive heart failure are bilateral in over 85% of patients (47). When pleural effusions occur unilaterally, right-sided effusions are twice as frequent as left-sided effusions (47,48). The right-sided pleural effusions tend to be larger in volume. In patients with left pleural effusions, congestive heart failure associated with pericardial disease is more common (49). Localized or loculated pleural effusion in the interlobar fissures may resemble a mass on the chest roentgenograph (Fig. 1) (50). A lateral view is helpful for clarification. The mass like abnormality, known as "vanishing tumor," disappears after the treatment of heart failure and resorption of the pleural fluid (50).

The diagnosis of pleural effusion due to congestive heart failure is generally based on the clinical history, physical findings, and chest roentgenograph. Common clinical features include acute or chronic dyspnea, orthopnea, paroxysmal nocturnal dyspnea, peripheral edema, distended neck veins, hepatojugular reflux, late inspiratory crackles in basal regions of lungs, and an S3 ventricular gallop. Dullness to percussion of the lungs with decreased lung sounds suggests presence of pleural effusion. Chest roentgenograph may show cardiomegaly, pulmonary venous congestion, Kerley-B lines, pulmonary edema, and pleural effusions. Echocardiography provides more information on the cardiac function.

When the clinical diagnosis of congestive cardiac failure is certain, there is little or no role for diagnostic thoracentesis. Optimization of medical therapy, primarily diuretics, may lead to decrease or resolution of the pleural effusion. If the pleural effusion is large and contributes to the symptoms, then a therapeutic thoracentesis is indicated. Diagnostic thoracentesis is indicated if there is doubt regarding the diagnosis. Persistent or unilateral pleural effusion despite appropriate medical therapy of heart failure also calls for a

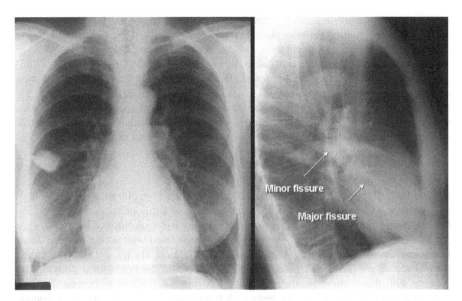

Figure 1 Loculated pleural effusion in the interlobar fissures may resemble a mass (pseudotumor) on the chest roentgenograph, as seen in the right-lung area (*left*); a lateral view (*right*) shows this to be an interlobar pleural effusion in a patient with heart failure. The mass-like abnormality, known as "vanishing tumor," disappears after treatment of heart failure and resorption of the pleural fluid.

diagnostic thoracentesis. If a contributing medical condition is suspected, for example, malignancy, empyema, or pleuropericarditis, a diagnostic thoracentesis is warranted.

Pleural fluid analysis in patients with congestive cardiac failure requires several special considerations. Generally, the results of pleural fluid studies satisfy the criteria for transudate (Tables 1 and 2). However, approximately 20% pleural fluids in patients with congestive heart failure meet exudative criteria (11,51). There are several reasons for this. The criteria for a transudate may not be fully reliable in patients who are on diuretic therapy because acute diuresis in this group of patients can elevate protein levels into an exudate range (17,52). Comorbid conditions or heart failure caused by or associated with certain disorders such as amyloidosis, hypothyroidism, malignancy, parapneumonic pleural effusion, and pulmonary embolism can increase the protein content of the pleural fluid to an exudate range. Compared to protein ratios (pleural/plasma), LDH ratios (pleural/plasma) may be more sensitive to repeated thoracentesis and diuretic therapy, and may convert the pleural fluid to an "exudate" (52).

When a pleural effusion meets exudative criteria in a patient with a clinically suspected transudate, the albumin gradient (the difference between the serum and pleural fluid albumin levels) can be used to separate a transudate from an exudate (11,27). If the albumin gradient exceeds 1.2 g/dL, then the effusion is considered a transudate. This criterion is not infallible, for in some patients with malignancy or infection, higher albumin gradient may misclassify an exudate as a transudate (53). Use of the albumin gradient along with the standard criteria (Tables 1 and 2) and clinical aspects should permit identification of a transudative pleural effusion. One study suggested that the measurement of N-terminal probrain natriuretic peptide (NT-proBNP) in pleural fluid may provide diagnostic differentiation between pleural effusion caused by congestive heart failure and other causes of transudative pleural effusion, such as hepatic hydrothorax (54).

Treatment of pleural effusion caused by congestive cardiac failure consists of optimizing the heart failure therapy. Improved cardiac function following the administration of diuretic and other drugs usually leads to gradual decrease in pleural effusion. The rapidity with which the pleural effusion responds varies from patient to patient. In patients with marked dyspnea, therapeutic thoracentesis, sometimes at regular intervals, is indicated. Refractory pleural effusions may require chest tube drainage and pleurodesis (55).

B. Hepatic Hydrothorax

Hepatic hydrothorax is a pleural effusion (usually greater than 500 mL) caused by hepatic cirrhosis and portal hypertension in the absence of cardiopulmonary disease (56–62). In the vast majority of cases, patients with hepatic hydrothorax have end-stage liver disease (62). Hepatic hydrothorax is usually associated with ascites but can occur in its absence (63,64). Usually, the pleural fluid is almost always a transudate unless there is secondary infection of the pleural fluid or ascitic fluid (65). In a study of 204 patients with transudative pleural effusions, 16% were secondary to hepatic cirrhosis (39). In a meta-analysis of 377 patients with transudates, 11% were caused by hepatic cirrhosis (8).

The accumulation of the fluid in the pleural space is the result of ascitic fluid transported through the diaphragmatic defects (diaphragmatic pores or "stomata" of von Recklinghausen) into the pleural space as a result of the negative intrapleural pressure. Negative intrapleural pressure creates sufficient pressure gradient across the diaphragmatic defects to enable the fluid in the peritoneal cavity to move up to the pleural space. Occasionally, the diaphragmatic defects can tear suddenly and lead to massive or tension hydrothorax (66). The diaphragmatic defects can be visualized at the time of thoracotomy or thoracoscopy. Radionuclide and other imaging techniques have been used to show their presence (63,66). Diaphragmatic lymphatics have no role in the pleural effusion as they drain peritoneal fluid to the mediastinal lymph nodes (67). Up to 10% of patients with cirrhosis develop hepatic hydrothorax. Pleural effusion is almost always right-sided; left-sided effusions occur in about 10% and bilateral effusions occur in up to 15% of patients (58,68).

The diagnosis of hepatic hydrothorax should be suspected in a patient with established cirrhosis and portal hypertension who presents with a unilateral pleural effusion, most commonly on the right side. The transudative nature of the pleural effusion is easily confirmed with diagnostic thoracentesis and estimation of the pleural fluid levels of protein and lactic dehydrogenase. Ascitic fluid and pleural fluid demonstrate identical biochemical profiles.

The natural course of patients with hepatic hydrothorax is dependent on the success of therapy for ascites. Other complications such as renal insufficiency and hypoalbuminemia contribute to the problem. Unless definitive therapy is undertaken to treat the ascites, pleural fluid accumulation persists. Vasoconstrictor therapy has been tried to minimize and treat hepatic hydrothorax (69). Transjugular intrahepatic portosystemic shunt (TIPS) has been used to treat hepatic hydrothorax (70). Among 28 patients who underwent TIPS placement for refractory hepatic hydrothorax, reduction in the volume of pleural effusion and improvement in clinical symptoms was observed in 68% while a complete radiological and echographic disappearance of hydrothorax was documented in 57%. Poor hepatic function was predictive of nonresponse to therapy (71).

Therapeutic thoracentesis for symptomatic relief of dyspnea has a temporizing effect. A large and symptomatic hydrothorax may require a combination of therapeutic thoracentesis and paracentesis. Successful diaphragmatic repair using video-assisted thoracoscopic surgery and repeated instillation of talc slurry to treat hepatic hydrothorax have been reported (72,73). A successful orthotopic liver transplantation is the best therapy to treat the hepatic cirrhosis as well the hydrothorax (62). Prognosis is poor without liver transplantation (74).

Large transudative pleural effusions are encountered in patients following liver transplant (75). These effusions are more common on the right side, develop three to seven days after transplant, and are not associated with cardiopulmonary disease.

C. Nephrotic Syndrome

Nephrotic syndrome is characterized by proteinuria, edema, and hypoproteinemia. Nephrotic syndrome is a well-known cause of transudative pleural effusion. The overall incidence is about 20% (14). In a study of 204 patients with transudative pleural effusions, 6% were caused by nephrotic syndrome (39). In a meta-analysis of 377 patients with transudates, 10% were caused by nephrotic syndrome (8). Pleural effusions in patients with nephrotic syndrome are usually bilateral (76). In many patients, pleural effusions are subpulmonic in location and the costophrenic angle may appear sharp. A chest roentgenograph in lateral decubitus may be necessary to ascertain this (Fig. 2). Pulmonary embolism occurs at a higher rate with the nephrotic syndrome and this etiology for the pleural effusion should be excluded in all patients with the nephrotic syndrome and a pleural effusion (77). All patients with chronic transudative pleural effusions should be evaluated for proteinuria and hypoproteinemia.

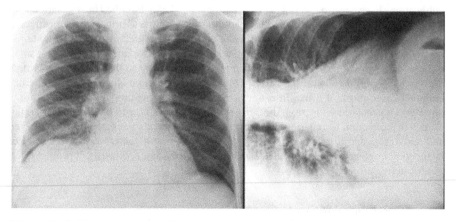

Figure 2 Subpulmonic pleural effusion on the right side is not apparent because of the sharp costophrenic angle on the right (*left*). A right lateral decubitus shows free layering of right pleural effusion (*right*). The subpulmonic pleural effusions are seen in nephrotic syndrome, congestive heart failure, and pleural effusions from other causes.

Treatment of pleural effusion caused by the nephrotic syndrome includes attempts to increase the level of serum protein by therapeutic attempts to stop or diminish proteinuria. Thoracentesis may be required if pleural effusion becomes symptomatic.

D. Hypoalbuminemia

Hypoalbuminemia per se is not a common cause of clinically significant transudative pleural effusion (78). In a meta-analysis of 377 patients with transudates, 7% were considered to be related to hypoalbuminemia (8). In patients with hepatic cirrhosis with hypoalbuminemia and absence of ascites, pleural effusion is seldom encountered. Even though hypoalbuminemia produces low serum osmolarity with resultant shifts in fluid balance and can lead to sequestration of fluid in the pleural space, collection of abnormal quantities of a transudate in the pleural space is not a common occurrence. However, a patient with Waldenström's macroglobulinemia who developed transudative pleural effusion after plasmapheresis has been described. The authors suspect that rapid removal of high–molecular-weight IgM led to an abrupt decrease in intravascular colloid oncotic pressure and transudation of fluid into the pleural space. When albumin was added to the apheresis, the pleural effusion resolved (79). Low serum osmolarity may favor formation of transudative pleural effusion due to other medical conditions (80–82). Of interest is the common finding of significant hypoalbuminemia in children with large parapneumonic exudative pleural effusions. The low serum albumin levels are explained in part by a shift of albumin from blood to pleural fluid (83).

E. Urinothorax

Urinothorax (or urothorax) denotes the presence of urine in the pleural space. This condition is usually secondary to ipsilateral obstructive uropathy. In most patients, the urinothorax resolves after the relief of obstructive uropathy. A subject review published in 2006 noted that there were 58 cases of urinothorax (84). Since then more than 10 publications have described it (84–93). Urinothorax has been described in association with urinary tract malignancy, renal calculi, postlithotripsy, trauma to urinary tract, obstructed or failed tube nephrostomy, hydronephrosis, and posterior urethral valve. Urinothorax occurs on the side of urinary obstruction, and the fluid accumulation can be rapid, small or large, and symptoms vary with the volume of urinothorax and the rapidity with which it accumulates in the pleural space. The color of the fluid and its biochemical properties are identical to those of urine. In patients without obstructive uropathy and urinothorax otherwise normal renal function, the concentration of creatinine in pleural fluid does not exceed that of serum (94). Urinothorax is usually a transudate unless the urine is infected and has significant protein content. Even though the protein content is low, the level of lactic dehydrogenase can be elevated. Treatment of urinothorax consists of prompt relief of obstructive uropathy.

F. Peritoneal Dialysis

Transudative pleural effusions are occasionally encountered in patients undergoing peritoneal dialysis (95–98). The pleural effusion accumulates as the dialysate instilled into the peritoneal cavity moves into to the pleural cavity through diaphragmatic defects. The mechanism and dynamics of fluid movement into the pleural space are similar to those in hepatic hydrothorax, described above. In a follow-up study of 3195 patients undergoing continuous ambulatory peritoneal dialysis, acute hydrothorax developed in 50 (1.6%) patients. The interval between onset of dialysis and hydrothorax ranged from one day to eight years and the majority of the pleural effusions were right-sided (88%), with four left-sided, and two bilateral hydrothoraces (99). The pleural effusion can occur during the first several sessions or later. Acute massive hydrothorax has been described in several cases (100–105). The occurrence of pleural effusion is dependent on the volume of dialysate instilled and the number and size of diaphragmatic defects. Recurrent or persistent symptomatic pleural effusion associated with peritoneal dialysis requires definitive therapy. To minimize pleural effusion, small-volume dialysate is recommended during each cycle with patient placed in a sitting or upright position (106). Repeated therapeutic thoracentesis is not a good option for long-term therapy. Acute hydrothorax can be prevented and treated using graduated cycle volumes (107). Surgical pleurodesis carries the highest success rate (98,108).

G. Trapped Lung

Trapped lung (or lung entrapment) denotes an unexpandable lung or part of the lung because of a restrictive visceral pleural peel or rind that surrounds it (109). This creates a negative pressure gradient, which promotes development of a chronic fluid-filled pleural space. A trapped lung also implies absence of an ongoing active pleural process, obstructing airway lesions, or pulmonary parenchymal pathology. Thoracentesis fails to expand the trapped lung. The increased negative intrapleural pressure that results after thoracentesis promotes reaccumulation of pleural effusion (effusions ex vacuo) or development of a loculated pneumothorax (pneumothorax ex vacuo) (Fig. 3).

In a group of 11 patients with trapped lung secondary to coronary artery bypass graft surgery, uremia, thoracic radiation, pericardiotomy, spontaneous bacterial pleuritis and repeated thoracentesis, and complicated parapneumonic effusion, the analysis of pleural fluid revealed a mean pleural fluid lactate dehydrogenase level 124 IU/L (range, 57–170 IU/L) and mean pleural fluid total protein of 2.9 g/dL (range, 2.0–4.2 g/dL); a pleural fluid total protein value >3.0 g/dL was observed in 5 of 11 patients (110).

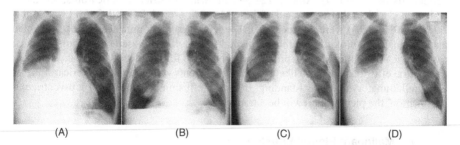

(A) (B) (C) (D)

Figure 3 A patient with chronic right pleural effusion and trapped lung following right-sided video-assisted thoracoscopic lung biopsy (**A**) underwent thoracentesis with aspiration of 1200 mL of a transudate. This failed to expand the trapped lung but resulted in hydropneumothorax ex vacuo (**B**). Within 4 days, the pleural effusion increased (**C**), and 10 days after thoracentesis, the pleural space was once again filled with fluid (pleural effusion ex vacuo) (**D**).

Most patients with small pleural effusions and those who are asymptomatic do not require therapy. As the visceral and parietal pleural surfaces cannot be brought together to achieve pleural adhesion, standard pleurodesis is rarely successful. In symptomatic patients with underlying normal lung parenchyma, pleural catheter drainage has been used to minimize or treat the pleural effusion (111). The definitive therapy of trapped lung is pleurectomy and decortication.

H. Atelectasis

Lobar or segmental atelectasis produces pleural effusion from various mechanisms. In the absence of an underlying inflammatory process, the pleural fluid is the result of excessive volume of the transudate entering the pleural space with diminished clearance of the same from the pleural space. In a study of 100 consecutive patients admitted to the medical intensive care unit, 62 patients had pleural effusions, and atelectasis was responsible for the effusion in 14 patients (23%) (80). Even though there were no other obvious causes for the effusions, the possibility that the atelectasis was the result of pleural effusion could not be refuted. Pleural effusions associated with chronic asymptomatic atelectasis are small and rarely cause symptoms by themselves. Acute atelectasis and resultant pleural effusion may cause sufficient symptoms to warrant further evaluation. An obstructive bronchial lesion (mucous plug, clot, tumor, or foreign body) should be excluded as the cause.

I. Constrictive Pericarditis

Constrictive pericarditis is a less-known cause of transudative pleural effusion. The mechanism of accumulation of a transudative pleural effusion includes diastolic dysfunction of the left ventricle, which leads to an elevated intravascular hydrostatic pressure. An identical mechanism may cause systemic venous congestion and ascites leading to a transudative pleural effusion through diaphragmatic defects (112). If the pericardial disease is severe, the resultant hepatic congestion and associated hepatic dysfunction with subsequent development of hypoproteinemia, contributes to the formation of pleural effusion (113–121).

Pleural effusion has been reported in up to 60% of patients with constrictive pericarditis (49,122–124). Among 124 patients with constrictive pericarditis, 35 (28%) patients had a pleural effusion, and of these 21 (60%) were left-sided, 2 (5%) were right-sided, and 12 (35%) were bilateral (49). The left-sided predominance is most likely the result of anatomic proximity of the left pleural space to the diseased pericardium. In such cases, pericardial inflammatory process is responsible for the pleural effusion. Transudative pleural effusions are more likely to occur in patients with constrictive pericarditis that is noninflammatory and long-standing. If pleural effusion is the result of left ventricular dysfunction, the pleural fluid will be a transudate.

J. Malignant Pleural Effusion

Malignant pleural effusions are usually exudates. However, 3% to 10% of malignant pleural effusions are transudates (19,125–127). The transient nature (change of transudate to an exudate) of malignant pleural effusions has been reported (127). The criteria of Light et al. may not be applicable in malignant pleural effusions because the effusions can result from comorbid conditions such as lymphatic obstruction, hypoalbuminemia, cirrhosis with ascites, pulmonary embolism, atelectasis, or chronic heart failure. Transudative malignant pleural effusions are likely to be cytologically negative.

K. Superior Vena Caval Syndrome

Superior vena caval (SVC) syndrome occurs when the venous blood flow through the superior vena cava is diminished or abolished. The pathogenesis is via either extrinsic compression or intrinsic blockage of the superior vena cava. The main etiologic entities include malignancies, benign processes, iatrogenic trauma, indwelling catheters, and thrombosis of the superior vena cava. Pleural effusion is among the several clinical manifestations of the SVC syndrome. Even though the pleural effusion is reported to occur in up to 25% of patients with SVC syndrome (128–134), it is much less commonly encountered in clinical practice. The precise mechanism of pleural fluid accumulation is unknown. It has been suggested that elevated pressure from SVC syndrome may impair lymphatic clearance and increase interstitial edema, with leakage of transudate into the pleural space (135). Many studies have reported that pleural effusions resulting from SVC syndrome are transudates. However, exudates and chylous effusions are also encountered in a significant number of patients (132).

L. Hypothyroidism

Hypothyroidism is an uncommon cause of pleural effusion (136–142). In a study of 60 patients who had chest roentgenograms at the time of documented hypothyroidism, 15 (25%) patients had roentgenographic evidence of pleural effusions. In 13 of the 15 patients, the etiology for the pleural effusions was unrelated to the hypothyroidism. Two patients had pleural effusions directly related to underlying hypothyroidism and the pleural effusions resolved after thyroid hormone replacement therapy (140).

The precise mechanism of transudative pleural fluid accumulation in hypothyroidism is unclear. It has been suggested that the extravascular accumulation of albumin, and presumably other plasma proteins, plays an important role in the generalized edema found in myxedema. In addition, inadequate lymphatic drainage may explain the formation of effusion in the pleural space (143). Pleural and pericardial effusions may occur simultaneously (142). Occurrence of pleural effusions demonstrating characteristics of an exudate has been described (140,141). Hypothyroidism-related pleural effusions can vary in volume and can be unilateral or bilateral (136). Very large effusions are uncommon. Most pleural effusions are small and of minor clinical importance.

M. Cerebrospinal Fluid in Pleural Space

Rare occurrences of cerebrospinal fluid (CSF) leaking into the pleural space with resultant pleural effusion have been reported. Most of these are secondary to trauma. The most common cause is the ventriculopleural shunting (144). Other causes have included penetrating injuries and fractures of the thoracic spine and thoracic spinal surgery (145–148). Computed tomography (CT) myelography may demonstrate the CSF–pleural fistula (147). The low protein levels in the pleural fluid match those in the cerebrospinal fluid.

N. Pulmonary Embolism

Pleural effusions occur in 20% to 50% of patients with pulmonary embolism (149–153). Pleural effusions are demonstrated by chest roentgenograph in approximately 30% of patients with pulmonary emboli. Nearly 50% of patients exhibit pleural effusions when computed tomography or ultrasonography is used. The pleural effusions are small to medium in volume, and more than 70% are unilateral (154). They can be loculated. The role for pleural fluid analysis in pulmonary thromboembolic disease is limited because the pleural fluid analysis does not help establish the diagnosis of pulmonary embolism. Previously, pleural effusions associated with pulmonary embolism were reported to be transudates (155). Others have shown that majority of pleural effusions in patients with pulmonary emboli are exudates (149,156).

O. Special Considerations

Pleural effusions are common in patients in the intensive care units. Up to 62% of patients admitted to the intensive care units have been found to have pleural effusions, and most of these tend to be transudates (80). Among a total of 1978 intensive care unit patients described in five publications (6,80,157–159), the most common cause of transudative pleural effusion was congestive cardiac failure (11–36%), followed less commonly by hepatic hydrothorax, and nephrotic syndrome (160). In a study of 62 patients with pleural effusion after admission to the medical intensive care unit, the main causes of transudative pleural effusions were as follows: heart failure in 22 (35%) patients, atelectasis in 14 (23%), hepatic hydrothorax in 5 (8%), and hypoalbuminemia in 5 (8%) (80). The documentation of the transudative nature of pleural effusion is particularly helpful in the patients in the intensive care unit in that it may preclude further diagnostic studies and assist the clinician to focus on treating the cause of the transudate.

P. Iatrogenic

Transudative pleural effusions from iatrogenic causes can be acute or gradual in onset, large or small, or unilateral or bilateral. Iatrogenic trauma in the form of misplaced catheters, tubes, and other medical devices may lead to transudative pleural effusion (80,161,162).

The Fontan procedure is the creation of an anastomosis is between the pulmonary artery and the right atrium, superior or inferior vena cava, to bypass the right ventricle in patients with tricuspid atresia or a univentricular heart. A transudative pleural effusion is a frequent finding after surgery, particularly in patients who have a large number of aortopulmonary collateral vessels (163–166). Pleural effusion may require chemical pleurodesis or insertion of a pleuroperitoneal shunt (163,165).

VI. Summary

Transudative pleural effusion is commonly encountered in clinical practice. Transudative pleural effusion is the result of increases in hydrostatic pressure or decrease in oncotic pressure, or a combination of these two factors. The separation of a transudate from an exudate is based on the biochemical analysis of pleural fluid. The criteria used to differentiate the transudate from the exudate are shown in Tables 1 and 2. Modifications to these criteria should be considered in certain special conditions.

The common etiologies include congestive cardiac failure, hepatic cirrhosis, hypoalbuminemia, and nephrotic syndrome. The primary therapy of transudative pleural effusions consists of optimal management of the underlying cause. This initial step alone may minimize or resolve the pleural effusion. Therapeutic thoracentesis is indicated if the pleural effusion is large and leads to lung compression and pulmonary symptoms. Pleurodesis should be considered in patients with recurrent or refractory pleural effusions.

References

1. Miserocchi G. Physiology and pathophysiology of pleural fluid turnover. Eur Respir J 1997; 10:219–225.
2. Broaddus VC, Light RW. What is the origin of pleural transudates and exudates? Chest 1992; 102:658–659.
3. Light RW. Diagnostic principles in pleural disease. Eur Respir J 1997; 10:476–481.
4. Light R. Transudative pleural effusions. In: Retford DC, ed. Pleural Diseases. Baltimore, MD: Willaims & Wilkins, 1995:83–93.
5. Courtney Broaddus V, Light R. Pleural effusion. In: Murray & Nadel's Textbook of Respiratory Medicine, 4th ed. Tokyo, Japan: Asia Pacific Society for Respirology, 2005.
6. Light RW, Macgregor MI, Luchsinger PC, et al. Pleural effusions: The diagnostic separation of transudates and exudates. Ann Intern Med 1972; 77:507–513.
7. Light RW. Useful tests on the pleural fluid in the management of patients with pleural effusions. Curr Opin Pulm Med 1999; 5:245–249.
8. Heffner JE, Brown LK, Barbieri CA. Diagnostic value of tests that discriminate between exudative and transudative pleural effusions. Primary Study Investigators. Chest 1997; 111:970–980.
9. Heffner JE. Discriminating between transudates and exudates. Clin Chest Med 2006; 27:241–252.
10. Gazquez I, Porcel JM, Vives M, et al. Comparative analysis of Light's criteria and other biochemical parameters for distinguishing transudates from exudates. Respir Med 1998; 92:762–765.
11. Burgess LJ, Maritz FJ, Taljaard JJ. Comparative analysis of the biochemical parameters used to distinguish between pleural transudates and exudates. Chest 1995; 107:1604–1609.
12. Romero S, Martinez A, Hernandez L, et al. Light's criteria revisited: Consistency and comparison with new proposed alternative criteria for separating pleural transudates from exudates. Respiration 2000; 67:18–23.
13. Vives M, Porcel JM, Vicente de Vera M, et al. A study of Light's criteria and possible modifications for distinguishing exudative from transudative pleural effusions. Chest 1996; 109:1503–1507.
14. Light RW. The undiagnosed pleural effusion. Clin Chest Med 2006; 27:309–319.
15. Agrawal V, Doelken P, Sahn SA. Pleural fluid analysis in chylous pleural effusion. Chest 2008; 133:1436–1441.
16. Sahn SA. The value of pleural fluid analysis. Am J Med Sci 2008; 335:7–15.
17. Romero-Candeira S, Hernandez L, Romero-Brufao S, et al. Is it meaningful to use biochemical parameters to discriminate between transudative and exudative pleural effusions? Chest 2002; 122:1524–1529.
18. Joseph J, Badrinath P, Basran GS, et al. Is the pleural fluid transudate or exudate? A revisit of the diagnostic criteria. Thorax 2001; 56:867–870.
19. Heffner JE, Klein JS. Recent advances in the diagnosis and management of malignant pleural effusions. Mayo Clin Proc 2008; 83:235–250.

20. Murphy MJ, Jenkinson F. Categorisation of pleural fluids in routine clinical practice: Analysis of pleural fluid protein and lactate dehydrogenase alone compared with modified Light's criteria. J Clin Pathol 2008; 61:684–685.

21. Atalay F, Ernam D, Hasanoglu HC, et al. Pleural adenosine deaminase in the separation of transudative and exudative pleural effusions. Clin Biochem 2005; 38:1066–1070.

22. Hamm H, Brohan U, Bohmer R, et al. Cholesterol in pleural effusions. A diagnostic aid. Chest 1987; 92:296–302.

23. Valdes L, Pose A, Suarez J, et al. Cholesterol: A useful parameter for distinguishing between pleural exudates and transudates. Chest 1991; 99:1097–1102.

24. Leers MP, Kleinveld HA, Scharnhorst V. Differentiating transudative from exudative pleural effusion: Should we measure effusion cholesterol dehydrogenase? Clin Chem Lab Med 2007; 45:1332–1338.

25. Meisel S, Shamiss A, Thaler M, et al. Pleural fluid to serum bilirubin concentration ratio for the separation of transudates from exudates. Chest 1990; 98:141–144.

26. Garcia-Pachon E, Padilla-Navas I, Sanchez JF, et al. Pleural fluid to serum cholinesterase ratio for the separation of transudates and exudates. Chest 1996; 110:97–101.

27. Roth BJ, O'Meara TF, Cragun WH. The serum-effusion albumin gradient in the evaluation of pleural effusions. Chest 1990; 98:546–549.

28. Gonlugur U, Gonlugur TE. The distinction between transudates and exudates. J Biomed Sci 2005; 12:985–990.

29. Yetkin O, Tek I, Kaya A, et al. A simple laboratory measurement for discrimination of transudative and exudative pleural effusion: Pleural viscosity. Respir Med 2006; 100:1286–1290.

30. Romero-Candeira S, Fernandez C, Martin C, et al. Influence of diuretics on the concentration of proteins and other components of pleural transudates in patients with heart failure. Am J Med 2001; 110:681–686.

31. Heffner JE. Diagnosis and management of malignant pleural effusions. Respirology 2008; 13:5–20.

32. Hirsch JH, Rogers JV, Mack LA. Real-time sonography of pleural opacities. AJR Am J Roentgenol 1981; 136:297–301.

33. Wu RG, Yuan A, Liaw YS, et al. Image comparison of real-time gray-scale ultrasound and color Doppler ultrasound for use in diagnosis of minimal pleural effusion. Am J Respir Crit Care Med 1994; 150:510–514.

34. Yang PC, Luh KT, Chang DB, et al. Value of sonography in determining the nature of pleural effusion: Analysis of 320 cases. AJR Am J Roentgenol 1992; 159:29–33.

35. Chen HJ, Tu CY, Ling SJ, et al. Sonographic appearances in transudative pleural effusions: Not always an anechoic pattern. Ultrasound Med Biol 2008; 34:362–369.

36. Zocchi L. Physiology and pathophysiology of pleural fluid turnover. Eur Respir Monogr 2002; 22(7):28–49.

37. Brandstetter RD, Velazquez V, Viejo C, et al. Postural changes in pleural fluid constituents. Chest 1994; 105:1458–1461.

38. Lee YC, Davies RJ, Light RW. Diagnosing pleural effusion: Moving beyond transudate-exudate separation. Chest 2007; 131:942–943.

39. Esquerda A, Trujillano J, Lopez de Ullibarri I, et al. Classification tree analysis for the discrimination of pleural exudates and transudates. Clin Chem Lab Med 2007; 45:82–87.

40. Wiener-Kronish JP, Berthiaume Y, Albertine KH. Pleural effusions and pulmonary edema. Clin Chest Med 1985; 6:509–519.

41. Wiener-Kronish JP, Matthay MA, Callen PW, et al. Relationship of pleural effusions to pulmonary hemodynamics in patients with congestive heart failure. Am Rev Respir Dis 1985; 132:1253–1256.

42. Wiener-Kronish JP, Broaddus VC. Interrelationship of pleural and pulmonary interstitial liquid. Annu Rev Physiol 1993; 55:209–226.

43. Broaddus VC, Wiener-Kronish JP, Staub NC. Clearance of lung edema into the pleural space of volume-loaded anesthetized sheep. J Appl Physiol 1990; 68:2623–2630.
44. Allen S, Gabel J, Drake R. Left atrial hypertension causes pleural effusion formation in unanesthetized sheep. Am J Physiol 1989; 257:H690–H692.
45. Wiener-Kronish JP, Goldstein R, Matthay RA, et al. Lack of association of pleural effusion with chronic pulmonary arterial and right atrial hypertension. Chest 1987; 92:967–970.
46. Light RW. Approach to the patient. Pleural Diseases, 3rd ed. Baltimore, MD: Williams and Wilkins, 1995:75–82.
47. Edwards JE, Race GA, Scheifley CH. Hydrothorax in congestive heart failure. Am J Med 1957; 22:83–89.
48. Weiss JM, Spodick DH. Laterality of pleural effusions in chronic congestive heart failure. Am J Cardiol 1984; 53:951
49. Weiss JM, Spodick DH. Association of left pleural effusion with pericardial disease. N Engl J Med 1983; 308:696–697.
50. Millard CE. Vanishing of phantom tumor of the lung; localized interlobar effusion in congestive heart failure. Chest 1971; 59:675–677.
51. Pillay VK. Total proteins in serous fluids in cardiac failure. S Afr Med J 1965; 39:142–143.
52. Broaddus VC. Diuresis and transudative effusions—Changing the rules of the game. Am J Med 2001; 110:732–735.
53. Ceyhan B, Celikel T. Serum-effusion albumin gradient in separation of transudative and exudative pleural effusions. Chest 1994; 105:974–975.
54. Porcel JM. The use of probrain natriuretic peptide in pleural fluid for the diagnosis of pleural effusions resulting from heart failure. Curr Opin Pulm Med 2005; 11:329–333.
55. Glazer M, Berkman N, Lafair JS, et al. Successful talc slurry pleurodesis in patients with nonmalignant pleural effusion. Chest 2000; 117:1404–1409.
56. Islam N, Sanaullah M, Khan AK. Hepatic hydrothorax. Am J Gastroenterol 1969; 52:213–217.
57. Islam N, Ali S, Kabir H. Hepatic hydrothorax. Br J Dis Chest 1965; 59:222–227.
58. Johnston RF, Loo RV. Hepatic hydrothorax; studies to determine the source of the fluid and report of thirteen cases. Ann Intern Med 1964; 61:385–401.
59. Morrow CS, Kantor M, Armen RN. Hepatic hydrothorax. Ann Intern Med 1958; 49:193–203.
60. Strauss RM, Boyer TD. Hepatic hydrothorax. Semin Liver Dis 1997; 17:227–232.
61. Kinasewitz GT, Keddissi JI. Hepatic hydrothorax. Curr Opin Pulm Med 2003; 9:261–265.
62. Roussos A, Philippou N, Mantzaris GJ, et al. Hepatic hydrothorax: Pathophysiology diagnosis and management. J Gastroenterol Hepatol 2007; 22:1388–1393.
63. Rubinstein D, McInnes IE, Dudley FJ. Hepatic hydrothorax in the absence of clinical ascites: Diagnosis and management. Gastroenterology 1985; 88:188–191.
64. Jimenez-Saenz M, Venero J, Castro J, et al. Hepatic hydrothorax without ascites: A rare form of a common complication. J R Soc Med 1990; 83:747–748.
65. Baylor PA, Bobba VV, Ginn PD, et al. Recurrent spontaneous infected pleural effusion in a patient with alcoholic cirrhosis, hepatic hydrothorax, and ascites. West J Med 1988; 149:216–217.
66. LeVeen HH, Piccone VA, Hutto RB. Management of ascites with hydrothorax. Am J Surg 1984; 148:210–213.
67. Broaddus VC. Transudative pleural effusions. Eur Respir Monogr 2002; 7 (Monograph 22):157–176.
68. Lieberman FL, Hidemura R, Peters RL, et al. Pathogenesis and treatment of hydrothorax complicating cirrhosis with ascites. Ann Intern Med 1966; 64:341–351.
69. Ibrisim D, Cakaloglu Y, Akyuz F, et al. Treatment of hepatic hydrothorax with terlipressin in a cirrhotic patient. Scand J Gastroenterol 2006; 41:862–865.
70. Perkins JD. Liver function determines success of transjugular intrahepatic portosystemic shunt in treating hepatic hydrothorax. Liver Transpl 2008; 14:382–383.

71. Wilputte JY, Goffette P, Zech F, et al. The outcome after transjugular intrahepatic portosystemic shunt (TIPS) for hepatic hydrothorax is closely related to liver dysfunction: A long-term study in 28 patients. Acta Gastroenterol Belg 2007; 70:6–10.

72. Ibi T, Koizumi K, Hirata T, et al. Diaphragmatic repair of two cases of hepatic hydrothorax using video-assisted thoracoscopic surgery. Gen Thorac Cardiovasc Surg 2008; 56:229–232.

73. Cerfolio RJ, Bryant AS. Efficacy of video-assisted thoracoscopic surgery with talc pleurodesis for porous diaphragm syndrome in patients with refractory hepatic hydrothorax. Ann Thorac Surg 2006; 82:457–459.

74. Cardenas A, Arroyo V. Management of ascites and hepatic hydrothorax. Best Pract Res Clin Gastroenterol 2007; 21:55–75.

75. Olutola PS, Hutton L, Wall WJ. Pleural effusion following liver transplantation. Radiology 1985; 157:594.

76. Jenkins PG, Shelp WD. Recurrent pleural transudate in the nephrotic syndrome. A new approach to treatment. JAMA 1974; 230:587–588.

77. Llach F, Arieff AI, Massry SG. Renal vein thrombosis and nephrotic syndrome. A prospective study of 36 adult patients. Ann Intern Med 1975; 83:8–14.

78. Eid AA, Keddissi JI, Kinasewitz GT. Hypoalbuminemia as a cause of pleural effusions. Chest 1999; 115:1066–1069.

79. Karlinsky J, Seder R, Corral R. Pleural effusion after plasmapheresis in Waldenstrom's macroglobulinemia. Chest 1986; 89:146–148.

80. Mattison LE, Coppage L, Alderman DF, et al. Pleural effusions in the medical ICU: Prevalence, causes, and clinical implications. Chest 1997; 111:1018–1023.

81. Joseph J, Strange C, Sahn SA. Pleural effusions in hospitalized patients with AIDS. Ann Intern Med 1993; 118:856–859.

82. Afessa B. Pleural effusion and pneumothorax in hospitalized patients with HIV infection: The pulmonary complications, ICU support, and prognostic factors of hospitalized patients with HIV (PIP) study. Chest 2000; 117:1031–1037.

83. Prais D, Kuzmenko E, Amir J, et al. Association of hypoalbuminemia with the presence and size of pleural effusion in children with pneumonia. Pediatrics 2008; 121:e533–e538.

84. Garcia-Pachon E, Romero S. Urinothorax: A new approach. Curr Opin Pulm Med 2006; 12:259–263.

85. Karkoulias K, Sampsonas F, Kaparianos A, et al. Urinothorax: An unexpected cause of pleural effusion in a patient with non-Hodgkin lymphoma. Eur Rev Med Pharmacol Sci 2007; 11:373–374.

86. Handa A, Agarwal R, Aggarwal AN. Urinothorax: An unusual cause of pleural effusion. Singapore Med J 2007; 48:e289–e292.

87. Deel S, Robinette E Jr. Urinothorax: A rapidly accumulating transudative pleural effusion in a 64-year-old man. South Med J 2007; 100:519–521.

88. Izzo L, Caputo M, De Toma G, et al. Urinoma and urinothorax: Report of a case. Am Surg 2008; 74:62–63.

89. Ziyade S, Ugurlucan M, Soysal O. Urinothorax: Urine discharge from thorax. Ann Thorac Surg 2008; 85:2141.

90. Garcia-Pachon E, Padilla-Navas I. Urinothorax: An unexpected cause of severe dyspnea. Emerg Radiol 2006; 13:55.

91. Shleyfer E, Nevzorov R, Jotkowitz AB, et al. Urinothorax: An unexpected cause of pleural effusion. Eur J Intern Med 2006; 17:300–302.

92. Tortora A, Casciani E, Kharrub Z, et al. Urinothorax: An unexpected cause of severe dyspnea. Emerg Radiol 2006; 12:189–191.

93. Garcia-Pachon E, Padilla-Navas I. Urinothorax: Case report and review of the literature with emphasis on biochemical diagnosis. Respiration 2004; 71:533–536.

94. Leung FW, Williams AJ, Guze PA. Lymphatic obstruction: A possible explanation for left-sided pleural effusions associated with splenic hematomas. AJR Am J Roentgenol 1982; 138:182.

95. Finn R, Jowett EW. Acute hydrothorax complicating peritoneal dialysis. Br Med J 1970; 2:94.

96. Edwards SR, Unger AM. Acute hydrothorax—A new complication of peritoneal dialysis. JAMA 1967; 199:853–855.

97. Benz RL, Schleifer CR. Hydrothorax in continuous ambulatory peritoneal dialysis: Successful treatment with intrapleural tetracycline and a review of the literature. Am J Kidney Dis 1985; 5:136–140.

98. Szeto CC, Chow KM. Pathogenesis and management of hydrothorax complicating peritoneal dialysis. Curr Opin Pulm Med 2004; 10:315–319.

99. Nomoto Y, Suga T, Nakajima K, et al. Acute hydrothorax in continuous ambulatory peritoneal dialysis—A collaborative study of 161 centers. Am J Nephrol 1989; 9:363–367.

100. Chow CC, Sung JY, Cheung CK, et al. Massive hydrothorax in continuous ambulatory peritoneal dialysis: Diagnosis, management and review of the literature. N Z Med J 1988; 101:475–477.

101. Milutinovic J, Wu WS, Lindholm DD, et al. Acute massive unilateral hydrothorax: A rare complication of chronic peritoneal dialysis. South Med J 1980; 73:827–828.

102. Rudnick MR, Coyle JF, Beck LH, et al. Acute massive hydrothorax complicating peritoneal dialysis, report of 2 cases and a review of the literature. Clin Nephrol 1979; 12:38–44.

103. Seebaran AR, Patel PL. Acute massive hydrothorax—A rare complication of peritoneal dialysis. A case report. S Afr Med J 1981; 60:827–828.

104. Singh S, Vaidya P, Dale A, et al. Massive hydrothorax complicating continuous ambulatory peritoneal dialysis. Nephron 1983; 34:168–172.

105. Suga T, Matsumoto Y, Nakajima K, et al. Three cases of acute massive hydrothorax complicating continuous ambulatory peritoneal dialysis (CAPD). Tokai J Exp Clin Med 1989; 14:315–319.

106. Grefberg N, Danielson BG, Benson L, et al. Right-sided hydrothorax complicating peritoneal dialysis. Report of 2 cases. Nephron 1983; 34:130–134.

107. Krishnan RG, Ognjanovic MV, Crosier J, et al. Acute hydrothorax complicating peritoneal dialysis. Perit Dial Int 2007; 27:296–299.

108. Lang CL, Kao TW, Lee CM, et al. Video-assisted thoracoscopic surgery in continuous ambulatory peritoneal dialysis-related hydrothorax. Kidney Int 2008; 74:136.

109. Moore PJ, Thomas PA. The trapped lung with chronic pleural space, a cause of recurring pleural effusion. Mil Med 1967; 132:998–1002.

110. Huggins JT, Sahn SA, Heidecker J, et al. Characteristics of trapped lung: Pleural fluid analysis, manometry, and air-contrast chest CT. Chest 2007; 131:206–213.

111. Pien GW, Gant MJ, Washam CL, et al. Use of an implantable pleural catheter for trapped lung syndrome in patients with malignant pleural effusion. Chest 2001; 119:1641–1646.

112. Ramar K, Daniels CA. Constrictive pericarditis presenting as unexplained dyspnea with recurrent pleural effusion. Respir Care 2008; 53:912–915.

113. Akdemir I, Davutoglu V, Aksoy M. Constrictive pericarditis localized to left ventricle presented with left pleural effusion: A case report. Echocardiography 2002; 19:329–332.

114. Akhter MW, Nuno IN, Rahimtoola SH. Constrictive pericarditis masquerading as chronic idiopathic pleural effusion: Importance of physical examination. Am J Med 2006; 119:e1–e4.

115. Amasyali B, Heper G, Akkoc O, et al. Chylous ascites and pleural effusion secondary to constrictive pericarditis presenting with signs of lymphatic obstruction. Jpn Heart J 2004; 45:535–540.

116. Cecconi M, Manfrin M, Berrettini U, et al. Constrictive pericarditis presenting as unexplained recurrent pleural effusion: A case report. Cardiologia 1998; 43:967–970.

117. Dell'Italia LJ, Walsh RA. Hemodynamic profile of constrictive pericarditis produced by a massive right pleural effusion. Cathet Cardiovasc Diagn 1984; 10:471–477.
118. Sadikot RT, Fredi JL, Light RW. A 43-year-old man with a large recurrent right-sided pleural effusion. Diagnosis: Constrictive pericarditis. Chest 2000; 117:1191–1194.
119. Tomaselli G, Gamsu G, Stulbarg MS. Constrictive pericarditis presenting as pleural effusion of unknown origin. Arch Intern Med 1989; 149:201–203.
120. Yamamoto N, Noda Y, Miyashita Y. A case of refractory bilateral pleural effusion due to post-irradiation constrictive pericarditis. Respirology 2002; 7:365–368.
121. Vladutiu AO. Cardiac Failure with Pleural Effusion. Pleural Effusion. New York, NY: Futura Publishing Co. Inc., 1986:173–174.
122. Plum GE, Bruwer AJ, Clagett OT. Chronic constrictive pericarditis; roentgenologic findings in 35 surgically proved cases. Proc Staff Meet Mayo Clin 1957; 32:555–566.
123. Light RW. Clinical practice. Pleural effusion. N Engl J Med 2002; 346:1971–1977.
124. Bertog SC, Thambidorai SK, Parakh K, et al. Constrictive pericarditis: Etiology and cause-specific survival after pericardiectomy. J Am Coll Cardiol 2004; 43:1445–1452.
125. Sahn SA. Malignant pleural effusions. Semin Respir Crit Care Med 2001; 22:607–616.
126. Sahn SA. Malignant pleural effusions. Clin Chest Med 1985; 6:113–125.
127. Fernandez C, Martin C, Aranda I, et al. Malignant transient pleural transudate: A sign of early lymphatic tumoral obstruction. Respiration 2000; 67:333–336.
128. Parish JM, Marschke RF Jr, Dines DE, et al. Etiologic considerations in superior vena cava syndrome. Mayo Clin Proc 1981; 56:407–413.
129. Bell DR, Woods RL, Levi JA. Superior vena caval obstruction: A 10-year experience. Med J Aust 1986; 145:566–568.
130. Rice TW. Pleural effusions in superior vena cava syndrome: Prevalence, characteristics, and proposed pathophysiology. Curr Opin Pulm Med 2007; 13:324–327.
131. Dhande V, Kattwinkel J, Alford B. Recurrent bilateral pleural effusions secondary to superior vena cava obstruction as a complication of central venous catheterization. Pediatrics 1983; 72:109–113.
132. Rice TW, Rodriguez RM, Barnette R, et al. Prevalence and characteristics of pleural effusions in superior vena cava syndrome. Respirology 2006; 11:299–305.
133. Walker RW. Recurrent pleural effusions following superior vena cava thrombosis. Anaesthesia 1991; 46:704.
134. Hussey HH. Superior vena caval syndrome. JAMA 1981; 246:1548.
135. Ando F, Arakawa M, Kambara K, et al. Effect of superior vena caval hypertension on alloxan-induced lung injury in dogs. J Appl Physiol 1990; 68:478–483.
136. Brown SD, Brashear RE, Schnute RB. Pleural effusion in a young woman with myxedema. Arch Intern Med 1983; 143:1458–1460.
137. Douglass RC. Pleural effusion with myxedema. Arch Intern Med 1983; 143:2334.
138. Locke W. Myxedema associated with pleural effusion and headache. Ochsner Clin Rep 1956; 2:32–36.
139. Schneierson SJ, Katz M. Solitary pleural effusion due to myxedema. J Am Med Assoc 1958; 168:1003–1005.
140. Gottehrer A, Roa J, Stanford GG, et al. Hypothyroidism and pleural effusions. Chest 1990; 98:1130–1132.
141. Hataya Y, Akamizu T, Kanamoto N, et al. A case of subclinical hypothyroidism developing marked pleural effusions and peripheral edema with elevated vascular endothelial growth factor. Endocr J 2007; 54:577–584.
142. Parker DR, Shaboury AH. Central hypothyroidism presenting with pericardial and pleural effusions. J Intern Med 1993; 234:429–430.
143. Parving HH, Hansen JM, Nielsen SL, et al. Mechanisms of edema formation in myxedema-increased protein extravasation and relatively slow lymphatic drainage. N Engl J Med 1979; 301:460–465.

144. Beach C, Manthey DE. Tension hydrothorax due to ventriculopleural shunting. J Emerg Med 1998; 16:33–36.
145. Gupta SM, Frias J, Garg A, et al. Aberrant cerebrospinal fluid pathway. Detection by scintigraphy. Clin Nucl Med 1986; 11:593–594.
146. Monla-Hassan J, Eichenhorn M, Spickler E, et al. Duropleural fistula manifested as a large pleural transudate: An unusual complication of transthoracic diskectomy. Chest 1998; 114:1786–1789.
147. Patel MR, Wehner JH, Soule WC, et al. Intracranial hypotension and recurrent pleural effusion after snow-boarding injury: A manifestation of cerebrospinal fluid–pleural fistula. Spine J 2005; 5:336–338.
148. Da Silva VF, Shamji FM, Reid RH, et al. Subarachnoid–pleural fistula complicating thoracotomy: Case report and review of the literature. Neurosurgery 1987; 20:802–805.
149. Porcel JM, Madronero AB, Pardina M, et al. Analysis of pleural effusions in acute pulmonary embolism: Radiological and pleural fluid data from 230 patients. Respirology 2007; 12:234–239.
150. Porcel JM, Light RW. Effusions from vascular causes. In: Light RW, Gary Lee YC, eds. Textbook of Pleural Diseases, 2nd ed. London, UK: Hodder Arnold, 2008:397–408.
151. Worsley DF, Alavi A, Aronchick JM, et al. Chest radiographic findings in patients with acute pulmonary embolism: Observations from the PIOPED Study. Radiology 1993; 189:133–136.
152. Monreal M, Munoz-Torrero JF, Naraine VS, et al. Pulmonary embolism in patients with chronic obstructive pulmonary disease or congestive heart failure. Am J Med 2006; 119:851–858.
153. Elliott CG, Goldhaber SZ, Visani L, et al. Chest radiographs in acute pulmonary embolism. Results from the International Cooperative Pulmonary Embolism Registry. Chest 2000; 118:33–38.
154. Porcel JM, Light RW. Pleural effusions due to pulmonary embolism. Curr Opin Pulm Med 2008; 14:337–342.
155. Bynum LJ, Wilson JE III. Characteristics of pleural effusions associated with pulmonary embolism. Arch Intern Med 1976; 136:159–162.
156. Romero Candeira S, Hernandez Blasco L, Soler MJ, et al. Biochemical and cytologic characteristics of pleural effusions secondary to pulmonary embolism. Chest 2002; 121:465–469.
157. Fartoukh M, Azoulay E, Galliot R, et al. Clinically documented pleural effusions in medical ICU patients: How useful is routine thoracentesis? Chest 2002; 121:178–184.
158. Colt HG, Brewer N, Barbur E. Evaluation of patient-related and procedure-related factors contributing to pneumothorax following thoracentesis. Chest 1999; 116:134–138.
159. Heffner JE, Brown LK, Barbieri C, et al. Pleural fluid chemical analysis in parapneumonic effusions. A meta-analysis. Am J Respir Crit Care Med 1995; 151:1700–1708.
160. Azoulay E. Pleural effusions in the intensive care unit. Curr Opin Pulm Med 2003; 9:291–297.
161. Jurivich DA. Iatrogenic pleural effusions. South Med J 1988; 81:1417–1420.
162. Duntley P, Siever J, Korwes ML, et al. Vascular erosion by central venous catheters. Clinical features and outcome. Chest 1992; 101:1633–1638.
163. Kiziltepe U, Eyileten ZB, Uysalel A, et al. Prolonged pleural effusion following Fontan operation: Effective pleurodesis with talc slurry. Int J Cardiol 2002; 85:297–299.
164. Korkut AK, Cetin G, Soyler I, et al. Pleural effusion and off-pump Fontan procedure. J Thorac Cardiovasc Surg 2004; 128:799.
165. Tansel T, Sayin OA, Ugurlucan M, et al. Successful bleomycin pleurodesis in a patient with prolonged pleural effusion after extracardiac Fontan procedure. J Card Surg 2006; 21:585–586.
166. Yun TJ, Im YM, Jung SH, et al. Pulmonary vascular compliance and pleural effusion duration after the Fontan procedure. Int J Cardiol 2008.

16
Management of the Undiagnosed Persistent Pleural Effusion

RICHARD W. LIGHT
Vanderbilt University, Nashville, Tennessee, U.S.A.

I. Introduction

On occasion, a patient will have a persistent pleural effusion that remains undiagnosed. This chapter assumes that the pleural effusion persists after the initial diagnostic workup, which includes measurement of a pleural fluid marker for tuberculosis such as adenosine deaminase (ADA) or gamma interferon.

II. Diseases That Cause Undiagnosed Persistent Pleural Effusions

When a patient with a persistent undiagnosed pleural effusion is encountered, the first thing to be considered is the list of the diseases most likely to be associated with this condition (Table 1). The first question to answer in a patient with a persistent undiagnosed pleural effusion is whether the effusion is a transudate or an exudate. For the past several decades, this differentiation has been made by measuring the levels of protein and lactate dehydrogenase (LDH) in the pleural fluid and in the serum (Light's criteria). If one or more of the following criteria are met, the patient has an exudative pleural effusion (1):

1. Pleural fluid protein/serum protein >0.5
2. Pleural fluid LDH/serum LDH >0.6
3. Pleural fluid LDH >two-thirds the normal upper limit for serum

Light's criteria are very sensitive at identifying exudates, but they also identify about 15% of transudative pleural effusions as being exudative pleural effusions (2,3). Usually, the transudates that are misclassified only minimally meet the exudative criteria, for example, the protein ratio is 0.52 or the LDH ratio is 0.63. If the pleural fluid LDH is more than the upper limit for the serum LDH or if the protein level is more than 4.0 g/dL, the patient does not have a transudate. Most of these transudates that are misclassified as exudates can be classified correctly if the gradient between the protein levels in the serum and the pleural fluid is measured. If this gradient is greater than 3.1 g/dL, the exudative classification by Light's criteria can be ignored because almost all such patients have a transudative pleural effusion (4). The protein gradient alone should not be used to separate transudates from exudates because, by itself, it will misidentify approximately 15% of exudates as transudates (4).

Table 1 Diseases Most Likely to Produce Persistent Undiagnosed Pleural Effusion

---

Transudative pleural effusions
  Congestive heart failure
  Cirrhosis
  Nephrotic syndrome
  Urinothorax
  Myxedema
  Cerebrospinal fluid leaks to the pleura
  Obstruction of the brachiocephalic vein
Exudative pleural effusions
  Malignancy
  Pneumonia (especially anaerobic)
  Tuberculosis
  Fungal infection
  Pancreatic pseudocyst
  Intra-abdominal abscess
  Post-coronary artery bypass graft surgery
  Postcardiac injury syndrome
  Pericardial disease
  Meigs' syndrome
  Rheumatoid pleuritis
  Lupus erythematosus
  Drug-induced pleural disease
  Asbestos pleural effusion
  Yellow nail syndrome
  Uremia
  Trapped lung
  Chylothorax
  Pseudochylothorax

A. Transudative Pleural Effusions

Congestive Heart Failure

Congestive heart failure is the most common cause of pleural effusion (5). At times in patients with persistent pleural effusion, it is not obvious that the heart failure is the cause of the effusion. Certainly, symptoms of congestive heart failure such as dyspnea on exertion, orthopnea, paroxysmal nocturnal dyspnea, and nocturia should be sought when the history is taken. In addition, signs of congestive heart failure such as basilar rales, S3 gallop, distended neck veins, and pedal edema should also be sought during the physical examination. If the patient clinically has congestive heart failure but the initial pleural fluid analysis reveals an exudate that just barely meets Light's criteria, the difference between the pleural fluid and serum protein should be measured as detailed above. If this gradient is above 3.1 g/dL, the effusion can be attributed to the congestive heart failure (4). If the patient has a transudative effusion but does not have obvious heart failure, further investigations of cardiac function such as echocardiography are indicated.

Measurement of the B-type natriuretic peptide (BNP) in the pleural fluid or serum is useful in the diagnosis of congestive heart failure (6). This hormone is synthesized by the cardiac ventricle in response to increased wall stress due to pressure or volume overload. It is synthesized as an inactive prohormone that is split into the active hormone BNP and the inactive N-terminal fragment (NT-proBNP). Recent data indicates that PF NT-proBNP levels >1500 pg/mL have more than 90% sensitivity and specificity for discriminating effusions caused by heart failure from those attributable to other causes [16]. Because of its comparable diagnostic accuracy at the same cutoff value, serum rather than pleural NT-proBNP measurement is preferable for making the diagnosis of heart failure (7,8). Additional advantages of using NT-proBNP are that it perfectly discriminates between transudates of hepatic and cardiac origin, and it also correctly identifies more than 80% of cardiac transudates mislabeled by Light's criteria (9). It should be noted that BNP, which is measured in many hospital laboratories, has different values than NT-proBNP and has not been evaluated for its accuracy in diagnosing pleural effusions due to congestive heart failure.

Cirrhosis with Hepatic Hydrothorax

If the patient has overt cirrhosis and massive ascites, the diagnosis of hepatic hydrothorax is easy. However, if the patient does not have ascites, the diagnosis of hepatic hydrothorax may be difficult to establish. In 1998, Kakizaki and associates reviewed the literature and were able to find 28 cases of hepatic hydrothorax without ascites (10). Of these 28 cases, 27 were on the right side. The only left-sided effusion occurred in a patient who had a tear in the left diaphragm as a result of a splenectomy. The mean serum albumin in these 28 cases was 2.7 g/dL with a range of 1.9 to 3.6 g/dL (10). The explanation for the pleural effusion in the absence of overt ascites is that the patients have defects in their diaphragm. When fluid is present in the peritoneal space, it flows immediately into the pleural space because the pleural pressure is negative compared to the peritoneal pressure. This diagnosis can be established by the intraperitoneal injection of technetium 99m (^{99m}Tc)-sulfur colloid (11) or indocyanine green (12) and their subsequent demonstration in the pleural fluid.

Nephrotic Syndrome

Another cause of a chronic transudative pleural effusion is the nephrotic syndrome. More than 20% of patients with the nephrotic syndrome have pleural effusions, which are usually bilateral (13). Therefore, all patients with chronic transudative pleural effusions should be evaluated for proteinuria and hypo-proteinemia. It should be remembered that the incidence of pulmonary emboli is high with the nephrotic syndrome (14), and this possibility should be considered in all patients with the nephrotic syndrome and a pleural effusion.

Urinothorax

A transudative pleural effusion can result when there is retroperitoneal urinary leakage secondary to bilateral obstruction or trauma to the urinary tract with subsequent dissection of the urine into the pleural space (15). This is a rare cause of pleural effusion as only 58 cases had been reported until 2006. This diagnosis is easy if it is considered as the pleural fluid looks and smells like urine. Confirmation of the diagnosis can be made by demonstrating that the pleural fluid creatinine is greater than the serum creatinine, but this finding is also present in 10% of patients with pleural effusions of other etiologies (16). The pleural fluid with urinothorax may also have a low glucose and a low pH. The only other instance in which a transudative pleural effusion has a low glucose or low pH is when there is systemic hypoglycemia or acidosis, respectively.

Cerebrospinal Fluid Leak to the Pleura

On rare occasions, cerebrospinal fluid (CSF) can collect in the pleural space and produce a pleural effusion. This most commonly occurs following ventriculopleural shunting (17), but can also occur after penetrating injuries and fractures of the thoracic spine and following thoracic spinal surgery (18,19). The diagnosis should be suggested by the appearance of the pleural fluid, which appears to be CSF. The protein levels are usually very low. If there is any doubt about the diagnosis, measurement of the pleural fluid β_2-transferrin is useful because only CSF contains this molecule (20). The diagnosis can also be confirmed by radionuclide cisternograph (19).

Obstruction of the Brachiocephalic Vein

A transudative pleural effusion can occur if the brachiocephalic vein is obstructed. The most common causes of brachiocephalic vein obstruction are thrombosis of a central venous or hemodialysis catheter or an intrathoracic goiter. The effusion is thought to result from high capillary pressure in the parietal pleural.

B. Exudative Pleural Effusions

Malignant Pleural Effusion

There is no doubt that malignancy causes more persistently undiagnosed exudative pleural effusions than any other disease. However, it should be emphasized that there is no huge hurry to establish this diagnosis, because (a) the presence of the effusion indicates that the patient has metastases to the pleura and the malignancy cannot be cured surgically, (b) most malignant pleural effusions are due to tumors that cannot be cured with chemotherapy, and (c) there is no evidence that attempts to create a pleurodesis early improve the quality of the patient's life.

Most patients who have a pleural malignancy usually have other characteristics suggesting malignancy. Ferrer and coworkers (21) prospectively studied 93 patients referred for thoracoscopy at a tertiary hospital. They found that the following four variables were associated with pleural malignancy in a multivariate model: (a) a symptomatic period of more than one month, (b) absence of fever, (c) blood-tinged or bloody pleural fluid, and (d) chest CT findings suggesting of malignancy. Twenty-eight patients had all the four criteria and all had malignancy. Twenty-one patients had at most one criterion and none had malignancy (21).

When patients with pleural effusions due to the most common types of tumors are analyzed, some interesting observations can be made. The tumor that causes the highest number of pleural effusions is lung cancer (5). When patients with lung cancer are first evaluated, about 15% have a pleural effusion (22), but 50% of patients with disseminated lung cancer develop a pleural effusion (5). The tumor that causes the second highest number of pleural effusions is breast cancer (5). Patients with breast carcinoma rarely present with pleural effusion. The mean interval between the diagnosis of the primary tumor and the appearance of a pleural effusion is two years (23). Hematological malignancies (lymphomas and leukemias) cause the third highest number of malignant pleural effusions (5). Approximately 10% of patients with Hodgkin's lymphoma and

25% of patients with non-Hodgkin's lymphoma have pleural effusions at presentation. Those that do almost invariably have intrathoracic lymph node involvement (24). If the patient has AIDS and cutaneous Kaposi' sarcoma, the likely diagnosis is a pleural effusion due to Kaposi's sarcoma. This diagnosis is usually established at bronchoscopy, which demonstrates erythematous or violaceus macules or papules in the respiratory tree (25).

There are several primary tumors of the pleura that should be considered if the patient has an undiagnosed pleural effusion. If the patient has a history of asbestos exposure, mesothelioma should be considered. Thoracoscopy or thoracotomy is usually necessary to make this diagnosis (5). If the patient has AIDS and has a lymphocytic pleural effusion with a very high LDH level, the diagnosis of primary effusion lymphoma is likely (26). This diagnosis can usually be established with pleural fluid cytology and flow cytometry (5). If the patient received an artificial pneumothorax many years previously, a likely diagnosis is pyothorax-associated lymphoma (27).

Parapneumonic Effusion
The diagnosis of parapneumonic effusion is easy in the patient with an acute febrile illness, purulent sputum, and pulmonary infiltrates. On occasion, however, particularly with anaerobic infections, the patient may present with a chronic illness. In one study of 47 patients with anaerobic parapneumonic effusions, the median duration of symptoms before presentation was 10 days and 60% of the patients had substantial weight loss (mean 29 lb) (28). Therefore, if the patient has a chronic illness with predominantly neutrophils in their pleural fluid, it is imperative to obtain anaerobic cultures of the pleural fluid. Since patients with actinomycosis and nocardiosis at times have a chronic pleural effusion with predominantly neutrophils, cultures for these organisms should be obtained in patients with chronic neutrophilic pleural effusions.

Tuberculous Pleural Effusion
Throughout the world, tuberculosis remains one of the principal causes of pleural effusion. It is important to make this diagnosis, because if the patient has pleural tuberculosis and is not treated, the effusion will resolve but the patient will have a greater than 50% chance of developing active pulmonary or extrapulmonary tuberculosis over the following five years (29). Therefore, all patients with a chronic undiagnosed pleural effusion should be evaluated for tuberculosis. The easiest way to do this is to measure the pleural fluid level of ADA or gamma interferon. If the level of ADA is below 40 IU/L or the level of gamma interferon is below 140 pg/mL, the diagnosis can be excluded (5). In one study, Ferrer et al. followed 40 patients with a chronic undiagnosed pleural effusion and a pleural fluid ADA level below 43 IU/L for a mean of five years, and none developed tuberculosis (30).

Fungal Pleural Effusions
Fungal disease is responsible for a very small percentage of pleural effusions (5). However, at times blastomycosis and coccidioidomycosis may cause a chronic lymphocytic pleural effusion (5). Accordingly, cultures for fungi should be obtained in the patient with a chronic undiagnosed pleural effusion with predominantly lymphocytes in the pleural fluid. It is unknown whether the lymphocytic effusions due to fungal diseases have a high ADA.

Chronic Pancreatic Pleural Effusion
This is one diagnosis that should always be considered in a patient with a chronic undiagnosed pleural effusion. Some patients with a pancreatic pseudocyst will develop a direct

sinus tract between the pancreas and the pleural space (31). The sinus tract will decompress the pancreas, and therefore the patient presents with symptoms usually referable only to the chest. The patient with a chronic pancreatic pleural effusion is usually chronically ill and looks like he or she has cancer. The diagnosis is virtually established if the level of amylase in the pleural fluid is greater than 1000 U/L (31). It is important to consider this diagnosis because the patient can be cured with appropriate surgery.

Intra-abdominal Abscess
A large percentage of patients with subphrenic, intrahepatic, intrasplenic, and intrapancreatic abscesses have an associated pleural effusion (5). Patients with intra-abdominal abscess are usually chronically ill with fever and weight loss. This diagnosis should be considered in any patient with a pleural effusion containing predominantly neutrophils but without pulmonary parenchymal abnormalities. The diagnosis can be made with CT scan or ultrasound of the abdomen.

Effusion Postcoronary Artery Bypass Graft (CABG) Surgery
Approximately 10% of patients who undergo CABG surgery have a pleural effusion that occupies more than 25% of their hemithorax 28 days postoperatively (32). Their primary symptom (if any) is dyspnea; chest pain and fever are distinctly unusual (32). The pleural fluid in these patients is an exudate characterized by a lymphocyte predominance and an LDH approximately equal to the upper limit of normal for serum (33). Although the pleural fluid characteristics are similar to those of patients with tuberculous pleuritis, these two entities may be differentiated by the pleural fluid level of ADA—the ADA level is below 40 U/L in patients with the post-CABG effusion (34). On rare occasions, these effusions can persist for years (35), and one must not be too aggressive in pursuing a diagnosis if the pleural fluid findings are as expected.

Postcardiac Injury Syndrome (PCIS)
PCIS, also known as Dressler's syndrome, is characterized by the development of fever, pleuropericarditis, and parenchymal pulmonary infiltrates in the weeks following trauma to the pericardium or myocardium (36). PCIS has been reported following myocardial infarction, cardiac surgery, blunt chest trauma, percutaneous left ventricular puncture, pacemaker implantation, and angioplasty. PCIS differs from pleural effusion post-CABG surgery because fever and chest pain invariably occur with the PCIS and are rare post-CABG. Following cardiac injury, symptoms usually develop between the first and third week, but can develop at any time between three days and one year (36). The pleural fluid is frankly bloody in about 30% of patients, and the differential cell count may reveal predominantly neutrophils or mononuclear cells depending upon the acuteness of the process (37).

Pericardial Disease
Approximately 25% of patients who have a pericardial effusion will have a concomitant pleural effusion (38). In patients with inflammatory pericarditis, the majority of the associated pleural effusions are unilateral and left-sided (38). The characteristics of the pleural fluid seen in conjunction with pericardial disease are not well described (5). The possibility of pericardial effusion should be evaluated in any patient with apparent cardiomegaly and an isolated left pleural effusion.

Approximately 60% of patients with constrictive pericarditis will have a concomitant pleural effusion (39). The associated pleural effusion is bilateral and symmetrical in the majority. In one report of four patients with constrictive pericarditis, the pleural fluid was transudative in one and exudative in three (39). We have reported one patient with constrictive pericarditis who had a pleural fluid protein of 4.0 g/dL (40). When a patient is seen with edema and an exudative pleural effusion, the diagnosis of constrictive pericarditis should be considered. It is important to realize that echocardiography may be normal in the patient with constrictive pericarditis and that cardiac catheterization may be necessary to establish the diagnosis (40).

Meigs' Syndrome

Meigs' syndrome is the constellation of a benign pelvic neoplasm associated with ascites and pleural effusion in which surgical extirpation of the tumor results in permanent disappearance of the ascites and pleural effusion (5). The pleural fluid is an exudate with a relatively low cell count, which at times may have an elevated CA125 (41). The importance of Meigs' syndrome is that not all patients with a pelvic mass, ascites, and a pleural effusion have metastatic disease.

Rheumatoid Pleuritis

Chronic pleural effusion may be a manifestation of rheumatoid pleuritis, and the diagnosis is usually straightforward. Classically, the effusion occurs in older males who have subcutaneous nodules. The pleural fluid is an exudate with a low glucose, a low pH, and a high LDH. The first manifestation of rheumatoid disease is virtually never a pleural effusion (5).

Systemic Lupus Erythematosus

In contrast to rheumatoid pleuritis, patients with systemic lupus erythematosus (SLE) may present with a pleural effusion. The possibility of drug-induced lupus should always be considered in the patient with an undiagnosed pleural effusion. Drugs that are most commonly implicated in drug-induced lupus are hydralazine, procainamide, isoniazid, phenytoin, and chlorpromazine (5). The diagnosis of SLE with pleural involvement is based on the usual criteria for the diagnosis of lupus. Measurement of the pleural fluid antinuclear antibody (ANA) levels (42) or performance of LE preparations on the pleural fluid (5) does not assist in the diagnosis.

Drug-Induced Pleural Disease

When a patient is evaluated with a chronic undiagnosed pleural effusion, the list of drugs that the patient is taking should be carefully reviewed as the ingestion of certain drugs can lead to the development of a pleural effusion. The primary drugs associated with the development of a pleural effusion are nitrofurantoin (a urinary antiseptic), dantrolene (a muscle relaxant), and the ergot alkaloids such as bromocriptine, which are used to treat Parkinson's disease (5). Other drugs that have been reported to induce pleural effusions include methysergide, amiodarone, procarbazine, methotrexate, clozapine, dapsone, metronidazole, mitomycin, isotretinoin, propylthiouracil, simvastatin, warfarin, and gliclazide (5). It is also important to scrutinize the list of drugs that the patient is taking to determine if any are associated with drug-induced lupus (5).

Asbestos Pleural Effusion

Exposure to asbestos can lead to the development of an exudative pleural effusion. In one series of 1135 asymptomatic asbestos workers, the prevalence of pleural effusion was 3% (43). In this series, all patients developed effusions within 20 years of the initial exposure and many had within 5 years of the initial exposure (43). The prevalence of pleural effusion was directly related to the total asbestos exposure. Patients with asbestos pleural effusions are usually asymptomatic (43,44). The effusion tends to last several months and then clears, leaving no residual disease. The pleural fluid is an exudate and can contain predominantly neutrophils or mononuclear cells (44). If a patient with a pleural effusion has a history of asbestos exposure and is asymptomatic, the patient can probably be observed to determine if the effusion disappears spontaneously.

Yellow Nail Syndrome

The yellow nail syndrome consists of the triad of deformed yellow nails, lymphedema, and pleural effusions (5). The three separate entities may become manifest at widely varying times. The pleural effusions are bilateral in about 50% of patients and vary in size from small to massive (5). Once a pleural effusion has occurred with this syndrome, it tends to persist and recur rapidly after a thoracocentesis. The pleural fluid is usually a clear yellow exudate with a normal glucose level and predominantly lymphocytes in the pleural fluid differential. The pleural fluid LDH tends to be low relative to the pleural fluid protein level.

Uremia

The prevalence of pleural effusions with uremia is approximately 3% (45). As many as 50% of patients on long-term hemodialysis have a pleural effusion (46). There is not a close relationship between the degree of uremia and the occurrence of a pleural effusion (45). More than 50% of the patients are symptomatic, with fever (50%), chest pain (30%), cough (35%), and dyspnea (20%) being the most common symptoms (45). The pleural fluid is an exudate, and the differential usually reveals predominantly lymphocytes (45). Tests of renal function should be obtained in every patient with an undiagnosed exudative effusion.

Trapped Lung

When there is intense inflammation in the pleural space, a fibrous peel may form over the visceral pleura. This peel can prevent the underlying lung from expanding, and therefore the lung is said to be trapped (47). The initial event producing the pleural inflammation is usually a pleural infection or a hemothorax, but it can be a spontaneous pneumothorax, thoracic operations (particularly CABG surgery) (35), uremia, or collagen vascular disease. The pleural fluid is usually clear yellow and is a borderline exudate with predominantly mononuclear cells. The diagnosis can be made by measuring the pleural pressure while fluid is withdrawn during a thoracocentesis. If the initial pleural pressure is below -10 cm H_2O or if the pleural pressure falls more than 20 cm H_2O per 1000 mL fluid removed, the diagnosis is confirmed provided that the patient does not have bronchial obstruction (47).

Chylothorax and Pseudochylothorax

When pleural fluid is found to be milky or very turbid, the possibility of a chylothorax or a pseudochylothorax should be considered. When turbid fluid is found, the first step is to centrifuge the fluid. If the supernatant remains turbid, then the turbidity is due to a high-lipid content in the pleural fluid and the patient has a chylothorax or a pseudochylothorax.

Chylothorax is usually easy to differentiate from pseudochylothorax on clinical grounds. Patients with a chylothorax have an acute illness and their pleural surfaces are normal on CT scan. In contrast, patients with a pseudochylothorax usually have had a pleural effusion for more than five years and their pleural surfaces are markedly thickened on CT scan. Measurement of the lipid levels in the pleural fluid is also useful in distinguishing these two conditions. Pleural fluid from a chylothorax has a triglyceride level above 110 mg/dL and the ratio of the pleural fluid to serum cholesterol is less than 1.0. In contrast, fluid from a pseudochylothorax has cholesterol crystals and/or cholesterol above 200 mg/dL and higher than the simultaneous serum level (5).

III. Tests to Consider for Patients with Persistent Undiagnosed Pleural Effusion

A. History

Certain points in the patient's history should receive special attention if the patient has a persistent undiagnosed pleural effusion. If a patient has a transudative pleural effusion, particular attention should be paid to symptoms of congestive heart failure such as dyspnea on exertion, orthopnea, paroxysmal nocturnal dyspnea, and nocturia. In addition, historical evidence of cirrhosis, alcoholism, or chronic hepatitis should be sought with the possibility of a hepatic hydrothorax in mind. A history of trauma or surgery to the thoracic spine should be sought with the diagnosis of a CSF leak in mind.

If the patient has a exudative pleural effusion, a history of malignancy should be sought. Malignant pleural effusions have been known to develop as long as 20 years after the primary tumor was diagnosed (48). A history of exposure to asbestos should be sought, as this would suggest mesothelioma or an asbestos pleural effusion. A history of fever suggests a chronic anaerobic, tuberculous, or fungal infection or an intra-abdominal abscess. A history of alcoholism or previous pancreatic disease raises the possibility of a chronic pancreatic pleural effusion. A history of CABG surgery or myocardial trauma suggests a post-CABG pleural effusion or postcardiac injury syndrome, respectively. A history of rheumatoid disease raises the possibility of rheumatoid pleuritis. The patient should be questioned carefully regarding the medications they are taking to determine whether they are taking a medication that causes a pleural effusion or is associated with drug-induced lupus erythematosus. The patient should be questioned carefully about previous pleural problems, which raise the likelihood of a pseudochylothorax or a trapped lung.

B. Physical Examination

In the patient with the chronic undiagnosed pleural effusion, it is worthwhile to repeat a careful physical examination. If the patient has a transudative pleural effusion, signs of congestive heart failure such as basilar rales, an S3 gallop, or distended neck veins should be sought. In addition, evidence of ascites should be carefully sought. The presence of pedal edema suggests congestive heart failure, cirrhosis with hepatic hydrothorax, nephrotic syndrome, pericardial disease, or the yellow nail syndrome.

If the patient has an exudative effusion, a careful search for lymphadenopathy or other masses, which would suggest malignancy, is indicated. In women, a careful breast and pelvic examination should be done to evaluate these locations for masses. Abdominal tenderness suggests an intra-abdominal abscess. Distant heart sounds, a pericardial friction rub, and/or Kussmaul's sign (increased jugular venous pressure that increases during inspiration) suggest pericardial disease. Ascites and a pelvic mass raise the possibility of Meigs' syndrome. Deformed joints and subcutaneous nodules make rheumatoid pleuritis likely. The presence of yellow nails establishes the diagnosis of the yellow nail syndrome.

C. Laboratory Examinations

Several blood tests should be routinely obtained in patients with a persistent undiagnosed pleural effusion. If the patient has a transudative pleural effusion, a serum BNP level should be measured to evaluate the possibility of congestive heart failure. The level of albumin and globulin should be measured to determine whether the patient has cirrhosis or the nephrotic syndrome, and liver function tests should be obtained to ascertain if there is chronic hepatitis. Additionally, I also obtain a CBC with differential. A serum ANA test should be obtained with the diagnosis of systemic lupus erythematosus in mind. A BUN and creatinine should be obtained to evaluate the possibility of uremia.

Several special tests on the pleural fluid are also indicated. The cheapest test is to smell the pleural fluid. If the pleural fluid smells like urine, the patient probably has a urinothorax, while if the pleural fluid smells feculent, the patient probably has an anaerobic pleural infection. As mentioned previously, either the ADA or the gamma interferon should be measured in the pleural fluid to assess whether the patient has pleural tuberculosis. Flow cytometry on the pleural fluid is indicated if lymphoma is suspected (49). If the pleural fluid is milky or cloudy, it should be centrifuged, and if the supernatant remains milky or cloudy, the pleural fluid should be sent for measurement of cholesterol and triglycerides. Every time a thoracocentesis is performed in a patient with a persistent undiagnosed pleural effusion, a pleural fluid LDH level should be determined. If this LDH tends to decrease with time, the pleural process is resolving and one can be conservative in his approach to the patient. Alternatively, if the LDH is increasing with time, the process is getting worse and one should be aggressive in pursuing a diagnosis (5).

D. Imaging Procedures

Most patients with an undiagnosed persistent pleural effusion should have a CT angiogram of the chest. With the CT angiogram, the diagnosis of pulmonary emboli can be established (50). In addition, parenchymal infiltrates and masses and mediastinal lymphadenopathy can be identified. Moreover, the thickening of the pleura can be demonstrated. Lastly, pericardial thickening and pericardial effusions can be identified on the CT scan. While the patient is receiving the CT scan, it is reasonable to obtain abdominal cuts also. These can demonstrate abdominal masses, lymphadenopathy, and ascites. An echocardiogram is indicated if congestive heart failure is suspected, but is not definitely established, and if a pericardial effusion is suspected. It is important to remember that the echocardiogram may not reveal any abnormality if the patient has constrictive pericarditis (40). If constrictive pericarditis is suspected, the patient should undergo right-heart catheterization.

E. Blind Needle Biopsy of the Pleura

For the past 50 years, most cases of tuberculous pleuritis have been diagnosed with blind needle biopsy of the pleura. However, in the past one year, it has been demonstrated that markers for tuberculosis obtained from the pleural fluid such as the ADA or the gamma interferon are very efficient at establishing this diagnosis. The other diagnosis that can be established with needle biopsy of the pleura is pleural malignancy. However, in most series, cytology is much more sensitive in establishing the diagnosis. Moreover, if the cytology of the fluid is negative, the pleural biopsy is usually nondiagnostic. In one series of 118 patients from the Mayo Clinic who had malignancy involving the pleural but negative pleural fluid cytology, the needle biopsy of the pleura was positive in only 20 (17%) patients (51). Since thoracoscopy is diagnostic in more than 90% of patients with pleural malignancy and negative cytology, it is the preferred diagnostic procedure in patients with a cytology-negative pleural effusion who are suspected of having pleural malignancy. Blind needle biopsy of the pleura is indicated if the patient has an undiagnosed pleural effusion that is not improving and thoracoscopy is not available. Blind needle biopsy of the pleura is also indicated if pleural tuberculosis is suspected and a pleural fluid marker for tuberculosis is unavailable or equivocal (5).

F. Image-Guided Needle Biopsy of the Pleura

It appears that image-guided biopsy of the pleural using either CT or ultrasound is a good way to obtain pleural tissue, particularly if there are pleural nodules or pleural thickening (52). In one study, 50 patients with pleural thickening or pleural nodules were randomly allocated to receive a blind needle biopsy of the pleura using an Abram's needle or a CT-guided cutting needle biopsy using a #18 needle (53). In this study, the cutting needle biopsy yielded the correct diagnosis of malignancy in 13 of 15 patients, while the blind needle biopsy yielded a correct diagnosis in only 8 of 17 patients (53). There have been less studies evaluating the utility of ultrasound (52). When image-guided needle biopsy is compared to thoracoscopy, image-guided needle biopsy is less invasive, but probably provides lower diagnostic yields. It is particularly useful when there is pleural thickening or pleural nodules.

G. Thoracoscopy

When one is dealing with patients with pleural effusions, thoracoscopic procedures should be used only when less-invasive diagnostic methods such as thoracocentesis with cytology and markers for tuberculosis have not yielded a diagnosis. In the series of 620 patients reported by Kendall and coworkers (54), only 48 (8%) patients required thoracoscopy for a diagnosis. The final diagnoses in these 48 patients were malignancy 24, parapneumonic effusion 7, rheumatoid pleural effusion 4, congestive heart failure 3, and pulmonary interstitial fibrosis 2. In eight patients, no diagnosis was established with the combination of the clinical presentation and thoracoscopy; six of these patients were subsequently diagnosed as having malignancy (mesothelioma 3, adenocarcinoma 3) (54).

In general, if the patient has malignancy, thoracoscopy will establish the diagnosis in about 90% (55–57). The diagnosis of tuberculous pleuritis can also be established with thoracoscopy (58,59). It should be emphasized, however, that thoracoscopy rarely establishes the diagnosis of benign disease other than tuberculosis (60). One advantage of thoracoscopy in the diagnosis of pleural disease is that pleurodesis can be performed at the time of the procedure. In general, thoracoscopy is indicated in the patient with an undiagnosed pleural effusion who is not improving spontaneously, provided that the patient has a significant likelihood of malignancy or tuberculosis.

H. Bronchoscopy

Bronchoscopy can be diagnostically useful in patients with pleural effusion if the patient has one of the following four characteristics (61), otherwise bronchoscopy is not indicated:

1. A pulmonary infiltrate is present on the chest radiograph or the chest CT. If an infiltrate is present, particular attention should be paid to the area with the infiltrate at the time of bronchoscopy.
2. Hemoptysis is present. The presence of hemoptysis in the patient with a pleural effusion increases the likelihood of malignancy with an endobronchial lesion or pulmonary embolus. The former can be diagnosed with bronchoscopy.
3. The pleural effusion is massive. The most common cause of a massive pleural effusion is malignancy, particularly lung cancer, and this diagnosis can be established at bronchoscopy. The other two leading causes of massive pleural effusion are hepatic hydrothorax and tuberculous pleuritis; these diagnoses cannot be established with bronchoscopy.
4. The mediastinum is shifted toward the side of the effusion. With this finding, an obstructing endobronchial lesion is probably responsible, and this can be identified and biopsied at bronchoscopy.

I. Open Biopsy

In most institutions, open thoracotomy with direct biopsy of the pleura has been replaced by video-assisted thoracoscopy. If both procedures are available, thoracoscopy is usually preferred because it is associated with less morbidity. The primary indication for open pleural biopsy is progressive undiagnosed pleural disease in an institution where thoracoscopy is not available.

One should realize that even with an open biopsy of the pleura, a diagnosis is not always obtained. In one study, the experience at the Mayo Clinic between 1962 and 1972 with open pleural biopsy for undiagnosed pleural effusion was reviewed. They found that no diagnosis was established at open biopsy in 51 patients (62). Thirty-one of the patients had no recurrence of their pleural effusion. However, 13 of these 51 patients were eventually found to have malignant disease (lymphoma 6, mesothelioma 4, other malignancy 3). In another study of 21 patients subjected to open pleural biopsy for undiagnosed pleural effusion, no diagnosis was obtained in 7 (33%) (63).

References

1. Light RW, MacGregor MI, Luchsinger PC, et al. Pleural effusions: The diagnostic separation of transudates and exudates. Ann Intern Med 1972; 77:507–514.
2. Romero S, Candela A, Martin C, et al. Evaluation of different criteria for the separation of pleural transudates from exudates. Chest 1993; 104:399–404.
3. Burgess LJ, Maritz FJ, Taljaard JJ. Comparative analysis of the biochemical parameters used to distinguish between pleural transudates and exudates. Chest 1995; 107:1604–1609.
4. Romero-Candeira S, Hernandez L, Romero-Brufao S, et al. Is it meaningful to use biochemical parameters to discriminate between transudative and exudative pleural effusions? Chest 2002; 122:1524–1529.
5. Light RW. Pleural Diseases, 5th ed. Baltimore, MD: Lippincott Williams and Wilkins, 2007.
6. Porcel JM. The use of probrain natriuretic peptide in pleural fluid for the diagnosis of pleural effusions resulting from heart failure. Curr Opin Pulm Med 2005; 11:329–333.

7. Kolditz M, Halank M, Schiemanck CS, et al. High diagnostic accuracy of NT-proBNP for cardiac origin of pleural effusions. Eur Respir J 2006; 28:144–150.
8. Porcel JM, Chorda J, Cao G, Esquerda A, et al. Comparing serum and pleural fluid pro-brain natriuretic peptide (NT-proBNP) levels with pleural-to-serum albumin gradient for the identification of cardiac effusions misclassified by Light's criteria. Respirology 2007; 12: 654–659.
9. Porcel JM. Effusions from cardiac failure. Int Pleural Newsl 2007; 5:16–17.
10. Kakizaki S, Katakai K, Yoshinaga T, et al. Hepatic hydrothorax in the absence of ascites. Liver 1998; 18:216–220.
11. Daly JJ, Potts JM, Gordon L, et al. Scintigraphic diagnosis of peritoneopleural communication in the absence of ascites. Clin Nuclear Med 1994; 19:892–894.
12. Umino J, Tanaka E, Ichijoh T, et al. Hepatic hydrothorax in the absence of ascites diagnosed by intraperitoneal spraying of indocyanine green. Intern Med 2004; 43:283–288.
13. Cavina C, Vichi G. Radiological aspects of pleural effusions in medical nephropathy in children. Ann Radiol Diagn 1958; 31:163–202.
14. Llach F, Arieff A1, Massry SG. Renal vein thrombosis and nephrotic syndrome: A prospective study of 36 adult patients. Ann Intern Med 1975; 83:8–14.
15. Garcia-Pachon E, Romero S. Urinothorax: A new approach. Curr Opin Pulm Disease 2006; 12:259–263.
16. Garcia-Pachon E, Padilla-Navas I. Urinothorax: Case report and review of the literature with emphasis on biochemical diagnosis. Respiration 2004; 71:533–536.
17. Beach C, Manthey DE. Tension hydrothorax due to ventriculopleural shunting. J Emerg Med 1998; 16:33–36.
18. Monla-Hassan J, Eichenhorn M, Spickler E, et al. Duropleural fistula manifested as a large pleural transudate: An unusual complication of transthoracic diskectomy. Chest 1998; 114: 1786–1789.
19. Gupta SM, Frias J, Garg A, et al. Aberrant cerebrospinal fluid pathway. Detection by scintigraphy. Clin Nucl Med 1986; 11:593–594.
20. Huggins JT, Sahn SA. Duro-pleural fistula diagnosed by beta2-transferrin. Respiration 2003; 70:423–425
21. Ferrer J, Roldan J, Teixidor J, et al. Predictors of pleural malignancy in patients with pleural effusion undergoing thoracoscopy. Chest 2005; 127:1017–1022.
22. Naito T, Satoh H, Ishikawa H, et al. Pleural effusion as a significant prognostic factor in non-small cell lung cancer. Anticancer Res 1997; 17:4743–4746.
23. Apffelstaedt JP, Van Zyl JA, Muller AG. Breast cancer complicated by pleural effusion: Patient characteristics and results of surgical management. J Surg Oncol 1995; 58:173–175.
24. Romano M, Libshitz HI. Hodgkin disease and non-Hodgkin lymphoma: Plain chest radiographs and chest computed tomography of thoracic involvement in previously untreated patients. Radiol Med (Torino) 1998; 95:49–53.
25. Huang L, Schnapp LM, Gruden JF, et al. Presentation of AIDS-related pulmonary Kaposi's sarcoma diagnosed by bronchoscopy. Am J Respir Crit Care Med 1996; 153:1385–1390.
26. Ascoli V, Scalzo CC, Danese C, et al. Human herpes virus-8 associated primary effusion lymphoma of the pleural cavity in HIV-negative elderly men. Eur Respir J 1999; 14: 1231–1234.
27. Taniere P, Manai A, Charpentier R, et al. Pyothorax-associated lymphoma: Relationship with Epstein-Barr virus, human herpes virus-8 and body cavity-based high grade lymphomas. Eur Respir J 1998; 11:779–783.
28. Bartlett JG, Finegold SM. Anaerobic infections of the lung and pleural space. Am Rev Respir Dis 1974; 110:56–77.
29. Roper WH, Waring JJ. Primary serofibrinous pleural effusion in military personnel. Am Rev Respir Dis 1955; 71:616–634.

30. Ferrer JS, Munoz XG, Orriols RM, et al. Evolution of idiopathic pleural effusion. A prospective, long-term follow-up study. Chest 1996; 109:1508–1513.
31. Rockey DC, Cello JP. Pancreaticopleural fistula. Report of 7 patients and review of the literature. Medicine 1990; 69:332–344.
32. Light RW, Rogers JT, Moyers JP, et al. Prevalence and clinical course of pleural effusions at 30 days post coronary artery bypass surgery. Am J Respir Crit Care Med 2002; 166:1563–1566.
33. Sadikot RT, Rogers JT, Cheng D-S, et al. Pleural fluid characteristics of patients with symptomatic pleural effusion after coronary artery bypass graft surgery. Arch Intern Med 2000; 160:2665–2668.
34. Lee YCG, Rogers JT, Rodriguez RM, et al. Adenosine deaminase levels in nontuberculous lymphocytic pleural effusions. Chest 2001; 120:356–361.
35. Lee YC (Gary), Vaz MAC, Ely KA, et al. Symptomatic persistent post-coronary artery bypass graft pleural effusions requiring operative treatment. Clinical and histologic features. Chest 2001; 119:795–800.
36. Light RW. Pleural effusions following cardiac injury and coronary artery bypass graft surgery. Sem Respir Crit Care Med 2001; 22:657–664.
37. Steizner TJ, King TE Jr, Antony VB, et al. The pleuropulmonary manifestations of the postcardiac injury syndrome. Chest 1983; 84:383–387.
38. Weiss JM, Spodick DH. Association of left pleural effusion with pericardial disease. N Engl J Med 1983; 308:696–697.
39. Tomaselli G, Gamsu G, Stulbarg MS. Constrictive pericarditis presenting as pleural effusion of unknown origin. Arch Intern Med 1989; 149:201–203.
40. Sadikot RT, Fredi JL, Light RW. A 43-year-old man with a large recurrent right-sided pleural effusion. Chest 2000; 117:1191–1194.
41. Timmerman D, Moerman P, Vergote I. Meigs' syndrome with elevated serum CA 125 levels: Two case reports and review of the literature. Gynecol Oncol 1995; 59:405–408.
42. Wang DY, Yang PC, Yu WL, et al. Serial antinuclear antibodies titre in pleural and pericardial fluid. Eur Respir J 2000; 15:1106–1110.
43. Epler GR, McLoud TC, Gaensler EA. Prevalence and incidence of benign asbestos pleural effusion in a working population. JAMA 1982; 247:617–622.
44. Hillerdal G, Ozesmi M. Benign asbestos pleural effusion: 73 exudates in 60 patients. Eur J Respir Dis 1987; 71:113–121.
45. Berger HW, Rammohan G, Neff MS, et al. Uremic pleural effusion: A study in 14 patients on chronic dialysis. Ann Intern Med 1975; 82:362–364.
46. Coskun M, Boyvat F, Bozkurt B, et al. Thoracic CT findings in long-term hemodialysis patients. Acta Radiol 1998; 40:181–186.
47. Light RW, Jenkinson SG, Minh V, et al. Observations on pleural pressures as fluid is withdrawn during thoracentesis. Am Rev Respir Dis 1980; 121:799–804.
48. Fentiman IS, Millis R, Sexton S, et al. Pleural effusion in breast cancer: A review of 105 cases. Cancer 1981; 47:2087–2092.
49. Moriarty AT, Wiersema L, Snyder W, et al. Immunophenotyping of cytologic specimens by flow cytometry. Diag Cytopath 1993; 9:252–258.
50. Goodman PC. Spiral CT for pulmonary embolism. Semin Respir Crit Care Med 2000; 21:503–510.
51. Prakash URS, Reiman HM. Comparison of needle biopsy with cytologic analysis for the evaluation of pleural effusion: Analysis of 414 cases. Mayo Clin Proc 1985; 60:158–164.
52. Rahman NM, Gleeson FV. Image guided pleural biopsy. Curr Opin Pulmon Dis 2008; 14:331–336.
53. Maskell NA, Gleeson FV, Davies RJO. Standard pleural biopsy verus CT-guided cutting-needle biopsy for diagnosis of malignant disease in pleural effusions: A randomized controlled trial. Lancet 2003; 361:1326–1331.

54. Kendall SW, Bryan AJ, Large SR, et al. Pleural effusions: Is thoracoscopy a reliable investigation? A retrospective review. Respir Med 1992; 86:437–440.
55. Hucker J, Bhatnagar NK, al-Jilaihawi AN, et al. Thoracoscopy in the diagnosis and management of recurrent pleural effusions. Ann Thorac Surg 1991; 52:1145–1147.
56. Menzies R, Charbonneau M. Thoracoscopy for the diagnosis of pleural disease. Ann Intern Med 1991; 114:271–276.
57. Hansen M, Faurshou P, Clementsen P. Medical thoracoscopy, results and complications in 146 patients: A retrospective study. Respir Med 1998; 92:228–232.
58. de Groot M, Walther G. Thoracoscopy in undiagnosed pleural effusions. S Afr Med J 1998; 88:706–711.
59. Emad A, Rezaian GR. Diagnostic value of closed percutaneous pleural biopsy vs pleuroscopy in suspected malignant pleural effusion or tuberculous pleurisy in a region with a high incidence of tuberculosis: A comparative, age-dependent study. Respir Med 1998; 92:488–492.
60. Daniel TM. Diagnostic thoracoscopy for pleural disease. Ann Thorac Surg 1993; 56:639–640.
61. Chang S-C, Perng RP. The role of fiberoptic bronchoscopy in evaluating the causes of pleural effusions. Arch Intern Med 1989; 149:855–857.
62. Ryan CJ, Rodgers RF, Unni KK, et al. The outcome of patients with pleural effusion of indeterminate cause at thoracotomy. Mayo Clin Proc 1981; 56:145–149.
63. Douglass BE, Carr DT, Bernatz PE. Diagnostic thoracotomy in the study of "idiopathic" pleural effusion. Am Rev Tuberc 1956; 74:954–957.

17
Drug-Induced Pleural Involvement

PHILIPPE CAMUS, CLIO CAMUS, and PHILIPPE BONNIAUD
Department of Pulmonary Disease and Intensive Care, University Medical Center—Hôpital du Bocage, Faculté de Médecine—Université de Bourgogne, Dijon, France

I. Introduction

With more than 400 specific drugs capable of injuring the respiratory system, drug-induced respiratory disease has become an important etiologic consideration in patients with interstitial lung disease (ILD), pulmonary edema, upper airway obstruction, and acute bronchospasm (1). Patients with drug-induced respiratory complications may present acutely with the sudden onset of cardiopulmonary failure or asphyxia, requiring prompt recognition and identification of the causal drug along with emergent management to secure the airway and/or to restore gas exchange (2).

Drug-induced pleural involvement is less common than is drug-induced ILD, and it took longer for the former to be recognized as a discrete clinical-pathologic entity (3). Ipsilateral pleural effusion was described as a complication of chest radiation therapy in the 1930s. In the 1940s, a mimic of systemic *lupus* with pleural or pleuropericardial effusions was recognized as a complication of treatments with hydralazine. In the 1960s, pleural thickening and/or effusion with or without pericardial pathology were described as a complication of chronic treatments with ergolines (methysergide, followed by other members of this family of drugs). Although several other drugs followed, it was not until the 1990s that the topic of drug-induced pleural involvement could be excellently reviewed (3–6).

About 80 drugs or families of drugs given via the oral, parenteral, or intrapleural route, or given topically can cause pleural insult. Of note, certain families of drugs such as β-receptor-blockers, ergolines, and virtually all *lupus*-inducing drugs can produce a similar pattern of pleural involvement. Recent additions to the list of causal drugs include thiazolidinedione oral antidiabetic agents, the ABL-kinase inhibitor dasatinib, and TNF-α antibody therapy (1). It is essential for the clinician to clue in on the drug etiology, so as the patient with pleural effusion does not undergo unnecessary and costly investigation.

Three major difficulties pave the way to diagnosing drug-induced pleural involvement:

(i) The lack of clinical, imaging, and histopathological individuality of pleural effusions.

(ii) A broad differential, with congestive heart failure, parapneumonic effusions, pleural involvement from solid or hematologic malignancies (7), and pleural manifestations of the underlying disease for which the drug was exactly given in the background (e.g., left ventricular dysfunction, rheumatoid arthritis, inflammatory bowel disease).

(iii)   An absence of reliable diagnostic features that would enable to unambigu-
        ously separate pleural effusions due to drugs from those of other causes
        (although some clinical, imaging, and laboratory characteristics may at times
        suggest the drug etiology, including the concomitance of pleural and blood
        eosinophilia, and antinuclear antibodies (ANA) in blood or pleural fluid along
        with an appropriate exposure to a compatible drug).
(iv)   The difficulty of evaluating the effect of drug withdrawal, because drug stop-
        page may influence pleural fluid *output* (a difficult-to-measure parameter),
        rather than fluid volume. Evacuation of the pleural space and/or corticosteroid
        therapy may hinder interpretation of drug stoppage.

The diagnosis of drug-induced pleural involvement is one of exclusion, and rests on
the cornerstone of exposure versus symptoms relationships (see below, under diagnostic
criteria).

The literature on iatrogenic pleural involvement totals 746 references and includes
case records, series of cases, and the "toxicity section" of randomized drug trials. Space
constraints do not permit inclusion of all of them (1,3,4,6,8).

The level of evidence for a drug as the cause of pleural involvement is wide-ranging,
from strong in randomized studies or case reports where recurrence followed rechallenge
to average where an accumulation of cases supports an association with a specific drug
(e.g., dantrolene, propylthiouracil, valproate) or circumstantial, enabling inference of the
drug etiology in isolated cases.

The present chapter covers pleural involvement secondary to treatments with therapy drugs, abused substances, and radiation therapy. Iatrogenic pleural injury due to
medical, imaging, or surgical procedures including esophageal sclerotherapy is considered elsewhere in this book. An updated list of drugs causing respiratory insult and the
corresponding patterns of involvement are depicted in Table 1 and on Pneumotox® (1).

II.   Definition—Pathophysiology

There is no consensual definition of drug-induced pleural pathology. The diagnosis is
entertained when (*i*) unilateral or bilateral, moderate, large or, less often, massive pleural
effusion/thickening develops in conjunction with a history of current or past exposure
to a compatible drug (1), (*ii*) if no underlying illness which can express itself in the
pleura is found after appropriate investigation, and (*iii*) in the absence of concomitant
drug-induced–pulmonary edema, heart failure or ILD such as methotrexate pneumonitis
or eosinophilic pneumonia, conditions in which pleural effusions can occur (nevertheless,
a section on pleural effusion associated with drug-induced ILD is considered below).

The mechanisms for drug-induced pleural insult include serosal edema, an inflammatory mononuclear cell infiltrate of the pleural membrane, which may be immune-
mediated in the drug *lupus*, chemokine (e.g., IL-5) gradient homing specific cell types
to the pleural space, altered osmotic and/or oncotic pressures in pleural space hindering
reabsorption of pleural fluid, altered lymph-flow dynamics organization of a an exudate,
coagulation, and organization of blood, disordered pleural fibrogenesis and deposition of
subpleural fat. Clinically, pleuritic chest pain, compression of lung, heart, or mediastinum
by space-occupying pleural fluid along with a decrease in pleural compliance combine
to hinder chest expansion and cause chest discomfort, pain, and dyspnea. Other possible

Table 1 Drugs Which Produce Pleural Involvement

Drugs / Families of drugs	Lone pleural effusion	Pleuropericardial effusion	Pleural effusion and pulmonary infiltrates	Eosinophilic pleural or pleuropericardial effusion	Pleural thickening	*Lupus* pleuritis w/wo pericardial effusion	Acute chest pain ± ECG changes	Hemothorax	Subpleural fat, lipomatosis	Pneumothorax	Chylothorax
Acebutolol	*					**					
ACE inhibitors											
Acrylate		*	*								
Acyclovir		*	*								
Adalimumab			*			*					
Alteplase								*			
Amiodarone	*		**			*					
Anticoagulants oral, parenteral								**			
Arsenic trioxide	*		*			*					
Beta receptor antagonists											
Bleomycin	*		*							*	
Bromocriptine	*			*	**		*				
Cabergoline	*				**						
Carbamazepine						**					
Carmustine (BCNU)			*		*					*	
Chrysotherapy/Gold	*										
Clomifen	***										
Clopidogrel								*			
Clozapine	*			*							
Corticosteroids									*		
Cyanoacrylate				*							
Cyclophosphamide	*				**						
Cytosine arabinoside (Ara-C)			*								
Dantrolene				**							
Dapsone	*										

Table 1 (*Continued*)

Drugs Families of drugs	Lone pleural effusion	Pleuropericardial effusion	Pleural effusion and pulmonary infiltrates	Eosinophilic pleural or pleuropericardial effusion	Pleural thickening	Lupus pleuritis w/wo pericardial effusion	Acute chest pain ± ECG changes	Hemothorax	Subpleural fat, lipomatosis	Pneumothorax	Chylothorax
Dasatinib	**										
Dextran	**	*									
Dihydroergocristine	*				**						
Dihydroergocryptine	*				**						
Dihydroergotamine	*				**						
Enoxaparine								*			
Ergolines	*	**			***						
Ergotamine	*				**						
Etanercept						**					
Ethchlorvynol			*								
Fenfluramine/ dexfenfluramine			*								
Fibrinolytic agents											
Fludarabine		*						*			
Fluorouracil							**				
Furazolidone	*						*				
Gliclazide				*							
Glitazones	**		**								
Gonadotropins	*		*								
G(M)-CSF			*								
HAART		**									
Heparin											
Hydralazine						***		*			
Imidapril				*							
Imatinib	*	*									
Infliximab			*	*		**					
Interleukin 2			**								
Isoniazid						*					

Table 1 (Continued)

Drugs Families of drugs	Lone pleural effusion	Pleuropericardial effusion	Pleural effusion and pulmonary infiltrates	Eosinophilic pleural or pleuropericardial effusion	Pleural thickening	Lupus pleuritis w/wo pericardial effusion	Acute chest pain ± ECG changes	Hemothorax	Subpleural fat, lipomatosis	Pneumothorax	Chylothorax
Isotretinoin	*										
Itraconazole		*	*								
IVIG											
Leuprorelin	*										
Lisuride	*	*			*			*			
Lupus-inducing drugs											
Mesalazine	*		*	*		****					
Mesulergine	*				*	*					
Methotrexate	**		**								
Methyldopa						**	**				
Methysergide	**	*	*		***						
Minocycline	*		*			*	*				
Minoxidil	*										
Mitomycin	*		*								
Nevirapine				*	**						
Nicergoline	*		**								
Nitrofurantoin	*		**	*							
Penicillamine						*					
Pergolide	*				*						
Phenytoin	*					*					
Pindolol							*				
Pioglitazone	*										
Practolol (recalled)	*				***						
Pravastatin	*										
Praziquantel				*							
Procainamide						***					
Procarbazine	*?		*	**							
Progesterone				*							
Propylthiouracil	*		*								
Prostacyclin	*										
Quinidine						*					

Table 1 (*Continued*)

Drugs / Families of drugs	Lone pleural effusion	Pleuropericardial effusion	Pleural effusion and pulmonary infiltrates	Eosinophilic pleural or pleuropericardial effusion	Pleural thickening	Lupus pleuritis w/wo pericardial effusion	Acute chest pain ± ECG changes	Hemothorax	Subpleural fat, lipomatosis	Pneumothorax	Chylothorax
Radiation therapy	*	**	***		***						*
Retinoic acid (ATRA)	**		**				*			*	
Simvastatin			*			*					*
Sulfamides-sulfonamides-sulfasalazine	*		**	*		**					
Sumatriptan							*				
TACE	*		*								
Talc			*		**						
Thiazolidinediones	**										
Tizanidine				*							
Trimipramine				*							
Troglitazone	**										
L-tryptophan (recalled)	*		***	*							
Valproate				*							
Vitamin B5											

Column 1: families of drugs, in which most specific drugs produce the adverse pleural effect are boldface.

Column 4: pleural effusion in association with infiltrative lung disease or pulmonary edema.

Column 6: pleural effusion, usually an exudate, may predate or occur in association with pleural thickening.

Column 7: *lupus* pleuritis, that is, the association of pleural effusion, or pericardial effusion, systemic symptoms (e.g., fever, rash, arthralgias) and positive antinuclear with or without anti-DNA antibodies (drugs which occasion the *lupus* syndrome do not all cause *lupus* pleuritis or pleural effusion).

The number of stars/asterisks reflects incidence. from * rare to **** common.

Abbreviations: ACE, angiotensin converting enzyme; ATRA, all-transretinoic acid; HAART, highly active antiretroviral therapy; IVIG, intravenous immunoglobulins; TACE, transhepatic arterial chemoembolization (in the treatment of hepatocellular carcinoma).

drug-induced consequences include blood loss causing anemia or cardiopulmonary failure if there is significant bleeding in the pleural space, pericardial tamponade if a large effusion or constriction is present, and concomitant underlying or drug-induced parenchymal lung involvement.

III. Clinical Presentation

The clinical presentation in moderate-sized drug-induced pleural effusion is similar to that in pleural involvement of other causes and is manifested by the insidious onset of dyspnea, chest discomfort, pleurodynia, and a nonproductive cough. Patients with massive and/or bilateral effusion(s) may present acutely with respiratory distress mandating prompt insertion of chest tube and extraction of pleural fluid. Patients on high-dose methotrexate or bleomycin may present with acute excruciating chest pain, causing diagnostic confusion with other thoracic emergencies. Chemotherapy-induced progressive pleural fibroelastosis manifests with unremitting dyspnea, chest pain, a restrictive lung function defect, and, sometimes, intervening episodes of pneumothorax.

Pleural involvement may occur in isolation, in the form of unilateral or bilateral effusion or thickening of pleuritis, or it occurs in association with pericardial effusion, tamponade, or polyserositis, with or without the clinical and laboratory features of the drug *lupus* (3,9), which include arthralgias, a malar rash, leukopenia, a positive ANA test, and less often anti–double-strand DNA antibodies or deep organ involvement. Rarely, pleural effusion(s) occur in the context of a drug-induced systemic reaction such as the "Drug Rash Eosinophilia and Systemic Symptoms" or DRESS or sulfone syndrome, the "Immune Reconstitution Inflammatory Syndrome" or IRIS, a condition seen in immunodepressed HIV-positive individuals who are being started on highly active antiretroviral therapy, or in the neuroleptic malignant syndrome (10).

IV. Imaging Features

Imaging studies indicate unilateral or bilateral pleural effusion, which can be from minimal to massive, although very large effusions causing compression are uncommon (3). Cardiomegaly raises the suspicion of pericardial effusion, a classical feature of drug-induced *lupus*. Cardiac ultrasound examination is indicated in the drug *lupus* and in patients with ergoline-induced pleural changes to detect pericardial thickening or valvular heart disease (11). The high-resolution CT (HRCT) is more sensitive than that of the chest radiograph to detect minimal pleural effusion (12). The specific merit and limits of pleural ultrasound and magnetic resonance imaging in drug-induced pleural involvement await further studies. Positron-emission tomography using ^{18}F-deoxyglucose (FDG-PET) may show tracer avid pleural areas, which appear localized rather than diffuse in patients with a history of talc pleurodesis (13,14). FDG-PET scanography is also used to rule out malignancy.

V. Laboratory Investigation—Pulmonary Physiology–Pathology

Pleural fluid should be examined macroscopically and microscopically when it is removed for diagnostic purpose or evacuation of the pleural space, because biochemistry and cellularity may change with time. Macroscopically, the pleural fluid can be clear, straw-colored, turbid, blood-stained, hemorrhagic, or milky. Biochemical evaluation includes the following: concomitant lactic dehydrogenase (LDH) in pleural fluid and blood to calculate the pleural fluid-to-serum LDH ratio, which is used along with total proteins to separate transudates from exudates. Amylase, hyaluronate, or lipids are evaluated to rule out other causes of pleural effusion. Microscopically, red and white cells and differential should be noted. Pathologic examination of pleural fluid and tissue for malignant cells, cultures, and special stains are also indicated to rule an infection or malignancy. Phospholipid-laden cells can be present in patients with amiodarone-induced pleuropulmonary toxicity, and LE-cells can be found in those with drug-induced *lupus*. High ANA titers in the pleural fluid contribute the diagnosis of *lupus erythematosus* and its levels should be compared to serum ANA.

The bronchoalveolar lavage (BAL) is indicated whenever there is the suggestion of concomitant ILD, when blood or pleural eosinophilia is present, or the patient is immunocompromised under the combined influence of therapy drugs (e.g., chemo agents, TNF-α antibody therapy) or the underlying condition, or both, to rule out an opportunistic infection. Its most important role is an exclusionary one.

A mildly restrictive pulmonary physiology is usually present in patients with pleural effusion or thickening, and the amount of restriction is typically less than the volume of fluid that can be extracted (15). Carbon monoxide (CO) transfer is slightly to moderately reduced, but the diffusing capacity for CO (KCO) is normal or is increased, except if parenchymal involvement is present concomitantly (15). Serial imaging and measurements of pulmonary function are used as a barometer to confirm improvement following drug discontinuation.

Pleural biopsy (closed or via thoracoscopy) and histopathological examination of pleural tissue are mainly indicated to rule out other pleural conditions. However, pathology may support the drug etiology when it shows acute inflammation, eosinophilic inflammation, or pleural fibrosis, along with vasculitis in *lupus* cases (16). An elastic fiber stain is indicated in chemotherapy-induced pleural thickening, to disclose fibroelastosis (17).

VI. Diagnosis

Diagnostic criteria include the following:

- Whenever available, pretherapy pulmonary imaging and physiology should be retrieved to check that the pleural changes were not evident earlier.
- Correct identification of the drug: History taking should include current and past exposure to (*i*) drugs (including batch number, dosage, and route of administration), (*ii*) abused/recreational substances, and (*iii*) radiation therapy to the chest, including portals and isodose mapping. An occupational history should also be taken, because exposure to asbestos may increase the risk of developing ergoline-induced pleural complications.
- Drug singularity. In patients exposed to more than one drug, the contribution of each drug taken in isolation should be specifically examined, as regards its propensity to cause pleural involvement. Sequential drug withdrawal, although cumbersome and time-consuming, may help sorting out the responsibility of each specific drug.
- Symptom–exposure relationship is the mainstay for diagnosing drug-induced pleural involvement:

- Pleural effusion/thickening should develop *after* (not *before*) the commencement of treatment with the drug under scrutiny although, at times, preexisting pleural pathology unrelated to drugs may by exacerbated by treatment with drugs.
- The interval between initiation of therapy with the causal drug and the development of symptoms corresponding to pleural involvement can be as short as a few hours in acute methotrexate-induced pleuritic chest pain, a few days in anticoagulant-induced hemothorax, or of months or years in most other drug- or radiation-induced pleural injury.
- Pleural changes may be diagnosed months or years after termination of treatment with ergolines, cyclophosphamide, intrapleural talc, or radiation therapy.
- Drug dechallenge (underlying illness permitting). Most patients with pleural effusion resolve their clinical, radiographic, and laboratory (ESR, ANA, ANCA) findings with discontinuation of the culprit drug. Symptoms disappear first in a few days or weeks, followed by diminution of pleural fluid amount over weeks. It takes longer for drug-induced pleural thickening to resolve. Antinuclear antibodies, if present, typically decrease over a few months or one year to low or undetectable levels. At variance with effusions, pleural fibrosis may progress despite cessation of exposure to the drug, causing progressive encasement of the lung. Evacuation of the pleural space to avoid long-term pleural complications should be discussed, as this may make the assessment of causality difficult.
- Recurrence with inadvertent or deliberate reexposure to the drug is taken as definite and definitive evidence for causality. This has been documented in a few cases where chest pain, pleural effusion, and/or peripheral eosinophilia returned after rechallenge with the drug. Rechallenge would be difficult to interpret in patients with drug-induced pleural fibrosis, and runs the risk of provoking further irreversible changes.
- The pattern of pleural reaction should be consistent with the literature on the specific drug. Interestingly, there is a tendency for drugs to produce a reproducible pattern of involvement. For instance, (*i*) dantrolene, propythiouracil, and valproate occasion an eosinophilic pleural or pleuropericardial effusion with or without blood eosinophilia, (*ii*) anticoagulants cause pleural bleeding, and (*iii*) ergot drugs cause pleural thickening with or without an effusion. Other features consistent with the drug etiology include (*i*) concomitant pleural and pericardial involvement, the latter in the form of an effusion or thickening [e.g., with the use of ATRA, clozapine, dantrolene, ergolines, imatinib, practolol (a drug recalled in 1976), valproate, and *lupus*-inducing drugs]; (*ii*) retroperitoneal (ergolines), (*iii*) mediastinal (corticosteroids, ergolines), and valvular heart disease (ergolines).
- Quality of evidence in the literature. The strength of the signal that a drug actually causes pleural involvement rests on incidence rate and clinical, imaging, and histopathological distinctiveness of the pleural reaction with the drug in question.
- Causes other than drugs should be ruled out. Several underlying or incidental infectious and noninfectious processes may manifest with pleural effusion, just as do the drugs used to treat them. An uncompromising discussion is required

to weigh the respective responsibility of drug versus the underlying disease, for instance, amiodarone or thiazolidinediones versus congestive heart failure, or dasatinib versus pleural involvement from myelogenous leukemia, or still TNF-α inhibitors versus pleural involvement from the underlying rheumatoid arthritis or inflammatory bowel disease.

– Laboratory investigation may help diagnose drug-induced pleural involvement. Concomitant eosinophilia in pleural fluid and blood is a useful marker for the drug etiology. Coagulation studies and platelet count are indicated in the patient with hemothorax suspected of being drug-induced. Elevated ANA and/or ANCAs suggest a drug-induced autoimmune condition. High titers of ANA or LE cells in pleural fluid are consistent with drug-induced *lupus*. In light of recent studies, lymphocyte proliferation assays may not be helpful to confirm the drug etiology (18).

VII. Lone Drug-Induced Pleural Effusion(S) [Table 1; (1,3,6)]

A. Lone Noneosinophilic Pleural Effusions (Fig. 1)

Main Features

Acebutolol, acyclovir, amiodarone, several β-blockers, clomifen, clozapine, cyclophosphamide, dapsone, dasatinib, dextran, most ergolines, gonadotropins, imatinib, intravenous immunoglobulins (IVIG), mesalazine, methotrexate, minoxidil, nitrofurantoin,

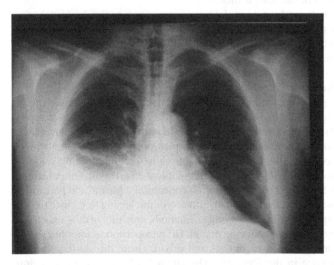

Figure 1 Drug-induced pleural exudate. A pleural neutrophilic and lymphocytic exudate developed in a patient on dihydralazine long term (the drug is generally unavailable any longer). Neutrophils were increased in blood. Although the drug can produce the *lupus* syndrome, ANA were negative in the present case. Symptoms improved and pleural effusion disappeared in a few weeks following drug discontinuance. The lists of drugs, which produce pleural exudate with or without pleural fluid eosinophilia, are depicted in Table 1 and in Pneumotox®. Positive dechallenge is expected in the majority of patients with drug-induced pleural effusion. Rechallenge is not advised.

penicillamine, pravastatin, propylthiouracil, sulfamides, sulfonamides, thiazolidinediones probably as a group and all-transretinoic acid or ATRA have been associated with otherwise unexplained unilateral or, less often, bilateral free-flowing pleural effusion (1,6). Results of pleural fluid analysis (though the pleural fluid was not analyzed in every patient) showed an exudate containing lymphocytes, or lymphocytes neutrophils and eosinophils in most, while in a few it was a transudate (3,6). Typically, the effusion resolves with drug therapy withdrawal, leaving little or no residual changes on imaging, although in a few patients, moderate pleural thickening persisted. The outcome of drug-induced pleural effusion is good following drug withdrawal. Persistence of the effusion is infrequent. Rechallenge was followed by recurrence in several patients.

Ergoline-Induced Effusion (Fig. 2)
Pleural effusions is less common a complication of treatments with ergolines than is pleural thickening in a ratio of 1 in 20 (11,19). Ergoline-induced free-flowing effusions were first described during treatments of migraine with methysergide. Among other ergots approved for the treatment or Parkinson's disease or restless leg syndrome, bromocriptine, cabergoline, nicergoline, and pergolide have been shown to cause a free-flowing pleural effusion on either side. Imaging studies indicate unilateral or bilateral moderate-to-large effusions. On HRCT, pleural thickening, rounded atelectasis, and trapped lung can be present underneath the pleural surface where it appears thickest. A raised ESR is a common laboratory finding. Analysis of the pleural fluid typically showed a lymphocyte-predominant (up to 99%) exudate. Pleural eosinophilia, a serosanguineous exudate, or a transudate are unusual findings (3). Ergoline-induced effusions usually resolve following drug withdrawal, with brief corticosteroid therapy indicated in symptomatic cases. Following drug dechallenge, chest symptoms and the effusion diminish. The ESR can be monitored following drug therapy withdrawal, supporting the drug etiology when it decreases together with drug holiday. Pleural thickening and rounded atelectasis decrease more slowly or, less often, persist unchanged.

Amiodarone (Fig. 3)
A moderate, more often unilateral pleural exudate develops in up to a third of patients with other evidence for amiodarone pulmonary toxicity (20). In contrast, a free-flowing effusion as the sole and primary manifestation of amiodarone toxicity is distinctly unusual. A pericardial effusion can be present. In one patient on high-dose amiodarone (1600 mg, followed by 1200 mg daily), there were bilateral exudates, which had the same biochemical characteristics and subsided after drug discontinuation (21). In another patient, a large bilateral serosanguineous effusion predated the onset of classic amiodarone pneumonitis (22). The pleural fluid in amiodarone-associated effusions is a lymphocyte-rich (23), or lymphocyte- and neutrophil-rich exudate with a range of protein concentration of 2.8 to 5.5 g/dL (21). Foam cells in the pleural fluid resembling those in the BAL fluid were evidenced in one case (22). Histopathologic examination of the pleura in one case revealed pleural thickening and dyslipidotic foam cells in pleural tissue (21). Causality assessment is problematic when pleural effusion develops during amiodarone treatment, because the diagnosis is against the background of heart failure, which can also manifest with pleural effusion. Cardiac effusions typically present as transudates, albeit exudates can also occur (24). It is unclear whether evaluation of natriuretic peptide B (BNP) may aid

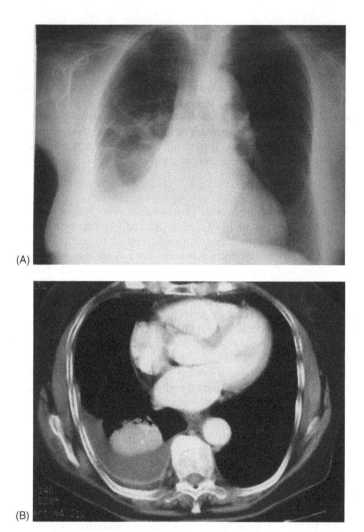

Figure 2 Ergoline-induced effusions. Right-sided lymphocytic pleural exudate developed insidiously during chronic treatment with an ergoline (**A**). Contrast-enhanced CT (**B**) shows pleural thickening, a right-sided free-flowing effusion with, surmounting it, rounded atelectasis. Both effusion and atelectasis diminished, without resolving completely upon drug withdrawal. The reason why drug-induced pleural effusion often is unilateral is unclear.

in the differentiation of amiodarone versus cardiac effusions, because heart failure may be present (25), and amiodarone suppresses BNP levels (26).

   A few cases of amiodarone-induced *lupus* have been reported, two of which manifested with pleural (27) or pleuropericardial effusion (28). Pleural fluid was examined in one of the two cases and was a lymphocytic exudate (27). Patients with amiodarone-induced *lupus* improved and ANA titers decreased upon discontinuance of the drug (see section, drug-induced *lupus erythematosus*).

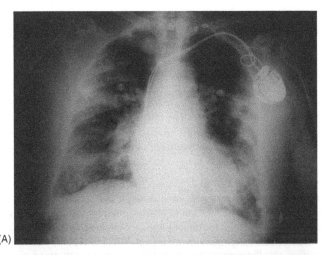

(A)

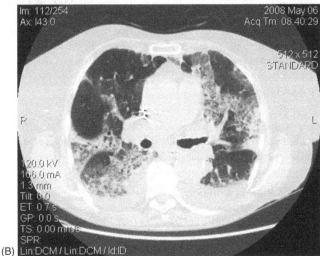

(B)

Figure 3 Amiodarone-associated effusions. Bilateral free-flowing effusion, more often an exudate, is common in patients with other evidence for amiodarone pulmonary toxicity, mainly raising the issue of cardiac dysfunction. Protein concentration of the pleural fluid, pulmonary physiology and diffusing capacity, cardiac ultrasound, diuresis, BNP levels, and prudent drug therapy withdrawal with or without corticosteroid therapy in severe cases are used to clarify the respective responsibility of amiodarone versus other causes. Upon drug withdrawal, amiodarone-related effusions diminish hand-in-hand with the parenchymal changes of amiodarone pulmonary toxicity.

Dasatinib

Dasatinib is an orally available Brc-Abl-kinase inhibitor that is used to treat patients with imatinib-resistant chronic myelogenous leukemia (CML). In a phase I study, 15 (18%) of 84 patients developed pleural effusions (29). Further studies confirmed a similar increase in the incidence of often asymptomatic pleural effusions with the use of this agent: in a study in 40 CML patients who were being treated with dasatinib 70 mg twice daily, six developed a blood-free pleural exudate that was bilateral in two, lymphocytic in five (up to 96% lymphocytes), and neutrophilic in one (7). Parenchymal infiltrates or septal lines were present on imaging in three patients. Most patients with dasatinb-induced pleural involvement exhibited a concomitant increase in BAL lymphocytes and, less often neutrophils (7). Pathologic examination of pleural tissue in two cases showed lymphocytic infiltration in one case, and leukemic infiltration in the other (7). Pleural effusion resolved after drug stoppage. Four patients were rechallenged to treat the underlying leukemia with the lower dosage of 40 mg dasatinib twice daily. The effusion returned in only one after five months to resolve again after drug withdrawal (7). A recent paper noted hemorrhagic or cloudy lymphocyte-rich effusion with chylomicrons present on both sides, in one case, suggesting a lymphatic network disorder (127).

Thiazolidinedione-Induced Effusions

The thiazolidinediones are insulin-sensitizing agents used for the treatment of type 2 *diabetes mellitus*. Treatment with these agents can be complicated by fluid retention and weight gain, which, sometimes, progresses to frank pulmonary edema that is refractory to diuretic therapy and responds specifically to drug withdrawal (30). The risk may be similar with all glitazones including troglitazone (31), which was recalled in 2000. In several patients with thiazolidinediones-induced pulmonary edema, small pleural effusion(s) were present on imaging, but pleural fluid was not examined (32). One report mentioned large bilateral effusions during treatment with pioglitazone (30). The pleural fluid had the characteristics of a transudate (total proteins: 2.5 g/dL; LDH: 79 UI/L). Treatment with furosemide and a 5-kg weight loss were without an effect, and only after pioglitazone was discontinued, did the effusions resolved (30).

Chylothorax

One case of chylothorax was diagnosed in a simvastatin-treated patient. The effusion resolved in conjunction with drug stoppage and a lipid-free diet (33). Chylous effusions were recently described following exposure to dasatinib.

B. Lone Eosinophilic Pleural Effusion

Eosinophilic pleural effusion is defined as >10% eosinophils in pleural fluid. Clozapine, cyanoacrylate, dantrolene, fluoxetine, gliclazide, G-CSF, imidapril, infliximab, isotretinoin, mesalasine, nitrofurantoin, praziquantel, propylthiouracil, simvastatin, sulfasalazine, tizanidine, trimipramine, L-tryptophan, valproate, and vitamin B5 can occasion lone eosinophilic pleural effusion (1,6). The effusion can be bilateral and occurs with or without pericardial effusion (1,34). The level of evidence for the drug etiology is the strongest with dantrolene and valproate and possibly propylthiouracil, with several well-documented cases each (34,35). With dantrolene, time to onset was 2 months to 12 years, and pleural eosiophilia ranged between 36% and 85% corresponding to absolute eosinophil numbers between 375 and 1840 per microliter (35). With valproate, the percentage of eosinophils was 40% to 75%. All effusions had resolved within six months of drug withdrawal (34).

Evidence for other drugs is less at the present time. Blood, BAL, or pleural eosinophilia can be present in conjunction with pleural eosinophilia. Rechallenge usually causes recurrence of symptoms and the pleural effusion. Of the above drugs, ACE inhibitors other than imidapril, clozapine, infliximab, isotretinoin, mesalazine, nitrofurantoin, praziquantel, propylthiouracil, sulfasalazine, trimipramine, and L-tryptophan can also occasion the syndrome of pulmonary infiltrates and eosinophilia (1). Interestingly and with no clear explanation, neither dantrolene nor valproate has produced pulmonary infiltrates and eosinophilia yet.

VIII. Pleural Effusion Associated With Drug-Induced Pneumonitis (Fig. 4)

Pleural effusions may occur in conjunction with acute or severe nitrofurantoin-, or methotrexate-induced pneumonitis, and in drug-induced eosinophilic pneumonias.

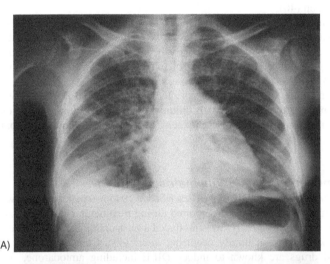

(A)

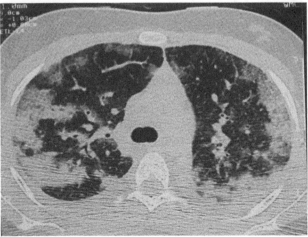

(B)

Figure 4 Pleural effusion as a related manifestation of acute drug–induced lung disease. Unilateral or bilateral exudate(s) or an eosinophilic pleural effusion can be a related manifestation of methotrexate pneumonia (**A**) or drug-induced eosinophilic pneumonia (**B**), when these conditions are acute or severe.

In acute *nitrofurantoin* lung, pleural effusions are present in up to 16% of patients. Pleural fluid amount ranged from minimal in the form of blunting of the costophrenic angles to a moderate volume effusion. Rechallenge in one patient occasioned recurrence of blood eosinophilia and of the pleural effusion, but the pleural fluid was not examined (36). In patients with subacute or chronic nitrofurantoin lung, the prevalence of pleural effusion is less with 6% (3,37).

With *methotrexate* pneumonitis, pleural effusion and/or thickening have a combined overall incidence of 2.9% to 10% (38,39).

A patient presented with a lymphocyte-predominant exudate while receiving therapy with *gold*, an antirheumatic drug that is less in use today. Pleural biopsy revealed nonspecific inflammation (40).

Pleural effusion was present in 2 out of 5 patients with *mitomycin* pneumonitis in the series by Gunstream et al. (41). Characteristics of the pleural fluid were not reported.

Peripheral opacities and lung shrinkage have been reported in patients exposed to *bleomycin*. Although the reaction was called "bleomycin pleuropneumonitis," a true effusion is unusual (42) (Fig. 5).

Pleural effusions with or without chest pain have been reported in patients with eosinophilic pneumonia due to ACEI, celecoxib, diflunisal, dapsone, fenfluramine, heroin, minocycline, nevirapine, progesterone, tosulofloxacin, trastuzumab, trypophan, herbals, or a health food (1).

IX.   Drug-Induced *Lupus Erythematosus* (Fig. 6)

Drug-induced *lupus erythematosus* (DILE) was described in 1945 in a patient treated with sulfadiazine. Then, many DILE cases were reported during treatments with hydralazine in the 1950s, and the clustering of early cases produced a measurable increase in prevalence above the background of naturally occurring *lupus* (43). Currently, about 100 chemically unrelated drugs are known to induce DILE including amiodarone, ACE inhibitors, anticonvulsants, β-blockers [mainly acebutolol]; DILE also occurred with topical ophthalmic β-blockers (9)], carbamazepine, chlorpromazine, oral contraceptives, dihydralazine, mesalazine, methyldopa, minocycline, nitrofurantoin, propylthiouracil, statins, sulfasalazine, ticlopidine, and, recently, TNF-α antibody therapy (44). Although the potent *lupus*-inducing drugs hydralazine and procainamide are less in use now, DILE is still prevalent with an incidence of 0.8 per 100,000 population, or 0.18% of patients exposed to anti-TNF biological drugs (45). Drugs may cause up to 30% of all *lupus* cases. Generally, drugs induce a form of *lupus* which is dissimilar to the idiopathic *lupus* both clinically (equal distribution in men and women, as opposed to the 90% female predominance in idiopathic *lupus*, milder course, absence of flares, rarity of renal or neurological involvement, reversal upon discontinuance of drug therapy) and biologically [anti–double-strand-DNA antibodies being a rare finding except with the novel anti–TNF-α biologicals (44,128); complement within the normal range]. Risk factors for the development of drug-induced *lupus* are drug- and patient-related and include (*i*) the type of drug (with arylamine and hydrazine drugs being potent *lupus*-inducing agents, and anti-TNF agents being capable of producing a form of DILE that is clinically and biologically closer to idiopathic *lupus erythematosus*), (*ii*) dose and duration of treatment with the drug, (*iii*) genotypic and phenotypic metabolic traits (patients with the slow hydralazine acetylator phenotype produce more oxidative and unconjugated metabolites have a higher liability to disease

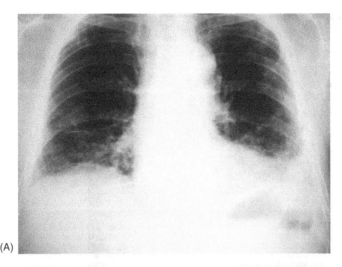

(A)

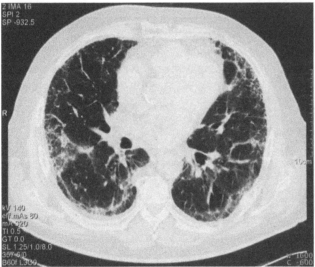

(B)

Figure 5 Bleomycin pleuropulmonary toxicity. Bibasilar shrinking is a common feature of bleomycin pleuropulmonary toxicity (**A**). Patients may present with acute intense chest pain. Basilar peripheral parenchymal infiltrates and pleural thickening can be seen on CT (**B**), and are presumably due to fibrinous pleural effusion or thickening. A true effusion is distinctly unusual.

and develop *lupus*-related symptoms earlier, as opposed to patients with the rapid acetylator phenotype, who preferentially metabolize hydralazine into less potent *lupus*-inducing conjugated metabolites), (*iv*) familial background (relatives of patients with DILE are prone to the development of idiopathic auto-immune conditions), and (*v*) ethnicity (the condition develops more often in whites than it does in dark-skinned people).

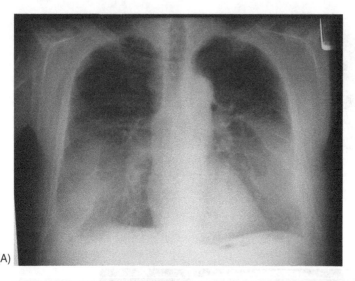

(A)

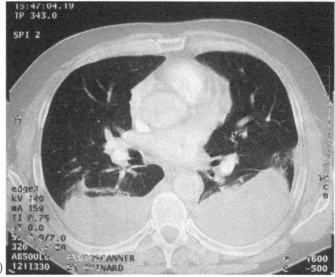

(B)

Figure 6 Drug-induced *lupus erythematosus* with bilateral pleural effusions. Modereate fever, a positive ANA test and free-flowing effusions (confirmed on one side as an exudate) developed in conjunction a patient with *lupus* induced by fluoxetine, one out of many *lupus*-inducing agents (**A,B**). Pericardial effusion, a cardinal manifestion of the drug *lupus* was not present in this particular patient. Stoppage of the *lupus*-inducing drug leads to disappearance of symptoms and the pleural effusion in a few weeks, as it did in the present case (**C**). Resolution of the abnormal ANA titers usually follows in a few months.

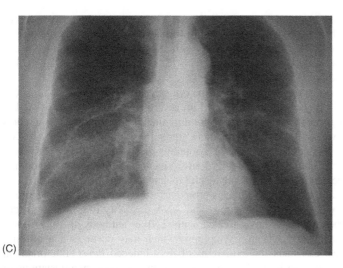

(C)

Figure 6 (*Continued*)

Onset of DILE is progressive after a few months to a few years into treatment, although it may manifest acutely with intense chest pain. Pleurodynia, cough, dyspnea, arthralgias, fever, skin changes alongside deep organ involvement during treatment with a compatible drug should prompt the diagnosis of DILE (9,44). When the disease develops insidiously, the diagnosis is made weeks or months after the clinical onset, and early evaluation of ANA titers is indicated in patients exposed to a compatible drug who develop symptoms consistent with DILE. Between 18% and 50% of patients with DILE present with pleuritis or pleural effusion, and up to a third do so with pericardial effusion (44). Rare DILE patients present with peripheral eosinophilia. By definition, circulating ANA are present in patients with DILE, with antibodies to histone and beta-2 glycoprotein 1 present in a portion of them. Antihistone antibodies are not specific for the drug etiology and demonstrate different specificity depending on the causal drug, for instance to H2A, H2B, or H2A–H2B complex in procainamide-induced *lupus*, and H3 and H4 in hydralazine-induced *lupus*, respectively (46). An antibody to histone may at times be the only antibody present and ANA are negative (47). Antibodies to double stand (ds)–DNA have been a rare finding, being described during treatments with acebutolol, hydralazine, penicillamine, procainamide, and anti–TNF-α antibody therapy (44). In a recent review of 33 ANA-positive DILE cases during treatment with TNF-α inhibitors (etanercept, infliximab, adalimumab), anti–ds-DNA antibody was found in 91%, hypocomplementemia in 59%, and antibody to histone in 57% (44). ANCA with myeloperoxidase specificity, antiphospholipid antibodies, and the *lupus* anticoagulant are unusual findings in DILE (48).

Drug-induced *lupus* manifests with unilateral or bilateral pleural effusion or pleuritis. An isolated pleural thickening has yet to be described in the drug *lupus*. As in idiopathic *lupus*, the pleural fluid in DILE is an exudate (9), with cell counts from 230 to 55,000 cells/μL, a percentage of neutrophils from 0% to 100% (3,49), and pleural LDH between 200 and 550 IU/L. The presence of ANA in the pleural fluid is a useful marker of *lupus*, regardless of the cause for it: 11 out of 13 patients (two drug-induced) with *lupus* pleuritis had pleural fluid ANA $\geq 1:160$. In 9 out of these 11, the pleural fluid-to-serum ANA ratio was greater than unity (49). ANA have been identified in the pleura of patients with drug-induced *lupus* pleuritis (50) and in the pericardial fluid in procainamide-induced *lupus* (51).

Treatment is mainly discontinuation of the drug. Nonsteroidal anti-inflammatory drugs or corticosteroid therapy is recommended for severe or symptomatic cases and/or if organ compromise is present. Upon stoppage of drug therapy, constitutional symptoms diminish over a few weeks, followed by the more gradual resolution of pleural effusion and ANA titers. In a few cases, ANA and/or symptoms persisted for longer periods of time. Rechallenging the patient with the drug leads to recurrence of symptoms within a shorter period of time, and it is not clinically useful to diagnose DILE.

The diagnosis of drug-induced *lupus* is problematic in patients whose underlying condition manifests with systemic symptoms and ANA positivity (e.g., inflammatory bowel disease or rheumatoid arthritis treated with TNF-α antibody therapy), inasmuch as pleural effusion and systemic symptoms, which may occur as a manifestation of these diseases, can meet the symptoms of drug-induced *lupus*. Interpretation of drug dechallenge may also be problematic, because the systemic manifestations of the underlying disease may return following drug therapy withdrawal, causing diagnostic confusion at a time when abatement of clinical symptoms is expected with drug discontinuation. Careful monitoring of the time course of symptoms, imaging, ANA, anti–ds-DNA, and anti-antihistone antibodies following drug withdrawal is used to sort out the respective responsibility of the drug, as opposed to the background condition.

If detected incidentally during treatment with a *lupus*-inducing drug, the presence and titers of ANA *per se* do not predict the likelihood of developing DILE nor the type or severity of the clinical presentation and are not an indication to withdraw the drug. Patients who develop subclinical ANA without evidence for pleural effusion or other organ involvement need watchful follow-up. The suspected drug need not be discontinued, unless signs or symptoms develop, or an alternate treatment is available (52).

X. Drug-Induced Pleural Thickening

Irradiation (See Below Under Radiation)

Amiodarone (Fig. 7)

Imaging studies, particularly HRCT, indicate smooth-edged crescent-shaped pleural thickening in up to two-thirds of patients with symptomatic amiodarone pulmonary toxicity (53). Pleural thickening is greatest en face the area where the pulmonary infiltrates are densest. Clinically, pleuritic chest pain and a friction rub can be present, but no study has correlated symptoms with location of pleural changes on imaging. Diagnosis of amiodarone pulmonary toxicity is aided when there is slate-grey color of the skin imparted by amiodarone, or if the lung parenchymal shadowing or the liver exhibit increased attenuation numbers on HRCT. The latter changes are thought to result from the sequestration of amiodarone in tissues, since two iodines are present on each amiodarone molecule (54). Upon amiodarone discontinuation, with corticosteroid therapy in symptomatic cases, pleural thickening may regress in concert with the pulmonary opacities

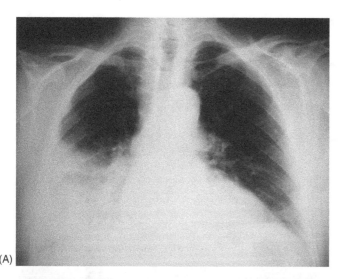

(A)

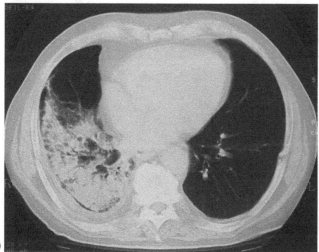

(B)

Figure 7 Pleural thickening in amiodarone pulmonary toxicity. In patients with amiodarone pulmonary toxicity (**A**), the HRCT (**B**) often shows smooth-edged crescent-shaped pleural thickening en face the areas of parenchymal involvement. Pleural changes may escape notice on the plain chest radiograph (**A**).

of amiodarone pulmonary toxicity, or it persists despite resolution of the pulmonary changes.

Ergolines (Fig. 8)

Ergolines produce fibrotic conditions, which may localize in the pleura, pericardium or retroperitoneum, and compress adjacent structures. Cardiac valve disease can also

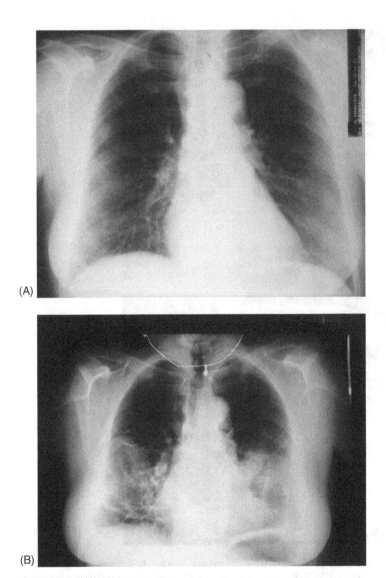

Figure 8 Pleural changes produced by chronic exposure to ergolines. Bromocriptine, ergotamine, methysergide, nicergoline as a group can produce distinctive pleural changes, mainly pleural thickening, and less often pleural effusion (Fig. 2). The pretherapy chest film (if done and available) is typically normal (**A**). In the full-blown condition, chest radiographs reveal marked, usually bilateral pleural thickening and plate-like or round atelectasis (**B**). Pleural thickening and areas of folded lung are best visualized on HRCT (**C**). Pulmonary physiology is notable for significant restrictive dysfunction. Rapid improvement in symptoms follows cessation of exposure. This is followed by slower improvement in imaging and physiology, which may remain suboptimal.

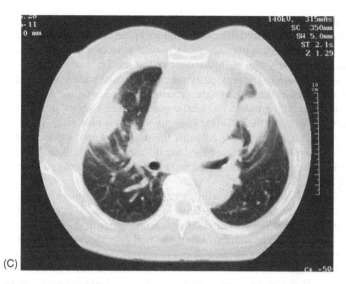

Figure 8 (*Continued*)

develop with ergolines (55). When ergoline-induced pleural fibrosis develops, this may be in association with any of the above fibrosing conditions, and appropriate tests should be used to detect them. Historically, the first ergoline associated with pleural fibrosis was methysergide used to treat migraine in the 1960s (56). Other ergolines followed (e.g., bromocriptine, cabergoline, dihydroergotamine, ergonovine, ergotamine, nicergoline, pergolide), suggesting that pleural injury is a class adverse effect of these agents. Incidence is high, 2% to 4% of the treated population and assiduous observation is required during therapy with these agents. Patients on high dosage of the drug and those with a history of exposure to asbestos may be at extra risk (57). Since onset is insidious, after a minimum of four months and up to 11 years into treatment, patients may be diagnosed after months and up to years of disabling symptoms or concerns, while drug discontinuation would have easily confirmed drug relatedness (11,58). The clinical presentation includes dyspnea, pleurodynia, a nonproductive cough, moderate fever, strange vibrating sounds in the chest that some patients describe as the noise of a rope in a hawse hole and that appears to be synchronous with inspiration and augmented by deep breaths. Clinical examination may reveal chest dullness, muffled breath sounds, and pleural friction rubs. Patients should be investigated for other possible fibrotic complications of ergolines, including pericardial effusion, tamponade or constriction, endomyocardial fibrosis, cardiac valvular regurgitation, urinary tract obstruction, or ascites. The erythrocyte sedimentation rate (ESR) is typically increased (59). Circulating ANA are typically absent. Imaging studies indicate bilateral pleural thickening laterally, anteriorly, posteriorly, and basally with, generally, sparing of the apices. HRCT appearances include smooth-edged pleural thickening which may contain a splitted pleura containing a loculated effusion, linear parenchymal streaks, lung shrinkage, and convoluted areas of trapped or atelectatic lung, assuming a whorled appearance, particularly in the areas where pleural thickness is greatest (59). Rarely is pleural involvement unilateral. When present as an associated feature, the pleural fluid can be a transudate or an exudate. Compared to asbestos-induced pleural thickening, to which ergoline-induced pleural involvement may resemble, pleural plaques and radiologically visible calcifications are typically absent in the drug condition. The rapid progression of pleural thickening or effusion in the previously asbestos-exposed patient should alert to the possibility of ergolines as the cause of the deterioration. A restrictive pulmonary dysfunction is almost universally present. The vital capacity can be reduced to less than 50% of predicted normal, whereas the diffusing capacity for CO is preserved. Thoracoscopic examination of the pleural cavity reveals that the parietal pleura is thickened in the form of a whitish glistening peel encasing the lung diffusely (59,60). Pleural biopsy indicates bland paucicellular pleural fibrosis with, sometimes, perivascular aggregates of inflammatory cells (59).

Most patients improve clinically following drug stoppage, with prompt abatement of systemic symptoms and diminution of the ESR in a few weeks. This is followed by slow improvement of pleural thickening on imaging and betterment of pulmonary physiology over months to years. The restrictive lung function defect may persist for long term (59). In some patients, pleural thickening does not improve after discontinuing the drug. Steroids have been used with clinical benefit in some cases. A trial is worthwhile in symptomatic patients. However, the contribution of long-term corticosteroid therapy to the overall management of ergoline-induced pleural pathology is unclear and probably unrewarding. Often, despite limited evidence for efficacy, patients receive long-term corticosteroid therapy with consequent complications. Surgical decortication was used in the past, but is not cited as being part of the management of this condition any longer. Rechallenge with the same ergot or another ergoline drug is not recommended, as this is likely to be followed by relapse, although a cross reaction will not occur in every patient (61).

Chemotherapeutic Agents

Early classic cyclophosphamide toxicity is in the form of the acute chemotherapy lung, an acute ILD with alveolar damage that may reverse following cessation of the drug and corticosteroid therapy (62). The peculiar features of late cyclophosphamide toxicity are in the form of pleural fibrosis, which involves the upper and lateral aspect of the pleura and the confines of the lung bilaterally (62). Pleural fibrosis tends to progress, causing substantial restrictive dysfunction and pneumothorax (63). When cyclophosphamide is given in childhood, late pleuropulmonary fibrosis causes progressive narrowing of the anteroposterior diameter of the chest during growth, a deformity known a platythorax (64).

Pleuroparenchymal fibroelastosis is a recently recognized entity, which has overlapping features with the above pattern, and may connote progression and severity (17) (Fig. 9). The condition can be idiopathic, familial, or it occurs in patients with a history of treatment with cyclophosphamide, or a chemotherapy regimen containing it. The patient described by Santamauro et al. (65), two of the five patients described by Frankel et al. (66), and one of the two patients reported by Becker et al. (17) had received chemotherapy, but no radiation therapy. The presentation includes the following: (i) pleural and parenchymal radiographic involvement with an upper lobe predominance, (ii) a peculiar HRCT pattern of dented or scalloping encroachment extending into the major fissures,

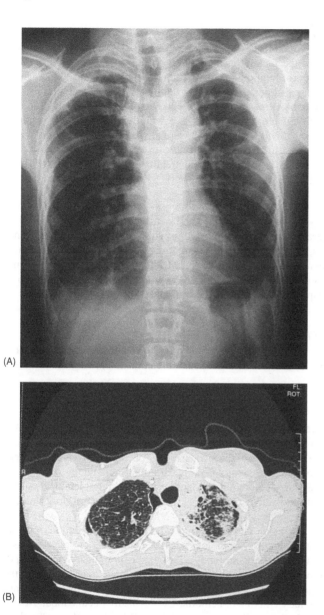

(A)

(B)

Figure 9 Chemotherapy-induced biapical pleural thickening. In a few patients with a history of exposure to cyclophosphamide or chemotherapy regimens containing it, biapical and paramediastinal pleural thickening develops (**A**). Marked restriction is present on pulmonary function tests. Histopathological examination demonstrates pleural fibrosis/fibroelastosis. The condition can be progressive and can be complicated by pneumothoraces (**B**). The bronchopleural fistula may be difficult to manage due to marked inward recoil of the lung and pleura. Similar changes can occur in a portion of patients who have received mantle (Y) radiation therapy for Hodgkin's disease or lymphoma, resulting in a Y-shaped area of pleural and mediastinal fibrosis on frontal views.

(*iii*) ubiquitous adhesions encasing the lung at pleuroscopy, (*iv*) the pathologic appearance of intense fibrosis of the visceral pleura (in contrast to the parietal pleura with ergolines) with an abrupt transition to the mostly normal underlying alveolated lung, (*v*) prominent subpleural elastic fiber proliferation on elastic stains, and (*vi*) propensity to develop "spontaneous" pneumothorax and persistent air leak that is difficult to treat, because the underlying pleuropulmonary block reexpands poorly. In one patient, transplantation was temporarily successful (65). Severe cases exhibit a downhill course that can result in death. Out of the above four patients, 2 died and 2 were alive at two years at the time of publication.

Pleural thickening has been reported following treatments with bleomycin (67) and BCNU (68), with pneumothorax as a complication (68).

Practolol

The β-blocker practolol was introduced in the 1970s in the United Kingdom. A few patients developed bilateral basilar pleural thickening with or without an effusion and, rarely elevated ANA titers, after a few months into treatment. A distinctive ocular inflammation or fibrosis, Lapeyronie's disease, or peritoneal fibrosis also developed in some patients and could persist despite drug withdrawal. Practolol was recalled in 1976 (69). Oxprenolol was once suspected of producing pleural abnormalities similar to those of practolol, but the drug was exonerated (70).

Corticosteroids (Fig. 10)

Rarely, fat deposits subpleurally, causing subpleural thickening, which exhibit low attenuation numbers on CT and can be mistaken for pleural thickening on the chest radiograph (71).

XI. Drug-Induced Hemothorax and Serosanguineous Effusions

Hemothorax is diagnosed when pleural fluid hematocrit is ≥50% of blood hematocrit (72). The pleura is a rare site of hemorrhage in patients on oral anticoagulants, heparin, enoxaparin, and thrombolytic agents (72,73). Anecdotal hemothorax cases have been reported with the use of clopidogrel, ticlopidine, aspirin, intrapleural alteplase, leuprorelide in women with thoracic endometriosis, and in the context of drug-induced thrombocytopenia.

Hemothorax may occur as an isolated complication of anticoagulation, with no detectable underlying pleuropulmonary pathology, or risk factors are present such as a history of recent chest trauma or cardiopulmonary resuscitation, pulmonary embolism, or infarction (72). Coagulation studies are within the therapeutic range in up to 70% of the patients, erroneously suggesting other etiologies (72). With the rupture of a pulmonary infarct complicating pulmonary embolism, hemothorax classically occurs about 7 to 10 days out, causing abrupt respiratory and/or circulatory failure. When hemothorax develops more progressively, this is more consistent with anticoagulant-induced bleeding from the pleural membrane (72). Cessation of drug or anticoagulation therapy is indicated in each case (underlying condition permitting), along with extraction of pleural fluid for the prevention of long-term pleural complications.

Serosanguineous effusions have been described during treatments with amiodarone and ergolines.

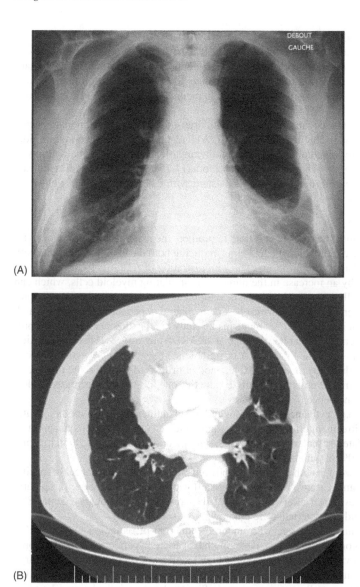

Figure 10 Subpleural corticosteroid-induced fat deposits—Lipomatosis. Long-term corticosteroid therapy (for rheumatoid arthritis in this patient) often leads to central fat distribution, which, in some patients, produces subpleural and paramediastinal deposits mimicking pleural "thickening" (**A**). Changes on HRCT are best seen with parenchymal window settings (**B**) and may be barely visible or are missed when using the mediastinal window settings owing to the low density and attenuation of fat. The condition is largely asymptomatic.

XII. Pleural Effusions Associated with Pulmonary Edema and Pulmonary Capillary Leak Syndrome

Pleural effusion is an unusual occurrence in patients with drug-induced pulmonary edema of moderate severity. For instance, when many cases of hydrochlorothiazide- and aspirin-induced pulmonary edema are considered, pleural effusion was noted in only one case (74).

Pleural effusion(s) occur(s) in patients with drug-induced severe pulmonary edema or ARDS induced by arsenic trioxide (As_2O_3), ATRA, GM-CSF, cytosine-arabinoside, ethchlorvynol, thiazolidinediones, novel chemotherapeutic agents and following transarterial chemoembolization of hepatocellular carcinoma (1,75). Postmortem studies indicate pleural effusion with a fibrinous exudate consistent with capillary leak (76). Following are the particulars of some drugs:

All-*trans*-retinoic acid (ATRA) is used to promote the maturation of promyelocytic cells in acute promyelocytic leukemia, reducing both the likelihood and intensity of hemorrhagic complications. The administration of ATRA is followed 2 to 21 days after by an increase in the number of circulating myeloid cells, which can be temporally associated with the development of weight gain, lower extremity edema, fever, dyspnea, pleuritic chest pain, pleural or pericardial effusion [which was present in 11 out of 15 patients in one study (77)], pulmonary infiltrates, pulmonary edema, alveolar hemorrhage or an ARDS picture (78). This constellation of symptoms is named the ATRA or retinoic acid syndrome. The condition can also be produced by arsenic trioxide, another drug used to treat acute promyelocytic leukemia. Pretreatment with dexamethasone has sharply decreased ATRA syndrome incidence (79).

Established (e.g., cytosine arabinoside) and novel antineoplastic chemotherapeutic agents, acitrecin, interleukin-2, and lymphokine-activated killer cells can produce a dose-related vascular leak syndrome, with pleural effusion present on imaging in 3% to 50% of patients (80,81).

About 5% of women with β2-agonist–induced pulmonary edema (a disease specific to the pregnant state), develop pleural effusion (82). In one case, the pleural effusion developed after resolution of the episode of pulmonary edema (83). Pleural fluid characteristics are unknown.

Women of childbearing age who undergo induction of ovulation with clomifen or other gonadotropins can develop the ovarian hyperstimulation syndrome (OHSS), a vascular leak syndrome which manifests with pleural effusion, large volume ascites, renal failure, thromboembolism, pulmonary edema, or an ARDS picture. Occasionally, massive pleural effusion develops in isolation. The pleural fluid is an exudate with a range of total protein concentration of 4.0 to 5.3 g/L. A transudate is a rare occurrence. Low LDH levels and cell counts are consistent with increased permeability of the pleural membrane. Abdominal ultrasound may aid in determining the size and severity of ascites and pleural effusion, and demonstrates the cystically enlarged ovaries. Repeated evacuation of large volume ascites (>40 L in one case) and pleural effusion is indicated.

Pulmonary edema and pleural effusions can occur during treatment of pulmonary hypertension or pulmonary veno-occlusive disease with calcium channel blockers or prostacyclin. Pleural fluid characteristics are unknown (84).

Patients with acute leukemia and high blast counts can develop acute respiratory failure and pleural effusions shortly after initiation of cytotoxic chemotherapy. In the two reported patients, the pleural fluid was an exudate containing blast cells and very high LDH levels (1787 and 3652 IU/L, respectively) (85).

XIII. Drug-Induced Pleuritic Chest Pain

Acute chest pain or a burning sensation with or without an audible friction rub can occur as a clinical manifestation of the drug *lupus*, or as a presenting feature of adverse pleuropulmonary reactions to carbamazepine, furazolidone, mesalazine, minocycline, or nitrofurantoin. Small volume pleural effusions can be present in the form of blunting of the costophrenic angles.

An excruciating pleuritic pain with sudden onset thought to reflect chemical pleuritis was the presenting feature in 18 out of 210 patients on high-dose methotrexate therapy in one study (86). The chest pain occurred after the third or fourth treatment course, and was of short duration (three to five days). Imaging revealed thickening of the intralobar pleura, which was most prominent on the right side. Pleural effusion was documented in about one-third of patients (87). Outcome under conservative treatment was good (86).

Severe chest pain suggesting acute cardiac or pulmonary events was observed after administration of bleomycin, with an incidence of 2.8% (88). The pain was sudden in onset, and described either as substernal pressure, or pleuritic in character. Electrocardiographic changes suggestive of pericarditis were found in two cases. Radiographic evidence of a small pleural effusion was seen in one patient. The syndrome was self-limited, or relieved with analgesics. Although an improvement was seen when the infusions were stopped, discontinuation of bleomycin was not necessary, as further courses of bleomycin did not lead to recurrent episodes in most patients (88).

Anterior constrictive chest pain with or without ECG changes suggestive of myocardial ischemia or actual myocardial infarction occurred in 0.7% of patients who were being treated with fluorouracil.

Acute chest pain developed in 1.6% of patients who underwent occlusion of brain arteriovenous malformation(s) with liquid acrylate (iso-butyl-2-cyanoacrylate, or *n*-butyl-2-cyanoacrylate) (89). Symptoms developed within 48 hours of injection and may correspond to emboli of the sealant material in the distal pulmonary circulation. Patients recovered with conservative treatment.

Chest pain without overt cardiac involvement has been reported during treatments with dihydro-5-azacytidine, polymethylmethacrylate, statins, and sumatriptan (1).

XIV. Drug-Induced Pneumothorax (See Also Under Drug Abuse)

Pneumothorax is a rare complication of therapy with drugs. Patients with rheumatoid nodules on methotrexate, metastatic lung tumors (e.g., germ cell tumor, sarcoma), or lymphoma can develop the complication following cytotoxic chemotherapy. The condition is thought to result from rupture of subpleural masses into the pleural space, causing bronchopleural fistula (90,129).

Difficult-to-treat pneumothorax can develop in patients with chemotherapy-induced pleural fibrosis or fibroelastosis (17,66).

Spontaneous pneumothorax with or without pneumomediastinum can develop in patients with drug-induced fibrosis (91,92), maybe just as it does in idiopathic pulmonary fibrosis.

Pneumothorax and pneumomediastinum have been described as a complication of *bronchiolitis obliterans* in recipients of bone marrow transplant (93).

XV. Pleural Involvement in Drug-Induced Systemic Conditions Other Than Drug-Induced *Lupus*

A. l-Tryptophan–Induced Eosinophilia-Myalgia Syndrome (EMS)

In the past, ethylene-bistryptophan, a contaminant formed during the manufacturing of L-tryptophan at one plant, was temporally and mechanistically associated with an epidemic of eosinophilia-myalgia syndrome or EMS. Patients presented with constitutional symptoms, myalgias, skin changes, fasciitis, and neurologic or cardiac involvement. Respiratory manifestations included pulmonary infiltrates, pulmonary hypertension, and acute respiratory failure. Small or moderate volume pleural effusions were present in about one-sixth of those patients with eosinophilic pneumonia (94). Although the effusions subsided following drug withdrawal, blood eosinophilia, skin, and neurologic changes, or pulmonary hypertension persisted or worsened in some patients (95). Despite the agent being recalled several years ago, L-tryptophan remains very popular in some countries (96). A sporadic case of EMS with acute eosinophilic pneumonia and a neutrophilic pleural exudate has been recently reported (96).

B. Drug-Induced Vasculitis

Bilateral pleural effusion corresponding to an eosinophilic exudate (proteins 4.3 g/L; LDH: 152 IU/L) was noted in a patient with montelukast-induced Churg–Strauss syndrome (97).

A patient developed hypersensitivity vasculitis, pulmonary infiltrates, and pleural effusion during treatment with propylthiouracil for Grave's disease (98). The pleural fluid was a transudate (total proteins 1.6 g/dL) containing 64 white cells per microliter, and 235 IU/L LDH. The pleuropulmonary manifestations improved with corticosteroid therapy upon drug therapy withdrawal.

Bilateral effusions were present in a patient with ulcerative colitis and c-ANCA–positive vasculitis, presumably induced by mesalasine (99).

C. Drug Rash and Eosinophilia with Systemic Symptoms (DRESS)

Pleural effusion is a rare manifestation of the DRESS syndrome, a systemic condition caused by anticonvulsants, dapsone, minocycline, sulfones, and other drugs. A pleural exudate containing 48% mononucleated cells and 666 IU/L LDH was noted in an adolescent treated for *acne vulgaris* with dapsone (100).

D. Antiretroviral Therapy-Related Immune Restoration Disorders (IRS)

Deeply immnocompromised individuals with human immunodeficiency virus infection who commence antiretroviral therapy are susceptible to immune reconstitution disorders. The condition corresponds to the restoration of a previously dysregulated immune response against pathogen-specific antigens such as *Mycobacterium tuberculosis* and *Mycobacterium avium* complex, and is characterized by clinical deterioration and organ dysfunction after initiation of highly active antiretroviral therapy. In a recent study, 1 and 2 out of 11 cases with IRS presented with pericardial or pleural effusion, respectively, in addition to involvement of other organs (101). There is evidence for the beneficial effect of corticosteroid therapy in severe cases.

XVI. Pleural Involvement as a Complication of Radiation Therapy

Pleural effusion is one of the many imaging features following radiation therapy to the chest (102). Radiation-induced pleural involvement is a dose-related complication, which raises the suspicion of progression or relapse of the underlying neoplastic condition, particularly lung or breast carcinoma.

A. Early Effusions

Early effusions, typically localize on the irradiated side, develop two to six months after radiation therapy to the chest or breast, and less commonly after mantle field irradiation for Hodgkin's disease or lymphoma. In the past, early pleural effusions developed in up to 10% of women who received radiation therapy for breast carcinoma, and in nearly all of them radiation pneumonitis was also present (103). Pleural effusion is not a feature of radiation-induced BOOP. Advances in targeting and conformal radiation therapy techniques have decreased the incidence of postirradiation pleural effusions. Early radiation effusions may be annunciated by chest pain and dyspnea. Imaging studies indicate a basilar tent-like appearance, particularly when there is retraction of the upper lung segments. The pleural fluid is an exudate containing reactive mesothelial cells (104). Early effusions generally follow an indolent course and rarely give rise to marked symptoms. Steroids and nonsteroidal anti-inflammatory drugs are used to control symptoms.

B. Late Effusions (Fig. 11)

Pleural effusions with or without pleural thickening can develop late after mediastinal or mantle field radiation therapy. Pleural fluid has the characteristics of an exudate containing neutrophils, lymphocytes, and a few eosinophils. Late radiation–induced effusions may develop in areas of the chest remote from the radiation beam, hence factors other than direct pleural injury may play a role. Mechanisms in addition to radiation-induced pleural insult include hemodynamic factors (e.g., pericardial constriction or myocardial fibrosis) and altered lymph flow (105). The effusion can be massive or recurrent, requiring repeated evacuation or pleurodesis (106), or it is associated with pleural or pleuropericardial thickening or calcification, causing severe cardiorespiratory dysfunction.

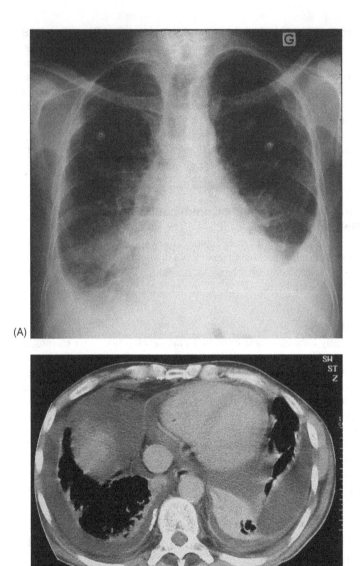

Figure 11 Late radiation-induced changes. Radiation therapy can produce irreversible and far-reaching changes in any organ in the chest, including lungs, pleurae, heart, cardiac valves, pericardium, and nerves. As for the pleura, late radiation changes are in the form of an effusion and/or thickening with or without pericardial effusion. This may cause severe cardiopulmonary compromise. Bilateral exudates (note pleural calcification on right) and pericardial effusion developed in this 60-year-old man 35 years after radiation therapy for Hodgkin's disease. Sadly, despite tracheostomy and home ventilation, he died from intractable cardiorespiratory failure.

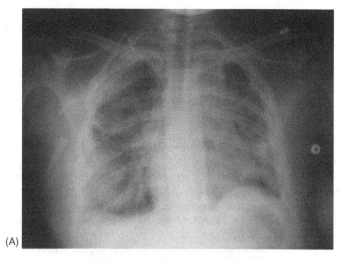

(A)

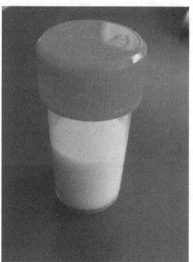

(B)

Figure 12 Iatrogenic chylothorax (**A**). Chylous effusion is unusual and is an elective complication of radiation therapy or thoracic surgery. Chylothorax may develop after chest radiation therapy. Inspection of the pleural fluid is suggestive (**B**), however, diagnosis must be confirmed by evaluation of the lipid profile and chyomicrons in pleural fluid.

C. Chylothorax (Fig. 12)

Chylothorax can develop late after radiation therapy to the chest [up to 23 years in one case (107)]. The lipidic interface may be spontaneously visible on unenhanced CT (108). Although the turbid or milky appearance of the pleural fluid is suggestive, confusion with cholesterol effusions is possible, and diagnosis by appearance is problematic. The diagnosis must be confirmed by the finding of elevated triglycerides and chylomicrons in the pleural fluid (109). Radiation-related chylothorax is thought to result from hindered lymph flow secondary to radiation-induced mediastinal fibrosis or retraction—rarely, it is secondary to a tear in the thoracic duct (110). Chylous ascites may be present in association with the chylothorax. Chylous effusions can be controlled by total parenteral nutrition followed by a low fat diet. In rare patients in whom a tear in the thoracic duct was evidenced, surgical repair controlled the effusion (110).

D. Pleural Thickening

Pleural thickening is a common finding on imaging in patients with prior radiation therapy to the chest (111) or breast (112) (Fig. 13). In a series of 39 patients with breast cancer or various intrathoracic malignancies, pleural thickening was evidenced in 9 on conventional chest radiographs, and in 15 on HRCT (113). After mantle-field or supraclavicular and cervical radiation therapy, localization of pleural fibrosis is typically in the apices or in paravertebral regions, causing complications analogous to fibrosing mediastinitis. A slight pleural effusion is sometimes present. In women who received radiation therapy for breast cancer, pleural thickening occurs in areas where the radiation dose was the highest (114). The impact of these changes in terms of volume restriction is usually modest. In 40 adult patients toxicity was evaluated following three courses of ABVD (cumulative dose of bleomycin 60 mg) and mediastinal irradiation at 40 Gy. Eight patients had a minor pericardial effusion—CT scan showed a small pleural effusion with pleural thickening in 19 patients and mediastinal or apical fibrosis in 15 (115). Rare cases of radiation-induced BOOP showed pleural thickening as an associated feature (112).

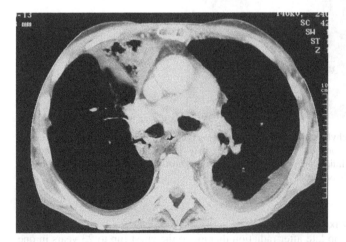

Figure 13 Localized pleural thickening following radiation therapy to the chest or breast. Thoracic changes following radiation therapy for breast or lung cancer are suggested when the distribution of the pleuropulmonary changes is along the radiation beam, which was oblique from right anterior to left posterior in the present case. Novel conformal radiation delivery techniques will alter the distribution of fibrotic pleural and pulmonary changes following radiation therapy.

E. Pneumothorax

Pneumothorax occasionally develops late after radiation therapy to the chest or mediastinum (116). The pneumothotax is usually ipsilateral to the side of irradiation and may be related to fibrosis of the underlying irradiated lung. Patients may recover spontaneously, or exsufflation is required.

F. Pleural Tumors

Patients can develop pleural or pericardial mesothelioma (117,118) or other malignant pleural tumors (119) late after chest radiation therapy.

XVII. Complications of Intrapleural Delivery of Drugs

The intrapleural instillation of talc, bleomycin, cisplatin, or etoposide can be complicated by pulmonary edema or an ARDS picture of rapid onset (120–122). Hemothorax has been described following intrapleural instillation of alteplase (118).

Talc pleurodesis or poudrage was performed for the management of persistent pneumothorax, or it is mainly used now to control relapsing malignant effusions. Calcified plaques, a splitted pleura, loculated effusion, and calcification can be seen as long-term changes following talc insufflation. In a study of nine patients, FDG-PET studies were performed on average 22 months after talc pleurodesis, and the CT was followed-up for an average of 25 months. There was linear or focal nodular-increased uptake of FDG in the pleura, with a mean SUV of 5.4. The uptake was diffuse in two patients and focal in seven, and on CT, high-density areas of pleural thickening or nodularity corresponded to regions of increased FDG uptake. The changes remained stable on serial imaging, enabling distinction from malignancy (13).

Intrapleural chemotherapy was deemed to be responsible for interstital pulmonary fibrosis (130).

XVIII. Pleural Disease in Drug Abusers

History taking is crucial, as not every patient will indulge in taking illicit drugs. Drug abusers turn to central sites of injection (e.g., the internal jugular or subclavian vein), when peripheral access has been sclerosed by long-term injection of abused drugs. Central injection may require the participation of a mate to perform the "pocket shot." The pleura can be lacerated during the attempt, with resultant pneumothorax. In a series of 12 drug abusers with various complications resulting from supra- or subclavicular drug injection, six presented with unilateral pneumothorax, and in one bilateral tension pneumothorax was present (123). In a large urban community, 113 pneumothorax episodes were diagnosed in 84 drug abusers, an alarming 21.5% rate of all causes of pneumothorax (124). In that study, nine patients developed bilateral lung collapse, as the consequence of bilateral attempts at injecting the drug, and 11 developed pneumothorax recurrence. Repeated Valsalva maneuvers or mouth-to-mouth breathing used to increase the "high" experienced during cocaine or marijuana inhalation may cause pneumothorax and/or pneumomediastinum (125,126). Lung bullae associated with marijuana abuse may increase the risk of developing this complication (126).

XIX. Conclusion

Man-made drug-induced pleural diseases are common enough to warrant evaluation of drug history in any patient with pleural effusion, hemothorax, pleural thickening, pneumothorax, or the *lupus* syndrome to avoid unnecessary and costly procedures. Rarely, is drug-induced pleural involvement a dire or life-threatening complication. Cessation of exposure to the drug is an effective clinical test, and it often translates into durable improvement of the pleural condition. An updated list of drugs causing pleural disease is available on Pnneumotox® (1).

References

1. http://www.pneumotox. com: Pneumotox®, 1997 (Web site). Producers: P Foucher & P Camus. Last update: July, 2009.
2. Bonniaud P, Camus C, Jibbaoui A, et al. Drug-induced respiratory emergencies. In: Fein A, Kamholz S, Ost D, eds. Respiratory Emergencies. London, UK: Edward Arnold, 2006: 269–290.
3. Morelock SY, Sahn SA. Drugs and the pleura. Chest 1999; 116:212–221.
4. Miller WT Jr. Drug-related pleural and mediastinal disorders. J Thorac Imaging 1991; 6: 36–51.
5. Antony VB. Drug-induced pleural disease. Clin Chest Med 1998; 19:331–340.
6. Huggins JT, Sahn SA. Drug-induced pleural disease. Clin Chest Med 2004; 25:141–154.
7. Bergeron A, Rea D, Levy V, et al. Lung abnormalities after dasatinib treatment for chronic myeloid leukemia: A case series. Am J Respir Crit Care Med 2007; 176:814–818.
8. Camus P. Drug-induced pleural disease. In: Bouros D, ed. Pleural Disorders. New York, NY: Mercel Dekker, 2004:317–352.
9. Rubin RL. Drug-induced lupus. Toxicology 2005; 209:135–147.
10. Eymin G, Andresen M, Godoy J, et al. Malignant neuroleptic syndrome and polyserositis associated to clozapine use: Report of one case. Rev Med Chil 2005; 133:1225–1228.
11. Agarwal P, Fahn S, Frucht SJ. Diagnosis and management of pergolide-induced fibrosis. Mov Disord 2004; 19:699–704.
12. Miles SE, Sandrini A, Johnson AR, et al. Clinical consequences of asbestos-related diffuse pleural thickening: A review. J Occup Med Toxicol 2008; 3:20.
13. Kwek BH, Aquino SL, Fischman AJ. Fluorodeoxyglucose positron emission tomography and CT after talc pleurodesis. Chest 2004; 125:2356–2360.
14. Abdalla AMH, White D. A 29-year-old woman with a remote history of osteosarcoma and positron emission tomography-positive pleurally based masses. Chest 2008; 134:640–643.
15. Gilmartin JJ, Wright AJ, Gibson GJ. Effects of pneumothorax or pleural effusion on pulmonary function. Thorax 1985; 40:60–65.
16. Abunasser J, Forouhar FA, Metersky ML. Etanercept-induced lupus erythematosus presenting as a unilateral pleural effusion. Chest 2008; 134:850–853.
17. Becker CD, Gil J, Padilla ML. Idiopathic pleuroparenchymal fibroelastosis: An unrecognized or misdiagnosed entity? Modern Pathol 2008; 21:784–787.
18. Matsuno O, Okubo T, Hiroshige S, et al. Drug-induced lymphocyte stimulation test is not useful for the diagnosis of drug-induced pneumonia. Tohoku J Exp Med 2007; 212:49–53.
19. Tintner R, Manian P, Gauthier P, et al. Pleuropulmonary fibrosis after long-term treatment with the dopamine agonist pergolide for Parkinson disease. Arch Neurol 2005; 62:1290–1295.
20. Siniakowicz RM, Narula D, Suster B, et al. Diagnosis of amiodarone pulmonary toxicity with high-resolution computerized tomographic scan. J Cardiovasc Electrophysiol 2001; 12:431–436.
21. Gonzalez-Rothi RJ, Hannan SE, Hood I, et al. Amiodarone pulmonary toxicity presenting as bilateral exudative pleural effusion. Chest 1987; 92:179–182.
22. Stein B, Zaatari GS, Pine JR. Amiodarone pulmonary toxicity. Clinical, cytologic and ultrastructural findings. Acta Cytol 1987; 31:357–361.

23. Akoun G, Milleron BJ, Badaro DM, et al. Pleural T-lymphocyte subsets in amiodarone-associated pleuropneumonitis. Chest 1989; 95:596–597.
24. Gotsman I, Fridlender Z, Meirovitz A, et al. The evaluation of pleural effusions in patients with heart failure. Am J Med 2001; 111:375–378.
25. Malhotra A, Muse VV, Mark EJ. An 82-year-old man with dyspnea and pulmonary abnormalities. Case Records of the Massachusetts General Hospital—Case 12–2003. N Engl J Med 2003; 348:1574–1585.
26. Troughton RW, Richards AM, Yandle TG, et al. The effects of medications on circulating levels of cardiac natriuretic peptides. Ann Med 2007; 39:242–260.
27. Susano R, Caminal L, Ramos D, et al. Amiodarone induced lupus. Ann Rheum Dis 1999; 58:655–656.
28. Sheikhzadeh A, Schafer U, Schnabel A. Drug-induced lupus erythematosus by amiodarone. Arch Intern Med 2002; 162:834–836.
29. Talpaz M, Shah NP, Kantarjian H, et al. Dasatinib in imatinib-resistant Philadelphia chromosome-positive leukemias. N Engl J Med 2006; 354:2531–2541.
30. Chen YW, Chen YC, Wu CJ, et al. Massive bilateral pleural effusion associated with use of pioglitazone. Clin Ther 2008; 30:1485–1489.
31. Koshida H, Shibata K, Kametani T. Pleuropulmonary disease in a man with diabetes who was treated with troglitazone. N Engl J Med 1998; 339:1400–1401.
32. Kermani A, Garg A. Thiazolidinedione-associated congestive heart failure and pulmonary edema. Mayo Clin Proc 2003; 78:1088–1091.
33. Volatron AC, Belleguic C, Polard E, et al. Chylothorax sous simvastatine. Rev Mal Respir 2003; 20:291–293.
34. Bullington W, Sahn SA, Judson MA. Valproic acid-induced eosinophilic pleural effusion: A case report and review of the literature. Am J Med Sci 2007; 333:290–292.
35. Lê-Quang B, Calmels P, Valayer-Chaleat E, et al. Dantrolene and pleural effusion: Case report and review of literature. Spinal Cord 2004; 42:317–320.
36. Israel HL, Diamond P. Recurrent pulmonary infiltration and pleural effusion due to nitrofurantoin sensitivity. N Engl J Med 1962; 266:1024–1026.
37. Holmberg L, Boman G. Pulmonary reactions to nitrofurantoin. 447 cases reported to the Swedish Adverse Drug Reaction Committee 1966–1976. Eur J Respir Dis 1981; 62: 180–189.
38. Massin F, Coudert B, Marot JP, et al. Methotrexate pneumonitis. Rev Mal Respir 1990; 7:5–15.
39. Tomioka H, King TEJ. Gold-induced pulmonary disease: Clinical features, outcome, and differentiation from rheumatoid lung disease. Am J Respir Crit Care Med 1997; 155: 1011–1020.
40. Baethge BA, Wolf RE. Gold-induced pneumonitis. J La State Med Soc 1988; 140:37–39.
41. Gunstream SR, Seidenfeld JJ, Sobonys RE, et al. Mitomycin-associated lung disease. Cancer Treat Rep 1983; 67:301–304.
42. Rimmer MJ, Dixon AK, Flower CDR, et al. Bleomycin lung: Computed tomographic observations. Br J Radiol 1985; 58:1041–1045.
43. Siegel M, Lee SL, Peress NS. The epidemiology of drug-induced systemic lupus erythematosus. Arthritis Rheum 1967; 10:407–415.
44. Costa MF, Said NR, Zimmermann B. Drug-induced lupus due to anti-tumor necrosis factor alpha agents. Semin Arthritis Rheum 2008; 37:381–387.
45. De Bandt M, Sibilia J, Le Loet X, et al. Systemic lupus erythematosus induced by anti-tumour necrosis factor alpha therapy: A French national survey. Arthritis Res Ther 2005; 7:R545–R551.
46. Portanova JP, Arndt RE, Tan EM, et al. Anti-histone antibodies in idiopathic and drug-induced lupus recognize distinct intrahistone regions. J Immunol 1987; 138:446–451.

47. Carter JD, Valeriano-Marcet J, Kanik KS, et al. Antinuclear antibody-negative, drug-induced lupus caused by lisinopril. South Med J 2001; 94:1122–1123.
48. Pape L, Strehlau J, Latta K, et al. Drug-induced lupus as a cause of relapsing inflammatory disease after renal transplantation. Pediatr Transplant 2002; 6:337–339.
49. Good JT Jr, King TE Jr, Antony VB, et al. Lupus pleuritis: Clinical features and pleural fluid characteristics with special reference to pleural fluid antibody titers. Chest 1983; 84: 714–718.
50. Chandrasekhar AJ, Robinson J, Barr L. Antibody deposition in the pleura: A finding in drug-induced lupus. J Allergy Clin Immunol 1978; 61:399–402.
51. Goldberg MJ, Husain M, Wajszczuk WJ, et al. Procainamide-induced lupus erythematosus pericarditis encountered during coronary bypass surgery. Am J Med 1980; 69:159–162.
52. Rubin RL, Nusinow SR, Johnson AD, et al. Serologic changes during induction of lupus-like disease by procainamide. Am J Med 1986; 80:999–1002.
53. Vernhet H, Bousquet C, Durand G, et al. Reversible amiodarone-induced lung disease: HRCT findings. Eur Radiol 2001; 11:1697–1703.
54. Kuhlman JE, Teigen C, Ren H, et al. Amiodarone pulmonary toxicity: CT findings in symptomatic patients. Radiology 1990; 177:121–125.
55. Pritchett AM, Morrison JF, Edwards WD, et al. Valvular heart disease in patients taking pergolide. Mayo Clin Proc 2002; 77:1280–1286.
56. Graham RG. Cardiac and pulmonary fibrosis during methysergide therapy for headache. Am J Med Sci 1967; 254:1–12.
57. De Vuyst P, Pfitzenmeyer P, Camus P. Asbestos, ergot drugs and the pleura. Eur Respir J 1997; 10:2695–2698.
58. Varsano S, Gershman M, Hamaoui E. Pergolide-induced dyspnea, bilateral pleural effusion and peripheral edema. Respiration 2000; 67:580–582.
59. Pfitzenmeyer P, Foucher P, Dennewald G, et al. Pleuropulmonary changes induced by ergoline drugs. Eur Respir J 1996; 9:1013–1019.
60. Danoff SK, Grasso ME, Terry PB, et al. Pleuropulmonary disease due to pergolide use for restless legs syndrome. Chest 2001; 120:313–316.
61. Törnling G, Unge G, Axelsonn G, et al. Pleuropulmonary reactions in patients on bromocriptine treatment. Eur J Respir Dis 1986; 68:35–38.
62. Malik SW, Myers JL, DeRemee RA, et al. Lung toxicity associated with cyclophosphamide use. Two distinct patterns. Am J Respir Crit Care Med 1996; 154:1851–1856.
63. Hamada K, Nagai S, Kitaichi M, et al. Cyclophosphamide-induced late-onset lung disease. Intern Med 2003; 42:82–87.
64. Alvarado CS, Boat TF, Newman AJ. Late-onset pulmonary fibrosis and chest deformity in two children treated with cyclophosphamide. J Pediatr 1978; 92:443–446.
65. Santamauro JT, Stover DE, Jules-Elysee K, et al. Lung transplantation for chemotherapy-induced pulmonary fibrosis. Chest 1994; 105:310–312.
66. Frankel SK, Cool CD, Lynch DA, et al. Idiopathic pleuroparenchymal fibroelastosis: Description of a novel clinicopathologic entity. Chest 2004; 126:2007–2013.
67. Tashiro M, Izumikawa K, Yoshioka D, et al. Lung fibrosis 10 years after cessation of bleomycin therapy. Tohoku J Exp Med 2008; 216:77–80.
68. Parish JM, Muhm JR, Leslie KO. Upper lobe pulmonary fibrosis associated with high-dose chemotherapy containing BCNU for bone marrow transplantation. Mayo Clin Proc 2003; 78:630–634.
69. Lombard JN, Bonnotte B, Maynadié M, et al. Celiprolol pneumonitis. Eur Respir J 1993; 9:588–591.
70. Page RL. Pleural thickening-oxprenolol exonerated. Br J Dis Chest 1979; 73:319.
71. Glazer HS, Wick MR, Anderson DJ, et al. CT of fatty thoracic masses. AJR Am J Roentgenol 1992; 159:1181–1187.

72. Ali HA, Lippmann M, Mundathaje U, et al. Spontaneous hemothorax: A comprehensive review. Chest 2008; 134:1056–1065.
73. Cafri C, Gilutz H, Ilia R, et al. Unusual bleeding complications of thrombolytic therapy after cardiopulmonary resuscitation. Three case reports. Angiology 1997; 48:925–928.
74. Reed CR, Glauser FL. Drug-induced non-cardiogenic pulmonary edema. Chest 1991; 100:1120–1124.
75. Lee-Chiong TLJ, Matthay RA. Drug-induced pulmonary edema and acute respiratory distress syndrome. Clin Chest Med 2004; 25:95–104.
76. Andersson BS, Luna BS, Yee C, et al. Fatal pulmonary failure complicating high-dose cytosine arabinoside therapy in acute leukemia. Cancer 1990; 65:1079–1084.
77. Jung JI, Choi JE, Hahn ST, et al. Radiologic features of all-trans-retinoic acid syndrome. AJR Am J Roentgenol 2002; 178:475–480.
78. Frankel SR, Eardley A, Lauwers G, et al. The "retinoic acid syndrome" in acute promyelocytic leukemia. Ann Intern Med 1992; 117:292–296.
79. Wiley JS, Firkin FC. Reduction of pulmonary toxicity by prednisolone prophylaxis during all-trans retinoic acid treatment of acute promyelocytic leukemia. Leukemia 1995; 9: 774–778.
80. Briasoulis E, Froudarakis M, Milionis H, et al. Chemotherapy-induced noncardiogenic pulmonary edema related to gemcitabine plus docetaxel combination with granulocyte colony-stimulating factor support. Respiration 2000; 67:680–683.
81. Saxon RR, Klein JS, Bar MH, et al. Pathogenesis of pulmonary edema during interleukin-2 therapy: Correlation of chest radiographic and clinical findings in 54 patients. AJR Am J Roentgenol 1991; 156:281–285.
82. Pisani RJ, Rosenow ECI. Pulmonary edema associated with tocolytic therapy. Ann Intern Med 1989; 110:714–718.
83. Milos M, Aberle DR, Parkinson BT, et al. Maternal pulmonary edema complicating beta-adrenergic therapy of preterm labor. AJR Am J Roentgenol 1988; 151:917–918.
84. Gugnani MK, Pierson C, Vanderheide R, et al. Pulmonary edema complicating prostacyclin therapy in pulmonary hypertension associated with scleroderma—A case of pulmonary capillary hemangiomatosis. Arthr Rheum 2000; 43:699–703.
85. Myers TJ, Cole SR, Klatsky AU, et al. Respiratory failure due to pulmonary leukostasis following chemotherapy of acute nonlymphocytic leukemia. Cancer 1983; 51:1808–1813.
86. Urban C, Nirenberg A, Caparros B, et al. Chemical pleuritis as the cause of acute chest pain following high-dose methotrexate treatment. Cancer 1983; 51:34–37.
87. Walden PA, Mitchell-Weggs PF, Coppin C, et al. Pleurisy and methotrexate treatment. Br Med J 1977; 2:867.
88. White DA, Schwartzberg LS, Kris MG, et al. Acute chest pain syndrome during bleomycin infusions. Cancer 1987; 59:1582–1585.
89. Pelz DM, Lownie SP, Fox AJ, et al. Symptomatic pulmonary complications from liquid acrylate embolization of brain arteriovenous malformations. Am J Neuroradiol 1995; 16: 19–26.
90. Mori M, Nakagawa M, Fujikawa T, et al. Simultaneous bilateral spontaneous pneumothorax observed during the administration of gefitinib for lung adenocarcinoma with multiple lung metastases. Intern Med 2005; 44:862–864.
91. Wilson KS, Brigden ML, Alexander S, et al. Fatal pneumothorax "BCNU lung". Med Pediatr Oncol 1982; 10:195–199.
92. Leeser JE, Carr D. Fatal pneumothorax following bleomycin and other cytotoxic drugs. Cancer Treat Rep 1985; 69:344–345.
93. Kumar S, Tefferi A. Spontaneous pneumomediastinum and subcutaneous emphysema complicating bronchiolitis obliterans after allogeneic bone marrow transplantation—Case report and review of literature. Ann Hematol 2001; 80:430–435.

94. Campagna AC, Blanc PD, Criswell LA, et al. Pulmonary manifestations of the eosinophilia-myalgia syndrome associated with tryptophan ingestion. Chest 1992; 101:1274–1281.

95. Pincus T. Eosinophilia-myalgia syndrome: Patient status 2–4 years after onset. J Rheumatol 1996; 23(suppl 46):19–24.

96. de Aurojo Guerra Grangeia T, Schweller M, Paschoal IA, et al. Acute respiratory failure as a manifestation of eosinophilia-myalgia syndrome associated with L-tryptophan intake. J Bras Pneumol 2007; 33:747–751.

97. Villena V, Hidalgo R, Sotelo MT, et al. Montelukast and Churg–Strauss syndrome. Eur Respir J 2000; 15:626.

98. Stankus SJ, Johnson NT. Propylthiouracil-induced hypersensitivity vasculitis presenting as respiratory failure. Chest 1992; 102:1595–1596.

99. Actis GC, Ottobrelli A, Baldi S, et al. Mesalamine-induced lung injury in a patient with ulcerative colitis and a confounding autoimmune background: A case report. Mt Sinai J Med 2005; 72:136–140.

100. Corp CC, Ghishan FK. The sulfone syndrome complicated by pancreatitis and pleural effusion in an adolescent receiving dapsone for treatment of acne vulgaris. J Pediatr Gastroenterol Nutr 1998; 26:103–105.

101. Rajeswaran G, Becker JL, Michailidis C, et al. The radiology of IRIS (immune reconstitution inflammatory syndrome) in patients with mycobacterial tuberculosis and HIV co-infection: Appearances in 11 patients. Clin Radiol 2006; 61:833–843.

102. Choi YW, Munden RF, Erasmus JJ, et al. Effects of radiation therapy on the lung: Radiologic appearances and differential diagnosis. Radiographics 2004; 24:985–997; discussion 998.

103. Gross NJ. Pulmonary effects of radiation therapy. Ann Intern Med 1977; 86:81–92.

104. Fentanes de Torres E, Guevara E. Pleuritis by radiation. Acta Cytol 1981; 25:427–429.

105. Whitcomb ME, Schwarz MI. Pleural effusion complicating intensive mediastinal radiation therapy. Am Rev Respir Dis 1971; 103:100–107.

106. Rodriguez-Garcia JL, Fraile G, Moreno MA, et al. Recurrent massive pleural effusion as a late complication of radiotherapy in Hodgkin's disease. Chest 1991; 100:1165–1166.

107. McWilliams A, Gabbay E. Chylothorax occurring 23 years post-irradiation: Literature review and management strategies. Respirology 2000; 5:301–303.

108. Kim FS, Bishop MJ. Cough during emergence from isoflurane anesthesia. Anesth Analg 1998; 87:1170–1174.

109. Agrawal V, Sahn SA. Lipid pleural effusions. Am J Med Sci 2008; 335:16–20.

110. Zoetmulder F, Rutgers E, Baas P. Thoracoscopic ligation of a thoracic duct leakage. Chest 1994; 106:1233–1234.

111. Logan PM. Thoracic manifestations of external beam radiotherapy. AJR Am J Roentgenol 1998; 171:569–577.

112. Cornelissen R, Senan S, Antonisse IE, et al. Bronchiolitis obliterans organizing pneumonia (BOOP) after thoracic radiotherapy for breast carcinoma—Art No. 2. Radiat Oncol 2007; 2:NIL_19–NIL_23.

113. Bell J, McGivern D, Bullimore J, et al. Diagnostic imaging of post-irradiation changes in the chest. Clin Radiol 1988; 39:109–119.

114. Srinivasan G, Kurtz DW, Lichter AS. Pleural-based changes on chest X-ray after irradiation for primary breast cancer: Correlation with findings on computerized tomography. Int J Radiat Oncol Biol Phys 1983; 9:1567–1570.

115. Brice P, Tredaniel J, Monsuez JJ, et al. Cardiopulmonary toxicity after three courses of ABVD and mediastinal irradiation in favorable Hodgkin's disease. Ann Oncol 1991; 2(suppl 2):73–76.

116. Epstein DM, Littman P, Gefter WB, et al. Radiation-induced pneumothorax. Med Ped Oncol 1983; 11:122–124.

117. Melato M, Rizzardi C. Malignant pleural mesothelioma following chemotherapy for breast cancer. Anticancer Res 2001; 21:3093–3096.
118. Small GR, Nicolson M, Buchan K, et al. Pericardial malignant mesothelioma: A latent complication of radiotherapy? Eur J Cardiothor Surg 2008; 33:745–747.
119. Henley JD, Loehrer PJ, Ulbright TM. Deciduoid mesothelioma of the pleura after radiation therapy for Hodgkin's disease presenting as a mediastinal mass. Am J Surg Pathol 2001; 25:547–548.
120. Rinaldo JE, Owens GR, Rogers RM. Adult respiratory distress syndrome following intrapleural instillation of talc. J Thorac Cardiovasc Surg 1983; 85:523–526.
121. Audu PB, Sing RF, Mette SA, et al. Fatal diffuse alveolar injury following use of intrapleural bleomycin. Chest 1993; 103:1638.
122. Tohda Y, Iwanaga T, Takada M, et al. Intrapleural administration of cisplatin and etoposide to treat malignant pleural effusions in patients with non-small cell lung cancer. Chemotherapy 1999; 45:197–204.
123. Lewis JWJ, Groux N, Elliott JPJ, et al. Complications of attempted central venous injections performed by drug abusers. Chest 1980; 78:613–617.
124. Douglass RE, Levison MA. Pneumothorax in drug abusers. An urban epidemic? Am Surg 1986; 52:377–380.
125. Miller WTJ. Pleural and mediastinal disorders related to drug use. Semin Roentgenol 1995; 30:35–48.
126. Newcomb AE, Clarke CP. Spontaneous pneumomediastinum: A benign curiosity or a significant problem? Chest 2005; 128:3298–3302.
127. Goldblatt M, Huggins JT, Doelken P, et al. Dasatinib-induced pleural effusions: A lymphatic network disorder? Am J Med Sci 2009; 338:414–417.
128. Wetter DA, Davis MD. Lupus-like syndrome attributable to anti-tumor necrosis factor alpha therapy in 14 patients during an 8-year period at Mayo Clinic. Mayo Clin Proc 2009; 84:979–984.
129. Ladoire S, Beynat C, Diaz P, et al. Spontaneous pyopneumothorax in patients treated with mTOR inhibitors for subpleural pulmonary metastases. Med Oncol 2009.
130. Zappa L, Savady R, Humphries GN, et al. Interstitial pneumonitis following intrapleural chemotherapy. World J Surg Oncol 2009; 7:17.

18

Parapneumonic Pleural Effusions and Empyema

DEMOSTHENES BOUROS

Democritus University of Thrace Medical School, and University Hospital of Alexandroupolis, Alexandroupolis, Greece

I. Introduction

Parapneumonic pleural effusions (PPE) present a frequently difficult diagnostic and therapeutic challenge in clinical practice because of their heterogeneity. Their spectrum ranges from a small pleural effusion that does not require specific therapy to multiloculated pleural empyema with pleural fibrosis, trapped lung, systemic sepsis, respiratory failure, and metastatic infection. Today, physicians are warranted to play an increasing role in the timely and modern management, with new available techniques, of the patients with PPE and pleural empyema (1).

This chapter reviews the epidemiological factors that influence their clinical course, the existing classification systems for PPE, and the current diagnostic and therapeutic options, and offers guidelines for treating the various stages of PPE and PE.

II. Definitions

Infectious pleural effusions are usually of parapneumonic origin; however, they may also have other causes, such as surgery, trauma, or esophageal perforation (Table 1). Any pleural effusion associated with bacterial pneumonia, lung abscess, or bronchiectasis is a parapneumonic effusion. An effusion is called an empyema when the concentration of leukocytes becomes macroscopically evident as a thick, highly viscous, whitish-yellow, opaque, and turbid fluid (pus). It consists of fibrin, cellular debris, and living or dead bacteria. There is no consensus on the white blood cell (WBC) count or the biochemistry for an empyema. The extent of the definition of empyema in a nonpurulent fluid with only the presence of a positive Gram stain or culture is not widely accepted (2).

Uncomplicated (simple) PPEs are usually small, not loculated, and not infected. Most often they resolve spontaneously under antibiotic treatment. Complicated PPEs are usually associated with pleural invasion of the infectious agent and require at least drainage and possibly further interventions. A loculated PPE is a nonfree-flowing pleural effusion. A multiloculated PPE is a pleural effusion with more than one loculus (3).

III. Epidemiology

The annual incidence of bacterial pneumonia is estimated to be 2 to 4 million in the United States, with approximately 20% of patients requiring hospitalization (3). It is estimated that 40% to 60% of patients with pneumonia develop PPE (4), which is associated with

Table 1 Causes of Bacterial Empyema

Pulmonary infection
Bacterial pneumonia
Lung abscess
Bronchiectasis
Septic pulmonary emboli
Postoperative
Thoracic surgery
Cardiac surgery
Esophageal surgery
Trauma
Mediastinitis
Esophageal perforation
Dental abscess
Epiglottitis
Abdominal infection
Subdiaphragmatic abscess
Peritonitis
Spontaneous pneumothorax
Thoracocentesis
Sepsis
Complicating rheumatoid pleurisy
Miscellaneous or unknown

an increased morbidity and mortality, despite the advent of potent antibiotics. Infection is the second leading cause of a pleural effusion after congestive heart failure in developed countries (3). Pleural infection caused by an underlying pneumonia is the most common cause of empyema and accounts for 70% of reported empyemas (2). Pleural empyemas occur in 5% to 10% of patients with PPE and seem to affect more frequently the elderly and debilitated and hospitalized patients with community-acquired pneumonia and men more than women (male-to-female ratio 1.8:1) (2). An important cause of PPE is the delayed diagnosis and initiation of proper antibiotic treatment or effective tube drainage in the course of a bacterial pneumonia.

Comorbidities include preexisting pulmonary diseases, such as bronchiectasis, chronic obstructive pulmonary disease (COPD), lung cancer, malignancy, previous tuberculosis (posttuberculous bronchiectasis), rheumatoid pleuropulmonary disease (drug immunosuppression, rupture of subpleural necrobiotic nodules, increased risk of infection because of impaired neutrophil function and altered bacterial clearance by a chemically inflamed pleura and low pleural fluid pH and glucose), acquired immunodeficiency syndrome (AIDS), and diabetes (65–10). Clinical factors that predict the presence of anaerobic pneumonia include poor dental hygiene, sedative drug use, alcoholism, seizures, mental retardation, and gastroesophageal reflux (6).

The majority of non-PPE and empyemas are iatrogenic either after thoracic surgery (about 20% of all causes of empyemas) or after thoracic surgical procedures. Trauma and esophageal perforation account for 5% each, while thoracocentesis is responsible for almost 2% of all causes of empyemas (Table 1). Rare causes of empyema include secondary pulmonary infarctions (11), postobstructive pneumonitis because of foreign body aspiration (12) and extension of head and neck infection from dental abscesses (more common in the preantibiotic era) (13).

The role of the pathogen in the underlying pneumonia and the likelihood of the patient to develop PPE is not clear since there are no comparative studies from a single institution. A cases series has shown that *Mycoplasma pneumoniae* (20%) (14) is less likely than *Streptococcus pneumoniae* (40–57%) to cause PPE (15). It is unusual for a loculation of a PPE or progress to empyema to occur after initiation of appropriate antibiotic therapy. Small patient series indicate that patients with pneumonia caused by gram-positive, gram-negative, or anaerobic bacteria have a 50% incidence of parapneumonic effusions when examined with decubitus chest radiographs (5).

Morbidity and mortality is higher in patients with PPE than in patients with pneumonia alone. Mortality from pleural empyema ranges from 5% to 30% (16). The mortality rate for immunocompromised patients can be as high as 40% (4).

In terms of the economic impact of PPE, little information is available. Patients with PPE or pleural empyema often have protracted duration of hospitalization. In a review of case series, the mean hospital stay for patients with empyema ranged from 12.3 to 56.8 days and the mortality rates ranged from 0% to 51% (17). It was found, in an NIH-sponsored study (18) that the presence of bilateral pleural effusions at the time of hospital admission is independently correlated with an increase in early (<7 days) and late (<30 days) mortality rates [total relative risk, 2.8; 95% confidence interval (CI), 1.4–5.8]. It is speculated that congestive heart failure as a comorbid condition played an additional role in the outcome.

IV. Pathophysiology

When a patient develops pneumonia, the pleura respond to the presence of microbes with a vigorous inflammatory response. The rate of pleural fluid formation, consisting of an exudate of WBC and proteins, is increased. The increase is mainly due to lung interstitial fluid, and secondary to increased permeability of the capillaries in the pleurae. When the amount of pleural fluid entering the pleural space exceeds the capacity of the pleural lymphatics to reabsorb the fluid, a pleural effusion develops. Initially, the pleural fluid has a normal glucose and pH and the lactate dehydrogenase (LDH) level and the WBC counts are low (3). Mesothelial cells are actively phagocytic, initiating inflammatory response when activated by the presence of bacteria, releasing a battery of chemokines (C-X-C group), cytokines (IL-1, IL-6, IL-8, TNF-α), oxidants, and proteases (19).

In some patients, the process progresses with bacteria invading the pleural fluid. Consequently, the pleural fluid glucose and pH become progressively lower, the LDH progressively higher, and the fluid increasingly more viscid. In addition, sheets of fibrin form loculi of fluid and cover the visceral pleura, which prevents the underlying lung from re-expanding if the fluid is removed. The process is reversible with the institution of proper antibiotic therapy during the early exudative phase. The evolution of a simple PPE to an empyema represents a continuous progression from a small amount of free flowing, noninfected pleural fluid to a large amount of frank pus, which is multiloculated and is associated with thick visceral pleura. In accordance, a PPE can be divided into four stages (Table 2), which are not sharply defined but gradually merge together.

Table 2 Pathophysiological Phases of Evolution of Parapneumonic Pleural Effusions and Empyema

---

Pleuritis sicca phase
   Pleural rub and pleuritic chest pain without pleural effusion
   Involvement of the pleura may be limited to this stage
Exudative phase
   Thin, free-flowing fluid
   Normal pleural fluid leukocytes, pH, LDH, glucose
Fibrinopurulent phase
   Increased viscosity of pleural fluid
   Fibrin deposition
   Bacteria may be present
   Increased leukocytes and LDH (>500 IU)
   Decreased pH (<7.2), glucose (<60 mg/dL)
Organizing phase
   Purulent fluid
   Increased leukocytes and LDH (>1000 IU)
   Decreased pH (<7.0), glucose (<40 mg/dL)
   Pleural peel

A. The Pleuritis Sicca Stage

In this stage, the inflammatory process of the lung extends to the visceral pleura, causing a local reaction. This leads to audible pleural rub and pleuritic chest pain, originating from the sensitive innervation of the adjacent parietal pleura. A significant number of patients with pneumonia report pleuritic chest pain without developing a pleural effusion (1,20), suggesting that the involvement of the pleura may be limited to this stage in many cases of pneumonia.

B. The Exudative Stage

The parapneumonic effusion that occurs in the initial hours tends to be small in volume and is a sterile, neutrophil predominant exudate. The ongoing inflammatory process leads to a mediator-induced increase of the permeability of local tissue and of regional capillaries. The following accumulation of fluid in the pleural space is probably the combined result of the influx of pulmonary interstitial fluid (21) and of a local microvascular exudate. This stage is the capillary leak or exudative stage. Typically, the pleural fluid is usually clear and sterile, the pH is >7.30, the glucose is >60 mg/dL, and the LDH is <500 U/L (1–3,22,23). Patients in this first stage can be treated successfully with antibiotics without the need for pleural space drainage.

C. The Fibropurulent Stage

If the pneumonia progresses, bacteria continue to multiply in the lung with invasion and persistence in the pleural space, while endothelial injury becomes more prominent with worsening pulmonary edema and increased pleural fluid formation. The pleural fluid in this bacterial invasion/fibrinopurulent stage is characterized by an increased number of polymorphonuclear cells (PMNs), by the effect of the major chemotactic factor interleukin-8 (IL-8), by a fall in pleural fluid pH and glucose, and by an increase in pleural fluid LDH (19). The pleural fluid/serum glucose ratio decreases to <0.5, with an absolute concentration of usually <40 mg/dL because of the increased rate of glycolysis from PMN phagocytosis and bacterial metabolism (1–3). As the end products of glucose metabolism, CO_2 and lactic acid accumulate in the pleural space and the pH falls (<7.2). The LDH increases (>1000 U/L), because of PMN lysis. The pleural fluid becomes clottable as procoagulants from the blood move into the pleural space in conjunction with a loss of pleural space fibrinolytic activity from mesothelial injury (20,24–28). Fibrin and collagen are deposited in a continuous sheet, covering the visceral and parietal pleura, and compartmentalize the pleural fluid into loculations by bridging the two pleural surfaces, making drainage increasingly difficult. In addition, pleural thickening limits lung expansion with deposition on the visceral pleura. Pleural fluid volume may increase further because of blockage of the parietal pleural stoma by fibrin and collagen and mesothelial swelling (25–28). Early in this stage, antibiotics alone may be effective, but later, pleural space drainage is usually required (29,30).

D. The Organizational/Empyema Stage

According to Hippocrates, "Pleurisy that does not clear up in 14 days, results in empyema" (31). Indeed, without treatment, this stage ensues over the next few weeks, characterized by the invasion of fibroblasts, leading to the transformation of intrapleural fibrin membranes into a thick and nonelastic pleural "peel," forming a single or multiple loculations. As a consequence, impairment of pleural fluid drainage and inhibition of lung expansion occurs. Functionally, gas exchange can be severely impaired on the side of the organizing empyema ("trapped lung"). Empyema fluid is a thick, purulent coagulum, which may not be adequately drained by tube thoracostomy. Pus is characterized by the coagulability of pleural fluid, the abundance of cellular debris, and increased fibrin and collagen deposition. Untreated empyema rarely resolves spontaneously. It may drain through the chest wall (empyema necessitatis) or into the lung (bronchopleural fistula) or may format lung abscess. Patients with empyema always require drainage for resolution of pleural sepsis.

V. Classification of Parapneumonic Effusion and Empyema

Numerous classification schemes (20,22,23,32–34) have been proposed to categorize the entire spectrum of PPE (Table 3). One common classification divides PPE into the following three categories:

1. Uncomplicated parapneumonic effusion: This corresponds to the exudative stage of a PPE. It is characterized by an exudative, predominantly neutrophilic effusion that occurs when the lung interstitial fluid increases during pneumonia. It resolves with the resolution of the pneumonia. No drainage is needed.

2. Complicated parapneumonic effusion: This corresponds to the fibrinopurulent stage of a PPE. Complicated effusions occur when there is persistent bacterial invasion of the pleural space. Bacterial invasion typically leads to an increased number of neutrophils and the development of pleural fluid acidosis, which results from anaerobic utilization of glucose by the neutrophils and bacteria. In addition, lysis of neutrophils increases the LDH concentration in the pleural fluid to values often in excess of 1000 1U/L. Complicated parapneumonic effusions

Table 3 Classification Schemes for Patients with Parapneumonic Pleural Effusion and Empyema and Key Characteristics

Early	Stage		Late	Ref.
Exudative	Fibrinopurulent		Organizing	32
Nonloculated	Loculated		Empyema	33
Uncomplicated/nonloculated	Complicated/loculated		Empyema	34
Uncomplicated	Complicated		Empyema	35
Nonsignificant typical borderline	Simple complex	Simple E	Complex E	36
Category 1	Category 2	Category 3 A2 or	Category 4	37
A0 + Bx + Cx	A1 + B0 + C0	B1 or C1	B2	

See Table 5 for details. E = empyema.

are often sterile because bacteria can be cleared rapidly from the pleural space (4). This occurs despite the deposition of a dense layer of fibrin on both the visceral and parietal pleurae that can lead to pleural loculation (4).

3. Thoracic empyema: This corresponds to the organizational/empyema stage of a PPE. It is characterized by bacterial organisms seen on Gram stain or by the aspiration of pus on thoracocentesis. A positive culture is not required for diagnosis. A negative bacterial culture may be due to anaerobic organisms, which are difficult to culture, sampling after antibiotic treatment, and aspiration adjacent to an infected loculus of infection. Table 4 shows the biochemical characteristics of a para-pneumonic effusion. Cases with borderline biochemical parameters on pleural fluid analysis characterize an undetermined PPE and need close follow-up. Table 5 presents a practical classification scheme introduced by Light.

The American College of Chest Physicians (ACCP) has developed a new classification system for PPE/PE (34), which is based upon the radiological characteristics of the effusion, the pleural fluid bacteriology, and the pleural fluid chemistry (Table 6). The key aspects are the characteristics that indicate that the patient has a moderate-to-high risk of a poor outcome without drainage. Radiological characteristics associated with a poor prognosis are an effusion that occupies >50% of the hemithorax, is loculated, or (paradoxically) is associated with thickened parietal pleura. However, pleural thickening is not related to the requirement for surgery (35). Bacteriological criteria associated with a poor prognosis are a positive culture and/or Gram stain or the presence of pus. The

Table 4 Biochemical Characteristics of the Stages of Parapneumonic Pleural Effusions and Empyema

Parameter	Uncomplicated	Undetermined	Complicated
pH	>7.3	7.3–7.1	<7.1
Glucose (mg/dL)	>60	60–40	<40
LDH (IU)	<500	<1000	>1000

Table 5 Classification, Characteristics and Treatment Scheme of Parapneumonic Pleural Effusion and Empyema

Category of PPE/PE	Characteristics/treatment
Class 1	<10 mm thick on decubitus radiograph
Nonsignificant	No thoracocentesis indicated
Class 2	10 mm thick
Typical PPE	Glucose >40 mg/dL, pH >7.2, Gram stain and culture negative; antibiotics alone
Class 3	7.0>pH <7.2 or LDH>500, and glucose >40 mg/dL
Borderline complicated PPE	Gram stain and culture negative Antibiotics plus serial thoracocentesis
Class 4	pH <7.0 or glucose <40 mg/dL, or Gram stain or culture positive
Simple complicated PPE	Not loculated, not frank pus
	Tube thoracostomy plus antibiotics
Class 5	pH <7.0 or glucose <40 mg/dL, or Gram stain or culture positive
Complex complicated PPE	Multiloculated
	Tube thoracostomy plus thrombolytics
	Thoracoscopy if above ineffective
Class 6	Frank pus present
Simple empyema	Single locule or free flowing
	Tube thoracostomy plus thrombolytics ± decortication
Class 7	Frank pus present
Complex empyema	Multiple locules
	Tube thoracostomy plus thrombolytics
	Usually require thoracoscopy or decortication

Source: Adapted from Ref. 33.

pleural fluid chemistry criterion associated with a poor prognosis is a pleural fluid pH of 7.20. Alternative pleural fluid chemistry criteria are a pleural fluid glucose <60 mL/dL or a pleural fluid LDH more than three times the upper limit of normal serum levels.

A schematic presentation of the classifications of parapneumonic pleural effusions is shown in Fig. 1.

VI. Etiology of PPE/PE

The bacteriology of PPE/PE is related to that of the pneumonic infection. Before the advent of modern antibiotics, the most common pleural infections occurred with streptococcal and staphylococcal species. Current series of empyemas support the continuing role of these organisms while documenting the emergence of anaerobes and gram-negative organisms as common pathogens. The reported spectra depend on the patient populations studied by various investigators. Animal models suggest that infection with a mixed bacterial flora containing aerobes and anaerobes is more likely to produce an empyema than a single organism infection (36,37). Anaerobic bacteria have been cultured in 36% to 76% of empyemas (38,39). According to many series (38–45), the majority of culture-positive effusions are due to aerobic organisms, while up to 15% are caused exclusively by

Table 6 Classification Scheme of Risk for Poor Outcome in Patients with Parapneumonic Pleural Effusion and Empyema and Drainage Recommendations

Pleural space anatomy	Pleural fluid bacteriology	Pleural fluid chemistry	Category	Risk of poor outcome	Drainage
A0: Minimal, free-flowing effusion (<10 mm on lateral decubitus)	and Bx culture and Gram stain results unknown	and Cx pH unknown	1	Very low	No
A1: Small to moderate free-flowing effusion (<10 mm and <1/2 hemithorax)	and B0 negative culture and Gram stain	and C0 pH>7.20	2	Low	No
A2: Large, free-flowing effusion (≥ 1/2 hemithorax), loculated effusion, or effusion with thickened parietal pleura	or B1 positive culture and Gram stain	or C1 pH<7.20	3	Moderate	Yes
	B2 pus		4	High	Yes

Source: Adapted from Ref. 34.

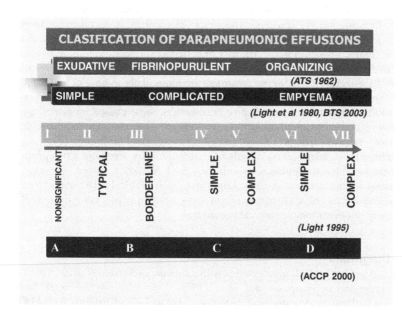

Figure 1 Schematic presentation of the classifications of parapneumonic pleural effusions.

anaerobic bacteria. This high incidence probably results from the indolent nature of these pneumonias, which permits pleural penetration of bacteria before antibiotics are instituted. The most frequent anaerobic isolates are *Bacteroides* species and *Peptostreptococcus.* Empyemas, particularly if they are multiloculated, may harbor multiple bacteria (29).

The remainder is usually due to a mixture of aerobic and anaerobic organisms. Streptococci (mostly *S. pneumoniae*) and staphylococci (mostly *S. aureus*) usually dominate gram-positive isolates, while *Escherichia coli, Klebsiella* species, *Pseudomonas* species, and *Haemophilus influenzae* are the most common gram-negative isolates (18,29). Particularly *E. coli* and anaerobic organisms are often found in combination with other organisms. Reports on viral, fungal (most frequently *Aspergillus*), and parasitic pleural infections are rare, although the incidence and awareness is increasing (46). Readers wanting further details are referred to a review article (46).

VII. Clinical Picture

The clinical presentation of patients with pneumonia with or without PPE is usually very much alike, with no significant differences between these two groups of patients regarding WBC count and occurrence of pleuritic chest pain (20). The clinical picture depends mainly on whether pneumonia is caused by aerobic or anaerobic bacteria. Patients with aerobic bacterial pneumonia usually suffer from an acute-onset fever, while anaerobic infections tend to present as a more subacute or chronic condition with longer duration of symptoms and weight loss (47). Anaerobic pleuropulmonary infections often follow aspiration of oral or gastric contents. These patients usually have poor oral hygiene *(fetor ex ore!)* with anaerobic colonization of the oropharynx and often suffer from conditions that predispose to aspiration like seizures, syncopes, or alcoholism. Alcoholism has been found to be associated in 29% (4) to 40% (41) of the cases. Leukocytosis (>20,000/mL) and anemia are common findings in the majority of patients (47).

In general, patients who have a longer history of symptoms before seeking medical attention or have received insufficient treatment are more likely to have complicated PPE/PE (29). Among gram-positive pneumonias, *S. pneumoniae* is even today responsible for most PPE. Among the gram-negative pneumonias, those caused by *E. coli* are more frequently related with complicated PPE (3). PPE are more common in anaerobic pneumonia, while some of them have no concomitant parenchymal infiltration (3).

The finding of a purulent effusion without pneumonia may represent a postpneumonic empyema in which the pulmonary infiltrates have already resolved. However, pleural empyemas are not necessarily caused by pneumonias (Table 1). The majority of nonpneumonic empyemas are of iatrogenic origin, most commonly as a complication of a pneumonectomy or other thoracic surgical procedures.

VIII. Diagnosis

Physicians should be alert for PPE in any patient with pulmonary infection who has a pleural effusion on presentation. Symptoms and signs of PPE—fever, pleurodynia, cough, and dyspnea—merge with those of underlying pneumonia. Up to 10% of patients with PPE and empyema are relatively asymptomatic, while 60% to 80% have underlying comorbidities (40,45). Prompt thoracocentesis is recommended before antibiotics are administered to improve the diagnostic yield of pleural fluid culture. A diagnostic thoracocentesis should usually be performed when clinical findings and/or imaging techniques suggest the presence of a significant pleural effusion. Smaller effusions can safely be reached, for example, by ultrasound guidance. Only very small (<10 mm), difficult-to-reach effusions may be observed.

A foul-smelling pleural fluid suggests the presence of anaerobic bacteria (47). Only 60% of anaerobic empyemas have feculent odor (47,48), because not all PPE have an acute presentation, and caution should be exercised for the possibility of PPE in all patients with a pleural effusion.

IX. Imaging Techniques

Radiology is central in the evaluation and proper management of PPE. Conventional radiographs, including decubitus films, and newer imaging techniques, including contrast enhanced computed tomography (CT) scans and real-time ultrasound, provide more detailed morphological information in terms of size and nature of the effusion, but they do not obviate the need for a thoracocentesis or other invasive diagnostic procedures (29,49).

A. Chest Radiograph

A chest radiograph showing a pleural-based opacity that has an abnormal contour or does not flow freely on lateral decubitus views first suggests the presence of a complicated PPE/PE. Conventional chest radiographs usually show a pulmonary infiltrate with ipsilateral pleural fluid. A lateral chest radiograph is particularly useful to detect blunting of the posterior costophrenic angle (Fig. 2). Accumulation of >200 mL of pleural fluid usually blunts the lateral costophrenic angle, although up to 500 mL may be present without blunting or other radiographic abnormalities (50). A meniscus sign is seen in nonloculated pleural effusions in excess of 500 mL. The lateral decubitus film can detect pleural effusion as small as 5 mL (51) and is used in the decision making of a thoracocentesis (3). A lateral decubitus radiograph with the diseased lung up is also useful since it allows for a better evaluation of the presence of pleural fluid loculi and the extent of pneumonia. Supine radiographs have sensitivity and specificity of about 70% compared with lateral decubitus films in demonstrating a pleural effusion (52). Increased opacity in the hemithorax without obscuration of the vascular markings, blunting of the costophrenic angle or apical cap indicates a pleural effusion in a supine radiograph (53). Interlobular loculation of pleural fluid is referred to as pseudotumor and has an oval shape and longitudinal orientation. The presence of consolidated or atelectatic lower lobe can obscure the silhouette of the diaphragm, concealing a PPE, and may require additional imaging examination by ultrasound or CT scan for detection (53,54).

B. Ultrasound

Ultrasonography (US) is a good method to confirm or rule out a pleural effusion in cases where chest radiographs are inconclusive. Also, it is the method of choice to guide a thoracocentesis or place a chest tube. It is especially useful for small effusions and in other difficult circumstances, which require precise targeting, for instance, loculated effusions. A distinct advantage of ultrasound is the ability to study the patient at the bedside. In patients with minimal pleural abnormalities on conventional radiographs, ultrasound can detect small amounts of pleural fluid and reliably distinguishes small effusions from

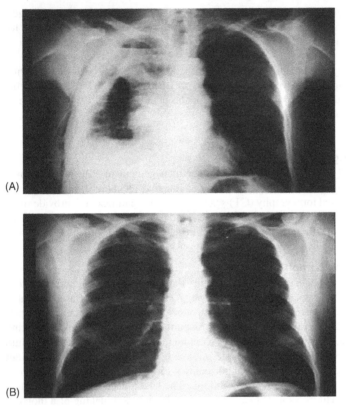

(A)

(B)

Figure 2 A posteroanterior chest radiograph of a patient with extensive multiloculated parapneumonic pleural effusion on the right before (**A**) and after treatment with intrapleural urokinase instillation for 5 days (**B**).

pleural thickening (55). When decubitus views fail to show layering of pleural fluid, sonography can significantly increase the diagnostic yield from thoracocentesis.

Pleural collections as seen on sonography are characterized as echo-free, complex septated, complex nonseptated, and homogeneously echogenic (56). Transudates are always anechoic, but exudates may also be anechoic. Effusions are usually exudates when they are septated or show a complex or homogeneously echogenic pattern. Dense echogenic patterns are most often associated with hemorrhagic effusions or empyemas (57) (Fig. 3). The real-time evaluation of the movement of pleural collections appears to be a more useful indicator of successful thoracocentesis than the echogenicity of the collection. However, the use of ultrasound guidance has been shown to be the single most significant factor in reducing the incidence of pneumothorax after thoracocentesis (58). Sonographic evaluation is more accurate in estimating pleural fluid volume than a decubitus radiograph (59), while it was found to expedite patient management in 49% of cases by either clarifying the nature of the pleural collection or identifying the most appropriate sites for thoracocentesis (60).

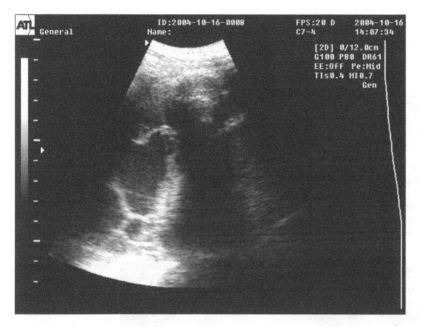

Figure 3 Ultrasonography showing a complex septated parapneumonic pleural effusion.

C. Computed Tomography

Although diagnosis can be facilitated by thoracocentesis under ultrasound guidance, optimal management requires a chest CT scan with contrast, which enhances the pleural surface and assists in delineating pleural fluid loculi (Fig. 4). CT scan may show pleural abnormalities at an earlier stage than other imaging modalities. It is useful in distinguishing pleural from parenchymal abnormalities; in detecting pleural fluid loculation in the mediastinal pleura, where ultrasound is usually negative (18); in determining the precise location and extent of pleural disease; and in occasionally providing information for the specific characterization of pleural fluid. It may also detect airway or parenchymal abnormalities (such as endobronchial obstruction), the extent of underlying pneumonia and its features (necrotizing pneumonia), or the presence of lung abscesses. Furthermore, chest CT can assess the position of chest tubes and give evidence for the presence of bronchopleural fistula or gas forming organisms. Contrast-enhanced chest CT aids in better outlining of the thick inflammatory pleura in empyema. However, it cannot differentiate inflammatory from malignant disease (61). Pleural thickening and thickening of extrapleural fat did not correlate with clinical stages or outcome (62). A chest CT scan performed after the intravenous administration of iodinated contrast that shows parietal and visceral pleural enhancement, thickening of the extrapleural subcostal tissues, and increased attenuation of the extrapleural fat is highly suggestive of an empyema (49,63). The combination of fluid between the enhancing thickened pleural layers has been termed the split pleura sign of empyema.

Mediastinal lymphadenopathy is a common finding (36%) in PPE/PE (64,65). Multiple sites may be involved, and node diameters may reach 2 cm. CT may also be used

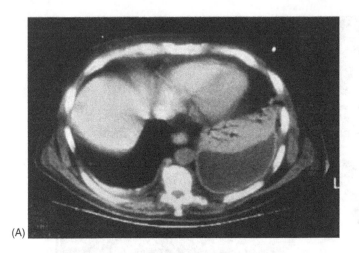

(A)

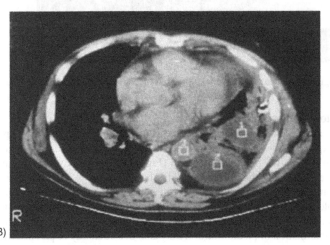

(B)

Figure 4 Chest computed tomographies showing a single loculus of pleural empyema (**A**) on the left, and a multiloculated parapneumonic pleural effusion on the left hemithorax (**B**).

for image-guided drainage and monitoring response to closed drainage or intrapleural fibrinolytic therapy.

D.   Magnetic Resonance Imaging

The role of magnetic resonance imaging (MRI) in the clinical evaluation of pleural infection is limited. Although MRI is able to show pleural fluid collections, it is severely limited in assessing lung parenchyma (49).

Sagittal T1–weighted MR images allow a detailed analysis of the layers of the chest wall and their possible infiltration by inflammatory or malignant processes. Uncomplicated parapneumonic effusions do not seem to induce visible changes of the chest wall, whereas malignant effusions are frequently associated with alterations of the peripleural fat layer and the innermost intercostal muscles (66,67). While these findings were interpreted as helpful in the differential diagnosis of benign and malignant effusions, it remains doubtful that complicated effusions and empyemas show infiltration of the chest wall similar to malignant disease. The use of MRI in the routine differentiation of transudates from exudates is not practical or cost-effective at the present time (68,69).

X. Pleural Fluid Analysis

All suspected PPE should undergo a thoracocentesis, unless they are very small (Table 5). The pleural fluid should be sent to microbiology lab for Gram stain and bacterial culture, WBC count and differential, and to biochemistry for determination of glucose, LDH, and pH.

A. Pleural Fluid Chemistry

Parapneumonic pleural effusions are exudates and are identified by application of Light's criteria (70) and/or the cholesterol level (71) and measuring the pleural fluid protein and LDH levels. If the pH is determined, it must be done with the same care, as is an arterial pH level. The fluid should be collected in a heparinized syringe and placed in ice for its transfer to the blood gas laboratory. pH meters and dip sticks do not provide sufficiently accurate pH measurements (3). In the case of frank empyema, a pH measurement is not useful, as the purulent material is at risk of filling the membrane of the arterial blood gas machine.

Several pleural fluid parameters have been described to assess the severity and to predict the future course of a PPE. Patients with complicated PPE/PE tend to have a lower pleural fluid pH and glucose level and a higher LDH activity (1,72–76). The glucose concentration correlates directly with the pH (76). The cause for pleural fluid acidosis and low glucose levels is the local metabolic activity of inflammatory cells and bacteria (77). The superiority of the pH over glucose or LDH measurements in PPE/PE has been confirmed in a meta-analysis of seven studies using receiver operating characteristic (ROC) statistical techniques (78). The decision threshold to identify complicated effusions ranged between pH 7.21 and 7.29. A pleural pH in this range appeared to represent the threshold for consideration of drainage of a complicated PPE. It should be noted, however, that other diseases are associated with pleural fluid acidosis, including malignancy, tuberculosis, rheumatoid pleurisy, and lupus pleuritis.

It may suffice to measure the pH alone, but it must be emphasized that there are still not enough large-scale studies that have firmly established the predictive and discriminative power of this parameter. Further, pH measurements are only valid when performed properly, which means (1) collection and transport under strict anaerobic conditions and (2) immediate measurement in a calibrated blood gas machine. It should also be kept in mind that the pleural fluid pH may not be useful in patients with systemic pH alterations (72) and in infections due to *Proteus* species, which can induce a local metabolic alkalosis due to ammonia production (79). Also, in loculated pleural effusions, it is possible to find pleural fluid with different macroscopic characteristics and pH values.

There is general clinical consensus that pleural fluid pH is the most important chemical parameter to predict the further course of a PPE/PE, and various recommendations have been made for the best cut-off point to distinguish complicated from uncomplicated cases (1,3,80,81). In a recently published consensus statement of the ACCP (34), a pH of <7.20 is recommended as one of the parameters that predict poor outcome and should lead to chest tube drainage (Table 2).

B. Pleural Fluid Cytology

PPE/PE are polymorphonuclear dominated effusions. Any other finding suggests another diagnosis (e.g., predominance of lymphocytes in an exudate is most often associated with tuberculosis or malignancy). The finding of food particles in the pleural fluid suggests the presence of esophageal–pleural fistula (82).

C. Bacteriology

Bacteriological studies should include Gram stain and aerobic and anaerobic cultures. Delayed thoracocentesis results in prolonged hospitalization (78,83). Pleural fluid cultures should be repeated if there is any alteration in the expected clinical status and radiological appearance, because new pathogens may be introduced in the pleural cavity via thoracocentesis needles, percutaneous catheters, intercostal tubes, or open thoracotomies.

XI. Differential Diagnosis

Fever, pulmonary infiltrates, and a pleural effusion are not invariably due to pneumonia or to a complication of some surgical procedure. Pulmonary embolism is a common disorder, and paraembolic effusions occur in about 25% to 50% of the cases (84). The effusions may become infected and will then require treatment identical to complicated PPE. Other disorders that should be considered include tuberculosis, lupus erythematosus, and other autoimmune disorders, acute pancreatitis and other diseases of the gastrointestinal-tract, and drug-induced pleuropulmonary disease. The turbid or milky aspect of empyemas may sometimes resemble the aspect of a chylothorax or pseudochylothorax.

XII. Treatment Strategy

The therapeutic options for a PPE depend on the particular type or stage of parapneumonic effusion. The best therapeutic approach for PPE and PE remains controversial (1,3,4,84–86). The development of new options for treatment further complicates decision making. There are only few prospective, randomized trials to guide intervention. A survey conducted at the 1991 ACCP Annual Scientific Assembly in order to record their personal management preferences reported heterogeneous approaches to management (87). The British Thoracic Society Research Committee conducted the first prospective multicenter study to document the present-day clinical course and management of empyema, which reported a great diversity in treatment approaches and outcomes of PPE and PE (6). Recently, the Health and Sciences Policy Committee (HSP) of the ACCP recognized the variability in clinical practice and convened a panel of experts in this field to develop a clinical practice guideline on the medical and surgical treatment of PPE (34). The rationale for effective management is to identify the pathophysiological stage and intervene quickly and appropriately to prevent progression to empyema.

Uncomplicated parapneumonic effusions resolve with antibiotics alone. Complicated parapneumonic effusions have a variable response to appropriate antibiotic therapy alone. Although some patients can be managed solely with antibiotics (18), there is a bias that early pleural fluid drainage of all loculi of fluid speeds clinical recovery and hospital discharge. Until clinical trials demonstrate the safety of alternative therapies, these patients are normally treated as though they have thoracic empyema. Thoracic empyema should be sterilized with appropriate antibiotics; at least four to six weeks of therapy are required, and a longer course may be necessary unless there is prompt resolution of fever and leukocytosis. Complete pleural fluid drainage with large-bore chest tube is sine qua non and evidenced by minimal chest tube output (<50 mL/24 hr) and US or CT documentation that no residual loculations persist. Obliteration of the empyema cavity by adequate lung expansion is also important (18).

When a patient with pneumonia is first evaluated, one should attempt first to determine whether a pleural effusion is present. A lateral radiograph should be obtained to screen. If both diaphragms cannot be seen throughout their entirety on the lateral chest radiograph, bilateral decubitus chest radiographs, chest CT scan, or US should be obtained. The amount of free pleural fluid can be estimated by measuring on the lateral chest radiograph the distance between the inside of the chest wall and the outside of the lung. If the thickness of the pleural fluid is >10 mm, thoracocentesis should be performed. One should perform the thoracocentesis as soon as the pleural effusion is recognized because a free-flowing, easily treated PPE can progress to a multiloculated PPE within a day (35,84).

It is important to realize that not all PPE and not all complicated PPE are the same. The classification outlined in Tables 3, 5, and 6 was developed to assist the practicing physician during the initial care of patients with parapneumonic effusions. A practical management plan is shown in Figure 5.

If the thickness of the pleural fluid is <10 mm, the effusion is nonsignificant and no thoracocentesis is indicated (3,84). If it appears from the standard radiographs that the patient has a loculated pleural effusion, this possibility should be evaluated with ultrasound. When a patient has a PPE of >10 mm in thickness on the decubitus radiograph, a thoracocentesis should be performed to determine the category of the effusion. It is reasonable to perform a therapeutic rather than a diagnostic thoracocentesis (18,33,35). If the fluid is removed completely with the therapeutic thoracocentesis and does not reaccumulate, no additional therapy is needed.

If the therapeutic thoracocentesis removes all the pleural fluid and the fluid recurs, the next step is guided by the initial pleural fluid findings (3). If none of the poor prognostic indicators are present (Table 7), a repeat thoracocentesis should be considered if the size of effusion is progressively increasing, while no invasive procedures are indicated if the patient is doing well clinically or the effusion is small. If any of the poor prognostic indicators were present at the initial thoracocentesis, a small 8–13-F chest tube should be inserted into the pleural space. The chest tube is removed if the drainage is <50 mL/24 hr. If the pleural fluid cannot be removed completely with a small chest tube, it is probably loculated. If the pleural fluid is loculated and if any of the poor prognostic factors listed in Table 7 are present, efforts should be made to break down the loculations in order to obtain complete drainage of the pleural space. Loculations can be broken down either chemically with intrapleural instillation of fibrinolytics or mechanically by thoracoscopy. If one selects intrapleural fibrinolytics, thoracoscopy should be performed if the fibrinolytics

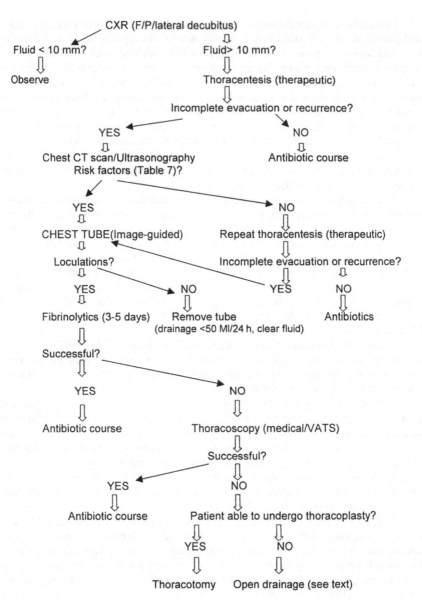

Figure 5 Management algorithm for patients with parapneumonic pleural effusion and empyema.

Table 7 Risk Predictors in Parapneumonic Effusions, Indicating the Need for Chest Tube Drainage and/or Further Invasive Procedures

Clinical signs
Prolonged symptoms
Comorbidity
Failure to respond to antibiotics
Pathogen (anaerobic, virulent pathogen)
Imaging signs
Large effusion ($\geq 1/2$ hemithorax)
Loculations (single or multiple, large)
Air-fluid level Pleural thickening
Complex sonographic pattern
Pleural fluid signs
Macroscopic signs (turbid fluid or frank pus, odorous)
Low pleural fluid pH (<7.20)
Low pleural fluid glucose (<40 mg/dL)
High pleural fluid LDH (>1000 IU)
Positive pleural fluid Gram stain/culture

are not successful within three to five days. If the lung does not expand at thoracoscopy, one should proceed to decortication unless the patient is too debilitated. In such a case, open drainage should be considered (Fig. 3). The primary mistake in the management of patients with complicated PPE/PE is that one progresses from one therapy to another too slowly. A definitive procedure should be done within 10 to 14 days after the patient is initially seen (3).

XIII. Methods for Treatment OF PPE/PE

Today, there are various medical and surgical methods for the treatment of PPE/PE (Table 8).

Table 8 Methods for Treatment of Parapneumonic Effusions and Pleural Empyema

Medical
Antibiotics
Daily thoracocentesis
Tube thoracostomy (standard chest tube)
Image-guided percutaneous catheter insertion
Intrapleural fibrinolytic debridement
Suction drainage
Medical thoracoscopy
Surgical
Video-assisted thoracoscopic surgery (VATS)
Standard thoracotomy
Open drainage

A. Medical Methods

A number of medical methods are available for the treatment of pleural space infection. The choice of therapy depends in part upon whether the PPE/PE is loculated.

Antibiotic Therapy

Antibiotic therapy is indicated for all patients with PPE and PE. Early institution of appropriate antibiotic therapy may prevent the development of PPE and clear small effusions before they become complicated.

The antibiotic selection depends primarily on whether the pneumonia is community or hospital acquired and not on the presence or absence of a PPE. Thus, initial treatment should follow the existing guidelines for treatment of community- or hospital-acquired pneumonia (4,88), but with the following in mind: antibiotics that exhibit satisfactory penetration into the pleural fluid include the penicillins, cephalosporins, aztreonam, clindamycin, and ciprofloxacin (3,89). The concentrations of parenterally administered aminoglycosides, particularly gentamicin, were found to be substantially lower in empyema pus than in sterile pleural fluid (see chap. 50) (89,90).

The recommended empiric treatment for a patient with community-acquired pneumonia that is not severe is a β-lactam-β-lactamase inhibitor with or without a macrolide (4). Alternatively, the newer generation fluoroquinolones, such as moxifloxacin and levofloxacin, can be used. The recommended treatment for severe community-acquired pneumonia is a macrolide or a new generation fluoroquinolone plus cefotaxime, ceftriaxone, or a β-lactam-β-lactamase inhibitor (4). Enteric gram-negative bacillii, or *S. aureus* with or without oral anaerobes frequently causes pneumonia acquired in institutions such as nursing homes or hospitals. If methicillin-resistant *S. aureus* infection is suspected, vancomycin should be administered. If gram-negative infection is suspected, the patient should be treated with a third-generation cephalosporin or a β-lactam-β-lactamase inhibitor plus an aminoglycoside.

Given the high incidence of anaerobic infection in empyema and the difficulty in isolating anaerobes in many clinical laboratories, most clinicians cover for anaerobes, even if cultures are negative. Options for empiric therapy, which also covers anaerobic organisms, include penicillin, metronidazole, clindamycin, extended spectrum penicillins (such as ticarcillin, piperacillin, ampicillin-sulbactam, or piperacillin-tazobactam), or imipenem.

There is still debate over the use of intrapleural antibiotics. Several studies have reported positive results, but none of them included a randomized control group (91,92).

Repeat Thoracocentesis

Repeat therapeutic thoracocentesis is the least invasive technique to treat PPE and PE. Nowadays it is used rarely as a mode of treatment. There is lack of controlled randomized trials to evaluate its efficacy. In the few reported nonrandomized series, the success rate ranged widely from 25% to 94%, and the mortality from 0% to 25%, probably due to variability in the PPE stage (85,87,92–95). Repeat thoracocentesis should be performed in cases where pleural fluid recurs or when the PPE is undetermined (Table 5; Fig. 3).

Storm et al. (92) in a retrospective study of 94 patients with PPE or PE compared patients who were treated with daily thoracocentesis, saline rinse, systemic antibiotics, and in some patients local antibiotics in the medical ward and patients with tube drainage and systemic antibiotics in the surgical ward. The thoracocentesis group had a lower frequency of complications and a shorter duration of hospital stay than the tube drainage group. The overall mortality was 8.5% with no difference between the two groups. The outcome, however, could be due to inclusion of more severe cases in the surgical group (92).

Standard Chest Tubes

In many centers even today relatively large (26–28 F) chest tubes are usually used to drain PPE, especially PE. The success rate ranges from 6% to 76% (mean 50%) (1,6,85,86,92,93,96–104). Their failure to drain PPE is usually due to misplacement, malfunctioning, or loculation of the pleural fluid. In a study by Huang et al., loculation and PPE leukocyte count >6.400/μL were independent predicting factors of poor outcome of tube thoracostomy drainage (103). The chest tube is removed when the daily drainage is <50 mL/24 hr and the fluid is clear and yellow. Complications include hemorrhage, pneumothorax, subcutaneous emphysema, or pain. The mortality ranges from 0% to 24% (mean 9.5%) (1,3,4,6,85,86,92,93,96–104).

Image-Guided Transcutaneous Catheters

Today image-guided transcutaneous catheter (IGTC) insertion is used increasingly as they are more comfortable for pleural drainage. Interventional radiologists or pneumonologists can easily and safely use IGTC under US or CT scan guidance. Their size ranges between 8 and 14 F (Malecot or pigtail). Their success rate ranges from 0% to 94% (mean 70%) (1,3,104–112). These wide differences are due to patient selection. IGTC drainage is successful if instituted early in the course of the disease process. They are indicated for small, inaccessible or multiloculated effusions, are not suitable for PE, and work better in free- or single-loculated effusion. They can also be used for fibrinolytic instillation. No major complications have been noted.

Intrapleural Instillation of Fibrinolytics

Intrapleural instillation of fibrinolytic agents [streptokinase (SK) or urokinase (UK)] has been shown, in a number of studies, to be an effective and safe mode of treatment in complicated PPE and PE, minimizing the need for surgical intervention.

Technique of Instillation

The optimum dose, frequency, and duration of instillation of fibrinolytics into the pleural space have not been determined. The most commonly used dose of SK is 250,000 IU and that of UK 100,000 (50,000–450,000 IU). The drug is usually diluted in 100 mL of normal saline. Dwell time varies from two to four hours, the duration of treatment from three to five days, and the chest tube size from 10 to 40 F. Duration of treatment is based on the presence of residual pleural fluid as determined by repeat chest radiograph, US, and/or CT scan.

Success Rate

The mean success rate in the published uncontrolled series of SK is about 85% (range 38–100%) and that of UK 88% (range 63–100%) (113).

Six controlled and/or randomized trials of the use of intrapleural fibrinolytics have been reported (Table 9). Bouros et al. (114) compared the efficacy and safety of SK and UK in the treatment of PPE. Fifty consecutive patients were randomly allocated to receive either SK (250,000 IU in 100 mL normal saline solution) or UK (100,000 IU in 100 mL normal saline) through tube thoracostomy in a double-blinded fashion. All patients had

Table 9 Success Rate in the Published Controlled Studies of Fibrinolytics in Parapneumonic Effusions and Pleural Empyema

SK, *n* (%)	UK, *n* (%)	CT+NS, *n* (%)	VATS, *n* (%)	CT, *n* (%)	Ref.
23/25 (92)	23/25 (92)				114
12 (100)		3/12 (25)			100
4/9 (44)			10/11 (91)		115
16/23 (70)				19/29 (66)	98
	13/15 (86.5)	4/16 (25)			116
	25 (60)	24 (29)			117

Abbreviations: CT, chest tube; SK, streptokinase; UK, urokinase; NS, normal saline; VATS, video-assisted thoracoscopic surgery.

inadequate drainage (<70 mL/24 hr) through a chest tube before fibrinolytic treatment. Pleural fluid drainage significantly increased with fibrinolytic therapy, and the increase in pleural fluid drainage was similar for patients treated with UK and SK. Most patients in both treatment groups had marked clinical improvement with fibrinolytic therapy. UK was suggested as the fibrinolytic of choice due to the lower incidence of drug-related adverse events and its only slightly higher cost (114).

In another randomized, prospective, controlled trial, Davies et al. (100) compared the efficacy of SK (250,000 IU in 20 mL of saline with a two-hour dwell time daily for three days) with normal saline flushes in 24 patients. Patients who received SK had greater daily and total pleural fluid drainage as well as more evidence of chest radiographic improvement at discharge. Three patients in the tube thoracostomy control group required a second intervention to effectively drain versus none in the fibrinolytic group. There were no significant differences between the two treatment groups in hospital length of stay, time to defervescence, and time to normalization of WBC (100).

Wait et al. (115) compared the results after fibrinolytic therapy with video-assisted thoracoscopic surgery (VATS) in the management of PPE. Twenty patients were randomly allocated to receive either SK (250,000 IU in 100 mL normal saline solution) administered daily for three days through tube thoracostomy or immediate VATS. They found that the VATS group had a significantly higher treatment success rate than the fibrinolytic group. The hospital length of stay and duration of chest tube drainage were significantly shorter in the VATS group (115).

Chin and Lim (98), in a controlled, nonrandomized trial, analyzed the treatment responses of PPE to either tube thoracostomy or fibrinolytics. A historical control group, studied from 1990 to 1992, of 29 patients was treated with tube thoracostomy and a second one of 23 patients, evaluated from 1992 to 1995, was given SK (250,000 IU in 100 mL normal saline solution) daily through tube thoracostomy. Decortication was done in 17% and the overall mortality rate was 15%. There were no differences between the two groups in time to defervescence, days of chest tube drainage, and hospital stay, although the fibrinolytic group did have a greater amount of total pleural fluid drainage. The death rate was lower for the group treated with fibrinolytics but the need for a second intervention to drain the pleural space was similar for the two treatment groups (98).

Bouros et al. (116) in a randomized, controlled double-blind trial compared UK (15 patients) to tube thoracostomy (16 patients) in managing PPE. No patients died in this series, but the fibrinolytic group needed a second intervention to manage the PPE less often (2 out of 15, or 13.5%) than the group receiving normal saline (12 out of 16, or 75%). From this study, it was suggested that UK is effective in the treatment of loculated pleural effusions through the lysis of pleural adhesions and not through the volume effect (116). Tuncozgur et al. in a recent randomized, controlled study confirmed the data of our own study (117).

Maskell et al. (118a) reported in 2005 the results of a UK multicenter controlled trial of streptokinase in 454 patients with pleural infection. The number of patients in the two groups who had died or needed surgical drainage at three months was compared (the primary end point); secondary end points were the rates of death and of surgery, the radiographic outcome, and the length of the hospital stay. They concluded that intrapleural administration of streptokinase does not improve mortality, the rate of surgery, or the length of the hospital stay among patients with pleural infection.

This article has been criticized for major protocol weaknesses (118b), including patients stratification, use of small chest tubes, no guidance for tube insertion, older patients with comorbidities, no standard protocol for interventions, the selection of the primary objective, etc.

Other fibrinolytics, like recombinant tissue plasminogen activator (r-TPA) alone or with Combined with Human Recombinant Deoxyribonuclease have been shown very effective in the treatment of PPE both in adults and children (118c,d).

Monitoring for Efficacy and Adverse Reactions

Fibrinolytic agents are most effective if used early in the evolution of PPE before significant collagen is deposited in the pleural space (early in the fibrinopurulent stage) (1). Factors to consider in evaluating whether intrapleural instillation of fibrinolytics is effective include an assessment of clinical response. Pre-position for clinical response is the installation via a patent, properly placed chest tube. Its use should be started early if after chest tube placement inadequate evacuation of pleural fluid is noted radiographically with no clinical improvement. Measurement of pleural fluid drainage, WBC count, chest radiographs, and US and/or CT could be used to monitor treatment efficacy.

In the face of fever persistence or pleural sepsis, a markedly elevated WBC with left sift, or unresponsiveness of the pleural process to drainage, the clinician should reevaluate whether alternative therapy should be employed. In this situation, further invasive intervention, such as thoracoscopy, is indicated (1,3,113,114,116,118).

Initial use of nonpurified solutions of SK and streptodornase had as a result frequent febrile reactions, general malaise, and leukocytosis. Newer preparations cause fewer allergic reactions. The most frequently observed adverse reaction is fever (0–20%), which in rare cases can be severe (1,113,118).

Anaphylactic intravenous reactions to UK have been rarely reported, which were usually mild. Only one possible case of ventricular fibrillation following IPUK has been reported in a patient with pleural empyema (119). A case of acute hypoxemic respiratory failure following intrapleural instillation of both SK and UK 24 hours apart for hemothorax has been described (120).

Table 10   Contraindications for Intrapleural Fibrinolytic Use

Absolute contraindications
History of allergic reaction to the agent
History of hemorrhagic stroke
Cranial surgery or head trauma within 14 days
Bronchopleural fistula
Trauma or surgery within 48 hr
Relative contraindications
Major thoracic or abdominal surgery within 7–14 days
Biopsy or invasive procedure in a location inaccessible to external compression
    within 7–14 days
Coagulation defects
Cerebrovascular accident (nonhemorrhagic)
Previous streptokinase thrombolysis
Streptococcal infection (?)

Source: Adapted from Ref. 118.

Intrapleural fibrinolytic treatment does not seem to have a measurable effect on systemic coagulation parameters (121). A case of major hemorrhage following intrapleural instillation SK in a dose of 500,000 IU, which is higher than the usual, has been reported (122) in a patient who was also taking carbenicillin and prophylactic heparin.

Although intravenous use of SK can potentially lead to anti-SK antibodies in the blood, which may lead to an allergic reaction if SK is readministered later (after an acute myocardial infarction), this has not been systematically studied in intrapleural instillation. It is possible that these antibodies may cause allergic reactions or neutralization in a further treatment with SK (122,123). Furthermore, its use is contraindicated in patients with recent streptococcal infection. Contraindications for intrapleural administration of fibrinolytics are not well known. However, caution should be exercised in certain situations (Table 10).

Timing of Decision for Additional Therapy
Failure of the pleural infection to resolve, both clinically and radiologically, within three to five days with the use of intrapleural fibrinolytics is considered as an indication for further intervention (1,118). Clinicians should be aware that patients with clinical improvement but with remaining radiographic pleural shadowing may have pleural peels that will resolve in a period of weeks (3).

In a recent study, Bouros et al. (124) reported that in 20 consecutive patients with complicated PPE/PE, intrapleural UK instillation failed to achieve complete drainage. This was achieved by applying VATS in 17 patients (85%). In the other 3 (15%) patients, the VATS procedure had to be con- verted to open thoracotomy due to a thickened visceral pleural peel. Therefore, in PPE patients who have failed to resolve with initial treatment with fibrinolytics, VATS could be the next procedure of choice.

Suction Drainage
Cummin et al. used strong suction (−100 mm Hg) with the catheter directed, under US guidance, into most parts of the infected cavity, permitting removal of septations and drainage of pus (125). However, others have not applied this technique up to now.

B. Surgical Methods

The various surgical methods used for patients with more advanced stages of PPE and PE are shown in Table 8 and discussed briefly in this chapter. For more details, see other chapters in this book.

Thoracoscopy

Today thoracoscopy (medical or surgical), conventional or video-assisted, for the breakdown of adhesions is considered as the procedure of choice and a major innovation when tube thoracostomy and intrapleural thrombolytic therapy fails (124). Medical thoracoscopy is performed under local anesthesia in the bronchoscopy suite (126). It is easy to learn and should be applied increasingly by pulmonologists. In one series the success rate was 75% (127).

Video-assisted thoracic surgery is being used increasingly (128–137). However, it needs one-lung ventilation, general anesthesia, expertise, availability, and is not suitable for chronic PE (success rate <50%). The conversion rate to thoracotomy ranges from 10% to 30% according to patient selection. In five retrospective studies and one prospective study, a mean success rate of 82% in a total of 212 patients has been reported (1,128–133) (Fig. 6).

Open Thoracotomy

With open thoracotomy the patient is submitted to debridement or decortication. The decision to proceed to open thoracotomy usually follows the failure of less-invasive methods to control pleural sepsis. Decortication is a major thoracic operation that is not indicated for markedly debilitated patients (1,3). Decortication in the acute phase of a PPE is performed in order to control pleural sepsis and not for pleural thickening. Pleural fibrosis usually begins to resolve once the pleural infection is controlled. Late decortication

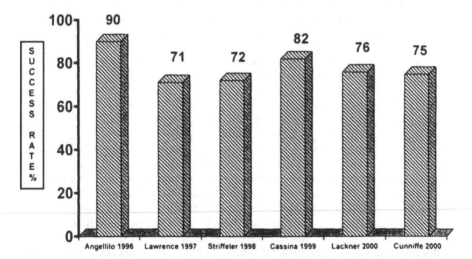

Figure 6 Success rate of video-assisted thoracoscopic surgery (VATS) in patients with parapneumonic effusions in six published series during the period 1995–2000. Mean success rate 78%. *Source*: Adapted from Ref. 1.

(>6 months) is indicated for persistent pleural thickening that leads to reduced pulmonary function and restrictive pulmonary function tests. Success and mortality rates range from 87% to 100% (mean 93.4%) and 0% to 9% (mean 2.5%), respectively (3,138–140). Comparative studies between VATS and thoracotomy showed similar rates of success, but VATS offered substantial advantages in terms of resolution of the disease, hospital stay, and cosmesis (128,140).

Open Drainage
Open drainage is an alternative to decortication in patients who are markedly debilitated. It involves rib resection and insertion of large-bore tubes to permit open drainage at the inferior border of the PE cavity. Daily irrigation with a mild antiseptic solution is necessary, while a colostomy bag can be used for drainage collection. In order for open drainage to be performed, fusion of the two pleural layers is required to avoid lung collapse. Early open drainage of pleural fluid before the fusion of the two pleural layers can lead to increased mortality, as happened during the Word War I (3). With this technique the patient is freed from the closed drainage system. A more complicated procedure is the Eloesser technique. A skin and muscle flap creates a skin-lined fistula, providing drainage without chest tubes. The time of healing, however, is lengthy (usually six months) (3,29).

XIV. Summary
PPE/PE are frequent complications of bacterial pneumonia and one of the oldest known diseases. Even today PPE/PE continue to be a significant medical problem, with high mortality in cases of late intervention. Their clinical presentation may vary from small, uncomplicated effusions to severe multiloculated empyemas. It is critical to assess the individual severity and risk of a PPE using imaging techniques and early thoracocentesis with pleural fluid analysis and bacteriology. Imaging techniques identify the size and the loculations of an effusion and may help to identify empyemas. There is widespread clinical consensus that the pleural fluid pH is the best chemical parameter to assess a PPE. A pH of <7.20 usually predicts a more complicated course. A positive Gram stain and/or culture of the pleural fluid, a low glucose (<40 mg/dL), a high LDH (>100 IU), large effusions ($\geq 1/2$ hemithorax), loculations, and the presence of frank pus are further important markers of severity and indications for chest tube drainage. These risk factors are associated with a complicated course. Small nonloculated effusions have a high probability of spontaneous resolution under appropriate antibiotic therapy and should be observed.

There are no general guidelines for the management of PPE/PE. The appropriate therapeutic approach should be individualized for each patient. The stage of the pneumonia and the PPE is critical to the outcome. Early detection and institution of adequate therapy are essential for the resolution of PPE/PE (141). The evolution from one stage to the other could progress quickly and an aggressive therapeutic modality is needed if less-invasive techniques fail ("the sun should never set on a PPE").

The pulmonologist should play a pivotal role, becoming increasingly active by the introduction of newer trends (intrapleural fibrinolytics, medical thoracoscopy, imaging-guided transcutaneous catheters) for the treatment of PPE. The application of these newer modalities protects patients from surgical intervention and its associated risks. These methods have been found to be efficient in the hands of experts in specialized centers. However, methodological weaknesses in the existing literature and lack of controlled, randomized trials relevant to the management of PPE do not permit the formulation of practical guidelines.

References

1. Bouros D, Hamm H. Infectious pleural effusions. Eur Respir Mon 2002; 22:204–218.
2. Strange C, Sahn SA. The definitions and epidemiology of pleural space infection. Semin Respir Infect 1999; 14:3–8.
3. Light RW. Pleural Diseases, 4th ed. Philadelphia, PA: Lippincott Williams & Wilkins, 2001.
4. Mandell LA, Wunderink RG, Anzueto A, et al. Infectious Diseases Society of America; American Thoracic Society. Infectious Diseases Society of America/American Thoracic Society consensus guidelines on the management of community-acquired pneumonia in adults. Clin Infect Dis 2007; 44(Suppl 2):S27–72.
5. Jerng JS, Hsueh PR, Teng LJ, et al. Empyema thoracic and lung abscess caused by viridans streptococci. Am J Respir Crit Care Med 1997; 156:1508–1514.
6. Ferguson AD, Prescott RJ, Selkon JB, et al. The clinical course and management of thoracic empyema. QJM 1996; 89:285–289.
7. Chin NK, Lim TK. Treatment of complicated parapneumonic effusions and pleural empyema: A four-year prospective study. Singapore Med J 1996; 37:631–635.
8. Densai GA, Mugala DD. Management of empyema thoracis at Lusaka Zambia. Br J Surg 1992; 79:537–538.
9. Hassan I, Mabogunje O. Adult empyema in Zaria, Nigeria. East African Med J 1992; 69:97–100.
10. Weissberg D, Refaely Y. Pleural empyema: 24-Year experience. Ann Thorac Surg 1996; 62:1026–1029.
11. Bashir Y, Benson MK. Necrotizing pneumonia and empyema due to clostridium perfringens complicating pulmonary embolus. Thorax 1990; 45:72–73.
12. Baethge GA, Eggerstedt JM, Olash FA. Group F streptococcal empyema from aspiration of a grass inflorescence. Ann Thorac Surg 1990; 49:319–320.
13. Zachariades N, Mezitis M, Stavrinidis P, et al. Mediastinitis, thoracic empyema, and pericarditis as complications of a dental abscess: Report of a case. Oral Maxillofac Surg 1988; 46:493–495.
14. Fine NL, Smith LR, Sheedy PF. Frequency of pleural effusions in mycoplasma and viral pneumonias. N Engl J Med 1970; 283:790–793.
15. Taryle DA, Potts DE, Sahn SA. The incidence and clinical correlates of parapneumonic effusions in pneumococcal pneumonia. Chest 1978; 74:170–173.
16. Sasse SA. Parapneumonic effusions and empyema. Curr Opin Pulm Med 1996; 2:520–526.
17. Hasley PB, Albaum MN, Li YH, et al. Do pulmonary radiographic findings at presentation predict mortality in patients with community-acquired pneumonia? Arch Intern Med 1996; 156:2206–2212.
18. Strange C, Sahn SA. Management of parapneumonic pleural effusions and empyema. Infect Dis Clin North Am 1991; 5:539–559.
19. Antony VB, Mohammed KA. Pathophysiology of pleural infections. Semin Respir Infect 1999; 14:9–17.
20. Light RW, Girard WM, Jenkinson SG, et al. Parapneumonic effusions. Am J Med 1980; 69:507–512.
21. Wiener-Kronish JP, Sakuma T, Kudoh I, et al. Alveolar epithelial injury and pleural empyema in acute P aeruginosa pneumonia in anesthetized rabbits. J Appl Physiol 1993; 75:1661–1669.
22. Potts DE, Levin DC, Sahn SA. Pleural fluid pH in parapneumonic effusions. Chest 1976; 70:328–331.

23. Potts DE, Taryle DA, Sahn SA. The glucose-pH relationship in parapneumonic effusions. Arch Intern Med 1978; 138:1378–1380.
24. Antony VB, Hadley KJ, Sahn SA. Mechanisms of pleural fibrosis in empyema: Pleural macrophage-mediated inhibition of fibroblast proliferation. Chest 1989; 95S:230–231.
25. Sahn SA, Taryle DA, Good JT Jr. Experimental empyema: Time course and pathogenesis of pleural fluid acidosis and low pleural fluid glucose. Am Rev Respir Dis 1979; 120:355–361.
26. Broaddus VC, Hebert CA, Vitangcol RV, et al. Interleukin-8 is a major neutrophil chemotactic factor in pleural liquid of patients with empyema. Am Rev Respir Dis 1992; 146:825–830.
27. Sahn SA, Reller LB, Taryle DA, et al. The contribution of leukocytes and bacteria to the low pH of empyema fluid. Am Rev Respir Dis 1983; 128:811–815.
28. Idell S, Girard W, Koenig KB, et al. Abnormalities of pathways of fibrin turnover in the human pleural space. Am Rev Respir Dis 1991; 144:187–194.
29. Hamm H, Light RW. Parapneumonic effusion and empyema. Eur Respir J 1997; 10:1150–1156.
30. Light RW, MacGregor M, Ball WCj, et al. Diagnostic significance of pleural fluid pH and PCO_2. Chest 1973; 64:591–596.
31. Hippocrates. Aphorisms. In: Jones WHS, trans-ed. Hippocrates Works, Vol. II. Cambridge, MA: Harvard University Press, 1967; Aphorisms No. VII, 87. [Hippocrates is the author; Jones is the translator-editor.]
32. Andrews NC, Parker EF, Shaw RR. Management of nontuberculous empyema. Am Rev Respir Dis 1962; 85:935–936.
33. Light RW. A new classification of parapneumonic effusions and empyema. Chest 1995; 108:299–301.
34. Colice GL, Curtis A, Deslauriers J, et al. Medical and surgical treatment of parapneumonic effusions. Chest 2000; 18:1158–1171.
35. Light RW. The management of parapneumonic effusions and empyema. Pneumonology 2002; 15:127–132.
36. Bhattacharyya N, Umland El, Kosloske AM. A bacteriologic basis for the evolution and severity of empyema. J Pediatr Surg 1994; 29:667.
37. Strange C. Pathogenesis and management of parapneumonic effusions and empyema. UpTo-Date 2002, March 2.
38. Brook I, Frazier EH. Aerobic and anaerobic microbiology of empyema: A retrospective review in two military hospitals. Chest 1993; 103:1502.
39. Bartlett JG, Gorbach SL, Thadepalli H, et al. Bacteriology of empyema. Lancet 1974; 1:338.
40. Alfagame I, Munoz F, Pena N, et al. Empyema of the thorax in adults. Etiology, microbiologic findings, and management. Chest 1993; 103:839–843.
41. LeMense GP, Strange C, Sahn SA. Empyema thoracis—Therapeutic management and outcome. Chest 1995; 107:1532–1537.
42. Yeh TJ, Hall DP, Ellison RG. Empyema thoracis: A review of 110 cases. Am Rev Respir Dis 1963; 88:785–790.
43. Snider GL, Saleh SS. Empyema of the thorax in adults: Review of 105 cases. Chest 1968; 54:12–17.
44. Smith JA, Mullerworth MH, Westlake GW, et al. Empyema thoracis: 14-Year experience in a teaching center. Ann Thorac Surg 1991; 51:39–42.
45. Kelly JW, Morris MJ. Empyema thoracis: Medical aspects of evaluation and treatment. South Med J 1994; 87:1103–1110.
46. Everts RJ, Reller LB. Pleural space infections: Microbiology and antimicrobial therapy. Semin Respir Infect 1999; 14:18–30.
47. Bartlett JG, Finegold SM. Anaerobic infections of the lung and pleural space. Am Rev Respir Dis 1974; 110:56–77.
48. Bartlett JG. Anaerobic bacterial infections of the lung. Chest 1987; 91:901–909.

49. Levin DL, Klein JS. Imaging techniques for pleural space infections. Semin Respir Infect 1999; 14:31–38.
50. Blackmore CC, Black WC, Dallas RV, et al. Pleural fluid volume estimation: A chest radiograph prediction rule. Acad Radiol 1996; 3:103–109.
51. Moskowitz H, Platt RT, Schachar R, et al. Roentgen visualization of minute pleural effusion. Radiology 1973; 109:33–35.
52. Ruskin JA, Gurney JW, Thorsen MK, et al. Detection of pleural effusion on supine chest radiographs. AJR 1987; 146:681–683.
53. Muller NL. Imaging of the pleura. Radiology 1993; 186:297–309.
54. McLoud TC, Flower CDR. Imaging the pleura: Sonography, CT, and MR imaging. AJR Am J Roentgenol 1991; 156:1145–1153.
55. Pugatch RD, Spirn PW. Radiology of the pleura. Clin Chest Med 1985; 6:17–32.
56. Hirsh JH, Rogers JV, Mack LA. Real-time sonography of pleural opacities. AJR 1981; 136:297–301.
57. Yang PC, Luh KT, Chang DB, et al. Value of sonography in determining the nature of pleural effusion: Analysis of 320 cases. AJR 1992; 159:29–33.
58. Raptopoulos V, Davis LM, Lee G, et al. Factors affecting the development of pneumothorax associated with thoracentesis. AJR 1991; 156:917–920.
59. Eibenberger KL, Dock WI, Ammann ME, et al. Quantification of pleural effusions: Sonography vs. radiography. Radiology 1994; 191:681–684.
60. Lipscomb DJ, Flower CDR, Hadfield JW. Ultrasound of the pleura: An assessment of its clinical utility. Clin Radiol 1981; 32:289–290.
61. Aquino SL, Webb WR, Gushiken BJ. Pleural exudates and transudates: Diagnosis with contrast-enhanced CT. Radiology 1994; 192:803–808.
62. Kearney SE, Davies CW, Davies RJ, et al. Computed tomography and ultrasound in parapneumonic effusions and empyema. Clin Radiol 2000; 55:542–547.
63. Arenas-Jimenez J, Alonso-Charterina S, Sanchez-Paya J, et al. Evaluation of CT findings for diagnosis of pleural effusions. Eur Radiol 2000; 10:681–690.
64. Haramati LB, Alterman DD, White CS, et al. Intrathoracic lymphadenopathy in patients with empyema. J Comput Assist Tomogr 1997; 21:608–611.
65. Kearney SE, Davies CW, Tattersall DJ, et al. The characteristics and significance of thoracic lymphadenopathy in parapneumonic effusion and empyema. Br J Radiol 2000; 73:583–587.
66. Bittner RC, Schnoy N, Schönfeld N, et al. High-resolution magnetic resonance tomography (HR-MRT) of the pleura and thoracic wall: Normal findings and pathological findings. Rofo Fortschr Geb Röntgenstr Neuen Bildgeb Verfahr 1995; 162:296–303.
67. Davis SD, Henschke CI, Yankelevitz DF, et al. MR imaging of pleural effusions. J Comput Assist Tomogr 1990; 14:192–198.
68. Himelman RB, Kallen PW. The prognostic value of loculations in parapneumonic pleural effusions. Chest 1986; 90:852–856.
69. Frola C, Cantoni S, Turtulici I, et al. Transudative vs. exudative pleural effusions: Differentiation using Gd-DTPA enhanced MRI. Eur Radiol 1997; 7:860–864.
70. Light RW, Macgregor MI, Luchsinger PC, et al. Pleural effusions: The diagnostic separation of transudates and exudates. Ann Intern Med 1972; 77:507–513.
71. Hamm H, Brohan U, Bohmer R, et al. Cholesterol in pleural effusions. A diagnostic aid. Chest 1987; 92:296–302.
72. Light RW, MacGregor M, Ball WCJ, et al. Diagnostic significance of pleural fluid pH and PCO_2. Chest 1973; 64:591–596.
73. Potts DE, Levin DC, Sahn SA. Pleural fluid pH in parapneumonic effusions. Chest 1976; 70:328–331.
74. Poe RH, Marin MG, Israel RH, et al. Utility of pleural fluid analysis in predicting tube thoracostomy/decortication in parapneumonic effusions. Chest 1991; 100:963–967.

75. Good JT, Taryle DA, Maulitz RM, et al. The diagnostic value of pleural fluid pH. Chest 1980; 78:55–59.
76. Potts DE, Taryle DA, Sahn SA. The glucose–pH relationship in parapneumonic effusions. Arch Intern Med 1978; 138:1378–1380.
77. Sahn SA, Reller LB, Taryle DA, et al. The contribution of leucocytes and bacteria to the low pH of empyema fluid. Am Rev Respir Dis 1983; 128:811–815.
78. Heffner JE, Brown LK, Barbieri C, et al. Pleural fluid chemical analysis in parapneumonic effusions. Am J Respir Crit Care Med 1995; 151:1700–1708.
79. Pine JR, Hollmann JL. Elevated pleural fluid pH in proteus mirabilis empyema. Chest 1983; 84:109–111.
80. Sahn SA. Management of complicated parapneumonic effusions. Am Rev Respir Dis 1993; 148:813–817.
81. Light RW, Rodriguez RM. Management of parapneumonic effusions. Clin Chest Med 1998; 19:373–382.
82. Massard G, Wihlm JM. Early complications. Esophagopleural fistula. Chest Surg Clin North Am 1999; 9:617–631.
83. Chu MW, Dewar LR, Burgess JJ, et al. Empyema thoracis: Lack of awareness results in a prolonged clinical course. Can J Surg 2001; 44:284–288.
84. Sahn SA. State of the art. The pleura. Am Rev Respir Dis 1988; 138:184–234.
85. Lemmer JH, Botham MJ, Orringer MB. Modern management of adult thoracic empyema. J Thorac Cardiovasc Surg 1985; 90:849–885.
86. Mandal AK, Thadepalli H. Treatment of spontaneous bacterial empyema thoracis. J Thorac Cardiovasc Surg 1987; 94:414–418.
87. Strange C, Sahn SA. The clinician's perspective on parapneumonic effusions and empyema. Chest 1993; 103:259–261.
88. American Thoracic Society; Infectious Diseases Society of America. Guidelines for the management of adults with hospital-acquired, ventilator-associated, and ealthcare-associated pneumonia. Am J Respir Crit Care Med 2005; 171:388–416.
89. Teixeira LR, Sasse SA, Villarino MA, et al. Antibiotic levels in empyemic pleural fluid. Chest 2000; 117:1734–1739.
90. Thys JP, Vanderhoeft P, Vanderlinden P, et al. Penetration of aminoglycosides in uninfected pleural exudates and in pleural empyemas. Chest 1988; 93:530–532.
91. Rosenfeldt FL, McGibney D, Braimbridge MV, et al. Comparison between irrigation and conventional treatment for empyema and pneumonectomy space infection. Thorax 1981; 36:272–277.
92. Storm HK, Krasnik M, Bang K, et al. Treatment of pleural empyema secondary to pneumonia: Thoracentesis regimen versus tube drainage. Thorax 1992; 47:821–824.
93. Heffner JE, Klein JS, Hampson C. Interventional Management of Pleural Infections *Chest* 2009; 136:1148–1159.
94. Vianna NJ. Nontuberculous bacterial empyema in patients with and without underlying disease. JAMA 1971; 215:69–75.
95. Wehr CJ, Adkins RB>Jr. Empyema thoracis: A ten-year experience. South Med J 1986; 79:171–176.
96. Ali I, Unruh H. Management of empyema thoracis. Ann Thorac Surg 1990; 50:355–359.
97. Berger HA, Morganroth ML. Immediate drainage is not required for all patients with complicated parapneumonic effusion. Chest 1990; 97:731–735.
98. Chin NK, Lim TK. Controlled trial of intrapleural streptokinase in the treatment of pleural empyema and complicated parapneumonic effusion. Chest 1997; 111:275–279.
99. Cohn LH, Blaisdell EW. Surgical treatment of nontuberculous empyema. Arch Surg 1970; 100:376–381.
100. Davies RJO, Traill ZC, Gleeson FV. Randomised controlled trial of intrapleural streptokinase in community acquired pleural infection. Thorax 1997; 52:416–421.

101. Hoover EL, Hsu HK, Webb H, et al. The surgical management of empyema thoracis in substance abuse patients: A 5-year experience. Ann Thorac Surg 1988; 46:563–566.
102. Roupie E, Bouabdallah K, Delclaux C, et al. Intrapleural administration of streptokinase in complicated purulent pleural effusion: A CT-guided strategy. Intensive Care Med 1996; 22:1351–1353.
103. Huang HC, Chang HY, Chen CW, et al. Predicting factors for outcome of tube thoracostomy in complicated parapneumonic effusion for empyema. Chest 1999; 115:751–756.
104. Manuel Porcel J, Vives M, Esquerda A, et al. Usefulness of the British Thoracic Society and the American College of Chest Physicians guidelines in predicting pleural drainage of non-purulent parapneumonic effusions. Respir Med 2006; 100:933–937.
105. Westcott JL. Percutaneous catheter drainage of pleural effusion and empyema. Am J Roentgenol 1985; 144:1189–1193.
106. Merriam MA, Cronan JJ, Dorfman GS, et al. Radiographically guided percutaneous catheter drainage of pleural fluid collections. Am J Roentgenol 1988; 151:1113–1116.
107. Silverman SG, Mueller PR, Saini S, et al. Thoracic empyema: Management with image-guided catheter drainage. Radiology 1988; 169:5–9.
108. VanSonnenberg E, Nakamoto SK, Mueller PR, et al. CT- and ultrasound-guided catheter drainage of empyemas after chest-tube failure. Radiology 1984; 151:349–353.
109. Moulton JS, Benkert RE, Weisiger KH, et al. Treatment of complicated pleural fluid collections with image-guided drainage and intracavitary urokinase. Chest 1995; 108:1252–1259.
110. Shankar S, Gulati M, Kang M, et al. Image-guided percutaneous drainage of thoracic empyema: Can sonography predict the outcome? Eur Radiol 2000; 10:495–499.
111. Ulmer JL, Choplin RH, Reed JC. Image-guided catheter drainage of the infected pleural space. J Thorac Imaging 1991; 6:65–73.
112. Maier A, Domej W, Anegg U, et al. Computed tomography or ultrasonically guided pigtail catheter drainage in multiloculated pleural empyema: A recommended procedure? Respirology 2000; 5:119–124.
113. Bouros D, Tzouvelekis A, Antoniou KM, et al. Intrapleural fibrinolytic therapy for pleural infection. Pulm Pharmacol Ther 2007; 20:616–626.
114. Bouros D, Schiza S, Patsourakis G, et al. Intrapleural streptokinase versus urokinase in the treatment of complicated parapneumonic effusions. A prospective, double-blind study. Am J Respir Crit Care Med 1997; 155:291–295.
115. Wait MA, Sharma S, Hohn J, et al. A randomized trial of empyema therapy. Chest 1997; 111:1548–1551.
116. Bouros D, Schiza S, Tzanakis N, et al. Intrapleural urokinase versus normal saline in the treatment of complicated parapneumonic effusions and empyema. Am J Respir Crit Care Med 1999; 159:37–42.
117. Tuncozgur B, Ustunsoy H, Sivrikoz MC, et al. Intrapleural urokinase in the management of parapneumonic empyema: A randomised controlled trial. J Clin Pract 2001; 55: 658–660.
118a. Maskell NA, Davies CW, Nunn AJ, et al. First Multicenter Intrapleural Sepsis Trial (MIST1) Group. U.K. Controlled trial of intrapleural streptokinase for pleural infection. N Engl J Med 2005; 352:865–874.
118b. Bouros D, Antoniou KM, Light RW. Intrapleural streptokinase for pleural infection. BMJ 2006; 332(7534):133–134.
118c. Froudarakis ME, Kouliatsis G, Steiropoulos P, et al. Recombinant tissue plasminogen activator in the treatment of pleural infections in adults. Respir Med 2008; 102:1694–1700.
118d. Zhu Z, Hawthorne ML, Guo Y, et al. Tissue plasminogen activator combined with human recombinant deoxyribonuclease is effective therapy for empyema in a rabbit model. Chest 2006; 129:1577–1583.
118. Bouros D, Schiza S, Siafakas N. Utility of fibrinolytic agents for draining intrapleural infection. Semin Respir Infect 1999; 14:39–47.

119. Alfageme I, Vazquez R. Ventricular fibrillation after intrapleural UK. Intensive Care Med 1997; 23:352.

120. Frye MD, Jarratt M, Sahn SA. Acute hypoxemic respiratory failure following intrapleural thrombolytic therapy for hemothorax. Chest 1994; 105:1595–1596.

121. Berglin F, Ekroth R, Teger-Nilsson A, et al. Intrapleural instillation of streptokinase effects on systemic fibrinolysis. Thorac Cardiovasc Surg 1981; 11:265–268.

122. Godley P1, Bell RC. Major hemorrhage following administration of intrapleural streptokinase. Chest 1984; 86:486–487.

123. Lee HS. How safe is the readministration of streptokinase? Drug Saf 1995; 13:76–80.

124. Bouros D, Antoniou KM, Chalkiadakis G, et al. The role of video-assisted thoracoscopic surgery in the treatment of parapneumonic empyema after the failure of fibrinolytics. Surg Endosc 2002; 16:151–154.

125. Cummin AR, Wright NL, Joseph AE. Suction drainage: A new approach to the treatment of empyema. Thorax 1991; 46:259–260.

126. Loddenkemper R. Thoracoscopy—State of the art. Eur Respir J 1998; 11:213–221.

127. Soler M, Wyser C, Bolliger T, et al. Treatment of early parapneumonic empyema by medical thoracoscopy. Schweiz Med Wochenschr 1997; 127:1748–1753.

128. Angelillo Mackinlay TA, Lyons GA, Chimondeguy DJ, et al. VATS debridement versus thoracotomy in the treatment of loculated postpneumonia empyema. Ann Thorac Surg 1996; 61:1626–1630.

129. Lawrence DR, Ohri SK, Moxon RE, et al. Thoracoscopic debridement of empyema thoracis. Ann Thorac Surg 1997; 64:1448–1450.

130. Striffleler H, Gugger M, Imhof V, et al. Video-assisted thoracoscopic surgery for fibrinopurulent pleural empyema in 67 patients. Ann Thorac Surg 1998; 65:319–323.

131. Cassina PC, Hauser M, Hillejan L, et al. Video-assisted thoracoscopy in the treatment of pleural empyema: Stage-based management and outcome. J Thorac Cardiovasc Surg 1999; 117:234–238.

132. Lackner RP, Hughes R, Anderson LA, et al. Video-assisted evacuation of empyema is the preferred procedure for the management of pleural space infections. Am J Surg 2000; 179:27–30.

133. Cunniffe MG, Maguire D, McAnena OJ, et al. Video-assisted thoracoscopic surgery in the management of loculated empyema. Surg Endosc 2000; 14:175–178.

134. Hornick P, Townsend ER, Clark D, et al. Videothoracoscopy in the treatment of early empyema: An initial experience. Ann Royal Coll Surg Eng 1996; 78:45–48.

135. Sendt W, Forster E, Hau T. Early thoracoscopic debridement and drainage as definite treatment for pleural empyema. Eur J Surg 1995; 161:73–623.

136. Waller DA, Rengarajan A. Thoracoscopic decortication: A role for video-assisted surgery in chronic postpneumonic pleural empyema. Ann Thorac Surg 2000; 71:1813–1816.

137. Silen ML, Naunheim KS. Thoracoscopic approach to the management of empyema thoracis. Indications and results. Chest Surg Clin North Am 1996; 6:491–499.

138. Mayo P. Early thoracotomy and decortication for nontuberculous empyema in adults with and without underlying disease. A twenty-five year review. Am Surg 1985; 51:230–236.

139. Muskett A, Burton NA, Karwande SV, et al. Management of refractory empyema with early decortication. Am J Surg 1988; 156:529–532.

140. Mackinlay TAA, Lyons GA, Chimondeguy DJ, et al. VATS debridement versus thoracotomy in the treatment of loculated postpneumonia empyema. Ann Thorac Surg 1996; 61:1626–1630.

141. Chu MW, Dewar LR, Burgess JJ, et al. Empyema thoracis: Lack of awareness results in a prolonged clinical course. Can J Surg 2001; 44:284–288.

19

Medical Thoracoscopy in the Management of Parapneumonic Pleural Effusions and Empyema

GIAN FRANCO TASSI and GIAN PIETRO MARCHETTI
Divisione di Pneumologia, Spedali Civili di Brescia, Brescia, Italy

With the advent of effective treatment with antibiotics, parapneumonic pleural effusions and empyema have become a less-frequent clinical problem. These complications do, however, remain a significant cause of mortality and morbidity in infectious pulmonary pathology. Late diagnosis and delayed treatment lengthen the duration of the illness and are very often the cause of invasive surgery.

Thoracocentesis or intrathoracic drains are often the preferred treatment, but they are not always able to provide a definitive cure. In these cases, it is advisable to use thoracoscopy, which is an appropriate alternative to thoracotomy, in particular if used in the initial stages of pleural complications.

However, the exact application of thoracoscopy in infections of the pleural cavity has yet to be established universally (1,2). Its use has been proposed prior to the positioning of a thoracic drain (3), while another application might be established only after the drain has determined a reduction in temperature or the complete evacuation of pleural fluid within a few days (4,5). Yet another approach makes reference to the loculate character of the effusion, and considers thoracoscopy appropriate in the presence of loculation both for parapneumonic effusion (6–8) and for empyema (7–13). The latter approach, when treating empyema, can be related to the well-known American Thoracic Society classification (14), which divides its evolution into three stages—exudative, fibrinopurulent, and organizing—and believes thoracoscopy as the indicated treatment in the fibrinopurulent form (7,9–13). More recently, in the surgical field, the treatment has been extended to chronic organizing empyema, both to clean the cavity prior to thoracotomic decortication (15) and for the actual decortication (16).

Given this situation, an attempt to clarify the approaches to medical and surgical treatment of parapneumonic effusions has been given in guidelines by the American College of Chest Physicians (ACCP) (17) using "evidence-based" criteria. They consider the role of surgical thoracoscopy—video-assisted thoracospic surgery (VATS)—and classify patients on the basis of the risk of unfavorable development. The guidelines limit VATS to patients defined as at high risk of unfavorable development (assigned to categories 3 and 4).

Category 3 includes effusions that occupy more than half of the hemothorax, which can be loculate and where there may be thickening of the parietal pleura.

Category 4 is characterized by the presence of pus in the pleural cavity. These recommendations are, however, based on a randomized study of just 20 patients (10) and retrospectively analyzed case studies of 60 patients (18). The paper makes no mention of medical thoracoscopy, even though the comments regarding VATS could be indirectly extended to it.

Apart from the ACCP indications (17), medical thoracoscopy may also be applied prior to the positioning of an intrathoracic drain (3) or with parapneumonic effusions and empyema when an ultrasound scan shows multiple loculations (8).

I. Instruments and Technique

Medical thoracoscopy and surgical thoracoscopy (VATS), both used to treat infections of the pleural space, are dissimilar in the type of anesthesia, instruments, and method used.

Medical thoracoscopy is defined as an endoscopic examination of the pleural cavity carried out by a pulmonologist, normally under local anesthesia or neuroleptanalgesia in an endoscopy room, after induced or spontaneous pneumothorax, using one or two points of entry and simple re-usable instruments (3,19–21).

Surgical thoracoscopy (VATS) is a mini-invasive technique carried out in an operating room under general anesthesia using double-lumen tracheal intubation (22,23).

With medical thoracoscopy, it is advisable to establish an entry point for the trocar after an ultrasound scan to identify where the accumulation is thickest and the position of the diaphragm, which is often elevated. The procedure is carried out step by step and comprises:

1. Aspiration of pus.
2. Exploration of pleural cavity to identify loculations and adhesions, as well as neoformations and foreign bodies.
3. Opening loculations.
4. Removal of fibrinous membranes (Figs. 1 and 2) from the cavity and from the parietal and visceral pleural surfaces.

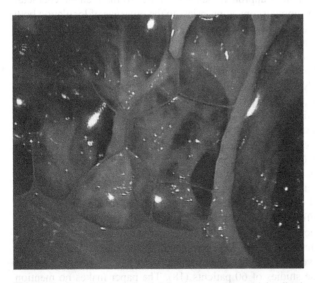

Figure 1 Loculations in bacterial empyema. *Note:* thick adhesions in the figure.

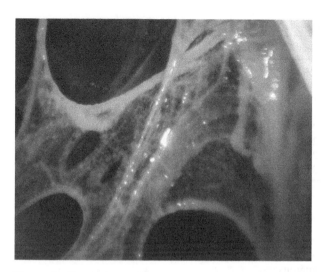

Figure 2   Fine fibrinous adhesions in parapneumonic effusion.

5. Pleural biopsy.
6. Washing the pleural space with saline solution.

After emptying the pleural cavity, there should be a careful inspection of the pleural surfaces (Fig. 3), followed by pleural biopsy and biopsy of any lesions discovered. Finally, a thoracic drain is introduced, with a calibre large enough (>24 F) to remove dense and viscous pus and fibrin detritus without blocking, if necessary under visual control.

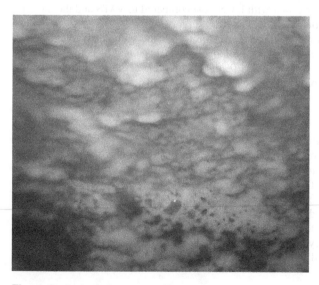

Figure 3   Parietal pleura covered by pus.

Table 1   Medical (M) and Surgical (S) Thoracoscopy in Parapneumonic Effusion and Empyema

References	M/S	Year	Patients	% Of success	% Of complications
(24)	M	1995	7	86	14
(8)	M	1997	16	73	0
(25)	S	1998	67	72	4
(26)	M	2004	5	100	0
(27)	M	2005	127	91	9
(28)	S	2005	234	86.3	8.3
(12)	S	2006	130	91	9
(13)	S	2007	120	91.8	11

II. Results

The case studies of the role of thoracoscopy in the infection of the pleural space (Table 1) deal principally with empyema and are both medical and surgical, the latter being undoubtedly more numerous.

In general, the figures demonstrate favorable results, with percentages of primary success (meaning complete cure without subsequent thoracotomy or conversion from VATS to thoracotomy) between 60% and 100%, and higher if the method was used without delay (2,11,13,29). However, the number of patients treated was generally small, and few authors (12,13,25,27,28) present case studies dealing with more than 50 patients.

In surgical thoracoscopy (9,11–13,14,18,25), there is total agreement about the advantages of VATS over thorocotomy, in terms of lower cost, shorter hospitalization, and better cosmetic results with less surgical sequelae.

The medical thoracoscopy experiences (1,3,7,8,24,26,27) outline the mini-invasive character of the procedure, together with lower cost compared to VATS and the fact that it can be used with frail patients at high risk from surgery.

Complications occurred in direct correlation with the complexity of the cases treated and were represented mainly by prolonged air leakage and bleeding, with very varied incidence, between 16% (18) and 0% (11). In some surgical series, including patients with severe comorbidity, deaths also occurred (10,18,30–32).

III. Conclusions

Thoracoscopy is undoubtedly useful in the treatment of infection of the pleural space, in particolar with multiloculate empyema, since it permits the treatment of the illness without thorocotomy, even though until now sufficiently large randomized studies on the method have not been carried out.

As an intermediate drain, procedure between positioning a drain tube and surgical thoracoscopy (VATS), medical thoracoscopy can play an important role and is characterized by its efficacy and low cost. It should be carried out without delay in the treatment of empyema and is recommended with patients in poor health and at high surgical risk.

References

1. Tassi GF, Davies RJ, Noppen M. Advanced techniques in medical thoracoscopy. Eur Respir J 2006; 28(5):1051–1059.
2. Waller DA. Thoracoscopy in management of postpneumonic pleural infections. Curr Opin Pulm Med 2002; 8(4):323–326.
3. Loddenkemper R. Thoracoscopy—State of the art. Eur Respir J 1998; 11(1):213–221.
4. Kohman LJ. Thoracoscopy for the evaluation and treatment of pleural space disease. Chest Surg Clin N Am 1994; 4(3):467–479.
5. Yim AP. Paradigm shift in empyema management. Chest 1999; 115(3):611–612.
6. Huang HC, Chang HY, Chen CW, et al. Predicting factors for outcome of tube thoracostomy in complicated parapneumonic effusion or empyema. Chest 1999; 115(3):751–756.
7. Casalini A, Cavaliere S, Consigli GF, et al. Standard operativi e linee guida in endoscopia toracica. Rass Patol App Resp 1997; 12(3):342–344.
8. Solèr M, Wyser C, Bolliger CT, et al. Treatment of early parapneumonic empyema by "medical" thoracoscopy. Schweiz Med Wochenschr 1997; 127(42):1748–1753.
9. Silen ML, Naunheim KS. Thoracoscopic approach to the management of empyema thoracis. Indications and results. Chest Surg Clin N Am 1996; 6(3):491–499.
10. Wait MA, Sharma S, Hohn J, et al. A randomized trial of empyema therapy. Chest 1997; 111(6):1548–1551.
11. Cassina PC, Hauser M, Hillejan L, et al. Video-assisted thoracoscopy in the treatment of pleural empyema: Stage-based management and outcome. J Thorac Cardiovasc Surg 1999; 117(2):234–238.
12. Wurnig PN, Wittmer V, Pridun NS, et al. Video-assisted thoracic surgery for pleural empyema. Ann Thorac Surg 2006; 81(1):309–313.
13. Solaini L, Prusciano F, Bagioni P. Video-assisted thoracic surgery in the treatment of pleural empyema. Surg Endosc 2007; 21(2):280–284.
14. Andrews NC, Parker EF, Shaw RP, et al. Management of nontuberculous empyema. A statement of the subcommittee on surgery. Am Rev Respir Dis 1962; 85(6):935–936.
15. Lawrence DR, Ohri SK, Moxon RE, et al. Thoracoscopic debridement of empyema thoracis. Ann Thorac Surg 1997; 64(5):1448–1450.
16. Waller DA, Rengarajan A. Thoracoscopic decortication: A role for video-assisted surgery in chronic postpneumonic pleural empyema. Ann Thorac Surg 2001; 71(6):1813–1816.
17. Colice GL, Curtis A, Deslauriers J, et al. Medical and surgical treatment of parapneumonic effusions. An evidence-based guideline. Chest 2000; 18(4):1158–1171.
18. Angelillo Mackinlay TA, Lyons GA, Chimondeguy DJ, et al. VATS debridement versus thoracotomy in the treatment of loculated postpneumonia empyema. Ann Thorac Surg 1996; 61(6):1626–1630.
19. Mathur PN, Astoul P, Boutin C. Medical thoracoscopy. Technical details. Clin Chest Med 1995; 16(3):479–486.
20. Rodriguez-Panadero F, Janssen JP, Astoul P. Thoracoscopy: General overview and place in the diagnosis and management of pleural effusion. Eur Respir J 2006; 28(2):409–421.
21. Technique of medical thoracoscopy. In: Buchanan DR, Neville E, eds. Thoracoscopy for Physicians. London, U.K.: Arnold, 2004:71–86.
22. Operative Technique. In: Inderbitzi R ed., Surgical Thoracoscopy. Berlin, Germany: Springer, 1994:12–46.
23. Demmy TL. Ovierview and general considerations for video-assisted thoracic surgery. In: Demmy TL, ed. Video-Assisted Thoracic Surgery (VATS). Georgetown, Washington, D.C.: Landes Bioscience, 2002:1–24.
24. Colt HG. Thoracoscopy. A prospective study of safety and outcome. Chest 1995; 108(2):324–329.

25. Striffeler H, Gugger M, Im Hof V, et al. Video-assisted thoracoscopic surgery for fibrinopurulent pleural empyema in 67 patients. Ann Thorac Surg 1998; 65(2):319–323.

26. Reynard C, Frey JG, Tschopp JM. Thoracoscopie en anesthésie locale dans le traitement des empyèmes: Une technique efficace et peu invasive. Med Hyg 2004; 62(6):2138–2143.

27. Brutsche MH, Tassi GF, Gjörik S, et al. Treatment of sonographically stratified multiloculated thoracic empyema by medical thoracoscopy. Chest 2005; 128(5):3303–3309.

28. Luh SP, Chou MC, Wang LS, et al. Video-assisted thoracoscopic surgery in the treatment of complicated parapneumonic effusions or empyemas: Outcome of 234 patients. Chest 2005; 127(4):1427–1432.

29. Sasse SA. Parapneumonic effusions and empyema. Curr Opin Pulm Med 1996; 2(4):320–326.

30. Lawrence DR, Ohri SK, Moxon RE, et al. Thoracoscopic debridement of empyema thoracis. Ann Thorac Surg 1997; 64(5):1448–1450.

31. Landreneau RJ, Keenan RJ, Hazelrigg SR, et al. Thoracoscopy for empyema and hemothorax. Chest 1996; 109(1):18–24.

32. Weissberg D, Refaely Y. Pleural empyema: 24-year experience. Ann Thorac Surg 1996; 62(4):1026–1029.

20
Postsurgical Pleural Infection

LESEK PUREK
Centre Valaisan de Pneumologie, Réseau Santé Valais, Montana, Switzerland
MARC LICKER
Département d'Anesthésiologie, Hôpitaux Universitaires Genevois, Geneva, Switzerland
JEAN MARIE TSCHOPP
Centre Valaisan de Pneumologie, Réseau Santé Valais, Montana, Switzerland

I. Effects of Thoracic Surgery on the Pleura

Normally, there is no pleural space because of the negative intrathoracic pressure generated by the opposing lung and thoracic recoil forces. A small amount of fluid results from the balance of fluid between parietal and visceral pleurae. Any thoracic operation either mini-invasive or by a classical open surgery constitutes a violation of the pleural space exposing it to ambient pressure and any potential source of infection. A simple primary spontaneous pneumothorax without any outside aggression of the thoracic wall provokes a strong pleural inflammation involving neutrophils, eosinophils, and lymphocytes as recently showed by De Smedt et al. (1). Not surprisingly, any thoracic surgery constitutes an aggression of the pleura, attracting inflammatory cells into the pleura and initiating a process of wound healing resulting in impaired fluid reabsorption within the pleural cavity. Accordingly, the pleura is thickened and adhesions occur between visceral and parietal pleurae leading sometimes to loculation of the pleural cavity. The thickening of the pleura (up to 10 times the normal size) gradually resolves over many weeks and the pleura recovers its single layer of mesothelial cells on both, the visceral and parietal pleurae (2).

In other words, after surgery, there are important changes in the pleura with the production of exudative fluid, potentially leading to serious systemic side effects when pleural infection occurs.

II. Prevention of Pleural Space Infection After Surgery

A. Residual Pleural Space

Residual space after pulmonary resection is mostly due to inefficient pleural drainage because of loculated and undrained spaces, restrictive lung disease, prolonged air leak or mediastinal fixation related to neoadjuvant radiotherapy.

Barker (3) and Wareham et al. (4) estimated that postoperative pneumothorax occurs in 20% of patients who underwent lobectomy, 40% in bilobectomy, and 5% to 10% in segmentectomy or wedge resection.

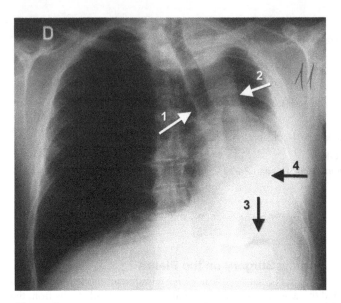

Figure 1 A 55-year-old patient having had 4 years ago a successful left pneumonectomy for non–small-cell cancer. This case illustrates the radiological changes occurring after complete lung resection. The remaining lung expands and partially fills the left cavity (→ 1), there is a mediastinal shift to the left (→ 2), and the left hemidiaphragm is elevated (→ 3). Despite these mechanisms, the pleural space is filled with exudative fluid that becomes serofibrinous over time (→ 4).

In the absence of pleural infection, the postoperative time course is usually unre-markable. Pneumonectomy is a special case—the pleural space is filled with air because three mechanisms are unable to compensate the important loss of an entire lung in the hemithorax: first, the mediastinum is shifted to the ipsilateral side; second, the hemidi-aphragm is elevated whereas the remaining contralateral lung is hyperinflated; third, the ipsilateral intercostal space shrinks. However, some air still remains within the ipsilateral chest, being slowly replaced by pleural fluid. Within approximately four months following pneumonectomy, the hemithorax is usually opacified to a large extent (5) (Fig. 1).

After thoracic surgery, the postoperative strategy is focused on avoiding infection of the remaining pleural space and/or occurrence of bronchopleural fistula (BPF).

In case of lung resection lesser than pneumonectomy, residual postoperative pneu-mothorax (RPP) may occur, resulting in prolonged hospital stay and pleural infection. Solak et al. (6) recently described the postoperative time course of 140 patients who under-went lesser than pneumonectomy pulmonary resection. RPP persisted in six patients after 12 weeks. Residuel spaces over the whole observation time were complicated in eight patients requiring four reoperations and four redrainages. Persistent air leakage and pleural infection were the main cause of complication.

Therefore, the medical approach to treat RPP uses negative suction through con-trolled and well-permeable chest tubes, chest physiotherapy, and bronchoscopy to remove impacted secretions, and bronchodilatator therapy combined with continuous positive pressure airway to allow expansion of the atelectatic lung areas and the elimination of any space and air leak in the operated chest cavity (2).

Occasionally, complete lung expansion is not possible and loculated pleural spaces filled with exudative fluid progressively disappear over time as far as no infectious pleural contamination or air leak persist (7,8).

B. Antibiotic Prophylaxis

The usual bacteria involved in postoperative pleural infection are correctly identified in only 70% of the cases (9). Both *Staphylococcus aureus* and *Hemophilus influenzae* constitute the main isolated pathogens playing a role in postoperative pleural infection (10,11). The choice of antibiotic should be guided either by microbiological cultures coupled with antibiograms or by the institutional prevalence pattern of bacterial infections (12).

Many centers use prophylactic antibiotic regimens for pulmonary surgery. Bernard et al. showed in a prospective randomized double blind trial that a 48-hour antibiotic prophylaxis regimen including second-generation cephalosporines was significantly more efficient than the flash therapy. They found that the overall infection rate was 46% in the 48-hour treatment group and 65% in the flash group. Even after treatment adjustment, a significant difference remained, for example, for the number of empyemas, which were 1% in the 48-hour group and 6% in the flash group (13).

III. Postpneumonectomy Empyema

A. Incidence and Etiology

Postsurgical empyema accounts for one-fifth of all empyemas (14), with pneumonectomy ranking as the leading cause of empyema after thoracic surgery.

Besides acute lung injury, postpneumonectomy empyema is the mostly feared postoperative complication in thoracic surgery. Its incidence ranges from 2% to ~13% of lung resections (15) and has been incriminated as a contributory factor in perioperative mortality (25%) that is further increased up to 70% in the presence of BPF (16–18). It is of note that patients who undergo pneumonectomy for suppurative lung diseases, such as tuberculosis, aspergillosis, and bronchiectasis are at higher risk of developing empyema in the immediate postoperative period. Indeed, Conlan et al. (19) reported a frequency of empyema of 15%, following pneumonectomy for chronic pulmonary infection, others 32% (20) or even 40% (21).

Major risk factors for postpneumonectomy empyema mainly includes the following factors: right pneumonectomy, completion pneumonectomy (22), immunosuppression as well as adjuvant or neoadjuvant chemo-radiotherapy (23).

Postpneumonectomy empyema can occur at any time in the postoperative period. Early empyema occurs within 10 to 14 days in the immediate postoperative period (11), however, late empyema has been reported to occur as long as 40 years after pneumonectomy (24). This complication is usually divided into early or late complication, the cutting point being three months after surgery (25). Weber et al. suggested that late empyemas represent 40% of all empyemas (26).

Empyema after pneumonectomy represents a "sanctuarized" space for bacterial growth and is a very serious infectious complication because the postpneumonectomy space is filled with liquid or organizing material, which constitutes an ideal nidus for contamination. The most common organisms causing postpneumonectomy empyema are *S. aureus* and *Pseudomonas aeruginosa* (11) and the infection is polymicrobial in 49% of the cases (10). In up to 27% cases, the purulent fluid collected from the postpneumonectomy space remains sterile (9).

Early postpneumonectomy empyema develops by several mechanisms (27). It may be due to not only contamination of the pleural space during surgery, but also due to the development of bronchopleural or esophagopleural fistulae. Late postpneumonectomy empyemas are thought to be the result of not only hematogenous dissemination from a distant sources (28), such as infected teeth (29), pneumonia, appendicitis (30), or dental work (28), but also very rarely due to the development of bronchopleural and esophagopleural fistulae (25).

B. Diagnosis

The diagnosis of postpneumonectomy empyema is confirmed by finding purulent material in the postpneumonectomy space by diagnostic thoracocentesis. Because of mediastinal shift and upward displacement of diaphragm, the procedure should, if performed by less-experienced hands, always be guided by US or CT imaging (31,32).

Signs and symptoms of postpneumonectomy empyema vary. In the immediate postoperative period, empyema is often associated with fever, cough, and this may be the only clinical finding. Classic signs such as expectoration of fluid or purulent drainage from the thoracotomy wound are not always present. Symptoms associated with late onset empyema are frequently nonspecific (flu-like illness, weight loss, low-grade fever), making sometimes the diagnosis very difficult. Chest X-ray may be helpful for diagnosis, showing shifting of mediastinal structures away from the postpneumonectomy space, failure of the mediastinum to shift to the postpneumonectomy empty space in the immediate postoperative period, development of new air–fluid levels, or change in preexisting air–fluid levels. Importantly, the sensitivity of chest X-ray in detecting empyema seems to be low (33).

Laboratory testings, like white blood cell count, are frequently elevated but are found to be nonspecific. Icard et al. (34) demonstrated that an elevated C-reactive protein level >100 mg/L in the postoperative period on day 12 had a 100% sensitivity and a 92% specificity for detecting postpneumonectomy empyema. On the other hand, a C-reactive protein level of <50 mg/L on postoperative day 12 had a 100% negative predictive value. However, diagnosis may be very difficult, especially in case of late empyema as symptoms of postpneumonectomy empyema are nonspecific and laboratory tests are often insensitive.

C. Treatment

Drainage of the postpneumonectomy space and adequate systemic antibiotics are the two key components of treatment of empyema postpneumonectomy. Simple postpneumonectomy empyema without BPF is quite uncommon. A repeated surgical intervention is often necessary in a patient in poor condition of health and with diminished pulmonary reserve due to pneumonectomy. The classical surgical approach is an open-window thoracostomy, which is plagued by a high mortality up to 29% (35) and a recurrence rate of empyema up to 38% (27). Such worst outcome led some surgeons to explore lesser invasive approaches.

In 1971, Provan (36) proposed antibiotic irrigation of the postpneumonectomy space via a single–chest tube drainage with a success rate of 50%. In an uncontrolled study, Rosenfeldt et al. found no real advantage of open-surgical management over simple irrigation of the pleural cavity (37). After successful eradication of empyema in 13 cases with simple irrigation and systemic antibiotics, Goldstraw concluded that this therapeutic approach might replace aggressive and invasive surgery in many instances (17). However, failure of pleural space irrigation does not preclude the use of other surgical procedures (38). It is postulated that irrigation through chest tube leaves membranes and debris in the pleural cavity therefore harboring germs that can cause recurrences and thus many surgeons prefer a thoracoscopic approach to prolonged chest drainage (39–41). Theoretically, thoracoscopy allows removal of false membranes and debris followed by washing and drainage of the pleural cavity under visual control. A randomized trial comparing chest tube pleural drainage plus streptokinase instillation with video-assisted thoracic surgery (VATS) demonstrated significantly less recurrences and shorter hospital stay in the video-assisted thoracoscopy group (42). Wait et al. (42) using thoracoscopy to remove infected tissue from the pleural space and continuous irrigation/drainage of the cavity had a success rate of 73%. However, they concluded that this approach should not be applied in case of BPF.

According to Hollaus et al., one of the reasons why VATS is not a well-accepted technique of treating this serious and potentially lethal complication, that is, postpneumonectomy empyema, is the difficulty to reach the costodiaphragmatic recessus (43). However, although video-assisted or simple thoracoscopy does not allow cleaning of the pleural space as well as thoracotomy, its success may depend on a decrease in bacterial load and inflammatory exudates below a critical level (42).

Surgical treatment of postpneumonectomy empyema by VATS (43–45) is reported in quite small and uncontrolled series, the largest one including only 9 patients (43). Another or combined therapeutic option in patients with persisting pleural infection could be to apply local irrigation with antibiotics, as proposed by Hollaus et al. (43). In case of small BPF (≤ 2 mm), local application of fibrin glue (Tissucol®) or sclerotherapy to close the BPF under VATS has been described (43,44). In 1963, Clagett and Geraci (45) described the classic two-step procedure for the treatment of postpneumonectomy empyema consisting in an open drainage via a fenestrated thoracostomy followed by daily irrigation of the postpneumonectomy space with antibiotics (or antiseptic solution) for 6 to 8 weeks, and then simple surgical closure of the window thoracostomy after sterilization of pleural space. Pairolero et al. (10) modified this procedure by reinforcing the closed bronchial stump with intrathoracic transposition of skeletal muscle and reported a definitive success rate of 84% but a high mortality rate of 13%.

Michaels et al. (46), using muscle transposition combined with thoracoplasty to reduce the postpneumonectomy space, had one recurrence in four treated patients. Wong and Goldstraw (9) reported 5 recurrences out of 13 patients treated by the two-step Clagett procedure.

More recently, Schneiter et al. (47) proposed a more aggressive and new approach, that is, repeated thoracotomy every two days to perform a radical debridement of the postpneumonectomy space with local application of antiseptic packing in the pleural space. They treated 20 patients with an average number of 3.5 interventions per patient and a success rate of 100% after a mean follow-up of 30 months, making such a new approach quite attractive.

However, in case of early postpneumonectomy empyema, we still do not know whether an initial aggressive surgical treatment is more effective than simple pleural drainage with systemic antibiotics. The Clagett procedure or other modified surgical procedures remain very risky especially in patients often in poor condition of health (9,10).

In conclusion, we have no evidence-based data on the best way to manage postpneumonectomy empyema. Currently, the treatment depends on the experience of local surgical teams. However, in case of large bronchopleural (> 2–3 mm) fistulae, some surgical treatment seems to be necessary.

IV. Postsurgical Bronchopleural Fistula

A. Definition and Incidence

Postsurgical BPF—a communication between pleural space and bronchial tree—is a rare but serious complication, occurring in 1.5% to 4.5% of pneumonectomies (48). After pulmonary resection, the occurrence of BPF can really be a life-threatening adverse event, with a high mortality, ranging from 29% to 79% and it is associated with prolonged hospital stay. Its incidence is variable depending on the etiology, surgical technique, and experience of the surgeon (49), being lower after surgical resection for benign than malignant conditions. Sirbu et al. (50) reported a series of 490 patients with lung resection for non–small-cell lung cancer. The incidence of BPF was 4.4%. It occurred in 12 patients (54.6%) after pneumonectomy, in 9 (40.9%) after lobectomy, and in 1 patient (4.5%) after sleeve resection. Postoperative BPF can be classified as acute (within 1 week after surgery), subacute (>2 weeks), and chronic (three months after surgery) (25). The acute form of BPF is mostly related to technical problems. It is not associated with empyema and requires immediate surgical closure. The subacute and chronic forms are mostly related to infection, in immuno-compromized or debilitated patients with many comorbidities.

B. Etiology

Most frequently, BPF is associated with pneumonectomy, its incidence being even higher in patients with right-sided procedures (50). Preoperative risk factors for development of BPF are persistent fever, steroids use, *H. influenzae* in sputum, anemia, tracheostomy, prolonged ventilation, and bronchoscopy for sputum suction or mucus plugging (51). In addition, residual tumor, large bronchial stumps ≥25 mm (52), concurrent radiotherapy or chemotherapy, tight sutures, and poor wound healing constitute risk factors favoring fistulization, as a result of ischemic necrosis and/or pooling of secretions with subsequent colonization and local bacterial overgrowth. Sonobe et al. (53) showed variable rates of BPF according to the type of surgical closure: 1.8% with a manual suture, 5% with a stapling device, 1.9% with a stapling device and reinforcement suture at the distal side of staplers, and 1% when the reinforcement suture was done at the proximal side of staplers. Other risk factors for development of BPF are found in patients with ARDS, pneumonia, lung abscess, or other ongoing infectious processes, and in patients with bullous lung disease, or other parenchymal pathologies like COPD (Table 1).

C. Diagnosis

Signs and symptoms are divided into acute/subacute and chronic forms. In the acute form, the presentation is characterized by the sudden appearance of dyspnea, hemoptysis, fever, subcutaneous emphysema, persistent air leak from a chest tube, productive cough, and

Table 1 Bronchopleural fistulae. Risk factors

Preoperative risk factors
  Fever
  Steroid use
  Anemia
Postoperative risk factors
  Fever
  Steroid use
  Tracheostomy
  Prolonged ventilation
  Bronchoscopy for sputum suction/mucus plugging
  Concurrent radio/chemotherapy
  Tight sutures
  Large bronchial stump diameter (> 25mm)
  Infections
    Hemophilus influenza
    Pseudomonas aeruginosa
    Staphylococcus aureus
    Klebsiella pneumoniae
    Aspergillus
  Malignancies
    Lung cancer
    Thyroid cancer
    Lymphoma
    Esophageal cancer
  Others
    ARDS
    Debilitated comorbidities
    Bullous lung disease
    Interstitial lung disease

---

shifting of the trachea and mediastinum to the contralateral side. The chronic form is suspected in case of nonspecific signs such as flu-like symptoms, subfebrile temperature, and weight loss. In case of esophagotracheal fistulae, the patient presents with coughing and shortness of breath when drinking or eating. On chest X-rays (48,54,55), a sudden drop of air–liquid level with shift of the mediastinum away from the pneumonectomy space, the development of a new air–liquid level or changes in existing air–liquid levels are highly suggestive of BPF. The mediastinum may be displaced to the opposite side because of an increase in air in the postpneumonectomy space. Clearing of fluid from the operated side with hemoptysis or productive cough of fluid strongly suggests a BPF. The BPF occurs at any time during the postoperative period but more often within 10 to 14 days after surgery (11). If seen within the first 4 postoperative days, the BPF is usually secondary to a technical failure in stump closure and requires surgical reexploration and reclosure. BPF can occur without associated empyema. The culture of pleural fluid is then sterile. Several methods have been used to diagnose BPF. Instillation of methylene blue into the postpneumonectomy space immediately followed by the appearance of bluish sputum is a simple, safe, and less-expansive diagnosis tool for BPF (55). Trapping of ^{133}Xe using

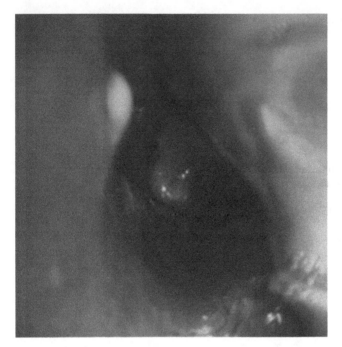

Figure 2   A 50-year-old patient with right-sided pneumonectomy for a non–small-cell lung cancer developing 15 days after surgery a bronchopleural fistula of the right stump with a diameter exceeding 6 mm as proven by bronchoscopy.

ventilation scintigraphy in pleural space has also been used (56). Bronchoscopy may be helpful in detecting larger fistulas, but its value in diagnosing small <1 to 2 mm fistulae is poor (Fig. 2). Ricci et al. (57) showed that the CT-scan was also useful in identifying and localizing the BPF in more than half of the patients requiring surgery. In fact, BPF was identified in 91% of the cases.

D.   Surgical Treatment
BPF is a serious postoperative complication of thoracic surgery. The correct diagnosis is often delayed in patients developing it after leaving the hospital. Once BPF is diagnosed, antibiotics and immediate drainage of the postpneumonectomy space are required. In the early postoperative period, direct surgical reclosure of the stump should be attempted. Other treatment options include the use of bronchoscopy with local application of glues, coils or sealants (51). Recently, West et al. (58) reviewed the current literature to know whether minimal approaches with bronchoscopy might be better than conventional re-thoracotomy to close BPF. Out of 1052 abstracts, they identified only six case series with more than two postpneumonectomy BPFs. In this small case series, there were 85 patients with postpneumonectomy BPF treated by bronchoscopic procedures, whatever the method of obliteration, with a success rate of 30% but a mortality rate of 40%. They concluded that bronchoscopic treatment should be reserved at present time for badly

ill patients unsuitable to undergo an open thoracotomy. A rare complication of BPF is the erosion of the pulmonary artery from bronchial stump inflammation occurring in about 4% of all BPFs (59). Hemoptysis or large amounts of blood draining into the chest tube are the presenting symptoms, followed by rapid hypotension or/and shock. Mortality exceeds 50% despite emergency thoracotomy.

The initial treatment of BPF (60) is aimed to control any life-threatening condition. If there is a tension pneumothorax, chest tube drainage has to be done urgently. In case of pulmonary flooding, airways control is required and in ventilated patients, limiting the tidal volume and reducing the respiratory rate will reduce the airway pressure and consequently the airflow through the fistula. When infectious etiologies like empyema is suspected, efficient drainage of the postpneumonectomy space is mandatory under appropriate systemic antimicrobial coverage. The patients are often debilitated due to the underlying process. Therefore, aggressive management of comorbidities and conditions is needed. High-caloric nutrition and intensive physical training is also necessary. Hollaus et al. (61) reviewed a retrospective series of 45 patients with BPF after pneumonectomy treated by bronchoscopy over more than 10 years. Only small fistulae (<3 mm) responded to primary endoscopic treatment. Sixteen (36%) patients required surgical intervention. Of 29 patients treated by bronchoscopy, 9 were cured after multiple firbrin glue or bone applications. Mortality was 20%. Scappaticci et al. (62) used methyl-2-cyanoacrylate glue in 12 patients with BPF after pneumonectomy. The resolution rate and survival were satisfactory in respectively 67% to 83%, but only 10% of empyemas resolved definitively. As summarized by Lois and Noppen (49), most of the studies about treatment of BPF by bronchoscopy after thoracic surgery are small series without controlled cases, or case reports using many different sealants (ethanol, polyethylene, glycol, cyanoacrylate glue, fibrin glue, blood, bone, etc.). Therefore, such minimal-invasive techniques should be reserved for patients unable to tolerate a new thoracotomy. Surgical management varies according to the size of the fistula using the Clagett procedure described above or other modified procedures (10,45).

References

1. De Smedt A, Vanderlinden E, Demanet C, et al. Characterisation of pleural inflammation occurring after primary spontaneous pneumothorax. Eur Respir J 2004; 23:896–900.
2. LoCicero J III. Postsurgical pleural infection. In: Bouros D, ed. Pleural Disease. New York and Basel: Marcel Dekker Inc., 2004:391–397.
3. Barker WL. Natural history of residual air spaces after pulmonary resection. Chest Surg Clin N Am 1996; 6:585–613.
4. Wareham EE, Barber H, McGoey JS, et al. The persistent pleural space following partial pulmonary resection. J Thorac Surg 1956; 31:593–600.
5. Christiansen KH, Morgan SW, Karich AF, et al. Pleural space following pneumonectomy. Ann Thorac Surg 1965; 122:298–304.
6. Solak O, Sayar A, Metin M, et al. Definition of postresectional residual pleural space. Can J Surg 2007; 50:39–42.
7. Brunelli A, Al Refai M, Muti M, et al. Pleural tent after upper lobectomy: A prospective randomized study. Ann Thorac Surg 2000; 69:1722–1724.
8. Nomori H, Horio H, Suemasu K. Mixing collagen with fibrin glue to strengthen the sealing effect for pulmonary air leakage. Ann Thorac Surg 2000; 70:1666–1670.
9. Wong PS, Goldstraw P. Post-pneumonectomy empyema. Eur J Cardiothorac Surg 1994; 8:345–349; discussion 9–50.

10. Pairolero PC, Arnold PG, Trastek VF, et al. Postpneumonectomy empyema. The role of intrathoracic muscle transposition. J Thorac Cardiovasc Surg 1990; 99:958–966; discussion 66–68.
11. Zumbro GL Jr, Treasure R, Geiger JP, et al. Empyema after pneumonectomy. Ann Thorac Surg 1973; 15:615–621.
12. Boldt J, Piper S, Uphus D, et al. Preoperative microbiologic screening and antibiotic prophylaxis in pulmonary resection operations. Ann Thorac Surg 1999; 68:208–211.
13. Bernard A, Pillet M, Goudet P, et al. Antibiotic prophylaxis in pulmonary surgery. A prospective randomized double-blind trial of flash cefuroxime versus forty-eight-hour cefuroxime. J Thorac Cardiovasc Surg 1994; 107:896–900.
14. Snider GL, Saleh SS. Empyema of the thorax in adults: Review of 105 cases. Dis Chest 1968; 54:410–415.
15. Miller J. Postsurgical empyemas. In: Shields T, ed. General Thoracic Surgery. Baltimore, MD: Williams & Wilkins, 1994:694–700.
16. Asamura H, Naruke T, Tsuchiya R, et al. Bronchopleural fistulas associated with lung cancer operations. Univariate and J Thorac Cardiovasc Surg 1992; 104:1456–1464.
17. Goldstraw P. Postpneumonectomy empyema. The cloud with a silver lining? J Thorac Cardiovasc Surg 1980; 79:851–855.
18. Patel RL, Townsend ER, Fountain SW. Elective pneumonectomy: Factors associated with morbidity and operative. Ann Thorac Surg 1992; 54:84–88.
19. Conlan AA, Lukanich JM, Shutz J, et al. Elective pneumonectomy for benign lung disease: Modern-day mortality and morbidity. J Thorac Cardiovasc Surg 1995; 110:1118–1124.
20. Massard G, Dabbagh A, Wihlm JM, et al. Pneumonectomy for chronic infection is a high-risk procedure. Ann Thorac Surg 1996; 62:1033–1037; discussion 7–8.
21. Odell JA, Henderson BJ. Pneumonectomy through an empyema. J Thorac Cardiovasc Surg 1985; 89:423–427.
22. Wright CD, Wain JC, Mathisen DJ, et al. Postpneumonectomy bronchopleural fistula after sutured bronchial closure: Incidence, risk factors, and management. J Thorac Cardiovasc Surg 1996; 112:1367–1371.
23. Frytak S, Lee RE, Pairolero PC, et al. Necrotic lung and bronchopleural fistula as complications of therapy in lung cancer. Cancer Invest 1988; 6:139–143.
24. Rogiers P, Van Mieghem W, Engelaar D, et al. Late-onset post-pneumonectomy empyema manifesting as tracheal stenosis with respiratory failure. Respir Med 1991; 85:333–335.
25. Kerr WF. Late-onset post-pneumonectomy empyema. Thorax 1977; 32:149–154.
26. Weber J, Grabner D, al-Zand K, et al. Empyema after pneumonectomy–empyema window or thoracoplasty? Thorac Cardiovasc Surg 1990; 38:355–358.
27. Van Raemdonck D, Kesteman J, Roekaerts F, et al. Treatment of postpneumonectomy empyema with or without bronchopleural fistula. Acta Chir Belg 1990; 90:59–66.
28. Schueckler OJ, Rodriguez MI, Takita H. Delayed postpneumonectomy empyema. J Cardiovasc Surg (Torino) 1995; 36:515–517.
29. DeMeester T, Lafontaine E. The pleura. In: Sabiston D, Spencer J, eds. Surgery of the Chest. Philadelphia, PA: Saunders WB, 1990:474–476.
30. Holden MP, Wooler GH. Pus somewhere, pus nowhere else, pus above the diaphragm. Postpneumonectomy empyema necessitates. Am J Surg 1972; 124:669–670.
31. Biondetti PR, Fiore D, Sartori F, et al. Evaluation of post-pneumonectomy space by computed tomography. J Comput Assist Tomogr 1982; 6:238–242.
32. Kopec SE, Conlan AA, Irwin RS. Perforation of the right ventricle: A complication of blind placement of a chest tube into the postpneumonectomy space. Chest 1998; 114:1213–1215.
33. Lams P. Radiographic signs in post pneumonectomy bronchopleural fistula. J Can Assoc Radiol 1980; 31:178–180.

34. Icard P, Fleury JP, Regnard JF, et al. Utility of C-reactive protein measurements for empyema diagnosis after pneumonectomy. Ann Thorac Surg 1994; 57:933–936.
35. Eckersberger F, Moritz E, Klepetko W, et al. Treatment of postpneumonectomy empyema. Thorac Cardiovasc Surg 1990; 38:352–354.
36. Provan JL. The management of postpneumonectomy empyema. J Thorac Cardiovasc Surg 1971; 61:107–109.
37. Rosenfeldt FL, McGibney D, Braimbridge MV, et al. Comparison between irrigation and conventional treatment for empyema and pneumonectomy space infection. Thorax 1981; 36:272–277.
38. Hakim M, Milstein BB. Empyema thoracis and infected pneumonectomy space: Case for cyclical irrigation. Ann Thorac Surg 1986; 41:85–88.
39. Waller DA, Rengarajan A. Thoracoscopic decortication: A role for video-assisted surgery in chronic postpneumonic pleural empyema. Ann Thorac Surg 2001; 71:1813–1816.
40. Lackner RP, Hughes R, Anderson LA, et al. Video-assisted evacuation of empyema is the preferred procedure for management of pleural space infections. Am J Surg 2000; 179: 27–30.
41. Cunniffe MG, Maguire D, McAnena OJ, et al. Video-assisted thoracoscopic surgery in the management of loculated empyema. Surg Endosc 2000; 14:175–178.
42. Wait MA, Sharma S, Hohn J, et al. A randomized trial of empyema therapy. Chest 1997; 111:1548–1551.
43. Hollaus PH, Lax F, Wurnig PN, et al. Videothoracoscopic debridement of the postpneumonectomy space in empyema. Eur J Cardiothorac Surg 1999; 16:283–286.
44. Urschel JD, Barnwell JM, Lipman BJ. Bronchoscopic sclerotherapy combined with thoracoscopic drainage for postpneumonectomy bronchial fistula and empyema. Surg Endosc 1999; 13:932–934.
45. Clagett OT, Geraci JE. A procedure for the management of postpneumonectomy empyema. J Thorac Cardiovasc Surg 1963; 45:141–145.
46. Michaels BM, Orgill DP, Decamp MM, et al. Flap closure of postpneumonectomy empyema. Plast Reconstr Surg 1997; 99:437–442.
47. Schneiter D, Cassina P, Korom S, et al. Accelerated treatment for early and late postpneumonectomy empyema. Ann Thorac Surg 2001; 72:1668–1672.
48. Kopec SE, Irwin RS, Umali-Torres CB, et al. The postpneumonectomy state. Chest 1998; 114:1158–1184.
49. Lois M, Noppen M. Bronchopleural fistulas: An overview of the problem with special focus on endoscopic management. Chest 2005; 128:3955–9365.
50. Sirbu H, Busch T, Aleksic I, et al. Bronchopleural fistula in the surgery of non-small cell lung cancer: Incidence, risk factors, and management. Ann Thorac Cardiovasc Surg 2001; 7:330–336.
51. Sato M, Saito Y, Fujimura S, et al. Study of postoperative bronchopleural fistulas—Analysis of factors related to bronchopleural fistulas. Nippon Kyobu Geka Gakkai Zasshi 1989; 37:498–503.
52. Hollaus PH, Setinek U, Lax F, et al. Risk factors for bronchopleural fistula after pneumonectomy: Stump size does matter. Thorac Cardiovasc Surg 2003; 51:162–166.
53. Sonobe M, Nakagawa M, Ichinose M, et al. Analysis of risk factors in bronchopleural fistula after pulmonary resection for primary lung cancer. Eur J Cardiothorac Surg 2000; 18:519–523.
54. Goodman LR. Postoperative chest radiograph: II. Alterations after major intrathoracic surgery. AJR Am J Roentgenol 1980; 134:803–813.
55. Hsu JT, Bennett GM, Wolff E. Radiologic assessment of bronchopleural fistula with empyema. Radiology 1972; 103:41–45.
56. Nielsen KR, Blake LM, Mark JB, et al. Localization of bronchopleural fistula using ventilation scintigraphy. J Nucl Med 1994; 35:867–869.

57. Ricci ZJ, Haramati LB, Rosenbaum AT, et al. Role of computed tomography in guiding the management of peripheral bronchopleural fistula. J Thorac Imaging 2002; 17:214–218.
58. West D, Togo A, Kirk AJ. Are bronchoscopic approaches to post-pneumonectomy bronchopleural fistula an effective alternative to repeat thoracotomy? Interact Cardiovasc Thorac Surg 2007; 6:547–550.
59. Khargi K, Duurkens VA, Knaepen PJ, et al. Hemorrhage due to inflammatory erosion of the pulmonary artery stump in postpneumonectomy bronchopleural fistula. Ann Thorac Surg 1993; 56:357–358.
60. Cooper WA, Miller JI Jr. Management of bronchopleural fistula after lobectomy. Semin Thorac Cardiovasc Surg 2001; 13:8–12.
61. Hollaus PH, Lax F, Janakiev D, et al. Endoscopic treatment of postoperative bronchopleural fistula: Experience with 45 cases. Ann Thorac Surg 1998; 66:923–927.
62. Scappaticci E, Ardissone F, Ruffini E, et al. As originally published in 1994: Postoperative bronchopleural fistula: Endoscopic closure in 12 patients. Updated in 2000. Ann Thorac Surg 2000; 69:1629–1630.

21
Surgical Management of Empyema

DEAN M. DONAHUE and DOUGLAS J. MATHISEN
Harvard Medical School, Division of Thoracic Surgery, Massachusetts General Hospital,
Boston, Massachusetts, U.S.A.

I. Introduction

Empyema thoracis develops when bacteria enters the sterile pleural space and overwhelms the normal pleural defense mechanisms. The most common mode of entry for these bacteria is migration across the visceral pleura from an area of pneumonia. Bacteria may also enter the pleural space from a thoracic surgical procedure or after the development of a bronchopleural fistula (BPF). Empyema can occur from extension across the diaphragm of a subphrenic abscess or with esophageal perforation. Identifying and correcting the underlying etiology of the empyema is critical to successful treatment.

The management of empyema is based on the surgical principles that pus should be drained, and an empty space should be obliterated. Treatment begins immediately with drainage of the pleural space. This can be done with closed-tube drainage or by opening the pleural space surgically. Once drainage is established there are two issues that must be addressed. First is the presence or absence of a BPF and second is the existence of a residual pleural space. A BPF can occur peripherally from a necrotizing pneumonia, or centrally with the dehiscence of a postresection bronchial closure. Either type may heal spontaneously following drainage and debridement of the pleural space, but more commonly a well-timed operative repair is required. Any residual pleural space after drainage must be addressed. One option for obliterating the space is filling it with viable tissue such as the underlying lung following decortication, or with a transposed flap of muscle or omentum. In rare situations, collapsing the chest wall with a thoracoplasty can eliminate this space.

II. Empyema without BPF

A. Etiology

Pneumonia with parapneumonic effusion remains the most common etiology for empyema. In the preantibiotic era, approximately 10% of patients with pneumonia developed empyema with *Streptococcus pneumoniae* being the predominant organism in two-thirds of all cases (1). With the advent of antibiotics Staphylococcus species became more prevalent. More recently, penicillin-resistant Staphylococcus, Gram-negative bacteria, and anaerobic organisms are increasing in incidence (2).

The second most common etiology for empyema is infection following a thoracic surgical procedure. This most frequently occurs after pneumonectomy, and is associated with a BPF from dehiscence of the bronchial closure in up to 80% of cases. However, it can occur following any thoracic surgical procedure with or without a pulmonary resection. Empyema following pulmonary resection is more complex because it is frequently associated with a BPF, and the potential of a residual space resulting from the resection. Empyema may also occur following esophageal injury or anastamotic leak. Bacterial migration across the diaphragm can result in empyema from intraperitoneal infections.

B. Pathophysiology of Parapneumonic Effusion
To determine both the timing and the extent of surgical intervention for parapneumonic pleural space infections, a thorough understanding of its pathophysiology is necessary. A pleural space infection due to pneumonia is a continuum of three stages: exudative (Stage I), fibrinopurulent (Stage II), and organizing (Stage III). The stage at presentation correlates with the length of time between the onset of the pneumonia and the initiation of antibiotic therapy.

The first stage begins as an exudative effusion. The infected lung parenchyma will develop a vascular endothelial injury mediated by migrating neutrophils. This vascular injury results in fluid leaking into the pleural space that is initially sterile. With progressive injury pleural fluid production exceeds the lymphatic drainage capacity, particularly when deposited fibrin obstructs the pleural lymphatic channels. The fluid is initially free flowing and turbid with a pH >7.30, a glucose >60, and LDH <500 IU/L. These early parapneumonic effusions occur to some degree in up to 50% to 60% of cases; however, most cases resolve with early initiation of appropriate antibiotic therapy.

If the pneumonia remains untreated, bacteria will enter the pleural space and the empyema progresses to the fibrinopurulent stage. Additional fibrin is deposited to act as scaffolding for white blood cell (WBC) migration. These WBC's utilize glucose and produce lactate and carbon dioxide resulting in a low glucose and pH in the pleural fluid. A high LDH results from cell death and lysis. Clinically, this second stage is characterized by purulent fluid with progressive loculations.

Unchecked, this progresses on to the sequelae of chronic inflammation with collagen deposition and organization. This organizing stage of an empyema results in an inelastic "peel" of collagen encasing the lung and chest wall, thus preventing their expansion. An empyema will rarely spontaneously resolve. If untreated, it will drain out of the chest wall (empyema necessitatis) or into the lung creating a BPF.

C. Diagnosis
Empyema in the absence of BPF typically presents as an extension of the symptoms of the underlying pneumonia. Patients most commonly present with symptoms of dyspnea, fever, cough, and chest pain (3). The duration of symptoms prior to initiating antibiotic treatment will correlate with the degree of pleural space contamination and severity of the symptoms. Bacterial invasion typically occurs several days after the formation of a pleural exudate.

A thoracocentesis draining as much of the pleural fluid as possible is the initial step in evaluation and treatment. Pleural fluid characteristics, as outlined in the preceding section, will stage the empyema and help in the initial decision on the need for chest tube drainage (Table 1).

Table 1 Indicators for Tube Drainage of Parapneumonic Effusion

Clinical
    Duration of pneumonia symptoms prior to initiation of antibiotic therapy
    Lack of clinical improvement with proper antibiotic
    Pneumonia due to virulent pathogen
Radiographic
    Chest X-ray
        Size of effusion
        Presence of air–fluid level
    Computerized tomography
        Presence of loculations
        Pleural thickening or enhancement on contrast scans
    Ultrasonography
        Presence of loculations or debris
Pleural fluid
    WBC >25,000 cells/mL
    Organisms seen on Gram stain or a positive culture
    pH < 7.30
    Glucose <50% serum level
    LDH > 1000 IU/L

D. Treatment of Empyema Without BPF

Understanding the stages of empyema formation helps guide surgical therapy. Following thoracocentesis, an early exudative stage with a small residual effusion can be observed if effective antibiotic treatment is followed by immediate clinical improvement with resolution of the effusion and expansion of the lung. The dilemma facing the clinician in the exudative phase is whether antibiotics alone are appropriate, or should the pleural space be drained with a chest tube. There are several clinical, radiographic, and pleural fluid features that suggest the need for pleural space drainage (Table 1). Early tube drainage is indicated for an effusion in a patient with pneumonia caused by a virulent organism such as an anaerobic organism or group A β-hemolytic streptococcus. Evidence of loculations on radiographic studies such as pleural thickening or enhancement, or debris in the pleural space is an indication for tube placement. Patients who fail to improve clinically soon after the initiation of appropriate antibiotic therapy should undergo tube drainage.

    Chest tube drainage often suffices in treating the exudative or early fibrinopurulent stage of parapneumonic effusion and empyema. This is because the low-viscosity fluid is easily drained, and the lung is able to expand and fill the pleural space. In patients who present later in the course, the fibrinopurulent debris may not be able to be drained through a closed-tube system. The options that exist in this scenario include instillation of a fibrinolytic agent through the chest tube, video-assisted thoracoscopy (VATS) for debridement, or open drainage with rib resection.

    A minimally invasive approach with VATS is particularly helpful in the fibrinopurulent or early organizing stage when tube placement has failed to expand the lung. Two or three 1 to 2 cm incisions are required for this procedure. This has the advantage of allowing a complete inspection of the pleural space with debridement and disruption of loculated collections. An early nonfibrous peel can be decorticated allowing re-expansion of the lung. Several series of VATS management of parapneumonic empyema have been reported (4,5). The likelihood of success depends upon the stage of empyema at operation. Recently, Cassina and associates reported a prospective series of 45 patients with nontuberculous empyema who had failed initial management with chest tube drainage and fibrinolytic therapy, and antibiotics (6). None of the patients had undergone prior thoracotomy or pulmonary resection. Persistent fever and chest pain were present in 60% of patients, and 47% continued to have bacteria in the empyema fluid in spite of antibiotics. All patients underwent VATS debridement, which successfully treated the empyema in 82% of patients. In the remaining eight (18%) patients, the underlying lung did not re-expand. This necessitated a thoracotomy and decortication in seven patients. Two of these patients required lung resection because of destroyed parenchyma with peripheral BPF. One patient was managed with open thoracostomy. Full re-expansion of the lung, which is critical to the success of the VATS approach, needs to be confirmed with the thoracoscope at the end of the procedure.

An alternative to a VATS approach is to convert a closed-tube thoracostomy to open drainage. This involves resecting a short segment of rib, leaving the wound open around a large bore tube for both drainage and irrigation. However, if this is done too early in the course of empyema formation then an open pneumothorax will be created. To insure that the lung will not collapse with open drainage, the patient's chest tube is disconnected from the drainage system and left open to air. If the patient's clinical condition and chest X-ray is unchanged, then open drainage can be performed. An extension of this procedure is an open thoracostomy using the techniques first described by Eloesser (7), and later modified by Symbas and associates (8). This "Eloesser flap" typically involves resecting a 4 to 6 cm segment of two ribs near a dependent portion of the empyema cavity. The skin is then sutured to the parietal pleura creating a window for irrigation or gauze dressing changes.

Following drainage of the pleural space, if the lung does not expand to fill the cavity then the surgeon can either attempt lytic therapy, or proceed to a thoracotomy for a decortication. A full discussion on the role of fibrinolytic therapy is beyond the scope of this chapter, but it is more successful when used in the earlier stages (9,10). In the later stage of empyema formation collagen is deposited and organized into a fibrothorax. This inhibits both lung and chest wall expansion resulting in restrictive physiology (11). Decortication of the lung involves removing the constricting layer from the parietal and visceral pleural surfaces, allowing the lung and chest wall to re-expand. The ease of freeing the entrapped lung depends upon the extent of fibrosis that has occurred over time. Preventing the development of fibrothorax is the basis for early and aggressive intervention in the management of pleural space infection. Before a decortication is performed, the quality of the underlying lung must be assessed. If the lung is densely consolidated, it may not expand. This will create the undesirable situation of a persistent pleural space with parenchymal air leaks.

The technique of decortication involves peeling the constricting rind off of the lung, chest wall, and diaphragm. This can be attempted with a VATS approach in the fibroproliferative or early organizing phase. With organized fibrosis, a posterolateral thoracotomy is usually required. An anesthetic technique allowing single-lung ventilation should be used; however, stripping the peel from the surface of the lung is frequently aided by intermittent positive pressure ventilation of the underlying lung. This helps delineate the fibrous peel from the lung tissue. Once the lung is fully expanded, the pleural space is drained with two or three chest tubes. If the underlying lung does not fill the remaining pleural space then further techniques are needed to fill the pleural space and to prevent recurrence. These techniques will be discussed later in this chapter.

III. Empyema with BPF

A. Etiology

The development of a communication between the bronchial tree and the pleural space provides access for bacteria to enter and develop an empyema. BPF can occur with the dehiscence of a bronchial closure following pulmonary resection. It can also develop from lung parenchyma following either necrotizing pneumonia or a spontaneous pneumothorax with a prolonged air leak.

Understanding and identifying the risk factors for postoperative bronchial dehiscence (Table 2) prior to resection allows for adjustment of operative strategy to prevent this complication. The most significant predictor for BPF in our own series of 256 consecutive pneumonectomy patients was the need for postoperative mechanical ventilation (12). The presence of residual infection within the pleural space such as a patient with preoperative supperative lung or pleural disease increases the risk of a postoperative empyema. All attempts should be made to control the infection preoperatively with adequate antibiotic therapy or drainage.

Several factors related to the technical aspects of the surgical resection can increase the risk of bronchial dehiscence. Patients undergoing a right pneumonectomy have been found to have a higher risk, as have patients with prior lung surgery that requires a completion pneumonectomy. Patients undergoing a mediastinal lymph node dissection or procedures that disrupt the bronchial blood supply are also at greater risk. The presence of carcinoma at the bronchial resection margins increases the possibility of fistula formation.

Table 2 Risk Factors for Postpneumonectomy Bronchopleural Fistula and Empyema

Preexisting supperative lung or pleural disease
Postobstructive pneumonia
Bronchiectasis
Empyema
Systemic factors
Age greater than 70 years
Corticosteroid therapy
Malnutrition
Associated treatment
Radiation therapy
Postoperative mechanical ventilation
Operative considerations
Completion pneumonectomy
Right pneumonectomy
Mediastinal lymph node dissection
Carcinoma at bronchial margin
Bronchial devascularization

Other groups at risk include patients with preoperative radiation therapy or systemic conditions such as malnutrition or corticosteroid therapy.

B. Clinical Presentation

Empyema from a peripheral BPF presents with the typical signs of empyema such as fever, dyspnea, cough, and chest pain. In addition, there will be radiographic evidence of an intrapleural air–fluid level.

Fistula formation from bronchial closure dehiscence following pneumonectomy occurs within the first week after surgery in one half of cases. During this time, a fistula is identified clinically by the production of thin watery sputum, or by a fall in the pleural cavity fluid level seen on an upright chest radiograph. The fistula causes varying degrees of respiratory distress depending upon the extent that the pleural fluid contaminates the remaining lung.

Delayed fistula formation and empyema has a more insidious presentation with chest pain, dyspnea, fatigue, cough, and weight loss. These symptoms can occur following any major thoracic surgical procedure, but they will worsen rather than getting improved in a patient with a BPF. Diagnosis is facilitated by having a high index of suspicion, particularly in patients with risk factors for the development of BPF and empyema (Table 2).

C. Initial Management

The potentially life-threatening nature of postpneumonectomy BPF requires immediate diagnostic and therapeutic maneuvers. Routine chest radiography is mandatory to evaluate the fluid level within the pneumonectomy space as well as the condition of the remaining lung. In the absence of BPF, a postpneumonectomy empyema may have an unremarkable chest radiograph. The clinical suspicion of a postpneumonectomy empyema or BPF mandates an immediate bronchoscopy to evaluate the bronchial closure. If the diagnosis remains uncertain, a CT scan of the chest should be performed. This may localize areas within the pleural space to guide a diagnostic thoracocentesis. In rare cases, a ventilation scan with xenon 133 can be obtained to look for ventilation into the empty pleural cavity.

In a patient with obvious clinical or radiographic features of BPF, immediate therapy is indicated to protect the remaining lung from contamination. The patient is positioned with the pneumonectomy space in a dependent position to minimize the amount of pleural fluid draining into the contralateral lung. A tube thoracostomy is performed above the level of the thoracotomy incision as the hemidiaphragm frequently rises to this level postoperatively. Immediate tube drainage is also the appropriate initial measure in BPF following pulmonary resection other than a pneumonectomy.

D. Closure of BPF

Successful management of a BPF depends upon the correct timing and technique of closure. The optimal time to close a BPF can be a difficult decision. It is determined by the presence of pleural space contamination and the patient's overall condition including the existence of risk factors for BPF that may be corrected prior to repair.

Repair should be considered in an early postoperative fistula that is identified immediately after it develops. This requires a pleural space free from contamination and a patient that was clinically well. Our group has reported successfully resuturing the bronchus and tissue flap coverage up to one month after pneumonectomy (12). Each of these cases was closed without recurrence or empyema formation. Critical to the success of a fistula closure is further resection of the anterior bronchial wall. This allows the membranous wall flap to be sutured to the anterior wall without tension. Equally as important is a completely clean pleural cavity with no sign of any purulence.

Immediate closure of a postoperative fistula should be avoided if there is any pleural space contamination. It should also be avoided if the patient is at high risk for recurrence of the BPF and if that risk factor can be corrected. In these instances an urgently placed tube thoracostomy is frequently present. This is converted to an open thoracostomy with an Eloesser flap (8). Gauze dressings are then applied and changed once or twice daily depending upon the degree of pleural contamination. This will debride the pleural space and allow for the formation of granulation tissue. This large wound creates a metabolic demand on the patient, and their nutritional status needs to be optimized and closely followed. Systemic antibiotic therapy is a critical component in the control of the initial sepsis. Once the pleural space begins to clear with dressing changes, the antibiotics can be discontinues.

By controlling the pleural sepsis, a small BPF may heal by secondary intention in up to one-third of cases (13). When this fails to occur, direct operative repair is required. Repair should only be considered when the pleural space is clean and lined with healthy granulation tissue.

Operative repair is typically approached through the initial thoracotomy incision. The bronchial stump is identified in the mediastinum and debrided back to viable tissue. A tension-free closure is accomplished by resecting a segment of anterior cartilaginous wall as previously described. It is our preference (12) as well as that of other groups (14–17) to reinforce the BPF closure with tissue flap transfer techniques detailed later in the chapter. This technique results in successful closure, which occurs in at least 75% of cases.

IV. Management of the Pleural Space

Definitive management of the pleural space in an empyema depends upon the presence or absence of a BPF. Regardless of the existence of a fistula, if there is a residual pleural space it will need to be obliterated. The options available are filling the space with either an antibiotic solution or with viable tissue, or collapsing it with thoracoplasty. A combination of these procedures may be required.

Once the pleural space contamination is cleared with drainage and irrigation or dressing changes, some small, early fistulae may spontaneously close. In the absence of a BPF, or following fistula closure, the technique described by Clagett and Geraci may be used to treat the residual pleural space (18). This involves filling the pleural space with an antibiotic solution and closing the soft tissue over the thoracostomy in a watertight fashion. The choice of antibiotic is adjusted to the cultured flora of the pleural space. This approach is successful in over 80% of cases (19). If a recurrent empyema develops, it is likely due to residual pleural space infection or an unsuspected BPF. This can be treated by re-establishing drainage followed by pleural irrigation or dressing changes. The identical procedure can be repeated with a similar success rate to the initial attempt. This technique has a low morbidity, and is a reasonable choice in the initial attempt to close a clean pleural space.

Table 3 Tissue Flaps Commonly Used for Filling
the Pleural Space

Tissue	Arterial supply
Muscle	
Latissimus dorsi	Thoracodorsal
Serratus anterior	Lateral thoracic
Pectoralis major	Thoracoacromial
Rectus abdominus	Superior epigastric
Omentum	Right gastroepiploic

Transposing healthy tissue into the pleural space is also an important component to both re-enforcing the closure of a BPF and filling space. A variety of muscle flaps exists with varying bulk and axis of rotation (Table 3). These can be selected based on the need to fill a specific area in the hemithorax. The flaps can be brought into the pleural space through the primary chest incision, but more frequently require a separate rib resection to create a window of entry. This window needs to be placed properly to minimize tension and kinking of the vascular pedicle, which would compromise the viability of the tissue flap.

The latissimus dorsi is an excellent muscle flap because of its proximity and size. It is our preferred muscle flap for intrathoracic procedures; however, it is frequently divided in patients who have had a prior thoracotomy. If this muscle is intact, it is harvested by raising tissue flaps over the muscle exposing its entire surface. Electrocautery is then used to divide the distal origin. If additional length is needed, the tendonous insertion to the humerus is divided avoiding the adjacent thoracodorsal artery. This muscle is brought into the chest by resecting a segment of the second or third rib. The serratus anterior muscle also has the advantage of proximity, and is useful in the upper half of the hemithorax. This is mobilized by raising it off of its origin along the chest wall. Some of the insertion to the scapula may need to be divided to increase the mobility of the flap.

Other tissue available includes the pectoralis major muscle. It is large, and is particularly useful for upper anterior cavities. The rectus abdominis may be used for lower thoracic spaces, but a modified transverse rectus abdominis myocutaneous (TRAM) flap with a deepithelialized pedicle has been used successfully up to the apex of the chest (17).

The omentum is an excellent treatment option, particularly in cases associated with a BPF. The pliable omentum will conform to the mediastinal contour and has the angiogenic property ideal for covering a fistula repair (20). We find it particularly useful in patients with prior high-dose radiation therapy (21). The omentum is first mobilized off of the transverse colon. The gastroepiploic branches along the greater curvature are divided as the omentum is removed from the stomach. The flap is based on the right gastroepiploic artery, and brought into the hemithorax substernally or through a small opening created in the peripheral hemidiaphragm.

An alternative means of obliterating the pleural space is the technique of thoracoplasty. This involves a series of subperiosteal rib resections allowing the soft tissues of the chest wall to collapse into the pleural space (22). The extent of thoracoplasty varies with the size of the cavity that needs to be ablated. It can be used alone, or in conjunction with tissue transposition. This procedure can be applied to the treatment of any pleural space problem including cavitary or drug-resistant tuberculosis, but in order to preserve chest wall integrity, our first preference is to fill the pleural space with muscle or omentum.

V. Conclusion

The two most common etiologies for empyema are parapneumonic and postoperative. The principle of therapy can be distilled down to two principles: complete drainage of the pleural cavity and obliteration of any residual pleural space. The management of a parapneumonic effusion depends upon many factors—most importantly the duration of symptoms prior to antibiotic therapy. A diagnostic thoracocentesis is strongly encouraged, and we would favor an aggressive approach to drainage. A residual pleural space following drainage can be treated with lytic therapy early in the patient's course. Failure to improve clinically, persistent loculations or incomplete lung re-expansion is an indication for decortication. This can be attempted with a minimally invasive VATS, but if unsuccessful a thoracotomy is mandated.

In cases of empyema where there is insufficient lung tissue present to fill the pleural space, the treatment begins with open drainage to clear the pleural space infection. If present, a reinforced closure of a BPF is performed. The timing of this repair is critical. It depends upon adequately clearing the pleural space contamination and correcting any underlying causative factors. Any residual pleural space can then be closed with a Claggett procedure, filled with tissue flap transfer or obliterated with a thoracoplasty.

References

1. Ehler AA. Non-tuberculous thoracic empyema: A collective review of the literature from 1934 to 1939. Int Abstr Surg 1941; 72:17.
2. Brook I, Frazier EH. Aerobic and anaerobic microbiology of empyema. A retrospective review in two military hospitals. Chest 1993; 103:1502.
3. Varkey B, Rose HD, Kutty CP, et al. Empyema thoracis during a ten-year period. Analysis of 72 cases and comparison to a previous study (1952 to 1967). Arch Intern Med 1981; 141:1771.
4. Angelillo Mackinlay T, Lyons G, Chimondeguy D, et al. VATS debridement versus thoracotomy in the treatment of loculated postpneumonia empyema. Ann Thorac Surg 1996; 61:1626–1630.
5. Weissberg D, Refaely Y. Pleural empyema: 24-year experience. Ann Thorac Surg 1991; 62:1026–1029.
6. Cassina P, Hauser M, Hillejan L, et al. Video-assisted thoracoscopy in the treatment of pleural empyema: Stage-based management and outcome. J Thorac Cardiovasc Surg 1999; 117:234–238.
7. Eloesser L. An operation for tuberculous empyema. Surg Gynecol Obstet 1935; 60:1096.
8. Symbas PN, Nugent JT, Abbott OA, et al. Nontuberculous pleural empyema in adults. The role of a modified Eloesser procedure in its management. Ann Thorac Surg 1971; 12:69–78.
9. Jerejes-Sanches C, Ramirez-Rivera A, Elizalde JJ, et al. Intapleural fibrinolysis with streptokinase as an adjunctive treatment in hemothorax and empyema: A multicenter trial. Chest 1996; 109:1514–1519.
10. Chin NK, Lim TK. Controlled trial of intrapleural streptokinase in the treatment of pleural empyema and complicated parapneumonic effusions. Chest 1997; 111:275–279.
11. Liu CT, Cellerino A, Baldi S, et al. Pulmonary function in patients with pleural effusion of varying magnitude and fibrothorax. Panminerva Med 1991; 33:86–92.

12. Wright C, Wain J, Mathisen D, et al. Postpneumonectomy bronchopleural fistula after sutured bronchial closure: Incidence, risk factors, and management. J Thorac Cardiovasc Surg 1996; 112:1367–1371.
13. Wain JC. Management of late postpneumonectomy empyema and bronchopleural fistula. Chest 1996; 6:529–541.
14. Miller JI, Mansour KA, Nahai F, et al. Single-stage complete muscle flap closure of the post pneumonectomy empyema space. A new method and possible solution to a disturbing complication. Ann Thorac Surg 1984; 38:227.
15. Regnard J, Alifano M, Puyo P, et al. Open window thoracostomy followed by intrathoracic flap transposition in the treatment of empyema complicating pulmonary resection. J Thorac and Cardiovasc Surg 2000; 120:270–275.
16. Francel T, Lee G, Mackinnon S, et al. Treatment of long-standing thoracostoma and bronchopleural fistula without pulmonary resection in high risk patients. Plastic and Recons Surg 1997; 99:1046–1053.
17. Serletti J, Feins R, Carras A, et al. Obliteration of empyema tract with de-epithelialized unipedicle transverse rectus abdominis myocutaneous flap. J Thorac Cardiovasc Surg 1996; 112:631–636.
18. Clagett OT, Geraci JE. A procedure for the management of post pneumonectomy empyema. J Thorac Cardiovasc Surg 1963; 45:141.
19. Zaheer S, Allen MS, Cassivi SD, et al. Postpneumonectomy empyema: Results after the Clagett procedure. Ann Thorac Surg 2006; 82:279–286.
20. Goldsmith H, Griffith A, Kupferman A, et al. Lipid angiogenic factor from omentum. JAMA 1984; 252:2034.
21. Mathisen DJ, Grillo HC, Vlahakes G, et al. The omentum in the management of complicated cardiothoracic problems. J Thorac Cardiovasc Surg 1988; 95:677–684.
22. Barker WL. Thoracoplasty. Chest Surg Clin N Am 1994; 4:593.

22
Tuberculous Pleuritis

BISWAJIT CHAKRABARTI
Aintree Chest Centre, University Hospital Aintree, Liverpool, U.K.

PETER D. O. DAVIES
The Cardiothoracic Centre, Liverpool NHS Trust, Liverpool, U.K.

I. Introduction

At the age of 65, Nelson Mandela, while imprisoned on Robbin Island off the coast of Cape Town, South Africa, developed tuberculous pleuritis. He gives a very graphic account of his diagnosis and treatment in his book: "Without any preliminaries he tapped me roughly on my chest and then said gruffly, there is water in your lung. He asked a nurse to bring him a syringe and without further ado he poked it into my chest and drew out some brownish liquid" (1). Tuberculous pleuritis can strike the old as well as the young, but once treated it does not usually affect the health or longevity of the individual.

II. Definition of Pleural Tuberculosis

Tuberculous pleurisy is the development of pleurisy and/or a pleural effusion as a result of infection with a bacterium of the *Mycobacterium tuberculosis* complex. It is a fairly benign form of tuberculosis, being usually self-limiting and only occasionally causing complications. It should always be treated, as nearly half of the patients will subsequently go on to develop postpleuritic tuberculosis. It may be difficult to confirm the diagnosis, but a strongly positive tuberculin test in the presence of symptoms and signs is highly suggestive. The isolation of *M. tuberculosis* from the fluid or pleural biopsy confirms the diagnosis. Treatment is with the standard six-month regimen, and the prognosis is generally good.

III. Epidemiology of Pleural Tuberculosis

The precise incidence of pleural tuberculosis is difficult to determine, as it is not routinely separated from other forms of respiratory tuberculosis when being notified. In 1993, a tuberculosis notification survey in England and Wales reported the incidence of pleural involvement at 9% (153 of 1699 cases) compared to 6% in previous surveys involving the same region undertaken in 1978–1979 and 1983 (2–4). These data compare with an incidence of 4.9% in a 20-year retrospective review of 1738 cases reported from the United States with a 2.2% incidence from New York (5,6). Meanwhile, in a large study of 5480 patients with pulmonary and pleural tuberculosis from Turkey, 6.3% had a pleural effusion while pneumothoraces were present in 1.5% (7).

In an extensive study of tuberculous pleurisy from Romania, the proportion of pleural involvement in respiratory disease was maintained at 13% to 15% for 1960–1980, with a subsequent diminution to 7.9% in 1989 (8). The proportion of pleural effusions presenting to clinicians attributable to tuberculosis varies in the literature. In a study of 642 pleural effusions in a high-incidence region of Spain, 25% were tuberculous in etiology (9). However, in a U.K. study conducted in Liverpool (a low-incidence area) following 75 patients with exudative pleural effusions that were undiagnosed following cytological analysis of pleural fluid, tuberculosis accounted for just 4% of cases (10).

Regarding age of presentation, tuberculous pleuritis has traditionally been regarded as a disease of young adults and adolescents. For example, the incidence of tuberculous pleurisy in a Romanian survey was at its highest level (19.1/100,000) at the age of 20 to 24 years in 1990 (8), while the peak age of pleural tuberculosis in a large study from Finland was at 18 years of age (11). In a study of 100 cases of pleural tuberculosis over a six-year period in Qatar, 84% of cases presented below the age of 45 years often with an acute febrile illness representing so-called "primary" tuberculous infection (12). However, there is evidence that patients with pleural tuberculosis in developed countries present at a more advanced age, perhaps reflecting a secondary "re-activation" phenomenon (13–15). In a U.S. study of 49 patients with tuberculous pleuritis, 20 were aged 35 years or above (13), while in another U.S. study examining 7549 cases of pleural tuberculosis over a 10-year period, pleural involvement occurred more often than pulmonary tuberculosis in those $\geq$65 years (30.4% vs. 23.3%) and less often in children <15 years (1.8% vs. 6.1%) (15).

Ethnicity may also be a factor in the development of pleural tuberculosis. In the United Kingdom, the proportion of pleural tuberculosis was found to be slightly higher in those of Indian subcontinent ethnic origin (patients originating from India, Pakistan, and Bangladesh). In the 1993 U.K. survey, 11% of tuberculosis cases arising in those from the Indian subcontinent exhibited pleural involvement contrasting to 7.1% in white Caucasians with a similar observation noted in the 1983 survey (2,3). In a U.S. survey, pleural tuberculosis patients were more likely to be born in the United States when compared to those with pulmonary disease (15), and a greater proportion of pleural tuberculosis cases were seen in Blacks when compared to those from other ethnic groups.

IV. Pleural Tuberculosis and the Impact of HIV

In modern times, perhaps the most significant factor to impact on the epidemiology of tuberculosis is that of human immunodeficiency virus (HIV). Co-infection with HIV in those individuals with latent tuberculosis results in a 10% annual risk of developing active tuberculosis compared to a 10% lifetime risk in those without HIV infection. Furthermore, the incidence of pleural involvement may be higher in the presence of HIV co-infection. In one U.S. study, cases of pleural tuberculosis in AIDS patients in South Carolina from 1988 through 1994 were reviewed. Twenty-two (11%) of the 202 AIDS patients with tuberculosis had pleural involvement compared to 6% in non-AIDS patients ($p = 0.01$). Associated features of AIDS tuberculous pleurisy included substantial weight loss (7.65 $\pm$ 1.35 kg) and lower lobe infiltrates (12/22; 55%). In the same study, no difference in pleural fluid characteristics were found when comparing AIDS patients with a serum CD4 count >200/µL to patients with CD4 count <200/µL. The overall response to treatment was good for most patients. Two (9%) of the 22 patients died of tuberculosis. Chest radiograph follow-up of 20 patients showed complete resolution in 7, improvement in 10, and no improvement in 3. The authors concluded that in South Carolina, pleural involvement is more common in AIDS patients than in non-AIDS patients with tuberculosis. Furthermore, the study noted that the clinical presentation of TB pleuritis was found to differ in AIDS patients compared to those without HIV co-infection in that the former group exhibited a greater frequency of lower-lobe infiltrates and weight loss (16). These findings were supported by a study of 112 pleural TB cases from Tanzania where 58% were found to be HIV positive (17). HIV-positive patients were more likely to present with breathlessness, night sweats, fatigue, fever, and diarrhea. On physical examination, there was also an increased frequency of hepatomegaly, splenomegaly, and lymphadenopathy. Tuberculin skin testing was found to be negative in 11.6% of HIV-negative cases compared with 47.2% of HIV-positive cases.

Meanwhile, in a prospective study, 94 patients presenting at two large Harare hospitals with clinically suspected pleural TB were enrolled over a 10-month period. Pleural TB was diagnosed in 90 individuals (median age 33 years; range 18–65 years; 64 males); the seroprevalence of HIV was 85%. HIV-positive patients were older than HIV-negative individuals and had a significantly lower median CD4+ count. A CD4+ count of $<200 \times 10^6$/L was associated with a length of illness >30 days, a positive–pleural fluid smear and a positive–pleural biopsy Ziehl–Neelsen stain. However, a relationship between CD4+ count and either pleural granuloma formation or radiological evidence of disseminated disease was not observed. The authors concluded that in sub-Saharan Africa, TB pleural effusions have become associated with older age, a chronic onset, an increased mycobacterial load, and a low CD4+ count (18).

In a study from Malawi assessing response to treatment in tuberculous pleuritis, 296 patients with smear-negative and 138 with pleural TB were enrolled of whom 366 (84%) of patients were HIV positive. A total of 220 (51%) patients completed treatment and 144 (33%) died by 12 months. Significantly higher case fatality rates were found in older patients, HIV-positive patients, and patients with pulmonary parenchymal lung disease. The treatment regimens compared three times weekly isoniazid, rifampicin, and pyrazinamide for two months followed by isoniazid and ethambutol or Thiacetazone for two months followed by isoniazid alone for four months, against the "standard" regimen of streptomycin, Thiacetazone (or ethambutol), and isoniazid for one month followed by isoniazid and ethambutol or Thiacetazone for 11 months. They found no difference in outcomes between the regimens. In resource-poor settings, the ability of a regimen that excludes rifampicin to cure the patient is an advantage in cost saving. However, in areas where HIV infection is high, ethambutol should be used instead of Thiacetazone to avoid serious adverse effects (19).

V. Pathophysiology of Pleural Tuberculosis

The etiology of pleural tuberculosis in so-called primary disease represents an immuno-logical phenomenon rather than the result of direct infection. Rupture of the Ghon focus into the pleural-cavity results in a delayed-type hypersensitivity reaction. Typically, such effusions occur three to six months following initial infection and the presence of rel-atively few bacilli in the pleural space results in a comparatively low diagnostic yield from microbiological analysis of pleural fluid (13,14,20,21). The clinical syndrome arises from the delayed-type hypersensitivity reaction in which plasma proteins are exuded into the pleural space and CD4+ cells accumulate, multiply, and release inflammatory mediators, particularly IFN-γ. These may provide a means of diagnosis (see below) (22–25). The occasional anergic response to purified protein derivative (PPD) in a patient suffering from tuberculous pleural effusion has been explained by the sequestration of the antigen-specific T cells into the pleural space, and so being unable to mount a peripheral hypersensitivity response; IL-2 is also released from macrophages within the pleural fluid (22,26,27). High vitamin D concentrations (cholecalciferol) have also been reported, representing enhanced macrophage activation (28).

In the absence of appropriate antituberculous therapy, the majority of these effusions resolve spontaneously over a period of several months only for half of such cases to develop pulmonary or extra-pulmonary disease in the future. This is illustrated in a comprehensive overview of TB pleuritis in a monograph by Patiala reviewing 2816 men with TB pleuritis from the Finnish army (11). Patiala was able to follow all but a few of these patients for a period of between seven and nine years. The great majority was between 18 and 20 years as they were mostly young recruits to the army. The main weakness of the paper is that tuberculous pleuritis was defined only as the presence of an exudative pleural effusion in the presence of a positive tuberculin test. During the follow-up period, 43.1% of the series developed postpleuritic tuberculosis, the great majority of who developed pulmonary (70%) or bone and joint (10%) tuberculosis. He found that the time interval between tuberculous pleurisy and the development of postpleuritic tuberculosis was short, 75% of patients proceeding to disease within two years. Progress to postpleuritic tuberculosis was more likely the older patient at age of onset of pleurisy. Development of postpleuritic tuberculosis was also more common in urban than in rural settings, as was the presence of a family history of tuberculosis. The prognosis of uncomplicated pleuritis was good. Within one year after the onset of the disease, three quarters of the group were considered fit for work, and at the end of the follow-up period only a few showed slight disabilities due to pleural thickening. Of the group with subsequent development of postpleuritic tuberculosis, only a quarter was fully fit for work nine years after the onset of pleuritis. The death rate for this group was 37.3%, while that for the entire pleuritis series was 15.6%.

Pleural tuberculosis may also occur in post-primary "re-activation" disease due to direct infection from cavitatory lung lesions, hilar lymph nodes or as a result of hematogenous dissemination from extra-pulmonary sources. In such cases, larger numbers of bacilli enter the pleural space, and the chest radiograph shows associated parenchymal and cavitatory abnormalities typically in the upper lobes in contrast to primary disease where such changes are absent. Recent evidence points to an increasing proportion of pleural tuberculosis occurring as a result of postprimary disease (29,30). In a Korean study examining 106 cases of pleural tuberculosis, 37% exhibited radiographic evidence of pulmonary tuberculosis, while sputum/bronchial washings yielded positive microbiology in 31%. The authors concluded that postprimary tuberculosis was responsible for 74% of cases with illness duration of 60 days compared to 14 days in primary disease (29). If post-primary disease is left untreated, the increasing bacillary load in the pleural space may lead to the development of tuberculous empyema. Rupture of a parenchymal cavity into the pleural space results in the formation of broncho-pleural fistula and subsequent pyo-pneumothorax.

VI. Case study 1: A Breathless Man

A. Presenting Complaint

A 47-year-old barman presented with a three-month history of breathlessness.

B. Medical History

The patient, who worked part-time in a social club bar, complained that for three months he had had progressive breathlessness. He had a persistent smoker's cough, which had not changed, and had lost no weight. There was no significant past history. He drank in excess of 50 units of alcohol a week.

C. Examination and Tests

He was obese (105 kg) and there was clinical evidence of a right-sided pleural effusion. He had a low-grade fluctuating pyrexia. The presence of an effusion was confirmed on chest X-ray (Fig. 1). A liter of straw-colored fluid was aspirated from the chest, which was an exudate. This was negative on direct smear for AAFB, but a pleural biopsy done at the same time showed a few granulomata. A Mantoux test was strongly positive (25 mm induration to 10 TU).

D. Outcome

He was started on triple antituberculous chemotherapy comprising isoniazid, rifampicin, and pyrazinamide. Initially, there was no apparent response. The pyrexia continued, and

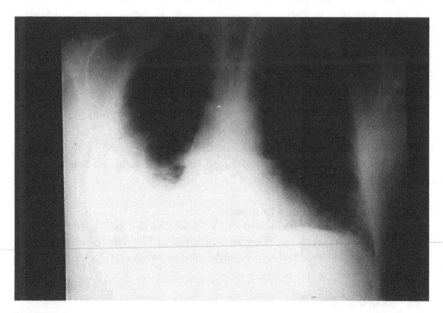

Figure 1 Chest X-ray of a 47-year-old British white barman showing a right-sided pleural effusion. See text for details.

he showed no symptomatic improvement. After a week of continuing pyrexia, he was started on oral prednisolone (60 mg). Within 24 hours, the temperature had returned to normal and he felt considerably better. He was discharged from hospital and continued on steroids in addition to full antituberculous chemotherapy for four months. The effusion had resolved by the end of the third month of treatment. Antituberculous drugs were continued for six months.

E. Comment

Depending on the epidemiological context, pleural effusions are usually associated with primary tuberculosis, as was the case in this man. Bacilli in the fluid are sparse so that smear is usually negative and negative culture is not uncommon. Rarely, they may become heavily contaminated with bacilli and a tuberculous empyema may result. This is usually the result of reactive, not primary disease. Histology and culture of the pleura are usually needed to make the diagnosis. If pleural fluid can be removed, then a pleural biopsy can and should be carried out. Standard chemotherapy for six months is sufficient, and steroids are said to speed the resorption of fluid, though recent evidence suggests that they make no difference to the final outcome.

This patient had continuing pyrexia despite several days of treatment. The fact that steroids immediately suppressed this suggests a hypersensitivity phenomenon, though whether this was due to the initial pathology or the antituberculous chemotherapy is not clear. Steroids have an important role in suppressing the hypersensitivity reaction of tuberculosis itself or of the drugs used in treatment and should be considered if pyrexia persists beyond a week of treatment in the presence of a firm diagnosis of tuberculosis.

The absence of weight loss or of any symptoms other than those caused by the effusion itself suggests a primary disease in this patient. In fact, he was one of several patients to be identified as part of an outbreak of tuberculosis around the bar in which he worked. Pleural effusion in the elderly is more likely to be due to reactivation of a primary infection, so-called post-primary disease, and in this situation weight loss and other symptomatology such as malaise is usual.

VII. Case study 2: A Febrile Immigrant with an Effusion

A. Presenting Complaint

An 18-year-old Pakistani woman presented with fever, dry cough, and breathlessness, which had persisted for two weeks.

B. History of Presenting Complaint

The patient had been in the United Kingdom for 12 months. She had experienced fever and "flu-like" symptoms for two weeks, with weight loss of 7 kg. She had also had a dry nonproductive cough and had developed breathlessness on moderate effort. There was no significant past history.

C. Examination

The patient was toxic, with a temperature of 39°C and signs of a large right pleural effusion.

D. Tests

The chest X-ray showed a left-sided pleural effusion (Fig. 2) Hemoglobin was 10.0 g/dL normochromic, and ESR was 123 mm/hr. Serum proteins showed an albumen level of 29 g/L and a globulin level of 37 g/L. The tuberculin test was strongly positive. Pleural aspiration, biopsy, and drainage were performed. The fluid showed an exudate

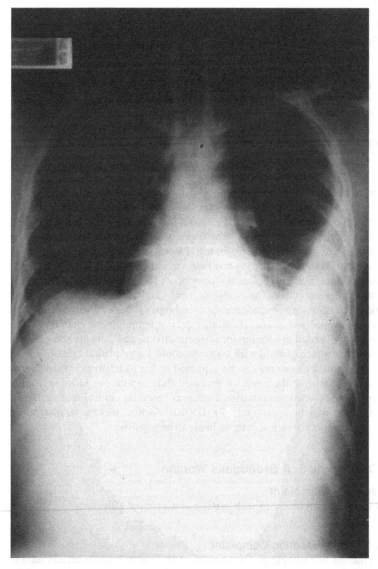

Figure 2   Chest X-ray of an 18-year-old immigrant Pakistani woman showing a left-sided pleural effusion. See text for details.

(protein 51 g/L), which was heavily lymphocytic on cytology. Pleural biopsy showed multiple necrotic granulomata with palisaded epithelioid histiocytes and lymphocytes. Pleural fluid was later culture positive at six weeks for *M. tuberculosis* fully sensitive to first-line drugs.

E. Progress

A total of 4 L of fluid was drained, and treatment recommended on the basis of the lymphocytic exudates. Treatment was started with rifampicin, isoniazid, and pyrazinamide orally. The patient remained toxic and was vomiting despite normal transaminases. Treatment with IV rifampicin and isoniazid, together with streptomycin and hydrocortisone, was given for four days. This stopped the vomiting and reduced the fever. Treatment was then switched back to oral rifampicin, isoniazid, and pyrazinamide with prednisolone (30 mg/day). Treatment with steroids was gradually withdrawn over two months. Pyrazinamide was stopped when full sensitivity was confirmed, and treatment was continued with rifampicin/isoniazid as combination tablets for a total of six months. At the end of treatment, the chest X-ray showed only minimal basal pleural reaction, and the ESR was 4 mm/hr.

F. Comment

The immediate working diagnosis here was tuberculosis. Any person in an ethnic minority group with a pleural effusion, particularly if a recent immigrant, should be regarded as having tuberculosis until proved otherwise. Treatment was commenced on the basis of a lymphocytic exudate and a positive tuberculin test. Pleural fluid is positive on culture in up to 50% of cases but is rarely microscopy positive, and it usually takes four to six weeks to yield a positive culture. Similarly, pleural biopsy is not positive in all cases due to the patchy distribution of granulomas. The biopsy is more likely to be positive if multiple samples are taken, the operator is experienced, or the biopsy is under direct vision (e.g., a thoracoscopy). Standard short-course chemotherapy is appropriate for pleural disease. Corticosteroids may be needed in addition for systemic effects, and there are some data to support more rapid clearance of fluid with corticosteroids. Large pleural effusions need to be drained, while smaller amounts can be aspirated or left to resolve on medication. Continued fluid production or the need for repeated fluid aspirations is an indication for corticosteroids. In low-income countries, treatment based on clinical findings and a positive tuberculin test may be appropriate. In HIV co-infection, there is an increase in pleural disease, but the tuberculin test is more likely to be negative.

VIII.   Case study 3: A Breathless Woman

A.   Presenting Complaint

A 69-year-old white woman was seen with malaise and a pleural effusion.

B.   History of Presenting Complaint

The patient had had flu-like symptoms four months earlier and had then been admitted to hospital eight weeks earlier with right pleuritic plan and fever. She had been treated for pneumonia and showed clinical improvement, but 50 mL of bloodstained fluid had been aspirated at that time. She had been a nonsmoker for over 20 years, but she had had some exposure to industrial asbestos 45 years earlier. Persistent pleural shadowing was seen on the chest X-ray, and the patient was referred to the chest clinic.

C. Past Medical History
Appendectomy and cholecystectomy were the only features of the history.

D. Examination
The patient's weight was 65 kg, with signs of a small right pleural effusion.

E. Tests
Chest X-ray showed right-basal shadowing, which was mainly pleural. Hemoglobin was 12.1 g/dL and ESR was 37 mm/hr. The pleural fluid that was removed several weeks earlier had shown no malignant cells and had a protein content of 46 g/L. Liver function and biochemical profile was normal.

F. Progress
A computed tomography (CT) scan of the thorax was arranged, but within a few days, the pleural fluid aspirated earlier was reported to be culture positive for AFB, later confirmed as *M. tuberculosis*, which was sensitive to all drugs. The CT was canceled, and treatment with Rifater was started. The patient now recalled that a cousin had died of tuberculosis 22 years earlier. Her treatment was uneventful until week 8, when vomiting and jaundice developed. Treatment was stopped with an alanine aminotransferase (ALT) concentration of 3690 IU/L. There had been considerable improvement in the chest X-ray. Liver function had returned to normal after three weeks, so rifampicin/isoniazid was restarted, but the ALT concentration decreased to 165 IU/L and bilirubin rose to 32 mmol/L within 10 days. The drugs were again stopped. Liver function returned to normal within five days, ethambutol (15 mg/kg) was started and isoniazid was reintroduced, initially at 50 mg/day for three days and then at 300 mg/day. Ethambutol was continued for a further seven months. The chest X-ray showed only minimal blunting of the right costophrenic angle on completion of treatment.

G. Comment
Tuberculosis was not suspected in the older white woman, and secondary malignancy or mesothelioma was considered more likely. However, pleural fluid had been sent for culture despite the small probability of infection. Pleural tuberculosis usually gives straw-colored lymphocyte-rich exudates, but the effusion can be heavily bloodstained. Pleural biopsy might have given the diagnosis, but may only yield granulomata in 50% of cases, multiple biopsies being more likely to give a positive result. Tuberculous pleural effusion is usually an immediate postprimary phenomenon, but can occur as a reactivation phenomenon in older age (30).

IX. Case study 4: A Case of Empyema

A. Presenting Complaint
A 38-year-old Pakistani man was seen with a five-day history of fever.

B. History of Presenting Complaint
The patient had returned one week earlier from a seven-week visit to Pakistan, and the fever had developed two days after his return. He had lost 4 kg in weight over a six-month period.

C. Past Medical History
The patient was a nonsmoker but admitted to drinking 90 units of alcohol a week until three months before presentation.

D. Examination
The patient was febrile at between 38.5 and 39.0°C, and showed signs of a right pleural effusion.

E. Tests
Hemoglobin was 11.7 g/dL normochromic and the white cell count was 6.1×10^6/mL. Bilirubin was normal, but ALT at 56 IU/L (normal range <45 IU/L) and alkaline phosphatase at 161 IU/L (normal range <145 IU/L) were slightly elevated. Chest X-ray showed a right pleural effusion with some widening of the upper mediastinum. Aspiration of the plural effusion showed 400 mL of purulent fluid, which was sent for culture.

F. Progress
Because of the purulent fluid, the patient was treated as an empyema case, with intravenous cefotaxime, gentamycin, and metronidazole. A right basal chest drain was inserted and a further 800 mL of purulent fluid were drained. His fever did not respond to seven days of the above antibiotics. The pleural fluid showed predominantly lymphocytes on cytology, was negative on standard and anaerobic cultures, and was an exudate (protein 55 mg/L). The pleural fluid was negative on direct microscopy for AFB. A trial of antituberculosis treatment with Rifater 5 tablets (for weight 63 kg) was given, and the fever responded within seven days. The drain was removed and the patient began to regain weight. His dose of Rifater was increased to 6 tablets when he reached 65 kg in weight. After five weeks, positive cultures were received for *M. tuberculosis*, later shown to be fully sensitive. Liver function monitoring because of the patient's history of abnormal liver function tests and previous excessive alcohol consumption showed improvement to normal over four weeks. The pyrazinamide was stopped when full sensitivity was confirmed. He was treated with a further four months of rifampicin/isoniazid and weighed 76 kg on completion of treatment. There was some residual pleural scarring, and the patient's spirometry showed a mild restrictive defect (FEV_1 2.35/2.75 L, compared to predicted value of 3.40/4.21 L).

G. Comment

In view of the short history and purulent pleural fluid, a nontuberculous empyema was first suspected. The lack of response to broad-spectrum antibiotics and particularly the finding of lymphocyte-predominant purulent fluid, rather than a polymorph leukocytosis, suggested tuberculosis. Pleural fluid was negative on microscopy, but was later culture positive. Tuberculous empyemas may be microscopy positive, whereas this is very rarely the case for "standard" tuberculous pleural effusions. A tuberculous empyema should be managed in the same way as any other empyema, with appropriate antibiotics, drainage of pus, and consideration of decortication. It is possible in this case that the lung function at the end of treatment might have been better if a decortication had been performed, but the patient was reluctant to consider surgery (31).

X. Case study 5: Untreated Tuberculous Pleuritis Leads to Something Worse

A. Presenting Complaint

A 29-year-old woman was seen in the TB contact clinic having been in close and frequent contact with an aunt who had developed pulmonary tuberculosis. The contact had a grade IV Heaf test but no follow-up was carried out. She presented to the same chest clinic six months later with a large right-sided pleural effusion.

B. Progress

The patient was seen on three occasions in the next two months and sputum taken for AFB. The effusion gradually resolved and the sputum was negative for AFB on smear and culture. The patient was discharged from the clinic. Five months later the patient presented with a month of increasingly severe headaches. When seen she had signs of meningitis. Within 48 hours she had a rapid deterioration in consciousness and required ventilation. A CSF sample was negative on direct smear but grew *M. tuberculosis*. Though the patient survived she remains severely handicapped.

C. Comment

The fact that the patient had tuberculous pleuritis was not recognized in the chest clinic. This was despite a previously strongly positive tuberculin test and a history of contact with a potentially infectious patient. The attempted exclusion of tuberculosis by sending sputum for smear and culture is often inappropriate in tuberculous pleuritis, which may be a complication of primary tuberculosis and will therefore have relatively few bacilli. The appropriate investigation would have been aspiration of the fluid and pleural biopsy for histology and culture. Even in the absence of a clear diagnosis by these means, a pleural effusion following TB contact and a positive tuberculin test in a relatively young person should have been treated as a case of tuberculous pleurisy with appropriate antibiotics. Had this been done, the subsequent development of tuberculous meningitis and the severe disability that resulted would have been avoided. The fact that this was not done was negligent on the part of the consulting doctor. This patient exhibited the classic sequence of primary disease manifesting initially as tuberculous pleuritis. This resolved spontaneously with no treatment, but as a result a much more serious form of tuberculosis, tuberculous meningitis, developed approximately six months later.

XI. Diagnosis of Pleural Tuberculosis

Perhaps the most valuable aid in diagnosing tuberculous pleuritis is for clinicians to maintain an index of suspicion when faced with a patient presenting with an exudative pleural effusion, particularly if lymphocyte predominant. Isolation of the organism from a sample taken from the patient is the only way to prove a diagnosis of a tuberculous pleural effusion. The problem is that bacteria may be scarce in this condition. The pleural fluid is very rarely smear-positive for organisms, and cultures may be negative. It is often necessary to rely on nonspecific diagnostic criteria, particularly while cultures are awaited.

A. Characteristics of the Pleural Fluid

Thoracocentesis of tuberculous pleural effusions characteristically yields clear yellow- or "straw"-colored fluid, although, rarely, fluid may be brown as a result of light bloodstaining or dark red due to heavy blood-staining (32). Typically, such effusions are exudative with pleural fluid-to-serum fluid ratio greater than 0.5, pleural fluid LDH (lactate dehydrogenase) greater than two-thirds the upper limit of normal for the serum LDH, pleural fluid-to-serum LDH ratio >0.6, usually with total pleural fluid LDH levels >200 U (33,34). Glucose concentration is usually low, under 60 mg/dL (35). Lymphocytes usually comprise more than half of the cellular material in over 85% of tuberculous pleuritis cases (36). The presence of a significant number of mesothelial cells in the pleural fluid (37) would suggest an alternative diagnosis. However, the above factors are not particularly useful in discriminating tuberculous pleural effusion from other causes, specifically malignant, parapneumonic, or rheumatoid (38,39).

Microbiological analysis of pleural fluid, that is, smears and culture carries limited diagnostic sensitivity due to paucity of bacilli in pleural fluid specimens. The proportion of positive pleural fluid cultures range from 7% to 70% (13,14,20,21,40). In a Brazilian study, only 9 (11%) of 84 cases were culture positive compared to 24% in an earlier U.S. cohort comprising 43 cases (13,20). In a study of 103 pleural effusions of which 27 were tuberculous in etiology, the diagnostic sensitivity of pleural fluid smear and culture was 11% and 33%, respectively (41).

Pleural biopsy represents the gold standard in terms of investigation for tuberculous pleuritis. Pleural biopsy specimens should be sent for both histology and culture. Histology may reveal granulomas exhibiting central caseous necrosis with identification of acid-fast bacilli or culture of tubercle bacilli being diagnostic. Pleural biopsy may be performed in a "blind" fashion using an Abrams needle (closed biopsy) or by using radiological guidance or under direct vision (thoracoscopy). Although, controversy exists regarding the role of closed pleural biopsy in the diagnosis of exudative pleural effusions secondary to malignancy, its role in diagnosing tuberculous pleuritis is well established. Histological examination of the pleura revealed granulomas in 60% of tuberculous effusions in one series with diagnostic yield rising to 90% if pleural biopsies are cultured (42,43). Meanwhile, in a small study comprising 30 cases, the diagnostic sensitivity of closed pleural biopsy reached 100% where six tissue specimens were taken (44). In a

South African study comparing the diagnostic approaches to pleural tuberculosis, the combined sensitivity of closed needle biopsy in terms of histology and culture reached 79%, while the sensitivity of thoracoscopy was higher at 100% (40). A small study from Egypt has suggested a role for polymerase chain reaction (PCR) techniques in the analysis of pleural biopsy specimens carrying a diagnostic sensitivity of 90% (45).

The utility of sputum samples as a diagnostic tool in tuberculous pleuritis has yielded conflicting results in the literature. Some authors distinguish between tuberculous pleuritis as a result of primary disease, where no lung infiltrates are present on chest X-ray, and reactivated disease, where infiltrates are present. In one series, a positive sputum was obtained from only 4 (11.4%) of 35 cases with no infiltrates but 31 (88.6%) of 35 cases with infiltrates. A positive culture result, however, was obtained from pleural fluid in 18 (60%) of 30 and from pleural biopsy in 6 (67%) of 9 noninfiltrate cases. Positive results from pleural fluid and biopsy specimens from those patients with infiltrates were similar (5). However, the use of sputum induction in a large Brazilian series carried a 55% yield in those patients with a normal chest radiograph compared to 45% where parenchymal abnormalities were noted on the chest radiograph (20). In another series from Spain with 129 patients, positive smear from sputum samples was obtained from 7% of the 98 patients with no infiltrates but 28% of the 31 with infiltrates. A positive microbiological culture was obtained from 64% to 63% of patients from the two groups, respectively (46). Results of diagnostic tests from a series of 88 patients from Malaysia showed a positive histological diagnosis (granulomas being present) in 80% of patients with no lung infiltrate designated primary disease and 70% of those with infiltrate designated reactive disease (29).

The delayed hypersensitivity response described earlier also occurs peripherally in areas such as the skin and bloodstream and forms the basis of a positive tuberculin skin test, an immunological response to infection with the *tubercle bacillus*. In a sample of 43 tuberculous pleural effusions, 93% of cases exhibited tuberculin skin test reactivity (5). It should be emphasized that tuberculin skin tests may be falsely negative in up to 30% of tuberculous pleural effusions, particularly in the elderly and in the context of HIV infection (17,46–49). However, repeat tuberculin testing after a six-week period may be subsequently positive in a number of tuberculous effusions, where these were initially negative (13,21).

B. Adenosine Deaminase and Interferon-γ Activity in Pleural Fluid

Despite 90% efficacy of diagnosis based on traditional histological and microbiological techniques, an enormous literature around less-invasive biochemical diagnostic tests for tuberculous pleurisy has evolved. The presence of high concentrations of adenosine deaminase (ADA) and interferon-γ in pleural fluid has received the most attention. ADA activity has been proposed as a diagnostic test for tuberculous pleurisy since 1978 (50). ADA is an enzyme involved in purine catabolism found in most cells, but particularly in lymphocytes, where its concentration is inversely related to the degree of differentiation. High levels of ADA have been found in patients with lung cancer and tuberculosis. Levels of ADA activity show a significant correlation with the number of CD4+ cells in the pleural effusion (51,52).

In a study of 218 pleural effusions of which 38% were tuberculous, the use of pleural fluid ADA levels (using a cut-off of 70 IU/L) showed a sensitivity of 98% with a specificity of 96%. Only 6 patients with non-tuberculous effusions had an ADA level

>70 IU/L, all of which were neoplastic in etiology (53). A Japanese paper examining various pleural fluid markers in 46 exudative effusions (10 being tuberculous) found that the level of ADA was significantly higher in the TB pleuritis cases (83 IU) in comparison to the non-tuberculous cases (25.8 IU). The level of interferon-γ in pleural fluid was also significantly higher (137 IU vs. 0.41 IU) in the tuberculous effusions. The authors concluded that interferon-γ was the most sensitive and specific indicator for TB pleuritis (54). A met analysis of 22 studies concluded that pleural fluid levels of interferon-γ carried a sensitivity of 89% and a specificity of 97% (55).

In a study of 410 non-tuberculous lymphocyte-predominant pleural effusions, ADA levels were ≥40 IU/L in only 7 (1.7%) cases (56). Meanwhile, in a study of 129 pleural effusions in Spain, 81 (62.8%) cases were tuberculous in etiology. All cases of tuberculous pleuritis were found to have pleural fluid ADA levels >47 IU/L but this was noted in 6 of the 7 empyema cases. ADA levels were also found to be elevated in pleural effusions due to lymphoma, adenocarcinoma, and rheumatological diseases (57,58). Clinicians must be cautious regarding data concerning such biomarkers taking into account the overall prevalence of tuberculosis in their own region of practice. In a region with a low prevalence of tuberculosis, the use of pleural fluid ADA levels in isolation should not be used to diagnose tuberculous pleuritis as false positives may often occur in the context of malignancy and parapneumonic effusions (59,60). Whether the use of pleural fluid ADA levels in conjunction with other parameters improves the diagnostic accuracy in tuberculous pleuritis has also been addressed. A pleural fluid ADA level >50 IU/L coupled with a lymphocyte/neutrophil ratio >0.75 carried a diagnostic specificity of 95% compared to a specificity of 81% when taking ADA levels alone (61). In this study, 130 of 143 tuberculous effusions exhibited a pleural fluid ADA level >50 IU/L. A few studies attempting to differentiate the isoenzymes of ADA as a diagnostic test for tuberculous pleurisy have yielded conflicting data and further research in this area is needed (41,62).

Despite a considerable body of evidence focusing on the role of T-cell interferon-γ release assays (TIGRA) in the diagnosis of latent tuberculosis infection, little exists examining the role of TIGRA specific to pleural tuberculosis when assessed both by peripheral blood and pleural fluid sampling of mononuclear cells (63,64). In a small study of 20 pleural tuberculosis cases and 21 controls (where there was an alternative etiology responsible for the pleural effusion), 90% and 95% were found to be positive on peripheral blood and pleural fluid sampling, respectively (65). Furthermore, in the control group, the interferon-γ release assay was only positive in 33% and 21% on sampling peripheral blood and pleural fluid, respectively. However, in this study, only eight patients had a diagnosis of pleural tuberculosis confirmed by culture. Furthermore, the diagnostic specificity of TIGRA was lower at only 67% in peripheral blood and just 76% in pleural fluid analysis. Further detailed studies are required in this area to better define the role of TIGRA and whether this offers any advantage to clinicians over and above the previously mentioned tests in the investigation of suspected pleural tuberculosis.

C. DNA Methods

DNA amplification techniques such as the PCR have been extensively studied in the diagnosis of pleural tuberculosis. The sensitivity of pleural fluid PCR ranges from 20% to 81% (66,67). In one study from Colombia, the sensitivity of PCR was found to be

73.8% in cases of definite pleural tuberculosis but this fell to just 31.6% in cases of "probable" pleural tuberculosis where there was an absence of a clear microbiological or histological diagnosis from pleural fluid or biopsy specimens. However, the overall diagnostic sensitivity of PCR rose to 90.2% in the overall sample when combined with analysis of pleural fluid ADA levels (68).

A more recent study on the sensitivity of PCR for DNA amplification to diagnose tuberculous pleuritis showed that, based on microbiological and histological diagnoses, the sensitivity could be improved to 89% and specificity to 100%. However, there were no cases in this series, which were undiagnosed by traditional methods, so it was not possible to determine whether PCR could be of use in the diagnosis of microbiologically and histologically negative tuberculous pleuritis (69).

In another recent study from Thailand, 98 patients with symptomatic exudative lymphocytic pleural effusion were enrolled in a study to evaluate the diagnostic sensitivity of PCR assay. Pleural fluid was sent for gram staining, AFB staining, aerobic culture, culture of *M. tuberculosis* on LJ media, and cytology. Additional fluid was used for a PCR assay of the 16 S–23 S rRNA gene spacer sequences and for a nested PCR of the 16 S rRNA gene as a blind control. Overall etiologies comprised malignancy 53.1%, tuberculosis 36.7%, lymphoma 2.0%, and chronic nonspecific inflammation 8.2%. The sensitivity and specificity of AFB staining were 6% and 79%, respectively; while cultures on LJ media were 17% and 100%, respectively. The sensitivity of the PCR assay was 50% and the specificity was 61%. When PCR was nested, the sensitivity was 72% and specificity was 53%. Two-thirds (26/36) of tuberculous pleural effusion cases underwent pleural biopsy, and 62% were diagnosed by histopathology. There were no complications from thoracocentesis or pleural biopsy in any of the patients. The authors concluded that PCR assay was more sensitive than AFB staining and mycobacteria culture for diagnosis tuberculous pleural effusion, but its specificity was quite low (70).

In practice, about 90% of cases of tuberculous pleural effusion can be diagnosed using the conventional techniques of pleural fluid and biopsy smear, culture, and histology. In the younger patient with a positive tuberculin test, a trial of therapy if the diagnosis remains unclear is probably warranted. In the older patient where malignancy is likely, further diagnostic procedures including thoracoscopy and even thoracotomy to obtain adequate tissue samples should be carried out.

D. Radiographic Diagnosis

The radiography of a tuberculous pleural effusion at presentation is essentially nonspecific. The absence of key radiological abnormalities, for example, cavitation, associated–lymph node enlargement, etc. should not dissuade clinicians from further investigation when the diagnosis is suspected. In a small pediatric study of 11 patients undergoing CT scanning, pleural thickening was seen in all along with associated-parenchymal abnormalities, while hilar or mediastinal lymph node enlargement was noted in 4 cases (71). Unusually, a nodular picture seen on CT scanning has been reported. Contrast-enhanced CT examination of a 22-year-old male with pleuritic chest pain showed pleural-based nodular thickening and masses without any parenchymal involvement or mediastinal lymphadenopathy. Pathological examination following right–parietal pleural decortication showed multiple granulomas with caseating necrosis typical of tuberculosis (72).

E. Differential Diagnosis of Pleurisy

The differential diagnosis of pleurisy will depend on the epidemiological circumstances.

Cardiac causes
Congestive cardiac failure (often bilateral and transudate)
Malignancy (malignant cells may be present in the fluid)
Bronchogenic carcinoma
Mesothelioma
Lymphoma
Autoimmune disease (may be a transudate, reduced glucose concentration)
Rheumatoid arthritis
Systemic lupus erythematosus
Polyserositis
Infections (parapneumonic)
Bacterial Tuberculosis
Any other bacteria
Viral
Bornholm disease
Circulatory
Pulmonary embolus
Renal disease (transudate)
Nephrotic syndrome
Peritoneal dialysis
Trauma

XII. Management and Sequelae of Tuberculous Pleural Effusion

All patients believed to be suffering from tuberculous pleurisy should be treated with antituberculous chemotherapy. The standard short-course chemotherapy of two months of isoniazid, rifampicin, pyrazinamide, and ethambutol followed by four months of isoniazid and rifampicin has shown to be adequate (73–75). It is now recommended that a fourth drug be added, usually ethambutol for the initial two months or until sensitivity results are available (73,76). Although using only two drugs for six months has also been shown to have no relapse, this approach can no longer be recommended because of the increased danger of drug resistance in recent years (77). Doses for children should be adjusted by weight (78). Patterns of drug resistance in pleural tuberculosis appear to be similar to that seen in pulmonary disease. However, a recent U.S. survey showed that tuberculous pleuritis was less likely to be resistant to isoniazid (6.0% to 7.5%) and one first line drug (9.9% vs. 11.9%) compared to pulmonary tuberculosis (15).

Controversy exists regarding the role of corticosteroid use in pleural tuberculosis. It is generally assumed that the addition of steroids speeds the time of resolution of the effusion but makes no difference to the overall outcome including the extent of residual pleural thickening and lung function abnormalities (79,80). Another study of 40 patients revealed that the addition of corticosteroid resulted in more rapid resolution of pleural effusion and clinical symptoms such as fever (81). A recent Cochrane review concluded that there was insufficient evidence to know whether steroids are effective in tuberculosis although only three small trials totaling 236 patients met the criteria for inclusion in the analysis (82). Paradoxical worsening of disease, in spite of effective chemotherapy for tuberculosis, has been reported to occur in cases of intracranial tuberculoma, lymph node, and pulmonary tuberculosis. However, only rare case reports describe such paradoxical response in tuberculosis pleurisy. Sixty-one patients with a proven tuberculous pleural effusion were retrospectively screened in Riyadh, Saudi Arabia. Paradoxical increase in the size of the effusion was detected in 10 of 61 patients. In 6 patients, the effusion became massive with worsening of dyspnea requiring the use of corticosteroids in five patients and therapeutic aspiration in all six. However, complete resolution occurred in all 10 patients within one to three months. Three out of the 10 patients developed residual pleural thickening (83).

When tuberculous pleuritis is recognized and appropriately treated, functional sequelae are infrequent. In a retrospective Spanish study of 81 cases of tuberculous pleuritis that were correctly managed, restrictive defects on spirometry were only noted in 10% of cases after follow up; being associated with pleural effusions containing a greater proportion of lymphocytes, cholesterol, and triglycerides with relatively lower levels of LDH. Furthermore, although 37% of the overall sample exhibited any degree of residual pleural thickening (RPT), this was only greater than 10 mm in 6% of cases (84). In another Spanish study of 56 cases, RPT >10 mm was noted in 19.6% of cases and here, this was associated with pleural effusions exhibiting lower glucose and pH levels and higher lysozyme and TNF-α levels (85). However, in this study, the presence of RPT was measured only up to 20 days following completion of medical therapy and resolution of such changes may take a longer period of time. This is shown in a Korean study of 77 cases where resolution of RPT occurred up to 24 months after presentation (86). Here, RPT ≥ 10 mm was noted at six months in 43 cases but only in 21 cases by 24 months. Interestingly, the presence of RPT ≥ 10 mm at 24 months was associated with loculation of the effusion at presentation.

Tuberculous empyema represents a chronic, active infection of the pleural space with a large number of *tubercle bacilli*. It is rare compared with tuberculous pleural effusions. The inflammatory process may be present for years with few symptoms. Patients often come to clinical attention at the time of a routine chest radiograph or after the development of bronchopleural fistula. The diagnosis of tuberculous empyema is suspected on CT imaging by finding a thick, calcific pleural rind and rib thickening surrounding loculated pleural fluid. The pleural fluid is grossly purulent and smear positive for acid-fast bacilli. Treatment consists of pleural space drainage and antituberculous chemotherapy. Problematic treatment issues include the inability to re-expand the trapped lung and difficulty in achieving therapeutic drug levels in pleural fluid, which can lead to drug resistance. Surgery, which is often challenging, should be undertaken by experienced thoracic surgeons (87). From a study in Saudi Arabia, 26 patients (23 male and 3 female) with an average age of 33.8 years (range 18–61 years) presented with tuberculous empyema. The empyema was right-sided in 13, left-sided in 12, and bilateral in 1 patient. Patients presented with respiratory symptoms for a mean duration of 4.43 months (range 1–48 months). In patients with exudative empyema ($n = 4$), the fluid was aspirated, but one patient required intercostal tube (ICT) drainage for six days. There were four patients with fibrinopurulent empyema treated with thoracoscopic drainage with a mean postoperative stay of eight days (range 4–12 days). In the organizing stage ($n = 18$), initial drainage with large ICT was performed. The pleura was less than 2 cm in thickness in eight patients, for which repeated installation of streptokinase was performed (3–7 times). Satisfactory results were achieved in 6 (75%) patients, and the remaining two required decortication.

Of the 10 patients with thick cortex, 1 required a window and 9 had decortication, 2 of which had additional lobectomy and 2 had pneumonectomy. All patients fully recovered with no mortality and with a mean duration of drainage of 18 days (range 3–61 days). The stage and the state of the underlying lung should guide surgical treatment for tuberculous empyema (88).

In another study, 12 patients suffering from posttuberculous chronic empyema were reviewed. There was an average latency period of 44.83 years between the acute tuberculous illness and the clinical manifestation of the empyema. Nine of the patients had been treated with collapse therapy, induced by artificial intrapleural pneumothorax, one with thoracoplasty, and two only with late and inadequate antimycobacterial chemotherapy. Eleven (91.6%) patients also had a cutaneous fistula (seven cases) and/or a bronchopleural fistula (four cases). Late tuberculous sequelae are significant not only from a numerical standpoint, but also for the seriousness of the caused pathological conditions, often posing problems for differential diagnosis. In essence, tuberculosis should never be neglected in the differential diagnosis of empyema and pyo-pneumothorax (89).

XIII. Recent Advances in the Diagnosis of Pleural Tuberculosis

The use of the microscopic-observation drug susceptibility (MODS) technique has shown promise in improving the diagnostic sensitivity of pleural biopsy and fluid specimens in pleural tuberculosis (90,91). In essence, the MODS assay involves the use of an inverted light microscope with culture in Middlebrook's 7H9 broth (90). In a study of 111 patients, the diagnostic sensitivity of pleural biopsy specimens was found to be significantly higher at 81% when using the MODS technique compared to 51% when cultured on standard Lowenstein-Jensen media (91). Furthermore, the use of MODS assay resulted in a shorter time to diagnosis at 11 days when compared to 24 days using Lowenstein-Jensen culture ($p < 0.001$). However, further studies are needed in this area prior to making definitive recommendations regarding use in routine clinical practice.

References

1. Mandela N. Long Walk to Freedom,1994 Abacus 646.
2. Kumar D, Watson JM, Charlett A, et al. Tuberculosis in England and Wales in 1993: Results of a national survey. Public Health Laboratory Service/British Thoracic Society/Department of Health Collaborative Group. Thorax 1997; 52:1060–1067.
3. Medical Research Unit Tuberculosis and Chest Diseases Unit. National Survey of Tuberculosis Notifications in England and Wales in 1983: Characteristics of disease. Tubercle 1987; 68: 19–32.
4. Medical Research Unit Tuberculosis and Chest Diseases Unit. National Survey of Tuberculosis Notifications in England and Wales 1978–9. Br Med J 1980; 281:895–898.
5. Seibert AF, Haynes J Jr, Middleton R, et al. Tuberculous pleural effusion—Twenty year experience. Chest 1991; 99:883–886.
6. Tuberculosis in New York City 1992. New York: Bureau of Tuberculosis Control, New York City Department of Health, 1993.
7. Aktogu S, Yorgancioglu A, Cirak K, et al. Clinical spectrum of pulmonary and pleural tuberculosis: A report of 5480 cases. Eur Respir J 1996; 9:2031–2035.
8. Didilescu C, Marica M, Jalba M. The epidemiological aspects of tuberculous pleurisy in Romania. Pneumoftiziologia 1992; 41:83–87.

9. Valdes L, Alvarez D, Valle JM, et al. The etiology of pleural effusions in an area with high incidence of tuberculosis. Chest 1996; 109:158–162.
10. Chakrabarti B, Ryland I, Sheard J, et al. The role of Abrams percutaneous pleural biopsy in the investigation of exudative pleural effusions. Chest 2006; 129:1549–1555.
11. Patiala J. Initial Tuberculous Pleuritis in the Finnish Armed Forces in 1939–45 with Special Reference to Eventual Postpleuritic Tuberculosis. Copenhagen, Denmark: Enjar Munksgaard, 1955.
12. Ibrahim WH, Ghadban W, Khinji A, et al. Does pleural tuberculosis disease pattern differ among developed and developing countries. Respir Med 2005; 99:1038–1045.
13. Berger HW, Mejia E. Tuberculous pleurisy. Chest 1973; 63:88–92.
14. Epstein DM, Kline LR, Albelda SM, et al. Tuberculous pleural effusions. Chest 1987; 91: 106–109.
15. Baumann MH, Nolan R, Petrini M, et al. Pleural tuberculosis in the United States: Incidence and drug resistance. Chest 2007; 131:1125–1132.
16. Frye MD, Pozsik CJ, Sahn SA. Tuberculous pleurisy is more common in AIDS than in non-AIDS patients with tuberculosis. Chest 1997; 112:393–397.
17. Richter C, Perenboom R, Mtoni I, et al. Clinical features of HIV-seropositive and HIV-seronegative patients with tuberculous pleural effusion in Dar es Salaam, Tanzania. Chest 1994; 106:1471–1475.
18. Heyderman RS, Makunike R, Muza T, et al. Pleural tuberculosis in Harare, Zimbabwe: The relationship between human immunodeficiency virus, CD4 lymphocyte count, granuloma formation and disseminated disease. Trop Med Intern Health 1998; 3:14–20.
19. Harries AD, Nyangulu DS, Banda H, et al. Efficacy of an unsupervised ambulatory treatment regimen for smear-negative pulmonary tuberculosis and tuberculous pleural effusion in Malawi. Int J Tuberc Lung Dis 1999; 3:402–408.
20. Conde MB, Loivos AC, Rezende VM, et al. Yield of sputum induction in the diagnosis of pleural tuberculosis. Am J Respir Crit Care Med 2003; 167:723–725.
21. Falk A. Tuberculous pleurisy with effusion. Diagnosis and results of chemotherapy. Postgrad Med 1965; 38:631–635.
22. Ellner JJ, Barnes PF, Wallis RS, et al. The immunology of tuberculous pleurisy. Semin Respir Infect 1988; 3:335–342.
23. Ribera E, Ocaana I, Martinez-Vazquez JM, et al. High levels of interferon gamma in tuberculous pleural effusions. Chest 1988; 93:308–311.
24. Shimakata K, Kishimoto H, Takagi E, et al. Determination of the T-cell subset producing gamma-interferon in tuberculous pleural effusion. Microbiol Immunol 1986; 30: 353–361.
25. Rossi GA, Balbi B, Manca F. Tuberculous pleural effusions. Am Rev Respir Dis 1987; 138:575–579.
26. Ota T, Okubo Y, Sekiguchi M. Analysis of immunological mechanisms of natural killer cell activity in tuberculous pleural effusions. Am Rev Respir Dis 1990; 142:29–33.
27. Ito M, Kojiro N, Shirasaka T, et al. Elevated levels of soluble interleukin-2 receptors in tuberculous pleural effusions. Chest 1990; 97:1141–1143.
28. Barnes PF, Modlin RL, Bikle DD, et al. Transpleural gradient of 1,25-dihydroxyvitamin D in tuberculous pleuritis. J Clin Invest 1989; 83:1527–1532.
29. Liam CK, Lim KH, Wong CM. Tuberculous pleurisy as a manifestation of primary and reactivation disease in a region with a high prevalence of tuberculosis. Int J Tuberc Lung Dis 1999; 3:816–822.
30. Moudgil H, Sridhar G, Leitch AG. Reactivation disease: The commonest form of tuberculous pleural effusion in Edinburgh, 1980–1991. Respir Med 1994; 88:301–304.
31. Davies PDO, Ormerod LP. Case Presentations in Clinical Tuberculosis. London, U.K.: Arnold, 1999.

32. Chakrabarti B, Davies PD. Pleural tuberculosis. Monaldi Arch Chest Dis 2006; 65:26–33.
33. Porcel JM, Light RW. Diagnostic approach to pleural effusion in adults. Am Fam Physician 2006; 73:1211–1220.
34. Light RW, Macgregor MI, Luchsinger PC, et al. Pleural effusions: The diagnostic separation of transudates and exudates. Ann Intern Med 1972; 77:507–513.
35. Light RW. Diagnostic principles in pleural disease. Eur Respir J 1997; 10:476–481.
36. Bothamley GH. Tuberculous pleurisy and adenosine deaminase. Thorax 1995; 50:593–594.
37. Spriggs AI, Boddington MM. Absence of mesothelial cells from tuberculous pleural effusions. Thorax 1960; 15:169–171.
38. Light RW, Erozan YS, Ball WC. Cells in pleural fluid: Their value in differential diagnosis. Arch Intern Med 1973; 132:854–860.
39. Yam LT. Diagnostic significance of lymphocytes in pleural effusions. Ann Int Med 1967; 66:972–982.
40. Diacon AH, Van de Wal BW, Wyser C, et al. Diagnostic tools in tuberculous pleurisy: A direct comparative study. Eur Respir J 2003; 22:589–591.
41. Perez-Rodriguez E, Perez Walton IJ, Sanchez Hernandez JJ, et al. ADA1/ADAp ratio in pleural tuberculosis: An excellent diagnostic parameter in pleural fluid. Respir Med 1999; 93:816–821.
42. Levine H, Metzger W, Lacera D, et al. Diagnosis of tuberculous pleurisy by culture of pleural biopsy specimen. Arch Intern Med 1970; 126:269–271.
43. Scharer L, McClement JH. Isolation of tubercle bacilli from needle biopsy specimens of parietal pleura. Am Rev Respir Dis 1968; 97:466–468.
44. Kirsch CM, Kroe DM, Azzi RL, et al. The optimal number of pleural biopsy specimens for a diagnosis of tuberculous pleurisy. Chest 1997; 112:702–706.
45. Hasaneen NA, Zaki ME, Shalaby HM, et al. Polymerase chain reaction of pleural biopsy is a rapid and sensitive method for the diagnosis of tuberculous pleural effusion. Chest 2003; 124:2105–2111.
46. Arriero JM, Romero S, Hernandez L, et al. Tuberculous pleurisy with and without radiographic evidence of disease. Is there a difference? Int J Tuberc Lung Dis 1998; 2:513–517.
47. Ferrer J. Pleural tuberculosis. Eur Respir J 1997; 10:942–947.
48. Korzeniewska-Kosela M, Krysl J, Muller N, et al. Tuberculosis in young adults and the elderly. A prospective comparison study. Chest 1994; 106:28–32.
49. Relkin F, Aranda CP, Garay SM, et al. Pleural tuberculosis and HIV infection. Chest 1994; 105:1338–1341.
50. Piras MA, Gakis C, Budroni M, et al. Adenosine deaminase activity in pleural effusions: An aid to differential diagnosis. Br Med J 1978; 2:1751–1752.
51. Baganha MF, Pego A, Lima MA, et al. Serum and pleural adenosine deaminase. Correlation with lymphocytic populations. Chest 1990; 97:605–610.
52. Nishihara H, Akedo H, Okada H, et al. Multienzyme patterns of serum adenosine deaminase by agar gel electrophoresis: An evaluation of the diagnostic value in lung cancer. Clin Chim Acta 1970; 30:251–258.
53. Banales JL, Pineda PR, Fitzgerald JM, et al. Adenosine deaminase in the diagnosis of tuberculous pleural effusions. A report of 218 patients and review of the literature. Chest 1991; 99:355–357.
54. Aoe K, Hiraki A, Murakami T, et al. Diagnostic significance of interferon-gamma in tuberculous pleural effusions. Chest 2003; 123:740–744.
55. Jiang J, Shi HZ, Liang QL, et al. Diagnostic value of interferon-gamma in tuberculous pleurisy: A metaanalysis. Chest 2007; 131:1133–1141.
56. Jimenez Castro D, Diaz Nuevo G, Perez-Rodriguez E, et al. Diagnostic value of adenosine deaminase in nontuberculous lymphocytic pleural effusions. Eur Respir J 2003; 21:220–224.
57. Ocana I, Ribera E, Martinez-Vazquez JM, et al. Adenosine deaminase activity in rheumatoid pleural effusion. Ann Rheum Dis 1988; 47:394–397.

58. Valdes L, Alvarez D, San Jose E, et al. Value of adenosine deaminase in the diagnosis of tuberculous pleural effusions in young patients in a region of high prevalence of tuberculosis. Thorax 1995; 50:600–603.
59. Maartens G, Bateman ED. Tuberculous pleural effusions: Increased culture yield with bedside inoculation of pleural fluid and poor diagnostic value of adenosine deaminase. Thorax 1991; 46:96–99.
60. van Keimpema AR, Slaats EH, Wagenaar JP. Adenosine deaminase activity, not diagnostic for tuberculous pleurisy. Eur J Respir Dis 1987; 71:15–18.
61. Burgess LJ, Maritz FJ, Le Roux I, et al. Combined use of pleural adenosine deaminase with lymphocyte/neutrophil ratio. Increased specificity for the diagnosis of tuberculous pleuritis. Chest 1996; 109:414–419.
62. Carstens ME, Burgess LJ, Martiz FJ, et al. Isoenzymes of adenosine deaminase in pleural fluid: A diagnostic tool? Int J Tuberc Lung Dis 1998; 2:831–835.
63. Lalvani A. Spotting latent infection: The path to better tuberculosis control. Thorax 2003; 58:916–918.
64. Lalvani A. Diagnosing tuberculosis infection in the 21st century: New tools to tackle an old enemy. Chest 2007; 131:1898–1906.
65. Losi M, Bossink A, Codecasa L, et al. Use of a T-cell interferon-gamma release assay for the diagnosis of tuberculous pleurisy. Eur Respir J 2007; 30:1173–1179.
66. De Wit D, Maartens G, Steyn L. A comparative study of the polymerase chain reaction and conventional procedures for the diagnosis of tuberculous pleural effusion. Tuberc Lung Dis 1992; 73:262–267.
67. De Lassence A, Lecossier D, Pierre C, et al. Detection of mycobacterial DNA in pleural fluid from patients with tuberculous pleurisy by means of the polymerase chain reaction: Comparison of two protocols. Thorax 1992; 47:265–269.
68. Villegas MV, Labrada LA, Saravia NG. Evaluation of polymerase chain reaction, adenosine deaminase, and interferon-gamma in pleural fluid for the differential diagnosis of pleural tuberculosis. Chest 2000; 118:1355–1364.
69. Takagi N, Hasegawa Y, Ichiyama S, et al. Polymerase chain reaction of pleural biopsy specimens for rapid diagnosis of tuberculous pleuritis. Int J Tuberc Lung Dis 1998; 2:338–341.
70. Reechaipichitkul W, Lulitanond V, Sungkeeree S, et al. Rapid diagnosis of tuberculous pleural effusion using polymerase chain reaction. Southeast Asian J Trop Med Public Health 2000; 31:509–514.
71. Moon WK, Kim WS, Kim IO, et al. Complicated pleural tuberculosis in children: CT evaluation. Pediatr Radiol 1999; 29:153–157.
72. Ariyurek OM, Cil BE. Atypical presentation of pleural tuberculosis: CT findings. Br J Radiol 2000; 73:209–210.
73. Joint Tuberculosis Committee of the British Thoracic Society. Chemotherapy and Management of Tuberculosis in the United Kingdom: Recommendations 1998. Thorax 1998; 53:536–548.
74. Ormerod LP, McCarthy OR, Rudd RM, et al. Short course chemotherapy for tuberculous pleural effusions and culture negative tuberculosis. Tuberc Lung Dis 1995; 76:25–27.
75. Ormerod LP, Horsfield N. Short-course antituberculosis chemotherapy for pulmonary and pleural disease: 5 years experience in clinical practice. Br J Dis Chest 1987; 81:268–271.
76. Migliori GB, Raviglione MC, Schaberg T, et al. Tuberculosis management in Europe. Recommendations of a working group of the European Respiratory Society (ERS), the World Health Organisation (WHO) and the International Union Against Tuberculosis and Lung Disease, European Region (IUATLD). Eur Respir J 1999; 14:978–992.
77. Dutt AK, Moers D, Stead WW. Tuberculous pleural effusion: Six-month therapy with isoniazid and rifampicin. Am Rev Respir Dis 1992; 145:1429–1432.
78. Donald PR, Byers N. Tuberculosis in childhood. In: Clinical Tuberculosis, 2nd ed. London, U.K.: Chapman and Hall, 1998.

79. Wyser C, Walzl G, Smedema JP, et al. Corticosteroids in the treatment of tuberculous pleurisy. A double-blind, placebo-controlled, randomized study. Chest 1996; 110:333–338.
80. Galarza I, Canete C, Granados A, et al. Randomised trial of corticosteroids in the treatment of tuberculous pleurisy. Thorax 1995; 50:1305–1307.
81. Lee CH, Wang WJ, Lan RS, et al. Corticosteroids in the treatment of tuberculous pleurisy. A double-blind, placebo-controlled, randomized study. Chest 1988; 94:1256–1259.
82. Matchaba PT, Volmink J. Steroids for Treating Tuberculous Pleurisy. Cochrane Database of Systemic Reviews DC0018876, 2000.
83. Al-Majed SA. Study of paradoxical response to chemotherapy in tuberculous pleural effusion. Respir Med 1996; 90:211–214.
84. Candela A, Andujar J, Hernandez L, et al. Functional sequelae of tuberculous pleurisy in patients correctly treated. Chest 2003; 123:1996–2000.
85. De Pablo A, Villena V, Echave-Sustaeta J, et al. Are pleural fluid parameters related to the development of residual pleural thickening in tuberculosis? Chest 1997; 112:1293–1297.
86. Han DH, Song JW, Chung HS, et al. Resolution of residual pleural disease according to time course in tuberculous pleurisy during and after the termination of antituberculosis medication. Chest 2005; 128:3240–3245.
87. Sahn SA, Iseman MD. Tuberculous empyema. Semin Respir Inf 1999; 14:82–87.
88. Al-Kattan KM. Management of tuberculous empyema. Eur J Cardiothor Surgery 2000; 17: 251–254.
89. Mancini P, Mazzei L, Zarzana A, et al. Post-tuberculosis chronic empyema of the "forty years after". Eur Rev Med Pharmacol Sci 1998; 2:25–29.
90. Caviedes L, Lee TS, Gilman RH, et al. Rapid, efficient detection and drug susceptibility testing of *Mycobacterium tuberculosis* in sputum by microscopic observation of broth cultures. The Tuberculosis Working Group in Peru. J Clin Microbiol 2000; 38:1203–1208.
91. Tovar M, Siedner MJ, Gilman RH, et al. Improved diagnosis of pleural tuberculosis using the microscopic-observation drug-susceptibility technique. Clin Infect Dis 2008; 46:909–912.

23
Pleural Effusions Secondary to Fungal, Nocardial, and Actinomycotic Infection

MARK WOODHEAD and IAIN CROSSINGHAM
Manchester Royal Infirmary, Manchester, U.K.

I. Introduction

The infections covered in this section are not common and are sometimes geographically isolated in their occurrence. The majority of these infections have their greatest pulmonary impact in the lung parenchyma, with pleural involvement occurring rarely and usually secondary to the parenchymal pathology. Likewise empyema is rarely due to fungal pathogens, for example, no cases of fungal empyema were identified in a recent series of 434 pleural infections (1).

There are two clinical and pathogenetic groupings: those "pathogenic" fungi that cause infections in the immunocompetent as well as the immunocompromised (e.g., histoplasmosis, actinomycosis) and those that are of low pathogenicity and are unusual other than as "opportunists" in hosts with depressed host defense (e.g., aspergillus, candida, cryptococcus). In almost all the cases pleural effusion occurs because of direct infection of the pleural space in the form of empyema. Most of such infections are difficult to treat and particularly in the immunocompromised group outcome is poor. This is not only because of the difficulty in treatment, but also because of the nature of underlying pathology and immune suppression. In a study of 67 patients with fungal empyema the mortality was 73% (2). The frequency of each fungal species is shown in Table 1. In this study, only 10% of cases had no significant underlying condition, with malignant disease (49%), diabetes mellitus (16%), long-term steroid use (15%), liver cirrhosis (12%), and organ transplantation (6%) being the most common underlying conditions. In 84% of cases the fungal empyema was judged to be nosocomial in origin.

II. *Aspergillus* Species

Aspergillus infection of the lung is unusual in the absence of a breakdown of the host defenses. This breakdown may be local (e.g., due to damage to lung tissue caused, e.g., by previous *Mycobacterium tuberculosis* infection) or generalized due to some form of immune suppression. The type of alteration of host defense determines the type of aspergillus infection. At one end of the spectrum, aspergillus may be found as a colonist in minimally damaged airways. In some individuals an allergic immune response to the aspergillus will lead to allergic bronchopulmonary aspergillosis. Local damage to the lung parenchyma may lead to local intracavitary saprophytic growth of fungal mycelia as a mycetoma or aspergilloma. Two clinicopathological manifestations of aspergillus infection occur with generalized immune suppression. Rarely an aspergillus

Table 1 Fungi Isolated from 73 Pleural Effusion Specimens
from 67 Patients[a] with Fungal Empyema in Taiwan

Fungal isolate	Number (%)
Candida species	47 (64)
C. albicans	28 (38)
C. tropicalis	13 (18)
C. parapsilosis	2 (3)
C. guilliermondii	2 (3)
C. humicola	1 (1)
C. famata	1 (1)
Torulopsis glabrata	13 (18)
Aspergillus species	9 (12)
Cryptococcus species	3 (4)
Rhizopus species	1 (1)

[a]Some had more than one species isolated.
Source: Ref. 1.

tracheobronchitis occurs, but more commonly invasive pulmonary aspergillosis (IPA) of
the lung parenchyma is found.

Aspergillus involvement of the pleura is uncommon and is only described as a
complication of local damage to the lung parenchyma, with or without aspergilloma, and
as a complication of IPA. In each situation, the common pathogenic factor appears to be
the occurrence at some point of a bronchopleural fistula. This may occur due to direct
pleural invasion by aspergillus infection, by rupture of chronically damaged lung, or be
iatrogenic. Iatrogenic pleural aspergillosis may be as a consequence of treatment directed
at pulmonary aspergillosis [e.g., surgery or pleural instrumentation either at intercostal
drainage or the percutaneous instillation of antifungal agents for the treatment of intracavitary aspergilloma (3)] or following surgery for other lung disease [e.g., lung cancer,
pneumothorax (4)]. Most older studies refer to pleural involvement following tuberculous
lung damage, either due to the disease itself or following artificial pneumothorax used in
treatment (5,6), while more recent studies more commonly relate to IPA as a consequence
of immunosuppression. Aspergillus pleural effusion has been described as a complication
in AIDS (7).

The absolute frequency of pleural involvement depends on the sensitivity of the
method used for detection and also on the origin of the patients. Many studies do not
make a clear distinction between pleural thickening and effusion. Although a CT study of
patients with pneumonia after lung transplantation found a frequency of pleural effusions
of 63% in eight patients with aspergillus pneumonia (8), and a study of 3284 unselected
autopsies found pleural involvement in 22% of 18 patients with various forms of pulmonary aspergillosis (9), these figures probably overestimate the frequency encountered
in clinical practice. Pleural effusion was seen on chest radiograph in only 1 (3%) of
30 patients with aspergillus pulmonary infection following lung transplantation (10), in
only one of 87 (1%) cases of IPA in hematology patients (11) and was not commented
on in a study of 595 cases of IPA of diverse origin in another (12). Local pleural thickening close to an aspergilloma within a lung cavity is a common phenomenon but the
development of pleural effusion as a consequence of this appears to be unusual (6).

Clinical presentations are diverse and may be acute with sudden onset of pleuritic chest pain and cough (13) or hemoptysis (4) or indolent with weeks or months of weight loss, malaise, fevers, and cough (6,14). Clinical presentation may occur shortly after breach of the visceral pleura where this is traumatic, for example, as a postoperative complication. However, this may, even in these circumstances, be delayed for months as in the two cases reported to have occurred four and six months after percutaneous instillation of antifungal agents into an intrapulmonary mycetoma (3). Presentation has been reported up to 25 years after the pleura was originally breached in patients with structural lung disease (4,6). In these circumstances, it is not clear whether the original pleural breach was responsible for the introduction of aspergillus into the pleural space or whether (as appears more likely) a subsequent clinically unrecognized breach occurred.

Radiographic appearances may be of an uncomplicated pleural effusion or a hydro(pyo)pneumothorax (15) (Fig. 1). Underlying lung disease (e.g., old tuberculous

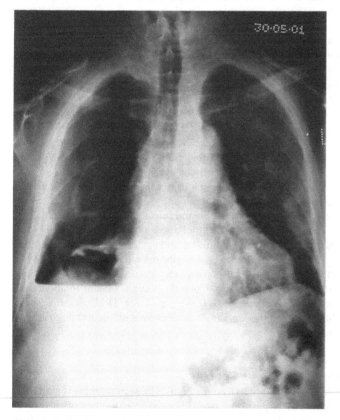

Figure 1   Patient with underlying Wegener's granulomatosis on cyclophosphamide with remission and on maintenance corticosteroids presents 9 months later with "pneumonia" and an empyema from which there is a pure growth of *Aspergillus fumigatus*. The *Aspergillus* infection had almost completely destroyed the right lung, leaving a pyopneumothorax. This chest radiograph was taken after response to itraconazole, but in the presence of a bronchopleural fistula, coinfected with β-hemolytic streptococci. (Courtesy of Dr. David Denning.)

changes, bullae, aspergilloma, or consolidation due to IPA) may also be visible. On CT, these appearances will be confirmed and in addition the pleura is usually seen to be thickened and may be nodular. Movement of the nodules with gravity when the CT is repeated in the prone position may confirm the presence of intrapleural mycetoma as in intracavitary disease (16,17). In those cases complicating chronic lung disease serial chest radiographs may reveal slowly progressing pleural thickening (4,6).

Laboratory investigations may show nonspecific abnormalities such as anemia and high erythrocyte sedimentation rate. Examination of pleural fluid usually reveals pus, which is odorless unless concomitant bacterial infection is present. The fluid has the characteristics of an exudate and cytological examination usually shows over 80% neutrophils. Using specific antifungal stains, mycelia may be seen in the aspirated fluid, which on culture will be confirmed as aspergillus. Fungi may, however, be scanty and multiple pleural fluid samples require examination before the diagnosis can be excluded (14). In some patients, aspergillus may also be found in sputum. In the immunocompetent where pleural involvement complicates chronic parenchymal involvement, aspergillus-precipitating antibodies may be present in high titer in the peripheral blood (5). Pleural biopsy may show nonspecific or granulomatous inflammation and may or may not contain fungal hyphae. *Aspergillus fumigatus* is the most common fungal species identified followed by *Aspergillus flavus* and *Aspergillus niger*. The frequency of coincident bacterial pleural infection is not clear, and may have been reduced by the widespread use of broad spectrum antibiotics. Older publications suggest from 70% to 25% (2,5,16), but these may be overestimates. *Staphylococcus aureus*, *Klebsiella*, *Pseudomonas* and *Mycobacteriam* are the most commonly reported coincident bacterial infections (5,15,16).

Guidelines for antifungal therapy in aspergillus infection are available in other texts and will not be repeated here (18). A combination of pleural drainage and antifungal treatment is the cornerstone of treatment, but a consensus on the best method of pleural drainage is not available. Patients affected by aspergillus effusion/empyema generally have comorbid conditions that render them unfit for surgery; however, closed drainage may not be adequate, especially where pleural infection is complicated by local aspergillus osteomyelitis of the ribs (15). Closed-tube drainage accompanied by local pleural instillation of antifungal agents (nystatin or amphoteracin) has been reported to be successful (2,5,13,19). Most reports, however, describe operative surgical drainage of the pleural cavity, accompanied variably by decortication, pleurectomy, pneumonectomy, omentoplasty and myoplasty (4,6,15,16,20,21). Complication rates occur in about 50% cases with recurrent empyema and hemorrhage being prominent. Death occurred postoperatively in 10% of 19 patients in the literature where those with pleural disease were separately defined (4,6,14,20).

III. *Candida* and *Torulopsis* Species

Lung infection (as opposed to colonization) by organisms of these two genera is extremely rare. They are normal colonists of the gastrointestinal tract and occur more frequently in the presence of chronic disease and following broad spectrum antibiotic therapy. In a study of fungal empyemas, these two organisms were the most common cause accounting for 82% of cases (Table 1) (2). In 84% of cases, the fungal empyema was judged to be nosocomial in origin, chronic underlying disease was present in 90% and 60% had received prior broad spectrum antibiotics. Occasionally, candida empyema may complicate subdiaphragmatic disease (22) or gastrointestinal tract pathology (23,24). *Candida albicans* occurs most frequently, followed by *Candida tropicalis* and *Torulopsis glabrata* (Table 1). As for aspergillus, drainage of the pleural space and antifungal therapy are required in treatment. Intrapleural instillation of fluconazole was reported to be successful in two patients (2).

IV. *Pneumocystis jiroveci*

Pleural disease due to *Pneumocystis jiroveci* [formerly *Pneumocystis carinii* (25)] is very rare. Pleural effusions were not recorded at all in the early radiographic series of pneumocystosis cases (26). Although the association of this infection with pneumothorax in 4% to 5% of cases (27,28) is now well recognized, the occurrence of pleural effusion remains a rare phenomenon. Pleural effusion occurred in 25% of episodes of *P. jiroveci* pneumonias in a series of cancer patients (29), with a suggestion that pleural effusion was more common in patients who had undergone hemopoietic stem cell transplantation compared with solid malignancy patients. While usually associated with *P. jiroveci* pneumonia, it may occur without apparent lung involvement (30). Bronchopleural fistula was present in 4 of 7 cases described up to 1993 (30,31), though not specifically mentioned in later series (29). *P. jiroveci* may be seen in pleural fluid with appropriate staining (30). Pleural fluid-to-serum LDH ratio is >1, but protein level may be below 3 g/dL, and glucose levels and pH are normal. Neutrophils or monocytes may predominate in the fluid (31).

Drug treatment is as for *P. jiroveci* pneumonia. Tube drainage has been described, however, the necessity for this is unknown (30).

V. *Cryptococcus* Species

Cryptococcus neoformans is an ubiquitous soil fungus. It is rarely found in the human lung. It can occur as a commensal organism or can cause infection, mainly in the immunocompromized, but also rarely in the immunocompetent. Lung infection can occur in isolation or be a manifestation of disseminated disease, the latter usually involving the meninges. Radiographically, it is usually manifested as consolidation or isolated pulmonary nodule(s). Presentation with a pleurally based mass has been described (32).

Pleural effusion is unusual especially in the immunocompetent (33). In the non-HIV immunocompromized, it was reported in 23% of 13 patients with *C. neoformans* pulmonary infection in one study (34). A review of eight studies in the HIV positive, each containing 18 patients or less, found pleural effusion in 14% of 92 cases. A study of 37 such patients in Rwanda found pleural effusion in only 5% cases. Isolated pleural effusion due to *C. neoformans* appears not to have been described, but a single such case of empyema due to *Cryptococcus albidus* (with coincident mucormycosis) has been described (35). There has also been one report of pneumonia and pleural effusion caused by *Cryptococcus laurentii* (36). Examination of pleural fluid may yield cryptococcal antigen or the organism on culture.

Treatment is of the underlying cryptococcal infection, which may be successful without the need for therapeutic pleural drainage (37).

VI. *Mucor* Species

These include *rhizopus*, *absidia*, and *mucor*. Disease caused by these saprophytic fungi is rare, usually occurs in the immunocompromized and presents as rhinocerebral or pulmonary disease. In the lung, it may be confined to the airways or be invasive. Pleuritic chest pain is common and pleural friction rubs may be heard. Pleural effusion may occur (38) and may be unilateral or bilateral (39). It has been suggested that the presence of pleural effusion on CT scanning can be used to differentiate pulmonary mucormycosis from invasive pulmonary aspergillosis (40).

VII. *Histoplasma capsulatum*

Histoplasma capsulatum is a soil-living fungus which is endemic to certain geographic regions, especially the Eastern United States, South and Central America, South East Asia, and India. Infection occurs through inhalation of microconidia from the mycelial form of the organism. The clinical pattern of illness varies according to the innoculum size and host factors, which include immune status. Illness may be acute or chronic. As many as 50% of infections may be asymptomatic (41).

Pleural thickening due to fibrosis is common in the chronic fibrocavitary form of the infection, but pleural effusion is very uncommon (42,43). The true frequency in patients presenting with clinical illness is probably close to the 0.4% found in a series of 269 cases reported in 1976 (44). Other series of more selected groups of patients report frequencies of 3.6% (45) and 6.3% (46). Pleural effusion may be more common in those with histoplasma pericarditis with a frequency of 44% in a small series of 16 such patients (47).

Pleural effusion may be asymptomatic (48), may occur both in the presence and absence (43) of underlying lung involvement and may be bloodstained (49) or empyematous (46). The infrequency of pleural effusion means that it is often investigated by surgical drainage and pleural biopsy. Pleural examination may show fibrosis (43) or subpleural granulomata (44).

In the absence of pleural fibrosis, resolution, either spontaneously or with treatment (41) normally occurs, but tube drainage or surgery may be required.

VIII. *Blastomyces dermatitidis*

Blastomyces dermatitidis is another soil-living fungus that occurs in South Eastern North America and is reported less commonly from Central and South America and occasionally from Africa and elsewhere. As with histoplasmosis, infection is acquired by inhalation and the clinical manifestations are varied. Many cases of infection are asymptomatic. Pleural effusion appears to be more common than with histoplasmosis. It was reported in 6% of 517 cases in seven series (50–56) ranging from 0% (51,52) to 20% (54) of cases in individual series (53). Large effusions have occasionally been reported (57,58).

In three patients, pleural fluid was described to have a high-protein content with normal glucose and raised cell count, with neutrophils predominating (53). The pleura may contain non-caseating granulomatous inflammation and yeasts may be visible (58).

IX. *Coccidioides immitis*

Coccidioidomycosis is a systemic fungal infection caused by *Coccidioides immitis* which is usually self-limiting. It is endemic in the South Western United States and parts of South and Central America. Outbreaks occur when the fungus is liberated from soil in dust storms, natural disasters, and earth excavation. The majority of infections are asymptomatic and most symptomatic cases have a flu-like illness. Occasionally, a chronic fibrocavitary lung infection develops and extrapulmonary dissemination can occur. Pyopneumothorax has been recorded following rupture of pulmonary cavities into the pleural space (59,60). In a series of 28 coccidioidal pleural effusions, the pleural disease was attributed to direct spread from pulmonary parenchyma in over 90% cases (61). Only two cases had evidence of disseminated infection.

X. *Paracoccidioides brasiliensis*

Paracoccidioides brasiliensis is endemic to South and Central America. Primary infection usually occurs in childhood with chronic adult infection occurring due to reactivation or reinfection. Pleural effusion has been described in primary infection in a child (62), but is unusual. The chronic form is associated with mid-zone interstitial lung shadowing and nodules, which may cavitate. Pleural effusion was recorded in 1 out of 12 patients with HIV and pulmonary paracoccidioidomycosis (63). The pleural effusion was adjacent to a pathological rib fracture also caused by *P. brasiliensis*.

XI. *Sporothrix schenkii*

Sporothrix schenkii is another soil fungus with worldwide distribution that occasionally causes human disease. This nearly always involves the skin, but primary lung infection can occur and disseminated disease can affect the lung. Consolidation and nodular (sometimes cavitating) shadowing occurs and pleural effusion has been reported (64). Of two cases where the pleural fluid characteristics were described, both were exudates, one with a mononuclear cell infiltrate and the other with a frank empyema containing granulocytes. Treatment is with amphotericin B and/or itraconazole (65).

XII. *Actinomyces israelii*

Both Actinomyces and Nocardia are Gram-positive bacteria which share a number of characteristics with the fungi (e.g., branching and mycelium formation). Actinomyces is a normal commensal organism of the oropharynx, which primarily causes disease in the cervico-dental region. Only 15% of cases are said to involve the thorax.

Disease characteristics are dependent on chronicity when the organism's unusual capacity to ignore anatomical boundaries and to directly invade contiguous tissues becomes manifest. In the thorax, early infection typically affects the lower lobes and lung periphery and takes the form of consolidation. The overlying pleura becomes fibrosed and thickened and local intrapleural abscesses and empyema may occur (66). Pleural shadowing typically occurs in one-third of cases (67) and notwithstanding the above comments may occur in isolation (68). A wavy periosteal reaction in the overlying ribs was said to be typical, but appears to be an unusual feature in recent reports (69). Direct invasion of contiguous tissues includes the chest wall (66,69,70), the diaphragm (71,72), and the mediastinum (73) [Figs. 2(A) and 2(B)].

Clinical features are nonspecific with cough, sputum, fever, chest pain, weight loss, dyspnea, hemoptysis, and night sweats all being common. The chronicity of symptoms may mimic those of tuberculosis. Similarly, the capacity for tissue invasion may imitate neoplasia.

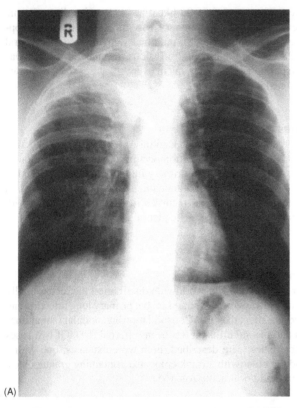

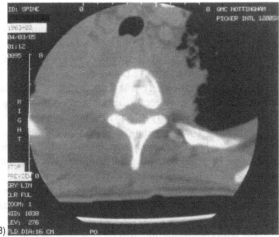

Figure 2 Patient with *Actinomyces israelii* lung infection. In addition to acute respiratory symptoms, the patient had a typical pustular overlying skin rash due to direct skin invasion and neurological features due to spinal cord compression. (a) Chest radiograph of right upper lobe pneumonia with pleural involvement. (b) CT scan showing direct invasion of adjacent structures including pleura, chest wall, contralateral lung, and spinal canal.

Diagnosis is based on isolation of the usual causative species, *A. israelii*, on culture from lung secretions or pleural fluid, but may be suspected from the presence of typical "sulfur granules" in pus or tissue including pleura (74). These particles are composed of an outer ring of neutrophils surrounding a central core of bacterial filaments. Concomitant infection with other microorganisms is not infrequent.

Treatment is with penicillin or other β-lactam antibiotics. Pleural drainage and/or surgery may be required, but does not appear to be mandatory (75).

XIII. *Nocardia* Species

Nocardia bacteria are common commensal organisms in soil and water. Infection is acquired by inhalation and in two-thirds or more of cases pulmonary involvement occurs. Dissemination occurs frequently and the organism has a predilection for involving the brain. Although the organism is Gram-positive, it is also weakly acid-fast which may lead to misdiagnosis as tuberculosis (76). *Nocardia asteroides* is the most common disease-causing species with other species (e.g., *Nocardia brasiliensis*, *Nocardia farcinica*) varying in frequency, probably according to their environmental prevalence. Infection usually occurs in the frankly immunocompromized, but those with mildly compromised host defenses [e.g., chronic steroid intake or bronchiectasis (77)] can be affected and ~10% of cases are immunocompetent. Pathologically, the infection can lead to suppuration or granulomatous inflammation depending on the integrity of the host immune response. This variability in pathology is in part responsible for the variable clinical and radiographic presentation. Cough and sputum, which may be bloodstained, are typically associated with fever and leucocytosis. Consolidation or nodules, which may be multiple, are typical radiographic features, with cavitation occurring frequently (77–80). Pleural changes may be seen in 12% (79) to 90% (80) of cases, but many studies are of small numbers of patients and often do not distinguish clearly between pleural thickening and fluid. Isolated empyema may occur (81) and simultaneous infection with other organisms [e.g., *P. jiroveci* (82), *Mycobacterium tuberculosis* (83)] has been reported. Direct spread into contiguous structures has been described, but appears to be less common than with Actinomyces infection.

Diagnosis is based on identification of the causative organism in affected tissues including pleural fluid and pleura. The bacterium grows slowly and cultures should be kept for three weeks if Nocardia is suspected.

Appropriate antibiotics (sulphonamides) are the mainstay of treatment, but drainage and or surgery may be required when the pleura is affected. Antibiotic therapy should be for a minimum of three months and possibly for as long as one year (78). The mortality may be as high as 80% in those with cerebral involvement, but in isolated pulmonary disease cure is usually achievable.

References

1. Maskell NA, Batt S, Hedley EL, et al. The bacteriology of pleural infection by genetic and standard methods and its mortality significance. Am J Respir Crit Care Med 2006; 174: 817–823.
2. Ko SC, Chen KY, Hsueh PR, et al. Fungal empyema thoracis: An emerging clinical entity. Chest 2000; 117(6):1672–1678.

3. Nakanishi Y, Wakamatsu K, Nomoto Y, et al. Empyema following the percutaneous instillation of antifungal agents in patients with aspergillosis. Intern Med 1996; 35(8):657–659.

4. Endo S, Sohara Y, Murayama F, et al. Late pleuropulmonary aspergillosis after the treatment of pneumothorax: Report of three cases. Surg Today 1999; 29(10):1125–1128.

5. Krakowka P, Rowinska E, Halweg H. Infection of the pleura by *Aspergillus fumigatus*. Thorax 1970; 25(2):245–253.

6. Hillerdal G. Pulmonary aspergillus infection invading the pleura. Thorax 1981; 36(10): 745–751.

7. Staples CA, Kang EY, Wright JL, et al. Invasive pulmonary aspergillosis in AIDS: Radiographic, CT, and pathologic findings. Radiology 1995; 196(2):409–414.

8. Collins J, Muller NL, Kazerooni EA, et al. CT findings of pneumonia after lung transplantation. AJR Am J Roentgenol 2000; 175(3):811–818.

9. Barth PJ, Rossberg C, Koch S, et al. Pulmonary aspergillosis in an unselected autopsy series. Pathol Res Pract 2000; 196(2):73–80.

10. Diederich S, Scadeng M, Dennis C, et al. Aspergillus infection of the respiratory tract after lung transplantation: Chest radiographic and CT findings. Eur Radiol 1998, 8(2):306–312.

11. Yeghen T, Kibbler CC, Prentice HG, et al. Management of invasive pulmonary aspergillosis in hematology patients: A review of 87 consecutive cases at a single institution. Clin Infect Dis 2000; 31(4):859–868.

12. Patterson TF, Kirkpatrick WR, White M, et al. Invasive aspergillosis. Disease spectrum, treatment practices, and outcomes. I3 Aspergillus Study Group. Medicine (Baltimore) 2000; 79(4):250–260.

13. Albelda SM, Gefter WB, Epstein DM, et al. Bronchopleural fistula complicating invasive pulmonary aspergillosis. Am Rev Respir Dis 1982; 126(1):163–165.

14. Kearon MC, Power JT, Wood AE, et al. Pleural aspergillosis in a 14 year old boy. Thorax 1987; 42(6):477–478.

15. Meredith HC, Cogan BM, McLaulin B. Pleural aspergillosis. AJR Am J Roentgenol 1978; 130(1):164–166.

16. Costello P, Rose RM. CT findings in pleural aspergillosis. J Comput Assist Tomogr 1985; 9(4):760–762.

17. Winer-Muram HT, Scott RL, Eastridge CE, et al. Pleural aspergillosis diagnosed by computerized tomography. South Med J 1987; 80(9):1193–1194.

18. Stevens DA, Kan VL, Judson MA, et al. Practice guidelines for diseases caused by Aspergillus. Infectious Diseases Society of America. Clin Infect Dis 2000; 30(4):696–709.

19. Stern JB, Girard P, Caliandro R. Pleural diffusion of voriconazole in a patient with *Aspergillus fumigatus* empyema thoracis. Antimicrob Agents Chemother 2004; 48(3):1065.

20. Wex P, Utta E, Drozdz W. Surgical treatment of pulmonary and pleuro-pulmonary Aspergillus disease. Thorac Cardiovasc Surg 1993; 41(1):64–70.

21. Lampo N, Spiliopoulos A, Licker M, et al. Management of postpneumonectomy Aspergillus empyema extending into the thoracic wall: A plea for radical surgery and caution when using liposomal amphotericin B. Interact Cardiovasc Thorac Surg 2003; 2(4):682–684.

22. Malik S, Giacoia GP. *Candida tropicalis* empyema associated with acquired gastropleural fistula in a newborn infant. Am J Perinatol 1989; 6(3):347–348.

23. Duffner F, Brandner S, Opitz H, et al. Primary *Candida albicans* empyema associated with epidural hematomas in craniocervical junction. Clin Neuropathol 1997; 16(3):143–146.

24. Weber KH, Wehmer W. Candida-Pleuraempyem nach Tonsillektomie. Thoracic empyema due to Candida after tonsillectomy. Munch Med Wochenschr 1970; 112(48):2170–2173.

25. Stringer JR, Beard CB, Miller RF, et al. A new name (*Pneumocystis jiroveci*) for pneumocystis from humans. Emerg Infect Dis 2002; 8(9):891–896.

26. DeLorenzo LJ, Huang CT, Maguire GP, et al. Roentgenographic patterns of *Pneumocystis carinii* pneumonia in 104 patients with AIDS. Chest 1987; 91(3):323–327.

Pleural Effusions Secondary to Fungal, Nocardial, and Actinomycotic Infection   *399*

27. Leoung GS, Feigal DW, Montgomery AB, et al. Aerosolized pentamidine for prophylaxis against *Pneumocystis carinii* pneumonia. The San Francisco community prophylaxis trial. N Engl J Med 1990; 323(12):769–775.
28. Pastores SM, Garay SM, Naidich DP, et al. Review: Pneumothorax in patients with AIDS-related *Pneumocystis carinii* pneumonia. Am J Med Sci 1996; 312(5):229–234.
29. Torres HA, Chemaly RF, Storey R, et al. Influence of type of cancer and hematopoietic stem cell transplantation on clinical presentation of *Pneumocystis jiroveci* pneumonia in cancer patients. Eur J Clin Microbiol Infect Dis 2006; 25(6):382–388.
30. Jayes RL, Kamerow HN, Hasselquist SM, et al. Disseminated pneumocystosis presenting as a pleural effusion. Chest 1993; 103(1):306–308.
31. Horowitz ML, Schiff M, Samuels J, et al. *Pneumocystis carinii* pleural effusion. Pathogenesis and pleural fluid analysis. Am Rev Respir Dis 1993; 148(1):232–234.
32. de Klerk AA, Bezuidenhout J, Bolliger CT. A young healthy woman presenting with acute meningitis and a large pleural-based mass. Respiration 2003; 70(6):655–657
33. Nunez M, Peacock JE, Chin R. Pulmonary cryptococcosis in the immunocompetent host. Therapy with oral fluconazole: A report of four cases and a review of the literature. Chest 2000; 118(2):527–534.
34. Aberg JA, Mundy LM, Powderly WG. Pulmonary cryptococcosis in patients without HIV infection. Chest 1999; 115(3):734–740.
35. Horowitz ID, Blumberg EA, Krevolin L. *Cryptococcus albidus* and mucormycosis empyema in a patient receiving hemodialysis. South Med J 1993; 86(9):1070–1072.
36. Shankar EM, Kumarasamy N, Bella D, et al. Pneumonia and pleural effusion due to *Cryptococcus laurentii* in a clinically proven case of AIDS. Can Respir J 2006; 13(5): 275–278.
37. Fukuchi M, Mizushima Y, Hori T, et al. Cryptococcal pleural effusion in a patient with chronic renal failure receiving long-term corticosteroid therapy for rheumatoid arthritis. Intern Med 1998; 37(6):534–537.
38. Bartrum RJ, Watnick M, Herman PG. Roentgenographic findings in pulmonary mucormycosis. Am J Roentgenol Radium Ther Nucl Med 1973; 117(4):810–815.
39. McAdams HP, Rosado-de-Christenson M, Strollo DC, et al. Pulmonary mucormycosis: Radiologic findings in 32 cases. AJR Am J Roentgenol 1997; 168(6):1541–1548.
40. Chamilos G, Marom EM, Lewis RE, et al. Predictors of pulmonary zygomycosis versus invasive pulmonary aspergillosis in patients with cancer. Clin Infect Dis 2005; 41(1):60–66.
41. George RB, Penn RL. Histoplasmosis. In: Sarosi GA, Davies SF, eds. Fungal Diseases of the Lung. New York, NY: Raven Press, 1993:39–50.
42. Brewer PL, Himmelwright JP. Pleural effusion due to infection with *Histoplasma capsulatum*. Chest 1970; 58(1):76–79.
43. Gluckman TJ, Corbridge T. Isolated pleural effusion with pleural fibrosis in a patient with subacute progressive disseminated histoplasmosis. Clin Infect Dis 1998; 26(6):1477–1478.
44. Connell JV, Muhm JR. Radiographic manifestations of pulmonary histoplasmosis: A 10-year review. Radiology 1976; 121(2):281–285.
45. Straus SE, Jacobson ES. The spectrum of histoplasmosis in a general hospital: A review of 55 cases diagnosed at Barnes Hospital between 1966 and 1977. Am J Med Sci 1980; 279(3):147–158.
46. Sutaria MK, Polk JW, Reddy P, et al. Surgical aspects of pulmonary histoplasmosis. A series of 110 cases. Thorax 1970; 25(1):31–40.
47. Picardi JL, Kauffman CA, Schwarz J, et al. Pericarditis caused by *Histoplasma capsulatum*. Am J Cardiol 1976; 37(1):82–88.
48. Swinburne AJ, Fedullo AJ, Wahl GW, et al. Histoplasmoma, pleural fibrosis, and slowly enlarging pleural effusion in an asymptomatic patient. Am Rev Respir Dis 1987; 135(2): 502–503.

49. Kilburn CD, McKinsey DS. Recurrent massive pleural effusion due to pleural, pericardial, and epicardial fibrosis in histoplasmosis. Chest 1991; 100(6):1715–1717.
50. Blastomycosis Cooperative Study of the Veterans Administartion. Blastomycosis I: A review of 198 collected cases in Veterans Administration hospitals. Am Rev Respir Dis 1964; 89: 659–672.
51. Sarosi GA, Hammerman KJ, Tosh FE, et al. Clinical features of acute pulmonary blastomycosis. N Engl J Med 1974; 290(10):540–543.
52. Rabinowitz JG, Busch J, Buttram WR. Pulmonary manifestations of blastomycosis. Radiological support of a new concept. Radiology 1976; 120(1):25–32.
53. Kinasewitz GT, Penn RL, George RB. The spectrum and significance of pleural disease in blastomycosis. Chest 1984; 86(4):580–584.
54. Sheflin JR, Campbell JA, Thompson GP. Pulmonary blastomycosis: Findings on chest radiographs in 63 patients. AJR Am J Roentgenol 1990; 154(6):1177–1180.
55. Patel RG, Patel B, Petrini MF, et al. Clinical presentation, radiographic findings, and diagnostic methods of pulmonary blastomycosis: A review of 100 consecutive cases. South Med J 1999; 92(3):289–295.
56. Vasquez JE, Mehta JB, Agrawal R, et al. Blastomycosis in northeast Tennessee. Chest 1998; 114(2):436–443.
57. Failla PJ, Cerise FP, Karam GH, et al. Blastomycosis: Pulmonary and pleural manifestations. South Med J 1995; 88(4):405–410.
58. Wiesman IM, Podbielski FJ, Hernan MJ, et al. Thoracic blastomycosis and empyema. JSLS 1999; 3(1):75–78.
59. Galgiani JN, Catanzaro A, Cloud GA, et al. Comparison of oral fluconazole and itraconazole for progressive, nonmeningeal coccidioidomycosis. A randomized, double-blind trial. Mycoses Study Group. Ann Intern Med 2000; 133(9):676–686.
60. Youssef SS, Ramu V, Sarubbi FA. Unusual case of pyopneumothorax in Tennessee. South Med J. 2005; 98(11):1139–1141.
61. Lonky SA, Catanzaro A, Moser KM, et al. Acute coccidioidal pleural effusion. Am Rev Respir Dis 1976; 114(4):681–688.
62. Benard G, Orii NM, Marques HH, et al. Severe acute paracoccidioidomycosis in children. Pediatr Infect Dis J 1994; 13(6):510–515.
63. Paniago AM, de Freitas AC, Aguiar ES, et al. Paracoccidioidomycosis in patients with human immunodeficiency virus: Review of 12 cases observed in an endemic region in Brazil. J Infect 2005; 51(3):248–252.
64. Fields CL, Ossorio MA, Roy TM. Empyema associated with pulmonary sporotrichosis. South Med J 1989; 82(7):910–913.
65. Kauffman CA, Hajjeh R, Chapman SW. Practice guidelines for the management of patients with Sporotrichosis. Clin Infect Dis 2000; 30(4):684–687.
66. Bates M, Cruickshank G. Thoracic actinomycosis. Thorax 1957; 12:99–124.
67. Kinnear WJ, MacFarlane JT. A survey of thoracic actinomycosis. Respir Med 1990; 84(1): 57–59.
68. Merdler C, Greif J, Burke M, et al. Primary actinomycotic empyema. South Med J 1983; 76(3):411–412.
69. Varkey B, Landis FB, Tang TT, et al. Thoracic actinomycosis. Dissemination to skin, subcutaneous tissue, and muscle. Arch Intern Med 1974; 134(4):689–693.
70. Webb WR, Sagel SS. Actinomycosis involving the chest wall: CT findings. AJR Am J Roentgenol 1982; 139(5):1007–1009.
71. Thompson AJ, Carty H. Pulmonary actinomycosis in children. Pediatr Radiol 1979; 8(1): 7–9.
72. Zeebregts CJ, van der Heyden AH, Ligtvoet EE, et al. Transphrenic dissemination of actinomycosis. Thorax 1996; 51(4):449–450.

73. O'Sullivan RA, Armstrong JG, Rivers JT, et al. Pulmonary actinomycosis complicated by effusive constrictive pericarditis. Aust N Z J Med 1991; 21(6):879–880.
74. Legum LL, Greer KE, Glessner SF. Disseminated actinomycosis. South Med J 1978; 71(4):463–465.
75. Skoutelis A, Petrochilos J, Bassaris H. Successful treatment of thoracic actinomycosis with ceftriaxone. Clin Infect Dis 1994; 19(1):161–162.
76. Olson ES, Simpson AJ, Norton AJ, et al. Not everything acid fast is *Mycobacterium tuberculosis*—A case report. J Clin Pathol 1998; 51(7):535–536.
77. Cremades MJ, Menendez R, Santos M, et al. Repeated pulmonary infection by *Nocardia asteroides* complex in a patient with bronchiectasis. Respiration 1998; 65(3):211–213.
78. Conant EF, Wechsler RJ. Actinomycosis and nocardiosis of the lung. J Thorac Imaging 1992; 7(4):75–84.
79. Buckley JA, Padhani AR, Kuhlman JE. CT features of pulmonary nocardiosis. J Comput Assist Tomogr 1995; 19(5):726–732.
80. Yoon HK, Im JG, Ahn JM, et al. Pulmonary nocardiosis: CT findings. J Comput Assist Tomogr 1995; 19(1):52–55.
81. Brechot JM, Capron F, Prudent J, et al. Unexpected pulmonary nocardiosis in a non-immunocompromised patient. Thorax 1987; 42(6):479–480.
82. Soubani AO, Ibrahim I, Forlenza S. Simultaneous nocardial empyema and *Pneumocystis carinii* pneumonia as an initial manifestation of HIV infection. South Med J 1993; 86(11):1318–1319.
83. Huang HC, Yu WL, Shieh CC, et al. Unusual mixed infection of thoracic empyema caused by *Mycobacteria tuberculosis*, nontuberculosis mycobacteria and *Nocardia asteroides* in a woman with systemic lupus erythematosus. J Infect 2007; 54(1):e25–e28.

24

Malignant Pleural Effusions

STEVEN A. SAHN
Division of Pulmonary, Critical Care, Allergy and Sleep Medicine, Medical University of South Carolina, Charleston, South Carolina, U.S.A.

I. Introduction

Malignant pleural effusions, a common consequence of malignancy, cause substantial morbidity for those inflicted. With the virtual epidemic of lung cancer and breast cancer, both in the United States and worldwide, clinicians will face the challenge of managing patients with malignant pleural effusions, as the aforementioned cancers are the most common cause of these effusions. For example, in the United States, there are approximately 160,000 deaths due to lung cancer and 44,000 deaths due to breast cancer annually (1). Based on the reported incidence of malignant pleural effusions in lung cancer (8–15%) and breast cancer (2–12%), clinicians in the United States can expect to care for approximately 75,000 patients a year with malignant pleural effusions due to lung cancer and 30,000 patients annually with breast cancer (1). With the estimated incidence of malignant pleural effusion of 7% in lymphoma and the contribution from non–lung primaries, more than 150,000 cases of malignant pleural effusions are diagnosed in the United States annually (1).

The primary goal of palliation in these patients is relief of breathlessness. Decisions relating to palliation should be determined only after global evaluation of the patient and should not be based on a single factor. This chapter discusses the pathogenesis, clinical manifestations, radiographic features, diagnostic techniques, prognosis, and management of patients with malignant pleural effusions.

II. Pathogenesis of Metastasis and Effusions

Autopsy studies report several mechanisms for pleural metastases including (*i*) pulmonary vascular invasion with tumor emboli to the visceral pleural surface (the major mechanism in lung cancer) with subsequent seeding of the parietal pleura, (*ii*) direct pleural tumor invasion (lung and breast cancer), (*iii*) hematogenous metastases to the parietal pleura from extra-pulmonary primaries, and (*iv*) lymphatic involvement (2–5).

The precise mechanisms of pleural metastasis have not been clearly delineated. However, it is clear that for tumor to metastasize to a distant site, such as the pleura, a succession of events needs to occur. Only if these sequential processes develop, will the tumor cells seed the pleura and result in independent growth. These processes—adhesion, migration, propagation, and angiogenesis—appear to be mediated by the interaction of mesothelial and neoplastic cells (6,7). Initially, the primary malignant cell must detach from the core tumor. Secondly, the malignant cell must adhere to and penetrate through the wall of the blood vessel. Third, migration must occur from the vasculature to the pleural surface. Lastly, for the potentiation of local growth and spread of the tumor, autocrine growth factors need to be operative and angiogenesis needs to be induced. Several systems may influence the remodeling with the stroma of neoplasms and growth of the tumor in the pleural space. Both the procoagulant and fibrinolytic systems (8,9) and the urokinase–urokinase receptor systems have been linked to the invasiveness of malignant mesothelioma cells and may be operative in other malignancies (10,11).

Tumors may produce specific growth, permeability, and adhesion-related factors. Vascular endothelial growth factor (VEGF), an important angiogenic factor, results in both new vessel formation and an alteration of mesothelial permeability (12). In addition, IL-8 functions as a growth factor for both malignant melanoma and mesothelial cells (13). The present evidence suggests that an interaction between the malignant cell, the mesothelial cell, and their extracellular matrix prevents the host from controlling the malignant cells and the independent growth and function of these cells on the pleura.

A malignant pleural effusion is defined by identifying malignant cells in pleural fluid. These effusions are developed by several mechanisms including increased capillary permeability, impaired lymphatic drainage from the pleural space, thoracic duct rupture, and pericardial involvement.

At times, a patient presents with a known malignancy and a pleural effusion but malignant cells cannot be documented in pleural fluid; these effusions are termed "paramalignant" and are usually related to the primary tumor but malignant cells have not been shed into the pleural space (14) (Table 1). Examples of paramalignant effusions include endobronchial obstruction with pneumonia and parapneumonic effusion or a transudative effusion from atelectasis, a transudative effusion from low oncotic pressure from severe malnutrition, and chylothorax from thoracic duct obstruction. Radiation and chemotherapy can also be causative. On occasion, a pleural effusion that may develop is unrelated to the malignancy, such as from congestive heart failure. Therefore, it is important to establish the precise cause of the effusion, as it will relate to prognosis (infra vide).

III. Clinical Features

Breathlessness is the most common presenting symptom in patients with malignant pleural effusions, occurring in more than half of the patients (4). Because malignant pleural effusions represent an advanced stage of the malignancy, patients may also have systemic manifestations, such as malaise, anorexia, and weight loss (4) (Table 2). The pathogenesis of dyspnea from a large pleural effusion has not been clearly defined; however, several factors may be operative including decreased chest-wall compliance, contralateral mediastinal shift, ipsilateral diaphragm depression, decreased ipsilateral lung volume, and reflex stimulation from receptors in the chest wall and lung parenchyma (15).

While dull, aching chest pain is common in malignant mesothelioma (16), it is relatively uncommon in the patient with lung cancer (4). In contrast, the patient with malignant pleural effusion and hemoptysis suggests that the underlying malignancy is bronchogenic cancer and not mesothelioma or an extra lung primary. A known history of malignancy is an important historical finding, as is occupational exposure, particularly asbestos, which should increase the suspicion for lung cancer or mesothelioma.

Table 1 Paramalignant Pleural Effusions

Cause	Comments
Local effects of tumor	
Lymphatic obstruction	Important mechanism for pleural fluid accumulation
Bronchial obstruction with pneumonia	Parapneumonic effusion; does not exclude operability in lung cancer
Bronchial obstruction with atelectasis	Transudate; does not exclude operability in lung cancer
Lung entrapment	An exudative effusion due to an unexpandable lung and malignant/fibrotic involvement of the pleura
Chylothorax	Disruption of thoracic duct; non-Hodgkin lymphoma most common cause
Superior vena cava syndrome	Transudate; due to an acute increase in systemic venous pressure
Malignant pericardial effusion	Transudative/exudative effusion due to increased pulmonary & systemic venous pressures
Systemic effects of tumor	
Pulmonary embolism	Hypercoagulable state associated with adenocarcinoma
Hypoalbuminemia	Serum albumin < 1.5 g/dL; associated with anasarca
Complications of therapy	
Radiation therapy	
Early	Pleuritis 6 wk to 6 mo after radiation completed; loculated exudative effusion to tends to resolve in 3–4 mo Fibrosis of mediastinum
Late	Constrictive pericarditis
	Mediastinal lymphatic fibrosis
	Myocardial fibrosis
	Vena caval obstruction
Chemotherapy	
Cyclophosphamide	Pleuropericarditis
Dasatinib	18–28% with effusions; may be dose related
Docetaxel	An exudate from increased capillary permeabililty
Imatinib	Pleuropericarditis
Methotrexate	Pleuritis or effusion; ± blood eosinophilia
Mitomycin/bleomycin	Associated with interstitial disease
Procarbazine	Blood eosinophilia; fever and chills

Adapted from Ref. 14.

Because most of the patients presenting with a malignant pleural effusion have a moderate volume of fluid in the pleural space, the typical physical findings of a pleural effusion are present (4). Lymphadenopathy and cachexia are seen in less than half of the patients at presentation (Table 2).

A malignant pleural effusion should be the primary consideration when an older individual (in the 6th or 7th decade) presents with a unilateral effusion or bilateral pleural effusions with a normal heart size and the insidious onset of dyspnea or a patient with a known malignancy develops a pleural effusion.

Table 2 Clinical Manifestations with Carcinomatous Pleural Effusions on Admission to Hospital ($n = 96$)

Symptoms	Patients No.	%	Physical findings	Patients No.	%
Dyspnea	55	57	Pleural effusion	88	92
Cough	41	43	Cachexia	35	37
Weight loss	31	32	Adenopathy	20	21
Chest pain	25	26	Fever	9	9
Malaise	21	22	Chest-wall tenderness	4	4
Anorexia	14	15	Clubbing	2	2
Fever	8	8	Pleural rub	2	2
Chills	5	5	Cyanosis	2	2
Asymptomatic	22	23			

Source: Adapted from Ref. 4.

IV. Radiologic Findings

At presentation, patients with metastatic carcinoma to the pleura typically have >1000 cm^3 of fluid in the pleural space (4). While small effusions (estimated <500 cm^3) are seen in about 10% of these patients, an additional 10% present with a massive pleural effusion, which involves the entire hemithorax (4). In the majority of patients who present with a massive pleural effusion, malignancy is the most likely diagnosis (17); this volume of fluid typically results in contralateral mediastinal shift, diaphragm depression, and outward movement of the chest wall (Fig. 1). The tumor responsible for this radiographic finding is usually from an extrapulmonic primary (18). However, when there is an absence of contralateral mediastinal shift with an apparent large pleural effusion, lung cancer involving the ipsilateral mainstem bronchus should be suspected (18) (Fig. 2). Other causes of the absence of contralateral mediastinal shift include malignant mesothelioma, fixation of the mediastinum due to malignant lymph nodes, or rarely marked tumor infiltration of the parenchyma.

The presence of bilateral pleural effusions with a heart of normal size makes malignancy a possible diagnosis, usually the result of an extrapulmonic primary (19) (Fig. 3). However, transudative effusions from nephrotic syndrome, hypoalbuminemia, hepatic hydrothorax, and constrictive pericarditis, and exudative effusions from lupus pleuritis and yellow nail syndrome can also cause the aforementioned radiographic findings. While patients with lung cancer and lymphoma often show other radiographic abnormalities in addition to the effusion, patients with extrathoracic primary malignancies usually present with a pleural effusion as the only radiographic abnormality.

Computed tomography (CT) of the chest may be helpful in the evaluation of patients with a malignant effusion by demonstrating mediastinal lymph node involvement, parenchymal disease, and airway involvement that cannot be detected on standard chest radiograph (20). In addition, CT scan can identify pleural abnormalities and distant metastases. If pleural plaques are noted as a sign of asbestos exposure, lung cancer and malignant mesothelioma need to be considered. Magnetic resonance imaging (MRI) may be helpful in evaluating chest-wall involvement (21). Positron emission tomography (PET scanning) may be helpful in evaluating the extent of pleural involvement in malignant

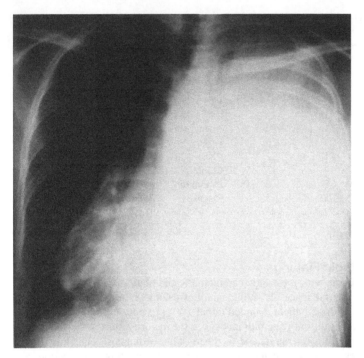

Figure 1 Posteroanterior chest radiograph of a woman with cervical carcinoma metastatic to the left pleura and mediastinum resulting in a massive pleural effusion with contralateral mediastinal shift. *Source*: Adapted from Ref. 140.

mesothelioma (22), and a PET–CT pattern of pleural uptake and increased effusion activity has a high predictive value for detecting a malignant effusion, and a negative PET–CT favors a benign effusion.

V. Diagnosis

A. Pleural Fluid Analysis

Virtually, all patients with an undiagnosed pleural effusion should undergo a diagnostic thoracocentesis. A total of 30 to 50 cm^3 of pleural fluid is all that is necessary for diagnostic studies. Malignant pleural effusions can be serous, hemorrhagic, or grossly bloody. The nucleated cell count is typically low (<3000/μL) and consists mainly of lymphocytes, macrophages, and mesothelial cells (4). About half of the time in carcinomatous pleural effusions, lymphocytes range from 50% to 70% of the nucleated cells and are typically >80% of the nucleated cells in lymphomatous effusions (23).

The pleural fluid is an exudate (4,24) but, on rare occasions, can be transudative, if the patient has a concomitant disease such as congestive heart failure, atelectasis from endobronchial obstruction, or is in the early phase of lymphatic obstruction (4,24,25). The absolute LDH value usually satisfies exudative criteria when compared to the upper

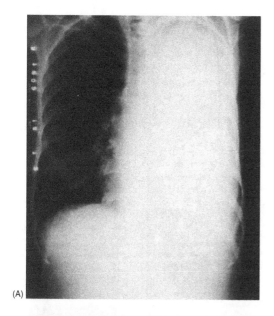

(A)

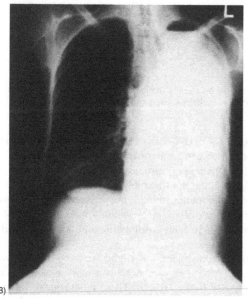

(B)

Figure 2 (**A**) Posteroanterior chest radiograph of a woman with small-cell lung cancer with total obstruction of the left mainstem bronchus. There is complete opacification of the left hemithorax with minimal ipsilateral mediastinal shift. (**B**) Posteroanterior chest radiograph following thoracentesis with resultant accentuation of ipsilateral mediastinal shift due to the increased intrapleural negative pressure from removal of pleural fluid in the setting of complete lung collapse. *Source*: Adapted from Ref. 141

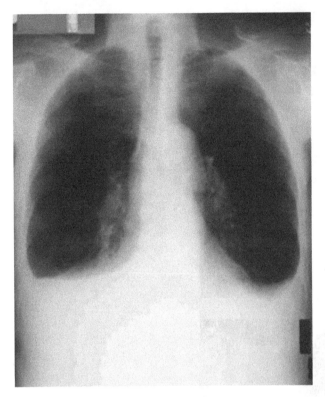

Figure 3 Posteroanterior chest radiograph of an elderly man with prostate cancer metastatic to mediastinum and pleura. Note bilateral effusions with a normal heart size.

limits of normal of the serum [either 0.45 (26), 0.67 (24), or 0.82 (27)]. Either the pleural fluid/serum protein ratio or the LDH criterion can be in the transudative range depending on the degree of capillary leak and the inflammatory process, respectively. However, in virtually all patients, the fluid is exudative if the fluid is solely from malignancy.

The presence of pleural fluid eosinophilia should not dissuade the clinician from pursuing the diagnosis of malignancy. Two investigations have demonstrated that the prevalence of malignancy is similar in both eosinophilic and non-eosinophilic effusions (28,29).

A low pleural fluid pH ($<$7.30) and a low pleural fluid glucose ($<$60 mg/dL) with a normal serum glucose or a PF/serum glucose ratio of $<$0.5 is a marker of advanced disease in the pleural space with increased tumor burden. These biochemical findings are associated with a decreased survival, a higher sensitivity of diagnosis by initial cytologic examination and pleural biopsy, and less-successful pleurodesis compared to those patients with a pH $\geq$7.30 and glucose $\geq$60 mg/dL (30–33).

A total of 10% to 14% of patients with malignant pleural effusions have an increased amylase concentration (34). Isoenzyme analysis demonstrates that the amylase is composed predominantly of the salivary type (34,35). Adenocarcinoma of the lung is the most common cause of a salivary amylase–rich pleural effusion with adenocarcinoma of the ovary being the next most frequent. A high–salivary amylase content has been found in tissue from adenocarcinoma of the lung. Clinically, the finding of an elevated pleural fluid amylase, in the absence of esophageal rupture, virtually establishes the diagnosis of a malignant pleural effusion.

B. Cytology

Pleural fluid cytology is the least invasive method for diagnosing a malignant pleural effusion. With improvement in cytological techniques and appropriate specimen handling, exfoliative cytology is diagnostic in 60% to 90% of patients with the sensitivity depending on the extent of pleural involvement and the primary malignancy (36–40); most malignant effusions are due to adenocarcinomas. However, it is problematic to determine the true sensitivity and specificity of malignancy in pleural fluid. The only "gold standard" would be a postmortem following thoracocentesis (41). While some investigators recommend the routine use of cell blocks and cytology smears (42,43), others have shown that the routine use of cell blocks is not cost-effective (41). It appears that the volume of fluid submitted to the cytology laboratory does not alter the diagnostic yield.

C. Pleural Biopsy

Percutaneous pleural biopsy is a blind sampling procedure whose sensitivity varies between 40% and 75% (39,40,44–46), depending on the extent of parietal pleural involvement, number and adequacy of biopsies obtained, and the experience of the operator. A reason for a low yield of percutaneous biopsy in early metastatic disease to the pleura is that the initial lesions tend to be established on the mediastinal and diaphragmatic pleurae with later progression cephalad along the costal parietal pleura (47).

D. Thoracoscopy

In a sequential study of pleural fluid cytology, percutaneous pleural biopsy and medical thoracoscopy in 208 consecutive patients, the diagnostic sensitivity of malignancy was 62%, 44%, and 95%, respectively (40). Similar results have been reported by others (48).

Medical thoracoscopy and video-assisted thoracic surgery (VATS) are clearly the most sensitive diagnostic procedures and approach 100% with experienced operators. Even in the early stages of pleural involvement, the yield with thoracoscopy can be high with a thorough examination by a skilled thoracoscopist. The reasons for false-negative thoracoscopies include operator inexperience (48), incomplete examination due to pleural adhesions (48,49), and insufficient and non-representative tissue samples.

Medical thoracoscopy, primarily a diagnostic procedure, can be performed using local anesthesia with conscious sedation in an endoscopy suite using non-disposable rigid instruments, making it less invasive and costly than VATS. In contrast, VATS requires general anesthesia and single-lung ventilation. A more extensive procedure can be accomplished with VATS compared to medical thoracoscopy and the treatment is often combined with diagnosis. Substantial adhesions, which may prevent thoracoscopy, can be suspected by chest radiograph, chest CT, or ultrasonography. When extensive adhesions are appreciated at the time of VATS, the surgeon can convert to an open procedure. Adhesions most commonly result from repeated thoracenteses or previous pleurodesis attempts (49).

E. Other Studies

With relatively low sensitivity and specificity, immunohistochemical staining with mono-clonal antibodies to tumor markers and chromosomal analysis are not reliable for diagno-sis. There are circumstances, however, where these tests may be useful, such as chromoso-mal analysis (50) in lymphomatous and leukemic effusions and flow cytometry (51) with identification of DNA aneuploidy for detection of a false negative with initial cytologic screen. Tumor markers, such as CEA, LEU-1, and mucin, may be helpful in differentiat-ing adenocarcinomas from mesothelioma (52–54). Elevated soluble mesothelin levels in serum and pleural fluid may be helpful in differentiating a malignant mesothelioma from benign disease; however, mesothelin can also be increased with carcinoma (55).

VI. Management

The major indication for palliation in patients with a malignant pleural effusion is relief of dyspnea. The degree of dyspnea is dependent not only on the volume of pleural fluid, but also on the underlying condition of the lungs and pleura. When palliation is considered, in addition to the patient's degree of breathlessness, their general health, functional status, and expected survival need to be assessed. The most favorable outcome with talc pleurodesis has been observed in women with an expandable lung, Karnofsky scores >60%, and those with BMI >25 kg/m^2 (56).

A. Therapeutic Thoracocentesis

Therapeutic thoracocentesis should be performed in virtually all dyspneic patients with a malignant pleural effusion to determine its effect on breathlessness and the rate and degree of recurrence. However, some clinicians choose to proceed directly to small-bore chest tube drainage and chemical pleurodesis or thoracoscopy with talc poudrage in dyspneic patients with large pleural effusions and contralateral mediastinal shift. Rapid recurrence (within two weeks) of the effusion following therapeutic thoracocentesis dictates the need for treatment, while stabilization with relief of dyspnea may warrant observation. When dyspnea is not relieved by thoracocentesis, other causes of breathlessness should be considered, such as lymphangitic carcinomatosis, atelectasis, tumor embolism, throm-boembolism, unilateral pulmonary edema, and lung entrapment. Those with significant unexpandable lung due to tumor involvement of the visceral pleura may not obtain sub-stantial relief and always develop significant anterior chest pain that can be relieved by allowing air entry into the pleural space to increase pleural pressure.

Therapeutic thoracocentesis may be the sole therapeutic option in patients with far-advanced disease, poor performance status, tumors associated with a poor survival, and very low pleural fluid pH. These patients can be managed with periodic outpatient thoracenteses or placement of an indwelling catheter rather than hospitalization for chest tube pleurodesis or VATS that are associated with morbidity and higher costs.

The volume of fluid that can be removed safely from the pleural space is unknown in an individual patient. Monitoring pleural fluid pressure during thoracocentesis would be optimal but is not routinely performed (57–63). Therefore, it is recommended, in the setting of contralateral mediastinal shift on chest radiograph, that a large volume (1–2 L) thoracocentesis can be accomplished, monitoring for the development of anterior chest pain or dyspnea (61,62). It is evident that the operator is not aware of a precipitous decrease in pleural pressure, and the first sign of an unexpandable lung is typically the development of significant anterior chest pain. However, if the pre-thoracocentesis chest radiograph shows ipsilateral or absence of mediastinal shift, the likelihood of an unexpandable lung is increased and caution should be exercised during thoracocentesis. Re-expansion pulmonary edema rarely occurs after rapid removal of either air or fluid from the pleural space and may not be related to the absolute level of negative pleural pressure. The mechanism of pulmonary edema is believed to be increased capillary permeability with the injury related to mechanical forces causing vascular stretching during re-expansion (64) or to ischemia reperfusion associated with oxidants (65).

B. Unexpandable Lung

In the setting of malignancy, an unexpandable lung occurs when a large tumor burden or tumor-induced fibrosis prevents partial or complete lung expansion to the chest wall. In the area where the lung cannot expand, a space in vacuo is created, which increases the pleural interstitial/pleural space pressure gradient, resulting in fluid movement from the interstitium of the parietal pleura and probably the lung into the pleural space to create a new steady state of formation and resorption of fluid (61,66,67). If fluid is withdrawn from the pleural space, the same volume will recur rapidly within 48 to 96 hours. An unexpandable lung is highly likely if any of the following criteria in the absence of endobronchial obstruction or chronic atelectasis is present: (1) failure of the lung to expand completely after most of the fluid has been removed by therapeutic thoracocentesis, as demonstrated by chest imaging; (2) an initial pleural fluid pressure of ≤ 5 cm H_2O (57,58,60,62,63); and (3) a decrease in pleural fluid pressure of ≥ 15 cm H_2O/L of fluid removed (60,62,63). It is futile to attempt pleurodesis in a patient with an extensive unexpandable lung. However, patients with unexpandable lung due to malignancy will have some relief of dyspnea with therapeutic thoracocentesis. In these patients, the fluid in the pleural space is produced both by the malignancy and the unexpandable lung (61). The patient has relief of breathlessness with removal of the "malignancy fluid" and subsequently develops severe anterior chest pain when pleural pressure decreases from the unexpandable lung.

C. Chemotherapy and Radiation

Malignant pleural effusions likely to respond favorably to chemotherapy include those from small-cell lung cancer (68), breast carcinoma (69–71), lymphoma, prostate cancer, ovarian cancer, germ cell tumor, and thyroid cancer. All other malignant pleural effusions are unlikely to be controlled by chemotherapy alone. In lymphomatous chylothorax, mediastinal radiation (72) may be effective and pleuroperitoneal shunt (73) may be helpful in failed therapy, as it can recirculate chyle. When chemotherapy is unavailable, contraindicated, or has become ineffective, local therapy such as pleurodesis should be considered.

D. Pleurodesis

Chemical pleurodesis is an accepted palliative treatment for patients with recurrent, symptomatic pleural effusions. A number of chemical agents have been used for pleurodesis; however, adequate assessment of the effectiveness of these agents has been problematic

Table 3 Success Rates of Commonly Used Agents for Pleurodesis in Malignant Pleural
Effusions (n = 952)

Chemical agent	Patients (n)	Complete successᵃ (n)	Complete success (%)	Dose
Talc	165	153	93	2.5–10 g
Corynebacterium parvum	169	129	76	3.5–14 mg
Doxycycline	60	43	72	500 mg (often multiple doses)
Tetracycline	359	240	67	500 mg–20 mg/kg
Bleomycin	199	108	54	15–240 units

ᵃComplete success: absence of re-accumulation of effusion (CXR or clinical).
Source: Adapted from Ref. 74.

because: (*i*) reported series have evaluated small numbers of patients, (*ii*) different pleurodesis techniques have been employed, (*iii*) different criteria for success have been used, and (*iv*) patients have been followed for varying time periods. In addition, there have been limited studies of direct comparisons between agents under similar conditions in similar patient populations. Furthermore, few studies have prospectively evaluated adverse effects.

Walker-Renard and colleagues (74) analyzed 1168 patients who received chemical pleurodesis as reported in the English language literature from 1966 through 1992. They found a complete response rate of 64% (752 of 1168), defined as no recurrence of the effusion determined by clinical examination or chest radiograph. Talc was the most effective agent with a complete response rate of 93% with *Corynebacterium parvum* being successful in 76%, doxycycline in 72%, tetracycline in 67%, and bleomycin in 54% (Table 3). The most commonly reported adverse effects with all agents in 1140 patients were chest pain (23%) and fever (19%) with the incidence varying between agents (74) (Table 4). Talc was found to be superior to both bleomycin and tetracycline in comparative studies of pleurodesis success (75–77).

Talc Pleurodesis

On literature review, when analyzed by method of administration, pleurodesis by poudrage (418 of 461) and slurry (168 of 185) had similar success rates of 91% (78). In a small

Table 4 Incidence of Chest Pain and Fever with Chemical Pleurodesis (n = 918)

Chemical agent	Patients (n)	Chest pain (%)	Fever (%)
Talc	131	7	16
Corynebacterium parvum	169	43	59
Doxycycline	60	40	31
Tetracycline	359	14	10
Bleomycin	199	28	24

Source: Adapted from Ref. 74.

series of 57 patients randomized to receive 5 g of either talc slurry through a chest tube or talc poudrage with thoracoscopy, no difference in recurrence was found between the two methods (79). A large, randomized multicenter trial also found no difference in the success rate between talc poudrage and talc slurry, but reported a lower efficacy of 70% (80).

The most common adverse effects of talc pleurodesis are fever (16%) and chest pain (7%) (74). Fever following talc pleurodesis typically occurs 4 to 12 hours after instillation or insufflation with a duration of up to 72 hours (81). It is rare for the fever to exceed 102.4°F. Empyema has been reported with talc slurry (0–11%) and with talc poudrage (0–3%) (81). Isolated cardiovascular events such as arrhythmias, cardiac arrest, chest pain, myocardial infarction, and hypotension have been documented, but it is unclear whether these complications are the result of the procedure itself, are related to talc per se, or the patient's comorbidities (81).

There has been concern about acute respiratory failure following talc pleurodesis. In a review of the English language literature from 1958 through 2001 in an attempt to determine the incidence and causality of acute respiratory failure following talc pleurodesis, the author found 3064 patients with malignant pleural effusions, 1009 with pneumothorax, and 178 patients with nonmalignant effusions treated with either talc slurry or talc poudrage (81–98). There were 43 patients who developed acute respiratory failure, 41 (1.3%) occurred in patients with malignant effusions, 2 (0.2%) patients with pneumothorax, and none with nonmalignant effusion. Therefore, of the 4252 patients who received talc poudrage and slurry pleurodesis, there was a 1% incidence of acute respiratory failure reported. After careful reading of these manuscripts, it was my opinion that approximately half of the reported cases of acute respiratory failure either provided no information that allowed determination of the cause of the acute respiratory failure, occurred in severely compromised patients (severe underlying COPD, widespread tumor involving the lung and mediastinum) (81), or received excess narcotics (81). In a report from de Campos and colleagues (89) of 614 patients who received talc pleurodesis, 7 (1.5%) of 457 patients with malignant pleural effusions developed acute respiratory failure; 2 of these patients had received multiple pulmonary and pleural biopsies prior to poudrage, 1 patient had lymphoma of the mediastinum and bilateral chylothoraces and had bilateral talc poudrage, and the other 4 patients were described as having "very limited pulmonary reserve." None of the 108 patients with nonmalignant effusions or 49 patients with pneumothorax developed respiratory failure following talc pleurodesis (89).

In a retrospective review of complications of talc pleurodesis from 1993 to 1997 with 78 patients who had 89 pleurodeses, a number of respiratory complications were noted (87). Seventy patients received talc slurry, with 5 g of talc used in 85 of the pleurodeses. Seven patients were reported with ARDS who had eight pleurodesis procedures. One of the patients with AIDS and *Pneumocystis carinii* (Jerovecii) pneumonia-induced pneumothorax had bilateral simultaneous talc pleurodeses preceded by a pleural abrasion. The other six patients all had malignant pleural effusions, two had pleural abrasion prior to talc poudrage, while the other four had only talc slurry pleurodesis. Therefore, it would have been more appropriate for the authors to state that with 89 pleurodeses, four patients developed ARDS, which may have been solely related to talc.

Recently, in a multi-center, open-label prospective cohort study, 558 patients with malignant pleural effusions were treated with thoracoscopic talc poudrage with 4 g of calibrated French large-particle talc. No patients developed ARDS. Seven (1.2%) patients had nonfatal postthoracoscopy complications, including one patient with respiratory failure from unexplained bilateral pneumothoraces (88).

Possible causes for acute respiratory failure following talc pleurodesis include a systemic inflammatory syndrome (SIRS) or ARDS from talc, re-expansion pulmonary edema, excess premedication, severe comorbidities, terminal malignancy, sepsis from unsterile talc or poor chest tube technique, and excess talc (high-dose or bilateral sequential pleurodesis). If talc is the culprit, it is likely caused by the talc preparation with a large percentage of very small talc particles <30 μm in diameter (97).

Long-term studies have not shown development of mesothelioma with the use of asbestos-free talc (98–101). In a short-term follow-up of patients receiving talc poudrage for pneumothorax, no difference in lung function was found when compared to patients who received a thoracotomy without talc poudrage (102,103). Twenty-two to 35 years following talc poudrage for pneumothorax, total lung capacity was 89% of predicted in 46 patients compared to 97% of predicted for 29 patients treated with tube thoracostomy alone (102). Although a minimal reduction in total lung capacity was found following talc poudrage, as well as pleural thickening observed on chest radiograph, these changes were not clinically significant. None of the 46 patients who received talc poudrage developed mesothelioma over the similar time of follow-up (102). Although a link has been found between talc and cancer in those who mine and process talc (103), the association has been attributed to asbestos exposure, which is commonly found with talc, rather than with talc per se. In a group of patients who received talc pleurodesis for pneumothorax and had long-term follow-up, there was no increased incidence of lung cancer (101).

Presently, with the available data on talc pleurodesis, the following conclusions are reasonable: (*i*) both poudrage and slurry are effective for treating malignant pleural effusions, nonmalignant effusions, and pneumothoraces; (*ii*) poudrage and slurry appear to be equally effective in the management of malignant pleural effusions; (*iii*) long-term (up to 35 years) safety has been documented; (*iv*) acute respiratory failure has been reported in approximately 1% of over 4200 patients, virtually all of whom had malignant pleural effusions; (*v*) in approximately half of the patients with acute respiratory failure, factors other than talc could be implicated, such as prior pleural abrasion or biopsies, bilateral pleurodeses were performed, or the patient had severe underlying pulmonary disease; and (*vi*) talc-induced acute respiratory failure is most likely attributed to the use of small-particle–size talc.

To virtually eliminate the possibility of talc-induced acute respiratory failure, the sterility of talc should be assured, a high percentage of talc particles should be >30 μm and only 10% should be <5 μm in diameter, the absence of endotoxin should be documented, not more than 4 g of talc should be used, pleural abrasion and multiple biopsies should be avoided prior to pleurodesis, and pleurodesis should not be attempted in terminal patients or those with marginal lung function.

Clinicians should be aware that following talc pleurodesis, pleural abnormalities are common and include pleural thickening, loculated effusions, pleural nodules, and pleural masses. Focal pleural lesions have been documented up to 3.7 cm in size, and these lesions commonly enhance on contrast CT. These lesions are typically not only observed in the posterior basilar regions of the chest but also may be observed in paravertebral and paramediastinal areas, and characteristically demonstrate high attenuation. As these "talcomas" continue to show growth for years and often raise concern for recurrent malignancy. Talcomas may be PET positive with a wide range of standard uptake values

(SUV) that may be greater than 15 units. The uptake, which can be diffuse or focal, can mimic malignancy. The uptake on PET scan is most likely related to the granulomatous reaction induced by talc. The findings of high attenuation pleural-based lesions and PET positivity in a patient with prior talc pleurodesis are highly suggestive of a talcoma. In the appropriate setting, the clinical presentation and imaging may be adequate for a confident clinical diagnosis without the need for biopsy (104–106).

Pleural Fluid pH and Glucose
Approximately 30% of patients on presentation with a malignant pleural effusion have a low pleural fluid pH (<7.30) and glucose (<60 mg/dL) (30); these patients have a greater pleural tumor burden than those with normal pH and glucose effusions. Pleural fluid pH and glucose are low in patients with far-advanced disease of the pleural space primarily because the end products of glucose metabolisms (CO_2 and lactic acid) are inhibited from effusing from the pleural space resulting in increased accumulation (107). There is a direct correlation between pleural fluid pH and survival with those patients with lower pH having a decreased survival (30–33,108). In addition, patients with a lower pleural fluid pH tend to have less-successful pleurodesis (30–33). However, a meta-analysis of 417 patients with malignant pleural effusion from multiple investigators from North America and Europe found that even in the lowest pH (6.70–7.26) quartile, 45% were still alive at three months (108). Furthermore, in the same low-pH quartile, only 35% failed chemical pleurodesis (109). Therefore, the clinician should not use pleural fluid pH in isolation but in conjunction with other variables, when deciding whether pleurodesis should be offered to the patient.

Technique of Pleurodesis
Proper technique is critical for successful pleurodesis, and several issues have been controversial. These include chest tube size, pain control, patient rotation, dwell time, timing of instillation of the pleurodesis agent, and chest tube removal. Twelve studies totaling 245 patients have been published on the response of small-bore (7–16 F) catheters with chemical pleurodesis (109–120). Fifty-five of the patients had pleurodesis with talc slurry, 50 with doxycycline, 94 with bleomycin, and 46 with tetracycline. Talc had the greatest success rate of 88%, followed by doxycycline (80%), bleomycin (75%), and tetracycline (75%). The overall success rate (complete or partial) of the 245 patients who had chemical pleurodesis using small-bore catheters was 78%. Small-bore catheters are as effective as standard chest tubes for pleurodesis and are associated with less patient morbidity.

In our experience, for pleurodesis, the administration of 2 to 3 mg of intravenous morphine and 2 to 3 mg of intravenous midazolam provides excellent pain control and amnestic response, respectively. These drugs should be administered 5 to 10 minutes prior to the instillation of the pleurodesis agent. If pain does occur, it is generally immediate and short lived.

We previously have demonstrated that radiolabeled tetracycline dispersed rapidly and completely throughout the pleural space when instilled through a chest tube (121). In a follow-up to the distribution study, we randomized patients who received tetracycline pleurodesis either to rotation or nonrotation following instillation (122). Although there was no difference in pleurodesis success suggesting that it was unnecessary to rotate patients when using a soluble agent such as tetracycline, the study was underpowered to definitively answer the null hypothesis. However, with the use of talc slurry, our current recommendation is to perform rotation over a one-hour period, moving the patient through right and left lateral decubitus positions, head of the bed at 45° to 60°, Trendelenburg, and supine because dispersion may not be as complete with a slurry as with a soluble agent.

Since the mesothelial cell initiates the inflammatory cascade that leads to a fibrotic response and mesothelial cell injury occurs virtually instantaneously after contact with the chemical agent (123), a one-hour (possibly two hours) dwell time would appear to be adequate, as the two pleural surfaces should be juxtaposed as soon as possible.

The dogma has been perpetuated over time that the chemical agent should be instilled into the pleural space when the lung is fully expanded on chest radiograph and there is <150 cm^3 of daily drainage through the chest tube. The "standard of care" also suggests that the chest tube be removed when there is <100 to 150 cm^3 of drainage over 24 hours. In a small, randomized study of 25 patients with malignant pleural effusions evaluating timely instillation and chest tube drainage, 15 patients were randomized to standard chest tube drainage and 10 patients to short-term chest tube drainage (124). Patients in the standard group had the chest tube in place until there was lung re-expansion on chest radiograph and the volume of fluid drained from the pleural space was <100 mL for 24 hours before 1500 mg of tetracycline was instilled. The chest tube was removed when fluid drainage was <150 mL for 24 hours following tetracycline. In the 10 patients in the short-term group, the same dose of tetracycline was instilled as soon as the chest radiograph showed lung re-expansion and the effusion was drained, which was usually within 24 hours, regardless of the volume of chest tube drainage; the chest tube was removed the day following instillation of tetracycline. Pleurodesis success was 80% in each group, but the duration of chest tube drainage was significantly shorter (median 2 days, range 2–9 days) in the short-term chest tube group compared with the standard group (median 7 days, range 3–19 days) ($p < 0.01$). This small, randomized study suggests that as soon as the lung is fully expanded on chest radiograph with an absence or minimal volume of fluid, the pleurodesis agent should be instilled, regardless of the volume of drainage through the chest tube. The chest tube probably can be removed shortly thereafter as long as the drainage is not excessive. The use of this technique could substantially shorten hospital stay or be accomplished as an outpatient, both minimizing cost. However, in our experience, if postpleurodesis chest tube drainage exceeds 250 to 300 cm^3 for 24 hours—the chest tube should not be removed, as success appears unlikely; in the latter situation, pleurodesis should be repeated if the lung is expanded.

Recommendations for Pleurodesis

Factors that should be considered before recommending pleurodesis to a patient with a malignant effusion include their response to therapeutic thoracocentesis, general health, performance status, expected survival, pleural space anatomy by chest radiograph or chest CT, pleural space elastance, primary malignancy, and pleural fluid pH. Absolute contraindications to pleurodesis include absence of relief of dyspnea with therapeutic thoracocentesis or an unexpandable lung from mainstem bronchial occlusion, visceral pleural restriction or chronic atelectasis. Relative contraindications to pleurodesis include a terminal patient, widespread metastatic disease, poor performance status, active air leak, low pleural fluid pH, severe comorbid disease, and following extensive pleural abrasion or multiple biopsies.

E. Short-Term Chest Tube Drainage

Five studies have evaluated the response of short-term (3–12 days) chest tube drainage for recurrent malignant pleural effusion (125–129). The range of reported successful pleurodeses in these five series was 0% to 77%. Of the total 126 patients who were treated with standard chest tube drainage without a pleurodesis agent, 78 (62%) patients had success. Although the response rate appears high, in several of the studies the observation period was not clearly defined. Furthermore, if a chest tube is placed in these patients and the lung expands with drainage, a pleurodesis agent should be instilled if no contraindication exists.

F. Chronic Indwelling Catheters

Two early studies with chronic indwelling catheters have shown that these 15.5 F catheters are effective in the relief of dyspnea, safe, as successful as pleurodesis with doxycycline or talc, and less costly than chemical pleurodesis (130,131). In a multicenter prospective trial, 144 patients were randomized in a 2:1 distribution to chronic indwelling silastic catheter ($n = 99$) or chest tube drainage with doxycycline pleurodesis ($n = 45$), respectively (132). Relief of dyspnea was equivalent in both groups after initial treatment and at 90 days. Patients with the indwelling catheter had significantly fewer hospital days, and no patient in the catheter group had symptomatic recurrence compared to 27% of patients who received doxycycline pleurodesis. Pleurodesis success was not different between the indwelling catheter group and the doxycycline group, both being low at 18% and 28%, respectively. Putnam and colleagues (133) retrospectively reviewed 100 consecutive indwelling pleural catheter patients, 60 treated as outpatients and 40 as inpatients, and compared them to 68 consecutive inpatients treated with chest tube drainage and doxycycline or talc pleurodesis who were treated for malignant pleural effusions. The median survival was 3.4 months and did not differ significantly between treatment groups. No deaths occurred in the chronic indwelling catheter group, and 81 (81%) of the 100 patients had no complications. In the other 19 patients, a malfunctioning catheter and an infected pleural space were complications. Those treated with the indwelling catheter as outpatients, as expected, had significantly lower costs than those treated with the catheter as inpatients treated with chest tube pleurodesis as inpatients. However, the cost of drainage bottles for the indwelling catheter must also be considered.

Tremblay and colleagues have reported on the use of 109 tunneled catheter procedures in 97 patients from a database of 250 tunneled catheter insertions (134). The criteria for patients included in the analysis were when pleurodesis was contraindicated based on expected short-term survival and unexpandable lung following drainage. The study subgroup included procedures where patient survival exceeded 90 days and there was ≤20% residual pleural fluid following two weeks of drainage. There were 109 procedures in 97 patients. Spontaneous pleurodesis was achieved in 70% of the procedures that correlated with symptom control; the mean time to spontaneous pleurodesis was 90 days. A repeat procedure was not required in 80% of all cases and in 92% of those who developed spontaneous pleurodesis. Complications included symptomatic loculation in 12 (11%), asymptomatic loculations in 8 (7%), re-accumulation of pleural fluid 4 (4%), empyema 5 (5%), pneumothorax, subcutaneous air or bronchopleural fistula 3 (3%), cellulitis 2 (2%), bleeding 1 (1%), tumor seeding 1 (1%), and dislodgement 1 (1%). There were no procedure-related deaths.

Chronic indwelling catheters should be strongly considered for all patients with an unexpandable lung and those who have failed pleurodesis. The patient with an indwelling catheter should be instructed to drain the pleural space when dyspnea develops and to discontinue drainage as soon as anterior chest pain occurs.

G. Pleuroperitoneal Shunting

Pleuroperitoneal shunt has been used in patients who have failed chemical pleurodesis, chemotherapy, or radiation therapy, and have an unexpandable lung or a malignant chylothorax. Petrou and colleagues (85) reported their 10-year experience with 180 patients who were referred for surgical palliation of a malignant pleural effusion. One hundred thirty-four patients (74%) had previous treatment, which included thoracocentesis, tube thoracostomy, pleurodesis, and pleurectomy. One hundred seventeen patients demonstrated full lung expansion at thoracoscopy or mini-thoracotomy and underwent talc pleurodesis, the remaining 63 patients had unexpandable lung and received a pleuroperitoneal shunt, which resulted in palliation in 98% of patients. Nine shunt occlusions occurred from several days to 2.5 months and were found to be infected. The occluded shunts were replaced in four, revised in two, and removed with open drainage in three. There were no intraoperative deaths. Pleuroperitoneal shunting can provide effective palliation in patients with an intractable chylothorax (73,135).

H. Parietal Pleurectomy

Parietal pleurectomy offers definitive treatment for patients with malignant pleural effusions but carries a high morbidity and mortality that is not justified in patients with a poor prognosis. Martini and coworkers (136) reported their results in 106 patients treated by pleurectomy for malignant pleural effusions. Sixteen (19%) of 83 patients were alive two years following pleurectomy with a survival range of two to six years. The primary postoperative complication was prolonged air leak in those requiring decortication. The overall 30-day postoperative mortality was 10%. Frye and Khandekar (137) performed parietal pleurectomy in 24 patients who did not respond to standard treatment for malignant pleural effusion using axillary thoracotomy. Three (13%) patients died in the postoperative period. In the remaining 21 patients, satisfactory control of their malignant pleural effusion was obtained with survival of 2 to 30 months (mean 10.6). Waller and colleagues (138) reported the use of VATS pleurectomy in 19 patients with malignant pleural effusions (13 mesothelioma and 6 metastatic adenocarcinoma). All patients were successfully extubated in the operating room without the need for mechanical ventilation and were discharged from the hospital with a median postoperative stay of five days (range 2–20). There were no postoperative deaths, six patients died of their underlying disease 4 to 17 months following surgery. Of the remaining 13 patients, two developed recurrent effusions. Because of its significant morbidity and mortality, parietal pleurectomy should only be considered if the malignant pleural effusion is found at the time of thoracotomy or VATS for resection of an intrathoracic tumor. The procedure should not be offered to patients who have a poor performance status and an expected survival of <6 months.

The goal of improving the quality of life of our patients is particularly germane in the setting of malignant pleural effusions where relief of breathlessness remains the primary objective. The least invasive, morbid, and costly treatment should be recommended for patients who have a limited survival. Hospitalization should be minimized for cost containment and separation from their family. Success of the initial procedure is important, as repeat procedures are associated with additional hospitalization, patient discomfort, and added expense. Therefore, the selection of patients for palliation and the specific procedure to be utilized needs to be chosen carefully, based on their general health, performance status, expected survival, and others. The clinician currently cannot rely on prospective, randomized, controlled trials that will help in these important therapeutic decisions. Prospective studies are needed that will evaluate the course of small, symptomatic, malignant pleural effusions, assess the potential of intrapleural immune modulators and epidermal growth factors receptors (EGFR) tyrosine kinase inhibitors (139), and compare ambulatory- and hospital-based management.

VII. Prognosis

In a combined series of 417 patients with malignant pleural effusions from nine investigators in the United States and Europe, lung cancer represented 43% and breast cancer 18% of the primary malignancies (99). Eighty percent were alive at one month, 54% at three months, 31% at six months, and 13% at one year. Lung cancer ($n = 146$) patients had a median survival of 3 months, GI cancers ($n = 18$) 2.3 months, and ovarian cancer ($n = 9$) 3.6 months. Those with breast cancer ($n = 60$) had a median survival of five months, mesothelioma ($n = 29$) six months, and lymphoma ($n = 7$) nine months.

VIII. Conclusion

Malignant pleural effusions are a common consequence of the primary tumor that cause substantial morbidity for the patient. There are an estimated 150,000 patients who develop a malignant pleural effusion in the United States annually with lung and breast cancer being the most common causes. Pleural metastases occur through pulmonary vascular invasion and embolization to the visceral pleural surface, direct invasion from lung and breast cancer, hematogenous metastases, and lymphatic involvement. Breathlessness, the most common presenting symptom, occurs in more than half of the patients. Bilateral pleural effusions with a normal heart size, a massive pleural effusion, and a large pleural effusion without contralateral mediastinal shift are suggestive of a malignant etiology. Malignant pleural effusions can be serous, hemorrhagic, or grossly bloody exudates with a low number of nucleated cells that commonly are lymphocyte predominant. The prevalence of malignancy is similar in both eosinophilic as well as non-eosinophilic pleural effusions. A pleural fluid pH <7.30 and a glucose <60 mg/dL are found in approximately 30% of patients who present with a malignant pleural effusion and are associated with increased diagnostic sensitivity and decreased survival. A total of 10% to 14% of patients with malignant effusions have an increased salivary amylase effusion, the most common cause being adenocarcinoma of the lung. Pleural fluid cytology is the least invasive method for diagnosis with a sensitivity of 60% to 90%. Percutaneous pleural biopsy has a sensitivity of 40% to 75%. The diagnostic sensitivity of the aforementioned procedures increases with the extent of pleural involvement. Thoracoscopy is the most sensitive diagnostic procedure approaching 100% with experienced operators. The major indication for palliative treatment for patients with a malignant effusion is relief of dyspnea. Therapeutic thoracocentesis is a therapeutic option in patients with far-advanced disease, poor performance status, a tumor associated with poor survival, and low pleural fluid pH. Malignant effusions from small-cell lung cancer, breast cancer, and lymphoma are likely to have a favorable response to chemotherapy. Mediastinal radiation may be effective for treating lymphomatous chylothorax. Chemical pleurodesis is an accepted palliative treatment for patients with recurrent, symptomatic pleural effusions. Talc, either as a poudrage or slurry, has been shown to be the most effective pleurodesis agent. The most common adverse effects of all pleurodesis agents are chest pain and fever. The incidence of acute respiratory failure associated with talc pleurodesis is approximately 1%. In about half of the patients reported with acute talc-associated respiratory failure, factors other than talc could be implicated. It would be highly unlikely for talc-induced acute respiratory failure to occur if the sterility of talc was assured, the majority of talc particles exceeded 30 μm in diameter, no more than 4 g of talc were used, pleural abrasion was not performed prior to the procedure, simultaneous bilateral pleurodeses were not attempted, and pleurodesis was not performed in terminal patients or those with marginal lung function. Factors that need to be considered prior to recommending pleurodesis include the response to therapeutic thoracocentesis, general health, performance status, expected survival, pleural space anatomy, pleural space elastance, primary malignancy, and pleural fluid pH. Absolute contraindications to pleurodesis include absence of relief of dyspnea with therapeutic thoracocentesis, extensive unexpandable lung, or mainstem bronchial occlusion. If patients are not candidates for or have failed chemical pleurodesis, an indwelling catheter should be strongly considered. In some centers, an indwelling catheter is the treatment of choice and can be performed as an outpatient. The least invasive, morbid and costly treatment should be recommended for these patients with a limited survival.

References

1. Antony VB, Loddenkemper R, Astoul P, et al. Management of malignant pleural effusions. Am J Respir Crit Care Med 2000; 162:1987–2001.
2. Rodriguez-Panadero F, Borderas-Naranjo F, Lopez-Mejias J. Pleural metastatic tumours and effusions. Frequency and pathogenic mechanisms in a post-mortem series. Eur J Respir Dis 1989; 2:366–369.
3. Meyer PC. Metastatic carcinoma of the pleura. Thorax 1966; 21:437–443.
4. Chernow B, Sahn SA. Carcinomatous involvement of the pleura. An analysis of 96 cases. Am J Med 1977; 63:695–702.
5. Kolin A, Koutoulakis T. Invasion of pulmonary arteries by bronchial carcinomas. Hum Pathol 1987; 18:1165–1171.
6. Jiang W. In vitro models of cancer invasion and metastasis: Recent developments. Eur J Surg Oncol 1994; 20:493–499.
7. Zetter B. Adhesion molecules in tumor metastasis. Sem Cancer Biol 1993; 4:219–229.
8. Shetty S, Kumar A, Johnson A, et al. Expression of the urokinase-type plasminogen activator receptor in human malignant mesothelial cells: Role in tumor cell mitogenesis and proteolysis. Am J Physiol Lung Cell Mol Physiol 1995; 12:L972–L982.
9. Idell S, Pueblitz S, Emri S, et al. Regulation of fibrin deposition by malignant mesothelioma. Am J Pathol 1995; 147:1318–1329.
10. Shetty S, Idell S. A urokinase receptor MRNA binding protein–MRNA interaction regulates receptor expression and function in human pleural mesothelioma cells. Arch Biochem Biophys 1998; 35:265–279.
11. Shetty S, Idell S. Post-transcriptional regulation of urokinase receptor gene expression in human lung carcinoma and malignant mesothelioma cells in vitro. Mol Cell Biochem 1999; 199:189–200.

12. Hott KW, Yu L, Antony VB. Role of VEGF in the formation of malignant pleural effusions. Am J Respir Crit Care Med 1999; 159:A212.
13. Galffy G, Mohammed KA, Ward MJ, et al. Interleuken 8—An autocrine growth factor for malignant mesothelioma. Am Cancer Res 1999; 59:367–371.
14. Sahn SA. Malignant pleural effusions. In: Light RW, ed. Pleural Diseases. Clinic Chest Medicine. Philadelphia, Pennsylvania: W.B. Saunders, 1985; 6:113–125.
15. Estienne M, Yeranult JC, DeTroyer A. Mechanism of relief of dyspnea after thoracentesis in patients with large pleural effusions. Am J Med 1983; 74:813–819.
16. Tammilehto L, Maasilita P, Kostianen S, et al. Diagnosis and prognostic factors in malignant pleural mesothelioma: A retrospective analysis of 65 patients. Respiration 1992; 52:129–135.
17. Maher GG, Berger HW. Massive pleural effusions: Malignant and non-malignant causes in 46 patients. Am Rev Respir Dis 1972; 105:458–460.
18. Liberson M. Diagnostic significance of the mediastinal profile in massive unilateral pleural effusions. Am Rev Respir Dis 1963; 88:176–180.
19. Rabin CB, Blackman NS. Bilateral pleural effusion. Its significance in association with a heart of normal size. J Mt Sinai Hosp 1957; 24:45–53.
20. O'Donovan PB, Eng P. Pleural changes in malignant pleural effusions: Appearance on computed tomography. Cleve Clin J Med 1994; 61:127–131.
21. Bittner RC, Felix R. Magnetic resonance (MR) imaging of the chest: State-of-the-art. Eur Respir J 1998; 11:1392–1404.
22. Benard F, Sterman D, Smith RJ, et al. Metabolic imaging of malignant pleural mesothelioma with fluorodeoxyglucose positron emission tomography. Chest 1998; 144:713–722.
23. Yam LT. Diagnostic significance of lymphocytes in pleural effusions. Ann Intern Med 1967; 66:972–982.
24. Light RW, MacGregor MI, Luchsinger PC, et al. Pleural effusions: The diagnostic separation of transudates and exudates. Ann Intern Med 1972; 77:507–513.
25. Fernandes C, Martin C, Aranda R, et al. Malignant transient pleural transudate: A sign of early lymphatic tumoral obstruction. Respiration 2000; 67:333–336.
26. Heffner JE, Brown LK, Barbieri CA. Diagnostic value of tests that discriminate between exudative and transudative pleural effusions. Chest 1997; 111:970–980.
27. Joseph J, Badrinath P, Basran G, et al. Is the pleural fluid transudate or exudate? A revisit of the diagnostic criteria. Thorax 2001; 56:867–870.
28. Rubins JB, Rubins HB. Etiology and prognostic significance of eosinophilic pleural effusions: A prospective study. Chest 1996; 11:1271–1274.
29. Martinez-Garcia MA, Cases-Viedma E, Cordero-Rodrigues PJ, et al. Diagnostic utility of eosinophils in the pleural fluid. Eur Respir J 2000; 15:166–169.
30. Sahn SA, Good JT Jr. Pleural fluid pH in malignant effusions: Diagnostic, prognostic, and therapeutic implications. Ann Intern Med 1988; 108:345–349.
31. Sanchez-Armengol A, Rodriguez-Panadero F. Survival and talc pleurodesis in metastatic pleural carcinoma, revisited. Chest 1993; 104:1482–1485.
32. Rodriguez-Panadero F, Lopez-Mejias L. Low glucose and pH levels in malignant effusions: Diagnostic significance and prognostic value in respect to pleurodesis. Am Rev Respir Dis 1989; 139:663–667.
33. Rodriguez-Panadero F, Lopez-Mejias L. Survival time of patients with pleural metastatic carcinoma predicted by glucose and pH studies. Chest 1989; 95:320–324.
34. Kramer MR, Saldana MJ, Cepro RJ, et al. High amylase in neoplasm-related pleural effusions. Ann Intern Med 1989; 10:567–569.
35. Joseph J, Viney S, Beck P, et al. A prospective study of amylase-rich pleural effusions with special reference to amylase isoenzyme analysis. Chest 1992; 102:1455–1459.
36. Johnston WW. The malignant pleural effusion: A review of cytopathological diagnoses of 584 specimens from 472 consecutive patients. Cancer 1985; 56:905–909.

37. Hsu C. Cytologic detection of malignancy in pleural effusion: A review of 5255 samples from 3811 patients. Diagn Cytopathol 1987; 3:8–12.
38. Molangraft FL, Fooijs GP. The interval between the diagnosis of malignancy and the development of effusions, with reference to the role of cytologic diagnosis. Acta Cytol 1988; 32:183–187.
39. Starr RL, Sherman ME. The value of multiple preparations in the diagnosis of malignant pleural effusions. Acta Cytol 1991; 35:533–537.
40. Loddenkemper R, Grosser H, Gabler A, et al. Prospective evaluation of biopsy methods in the diagnosis of malignant pleural effusions: Intra-patient comparison between pleural fluid cytology, blind needle biopsy, and thoracoscopy. Am Rev Respir Dis 1983; 127(Suppl. 4):S114.
41. Jonasson JG, Ducatman BS, Wang HH. The cell block for body cavity fluids: Do the results justify the cost? Mod Pathol 1990; 3:667–670.
42. Dekker A, Bupp PA. Cytology of serous effusions: An investigation into the usefulness of cell blocks versus smears. Am J Clin Pathol 1978; 70:855–860.
43. Irani DR, Underwood RD, Johnson EH, et al. Malignant pleural effusions. A clinical cytopathologic study. Arch Intern Med 1987; 147:1133–1136.
44. Prakash UBS, Reiman HM. Comparison of needle biopsy with cytologic analysis for the evaluation of pleural effusions: Analysis of 414 cases. Mayo Clin Proc 1985; 60:158–164.
45. Poe RH, Israel RH, Utell MJ, et al. Sensitivity, specificity, and predictive values of closed pleural biopsy. Arch Intern Med 1984; 144:325–328.
46. Escudero BC, Garcia CM, Cuesta CB, et al. Cytological and bacteriologic analysis of fluid and pleural biopsy specimens with Cope's needle. Arch Intern Med 1990; 150:1190–1194.
47. Canto A, Rivis J, Saumench J, et al. Points to consider when choosing a biopsy method in cases of pleurisy of unknown origin. Chest 1983; 83:176–179.
48. Boutin C, Viallat JR, Cargaino P, et al. Thoracoscopy in malignant pleural effusions. Am Rev Respir Dis 1981; 124:588–592.
49. Loddenkemper R, Boutin C. Thoracoscopy: Diagnostic and therapeutic indications. Eur Respir J 1993; 6:1544–1555.
50. Mentintas M, Ozdemir N, Solak M, et al. Chromosome analysis in pleural effusions: Efficiency of this method in the diagnosis of pleural effusions. Respiration 1994; 61:330–335.
51. Rijken A, Dekker A, Taylor S, et al. Diagnostic value of DNA analysis in effusions by post-cytometry and image analysis. Am J Clin Pathol 1991; 95:6–12.
52. Sheibani K, Esteban J, Bailey A, et al. Immunopathologic and molecular studies as an aid in the diagnosis of malignant mesothelioma. Hum Pathol 1992; 23:107–116.
53. Shield PW, Callan JJ, Devine PL. Markers for metastatic adenocarcinoma in serous effusion specimens. Diagn Cytol 1994; 11:237–245.
54. Mezger J, Stotzer O, Schilli G, et al. Identification of carcinomas cells in acidic and pleural fluid: Comparison of 4 panepithelial antigens with carcinoembryonic antigen. Acta Cytol 1992; 36:758–781.
55. Creaney J, Yeoman D, Maumoff LK, et al. Soluble mesothelin in effusions: A useful toll for the diagnosis of malignant mesothelioima. Thorax 2007; 62:569–576.
56. Steger V, Mika U, Toomes H, et al. Who gains most? A 10-year experience with 611 thorasoscopic talc pleurodesis. Ann Thorac Surg 2007; 83:1940–1945.
57. Light RW, Jenkinson SG, Minh V-D, et al. Observations on pleural fluid pressures as fluid is withdrawn during thoracentesis. Am Rev Respir Dis 1980; 121:799–804.
58. Light RW, Stansbury DW, Brown SE. The relationship between pleural pressures and changes in pulmonary function after therapeutic thoracentesis. Am Rev Respir Dis 1986; 133:658–661.
59. Lan R, Singh KL, Chuang M, et al. Elastance of the pleural space: A predictor for the outcome of pleurodesis in patients with malignant effusion. Ann Intern Med 1997; 126:768–774.

60. Villena V, Lopez-Encuentra A, Pozo F, et al. Measurement of pleural pressure during therapeutic thoracentesis. Am J Respir Crit Care Med 2000; 162:1534–1538.
61. Doelken P, Sahn SA. In: Sahn SA, ed. Trapped Lung in Management of Pleural Disease. Semin Respir Crit Care Med 2001; 22(6):631–636.
62. Doelken P, Huggins JT, Pastis NJ, et al. Pleural manometry: Technique and clinical implications. Chest 2004; 126:1764–1769.
63. Huggins JT, Sahn SA, Heidecker J, et al. Characteristics of trapped lung: Pleural fluid analysis, manometry, and air-contrast chest computed tomography. Chest 2007; 131:206–213.
64. Sprung CL, Loewenherz JW, Baier H, et al. Evidence of increased permeability in re-expansion pulmonary edema. Am J Med 1981; 71:497–500.
65. Heffner JE, Fracica P. Nitric oxide and radical in the pulmonary vasculature. In: Weir EK, Archer SL, Reeves JT, eds. Armonk, New York: Futura, 1996:105–133.
66. Black LF. The pleural space and pleural fluid. Mayo Clin Proc 1972; 47:493–506.
67. Lai-Fook SJ. Mechanics of the pleural space: Fundamental concepts. Lung 1987; 165:249–267.
68. Livingston RV, McCracken JD, Trauth CJ, et al. Isolated pleural effusion in small cell lung cancer: Favorable prognosis. Chest 1982; 81:208–210.
69. Fentiman IS, Reubens RD, Hayward JL. Control of pleural effusions in a patient with breast cancer. Cancer 1983; 52:737–739.
70. Lees AW, Hoy W. Management of pleural effusions in breast cancer. Chest 1979; 75:51–53.
71. Poe RH, Qazi R, Israel RH, et al. Survival of patients with pleural involvement by breast carcinoma. Am J Clin Oncol 1983; 6:523–527.
72. Xaubet A, Diumenjo MC, Masin A, et al. Characteristics and prognostic value of pleural effusions in non-Hodgkin's lymphomas. Eur J Respir Dis 1985; 6:135–140.
73. Murphy MC, Newman BM, Rodgers BM. Pleuroperitoneal shunts in the management of persistent chylothorax. Ann Thorac Surg 1989; 48:195–200.
74. Walker-Renard PB, Vaughan LM, Sahn SA. Chemical pleurodesis for malignant pleural effusions. Ann Intern Med 1994; 120:56–64.
75. Hamed H, Fentiman IS, Chaudary MA, et al. Comparison of intracavitary bleomycin and talc for control of pleural effusions secondary to carcinoma of the breast. Br J Surg 1989; 76:1266–1267.
76. Hartman DL, Gaither JM, Kesler MA, et al. Comparison of insufflated talc under thoracoscopic guidance with standard tetracycline and bleomycin pleurodesis for control of malignant pleural effusions. J Thorac Cariovasc Surg 1993; 105:743–748.
77. Fentiman IS, Reubens RD, Hayward JL. A comparison of intracavitary talc and tetracycline for the control of pleural effusions secondary to breast cancer. Eur J Cancer Clin Oncol 1986; 22:1079–1081.
78. Kennedy L, Sahn SA. Talc pleurodesis for the treatment of pneumothorax and pleural effusion. Chest 1994; 106:1215–1222.
79. Yim AP, Chan AT, Lee TW, et al. Thoracoscopic talc insufflation versus talc slurry for symptomatic malignant pleural effusions. Ann Thorac Surg 1996; 62:1655–1658.
80. Dresler CM, Olak J, Herndon JE, et al. Phase III intergroup study of talc poudrage vs talc slurry sclerosis for malignant pleural effusion. Chest 2005; 127:900–915.
81. Kennedy L, Rusch VW, Strange C, et al. Pleurodesis using talc slurry. Chest 1994; 106:342–346.
82. Sahn SA. Talc should be used for pleurodesis. Am J Respir Crit Care Med 2001; 62:2024–2025.
83. Viallat J-R, Rey F, Astoul P, et al. Thoracoscopic talc poudrage pleurodesis for malignant effusions. A review of 360 cases. Chest 1996; 110:1387–1393.
84. Campos JR, Werebe EC, Vargas FS, et al. Respiratory failure due to insufflated talc. Lancet 1997; 349:251–252.

85. Petrou M, Kaplan D, Goldstraw P. Management of recurrent malignant pleural effusions. The complementary role of talc pleurodesis and pleuroperitoneal shunting. Cancer 1995; 75:801–805.

86. Weissberg D, Ben-Zeev I. Talc pleurodesis: Experience with 360 patients. J Thorac Cardiovasc Surg 1993; 106:689–695.

87. Rehse DH, Aye RW, Florence MG. Respiratory failure following talc pleurodesis. Am J Surg 1999; 177:437–440.

88. Janssen JP, Collier G, Astoul P, et al. Safety of pleurodesis with talc poudrage in malignant pleural effusion: A prospective cohort study. Lancet 2007; 369:1435–1539.

89. de Campos JRM, Vargas FS, de Campos Werebe E, et al. Thoracoscopy talc poudrage. A 15-year experience. Chest 2001; 119:801–806.

90. Glazer MM, Berkman N, Lafair JS, et al. Successful talc slurry pleurodesis in patients with non-malignant pleural effusion. Report of 16 cases and review of the literature. Chest 2000; 117:1404–1409.

91. Sudduth CD, Sahn SA. Pleurodesis for nonmalignant pleural effusions: Recommendations. Chest 1992; 102:1855–1860.

92. Cardillo G, Facciolo F, Guinti R, et al. Videothoracoscopic treatment of primary spontaneous pneumothorax: A six year experience. Ann Thorac Surg 2000; 69:357–362.

93. Mares DC, Mathur PN. Medical thoracoscopic talc pleurodesis for chylothorax due to lymphoma. Chest 1998; 114:731–735.

94. Rinaldo JE, Owens GR, Rodgers RM. Adult respiratory distress syndrome following intrapleural instillation of talc. J Thorac Cardiovasc Surg 1983; 85:523–526.

95. Bouchama A, Chastre J, Gaudichet A, et al. Acute pneumonitis with bilateral pleural effusion after talc pleurodesis. Chest 1984; 86:795–797.

96. Lineau C, Le Coz A, Quinquenel ML, et al. Acute respiratory insufficiency after pleural talcage of pneumothorax. Apropos of a case. Rev Pneumol Clin 1993; 49:153–155.

97. Ferrer J, Villarino MA, Tura JM, et al. Talc preparations used for pleurodesis vary markedly from one preparation to another. Chest 2001; 119:1901–1905.

98. Shaffer JP, Allen JN, Prior RB. Detection of endotoxin in talc preparations used for pleurodesis. Chest 2000; 118:130S.

99. Chappell AG, Johnson A, Charles WJ, et al. A survey of the long-term effects of talc in kaolin pleurodesis. Br J Dis Chest 1979; 73:285–288.

100. Lange P, Mortensen J, Groth S. Lung function 22–25 years after treatment of idiopathic spontaneous pneumothorax with talc poudrage with simple drainage. Thorax 1988; 43:559–561.

101. Viskum K, Lange P, Mortensen J. Long-term sequelae after talc. Pneumonolige 1989; 43:105–106.

102. Paul JS, Geatiee EJ, Blades B. Lung function studies in poudrage treatment of recurrent spontaneous pneumothorax. J Thorac Surg 1951; 22:52–61.

103. Knowles JH, Storey CF. Effects of talc poudrage on pulmonary function. J Thorac Surg 1957; 340:250–256.

104. Kleinfeld M, Messite J, Kooyman O, et al. Mortality among talc miners and millers in New York state. Arch Environ Health 1967; 14:663–667.

105. Murray JG, Patz EF Jr, Eramus AJ, et al. CT appearance of the pleural space after talc pleurodesis. AJR 1997; 169:89–91.

106. Weiss MN, Solomon SB. Talc pleurodesis mimics pleural metastases: Differentiating with positron emission tomography/computed tomography. Clin Nucl Med 2003; 28:811–814.

107. Narayanaswamy S, Kamath S, Williams M. CT appearances of talc pleurodesis. Clin Rad 2007; 62:233–237.

108. Good JT Jr, Taryle DA, Sahn SA. The pathogenesis of low glucose, low pH malignant effusions. Am Rev Respir Dis 1985; 131:737–741.

109. Heffner JE, Nietert PJ, Barbieri C. Pleural fluid pH as a predictor of survival of patients with malignant pleural effusions. Chest 2000; 117:79–86.
110. Heffner JE, Nietert PJ, Barbieri C. Pleural fluid pH as a predictor of pleurodesis failure. Chest 2000; 117:87–95.
111. Walsh FW, Alberts M, Solomon DA, et al. Malignant pleural effusions: Pleurodesis using small-bore catheter. So Med J 1989; 82:963–972.
112. Parker LA, Charnock GC, Delany DJ. Small-bore catheter drainage and sclerotherapy for malignant effusions. Cancer 1989; 64:1218–1221.
113. Morrison MC, Mueller PR, Lee MJ, et al. Sclerotherapy of malignant pleural effusion through sonographically placed small-bore catheters. AJR 1992; 158:41–43.
114. Goff BA, Mueller PR, Muntz HG, et al. Small chest-tube drainage followed by bleomycin sclerosis from malignant pleural effusions. Obstet Gynecol 1993; 84:993–996.
115. Seaton KG, Patz EF Jr, Goodman PC. Palliative treatment of malignant pleural effusions: Value of small-bore catheter thoracostomy and doxycycline sclerotherapy. AJR 1995; 164:589–591.
116. Patz EF Jr, McAdams HP, Goodman PC, et al. Ambulatory sclerotherapy for malignant pleural effusions. Radiology 1996; 199:133–135.
117. Hsu WH, Chiang CD, Chen CY, et al. Ultrasound-guided small-bore Elecath tube insertion for the rapid sclerotherapy of malignant pleural effusion. Jpn J Clin Oncol 1998; 28:187–191.
118. Patz EF Jr, McAdams HP, Erasmus JJ, et al. Sclerotherapy for malignant pleural effusions. A prospective randomized trial of bleomycin versus doxycycline with small-bore catheter drainage. Chest 1998; 113:1305–1311.
119. Thompson RL, Yau JC, Donnelly RF, et al. Pleurodesis with iodized talc for malignant effusions using pigtail catheters. Ann Pharmacother 1998; 32:739–742.
120. Marom EM, Patz EF Jr, Erasmus JJ, et al. Malignant pleural effusions. Treatment with small-bore-catheter thoracostomy and talc pleurodesis. Radiology 1992; 210:277–281.
121. Bloom AI, Wilson MW, Kerlan RK Jr, et al. Talc pleurodesis through small-bore percutaneous tubes. Cardiovasc Interv Radiol 1999; 22:433–438.
122. Saffran L, Ost DE, Fein AM, et al. Outpatient pleurodesis of malignant pleural effusions using a small-bore pigtail catheter. Chest 2000; 118:417–421.
123. Lorch BG, Gordon L, Wooten S, et al. The effect of patient positioning on the distribution of tetracycline of pleural space during pleurodesis. Chest 1988; 93:527–529.
124. Dryzer S, Allen ML, Strange C, et al. A comparison of rotation and non-rotation in tetracycline pleurodesis. Chest 1993; 104:1763–1766.
125. Van Den Heuvel MM, Smit HJ, Barbierato SB, et al. Talc-induced inflammation in the pleural cavity. Eur Respir J 1998; 12:1419–1423.
126. Villaneuva AG, Gray AW Jr, Shahian DM, et al. Efficacy of short-term versus long-term tube thoracostomy drainage of tetracycline pleurodesis in the treatment of malignant pleural effusions. Thorax 1994; 49:23–25.
127. Lambert CJ, Shah HH, Urshel HC Jr, et al. Treatment of malignant pleural effusions by closed trocar tube drainage. Ann Thorac Surg 1967; 3:1–5.
128. Anderson CB, Philpott GW, Ferguson TB. The treatment of malignant pleural effusions. Cancer 1974; 33:916–922.
129. Izbicki R, Weyhing BT III, Baker L, et al. Pleural effusion in cancer patients. A prospective randomized study of pleural drainage with the addition of radioactive phosphorus to the pleural space versus pleural drainage alone. Cancer 1975; 36:1511–1518.
130. Sorensen PG, Svendsen TL, Enk B. Treatment of malignant pleural effusion with drainage with and without instillation of talc. Eur J Respir Dis 1984; 65:131–135.
131. Groth G, Gatzemeier U, Haussigen K, et al. Intrapleural palliative treatment of malignant pleural effusion with mitoxantrone versus placebo (pleural tube alone). Ann Oncol 1991; 2:213–215.

132. Putnam JB Jr, Light RW, Rodrigues RM, et al. A randomized comparison of indwelling pleural catheter and doxycycline pleurodesis in the management of malignant pleural effusions. Cancer 1999; 86:1992–1999.

133. Putnam JB Jr, Walsh GL, Swisher SG, et al. Outpatient management of malignant pleural effusion by chronic indwelling pleural catheter. Ann Thorac Surg 2000; 69:369–375.

134. Tremblay A, Mason C, Michaud G. Use of tunneled catheters for malignant pleural effusions in patients fit for pleurodesis. Eur Respir J 2007; 30:759–762.

135. Rheuban KS, Kron IL, Carpenter MA, et al. Pleuroperitoneal shunts for refractory chylothorax after operation for congenital disease. Ann Thorac Surg 1992; 53:85–87.

136. Martini N, Bains M, Beattie EJ Jr. Indications for pleurectomy in malignant effusions. Chest 1975; 35:734–738.

137. Frye WA, Khandekar JD. Parietal pleurectomy for malignant pleural effusion. Ann Thorac Oncol 1995; 2:160–164.

138. Waller DA, Morritt GN, Forty J. Video-assisted thoracoscopic pleurectomy in the management of malignant pleural effusion. Chest 1995; 107:1454–1456.

139. Kimura H, Fujiwara Y, Sone T, et al. EGFR mutation status in tumour-derived DNA from pleural effusion fluid is a practical basis for predicting the response to gefitinib. Br J Cancer 2006; 10:1390–1395.

140. Sahn SA. Malignant pleural effusions. In: Fishman AP, Elias JA, Fishman JA, Grippi MA, Kaiser LR, Senior R, eds. Pulmonary Diseases and Disorders, 3rd ed. New York, New York: McGraw Hill, 1998:1429–1438.

141. Sahn SA. Pleural effusion in lung cancer. In: Matthay RA, ed. Lung Cancer: Recent Advances. Philadelphia, Pennsylvania: W.B. Saunders, 1982; 3:443–452.

25
Diagnosis and Management of Pleural Effusion in Lung Cancer

MARIOS E. FROUDARAKIS
Department of Pneumonology, Democritus University of Thrace Medical School,
Alexandroupolis, Greece

I. Introduction

Carcinoma of the lung is the most common cause of malignant pleural effusion. Thus, the incidence of pleural effusion due to lung carcinoma was reported in 641 (36%) cases out of 1783 patients, while the second most common cause was breast carcinoma in 449 (25%) cases (1). The incidence of pleural effusion in patients with lung carcinoma is ranging between 7% (280 out of 4000 cases) (2) to 23% (5888 out of 25,464 cases) (3). All histological types of bronchogenic carcinomas are likely to present pleural effusion (3). However, the most frequent histological type seems to be adenocarcinoma in about 40% of the cases, as it is more likely to arise in the periphery next to the pleura, which may be invaded by the tumor. The second most common tumor is small cell lung carcinoma, which is a tumor with high-invasive potential, with about 25% of the cases (3).

Pleural effusion is mostly diagnosed by a simple chest radiograph and/or computed tomography. In lung cancer, its presence is associated with advanced-stage disease and therefore with poor prognosis (4). However, in some cases, pleural effusion is due to postobstructive pneumonia or atelectasis, venous obstruction by tumor compression, or lymphatic obstruction by mediastinal lymph nodes, and are not associated with direct pleural involvement (5). In case of negative pleural cytology, medical or surgical video-assisted thoracoscopy must be performed in order to evaluate the extension of the disease and prove the possible malignant infiltration of the pleura (6).

II. Pathogenesis

Mechanism of occurrence of pleural effusion in malignancy is mainly due to any obstacle of lymphatic drainage from the pleural space, such as pleural thickening by widespread carcinomatosis, obstruction caused by infiltration of mediastinal lymph nodes, obstruction caused by tumor emboli (7–9). Also, local response with inflammatory reaction to tumors next to the pleura might play an important role in pleural effusion development, by increasing capillary permeability (10). These mechanisms explain the existence of the lymphocyte predominance in malignant pleural effusion, although their role is still unclear. However, some authors believe that T-lymphocytes have an important role in host versus tumor local defense in malignant pleural effusions (11).

Pathogenetic mechanisms of pleural effusion due to lung carcinoma have been reported in postmortem studies (7,8). Most of the patients have both parietal and visceral pleurae infiltrated. It was shown that invasion of parietal pleura is due to neoplastic spread across the pleural cavity from visceral pleural sites along pleural adhesions that are preformed or secondary to the malignant process. Also, parietal pleura is invaded by the attachment of exfoliated cells from the visceral pleura. Visceral pleura might be invaded primarily by pulmonary arterial invasion and embolization (8).

When the tumor directly infiltrates blood vessels, and/or occludes venules, a bloody pleural effusion may occur. Another mechanism of hemorrhagic pleural effusion might be the capillary dilatation occurring due to release of vasoactive substances (8,9). Bilateral pleural metastases from lung carcinoma are due to hematogenous spread to the contralateral hemithorax secondary to the presence of liver metastases (8). Nonmalignant pleural effusions (paramalignant) may occur due to bronchial obstruction causing atelectasis or pneumonia with parapneumonic effusion. This circumstance is purely a mechanic obstruction without malignant-cell infiltration of lymphatics or blood vessels. Lung carcinoma is also frequently associated with heart failure, as both bronchogenic carcinoma and heart disease have the same terrain of occurrence. Thus, pleural effusion may be a transudate due to heart failure. The same finding is observed in patients associated with bronchogenic carcinoma with hepatic insufficiency. In some cases, there is also association of pulmonary embolism and pneumothorax (12) in patients with bronchogenic carcinoma.

III. Diagnostic Approach

A. Clinical Presentation

Pleural effusion in patients with lung carcinoma may be present in two situations: as a presenting syndrome revealing, during the work up, an unknown previously lung carcinoma, or as a pleural effusion in the evolution of a known carcinoma. The diagnostic approach, although basically the same, must be specific to each case as the patient's prognosis relies on this. In the first case, the pleural effusion is discovered after the patient consults his physician for worsening progressively dyspnea, dry cough, lateral thoracic pain, or hemoptysis. General symptoms such as fever, weight loss, loss of appetite, and restriction of the daily activity (13–15) may be associated. Only about 25% of the patients are totally asymptomatic, and pleural effusion is discovered after a routine chest radiograph (15,16). Typically, on physical examination, there is a pleural syndrome confirmed by the chest radiograph, which shows the extent of the pleural effusion (13–15).

B. Imaging

Pleural effusion may be free-flowing or loculated (17). The chest radiograph may also show the cause of the pleural effusion, such as peripheral lesion [Figs. 1(A) and 1(B)] in contact with the thoracic wall, central lesion with atelectasis, or obstructive pneumonia (18,19). It also provides useful information about associated findings, such as pericardial effusion, air in the pleural space, and mediastinal lymph node enlargement (17–19). In 15% of the cases, however, chest radiograph is negative because of the location of the tumor (in the pleural effusion, or cardiac, or diaphragmatic shadows, or endobronchially). A profile chest radiograph must be performed in order to help diagnosis (17).

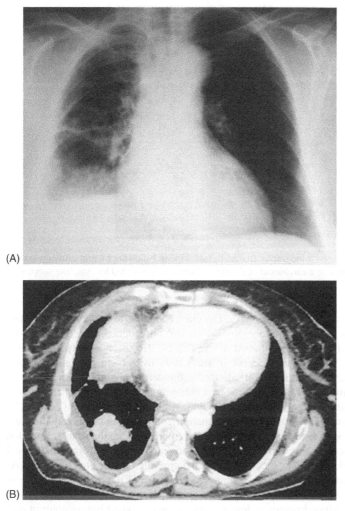

Figure 1 (**A**) Chest radiograph showing right pleural effusion and (**B**) the chest computed tomography association of peripheral lung carcinoma invading the visceral pleura.

Spontaneous pneumothorax is a rare manifestation of lung cancer and may be associated with pleural effusion (Fig. 2). It was estimated that the occurrence of air in the pleural space is less than 1% of patients with lung cancer (12,20,21). Also, lung cancer causes only about 0.05% of cases of pneumothorax (20). Pneumothorax may develop as a complication of bronchopleural fistula due to both pleural and bronchial infiltration from the tumor, of peripheral necrotizing tumor invading the pleura, and of obstructive hyperinflation due to central obstruction (20,21). In most of the cases, pneumothorax occurs while lung cancer is already in an advanced stage (21).

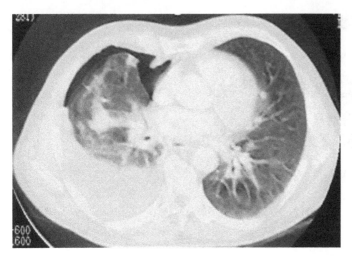

Figure 2 Chest computed tomography (parenchymal window) showing pleural effusion associated to pneumothorax due to a carcinoma of the right lower lobe associated to a satellite subpleural nodule.

Pleural extension must also be assessed by chest computed tomography [Figs. 3(A) and 3(B)] (4). Chest computed tomography is sensitive in recognizing pleural effusion, but cannot identify its possible malignant nature (22,23). However, some patterns may indicate malignancy, such as a thickness of the pleura over 1 cm indicating pleural carcinomatosis (24). It is controversial whether computed tomography is sensitive in associated findings missed by the standard chest radiograph, such as a peripheral nodule and/or mass infiltrating the thoracic wall, the diaphragm, or the mediastinum (23,25,26), as soft tissue swelling may be due to inflammation and/or fibrosis rather than direct infiltration (27). Also, it seems that focal chest pain is more accurate than chest computed tomography in predicting chest wall invasion (28). Computed tomography may also reveal mediastinal lymphadenopathy or localizations at the opposite lung or pleura [Figs. 4(A) and 4(B)]. The presence of these findings may be indicative of the malignant nature of the pleural effusion (21,24,28).

Magnetic resonance imaging is less sensitive than computed tomography in recognizing pleural effusion (22,29). On T1-weighted images, the signal from the fluid is very low and may not be detected, although characteristic brightening on T2-weighted images allows detection (29,30). In addition, magnetic resonance imaging has the same problems as computed tomography in recognizing chest wall, mediastinal, pericardial, or diaphragmatic infiltration (23,29,30).

In malignant pleural disease, chest imaging with positron emission tomography (PET) with fluorine 18–labeled fluorodeoxyglucose (FDG) has a sensitivity ranging from 93% to 100%, and specificity from 67% to 89%. The PET negative predictive value is ranging from 94% to 100%, and its positive predictive value varies from 63% to 94% (31–33). False-positive results occur in patients with any other inflammatory process such as parapneumonic effusions, pleurodesis after talc instillation (34). When PF cytology is negative, a negative PET-FDG scan provides the most useful clinical information for ruling out a pleural effusion of malignant etiology (negative predicted value).

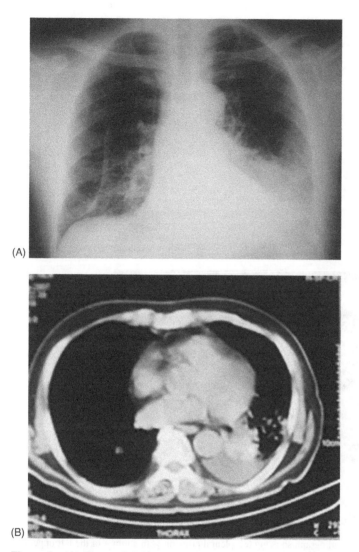

Figure 3 (**A**) Chest radiograph showing left pleural effusion and (**B**) the chest computed tomography association of lung carcinoma of the apical segment of the left lower lobe.

Ultrasound is another noninvasive method to investigate the pleura. Although its major indication is loculated pleural effusions mostly due to infection, it may be helpful in patients with low-performance status who are unable to perform a more sophisticated examination, such as computed tomography of the thorax (35,36). Ultrasound sensitivity in case of pleural effusion is 92% alone, and combined with the standard chest radiograph is 98% (36,37). It also helps in diagnosis of associated findings such as pleural thickness, pleural or subpleural tumors, and parenchymal masses (38).

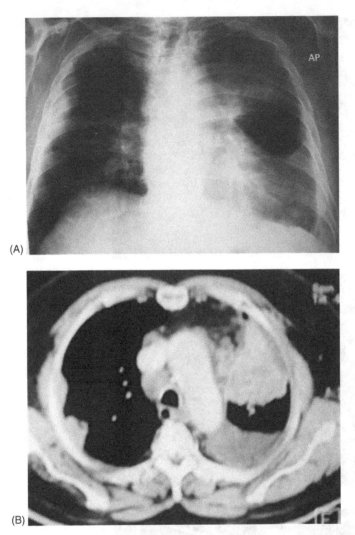

Figure 4   (**A**) Chest radiograph showing left pleural effusion with a tumor of the left upper lobe and left pleural thickening and (**B**) the chest computed tomography the lung carcinoma invades the thoracic wall and is associated despite to a left pleural effusion, to mediastinal controlateral adenopathy (N3) and to metastatic localizations of the left pleura.

C.   Pleural Thoracocentesis

Chemistry of pleural fluid was the subject of many reports in patients with malignancy. There is nothing specific in pleural fluid chemistry data of patients with lung carcinoma compare to those with metastatic malignancy to the pleura (1,39). Thus, as in other malignant pleural effusions, we expect an exudative fluid, with protein concentration >3 g/dL (or pleural-to-serum protein ratio >0.5), levels of lactate dehydrogenase (LDH)

>200 IU/L (or pleural-to-serum LDH ratio >0.6) (40,41). In about 30% of the cases, pH is less than 7.30, glucose levels less than 0.6 mg/dL (or the ratio of pleural-to-serum glucose <0.5) (41–45). In rare occasions pleural fluid is a transudate due to associated diseases such as congestive heart failure, atelectasis from bronchial obstruction, or hypoalbuminemia (9,39). Exudate–transudate tests are not pathognomonic, but provide a probabilistic statement as to the likely nature of a pleural effusion (46).

Leukocytes in the malignant pleural fluid are relatively low with mean value ranging from 2000 to 2500 cells/mL with a huge range (1,9). While the total amount of leukocytes is not helpful in differential diagnosis, the type is important as in malignant pleural effusions we find lymphocytes in a rate over 50% (9,11). Neutrophils usually represent less than 25% (1), while eosinophils are low (7–10%) (47,48). Other nucleated cells may be found, such as macrophages and mesothelial cells. Erythrocytes average about 40,000 to 50,000 cells/mL with also a wide range, from none to hemothorax (9).

Several tumor markers, such as carcinoembryonic antigen (CEA), CA-125, CA-19-9, CYFRA 21-1, NSE, have been tested in patients with malignant pleural effusion (49,50). Although results seem to be controversial as to the usefulness of these tumor markers in the differential diagnosis of pleural effusions, even between malignant and nonmalignant, some authors propose specific tumor markers for the diagnosis of pleural effusions due to bronchogenic carcinoma (51). A reasonable attitude may be that tests should be performed in a selected population of patients with negative cytology and "suspect" clinical outcome (52). Recently, a number of reports have been emerged, studying various novel markers, such as oncogenes (53), cytokines involved in inflammation (54), matrix metalloproteinases (55), in differential diagnosis and prognosis of malignant pleural effusions. Until now, none of these markers proved their usefulness even in differentiating malignant from benign pleural effusions. Generally, biochemical or biological markers in malignant pleural effusions, as well as in the serum, cannot replace the routine cytopathologic examination in the diagnosis of the disease and predict the outcome of the patient without firm diagnosis (56).

Diagnosis of lung cancer pleural effusion can be made only by finding cancer cells in the pleural fluid, as in any other malignant pleural effusion. Cytologic examination of pleural fluid taken after thoracocentesis is the first step in the diagnosis of pleural effusion (1,5). Cytologist faces two major problems: to prove the malignant origin of the pleural effusion by the existence of malignant cells and to prove the organ originated of those malignant cells. Thus, diagnostic accuracy of cytological examination of the pleural fluid varies from series to series. It is very low for some authors ranging from 15% to 35% (57,58), while is very high for others ranging from 80% to 90% (3,59).

D. Minimally Invasive Techniques

The blind pleural biopsy has similar results with pleural cytology (58). Combination of both techniques seems to improve diagnostic yield (5,60,61). The low diagnostic yield of closed pleural biopsy is due to factors such as small pleural extension, localization of tumors is unreachable by the needle areas of the pleura, including the visceral pleura (62), as well as to the physician's inexperience (63). Also, diagnostic yield of blind biopsy increases with the number of specimens taken in malignant pleural effusion (64). We need at least four biopsy samples (64). Because the pleural invasion is preferentially located in the bases of the hemithorax, it is recommended that the sample be taken from the lowest part in the costal pleura in order to achieve a higher diagnostic success (62,65).

When the pleural thoracocentesis and/or biopsy does not show any malignant cell and lung carcinoma is highly suspected, it is reasonable to perform fiberoptic bronchoscopy, as it may help in diagnosis (66). Indeed, pleural effusion of unknown origin after initial work up is associated with bronchogenic carcinoma in about 30% of the cases (66,67). Also, fiberoptic bronchoscopy is useful in assessing the extent of the disease in the tracheobronchial tree, which is important for the patient's treatment and prognosis (66).

Thoracoscopy is a simple and safe method of choice in the diagnosis of the cause of pleural effusion (68,69) and the assessment of the extent of lung carcinoma (6,70,71) (Fig. 5). This minimal invasive method can be performed by the pneumonologists under local anesthesia in the endoscopy suite, or by the thoracic surgeons [video-assisted thoracic surgery (VATS)] under general anesthesia and selective ventilation in the operating theater. Its sensitivity is ranging from 92% to 97% (72,73) and its specificity from 99% to 100% (70,72,73) in patients with malignant pleural effusion. If thoracocentesis is negative and there is suspicion of lung cancer, thoracoscopy can be performed to diagnose and to detect localized or diffused pleural infiltration (74), determining in case of non–small-cell lung carcinoma (NSCLC), the unresectable character of the tumor (Fig. 6) (6,75). Several series have been published in the last decades, showing the utility of thoracoscopy in staging NSCLC. Generally, these series confirm the low rate of resectability ranging from 0% to 36% (2,6) and so the poor prognosis in patients with lung cancer and pleural effusion. Many patients, even with paramalignant pleural effusions, may be unresectable, due to the extent of the intrathoracic tumor. This technique has limitations in recognizing a possible intrapleural extent of the disease, because localized disease may be missed and areas such as costodiaphragmatic angles and/or mediastinal pleura may be difficult to explore (75).

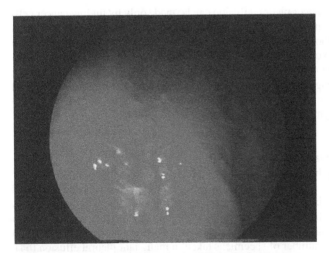

Figure 5   Metastatic nodules on the parietal pleura discovered during thoracoscopy in a patient with lung adenocarcinoma associated with a small costodiaphragmatic effusion.

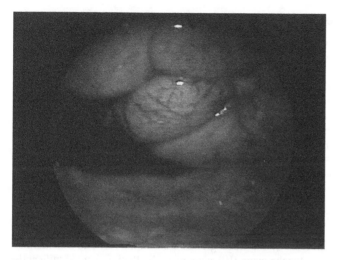

Figure 6   Lung adenocarcinoma of the lower lobe associated with satellite nodule and metastatic pleural effusion with secondary nodules on the parietal pleura.

Concluding diagnostic approach in patients with pleural effusion and suspected lung cancer, major investigations for diagnosis are cytopathologic examination from pleural combined to closed pleural biopsy puncture or thoracoscopy in case of failure and fiberoptic bronchoscopy (74). These examinations will also be useful in staging the disease and in prognosis or will condition for further investigations in case of lung cancer exclusion (Fig. 7).

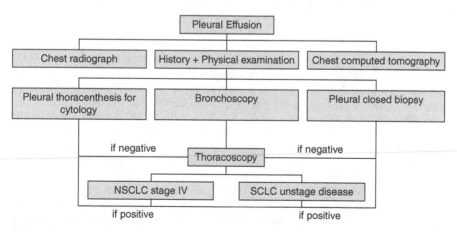

Figure 7   Diagnostic approach in a patient with pleural effusion and suspected lung cancer.

IV. Management

A. Stage of Patients with Lung Cancer and Pleural Effusion

Patients with NSCLC and confirmed malignant pleural effusion were classified as IIIB-T4, unresectable disease, according to the Mountain revised classification (4), although it was known already since 1974 that NSCLC patients with malignant pleural effusion presented a particularly poor prognosis (76,77). The reason of this classification was purely anatomic, as all situations within the hemithorax of the primary tumor should belong to the T component, except for nodules in another ipsilateral lobe.

For both 1986 (78) and 1997 (4) staging system revisions, NSCLC with malignant pleural effusion was classified IIIB-T4 disease, suggesting a more favorable prognosis for those patients than those with M1 disease. However, in the last decade, many authors raised the question, whether those patients should be classified as T4 disease since their survival seems to be significantly poorer than other IIIB-T4 (79–81).

Sugiura et al. (81) compared the survival of 197 patients with stage IIIB disease without pleural effusion, stage IIIB with pleural effusion, and stage IV disease. They found that the median survivals of the three groups were 15.3, 7.5, and 5.5 months, respectively. Survival curves for the stage IIIB patients with effusion were significantly worse than those for stage IIIB patients without effusion, but not significantly different from stage IV patients. Also, they found no significant difference in survival when pleural fluid cytology was positive or negative when negative effusion was exudative and/or bloody, and clinically judged malignant (81). Recently, the IASLC Lung Cancer Staging Project has reviewed the T and M stage of 18,198 NSCLC patients (82,83). Number of patients with pleural dissemination classified T4 according to the Mountain's revised classification were 471. Five year and median survival for those patients were 2% and 8 months, respectively, versus 14% and 13 months for clinical T4 disease other than pleural effusion ($p < 0.0001$).

Based on these observations, it is more appropriate to classify patients with pleural effusion as having stage IV rather than T4 stage IIIB disease, as both prognosis and management for these patients are similar to that for stage IV disease. Therefore, the latest IASLC proposals of the seventh classification suggest that patients with NSCLC and malignant pleural effusion are not classified as stage IIIB-T4, but are classified as stage IV-M1 (84,85).

In SCLC, survival and disease-free interval of patients with ipsilateral malignant pleural effusion seemed to be worse than the patients with limited-stage disease (LD) without pleural effusion, but better than those with extensive disease (ED), identical of those with limited disease without pleural effusion (86–88). However, it has been suggested that these patients should benefit the same treatment as LD (87).

Shepherd et al. (89) have reviewed the data of the SCLC database. Information concerning the presence or the absence of pleural effusion or other distant sites was available for 1258 patients with otherwise LD (1113 of whom were without pleural effusion, 145 with pleural effusion) and 4500 patients with ED with other metastatic sites. Of the 145 cases of limited disease with pleural effusion, 81 were actually designated as ED without any other metastatic sites. These 81 were assumed to have LD with pleural effusion. Surgically managed cases were excluded. The survival of patients with LD with effusion (median survival 12 months) is intermediate between those of patients with LD without effusion (median survival 18 months) and patients with ED (median survival

7 months) ($p = 0.0001$) (89). The result of cytologic examination of the pleural effusion was availabel for only 68 patients in the database. The survival of patients with LD with effusion, whether cytologically negative (median survival 13 months) or positive (median survival 12 months), remained intermediate between those of patients with LD without effusion (median survival 18 months) and patients with ED (median survival 7 months) ($p = 0.0001$) (89).

Their analysis showed that patients who have pleural effusion without extrathoracic metastases (M1a) have a survival that is intermediate between that of stage I–III without effusion and stage IV (89). Perng et al. reported a similar observation in a series of patients treated in Taiwan (88). Therefore, they recommended that pleural effusion should be a stratification parameter in clinical trials for both LD and ED SCLC (89). Having even a small proportion of patients with pleural effusion in LD trials could affect outcome significantly if they are not balanced between the arms, as could patients with only a pleural effusion in ED trials. The authors did not make a clear statement concerning cytology-positive or -negative effusions since they did not have enough patients in their analysis (89).

B. Therapeutic Approach

Parameters, other than the stage of the disease, taken under consideration before therapy in a lung cancer patient with pleural effusion are: the patient's performance status (90,91), the cell type of the lung carcinoma (92), the patient's expected survival, the patient's symptoms palliation with preservation of quality of life after therapy (93,94). All the above questions must be raised in each patient individually, before treatment initiation.

An important point is the patient's performance status (90,91). In patients with stage IV disease, if chemotherapy is to be given, it should be initiated while the patient still has good performance status. Delaying chemotherapy until performance status worsens or weight loss develops may negate the survival benefits of the treatment (93).

In good performance status NSCLC patients with resectable tumor and pleural effusion, surgical resection may be an option after repeated negative cytologic specimen of the pleural fluid, and negative thoracoscopy (6,71,95). However, resectability rate of patients with NSCLC and negative pleural effusion is low even after exploratory thoracotomy (2,7,45,72). This is due to the low rate of confirmed pathologically nonmalignant pleural effusion, and to the extent of the tumor in the chest wall, the mediastinum, and the mediastinal lymph nodes.

When a malignant pleural effusion is present in a patient with NSCLC at diagnosis, surgical resection is not possible (4,82,85). Systemic chemotherapy is indicated in unresectable NSCLC of good performance status (93,94), because meta-analysis has shown its benefits versus best supportive care (96,97). However, despite chemotherapy, survival of patients with stage IV disease and pleural effusion is poor ranging from 6.9 (98) to 12 months (99). Even the new chemotherapeutic agents have not yet proven a significant benefit in survival in large phase III trials (100,101), despite a better response rate reported in phase II trials (102–104). However, this response may be translated in gain of quality of life (96,97,105), especially in case of pleural effusion, with improvement of dyspnea (106). First-line chemotherapy should be a platinum-based combination, because survival improvement has been shown in it compare to nonplatinum doublets (94,105,107). Neither particular two-drug, platinum-based combination has been identified as superior in terms of efficacy, nor have three-drug combinations proven superior despite increased toxicity (100,108,109). Second-line chemotherapy should be addressed in patients with conservation of performance status (93,94).

Radiation therapy in NSCLC patients with pleural effusion is not indicated, since it did not prove any benefit in response rate nor in survival (110–112). However, in some cases, the combination of irradiation to chemotherapeutic agents as radiosensitizers (113), or as a part of multimodality treatment associating concomitant or alternating chemotherapy and irradiation, may offer local control (110,114–116).

In patients with SCLC and malignant pleural effusion, the treatment of choice is systemic chemotherapy (117), as untreated patients lived only four to six months (118). Platinum-based chemotherapy remains the mainstay of treatment for extensive SCLC (94). Pujol and associates published a meta-analysis of 19 trials randomizing 4054 assessable patients comparing cisplatin-based regimen with a non-cisplatin regimen. Patients randomized to regimens containing cisplatin had significantly increased survival rates of 2.6% and 4.4% at 6 and 12 months, respectively, without an increase in toxicity. These patients also had a significant lower risk of death at 6 (OR $= 0.87, p = 0.03$) and 12 months (OR $= 0.80, p = 0.002$) compare to patients treated in the non-platinum arm. The Mascaux et al. meta-analysis of 36 trials (119) confirmed the Pujol's results concerning the platinum-based chemotherapy, and indicated that the combination with etoposide offers significant better results than any other platinum-based combination. Concerning the platinum combinations with new drugs, a phase III trial randomizing 331 patients in two arms comparing cisplatin–irinotecan to cisplatin–etoposide, failed to show a survival, time to progression, or response-rate benefit (120). However, fewer patients treated with CDDP–irinotecan had grade 3/4 myelotoxicity, but more had grade 3/4 diarrhea and emesis (120).

Quality of life in cancer patients is an important factor of treatment (121–123). Dyspnea is a frequent and devastating symptom among advanced cancer patients and is often difficult to control (106). Lung cancer patients with dyspnea have shorter survival than patients with other types of cancer. Palliative care assessment should be focused on dyspnea (106,123). Management of symptomatic MPE begins with therapeutic thoracocentesis, which assesses the response of dyspnea to fluid removal (124). Although symptoms can improve after thoracocentesis, 98% to 100% of patients with MPE experience reaccumulation of fluid and recurrence of symptoms within 30 days. Repeated thoracocentesis, therefore, should be reserved for patients who reaccumulate pleural fluid slowly after each thoracocentesis; have cancers that commonly respond to therapy with resolution of the associated effusions; appear unlikely to survive beyond one to three months; and cannot tolerate other more interventional procedures to control pleural fluid, such as pleurodesis (124).

We should consider pleurodesis in patients with significant and/or invalidating pleural effusion whose general condition is good and whose expected survival is prolonged (39,125,126). Pleurodesis may be followed by systemic chemotherapy if necessary, in order to palliate lung carcinoma. Several modalities of pleurodesis are possible, such as chemical pleurodesis through a simple thoracic drain tube or during medical thoracoscopy, VATS, thoracoscopic or surgical pleural abrasion or pleurectomy (126,127).

Criteria for successful pleurodesis are reexpandable lung, complete removal of the pleural fluid (<100 mL drainage/24 hr). Although low pleural fluid pH (<7.20) may indicate trapped lung, short expected survival, and ineffective pleurodesis (126,128,129); Aelony et al. reported that thoracoscopic talc poudrage was successful in 88% of patients with malignant pleural effusion despite low pH (130). The choice of the sclerosing agent has been the subject of many publications. More than 30 agents have been proposed as sclerosants to induce pleurodesis through the last decades (1,5,126,127). Cyclins (doxy-cycline, minocycline, tetracycline hydrocloride) are instilled intrapleurally in a saline solution through a chest tube (131–133). Their effectiveness in malignant pleural effusion is ranging from 25% (134) to 88% (135). Their advantages are the mild and rare side effects (chest pain, fever) and low cost. Since few years, tetracycline is not available but minocycline and doxycycline are good alternatives (136,137).

Bleomycin has a success rate comparable to cyclins, ranging from 35% (134) to 90%, with the same side effects. However, the cost of pleurodesis with bleomycin was evaluated about 80 times the cost of talc slurry (138). New cytostatics instilled in the pleura such as taxans has also been used as sclerosing agents (139). Antimitotic drugs were not only used for pleurodesis, but also to treat locally the underlying disease (140). However, the toxicity and current high cost of the use of cytostatics limits considerably their utilization (141–144).

Talc is the agent most commonly used, as it is the most effective (over 90% of success rate) and cheap (about $13) at the present time for pleurodesis in malignant pleural effusions (1,125–127,145,146). Administration of talc in the pleura may be performed through a chest tube diluted in a saline solution (talc slurry) (136,138), or aerosolized powder during medical (5,73,75,147) or surgical thoracoscopy (148,149), initiating an inflammatory reaction that produces pleurodesis (150,151). Both methods seem to be effective (median success rate 90%), although it seems that thoracoscopic method has an advantage (130,141,145,152–155). Tan and associates have reviewed 2053 lung cancer patients with pleural effusion, from different databases included in randomized trials (156). They concluded that talc should be the agent of choice for pleurodesis since it is associated with fewer rate of recurrences versus bleomycin or versus tetracycline. Also, thoracoscopy talc insufflation is associated with less possibilities of effusion recurrence than talc slurry, although there is lack of large number of studies and patients (156).

Side effects of talc are not different from other agents. Some authors do not rec-ommend talc for pleurodesis as cases of respiratory insufficiency have been reported (157–159). However, various bias exist explaining, in a part, the respiratory complica-tions from talc such as the patient's poor performance status, his respiratory comorbidities (COPD), and the extent of the pleural effusion, suggesting that earlier the pleurodesis is performed, lower is the frequency of occurrence of such manifestations (160). Another important point is the choice of the right powder in the right dose, suggesting that respi-ratory complications may be avoided (146). Recently, Janssen et al. reported a study in more than 500 patients with malignant pleural effusion, showing that the French talc is safe with no case of ARDS reported (161). Talc is also the less-expensive agent for pleu-rodesis currently commercialized (141,142,146,162). *Corynebacterium parvum* injected intrapleurally without chest tube drainage has been tested as a sclerosing agent with good results and no specific side effects (163,164). Other compounds used as scleros-ing agents are interferon (165), quinacrine (166). Pleural abrasion by gauze may be an alternative when no talc is availabel. The method is performed during medical or surgical thoracoscopy, which means a knowledge of the procedure (148,152,157). Pleurectomy may also be an alternative (164,167,168), but this method is aggressive in patients with advanced malignancy, considering the great number of noninvasive chemical pleurodesis possibilities.

V. Conclusion

Pleural effusion in patients with lung cancer represents an important clinical condition. Considerable advances have been made in the diagnosis of lung cancer patients with malignant pleural effusion through specialized imaging and minimally invasive techniques. Although therapy is directed towards palliation of symptoms, appropriate management may improve survival, functional capacity, and quality of life. Pleurodesis, especially thoracoscopic talc poudrage, when is indicated offers an important palliation of symptoms. Based on survival data, the new (seventh) revised classification of lung cancer proposed the switch of malignant pleural effusion into stage IV-M1 disease for NSCL. No clear stage is actually available for patients with SCLC and pleural effusion. Chemotherapy with a platinum combination is actually indicated in patients with good performance status. Through careful assessment of the patient's stage and physical condition, combined with an evaluation of the pleural effusion, an effective intervention exists to provide effective palliation in almost every clinical circumstance.

References

1. Sahn SA. Malignancy metastatic to the pleura. Clin Chest Med 1998; 19:351–361.
2. Le Roux BT. Bronchial Carcinoma. London, U.K.: E & S Livingstone, 1968.
3. Johnston WW. The malignant pleural effusion. A review of cytopathologic diagnoses of 584 specimens from 472 consecutive patients. Cancer 1985; 56:905–909.
4. Mountain CF. Revisions for the international system for staging lung cancer. Chest 1997; 111:1710–1715.
5. Antony VB, Loddenkemper R, Astoul P, et al. Management of malignant pleural effusions. Eur Respir J 2001; 18:402–419.
6. Rodriguez Panadero F. Lung cancer and ipsilateral pleural effusion. Ann Oncol 1995; 6:S25–S27.
7. Rodriguez-Panadero F, Borderas Naranjo F, Lopez Mejias J. Pleural metastatic tumours and effusions. Frequency and pathogenic mechanisms in a post-mortem series. Eur Respir J 1989; 2:366–369.
8. Meyer PC. Metastatic carcinoma of the pleura. Thorax 1966; 21:437–443.
9. Chernow B, Sahn SA. Carcinomatous involvement of the pleura: An analysis of 96 patients. Am J Med 1977; 63:695–702.
10. Leff A, Hopewell PC, Costello J. Pleural effusion from malignancy. Ann Intern Med 1978; 88:532–537.
11. Domagala W, Emeson E, Kass LG. Distribution of T-lymphocytes and B-lymphocytes in peripheral blood and effusions in patients with cancer. J Natl Cancer Inst 1978; 61:295–301.
12. Kabnick EM, Sobo S, Steinbaum S, et al. Spontaneous pneumothorax from bronchogenic carcinoma. J Natl Med Assoc 1982; 74:478–479.
13. Hyde L, Hyde CI. Clinical manifestations of lung cancer. Chest 1974; 65:299–306.
14. Cohen MH. Signs and symptoms of bronchogenic carcinoma. Semin Oncol 1974; 1:183–189.
15. Scagliotti GV. Symptoms and signs and staging of lung cancer. Eur Respir Mon 1995; 1:91–136.
16. Grippi MA. Clinical aspects of lung cancer. Semin Roentgenol 1990; 25:12–24.
17. White CS, Templeton PA, Belani CP. Imaging in lung cancer. Semin Oncol 1993; 20:142–152.

18. Romney BM, Austin JHM. Plain film evaluation of carcinoma of the lung. Semin Roentgenol 1990; 25:45–63.

19. Woodring JH. Pitfalls in the radiologic diagnosis of lung cancer. AJR Am J Roentgenol 1990; 154:1165–1175.

20. Steinhausling CA, Cuttat JF. Spontaneous pneumothorax a complication of lung cancer? Chest 1985; 88:709–713.

21. Woodring JH. Unusual radiographic manifestations of lung cancer. Radiol Clinics North Am 1990; 28:599–618.

22. McLoud TC. CT and MRI in pleural space. Clin Chest Med 1998; 19:261–276.

23. Armstrong P, Reznek RH, Phillips RR. Diagnostic imaging of lung cancer. Eur Respir Mon 1995; 1:137–187.

24. Leung AN, Müller NL, Miller RR. CT in differential diagnosis of diffuse pleura disease. AJR Am J Roentgenol 1990; 154:487–492.

25. Glazer HS, Kaiser LR, Anderson DJ, et al. Indeterminate mediastinal invasion in bronchogenic carcinoma: CT evaluation. Radiology 1989; 173:37–42.

26. Rato GB, Piacenza G, Frola C, et al. Chest wall involvement by lung cancer: Computed tomography detection and results of operation. Ann Thorac Surg 1991; 51:182–188.

27. Pearlberg JL, Sandler MA, Beute GH. Limitations of CT in evaluation of neoplasms involving chest wall. J Comput Assist Tomogr 1987; 11:290–293.

28. Glazer HS, Duncan-Meyer J, Aronberg DJ, et al. Pleural and chest wall invasion in bronchogenic carcinoma: CT evaluation. Radiology 1985; 157:191–194.

29. Webb WR. The role of magnetic resonance imaging in the assessment of patients with lung cancer. A comparison with computed tomography. J Thorac Imaging 1989; 4:65–75.

30. Templeton PA, Caskey CI, Zerhouni EA. Current uses of CT and MR imaging in the staging of lung cancer. Radiol Clin North Am 1990; 28:631–646.

31. Duysinx B, Nguyen D, Louis R, et al. Evaluation of pleural disease with 18-fluorodeoxyglucose positron emission tomography imaging. Chest 2004; 125:489–493.

32. Erasmus JJ, McAdams HP, Rossi SE, et al. FDG PET of pleural effusions in patients with non-small cell lung cancer. AJR Am J Roentgenol 2000; 175:245–249.

33. Schaffler GJ, Wolf G, Schoellnast H, et al. Non-small cell lung cancer: Evaluation of pleural abnormalities on CT scans with 18F FDG PET. Radiology 2004; 231:858–865.

34. Kwek BH, Aquino SL, Fischman AJ. Fluorodeoxyglucose positron emission tomography and CT after talc pleurodesis. Chest 2004; 125:2356–2360.

35. O'Moore PV, Mueller PR, Simeone JF, et al. Sonographic guidance in diagnostic and therapeutic interventions in the pleural space. AJR Am J Roentgenol 1987; 149:1–5.

36. Lipscomb DJ, Flower CD, Hadfield JW. Ultrasound of the pleural: An assessment of its clinical value. Clin Radiol 1981; 32:289–290.

37. Henschke CI, Davis SD, Romano PM, et al. Pleural effusions: Pathogenesis, radiologic evaluation and therapy. J Thorac Imag 1989; 4:49–60.

38. Yang PC, Luh KT, Chang DB, et al. Value of sonography in determining the nature of pleural effusion: Analysis of 320 cases. AJR Am J Roentgenol 1992; 159:29–33.

39. Sahn SA. Pleural effusion in lung cancer. Clin Chest Med 1982; 3:443–452.

40. Light RW, Macgregor MI, Luchsinger PC, et al. Pleural effusions: The diagnostic separation of transudates and exudates. Ann Intern Med 1972; 77:507–513.

41. Light RW. Pleural Disease, 3rd ed. Baltimore, Maryland: Williams & Wilkins, 1995:36–74.

42. Light RW, MacGregor MI, Ball WC Jr, et al. Diagnostic significance of pleural fluid pH and PCO_2. Chest 1973; 64:591–596.

43. Berger HW, Maher G. Decreased glucose concentration in malignant pleural effusions. Am Rev Respir Dis 1971; 103:427–429.

44. Chavalittamrong B, Angsusingha K, Tuchinda M, et al. Diagnostic significance of pH, lactic acid dehydrogenase, lactate and glucose in pleural fluid. Respiration 1979; 38:112–120.

45. Good JT Jr, Taryle DA, Sahn SA. The pathogenesis of low glucose, low pH malignant effusions. Am Rev Respir Dis 1985; 131:737–741.
46. Heffner JE. Evaluating diagnostic tests in the pleural space. Clin Chest Med 1998; 19:277–293.
47. Kuhn M, Fitting JW, Leuenberger P. Probability of malignancy in pleural fluid eosinophilia. Chest 1989; 96:992–994.
48. Rubins JB, Rubins HB. Etiology and prognostic significance of eosinophilic pleural effusions. A prospective study. Chest 1996; 110:1271–1274.
49. Cascinu S, Del Ferro E, Barbanti I, et al. Tumor markers in the diagnosis of malignant serous effusions. Am J Clin Oncol 1997; 20:247–250.
50. Alatas F, Alatas O, Metintas M, et al. Diagnostic value of CEA, CA 15-3, CA 19-9, CYFRA 21-1, NSE and TSA assay in pleural effusions. Lung Cancer 2001; 31:9–16.
51. Menard O, Dousset B, Jacob C, et al. Improvement of the diagnosis of the cause of pleural effusion in patients with lung cancer by simultaneous quantification of carcinoembryonic antigen (CEA) and neuron-specific enolase (NSE) pleural levels. Eur J Cancer 1993; 13:1806–1809.
52. Falcone F, Marinelli M, Minguzzi L, et al. Tumor markers and lung cancer: Guidelines in a cost-limited medical organization. Int J Biol Markers 1996; 11:61–66.
53. Stoetzer OJ, Munker R, Darsow M, et al. P53-immunoreactive cells in benign and malignant effusions: Diagnostic value using a panel of monoclonal antibodies and comparison with CEA-staining. Oncol Rep 1999; 6:455–458.
54. Alexandrakis MG, Coulocheri SA, Bouros D, et al. Evaluation of inflammatory cytokines in malignant and benign pleural effusions. Oncol Rep 2000; 7:1327–1332.
55. Hurewitz AN, Zucker S, Mancuso P, et al. Human pleural effusions are rich in matrix metalloproteinases. Chest 1992; 102:1808–1814.
56. Marel M, Stastny B, Melinova L, et al. Diagnosis of pleural effusions. Experience with clinical studies, 1986 to 1990. Chest 1995; 107:1598–1603.
57. Storey DD, Dines DE, Coles DT. Pleural effusion: A diagnostic dilemma. JAMA 1976; 236:2183–2186.
58. Salyer WA, Eggleston JC, Erozan YS. Efficacy of pleural needle biopsy and pleural fluid cytopathology in the diagnosis of malignant neoplasm involving the pleura. Chest 1975; 67:536–538.
59. Light RW, Erozan YS, Ball WC. Cells in pleural fluid. Their value in differential diagnosis. Arch Intern Med 1973; 132:854–860.
60. Antony VB, Loddenkemper R, Astoul P, et al. Management of malignant pleural effusions. Eur Respir J 2001; 18:402–419.
61. Edmondstone WM. Investigation of pleural effusion: Comparison between fiberoptic thoracoscopy, needle biopsy and cytology. Respir Med 1990; 84:23–26.
62. Canto A, Rivas J, Saumench J, et al. Points to consider when choosing a biopsy method in cases of pleurisy of unknown origin. Chest 1983; 84:176–179.
63. Walshe AD, Douglas JG, Kerr KM, et al. An audit of the clinical investigation of pleural effusion. Thorax 1992; 47:734–737.
64. Jimenez D, Perez-Rodriguez E, Diaz G, et al. Determining the optimal number of specimens to obtain with needle biopsy of the pleura. Respir Med 2002; 96:14–17.
65. Rodriguez-Panadero F, Borderas Naranjo F, Lopez Mejias J. Pleural metastatic tumours and effusions. Frequency and pathogenic mechanisms in a post-mortem series. Eur Respir J 1989; 2:366–369.
66. Vergnon JM, Froudarakis M. Bronchoscopy. In: Grassi C, ed. Pulmonary Diseases. London, U.K.: McGraw-Hill International, 1999:39–43.
67. Poe RH, Levy PC, Israel RH, et al. Use of fiberoptic bronchoscopy in the diagnosis of bronchogenic carcinoma. A study in patients with idiopathic pleural effusions. Chest 1994; 105:1663–1667.

68. Mathur PN, Astoul P, Boutin C. Medical thoracoscopy: Technical details. Clin Chest Med 1995; 16:479–486.
69. Boutin C, Astoul P. Diagnostic thoracoscopy. Clin Chest Med 1998; 19:295–309.
70. Roeslin N, Kessler R. Quelle est la place de la thoracoscopie dans le bilan d'extension pré-opératoire du cancer bronchique non à petites cellules? Rev Mal Respir 1992; 9:R247–R251.
71. Canto A, Ferrer G, Romagosa V, et al. Lung cancer and pleural effusion. Clinical significance and study of pleural metastatic locations. Chest 1985; 87:649–652.
72. Boutin C, Viallat JR, Cargnino P, et al. Indications actuelles de la thoracoscopie. Compte rendu du Symposium de Marseille. Rev Fr Mal Respir 1981; 9:309–318.
73. Boutin C, Loddenkemper R, Astoul P. Diagnostic and therapeutic thoracoscopy: Techniques and indications in pulmonary medicine. Tuber Lung Dis 1993; 74:225–239.
74. Froudarakis ME. Diagnostic work-up of pleural effusion. Respiration 2008; 75:4–13.
75. Colt HG. Thoracoscopic management of malignant pleural effusions. Clin Chest Med 1995; 16:505–518.
76. Carr DT, Mountain CF. The staging of lung cancer. Semin Oncol 1974; 1:229–234.
77. Mountain CF, Carr DT, Anderson WA. A system for the clinical staging of lung cancer. Am J Roentgenol Radium Ther Nucl Med 1974; 120:130–138.
78. Mountain CF. A new international staging system for lung cancer. Chest 1986; 89:225S–233S.
79. Alon BN, Anson BL. Pleural effusion in patients with non-small cell carcinoma—Stage IV and not T4. Lung Cancer 2007; 57:123.
80. Leong SS, Rocha Lima CM, Sherman CA, et al. The 1997 International Staging System for non-small cell lung cancer: Have all the issues been addressed? Chest 1999; 115:242–248.
81. Sugiura S, Ando Y, Minami H, et al. Prognostic value of pleural effusion in patients with non-small cell lung cancer. Clin Cancer Res 1997; 3:47–50.
82. Rami-Porta R, Ball D, Crowley J, et al. The IASLC Lung Cancer Staging Project: Proposals for the revision of the T descriptors in the forthcoming (seventh) edition of the TNM classification for lung cancer. J Thorac Oncol 2007; 2:593–602.
83. Postmus PE, Brambilla E, Chansky K, et al. The IASLC Lung Cancer Staging Project: Proposals for revision of the M descriptors in the forthcoming (seventh) edition of the TNM classification of lung cancer. J Thorac Oncol 2007; 2:686–693.
84. Goldstraw P, Crowley J, Chansky K, et al. The IASLC Lung Cancer Staging Project: Proposals for the revision of the TNM stage groupings in the forthcoming (seventh) edition of the TNM Classification of malignant tumours. J Thorac Oncol 2007; 2:706–714.
85. Groome PA, Bolejack V, Crowley J, et al. The IASLC Lung Cancer Staging Project: Validation of the proposals for the revision of the TNM stage groupings in the forthcoming (seventh) edition of the TNM classification of malignant tumours. J Thorac Oncol 2007; 2:694–705.
86. Shepherd FA, Ginsberg RJ, Haddad R, et al. Importance of clinical staging in limited small-cell lung cancer: A valuable system to separate prognostic subgroups. The University of Toronto Lung Oncology Group. J Clin Oncol 1993; 11:1592–1597.
87. Livingston RB, McCracken JD, Trauth CJ, et al. Isolated pleural effusion in small cell lung carcinoma: Favorable prognosis. A review of the Southwest Oncology Group experience. Chest 1982; 81:208–211.
88. Perng RP, Chen CY, Chang GC, et al. Revisit of 1997 TNM staging system—survival analysis of 1112 lung cancer patients in Taiwan. Jpn J Clin Oncol 2007; 37:9–15.
89. Shepherd FA, Crowley J, Van Houtte P, et al. The IASLC Lung Cancer Staging Project: Proposals regarding the clinical staging of small cell lung cancer in the forthcoming (seventh) edition of the TNM classification for lung cancer. J Thorac Oncol 2007; 2:1067–1077.
90. Stanley KE. Prognostic factors for survival in patients with inoperable lung cancer. JNCI 1980; 65:25–32.
91. Albain KS, Crowley JJ, LeBlanc M, et al. Survival determinants in extensive-stage non-small cell lung cancer: The Southwestern Oncology Group experience. J Clin Oncol 1991; 9:1618–1626.

92. Mountain CF, Lukeman JM, Hammar SP, et al. Lung cancer classification: The relationship of disease extent and cell type to survival in a clinical trials population. J Surg Oncol 1987; 35:147–156.

93. Pfister DG, Johnson DH, Azzoli CG, et al. American Society of Clinical Oncology treatment of unresectable non-small-cell lung cancer guideline: Update 2003. J Clin Oncol 2004; 22:330–353.

94. Socinski MA, Crowell R, Hensing TE, et al. Treatment of non-small cell lung cancer, stage IV: ACCP evidence-based clinical practice guidelines (2nd edition). Chest 2007; 132:277S–289S.

95. Decker DA, Dines DE, Payne WS, et al. The significance of cytologically negative pleural effusion in bronchogenic carcinoma. Chest 1978; 74:640–642.

96. Souquet PJ, Chauvin F, Boissel JP, et al. Polychemotherapy in advanced non small cell lung cancer: A meta-analysis. Lancet 1993; 342:19–21.

97. Souquet PJ, Chauvin F, Boissel JP, et al. Meta-analysis of randomised trials of systemic chemotherapy versus supportive treatment in non-resectable non-small cell lung cancer. Lung Cancer 1995; 12(Suppl. 1):S147–S154.

98. Albain KS, Hoffman PC, Little AG, et al. Pleural involvement in stage IIIM0 non-small-cell bronchogenic carcinoma. A need to differentiate subtypes. Am J Clin Oncol 1986; 9:255–261.

99. Fujita A, Takabatake H, Tagaki S, et al. Combination chemotherapy in patients with malignant pleural effusions from non-small cell lung cancer: Cisplatin, ifosfamide, and irinotecan with recombinant human granulocyte colony-stimulating factor support. Chest 2001; 119:340–343.

100. Schiller JH, Harrington D, Belani CP, et al. Comparison of four chemotherapy regimens for advanced non-small-cell lung cancer. N Engl J Med 2002; 346:92–98.

101. Comella P, Frasci G, Panza N, et al. Randomized trial comparing cisplatin, gemcitabine, and vinorelbine with either cisplatin and gemcitabine or cisplatin and vinorelbine in advanced non-small-cell lung cancer: Interim analysis of a phase III trial of the Southern Italy Cooperative Oncology Group. J Clin Oncol 2000; 18:1451–1457.

102. Jett JR, Kirschling RJ, Jung SH, et al. A phase II study of paclitaxel and granulocyte colony-stimulating factor in previously untreated patients with extensive-stage small cell lung cancer: A study of the North Central Cancer Treatment Group. Semin Oncol 1995; 22:75–77.

103. Lilenbaum RC, Green MR. Novel chemotherapeutic agents in the treatment of non-small-cell lung cancer. J Clin Oncol 1993; 11:1391–1402.

104. Mattson K, Saarinen A, Jekunen A. Combination treatment with docetaxel (Taxotere) and platinum compounds for non-small cell lung cancer. Semin Oncol 1997; 24:S14-5-S-8.

105. Non-Small-Cell Lung Cancer Cooperative Group. Chemotherapy in non-small cell lung cancer: A meta-analysis using updated data on individual patients from 52 randomised clinical trials. BMJ 1995; 311:899–909.

106. Ripamonti C. Management of dyspnea in advanced cancer patients. Support Care Cancer 1999; 7:233–243.

107. Socinski MA, Morris DE, Masters GA, et al. Chemotherapeutic management of stage IV non-small cell lung cancer. Chest 2003; 123:226S–243S.

108. Masutani M, Akusawa H, Kadota A, et al. A phase III randomized trial of cisplatin plus vindesine versus cisplatin plus vindesine plus mitomycin C versus cisplatin plus vindesine plus ifosfamide for advanced non-small-cell lung cancer. Respirology 1996; 1:49–54.

109. Greco FA, Gray JR Jr, Thompson DS, et al. Prospective randomized study of four novel chemotherapy regimens in patients with advanced nonsmall cell lung carcinoma: A Minnie Pearl Cancer Research Network trial. Cancer 2002; 95:1279–1285.

110. Werner-Wasik M, Scott C, Cox JD, et al. Recursive partitioning analysis of 1999 Radiation Therapy Oncology Group (RTOG) patients with locally-advanced non-small-cell lung cancer

(LA-NSCLC): Identification of five groups with different survival. Int J Radiat Oncol Biol Phys 2000; 48:1475–1482.

111. Wigren T, Kellokumpu-Lehtinen P, Ojala A. Radical radiotherapy of inoperable non-small cell lung cancer. Irradiation techniques and tumor characteristics in relation to local control and survival. Acta Oncol 1992; 31:555–561.

112. Scott C, Sause WT, Byhardt R, et al. Recursive partitioning analysis of 1592 patients on four Radiation Therapy Oncology Group studies in inoperable non-small cell lung cancer. Lung Cancer 1997; 17(Suppl. 1): S59–S74.

113. Koukourakis MI, Bahlitzanakis N, Froudarakis M, et al. Concurrent conventionally fractionated radiotherapy and weekly docetaxel in the treatment of stage IIIb non-small-cell lung carcinoma. Br J Cancer 1999; 80:1792–1796.

114. Marino P, Preatoni A, Cantoni A. Randomized trials of radiotherapy alone versus combined chemotherapy and radiotherapy in stages IIIa and IIIb nonsmall cell lung cancer. A meta-analysis. Cancer 1995; 76:593–601.

115. Baldini E, Silvano G, Tibaldi C, et al. Sequential chemoradiation therapy with vinorelbine, ifosfamide, and cisplatin in stage IIIB non-small cell lung cancer: A phase II study. Semin Oncol 2000; 27:28–32.

116. Eberhardt W, Bildat S, Korfee S. Combined modality therapy in NSCLC. Ann Oncol 2000; 11:85–95.

117. Rawson N, Peto J. An overview of prognostic factors in small-cell lung cancer. Br J Cancer 1990; 61:597–604.

118. Zelen M. Keynote address on biostatistics and data retrieval. Cancer Chemoth Rep 1973; 4:31–42.

119. Mascaux C, Paesmans M, Berghmans T, et al. A systematic review of the role of etoposide and cisplatin in the chemotherapy of small cell lung cancer with methodology assessment and meta-analysis. Lung Cancer 2000; 30:23–36.

120. Hanna N, Bunn PA Jr, Langer C, et al. Randomized phase III trial comparing irinotecan/cisplatin with etoposide/cisplatin in patients with previously untreated extensive-stage disease small-cell lung cancer. J Clin Oncol 2006; 24:2038–2043.

121. Aaronson NK. Methodologic issues in assessing the quality of life of cancer patients. Semin Oncol 1991; 67:844–850.

122. Muers MF. Quality of life and symptom control. Eur Respir Mon 2001; 17:305–329.

123. Heffner JE. Diagnosis and management of malignant pleural effusions. Respirology 2008; 13:5–20.

124. Heffner JE, Klein JS. Recent advances in the diagnosis and management of malignant pleural effusions. Mayo Clin Proc 2008; 83:235–250.

125. Sahn SA. Pleural effusion in lung cancer. Clin Chest Med 1993; 14:189–200.

126. Rodriguez-Panadero F, Antony VB. Pleurodesis: State of the art. Eur Respir J 1997; 10:1648–1654.

127. Rodriguez-Panadero F. Current trends in pleurodesis. Curr Opin Pulm Med 1997; 3:319–325.

128. Sanchez-Armengol A, Rodriguez-Panadero F. Survival and talc pleurodesis in metastatic pleural carcinoma, revisited. Report of 125 cases. Chest 1993; 104:1482–1485.

129. Sahn SA. Malignancy metastatic to the pleura. Clin Chest Med 1998; 19:351–361.

130. Aelony Y, King RR, Boutin C. Thoracoscopic talc poudrage in malignant pleural effusions: Effective pleurodesis despite low pleural pH. Chest 1998; 113:1007–1012.

131. Antony VB, Rothfuss KJ, Godbey SW, et al. Mechanism of tetracycline-hydrochloride-induced pleurodesis. Tetracycline-hydrochloride-stimulated mesothelial cells produce a growth-factor-like activity for fibroblasts. Am Rev Respir Dis 1992; 146:1009–1013.

132. Herrington JD, Gora-Harper ML, Salley RK. Chemical pleurodesis with doxycycline 1 g. Pharmacotherapy 1996; 16:280–285.

133. Mansson T. Treatment of malignant pleural effusion with doxycycline. Scand J Infect Dis Suppl 1988; 53:29–34.
134. Emad A, Rezaian GR. Treatment of malignant pleural effusions with a combination of bleomycin and tetracycline. A comparison of bleomycin or tetracycline alone versus a combination of bleomycin and tetracycline. Cancer 1996; 78:2498–2501.
135. Robinson LA, Fleming WH, Galbraith TA. Intrapleural doxycycline control of malignant pleural effusions. Ann Thorac Surg 1993; 55:1115–1121; discussion 21–22.
136. Grasela TH, Walawander CA, Jolson HM, et al. Alternatives to intravenous tetracycline hydrochloride for malignant pleural effusions. Ann Pharmacother 1994; 28:968–969.
137. Light RW, Wang NS, Sassoon CS, et al. Comparison of the effectiveness of tetracycline and minocycline as pleural sclerosing agents in rabbits. Chest 1994; 106:577–582.
138. Zimmer PW, Hill M, Casey K, et al. Prospective randomized trial of talc slurry vs bleomycin in pleurodesis for symptomatic malignant pleural effusions. Chest 1997; 112:430–434.
139. Perng RP, Chen YM, Wu MF, et al. Phase II trial of intrapleural paclitaxel injection for non-small-cell lung cancer patients with malignant pleural effusions. Respir Med 1998; 92:473–479.
140. Rusch VW, Figlin R, Godwin D, et al. Intrapleural cisplatin and cytarabine in the management of malignant pleural effusions: A Lung Cancer Study Group trial. J Clin Oncol 1991; 9:313–319.
141. Diacon AH, Wyser C, Bolliger CT, et al. Prospective randomized comparison of thoracoscopic talc poudrage under local anesthesia versus bleomycin instillation for pleurodesis in malignant pleural effusions. Am J Respir Crit Care Med 2000; 162:1445–1449.
142. Aelony Y. Cost-effective pleurodesis. Chest 1998; 113:1731–1732.
143. Martinez-Moragon E, Aparicio J, Rogado MC, et al. Pleurodesis in malignat pleural effusions: A randomized study of tetracycline versus bleomycin. Eur Respir J 1997; 10:2380–2383.
144. Ong KC, Indumathi V, Raghuram J, et al. A comparative study of pleurodesis using talc slurry and bleomycin in the management of malignant pleural effusions. Respirology 2000; 5:99–103.
145. Rodriguez-Panadero F. Malignant pleural diseases. Monaldi Arch Chest Dis 2000; 55:17–19.
146. Bouros D, Froudarakis M, Siafakas NM. Pleurodesis: Everything flows. Chest 2000; 118:577–579.
147. Mathur PN, Loddenkemper R. Medical thoracoscopy. Role in pleural and lung diseases. Clin Chest Med 1995; 16:487–496.
148. Perrault LP, Gregoire J, Page A. Video-assisted thoracoscopy and thoracic surgery: The first 50 patients. Ann Chir 1993; 47:838–843.
149. Schulze M, Boehle AS, Kurdow R, et al. Effective treatment of malignant pleural effusion by minimal invasive thoracic surgery: Thoracoscopic talc pleurodesis and pleuroperitoneal shunts in 101 patients. Ann Thorac Surg 2001; 71:1809–1812.
150. Ferrer J, Montes JF, Villarino MA, et al. Influence of particle size on extrapleural talc dissemination after talc slurry pleurodesis. Chest 2002; 122:1018–1027.
151. Froudarakis ME, Klimathianaki M, Pougounias M. Systemic inflammatory reaction after thoracoscopic talc poudrage. Chest 2006; 129:356–361.
152. Colt HG, Russack V, Chiu Y, et al. A comparison of thoracoscopic talc insufflation, slurry, and mechanical abrasion pleurodesis. Chest 1997; 111:442–448.
153. Yim AP, Chan AT, Lee TW, et al. Thoracoscopic talc insufflation versus talc slurry for symptomatic malignant pleural effusion. Ann Thorac Surg 1996; 62:1655–1658.
154. Cohen RG, Shely WW, Thompson SE, et al. Talc pleurodesis: Talc slurry versus thoracoscopic talc insufflation in a porcine model. Ann Thorac Surg 1996; 62:1000–1002; discussion 3-4.
155. Aelony Y. Talc pleurodesis. Talc slurry vs talc poudrage. Chest 1995; 108:289.
156. Tan C, Sedrakyan A, Browne J, et al. The evidence on the effectiveness of management for malignant pleural effusion: A systematic review. Eur J Cardiothorac Surg 2006; 29:829–838.

157. Light RW. Diseases of the pleura: The use of talc for pleurodesis. Curr Opin Pulm Med 2000; 6:255–258.
158. Brant A, Eaton T. Serious complications with talc slurry pleurodesis. Respirology 2001; 6:181–185.
159. de Campos JR, Vargas FS, de Campos Werebe E, et al. Thoracoscopy talc poudrage: A 15-year experience. Chest 2001; 119:801–806.
160. Viallat JR, Rey F, Astoul P, et al. Thoracoscopic talc poudrage pleurodesis for malignant effusions. A review of 360 cases. Chest 1996; 110:1387–1393.
161. Janssen JP, Collier G, Astoul P, et al. Safety of pleurodesis with talc poudrage in malignant pleural effusion: A prospective cohort study. Lancet 2007; 369:1535–1539.
162. Belani CP, Pajeau TS, Bennett CL. Treating malignant pleural effusions cost consciously. Chest 1998; 113(1Suppl):78s–85s.
163. Walker-Renard PB, Vaughan LM, Sahn SA. Chemical pleurodesis for malignant pleural effusions. Ann Intern Med 1994; 120:56–64.
164. Vargas FS, Teixeira LR. Pleural malignancies. Curr Opin Pulm Med 1996; 2:335–340.
165. Parulekar W, Di Primio G, Matzinger F, et al. Use of small-bore vs large-bore chest tubes for treatment of malignant pleural effusions. Chest 2001; 120:19–25.
166. Banerjee AK, Willetts I, Robertson JF, et al. Pleural effusion in breast cancer: A review of the Nottingham experience. Eur J Surg Oncol 1994; 20:33–36.
167. Keller SM. Current and future therapy for malignant pleural effusion. Chest 1993; 103:63S–67S.
168. Ruckdeschel JC. Management of malignant pleural effusion: An overview. Semin Oncol 1988; 15:24–28.

26

Benign Tumors of the Pleura

CAMERON D. WRIGHT and EUGENE J. MARK
Harvard Medical School and Massachusetts General Hospital, Boston, Massachusetts, U.S.A.

Localized fibrous tumors of the pleura (LFTP) are rare, usually benign neoplasms of the pleura. This tumor has received many names including fibrous mesothelioma, benign mesothelioma, localized mesothelioma, subpleural fibroma, solitary fibrous tumor of the pleura, and LFTP, which reflect clinical and pathological characteristics of this tumor (1). Recently, the term fibrous tumor of the pleura has been preferred as it emphasizes its distinct separation from malignant mesothelioma. In contradistinction to LFTP, malignant mesothelioma is causally related to asbestos exposure, is usually diffuse in gross appearance, is of mesothelial origin and stains for cytokeratin, and is rapidly fatal. LFTP is the preferred description of this tumor rather than solitary fibrous tumors of the pleura (SFTP) because several reports have documented multiple LFTP within the same patient (2,3).

I. History

The first LFTP was probably described by Wagner in 1870 (4). In 1931, Klemperer and Rabin divided primary tumors of the pleura into two types: localized and diffuse (5). The diffuse form (malignant mesothelioma) was purported to arise from the mesothelial cells whereas the localized form (LFTP) was thought to arise from the submesothelial fibrous connective tissue. Clagett et al. reported the first large (24 patients) surgical series in 1952 from the Mayo Clinic and stressed their difference from malignant mesothelioma and the importance of resection for cure (6). Two large classic review articles have summarized the clinicopathologic features of fibrous tumors of the pleura, a decade apart. Briselli et al. from the Massachusetts General Hospital reviewed 368 cases in 1981—88% of the cases behaved in a benign fashion, nuclear pleomorphism and a high mitotic rate were harbingers of malignancy and the best predictor of a good prognosis was a pedicle supporting the tumor (1). England et al. in 1989 reviewed 223 cases from the Armed Forces Institute of Pathology in which 58% were histologically malignant, patients with malignant tumors that were cured had pedunculated or well-circumscribed tumors and the best predictor of a good outcome was resectability (7).

II. Incidence

LFTP are rare with only 600 cases reported up to 1989 (7). In large series of pleural tumors, about 10% will be LFTP and 90% will be malignant mesotheliomas (8). The Mayo Clinic reported on 60 cases over 25 years, an incidence of 3 cases per 100,000 admissions (9). Most modern series of LFTP from thoracic surgical units report about one case per year emphasizing the rarity of this tumor (3,10–15). The most recent review of LFTP reviewed 800 cases up to 2005 (16).

III. Etiology

Unlike mesothelioma, asbestos is not associated with LFTP (1,7). There are no known predisposing factors for LFTP.

IV. Demographics

LFTP are the most common in the sixth decade of life with more than one-half of the cases over the age of 50 (1,7). A few cases have been reported in children as young as the age of 5 (1). LFTP are evenly distributed among men and women.

V. Clinical Features

Many patients are asymptomatic and come to medical attention because of an abnormal chest radiograph. Recent series report the incidence of symptoms from 42% to 88% (Table 1) (3,10–15). The common reported symptoms are chest pain, cough, and dyspnea. Constitutional symptoms such as fever, night sweats, and weight loss are rare. Symptoms of hypoglycemia are rare but can be dramatic and lead to an accurate clinical diagnosis if there is a known circumscribed mass in the chest. Patients with malignant and/or large tumors are more likely to be symptomatic (7). Rare patients report the sensation of a mass moving in the chest, which is highly suggestive of this tumor since many are pedunculated. Signs of a pleural effusion may be evident on chest examination and is more common in malignant than benign tumors (7). Clubbing or other manifestations of hypertrophic pulmonary osteoarthropathy are occasionally seen and were more common in older series (probably due to delayed diagnosis) than in recent reports (Table 1). Clubbing resolves with complete resection of the mass.

VI. Laboratory Features

Hypoglycemia may be rarely present (0–14%) due to the tumor-secreting insulin-like growth factor II (IGF-II) (Table 1) (17). The hypoglycemia resolves after the complete

Table 1 Clinical Features of Patients with LFTP

References	Patients	Symptomatic (%)	Clubbing (%)	Hypoglycemia (%)	Malignant (%)
(15)	27	63	7	4	37
(14)	18	44	6	0	11
(13)	63	57	1	0	30
(12)	21	43	14	14	38
(3)	55	42	ns	2	7
(11)	11	70	0	0	20
(10)	15	88	7	7	60
(1)	360	64	35	4	13
(7)	223	48	4	6	58

ns: not stated.

resection of the tumor. The pleural effusion associated with LFTP is usually clear yellow transudates, which are cytologically negative (6,12). Exudative and bloody effusions have been rarely reported (6,12). Although most effusions are small, there have been case reports of massive effusions (18).

VII. Radiographic Features

Chest radiographs usually show a well delineated, round, oval or lobulated mass (Figs. 1–3). The average size of the mass is often rather large, with two series reporting the average

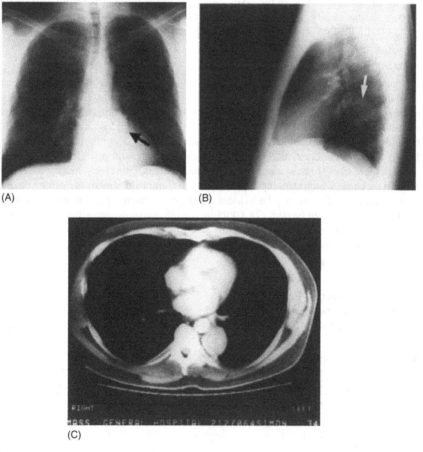

(A)   (B)

(C)

Figure 1 LFTP simulating a benign neurogenic tumor. The patient is a 51-year-old man who was asymptomatic. (**A**) PA chest radiograph demonstrates a 4-cm sharply defined retrocardiac density (*black arrow*). (**B**) Lateral chest radiograph confirms posterior paravertebral gutter location and sharply defined borders (*white arrow*) suggest a benign etiology. (**C**) CT scan confirms moderately enhancing sharply defined 4-cm paravertebral mass. The preoperative diagnosis was a benign neurogenic tumor. Resection was by thoracotomy, which revealed the origin was the posterior pleura. Pathology revealed a bland LFRP and the patient is free of recurrence 18 years after resection.

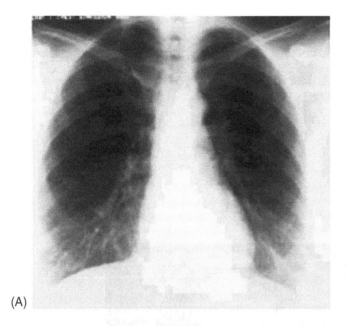

(A)

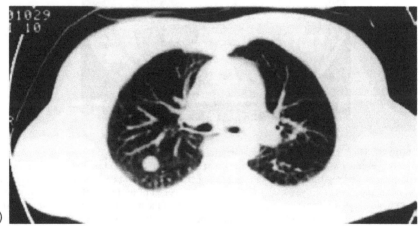

(B)

Figure 2 LFTP simulating a solitary pulmonary nodule (inverted fibroma). The patient is a healthy 41-year-old woman who was asymptomatic. The patient underwent thoracotomy and resection with a preoperative diagnosis of a solitary pulmonary nodule. (**A**) PA chest radiograph shows a 1.5-cm (*black arrow*) sharply demarcated round mass. (**B**) CT scan shows a 1.5-cm sharply defined mass in the posterior segment of the right upper lobe close to the major fissure. The lesion originated from the visceral pleura within the major fissure and grew into the lung (inverted fibroma). Pathology revealed a benign appearing LFTP and follow-up has demonstrated no recurrence.

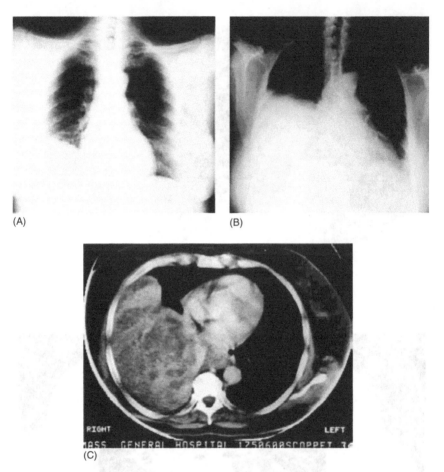

(A)   (B)

(C)

Figure 3   Huge LFTP with an unusual natural history. The patient is a 67-year-old woman who initially presented in 1991 with vague right chest discomfort. (**A**) PA chest radiograph revealed an apparent elevated right hemidiaphragm and an abnormal diaphragm contour. Further investigation was not undertaken. Two years later (1983), she complained of dyspnea. (**B**) PA chest radiograph shows a huge right chest mass occupying about one-half of the hemithorax. (**C**) CT scan confirms a huge heterogeneous tumor with areas of central low density consistent with hemorrhage or necrosis. The borders of the mass are sharp and there is no evidence of lung or chest-wall invasion suggesting an encapsulated tumor. Resection revealed a tumor based on the visceral pleura of the base of the right lower lobe and was a benign LFTP. Sixteen years later (1999), she represented with an apparent local recurrence on the diaphragm and she underwent re-resection.

size to be 8.5 or 10 cm (Table 2) (1,7). If the mass is based on the parietal pleura, the angle between the mass and chest wall is characteristically obtuse. If the lesion is pedunculated, a change in patient position may lead to a change in tumor position. Evidence of a pleural effusion is present in 1% to 19% of the patients (Table 2). Computed tomography (CT) of the chest is the next step in diagnostic evaluation and is indicated in all patients

Table 2 Radiologic Features of Patients with LFTP

References	Size (cm)	Multiple tumors (%)	Pleural effusion (%)	Sharp borders (%)	Calcification (%)	Correct FNA diagnosis (%)
(15)	8 (2–23)	0	4	4	11	40
(14)	10 (0.8–30)	0	33	All	ns	38
(12)	ns	0	19	76	ns	38
(3)	8.5 (1–28)	2	5	All	ns	36
(11)	10 (2.5–23)	0	0	All	27	33
(10)	ns	7	5	80	ns	20
(7)	≤5 cm, 34% ≥6 cm, 60%	ns	17	93	ns	ns

ns: not stated.

(19–21). CT typically shows a sharply defined homogenous soft tissue mass adjacent to some aspect of the pleura (Fig. 4). Calcification is occasionally noted in the mass. Heterogeneous tumors with areas of low density (which may represent areas of cystic change, hemorrhage, or necrosis) are more common in larger and malignant tumors. These tumors markedly enhance with intravenous contrast as would be expected given their gross and microscopic findings of hypervascularity. The finding of marked enhancement with contrast can suggest the correct diagnosis of a LFTP in an unknown chest mass to the discriminating radiologist. Rarely more than one tumor is present (2,3). About two-thirds of the tumors originate from the visceral pleura and one-third from the parietal pleura (7). Tumors can rarely present as intraparenchymal lung tumors—the so-called inverted fibroma (Fig. 2). Magnetic resonance imaging (MRI) can be helpful in selected cases (22–24). Low-signal intensity is typically seen in T1- and T2-weighted sequences, which reflects their fibrous nature (Figs. 5 and 6). The tumor markedly enhances with gadolinium contrast reflecting hypervascularity of the tumor. MRI is useful in assessing large tumors, tumors with extensive chest wall or diaphragm abutment or apical tumors to better define extent of invasion and potential resectability. There are very few reports on the use of positron emission tomography (PET) with 18 fluorine fluorodeoxyglucose (FDG) performed in these tumors. A recent report indicated that the FDG-PET was negative in all the three patients with benign LFTP and was positive in all the three malignant cases of LFTP (15). PET scans may prove useful in predicting malignancy in cases of suspected malignant LFTP. Angiography has been reported to be useful in defining the origin of the vasculature of huge tumors and also to embolize the feeding vessels to facilitate resection (25). Massive hemorrhage has been reported during resection of large tumors, so it is prudent to consider embolization of massive tumors preoperatively.

The role of CT-guided fine needle aspiration (FNA) is controversial and the diagnostic yield is rather low with this tumor with a reported accuracy of 10% to 38% in recent reports (Table 2) (3,10–15). A recent report by Okada and colleagues reported on 10 patients with LFTP of which five had attempted preoperative FNA diagnosis (26). All five biopsies were nondiagnostic due to a paucity of diagnostic tumor cells recovered. At operation, intraoperative scratch cytology was performed on all patients and a variety of cells were recovered, including spindle (bipolar, dendritic/stellate, and intermediate cells). They concluded that it was difficult to diagnose LFTP by FNA with certainty in

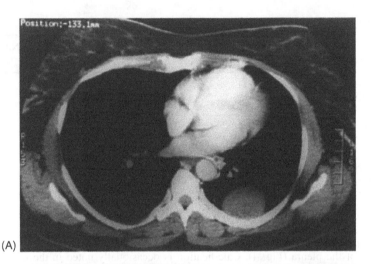

(A)

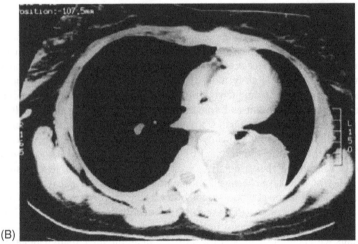

(B)

Figure 4   Recurrent invasive malignant LFTP. The patient is a 40-year-old woman who presented initially with an asymptomatic 8-cm left chest mass. Thoracotomy revealed a mediastinal pleural-based mass extending over to the lateral chest wall and adherent to the left lower lobe. Extrapleural resection of the mass with wedge resection of the lung was performed. The tumor was very cellular, had focal areas of necrosis, had minimal cytologic atypia, and had 5 mitoses per 10 high-power fields. Resection margins were negative. Three years later, she developed left chest pain. A CT scan was performed (**A**) which confined a 4-cm local recurrence in the posterior chest wall. The CT scan shows a homogeneous tumor, which does not avidly take up contrast. The patient refused surgery. Three months later, the pain worsened and a repeat CT scan (**B**) showed marked enlargement of the tumor to 8 cm with areas of heterogeneity. Centrally, the tumor now avidly takes up contrast and there is a peripheral rim of lower density. She now consented to re-resection which involved en-bloc resection of the mass with three attached ribs and the entire left lower lobe. Pathology revealed a cellular tumor with 2 mitoses per 10 high-power fields with about 25% of the tumor necrotic. Resections margins were negative.

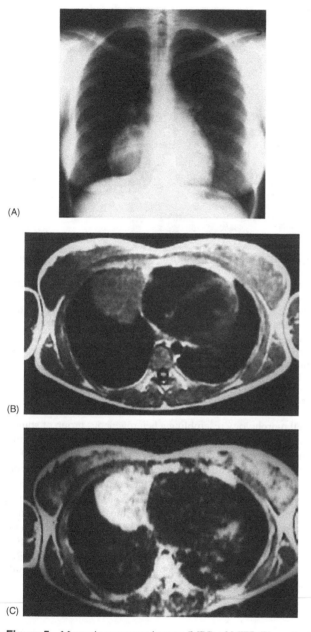

Figure 5 Magnetic resonance images (MRI) of LFTP. The patient is a 31-year-old woman who presented with a cough. (**A**) PA chest radiograph demonstrates a right paracardiac mass with sharp lateral borders. (**B**) T1-weighted sequence of MRI exam shows a homogenous lesion of muscle (soft tissue) density. (**C**) T2-weighted sequence of MRI exam demonstrates some inhomogeneity with several low-density areas. Resection showed the tumor to be based on the anterior sulcus between the chest wall and pericardium. Pathology revealed a benign LFTP.

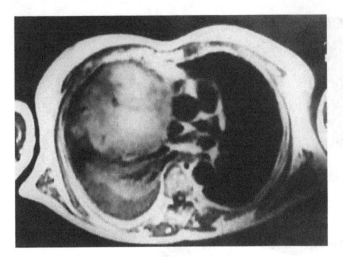

Figure 6 Huge LFTP with pleural effusion. The patient is a 56-year-old man with dyspnea and cough. A huge chest mass and a small pleural effusion was seen. The pleural effusion was tapped and was cytologically negative. Attempted resection at another hospital by a small anterior thoracotomy was met with massive bleeding and was abandoned. (**A**) MRI exam (T1 image) shows a large anterior 10-cm tumor, which is heterogeneous. Compression of the lung with a dependent pleural effusion is seen. The mediastinum and great vessels are shifted to the opposite side and there is extensive abutment (invasion indeterminent) of the great vessels. Preoperative angiographic embolization of internal thoracic and phrenic artery branches was performed in view of the previous operative experience. Exploration through an extended posterolateral thoracotomy incision allowed easy resection of a tumor based on the mediastinal pleura. The patient remains free of recurrence 13 years after resection.

part due to the presence of cell morphology resembling a heterogeneous group of spindle cell tumors and the difficulty in obtaining enough cells to review. Reports of core-cutting needle biopsies suggest a higher diagnostic yield (27,28). For the routine case of an undiagnosed readily resectable chest mass, an expeditious surgical resection for diagnosis and treatment is the correct approach as the results of the needle biopsy, whether it is diagnostic or not, would not change the need for resection. Complex cases, including those that are quite large, potentially difficult to resect tumors or those where other tumors that would require a different treatment strategy (i.e., induction treatment) are high in the differential diagnosis would probably be benefited by a preoperative diagnosis. If LFTP is in the differential diagnosis of a lesion that is to be sampled preoperatively, both a FNA and a core biopsy should be requested. If the result is nondiagnostic, the clinician should remember that a LFTP is not excluded.

VIII. Pathology

A. Gross Pathology of Benign LFTP

As the name localized fibrous tumor of the pleura indicates, the typical lesion is round or oval and well circumscribed (1,7,29). The lesions may range from several millimeters to

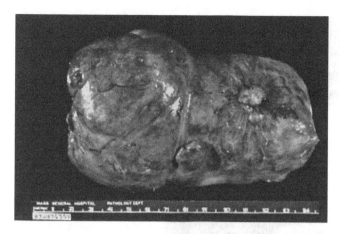

Figure 7 External surface of large localized fibrous tumor arising in the parietal pleura and presenting as a smooth bosselated mass 14 cm in greatest diameter.

many centimeters in diameter, including examples measuring up to 36 cm and weighing up to 5000 g (Fig. 7). Larger lesions may be multilobulated. The cut surface of a resected specimen is rubbery and firm with a whorled pattern (Figs. 8 and 9). Central myxoid change and hemorrhage may occasionally be seen and are more commonly encountered in large tumors. Tumors arise more commonly from the parietal than the visceral pleura. Rarely tumors arise from the thoracic surface of the diaphragm, from the mediastinum, or in the lung, where they are thought to arise from a pleural invagination in a lobular fissure. A vascular pedicle may be present, particularly on those arising from the parietal pleura.

B. Microscopic Pathology of Benign LFTP

The neoplastic cell is derived from a submesothelial fibroblast. Dark spindled nuclei may have stippled or homogeneously dense chromatin with occasional vacuolar change and inconspicuous nucleoli. Density of the nuclei varies from richly cellular to poorly cellular. The nuclei are separated by fibrillar collagen. The cells form fascicles or storiform arrays and also grow without any reproducible pattern (Figs. 10–12). Mitoses are very rare in benign tumors (30). Regions with numerous large blood vessels are common (Figs. 13 and 14). Entrapment of surface epithelioid mesothelial cells or pneumocytes as the tumor grows within the lung may cause gland-like spaces, but these are not intrinsic parts of the neoplasm.

C. Electron Microscopy of Benign LFTP

The neoplastic cells have spindled nuclei with heterochromatin and occasional admixed polygonal cells (30). Nuclei may be mildly indented. Nucleoli are not prominent. Cytoplasm contains microfilaments and rough endoplasmic reticulum with cisternae. Mitochondria are generally scarce. The cells are arranged in groups and surrounded by collagen. Intercellular junctions are often discernible. The cells do not produce basement membrane.

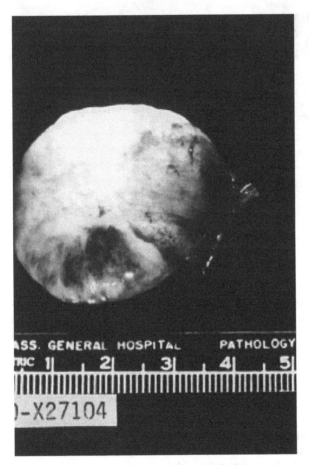

Figure 8 Cut surface of localized fibrous tumor of the pleura with a smooth homogeneous fleshy surface and focal cystic degeneration.

D. Differential Diagnosis of Benign LFTP

Depending on the variety of patterns seen on routine staining, the differential diagnosis includes diffuse malignant mesothelioma of the fibrosarcomatous pattern, hemangiopericytoma, schwannoma, leiomyoma, sclerosing epithelioid fibrosarcoma, sclerosing epithelioid hemangioendothelioma, inflammatory myofibroblastic tumor, desmoid tumor, fibrous histiocytoma, sclerosing hemangioma, carcinoid tumor with sclerosis or metastases. Immunochemistry is not usually necessary for diagnosis, but it may be useful in cases with one or more of these differential diagnoses and in diagnosis based on needle biopsy specimen. Typically, the cells of the solitary fibrous tumor stain for vimentin, which is a general but non-specific marker for mesenchymal cells, and for CD34, which is a marker for fibroblasts (31,32). Some tumors stain for bcl-2 protein. The cells generally do not stain for keratin or other epithelial, endothelial, or histiocytic markers.

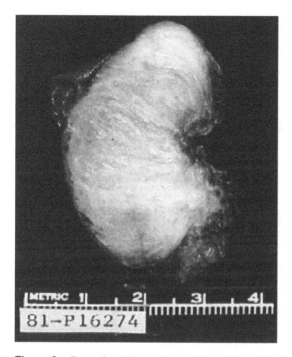

Figure 9   Cut surface of localized fibrous tumor of the pleura with dense gritty white fibrous cut surface.

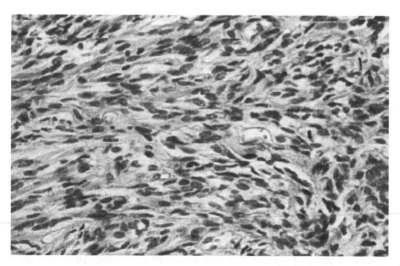

Figure 10   Localized fibrous tumor of the pleura with spindle cell proliferation, where the spindled nuclei form fascicles.

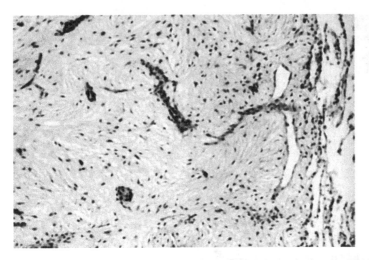

Figure 11   Localized fibrous tumor of the pleura with loose myxomatous pattern.

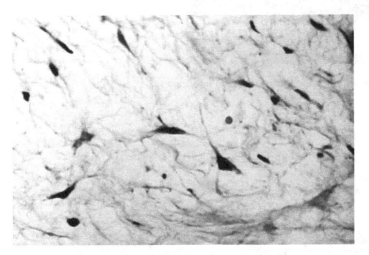

Figure 12   Individual spindled and stellate cells in myxoid region of localized fibrous tumor of the pleura.

IX.   Pathology of Malignant Fibrous Tumor of the Pleura

Approximately one-third of fibrous tumors of the pleura have histological characteristics indicative of potentially malignant behavior (1,7,33). These tumors are generally grouped with fibrous tumors of the pleura and thought to be on a spectrum of variable malignancy developing either in a benign tumor or as a progression of malignancy over time. The tumor has also been termed fibrosarcoma of the pleura. Resectability is the best predictor of prognosis. Approximately one-half of patients whose tumors have histologic features of malignancy die with locally invasive, recurrent or metastatic disease.

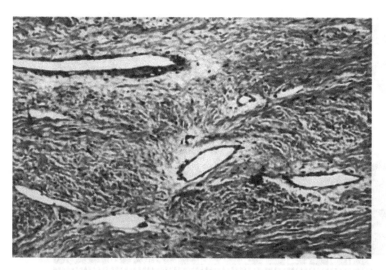

Figure 13 Ectatic thin-walled blood vessels amid proliferating spindled cells creating a pattern of angiofibroma.

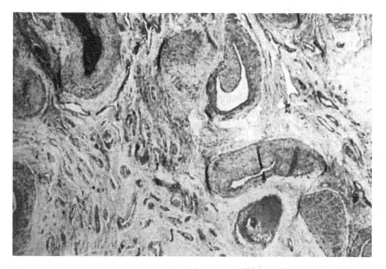

Figure 14 Large thick-walled blood vessels in the pedicle of a localized fibrous tumor attached to the parietal pleura.

A. Gross Pathology of Malignant LFTP

Necrosis and hemorrhage are visible in slightly more than half of the cases of malignant fibrous tumor, while it is uncommon in lesions with benign histology (Fig. 15). Malignant fibrous tumors of the pleura appear generally similar to solitary fibrous tumor. Malignant fibrous tumors are twice as likely to be greater than 10 cm in size, with approximately

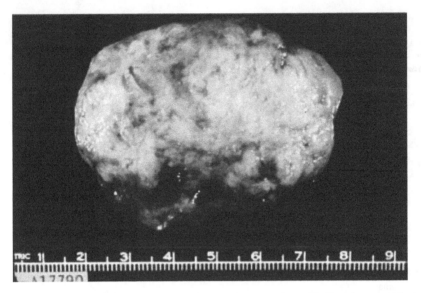

Figure 15   Malignant fibrous tumor of the pleura has cut surface with glistening myxoid gelatinous tissue and focal hemorrhagic necrosis.

50% of malignant fibrous tumor reaching this size as compared to 25% of localized fibrous tumor.

B.   Microscopic Pathology of Malignant LFTP

There are three specific criteria for malignancy: (*i*) increased cellularity, (*ii*) nuclear pleiomorphism, and (*iii*) mitoses. Increased cellularity consists of areas where the tumor appears solid with closely packed dark cells, which may be so dense as to suggest small-cell carcinoma (Fig. 16). Very high cellular regions are seen in three-fourths of malignant tumors. Nuclear pleiomorphism is characterized by irregularity of the nuclei. It is seen in the great majority of cases. Mitoses are the most specific feature in the diagnosis of malignant fibrous tumor. A mitotic count of greater than 4 mitoses per 10 high-power fields has been used as a line of demarcation. By this criterion, approximately 75% of malignant fibrous tumors have this many mitoses, in contrast to 1% of solitary fibrous tumors.

C.   Differential Diagnosis of Malignant LFTP

The differential diagnosis includes localized fibrous tumor, sarcomas in general, and the sarcomatous variant of diffuse malignant mesothelioma (34,35). The latter is sometimes referred to as desmoplastic diffuse malignant mesothelioma, which is an entirely different tumor and the most important conceptual and clinicopathological differentiation to be made (36,37).

When one is dealing with a biopsy only and is not aware of whether a tumor is radiographically or clinically diffuse or localized, delineation of a spindle-cell neoplasm may be difficult. Storiform patterns can be seen in both malignant fibrous tumor and

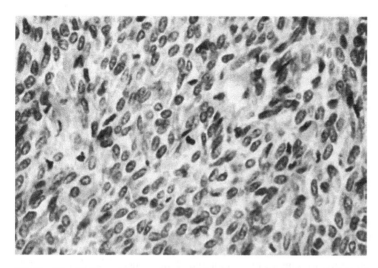

Figure 16 Malignant fibrous tumor of the pleura with closely packed, hyperchromatic, small, oval nuclei, and containing several mitoses.

sarcomatous forms of diffuse malignant mesothelioma. Nuclear pleiomorphism may not be prominent in either. Ectatic blood vessels surrounded by proliferating spindled cells creating a pattern resembling angiofibroma favor localized fibrous tumor. Any epithelioid characteristic favors a diffuse malignant mesothelioma. Immunopathology is valuable. Positive staining for broad-spectrum keratin, cytokeratin 5/6, calretinin, Wilm's tumor-1, and D240 favor a diffuse malignant mesothelioma, but spindled forms of diffuse malignant mesothelioma often fail to stain with any of these markers. Positive staining for CD31 favors malignant fibrous tumor.

D. Surgery

Large tumors are approached through a standard posterolateral thoracotomy. Small lesions can be adequately removed by video-assisted thoracic surgery (VATS) techniques if the surgeon is experienced in VATS (3). A thorough exploration should be done at the time of resection, as rarely additional synchronous tumors not seen on preoperative imaging may be present (3,38). In the classic case of a pedunculated tumor of the visceral pleura, a wedge resection of normal lung should be performed to obtain an adequate margin. Local recurrences have been reported even in cases with a pedicle, so that a margin of normal lung should be removed and checked with intraoperative frozen section to confirm that the resection is complete (3,10–15). Pleural-based lesions are more difficult to deal with because of the difficulty in obtaining a clear margin along the chest wall. For smaller tumors that are clinically and radiologically benign, a preliminary attempt at extrapleural dissection should be performed and if the normal areolar tissue plane is present the mass should be removed in the extrapleural plane. Intraoperative frozen section evaluation should be done to asses for malignancy, evaluate the peripheral characteristics of the tumor (encapsulated or invasive), and to check the true deep margin along the extrapleural plane. If a benign encapsulated tumor is found, chest-wall resection is not indicated.

Patients with invasive or malignant tumors should have a chest-wall resection performed. Patients with large tumors that are pleural-based and that do not appear invasive by CT or intraoperative findings should also have a trial of extrapleural dissection, as previously mentioned. Intraoperative core-cutting biopsies should be considered in doubtful cases as the finding of atypical histologic features support more aggressive surgery. Careful evaluation of the margins is again mandatory as the completeness of the resection is the most important factor in a favorable long-term prognosis (7). Complete parietal pleurectomy is not indicated. Resection of massive tumors can be quite challenging and incisional approaches may need to be modified to fit the location of the tumor. Two incisions (i.e., median sternotomy and lateral thoracotomy) and the clamshell incision may be of use in such cases (39). Preoperative embolization has been used with success to minimize bleeding in formidable tumors (25).

E. Results

Operative mortality is zero in almost all series reflecting the straightforward nature of most resections (Table 3). Essentially, all benign and most invasive tumors are resectable. Chest wall or diaphragm resections are rarely required. Benign-encapsulated tumors rarely recur if adequately resected. Recurrences of benign tumors have been noted up to 18 years after the primary resection, reflecting an indolent tumor biology in these patients (10). Re-resection of benign tumors for apparent cure has been reported several times and suggests the need for very long-term follow-up (3,10–15). Recurrences after resection of LFTP with benign histology have been noted sometimes to be histologically bland but sometimes are histologically malignant (3,10–15). Return of the original symptoms of

Table 3 Results of Surgical Treatment of LFTP

References	Number	% Malignant	Recurrence	Follow-up
(15)	27	37	4 (6–122 mo)	All benign LFTP alive and well 5 yr survival 90%
(14)	18	11	2	All benign LFTP alive and well 5 year survival 80%
(13)	63	30	11 (3 local, 8 distant)	All benign LFTP alive and well and median survival malignant LFTP 24 months
(12)	21	38	1 (10 yr postop)	All alive and well, median 68 months
(3)	55	7	1 (1 yr postop)	All alive and well, median 53 months
(11)	10	30	1 (6 yr postop)	All alive and well, median 53 months
(10)	15	56	5 (5 mo, 10 mo, 4yr, 6yr, 18yr)	2 died with disease, rest alive and well, mean 9 yr
(7)	223	37	Benign 140: 2 recurrences; malignant 77: 39 recurrences	Survival at 15 yr, benign 85%, malignant without invasion 25%, malignant with invasion 15%

Table 4 Clinical, Radiologic, and Gross Pathologic Features That Affect Prognosis

Benign	Malignant
Asymptomatic	Symptomatic
Small	Large
No pleural effusion	Pleural effusion
Pedunculated	Broad-based
Visceral pleural origin	Origin from fissure, mediastinum or parietal pleura
Homogeneous CT appearance	Heterogeneous (necrosis and hemorrhage) CT appearance

either clubbing or hypoglycemia has been noted in patients with recurrent tumors. Death from recurrent tumors is extremely rare after complete resection of histologically benign tumors.

Patients with malignant or invasive tumors do not fare as well and have a more variable prognosis. Many patients with worrisome histology have encapsulated tumors, which portend an intermediate prognosis (7). In England's large series, about one-half of the patients in this category were apparently cured by complete resection (7). Patients with malignant histologic features and invasive tumors had the worst prognosis. Table 4 contrasts clinical, radiologic, and pathologic prognostic factors identified in collected series (1,3,7,10–15).

X. Calcifying Fibrous Pseudotumor of the Pleura

Calcifying fibrous pseudotumor is a recently described entity, which generally occurs in the extremities, scrotum, groin, neck, and axilla. A few cases have presented in the pleura (40–42). The lesion is benign. The histology is distinctive. Calcifying fibrous pseudotumor is characterized by dense hyalinized collagen with interspersed benign spindled cells, a sparse inflammatory infiltrate, and randomly distributed psammoma bodies, as well as dystrophic calcification. The psammoma bodies and dystrophic calcification distinguish calcifying fibrous pseudotumor of the pleura from solitary fibrous tumor of the pleura and from desmoid tumor of the pleura.

XI. Pleural Hibernoma

Pleural hibernoma is a very rare benign tumor originating from fetal brown fat. It is rarely found in the pleura. It is very difficult to diagnosis preoperatively and is usually diagnosed on the excised specimen. It is a very benign lesion but must be differentiated from liposarcoma (43).

References

1. Briselli M, Mark EJ, Dickersin GR. Solitary fibrous tumors of the pleura: Eight new cases and review of 360 cases in the literature. Cancer 1981; 47:2678–2689.
2. Tastepe I, Alper A, Ozaydin HE, et al. A case of multiple synchronous localized fibrous tumor of the pleura. Eur J Cardiothorac Surg 2000; 18:491–494.
3. Cardillo G, Facciolo F, Cavazzana AO, et al. Localized (solitary) fibrous tumors of the pleura: An analysis of 55 patients. Ann Thorac Surg 2000; 70:1808–1812.

4. Wagner E. Das tuberkelahnliche lymphadenom (der cytogene oder reticulite tuberkel). Arch Heilk 1870; 11:497.
5. Klemperer P, Rabin CB. Pulmonary neoplasm of the pleura: A report of five cases. Arch Pathol 1931; 11:385–412.
6. Clagett OT, McDonald JR, Schmidt HW. Localized fibrous mesothelioma of the pleura. J Thorac Surg 1952; 24:213–230.
7. England DM, Hochholzer L, McCarthy M. Localized benign and malignant fibrous tumors of the pleura. A clinicopathologic review of 223 cases. Am J Surg Pathol 1989; 13:640–658.
8. Martini N, McCormack PM, Bains MS, et al. Pleural mesothelioma. Ann Thorac Surg 1987; 43:113–120.
9. Okike N, Bernatz E, Woolner B. Localized mesothelioma of the pleura. J Thorac Cardiovasc Surg 1978; 75:363–372.
10. Suter M, Gebhard S, Boumghar M, et al. Localized fibrous tumours of the pleura: 15 new cases and review of the literature. Eur J Cardiothorac Surg 1998; 14:453–459.
11. De Perrot M, Kurt A, Robert JH, et al. Clinical behavior of solitary fibrous tumors of the pleura. Ann Thorac Surg 1999; 67:1456–1459.
12. Rena O, Filosso PL, Papalia E, et al. Solitary fibrous tumour of the pleura: Surgical treatment. Eur J Cardiothorac Surg 2001; 19:185–189.
13. Sung SH, Chang JW, Kim J, et al. Solitary fibrous tumors of the pleura: Surgical outcome and clinical course. Ann Thorac Surg 2005; 79:303–307.
14. Carreta A, Bandiera A, Melloni G, et al. Solitary fibrous tumors of the pleura: Immunohisto-chemical analysis and evaluation of prognostic factors after surgical treatment. J Surg Oncol 2006; 94:40–44.
15. Kohler M, Clarenbach CF, Kestenholz P, et al. Diagnosis, treatment and long-term outcome of solitary fibrous tumors of the pleura. Eur J Cardiothorac Surg 2007; 32:403–408.
16. Robinson LA. Solitary fibrous tumor of the pleura. Cancer Control 2006; 13:264–269.
17. Kishi K, Homma S, Tanimura S, et al. Hypoglycemia induced by secretion of high molecular weight insulin-like growth factor-II from a malignant solitary fibrous tumor of the pleura. Intern Med 2001; 40:341–344.
18. Ulrik CS, Viskum K. Fibrous pleural tumor producing 171 liters of transudate. Eur Respir J 1998; 12:1230–1232.
19. Lee KS, Im JG, Choe KO, et al. CT findings in benign fibrous mesothelioma of the pleura: Pathologic correlation in nine patients. Am J Roentgenol 1992; 158:983–986.
20. Qureshi NR, Gleeson FV. Imaging of pleural disease. Clin Chest Med 2006; 27:193–213.
21. Chong S, Kim TS, Cho EY, et al. Benign localized fibrous tumor of the pleura: CT features with histopathological correlations. Clin Radiol 2006; 61:875–882.
22. Harris GN, Rozenshtein A, Schiff MJ. Benign fibrous mesothelioma of the pleura: MR imaging findings. Am J Roentgenol 1995; 165:1143–1144.
23. Padovani B, Mouroux J, Raffaelli C, et al. Benign fibrous mesothelioma of the pleura: MR study and pathologic correlation. Eur Radiol 1996; 6:425–428.
24. Ferretti GR, Chiles C, Cox JE, et al. Localized benign fibrous tumors of the pleura: MR appearance. J Comput Assist Tomogr 1997; 21:115–120.
25. Khan JH, Rahman SB, Clary-Macy C, et al. Giant solitary fibrous tumor of the pleura. Ann Thorac Surg 1998; 65:1461–1464.
26. Okada S, Ebihara Y, Kudo M, et al. Scratch cytologic findings on surgically resected solitary fibrous tumors of the pleura. Acta Cytol 2001; 45:372–380.
27. Bicer M, Yaldiz S, Gursoy S, et al. A case of giant benign localized fibrous tumor of the pleura. Eur J Cardiothorac Surg 1998; 14:211–213.
28. Weymand B, Noel H, Goncette L, et al. Solitary fibrous tumor of the pleura. A report of five cases diagnosed by transthoracic cutting needle biopsy. Chest 1997; 112:424–428.
29. Scharifker D, Kaneko M. Localized fibrous "mesothelioma" of pleura (submesothelial fibroma). A clinicopathologic study of 18 cases. Cancer 1979; 43:627–635.

30. Keating S, Simon GT, Alexopoulou I, et al. Solitary fibrous tumor of the pleura: An ultrastructural and immunohistochemical study. Thorax 1987; 42:976–979.

31. Westra WH, Gerald WL, Rosai J. Solitary fibrous tumor. Consistent CD34 immunoreactivity and occurrence in the orbit. Am J Surg Pathol 1994; 18:992–998.

32. Van de Rijn M, Lombard CM, Rouse RV. Expression of CD34 by solitary fibrous tumors of the pleura, mediastinum, and lung. Am J Surg Pathol 1994; 18:814–820.

33. Hanau CA, Mietinen M. Solitary fibrous tumor: Histochemical spectrum of benign and malignant variants presenting at different sites. Hum Pathol 1995; 26:440–449.

34. Flint A, Weiss SW. CD-34 and keratin expression distinguishes solitary fibrous tumor (fibrous mesothelioma) of pleura from desmoplastic mesothelioma. Hum Pathol 1995; 26:428–431.

35. Bai H, Aswad BI, Gaissert H, et al. Malignant solitary fibrous tumor of the pleura with liposarcomatous differentiation. Arch Pathol Lab Med 2001; 125:406–409.

36. Cagle PT, Churg A. Differential diagnosis of benign and malignant mesothelial proliferations on pleural biopsies. Arch Pathol Lab Med 2005; 129:1421–1427.

37. Granville L, Allen TC, Dishop M, et al. Review and update of uncommon primary pleural tumors. Arch Pathol Lab Med 2005; 129:1428–1443.

38. Tastepe I, Alper A, Ozaydin HE, et al. A case of multiple synchronous localized fibrous tumors of the pleura. Eur J Cardiothorac Surg 2000; 18:491–494.

39. Veronesi G, Spaggiari L, Massarol G, et al. Huge malignant localized fibrous tumor of the pleura. J Cardiovasc Surg 2000; 41:781–784.

40. Fetsch JF, Montgomery EA, Meis JM. Calcifying fibrous tumor. Am J Surg Pathol 1993; 17:502–508.

41. Pinkard NB, Wilson RW, Lawless N. Calcifying fibrous pseudotumor of the pleura: A report of three cases of a newly described entity involving the pleura. Am J Clin Pathol 1996; 105:189–194.

42. Shibata K, Yuki D, Sakata K. Multiple calcifying fibrous pseudotumors disseminated in the pleura. Ann Thorac Surg 2008; 85:e3–e5.

43. Congregado M, Jimenez-Merchan R, Arroyo A, et al. Pleural hibernoma: Treatment by videothoracoscopic surgery. Interact Cardiovasc Surg 2004; 3:83–85.

27
Malignant Pleural Mesothelioma

CHARLES-HUGO MARQUETTE
Service de Pneumologie, Oncologie Thoracique et Soins Intensifs Respiratoires,
Hôpital Pasteur, Centre Hospitalier Universitaire de Nice, France

ANTOINE DELAGE
Departement Multidisciplinaire de Pneumologie, Institut Universitaire de Cardiologie et de
Pneumologie de Quebec—Hôpital Laval, Quebec, Canada

PHILIPPE ASTOUL
Département des Maladies Respiratoires, Unité d'Oncologie
Thoracique—Hôpital Sainte-Marguerite, Marseille, France

ARNAUD SCHERPEREEL
Service de Pneumologie et Oncologie Thoracique—Hôpital Calmette,
Centre Hospitalier Universitaire de Lille, France

I. Introduction

Malignant pleural mesothelioma (MPM) is an aggressive tumor, which originates from mesothelial cells of the pleura. Once considered rare, its worldwide incidence has been steadily rising due to massive asbestos use in the past decades. Asbestos is the main etiologic factor for MPM and a thorough search for exposure should be done in face of a suspected or confirmed MPM diagnosis. Attention for this disease is on the rise for many reasons including its forecasted increase in incidence in the next two decades, its widespread workplace-related exposure in various professions and the associated professional disease compensations and other potential medicolegal aspects related to this, the notion of environmental exposure linked to the absence of a known safe threshold of asbestos exposure, and the widespread media attention it has received (more the 3 million internet web pages are devoted to mesothelioma). There has also been a shift in paradigm in the treatment of mesothelioma in recent years. What used to be a rapidly lethal disease now sees a real investment in medical care including better acceptance of surgery, use of new and more effective cytotoxic drug combinations, emerging biotherapies, and new radiotherapy schedules. Most importantly, the recent development of multidisciplinary approaches has allowed the design of prospective randomized-controlled studies, which were critically lacking in this field of oncology (1).

II. Epidemiology

Mesothelioma, a rare cancer before the industrial era, has become a major public health issue because of its rising incidence since the Second World War. This has been linked to massive use of asbestos in various fields of industry (transformation industry, steelwork, shipyard, construction, mining, etc.) (Table 1) (2), especially until its use was banned

Table 1 Incidence of Mesothelioma in 11 Industrialized Countries

Country	Cases	Year	Case/million/year
Australia	490	2000	35
Finland	74	1999	18
France	750	1996	16
Germany	1007	1997	15
United Kingdom	1595	1999	33
Italy	930	1995	19
The Netherlands	377	1997	30
New Zealand	50	1996	18
Norway	48	1995	14
Sweden	105	2000	15
United States	2800	2000	14
All countries	8236		18

Source: Adapted from Ref. 2.

in France (1997), Australia (2003), and the European Union (2005). Although it has been clearly established since 1960 (3) that exposure to asbestos fibers is the main etiologic factor responsible for mesothelioma, asbestos still remains partially in use in North America and is widely used in some developing or emerging countries (Asia, South America) and parts of the former Soviet Union. Thus, epidemiology of MPM is closely linked to asbestos use in industry, although endemic exposure, particularly in certain regions of Turkey by environmental erionite, has been described (4). Although short incubation periods have been reported, the exponential curve between mesothelioma appearance and elapsed time since asbestos exposure is explained by the long latency for this tumor (20–40 years). MPM is also two to sixfold more frequent in men, classically being diagnosed at ages of 50 to 70 years. In comparison with lung cancer, MPM has not been associated to tobacco smoke exposure, likely because carcinogens in tobacco smoke do not reach the mesothelium and, unlike the lung cancer–smoking risk relationship which decreases with time after exposure has stopped, the risk of MPM is close to none in the first 15 years after asbestos exposure and increases thereafter throughout life (5).

Essentially three groups of asbestos exposed subjects can be defined: (*i*) subjects directly exposed to massive quantities of asbestos (in mines, for example, or in factories which use asbestos or its derived products); (*ii*) workers of various fields who manipulate these products containing asbestos, as demonstrated by a recent French public health study (6) (Tables 2 and 3); (*iii*) subjects exposed to asbestos in multiple situations that are accidental or unknown (represent 20–30% of the total cases) (7). It is noteworthy that a clear history of asbestos exposure is found in only 50% of females diagnosed with mesothelioma (in comparison with more than 90% of male subjects).

The number of patients suffering from mesothelioma is thus on the rise. Accordingly, a 25% increase every third year in mesothelioma cases in the United Kingdom was observed between 1979 and 1990. This translates to an estimated 3000 attributable deaths per year in this country by 2020. In France, where the annual MPM incidence was estimated between 632 and 844 cases in 1998, a peak incidence of 1550 annual

Table 2 Pleural Mesothelioma Risk According to Occupation (879 Men: 360 Cases and 519 Controls) (PNSM, 2003) (6)

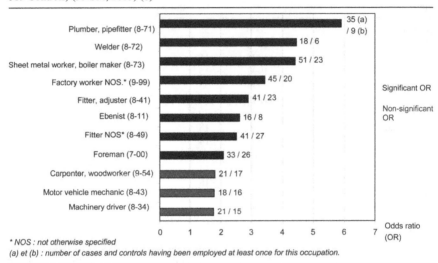

* NOS : not otherwise specified
(a) et (b) : number of cases and controls having been employed at least once for this occupation.

deaths in males born after 1950 is forecasted for the 2015 to 2020 period. In Western Europe, estimates based on data from 1994 predicted up to 250,000 deaths from mesothelioma in the next 35 years. However, the same authors recently lowered their estimates in accordance with the 2003 data from the WHO, at least for France, Italy, and Germany (8).

Table 3 Pleural Mesothelioma Risk According to Activity Sector (879 Men: 360 Cases and 519 Controls) (PNSM, 2003) (6)

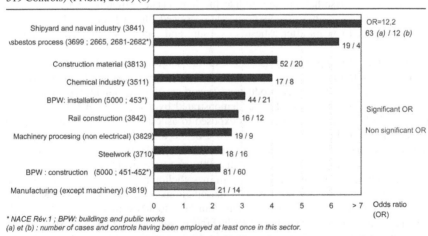

* NACE Rév.1 ; BPW: buildings and public works
(a) et (b) : number of cases and controls having been employed at least once in this sector.

III. Etiology of Mesothelioma

Asbestos is the main causal agent associated with MPM. Two types of asbestos fibers exist: amphibole (elongated and fine) and chrysotile. Both are considered oncogenic although chrysotile fibers are so to a lesser degree (9). MPM initially develops at the mesothelial surface of the parietal pleura rather than the visceral pleura. The hypothesis for this is the passage of asbestos fibers through the visceral pleura which repeatedly erodes the parietal pleura, creating inflammation in the latter and stimulating repair mechanisms, eventually leading to oncogenesis (10). Simian virus 40 (SV40) has been implied as a cofactor in the development of MPM. This virus blocks tumor-suppressing genes and is a potential oncogenic agent in human and murine cells. DNA sequences of SV40 have been found in certain bone and cerebral tumors, lymphomas, malignant pleural mesotheliomas as well as other atypical proliferative and noninvasive lesions of the mesothelium (11). It is believed that this virus could have been transmitted by contaminated batches of antipoliomyeletic vaccine administered in the United Stated 35 to 50 years ago. Its role in the genesis of MPM is, however, still not clearly demonstrated and thus controversial. It is also thought that ionizing radiation exposure could be linked to MPM in rare cases. Finally, genetic predisposition could lead to mesothelioma as evidenced by the study of familial clusters in environmental mesothelioma series in Turkey, which suggested a very probable genetic factor following an autosomal dominant transmission pattern. However, no candidate gene predisposing to mesothelioma has been identified up to now.

Many hypotheses have been formulated to explain the pathogenesis of MPM. Mechanical criteria are first and foremost: longer and finer fibers are believed to be more dangerous because they can penetrate lung tissue deeper and erode into the mesothelial surface, triggering multiple events in the parietal pleura where damage, repair, and local inflammation alternate (10,12). These changes eventually lead to scar tissue formation, which manifests as pleural plaques or malignant tumors (MPM). Asbestos fibers also interfere with cell mitosis leading to aneuploidy and other chromosomal damages that characterize MPM (13). Toxic oxygen free radicals are also released by damaged mesothelial cells, creating genetic alterations (14). Finally, asbestos fibers, by inducing phosphorylation reactions, increase the expression of many proto-oncogenes in the mesothelial cell (15). Animal and human molecular studies show an increased genetic susceptibility to the development of an asbestos-induced tumor. Cytogenetic analyses show caryotypic anomalies such as aneuploidy and complex structural rearrangement (see Ref. 16 for more detail).

IV. Pathology

Diagnosis of mesothelioma, a malignant tumor stemming from cells lining the serous cavities, is essentially pathological. It is a difficult diagnosis, which is reputed to often be mistaken. Macroscopic aspect is usually suggestive but other malignant tumors can also present a pseudo-mesothelioma aspect (thymoma, carcinoma, lymphoma, angiosarcoma). Histologic presentation is defined by the new 2004 WHO international classification for tumors of the pleura (Table 4) (17), but it is common knowledge that this tumor can have various and confounding aspects and can resemble benign pleural lesions or malignant pleural metastases, which are more frequent than MPM (incidence ratio of 1:50 compared to that of MPM). Bronchopulmonary and breast cancer are the two most common types of tumor, which metastasize to the pleura (respectively 7–15% and 7–11% of cases) and their morphology can often be confused with that of MPM. Benign inflammatory lesions of the

Table 4   Classification of Pleural Tumors—WHO 2004 (17)

Primitive pleural tumors of mesothelial origin
    Diffuse malignant mesothelioma
        Epithelioid malignant mesothelioma
        Sarcomatoid malignant mesothelioma
        Desmoplastic malignant mesothelioma
        Biphasic malignant mesothelioma
    Localized malignant mesothelioma
Other primary pleural tumors of mesothelial origin
    Adenomatoid tumor
    Well-differentiated papillary mesothelioma
Primary pleural tumors of mesenchymal origin
    Epithelioid hemangioendothelioma
    Angiosarcoma
    Synovial sarcoma (monophasic/biphasic)
    Solitary fibrous tumor
    Calcified pseudotumor of the pleura
    Desmoplastic small round cell tumor/Ewing sarcoma
Lymphoproliferative syndromes

pleura can also pose diagnostic challenges. These lesions are quite common and are found for the most part in patients belonging to the same age group as those affected by MPM (postcardiac, inflammatory, or infectious pleurisies, for example). These are frequently recurring lesions and can cause atypical mesothelial hyperplasia, which can lead to an erroneous diagnosis. These mistakes account for 13% of cases excluded after the diagnostic certification protocol started by the Mesopath group (an expert pathology panel for MPM initiated by the French national mesothelioma surveillance program) (18). According to data from this group, the pleura is the most frequent site for MPM (90% of cases), the peritoneum, tunica vaginalis or pericardium being rarer (respectively 6%, 3%, and 1% of cases of MPM) (9,19). Pleural endoscopic anomalies can range from small granulations to extensive thickening of the parietal and/or visceral pleura. Because patients often present at an evolved stage of disease, a pleural effusion is often associated with isolated or disseminated pleural nodularities. These nodules gradually coalesce to form larger tumoral masses, which can encroach on the lung. Gross cuts of MPM show a fleshy white consistency but some tumors can produce large quantities of hyaluronic acid making them more viscous in appearance. Desmoplastic MPM is a rare histological variant presenting macroscopically as diffuse pleural fibrosis, sometimes calcified. Exceptionally, MPM can mimic fibrosing mediastinitis. Recently, localized variants of MPM have been described and are included in the 2004 WHO classification (17). It is of utmost importance for pathologists to identify these variants as they can be amenable to surgical excision and have a better prognosis.

Malignant pleural mesothelioma initially does not invade the lung but rather spreads along the interlobular and lobular septae. Exceptionally, it can present as a parenchymal mass. At later stages, it can invade hilar lymph nodes, large vessels, and other mediastinal structures. The parietal pericardium is involved in one-third of cases, with the visceral pericardium and myocardium being so more rarely. Distant metastases are found in more than 50% of cases at autopsy, in sites often similar to bronchopulmonary cancer (19). Metastatic spread is through the lymphatic system toward hilar and mediastinal lymph nodes, to the visceral pleura and contralateral lung. Peritoneal dissemination happens through the diaphragm.

Fibrohyaline plaques have been associated with a number of MPM cases [up to 70% of cases in the series by Roggli et al. (20)], although pleural plaques usually demonstrate past asbestos exposure and are not to be considered as precancerous lesions. However, MPM usually arises from plaque borders, which should incite clinicians to biopsy in this zone when looking for an early tumor. Finally; 25% of patients with mesothelioma have asbestos lung fibrotic lesions.

Pleural effusion being a common clinical presentation, pleural fluid cytology is often one of the first diagnostic tests done but is not of diagnostic certitude. As a matter of fact, well-differentiated malignant pleural cells can be difficult to distinguish from reactive mesothelial cells. MPM cells can also have a pseudo-carcinomatous appearance, frequently being misdiagnosed as metastatic carcinoma. Finally, sarcomatoid forms of MPM do not desquamate and pleural fluid cytology is poorly sensitive in these cases.

The 2004 World Health Organization classification identifies two groups of MPM (diffuse and localized) as well as other primitive pleural tumors of mesothelial origin (17). Diffuse and localized MPM are subdivided into four histological subtypes: epithelial forms known as epithelioid, sarcomatous appearing forms known as sarcomatoid, the desmoplastic form being fibrous and containing few fusiform cells (often misdiagnosed as organizing pleurisy), and the biphasic form containing both epithlioid and sarcomatoid appearing cells. Diagnosis of the latter subtype requires that each type of cells represent at least 10% of the tumor. Hence, diagnosis of biphasic MPM is dependent on specimen size and its frequency increases with increasing number and size of biopsy specimens. Precancerous lesions, specifically atypical mesothelial hyperplasia, are not included in the WHO classification, because their prognostic significance and their treatment remain to be defined. Well-differentiated papillary superficial MPM is new concept of superficial mesothelial proliferation, containing very few cytonuclear atypias and showing a propensity to spread along the pleural surface without infiltrating the underlying pleural tissues. Associated with prolonged survival, this lesion is considered an indolent pleural disease and must interpreted as an intermediate malignant proliferation. However, deeper tissue invasion is associated with a more aggressive clinical course. Solitary fibrous tumor of the pleura, a pleural fibroma formerly called local fibrous MPM; must be differentiated from localized sarcomatoid MPM. The former represents more a pleural fibroma and does not appear to be associated with asbestos exposure (21). Pathological diagnosis is discussed in the next section.

V. Diagnosis

A. Clinical Presentation

MPM typically presents as a nonspecific pleurisy with or without vague thoracic pain in a male subject. Weight loss and fatigue are usually late signs and suggest an advanced disease stage, as are ascites, superior vena cava obstruction, and extra-thoracic metastases. The latter are rarely seen but commonly found on postmortem studies (22). In approximately 80% of cases, a history of asbestos exposure can be traced back.

B. Imaging

Radiological manifestations of MPM are most often unilateral, presenting as a pleural effusion with or without mediastinal shift [Fig. 1(A) and 1(B)]. Only 5% present with

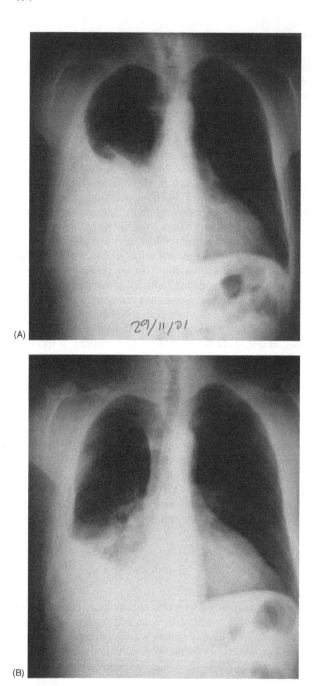

Figure 1 Malignant pleural mesothelioma often presents as a unilateral pleural effusion on chest radiograph with or without mediastinal shift (**A**). After thoracoscopic, pleurodesis using talc has been performed, the classical retractile pleural thickening is better visualized in this patient with MPM (**B**).

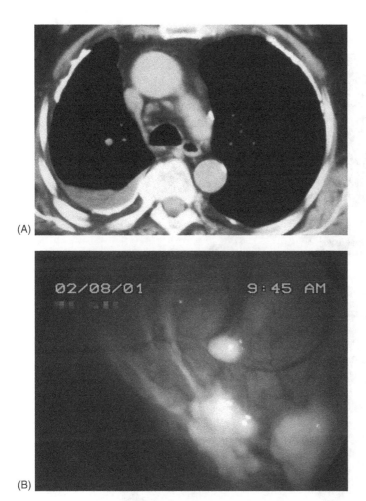

(A)

(B)

Figure 2 In patients with previous asbestos exposure, multiple pleural plaques are often found on CT examination (**A**) and during pleuroscopy (**B**).

bilateral disease. On occasion, it can present as a pleural mass or thickening without an associated pleural effusion. Whereby only 20% of patients will show radiological signs of asbestosis (bilateral basal interstitial fibrosis), pleural plaques are on the other hand quite common [Fig. 2(A) and 2(B)]. In advanced stages, ipsilateral mediastinal shift is due to encroachment of the lung by the tumor mass and secondary atelectasis. Mediastinal widening can be seen in advanced stage disease secondary to local spread, lymph node involvement, or pericardial effusion. Rib erosion and thoracic cage involvement are also seen in later stages.

Computed tomography (CT) of the chest is superior to plain chest radiographs and helps in disease staging (23). Ideally, it should be performed after drainage of the pleural effusion (24). CT can show pleural thickening (92%) most often localized and in the lower

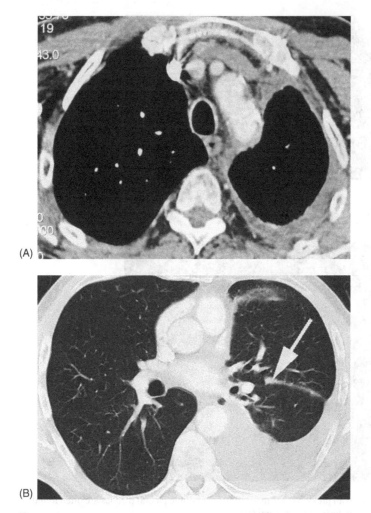

Figure 3 Ideally performed after pleural fluid drainage, thoracic CT can show pleural thickening (**A**), often in the lower part of the thoracic cavity, fissural thickening (**B**, *white arrow*), pleural nodules or masses which can evolve to encroach on the entire lung. With disease evolution, intraparenchymal masses (**C**), mediastinal involvement, with or without pericardial effusion (**D**) and or contralateral extension (**C,D**) can be seen.

part of the thorax with thickening of the fissure (86%), pleural nodules or masses which can evolve to large tumoral mass encircling the lung parenchyma [Fig. 3(A) to 3(D)]. CT is useful for initial local staging of disease and to better define a therapeutic strategy by looking for local invasion of the ribcage—pericardium, diaphragm, or mediastinum. Mediastinal lymphadenopathy (N2-N3; IMIG staging, Table 5) is seen in 34% to 50% of cases (25). Mediastinal pleural involvement can mask its presence.

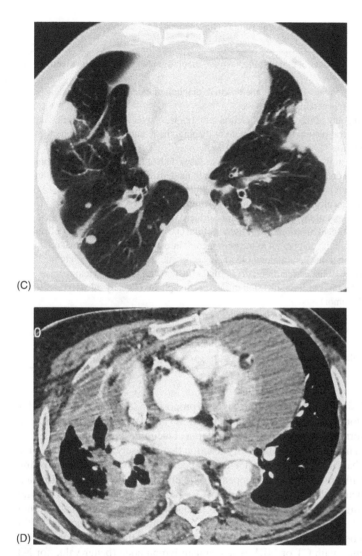

Figure 3 (*Continued*)

Magnetic resonance imaging (MRI) of the chest shows a large increase in signal in T1 sequences and a moderate increase in T2, allowing distinction of MPM from the neighboring thoracic cage and detecting its involvement. MRI can also evaluate diaphragmatic and mediastinal invasion with sagittal and coronal images. Gadolinium contrast injection allows for better characterization of T3 and T4 stages. However, CT and MRI do not allow for precise differentiation of tumor invasion from nonspecific tissue inflammation (23).

Table 5   TNM Staging System for Pleural Tumors (International Mesothelioma Interest Group—IMIG) (25)

T1a	Tumor limited to ipsilateral parietal, mediastinal, diaphragmatic pleura; no involvement of visceral pleura
T1b	Tumor involving ipsilateral parietal, mediastinal, diaphragmatic pleura, with focal involvement of viscera pleural surface
T2	Tumor involving any of the ipsilateral pleural surfaces with at least one of the following: confluent visceral pleural tumor, invasion of diaphragmatic muscle, or invasion of lung parenchyma
T3	Tumor involving any of the ipsilateral pleural surfaces with at least one of the following: invasion of the endothoracic fascia, invasion into mediastinal fat, solitary focus of tumor invading the soft tissues of the chest wall, or nontransmural involvement of the pericardium (Locally-advanced, but resectable tumor)
T4	Tumor involving any of the ipsilateral pleural surfaces, with at least one of the following: diffuse or multifocal invasion of soft tissues of the chest wall, any involvement of rib, invasion through the diaphragm to the peritoneum, invasion of any mediastinal organ, direct extension to the contralateral pleura, invasion into the spine, extension to the internal surface of the pericardium, pericardial effusion with positive cytology, invasion of the myocardium, invasion of the brachial plexus (Locally-advanced, unresectable tumor)
N1	Metastases in the ipsilateral bronchopulmonary or hilar lymph nodes
N2	Metastases in the subcarinal or ipsilateral mediastinal lymph nodes
N3	Metastases in the contralateral mediastinal or internal mammary lymph nodes, or any supraclavicular node metastasis

Positron emission tomography (PET) has been proposed in screening and staging for MPM. ^{18}FDG fixation is significantly increased in MPM (Fig. 4). As much as possible, it is important to perform this examination before chemical pleurodesis is done because this procedure triggers a nonspecific inflammatory reaction that intensely fixates ^{18}FDG. PET has been shown to have a sensitivity of 91% and a specificity of 100% in distinguishing MPM from benign pleural lesions. TEP appears to be efficient in detecting a malignant pathology when pleural thickening is found on CT. Benign asbestos–induced pleural lesions, such as benign asbestos pleurisy, pleural plaques, or rounded atelectasis do not capture ^{18}FDG (23). Standard uptake value (SUV) is significantly increased in MPM when compared to benign lesions of the pleura (26). However, the most important role of TEP, in conjunction with CT or MRI, is to evaluate lymph node (better value for N3 than N2 disease, however) and extrathoracic metastatic involvement. On the other hand, studies have shown conflicting results for locoregional extension of MPM using PET imaging (27).

C.   Pleural Fluid Drainage and Closed Pleural Biopsy

Pleural effusion in MPM is usually exudative, showing elevated pleural fluid protein concentration and lymphocytic pleiocytosis. Pleural LDH levels often exceed that of metastatic pleural effusion, with concentrations higher than 600 IU/L. Pleural fluid often has a viscous aspect due to high concentrations of hyaluronic acid. Elevated levels suggest

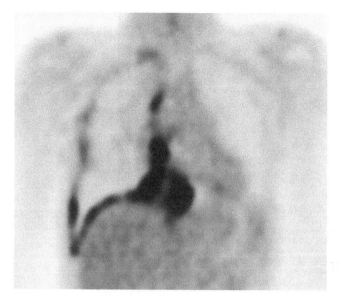

Figure 4 [18]FDG fixation is significantly increased in MPM, which can appear as "drawing" the pleural contour down to the pleural recesses. However, the main utility of PET imaging is evaluating for lymph nodal involvement (especially stage N3) and metastatic disease.

MPM but are not diagnostic. Pleural fluid drainage or percutaneous pleural biopsy can be diagnostic but often do not yield enough material to confirm a diagnosis of MPM. Pleural fluid cytology is useful to diagnose cancer but rarely differentiates mesothelioma from adenocarcinoma or, for sarcomatoid MPM, between fibrosarcoma and hemangiopericytoma (28). Diagnosis is made in only 20% to 30% of cases using cytology alone and in 20% to 23% of cases using closed pleural biopsy. Combination of both techniques has a 35% to 40% yield. The combined sensitivity of pleural and closed pleural biopsy averages 40% when guided by imaging (29). Of course, this depends on tumor size and becomes more sensitive in later stages of disease. Immunohistochemical markers and use of monoclonal antibodies can also be of help in the diagnosis (28).

D. Pleuroscopy

Pleuroscopy or medical thoracoscopy, a simple procedure done under local or general anesthesia, is the most sensitive mean of diagnosing MPM (28). The main indication for pleuroscopy is investigation of an exudative effusion in a subject with previous asbestos exposure. Pleuroscopy is also useful for distinguishing early stage disease, involving exclusively the parietal or diaphragmatic pleura and showing in inflammatory aspect, from visceral pleural involvement [Fig. 5(A) to 5(C)]. This represents an important marker for prognosis.

Medical thoracoscopy is essential in MPM management for various reasons. It helps in explaining the natural evolution of disease by showing accumulation of asbestos fibers in certain sites of the parietal pleura, which can show oncogenic characteristics. These

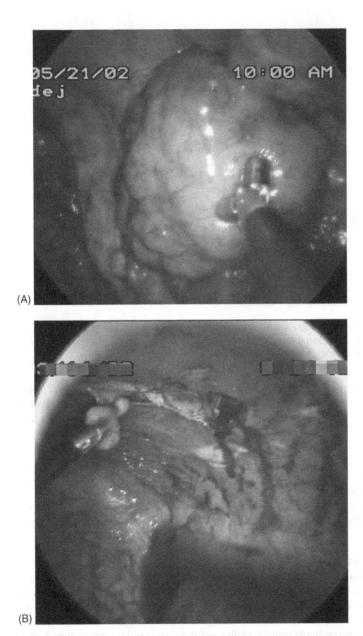

Figure 5   Medical thoracoscopy allows for distinction of early stage mesothelioma whereby only the costal or diaphragmatic pleura is involved, an important prognostic marker. Nodules and masses are often seen and are biopsied (**A**). The "grape-like" characteristic appearance is only seen in 10% to 15% of cases. Note that, if pleural plaques themselves do not evolve into mesothelioma, biopsy specimen should be sampled from their edges where malignant mesothelioma can form (**B**).

are often associated with anthracosic deposits, also called "dark spots," which should be targeted for biopsy (30). On clinical grounds its main value is:

(i) *Diagnostic*: showing higher sensitivity and sensibility when compared to other methods. It is also more cost-effective than surgery.
(ii) *Prognostic*: it can show visceral pleural involvement, a marker for poor prognosis.
(iii) *Therapeutic*: it allows for chemical pleurodesis with talc in cases of recurring effusion or, in earlier stages and in selected centers, for intrapleural neoadjuvant therapy to be administered.

Pleuroscopy shows a similar diagnostic yield to surgery and is much higher than cytology or closed pleural biopsy. It is thus indicated in almost all cases of suspected mesothelioma. In most cases, the pleural space is free or shows small fibrous adhesions, which do not interfere with endoscopic pleural examination. Larger, vascularized adhesions can, however, necessitate lysis using electrocoagulation in order to have adequate space for visualization of the pleural cavity. The main goal is to free the inferoposterior part of the pleural cavity where most malignant tumors originate.

Mesothelioma can show many nonspecific appearances on pleuroscopy. Most often, it presents as nodules and masses of more or less important size. The characteristic "grape-like" appearance is found in only 10% to 15% of cases [Fig. 5(B)]. Pleural thickening can be the only anomaly. It can be more or less regular and can be a simple, whitish, hard pleural elevation, which suggests malignancy. In one-third of cases, a neoplastic appearing pachypleuritis associated with multiple nodules and masses is found. Finally, a nonspecific inflammation with fine granulations, lymphanigitis, or a congestive and hypervascularized aspect of the pleura with local thickening can also be seen.

Sensitivity of pleuroscopic examination exceeds 95%. Failure to obtain a diagnosis is most often secondary to inability for the operator to obtain an adequate pleural space because of adhesions, which prevent lung deflation via an artificial pneumothorax. In these cases, surgical open pleural biopsy, although a more aggressive procedure, is another option.

E. Pathological Findings

Mesothelioma is famous for being a pleiomorphic tumor. Its propensity to have various aspects explains the diagnostic challenge that pathologists face in making such a diagnosis. Hence, the terms epitheloid and sarcomatoid are used rather than epithelial and sarcomatous to better emphasize the different appearances this tumor can show. Although multiple histological variants exist, the 2004 WHO classification has been voluntarily simplified to keep only those histological types which pathologists would agree upon. The 2004 WHO classification distinguishes malignant mesothelioma from other mesothelium originating tumors (Table 6) (17). Characteristic markers for MPM include EMA (epithelial membrane antigen), calretinin (essentially a nuclear marker), WT1, cytokeratin 5/6, HBME-1 (an antibody directed against mesothelial cells), and mesothelin. It also typically shows negativity for CEA, TTF-1, B72.3, MOC-31, Ber-EP4, and glycoprotein BG8. These markers are, however, of variable sensitivity and specificity. Electron microscopy, a costly examination, is not routinely used to validate diagnosis but can be useful in distinguishing MPM from adenocarcinoma or distinguishing desmoplastic or sarcomatoid

Table 6 Criteria for Evaluating Therapeutic Response in MPM

	Measurement	Partial response	Disease progression
OMS	$L \times l$	↘ ≥ 50% Σ $(L \times l)$	↗ ≥ 25% Σ $(L \times l)$
RECIST	L	↘ ≥ 30% Σ (L)	↗ ≥ 20% Σ (L)

Abbreviations: L, maximal axial diameter; l, largest perpendicular diameter.

tumors from fibrous pleurisy (23). A finding of elongated fine microvillae is a strong argument for a diagnosis of mesothelioma.

In the presence of fibrohyaline plaques, it is recommended to obtain biopsy specimen on the border of these plaques during thoracoscopy. If the pleura shows a uniform aspect, peeling biopsies should be obtained after thorough examination. A diagnosis in a MPM should not be done on gross pathological examination and should be based on immunohistochemical markings. The International Mesothelioma Interest Group has proposed guidelines for the diagnosis of MPM. They recommend validating the diagnosis with the presence two positive markers for mesothelioma and the absence of staining for two markers that are typically negative in MPM (as cited above). For sarcomatoid forms, two types of wide-spectrum anticytokeratin antibody markers should be used (negative staining with one type does not exclude such a diagnosis) paired with absence of staining for two typically negative markers (anti-CD34, BCL2, anti-desmin, or anti-PS100) (1). The 2004 WHO classification should be used as reference for diagnosis and, when diagnosis is uncertain or as part of a controlled trial, an expert panel should be consulted.

F. Biological Markers

MPM has a poor prognosis, due in part to its insidious initial course and late presentation, preventing curative therapy. Hence, biological markers have been studied to allow screening and early diagnosis. Measuring levels of CA 125, CA 15–3, and hyaluronic acid have not shown clinical utility for this. More recently, soluble mesothelin–related peptides (SMRP) (31), osteopontin (32), and megakaryocyte potentiation factor (MPF) (33) have been proposed as potential serum markers for MPM. Mesothelin, a glycoprotein found on the surface of normal mesothelial cells, is strongly expressed in mesothelioma and other carcinomas (34). Elevated serum levels of SMRP have been demonstrated in patients with MPM or ovarian tumors. A study using serum SMRP levels as a diagnostic marker for MPM suggested an excellent sensitivity (84%) and specificity (close to 100%) using this test. Serum levels were low in patients with lesions of the pleura or lung other than MPM, and patients with previous asbestos exposure (31). Measuring serum and pleural fluid levels of SMRP in MPM have some clinical interest and could help distinguishing MPM from benign pleural lesions linked to asbestos or pleural metastasis (35). Using a threshold SMRP serum level of 0.93 μM/L, a diagnostic sensitivity of 80% and specificity of 83% is obtained. Pleural SMRP levels did not, however, add significant value when compared to serum levels.

In subjects with asbestos exposure, it has been suggested that an elevation in serum SMRP could predict future development of MPM (31). Although there are methodological caveats to these results, it has been proposed that patients with previous asbestos exposure presenting with pleural anomalies and elevated SMRP serum dosage be "aggressively" investigated to rule out MPM or pleural metastases. This approach still remains controversial, as SMRP serum levels alone seem insufficient for MPM screening due to specificity below 50% when sensitivity is greater than 90% (35). This likely is linked to the fact that SMRP levels are elevated in epithelioid but not in sarcomatoid MPM (31,35). Finally, serum SMRP and MPF levels have been proposed to evaluate therapeutic response in peritoneal mesothelioma (33,36).

To conclude, measurement of serum SMRP alone probably has an inadequate sensitivity and specificity for MPM screening but could guide clinicians in diagnosing this tumor and evaluating its prognosis. Its use should, however, not be dissociated from histological and cytological considerations. Combinations of other serum markers could possibly increase its sensitivity and specificity as a screening test but further studies will be needed to validate SMRP or other molecules as markers for MPM.

G. Prognosis and Staging

Median survival in MPM is short (below one year) but varies depending on prognostic factors and disease extension. The latter is the principal prognosticator with longer survival in cases of earlier stage disease diagnosed via thoracoscopy (IMIG stage Ia; Table 5) (25). Various prognosis factors have been validated by study groups (CALBG/EORTC) that have lead to the elaboration of prognostic scoring systems, either clinical (sex, performance status, body weight, age) or biological (histology, inflammatory markers, LDH, blood cell count). Although these prognostic scores are of limited value in daily clinical practice and on an individual basis, they should be used as part of clinical research protocols to classify patients into similar groups and compare results of separate studies.

VI. Therapeutic Management of Malignant Pleural Mesothelioma

A. Surgical Therapy

Three surgical approaches can be envisioned for patients with MPM: diagnostic (surgical thoracoscopy, surgical pleural biopsy, mediastinoscopy), palliative (pleurectomy, thoracoscopic pleurodesis, or rarely pleuroperitoneal shunt), or curative (pleurectomy/decortication and extrapleural pleuropneumonectomy) (36,37). Of these modalities, only extrapleural pleuropneumonectomy (EPP) aims for total resection of the tumor. Perioperative mortality for EPP averages 6% in selected patients, mainly based on preoperative cardiac function and overall performance status (38). This procedure is usually followed by adjuvant radiotherapy and/or chemotherapy to eliminate residual microscopic disease. Prolonged survival has been seen using this approach (36). This therapy, however, remains controversial because it has not been studied in controlled trials.

Most experts recommend avoiding pleurectomy, except in patients with stage Ia disease. Also, decortication pleurectomy is not considered an acceptable approach in MPM by many experts. EPP is the sole recommended surgical approach for patients with stages other than Ia and should ideally be undertaken as part of a controlled trial. Whatever therapy is planned, surgical treatment of MPM should always be via a concerted multidisciplinary approach.

B. Chemotherapy

No chemotherapeutic agent has been shown to be curative in MPM but many combination regimens have shown an improvement in quality of life when used in a palliative goal

(39). The association of cisplatin with an antifolate agent (permetrexed or ralitrexed) has, however, shown significant improvement in survival when compared with cisplatin alone (40,41). For patients with good performance status, these therapeutic regimen should be considered in first intention rather than waiting for the appearance of systemic symptoms. Ideally, chemotherapy for MPM should be administered as part of a controlled trial. No second line of chemotherapy can be recommended to date. Evidence in the medical literature supporting the use of chemotherapy early after diagnosis is weak, but it is recommended to start therapy before systemic symptoms appear. Chemotherapy should be ceased if disease shows progression or if grade 3 or 4 toxicity is seen. A total of no more than six cycles should be given in patients who show tumor response or stability.

C. Immunotherapy

Animal studies and clinical trials on immunotherapy suggest that MPM is sensitive to these agents. Studies of interferon-alpha, intrapleural interleukin-2, and certain other intrapleural growth factors have demonstrated tumor shrinkage (42,43). These therapies should, however, not be administered outside of clinical trials.

A small trial has shown promising results with the administration of Mycobacterium Vaccae but more results are needed before recommending its use. Finally, ranpirnase, and antineoplastic ribonuclease, has not been shown to be efficient in MPM.

D. Targeted Therapies

So far, few studies have been done in MPM using "targeted" agents:

- Thalidomide, a potential inhibitor of angiogenesis, has not shown improvement in a small phase I/II study of 40 patients with MPM (only 11/40 patients remained stable for more than six months with a median survival of 230 days) (44).
- Bevacizumab, a monoclonal antibody directed against VEGF, is being studied in a phase II randomized trial in combination with cisplatine-gemcitabine–based chemotherapy (45). An association with cisplatin and permetrexed remains yet to be studied.
- Gefitinib, an EGF receptor inhibitor, has not been shown to be efficacious in a phase II trial of 42 patients with MPM (46).
- Imatinib mesylate, targeting the PDGF receptor, has not been proven efficacious in on published phase II study (47) and two subsequently presented trials (48,49).
- Suberoylanilide hydroxamique acid (also known as SAHA), a pro-apoptotic histone deacetylase inhibitor, is showing promising results in an ongoing phase III randomized placebo controlled trial.

E. Gene and Cellular Therapy

Although the first attempts made with gene therapy in oncology have yet to show curative benefits, there are arguments favoring these approaches with higher dosages in localized tumors. With the advent of newer and better vectors for genes, gene therapy could quickly become a cornerstone in the treatment of MPM. Hence, tumor responses have been shown in murine models of MPM and in preliminary studies in human subjects using intrapleural administration of adenoviral vectors (Ad) containing thymidine kinase and IFN-β genes (50,51). Tumoral response to Ad.IFN-β varies according to tumor type and anatomical localization. This model shows that CD4+ and CD8+ T lymphocytes specific to tumor cells are key agents in tumor eradication (52), arguing for the use of cell therapy in combination with gene therapy. Experimental animal models have also shown promising results with the transfection of p53, Bak, p14^{arf}, CD40 ligand, or antisense oligonucleotides that block messenger RNA expression of certain growth factors (PDG α, PDG β, IGF I, TGF-β) (53–55).

Another potential approach for the future is cell therapy. If chemotherapy and radiotherapy have improved the rate of complete remission and survival in patients with inoperable cancer, there remains a contingent of tumor cells resistant to chemotherapy and the immune system. It is thus suggested that the organism's immune cells (NK cells, T cytotoxic lymphocytes, CTL lymphocytes, etc.) could be "taught" to eliminate such resistant cancerous cells. This potential antitumoral immune response can be triggered directly via these effector cells or by using antigen presenting cells such as dendritic cells. Combined with other treatment modalities, this allows one to envision MPM therapy using CTL lymphocytes activated ex vivo with tumor antigens and cytokines or via dendritic cells as part of an antitumor vaccine (56,57).

F. Radiation Therapy

MPM is known to be resistant to radiotherapy although studies have shown that radiosensitivity depends on the degree of tumor cell ploidy (58). The challenge is essentially ballistic due to disease configuration and the presence of underlying lung parenchyma. Radiation therapy is often used in preventive situations by targeting puncture or drainage sites to prevent tumor seeding. It can also be aimed at controlling pain in situations of ribcage invasion or bony metastases (59). Intensity modulated radiotherapy (IMRT) following EPP seems well tolerated but its role remains to be precised (60).

G. Palliative Care

Recurring pleural effusion should be controlled with pleural fluid drainage and chemical pleurodesis, ideally using talc poudrage via thoracoscopy (61). Pain is usually of various causes, being either caused by local tumor spread or via nerve or bony involvement. Obtaining adequate analgesia can be challenging, and fast-acting opiates are titrated for this purpose. Somatic pain also responds to nonsteroidal anti-inflammatory agents. Anticonvulsivant drugs have been used as part of pain control regimen, and psychological factors should always be taken into consideration by caretakers (62).

Figure 6 shows a simplified decisional scheme for care of mesothlioma.

H. Evaluating Response to Therapy

Efficacy of therapy can be evaluated on multiple grounds. Clinical criteria such as quality of life and symptomatic improvement as well as survival can be used. Also, imaging studies such as CT and PET can be of use in evaluating response to treatment. As a general rule, appreciating response by using thoracoscopy is not routinely undertaken and not recommended.

For radiological evaluation of tumor response, the use of plain chest radiographs alone is not valuable and CT should be considered a key examination, especially after pleural symphysis has been performed. For this purpose, many criteria have been suggested

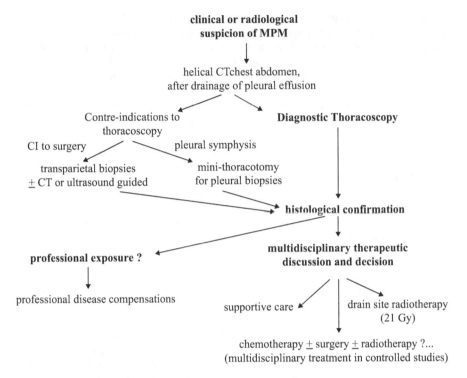

Figure 6 Simplified decisional tree for care of malignant mesothelioma.

but the most commonly used are the WHO criteria (product of two perpendicular measures) or RECIST (unidimensional measurement) (Table 4). Comparison of the latter two methods shows less notification of disease progression using the RECIST criteria (63). However, these two methods are not adapted to the circumferential growth pattern that mesotheliomas often exhibit (64). "Modified RECIST" criteria have thus been suggested using the sum of measurements of the longest pleural thickening at two different sites and on three different CT slices (64–66). Van Klaveren suggests using the WHO criteria for bidimensional tumors, RECIST criteria for unidimensional tumors, and modified RECIST criteria for circumferential disease (64).

Because postchemotherapy scarring can be hard to differentiate from tumor on CT, PET scanning can also be useful in evaluating the therapeutic response. PET allows for better evaluation of tumor size changes and fixation intensity. Preliminary results suggest that automated PET scanning is reproducible and faster than the modified RECIST criteria in appreciating response to therapy (67). Combination of PET and CT scanning (PET–CT) probably allows for better correlation but its role remains to be determined.

Overall survival is considered the only valuable study endpoint in evaluating efficacy of a chemotherapeutic regimen. Quality of life and symptoms should, however, be also evaluated properly to better quantify the clinical benefit (efficacy over tolerance) for diseases in which prognosis is poor and impact of therapy on survival is marginal or not clearly demonstrated. Of all scoring systems available to evaluate quality of life, none is particularly recommended although the Lung Cancer Symptom Scale (LCSS) is most often used in patients with mesothelioma (68). In the three arm study design done by Muers and colleagues (69), palliative treatment alone allowed for better symptom control in a non-negligible number of patients. Adding chemotherapy to this symptomatic treatment did, however, improve symptom control.

Finally, no biological marker has proven to be useful in evaluating response to therapy in MPM and their use is thus not recommended.

VII. Conclusion

The relationship between asbestos exposure and all forms of MPM is so strong that epidemiology of this disease may be superimposed to it, although other rare etiologies have been suggested. With an expected peak incidence in the next two decades, MPM is a classical model of workplace-related disease, and although a rare diagnosis, its social and medicolegal aspects are significant. Thus, for each rare patient who will get this disease, thousands exposed to asbestos live in the fear of this "Sword of Damocles" hanging over their head. The search for biological markers, which could be used as screening tests for individuals labeled "at risk," is not only offering hope but also could amplify this anguish that such patients live with.

Although still considered an incurable tumor, the past years have seen real advances in all aspects of care for mesothelioma. On epidemiological grounds, populations exposed to asbestos are better screened. On a molecular and etiological standpoint, pathogenesis of this disease is becoming better understood. Early diagnosis is due to rapid indication for thoracoscopy, which allows for more precise evaluation of the pleural cavity and better samples for pathological diagnosis using immunohistochemical markers. When combined with thoracoscopy, modern imaging techniques allow for better disease quantitation before therapy is undertaken. Besides newer radiation therapy approaches and emerging chemotherapy drugs, surgery is making a comeback as a therapy for selected mesothelioma patients.

Without a doubt, the most important recent advance is the concerting of all actors involved in the care of this disease from diagnosis to treatment as part of a multidisciplinary approach. From this point of view, care of MPM is a collaborative model involving physicians and surgeons, not unlike bronchopulmonary cancer (70). Finally, if guidelines have recently been elaborated for the care of patients with MPM, they also pointed out the poverty of literature in the treatment of this tumor (1,21). It is thus of utmost importance to implement therapy in MPM as part of clinical studies to allow future advances in knowledge of this rare and lethal disease.

References

1. Conférence d'experts de la Société dePneumologie deLangue Française (SPLF). Recommandations de la Société de Pneumologie de Langue Française sur le Mésothéliome pleural. Rev Mal Respir 2006; 23:6S78–6S92 [French].
2. Tossavainen A. Global use of asbestos and the incidence of mesothelioma. Int J Occup Environ Health 2004; 10:22–25.
3. Wagner JC, Sleggs CA, Marchand P. Diffuse pleural mesothelioma and asbestos exposure in the North Western Cape Province. Br J Ind Med 1960; 17:260–271.

4. Baris YL, Simonato L, Artvinli M. Epidemiological and environmental evidence of health effects of exposure to erionite fibres. Int J Cancer 1987; 39:10–17.

5. Berry G, de Klerk NH, Reid A, et al. Malignant pleural and peritoneal mesotheliomas in former miners and millers of crocidolite at Wittenoom, Western Australia. Occup Environ Med 2004; 61:14.

6. Gilg Soit Ilg A, Rolland P, Brochard P, et al. Estimation de l'incidence nationale du mésothéliome pleural à partir du Programme national de Surveillance du Mésothéliome, 1998–1999. BEH 2003;40:185–188 [French].

7. de Klerk NH, Musk AW. Epidemiology of mesothelioma. In: Robinson BWS, Chahinian PA, eds. Mesothelioma. London, UK: Martin Dunitz, 2002:339–350.

8. Pelucchi C, Malvezzi M, La Vecchia C, et al. The Mesothelioma epidemic in Western Europe: An update. Br J Cancer 2004; 90(5):1022–1024.

9. Roggli VL, Sharma A, Butnor KJ, et al. Malignant mesothelioma and occupational exposure to asbestos: A clinicopathological correlation of 1445 cases. Ultrastruct Pathol 2002; 26: 55–65.

10. Boutin C, Rey F. Thoracoscopy in pleural malignant mesothelioma: A prospective study of 188 consecutive patients. Part 1: Diagnosis. Cancer 1993; 72:389–393.

11. MacLachlan DS. SV40 in human tumors: New documents shed light on the apparent controversy. Anticancer Res 2002; 22:3495–3499.

12. Pott F, Ziem U, Reiffer FJ, et al. Carcinogenicity studies on fibres, metal coumpounds and some others dust in rats. Exp Pathol 1987; 32:129–152.

13. Ault JG, Cole RW, Jensen CG, et al. Behavior of crocidolite asbestos during mitosis in living vertebrate lung epithelial cells. Cancer Res 1995; 55:792–798.

14. Shatos MA, Doherty JM, Marsh JP, et al. Prevention of asbestos-induced cell death in rat lung fibroblasts and alveolar macrophages by scavengers of active oxygen species. Environ Res 1987; 44:103–116.

15. Manning CB, Cummins AB, Jung MW, et al. A mutant epidermal growth factor receptor targeted to lung epithelium inhibits asbestos-induced proliferation and proto-oncogene expression. Cancer Res 2002; 62:4169–4175.

16. Robinson BWS, Lake RA. Advances in malignant mesothelioma. N Engl J Med 2005; 353:1591–1603.

17. Beasley MB, Brambilla E, Travis WD. Semin Roentgenol 2005; 40:90–97.

18. Goldberg M, Imbernon E, Rolland P, et al. The French National Mesothelioma Surveillance Program. Occup Environ Med 2006; 63(6):390–395.

19. Galateau-Sallé F, Brambilla E, Cagle P, et al. Pathology of Malignant Mesothelioma: An Update of the International Mesothelioma Panel. 1st ed. In: Galateau-Sallé, ed. New York, NY: Springer-Verlag, 2005.

20. Roggli VL, Oury TD, Sporn TA. Pathology of Asbestos-Associated Diseases. 2nd ed. In: Roggli VL, Oury TD, Sporn TA, eds. New York, NY: Springer-Verlag, 2004.

21. Scherpereel A et le groupe de la Conférence d'experts de la Société dePneumologie de Langue Française (SPLF). Recommandations de la Société de Pneumologie de Langue Française sur le Mésothéliome pleural. Rev Mal Respir 2006; 23:7–104.

22. Musk AW. More cases of military mesothelioma. Chest 1995; 108:587–563.

23. Wang ZJ, Reddy GP, Gotway MB, et al. Malignant pleural mesothelioma: Evaluation with CT, MR imaging, and PET. Radiographics 2004; 24:105–119.

24. Garg K, Lynch DA. Imaging of thoracic occupational and environmental malignancies. J Thorac Imaging 2002; 17:198–202.

25. Rusch VW. A proposed new international TNM staging system for malignant pleural mesothelioma. From the International Mesothelioma Interest Group. Chest 1995; 108:1122–1128.

26. Carretta A, Landoni C, Melloni G, et al. 18-FDG positron emission tomography in the evaluation of malignant pleural diseases—A pilot study. Eur J Cardiothorax Surg 2000; 17:377–383.

27. Flores RM, Akhurst T, Gonen M, et al. Positron emission tomography defines metastatic disease but not locoregional disease in patients with malignant pleural mesothelioma. J Thorac Cardiovasc Surg 2003; 126:11–16.

28. Astoul P. Pleural mesothelioma. Curr Opin Pulm Med 1999; 5:259–268.

29. Maskell NA, Gleeson FD, Davies RJ. Standard pleural biopsy versus CT-guided cutting-needle biopsy for diagnosis of malignant disease in pleural effusions: A randomised controlled trial. Lancet 2003; 361: 1326–1330.

30. Boutin C, Dumortier P, Rey F, et al. Black spots concentrate oncogenic asbestos fibers in the parietal pleura. Am J Respir Crit Care Med 1996; 153: 444–449.

31. Robinson BWS, Creaney J, Lake RA, et al. Mesothelin-family proteins and diagnosis of mesothelioma. Lancet 2003; 362:1612–1616.

32. Pass HI, Lott D, Lonardo F, et al. Asbestos exposure, pleural mesothelioma, and serum osteopontin levels. N Engl J Med 2005; 353:1564–1573.

33. Onda M, Nagata S, Ho M, et al. Megakaryocyte potentiation factor cleaved from mesothelin precursor is a useful tumor marker in the serum of patients with mesothelioma. Clin Cancer Res 2006; 12:4225–4231.

34. Ordonez NG. The immunohistochemical diagnosis of mesothelioma: A comparative study of epithelioid mesothelioma and lung adenocarcinoma. Am J Surg Pathol 2003; 27: 1031–1051.

35. Scherpereel A, Grigoriu BD, Conti M, et al. Soluble mesothelin-related protein in the diagnosis of malignant pleural mesothelioma. Am J Respir Crit Care Med 2006; 173:1155–1160.

36. Rusch VW. Pleurectomy/decortication for palliation in the setting of multimodality treatment for diffuse malignant pleural mesothelioma. Semin Thorac cardiovasc Surg 1997; 9:367–372.

37. Sugarbaker DJ, Flores RM, Jaklitsch MT, et al. Resection margins, extrapleural nodal status, and cell type determine postoperative long-term survival in trimodality therapy of malignant pleural mesothelioma: Results in 183 patients. J Thorac Cardiovasc Surg 1999; 117:54–63.

38. Sugarbaker DJ, Jaklitsch MT, Bueno R, et al. Prevention, early detection, and management of complications after 328 consecutive extrapleural pneumonectomies. J Thorac Cardiovasc Surg 2004; 128:138–146.

39. Nowak AK, Byrne MJ, Williamson R, et al. A multicentre phase II study of cisplatin and gemcitabine for malignant mesothelioma. Br J Cancer 2002; 87(5):491–496.

40. Vogelzang NJ, Rusthoven JJ, Symanowski J, et al. Phase III study of pemetrexed in combination with cisplatin versus cisplatin alone in patients with malignant pleural mesothelioma. J Clin Oncol 2003; 21:2636–2644.

41. van Meerbeeck JP, Gaafar R, Manegold C, et al; European Organisation for Research and Treatment of Cancer Lung Cancer Group; National Cancer Institute of Canada. Randomized phase III study of cisplatin with or without raltitrexed in patients with malignant pleural mesothelioma: An intergroup study of the European Organisation for Research and Treatment of Cancer Lung Cancer Group and the National Cancer Institute of Canada. J Clin Oncol 2005; 23:6881–6889.

42. Mukherjee S, Robinson BWS. Immunotherapy of malignant mesothelioma. In: Robinson BWS, Chahinian AP, eds. Mesothelioma. London, UK: Martin Dunitz, 2002:325–338.

43. Robinson BWS, Bowman R, Christmas T, et al. Immunotherapy for malignant mesothelioma: Use of interleukin-2 and interferon alpha. Interferons Cytokines 1991; 18:5–7.

44. Baas P, Boogerd W, Dalesio O, et al. Thalidomide in patients with malignant pleural mesothelioma. Lung Cancer 2005; 48(2):291–296.

45. Kindler HL, Karrison T, Lu C, et al. A multicenter, double-blind, placebo-controlled randomized phase II trial of gemcitabine/cisplatin plus bevacizumab or placebo in patients with malignant mesothelioma. J Clin Oncol 2005; 23(16 S):625.

46.   Govindan R, Kratzke RA, Herndon JE, et al. Gefitinib in patients with malignant mesothelioma: A phase II study by the Cancer and Leukemia Group B. Clin Cancer Res 2005; 11(6):2300–2304.

47.   Mathy A, Baas P, Dalesio O, et al. Limited efficacy of imatinib mesylate in malignant mesothelioma: A phase II trial. Lung Cancer 2005; 50:83–86.

48.   Millward M, Parnis F, Byrne M, et al. Phase II trial of imatinib mesylate in patients with advanced pleural mesothelioma. Proc ASCO 2003; 22:228.

49.   Villano JL, Husain AN, Stadler WM, et al. A phase II trial of imatinib mesylate in patients with malignant mesothelioma. Proc ASCO 2004; 23:663.

50.   Sterman DH, Recio A, Vachani A, et al. Long-term follow-up of patients with malignant pleural mesothelioma receiving high-dose adenovirus herpes simplex thymidine kinase/ganciclovir suicide gene therapy. Clin Cancer Res 2005; 11(20):7444–7453.

51.   Kruklitis RJ, Singhal S, Delong P, et al. Immuno-gene therapy with interferon-beta before surgical debulking delays recurrence and improves survival in a murine model of malignant mesothelioma. J Thorac Cardiovasc Surg 2004; 127(1):123–130.

52.   Odaka M, Sterman DH, Wiewrodt R, et al. Eradication of intraperitoneal and distant tumor by adenovirus-mediated interferon-beta gene therapy is attributable to induction of systemic immunity. Cancer Res 2001; 61(16):6201–6212.

53.   Hopkins-Donaldson S, Cathomas R, Simoes-Wust AP, et al. Induction of apoptosis and chemosensitization of mesothelioma cells by Bcl-2 and Bcl-xL antisense treatment. Int J Cancer 2003; 106(2):160–166.

54.   Yang CT, You L, Lin YC, et al. A comparison analysis of anti-tumor efficacy of adenoviral gene replacement therapy (p14ARF and p16INK4 A) in human mesothelioma cells. Anticancer Res 2003; 23(1A):33–38.

55.   Friedlander PL, Delaune CL, Abadie JM, et al. Efficacy of CD40 ligand gene therapy in malignant mesothelioma. Am J Respir Cell Mol Biol 2003; 29:321–330.

56.   Gregoire M, Ligeza-Poisson C, Juge-Morineau N, et al. Anti-cancer therapy using dendritic cells and apoptotic tumour cells: Pre-clinical data in human mesothelioma and acute myeloid leukaemia. Vaccine 2003; 21(7–8):791–794.

57.   Hegmans JP, Hemmes A, Aerts JG, et al. Immunotherapy of murine malignant mesothelioma using tumor lysate-pulsed dendritic cells. Am J Respir Crit Care Med 2005; 171(10):1168–1177.

58.   Häkkinen AM, Laasonen A, Linnainmaa K, et al. Radiosensitivity of mesothelioma cell lines. Acta ncologica 1996; 4:451–456.

59.   Baldini EH. External beam radiation therapy for the treatment of pleural mesothelioma. Thorac Surg Clin 2004; 14:543–548.

60.   Ahamad A, Stevens CW, Smythe WR, et al. Promising early local control of malignant pleural mesothelioma following postoperative intensity modulated radiotherapy (IMRT) to the chest. Cancer J 2003; 9:476–484.

61.   Shaw P, Agarwal R. Pleurodesis for malignant pleural effusions. Cochrane Database Syst Rev 2004: CD002916.

62.   Lee YC, Thompson RI, Dean A, et al. Clinical and palliative care aspects of malignant mesothelioma. In: Robinson BWS, Chahinian AP, eds. Mesothelioma. London, UK: Martin Dunitz, 2002:111–126.

63.   Mazumdar M, Smith A, Schwartz LH. A statistical simulation study finds discordance between WHO criteria and RECIST guideline. J Clin Epidemiol 2004; 57(4):358–365.

64.   van Klaveren RJ, Aerts JG, de Bruin H, et al. Inadequacy of the RECIST criteria for response evaluation in patients with malignant pleural mesothelioma. Lung Cancer 2004; 43(1):63–69.

65.   Byrne MJ, Nowak AK. Modified RECIST criteria for assessment of response in malignant pleural mesothelioma. Ann Oncol 2004; 15(2):257–260.

66. Nowak AK. CT, RECIST, and malignant pleural mesothelioma. Lung Cancer 2005; 49 Suppl 1:S37-S40.
67. Byrne M, Francis R, van des Schaaf A, et al. Comparison of FDG-PET and CT scans to assess response to chemotherapy in patients with malignant mesothelioma. Lung Cancer 2005; 49(Suppl 2):S27.
68. Hollen PJ, Gralla RJ, Liepa AM, et al. Measuring quality of life in patients with pleural mesothelioma using a modified version of the Lung Cancer Symptom Scale (LCSS): Psychometric properties of the LCSS-Meso. Support Care Cancer 2006; 14:11–21.
69. Muers MF, Rudd RM, O'Brien ME, et al. BTS randomised feasibility study of active symptom control with or without chemotherapy in malignant pleural mesothelioma: ISRCTN 54469112. Thorax 2004; 59(2):144–148.
70. Astoul P. Introduction: Mésothéliome pleural. In: Astoul Ph, ed. Mésothéliome pleural. Paris: Elsevier SAS, 2005 [French].

28

Extrapleural Pneumonectomy for Early-Stage Diffuse Malignant Pleural Mesothelioma

LAMBROS ZELLOS and DAVID J. SUGARBAKER
Harvard Medical School, Brigham & Women's Hospital, Boston, Massachusetts, U.S.A.

I. Introduction

Diffuse malignant pleural mesothelioma (DMPM) is a rare, insidious disease that poses unique challenges in every aspect of its management, from diagnosis and staging to treatment and follow-up. The actual incidence of this rare disease is difficult to quantify in the United States given the lack of a national registry. The SEER (Surveillance Epidemiology and End Results) database reports a steady incidence for women and a decreasing incidence for men. Whether the SEER database captures the actual rate or misses geographic regions where the incidence is much higher, however, is debatable. On average an incidence of 2000 to 3000 cases each year can be anticipated (1,2). The average physician does not see such cases routinely, and the index of suspicion is not high when a patient presents with a pleural effusion, alone. Consequently, there is often a delay of months from initial visit to eventual diagnosis. Radiographic studies do not reliably predict pathologic staging. In addition, universally accepted and validated pathologic staging systems are lacking. To complicate matters further, consensus treatment guidelines do not exist. Surgery, chemotherapy, radiotherapy, and immunotherapy alone or in various combinations have been applied over the years but rarely in the context of a randomized phase III trial. Surgery is usually offered in the setting of a multimodality treatment approach. Over the last several years, enthusiasm has grown for neoadjuvant chemotherapy given prior to extrapleural pneumonectomy (EPP) or pleurectomy/decortication (P/D). On the other hand, surgical intervention for nonepithelial tumors has waned because of limited survival in patients with nonepithelial histology, even in the setting of the most aggressive protocols.

II. Clinical Presentation

Most patients are male over the age of 55 because the primary risk factor for mesothelioma remains occupational exposure to asbestos, which occurs traditionally in male-dominated professions (3:1 male-to-female ratio). Right-sided disease is more common; only 5% of patients present with bilateral disease (3). Patients usually have symptoms related to the presence of pleural effusion or chest wall invasion by the tumor. However, chest pain, cough, dyspnea, fever, fatigue, and night sweats (3) are nonspecific symptoms and a high index of suspicion is required to proceed with imaging and biopsy to diagnose DMPM. Therefore, the average time from onset of symptoms (initial visit) to diagnosis is about three months (3).

III. Diagnosis

The initial procedure is thoracocentesis. The typical effusion is more viscous than serous and has an oily appearance and color (gray). All of the effluent produced by thoracocentesis should be sent for cytology and other usual analysis. The effusion usually recurs and the diagnosis is often still lacking, since cytological examination has a low yield and high false-negative rate. Signs of recurrent effusion should be worked up with CT of the chest. Pleural biopsy should be considered, guided either by CT or VATS (4–6). Adequate tissue must be obtained for numerous diagnostic studies, since it can be difficult to differentiate mesothelioma from other malignancies (Table 1) (7).

VATS has the advantage of providing a more comprehensive survey of the entire chest; biopsy should be performed at several sites to reduce sampling error. VATS has a 90% diagnostic yield (8). In addition, VATS permits drainage of the entire pleural fluid, it can break loculations, and there is better re-expansion of the lung. In nonoperative candidates, talc can be used for pleurodesis and palliation. Since mesothelioma is capable of seeding thoracocentesis and thoracoscopic sites, biopsy incisions should be placed along the path of future thoracotomy incision to minimize potential sites of chest wall recurrence.

IV. Staging

Mesothelioma lacks a user friendly and accurate clinical staging system. Several staging systems have been proposed from the less-complex Butchart (Table 2) or Brigham (Table 3) to the rather detailed TNM-based system endorsed by the International Mesothelioma Interest Group (Table 4) (9–11).

Table 1 Staining and Microscopic Profiles of Malignant Pleural Mesotheliomas, Adenocarcinomas, and Localized Fibrous Tumors of the Pleura

Marker	MPM	AC	LFTP
Diastase-PAS	−	+ (50%)	−
Hyaluronic acid	+++	±	−
Mucicarmine	−	+ (50%)	−
CD34	−	−	+ (80%)
CEA	± (10%)	+ (>75%)	−
Cytokeratins	Diffuse cytoplasmic or perinuclear	Peripheral cytoplasmic or membrane-associated	−
EMA	Membrane	Diffuse, cytoplasmic	−
Leu-M1 (CD15)	−	+ (60–70%)	
Desmosomes/tonofilaments	Abundant	−	Few
Secretory granules, glycocalyceal bodies	−	+	
Villi	Long, thin, curved, branched		
(LDR >15)	Short, thick, straight, sparse (LDR < 10)	Absent	
Vimentin	−	−	++

Source: Adapted from Ref. 7.

Table 2   The Butchart Staging System

Stage	Definition
I	Tumor is confined to the capsule of the parietal pleura (i.e., involves only the ipsilateral lung, pleura, pericardium, and/or diaphragm)
II	Tumor invades the chest wall or mediastinal structures (e.g., esophagus, heart, and/or contralateral pleura), or
	Tumor involves intrathoracic lymph nodes
III	Tumor penetrates the diaphragm to involve peritoneum, or
	Tumor involves the contralateral pleura, or
	Tumor involves extrathoracic lymph nodes
IV	Distant blood-borne metastases

Source: Adapted from Ref. 11.

The 1976 Butchart staging system is based on 29 patients who underwent EPP (11). Even among stage I patients, the median survival varies widely, ranging from 7 to 33 months based on the degree of parietal pleural involvement (12). The Brigham staging system is based on 183 patients who underwent EPP followed by adjuvant chemoradiation. Positive resection margins, NI or N2+ disease, or tumor extending into the pericardium, diaphragm, chest wall, or surrounding structures are the factors used to stratify disease into the first three stages, while metastatic disease is classified as stage IV (9). When applied to this cohort of 183 patients, the Brigham staging system more accurately stratified survival based on stage in comparison with the Butchart and International Mesothelioma Interest Group (IMIG) systems (9). Specifically, the median survival of stages I, II, and III in the Brigham staging system was 25, 20, and 16 months, respectively (9). Other preoperative tests commonly obtained for staging purposes include chest CT, MRI, and PET-CT. CT and MRI are used to assess local extension, and PET-CT (13,14) is used to rule out occult metastatic disease, which occurs in a minority of patients. MRI provides a more accurate assessment of diaphragmatic or chest wall involvement (14). PET-CT is valuable for detecting occult mediastinal lymph node involvement as well as distant metastasis. Tumor activity, measured by the standard uptake value (SUV), can also provide prognostic information. A high SUV (mean SUV 6.6 vs. 3.2) is a negative

Table 3   Brigham Staging System for Malignant Pleural Mesothelioma

Stage	Definition
I	Disease completely resected within the capsule of the parietal pleura without adenopathy: ipsilateral pleura, lung, pericardium, diaphragm, or chest-wall disease limited to previous biopsy sites
II	All of stage I with positive resection margins and/or intrapleural adenopathy
III	Local extension (1) into the chest wall or mediastinum, into the heart or through the diaphragm or peritoneum, or with extrapleural lymph node involvement
IV	Distant metastatic disease

Note: Patients with Butchart stages II and III disease (9) are combined into stage III. Stage I represents patients with resectable disease and negative nodes. Stage II indicates resectable disease but positive nodes.
Source: Adapted from Ref. 9.

Table 4 Staging System of the International Mesothelioma Interest Group (IMIG)

Tumor (T) staging	
T1a	Tumor limited to the ipsilateral parietal pleura, including the mediastinal and diaphragmatic pleura, without involvement of the visceral pleura
T1b	T1a + scattered foci of tumor involving the visceral pleura
T2	Tumor involving each of the ipsilateral pleural surfaces (parietal, mediastinal, diaphragmatic, and visceral pleura) with at least one of the following features: Involvement of diaphragmatic muscle Confluent visceral pleural tumor (including the fissures) or extension of tumor from the visceral pleura into the underlying pulmonary parenchyma
T3	Locally advanced but potentially resectable tumor. The tumor involves all of the ipsilateral pleural surfaces with at least one of the following features: Involvement of the endothoracic fascia Extension into the mediastinal fat A solitary, completely resectable focus of tumor extending into the soft tissues of the chest wall Nontransmural involvement of the pericardium
T4	Locally advanced, technically unresectable tumor. The tumor involves all of the ipsilateral pleural surfaces with at least one of the following features: Diffuse extension or metastatic spread to the chest wall with or without rib destruction Direct trans-diaphragmatic extension to the peritoneum Direct extension to the contralateral pleura Direct extension to any mediastinal organ Direct extension to the spine
Lymph node (N) staging	
Nx	Regional lymph nodes (LNs) cannot be assessed
N0	No regional LN metastases
N1	Involvement of ipsilateral bronchopulmonary or hilar LNs
N2	Involvement of subcarinal or ipsilateral mediastinal LNs (including the internal mammary LNs)
N3	Involvement of the contralateral mediastinal or internal mammary LNs or any supraclavicular LNs
Metastases (M) staging	
Mx	Presence of distant metastases cannot be assessed
M0	No distant metastases
M1	Distant metastases present
Overall staging	
Stage I	Ia: T1a N0 M0 Ib: T1b N0 M0
Stage II	T2 N0 M0
Stage III	Any T3 M0 Any N1 M0 Any N2 M0
Stage IV	Any T4 Any N3 Any M1

Source: Adapted from Ref. 10.

prognostic factor for survival (15). Cervical mediastinoscopy can be used to rule out N2 disease. It is less accurate for mesothelioma than lung cancer, since the diffuse nature of mesothelioma often affects nodes that are not accessible to mediastinoscopy including levels 5, 6, deep level 7, 8, 9, and mammary or diaphragmatic nodes. Nevertheless, it can identify preoperatively those patients with positive nodes at levels 2, 4, and 7 who would not benefit from EPP.

V. EPP vs. P/D

Although there are strong opinions regarding the procedure of choice for cytoreduction of the tumor [(P/D) vs. EPP], there are no randomized studies to compare these procedures for each subtype of mesothelioma and stage of disease. The principal differences between EPP and P/D are lung preservation, postoperative functional status, and type of adjuvant therapies that can be applied. EPP involves the en bloc resection of tumor along with parietal pleura, lung, pericardium, and diaphragm. The pericardium and diaphragm are reconstructed with Gore-Tex (W. L. Gore, Flagstaff, AZ, U.S.A.) (16). Generally speaking, EPP is recommended when the goal is aggressive cytoreduction (macroscopic complete resection), but to be eligible, patients must have good functional status (i.e., younger patients). P/D is recommended for early stage, less bulky disease, or for patients unable to tolerate the physiologic demands of EPP (i.e., older patients or patients with limited cardiopulmonary reserve). During P/D, the lung is preserved and the visceral and parietal pleurae, pericardium, and diaphragm are resected. The lung should be free of disease, although the presence of one or several nodules that are amenable to excision without major loss of parenchyma does not preclude surgery. In addition, the decorticated lung must be capable of re-expanding. If chronic entrapment has impaired the lung such that re-expansion is not feasible, P/D is not advised and an EPP should be performed. By definition, P/D patients have less bulky disease than patients undergoing EPP. Retrospective or prospective comparisons that do not account for this difference can be misleading. A recent retrospective study comparing EPP to P/D found no statistical difference in survival between cohorts when procedures were compared stage for stage; however, staging did not account for bulkiness of disease (17). Despite the limitations of such studies, pleurectomy can be the indicated surgery for many patients. The decreased postoperative physiological strain on the patient also translates into a lower mortality rate than observed with EPP, in the range of 1.5% to 5% (Table 5). On the other hand, constant improvement in surgical technique and early aggressive management of complications has reduced mortality after EPP, from a high of 30% to less than 4% at experienced centers (9,11,18,29–35) (Table 6).

Local recurrence is the most common site of failure after surgery (29,37). Use of adjuvant therapy to decrease this local recurrence rate is therefore important. The options for adjuvant therapy after EPP include chemotherapy and high-dose radiation to the hemithorax. Adjuvant therapy after pleurectomy is generally limited to chemotherapy, as the preserved lung cannot withstand high doses of radiation. Hence, local recurrence is more prevalent after P/D than EPP. More advanced radiation techniques, such as intensity-modulated radiation therapy (IMRT), may in future be capable of delivering meaningful adjuvant radiation after P/D, as well. Because patients undergoing P/D have improved postoperative functional capacity, a larger pool of these patients can tolerate adjuvant chemotherapy as compared with EPP.

Table 5 Results of Pleurectomy

			Survival			
N	% Morbidity	% Mortality	1-Year (%)	2-Year (%)	Median (mo)	References
56	26.8	5.4	30.4	8.9	9.0	(18)
45	16.0	2.2	58.0	21.0	16.0	(19)
105	NS	NS	52.0	23.0	12.6	(20)
26	NS	0	NS	NS	10.9	(21)
63	NS	NS	NS	NS	9.8	(22)
64	25.0	1.5	49.0	NS	NS	(23)
30	NS	0	57.0	27.0	13.0	(24)
13	NS	NS	NS	NS	17.0	(25)
28	NS	11.0	82.0	32.0	20.0[a]	(26)
17[b]	NS	NS	NS	NS	21.0	(27)
16[b]	NS	NS	NS	NS	11.0	(27)

NS: not stated.
[a] Survival calculated from onset of symptoms rather than date of operation.
[b] Patients divided into epithelium (*n* = 17) and mixed (*n* = 16) histopathological findings.
Sources: Adapted from Refs. 18–28.

Success with surgical resection after neoadjuvant chemotherapy in stage IIIA lung cancer prompted several groups to apply this approach in MPM (49,50). Whether the risks outweigh the benefits has not been established. Although several studies have reported overall median survival of 23 months with no perioperative mortality, patient numbers remain too small to make meaningful comparison between the adjuvant and neoadjuvant

Table 6 Reported Mortality with Extrapleural Pneumonectomy

			Survival (%)		
N	Epithelial cell type	Operative mortality (%)	2-Year	5-Year	References
62	–	–	37	10	(31)
29	11	31	10	3	(11)
11	9	0	27	–	(32)
33	20	9	24	6	(33)
20	–	15	33	–	(34)
40[a]	26	7.5	22.5	10	(18)
183[b]	103	3.8	37	14	(9)
54	–	7.9	–	–	(36)

[a] Extrapleural pneumonectomy followed by chemotherapy [cyclophosphamide, adriamycin (doxorubicin), and prednisone (cisplatin) (CAP)].
[b] Extrapleural pneumonectomy followed by adjuvant radiation therapy (40.5 ± 14.4 Gy boost dose to areas of residual disease, localized lymph nodes and/or localized positive resection margins) and chemotherapy [doxorubicin (9 patients), CAP (80 patients), and carbo-platin/paclitaxel (94 patients)]. The 2- and 5-year survival for 176 patients who survived surgery was 38% and 15%, respectively.
Sources: Adapted from Refs. 9, 11, 18, 29–36.

approach. Moreover, neoadjuvant chemotherapy can alter the surgical planes, and patients with aggressive tumors may progress on chemotherapy, precluding a potentially successful surgical resection (51,52).

VI.   EPP with Adjuvant Systemic Chemoradiation

At the authors' institution, EPP is the procedure of choice for patients who have good functional status. Eligible patients should have resectable disease documented by CT and MRI studies that show an absence of mediastinal, transdiaphragmatic, or chest wall involvement. Adequate postoperative cardiopulmonary capacity is determined by Karnofsky score greater than 70 (35,38,39), predicted postoperative forced expiratory volume in one second (FEV1) greater than 0.8 L, and ejection fraction greater than 45% (9,39). En bloc resection of the tumor with the parietal pleura, lung, pericardium, and diaphragm is performed. The pericardium and diaphragm are reconstructed with Gore-Tex (W. L. Gore) (16).

The role of neoadjuvant chemotherapy is evolving. Patients who are clearly unre-sectable, or who have N2+ disease identified preoperatively, are given neoadjuvant ther-apy. However, the response to currently available agents is not sufficient to warrant neoadjuvant chemotherapy in all patients. This approach can also render those patients who do not respond to chemotherapy unresectable. Rather we select a priori those patients who are clearly not resectable from an oncologic or technical standpoint and offer them neoadjuvant chemotherapy. Six weeks after surgery, adjuvant therapy is offered to any patient who is capable of tolerating the regimen. Between 1980 and 1997, 183 patients underwent EPP. There were 7 (3.8%) deaths (9).

A proportion of the 176 surviving patients received adjuvant therapy. From 1980 to 1985 doxorubicin and cyclophosphamide were prescribed while cisplatin was added from 1985 to 1994. After 1994, the protocol was revised again to carboplatin [area under the curve (AUC) of 6 mg/m^2] and paclitaxel (AUC 200 mg/m^2) for two cycles, followed by concurrent radiotherapy and weekly paclitaxel (60 mg/m^2). The protocol was concluded with two additional cycles of chemotherapy. Radiation was given at a dose of 30 Gy to the hemithorax, 40 Gy to the mediastinum with an additional 14 Gy given to positive microscopic margins or positive nodes (9). The two- and five-year survival rates were 38% and 15%, respectively (Fig. 1) (9). Histology (epithelial vs. nonepithelial subtype), lymph node status (N0 vs. N1+ vs. N2+), resection margins, and invasion beyond the pleural envelope (invasion into diaphragm or pericardium) were important prognostic factors (9). The subset of patients with epithelial histology and stage I disease had a median survival of 51 months with a five-year survival of 46%. However, patients with nonepithelial histology and positive N2 nodes or positive margins did not survive to five years (9) (Fig. 1).

As stated above the Butchart and IMIG staging systems were also applied to this cohort of 176 patients. While the Brigham system stratified patient survival by stage ($p = 0.0011$), the Butchart ($p = 0.09$) and IMIG systems ($p = 0.31$) did not. Patterns of recurrence were analyzed on a subset of 46 patients who underwent trimodality therapy between 1987 and 1993. Median follow-up was 18 months; 25 (54%) patients had recurrence (ipsilateral 35%, abdominal 26%, and contralateral chest 17%) (37). Isolated distant disease was rare.

Since this report the adjuvant protocol has been revised. Most patients cannot tolerate both chemotherapy and radiation postoperatively. Therefore, a more selective

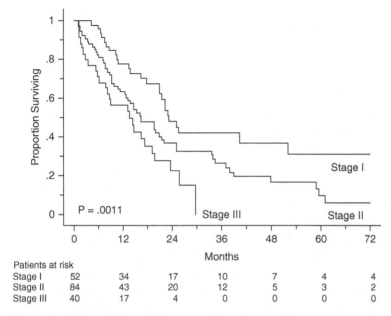

Figure 1 Kaplan–Meier survival curves of all patients surviving surgery: stage I, $n = 52$; stage II, $n = 84$; and stage III, $n = 40$. Brigham staging system ($n = 176$; $p = 0.0011$). *Source*: Adapted from Ref. 9.

approach is chosen. Patients at high risk for early regional, abdominal or distant recurrence such as those with N2+ disease are given chemotherapy while those who are N2− are given high-dose hemithorax radiation to reduce local recurrence, with chemotherapy given when recurrent disease is detected. In addition, the chemotherapy given currently is cisplatin and alimta for 2 to 4 cycles, as this is the most active regimen that has been tested in North America (40).

Adjuvant radiotherapy has also changed in the last several years. Rusch et al. reported a phase II trial of EPP and P/D followed by high-dose adjuvant radiation (36). Between 1995 and 1998, 88 patients were enrolled, and 54 patients underwent EPP followed by 54 Gy median dose of adjuvant radiotherapy to the hemithorax. Operative mortality was 7.9%. The median survival for patients with IMIG stages I or II disease was 33.8 months, and for patients with stage III and IV disease, it was 10 months (36). In regards to radiotherapy, we have adopted the Sloan-Kettering protocol at our institution. Attempts to incorporate IMRT in patients post-EPP have not been successful, with a postradiation mortality that exceeds even the operative mortality (41). Therefore, IMRT has been abandoned by our group.

VII. EPP with Adjuvant Regional Modalities

In efforts to decrease local recurrence rates, several protocols have combined aggressive cytoreduction with EPP and loco-regional administration of adjuvant therapy such as intracavitary chemotherapy or photodynamic therapy (PDT). A Cleveland Clinic protocol treated 19 patients, 10 of whom underwent EPP and 9 P/D. Intrapleural cisplatin and mitomycin C were administered immediately after P/D, and one to two weeks after EPP, followed by systemic adjuvant chemotherapy. Perioperative mortality was 5%. Median survival was 13 months (42). Hyperthermia is known to increase the effectiveness of chemotherapeutic agents and a few centers have studied hyperthermic intracavitary perfusion of cisplatin after EPP (43). Ratto et al. reported a study of P/D with normothermic cisplatin perfusion ($n = 3$), P/D with hyperthermic cisplatin ($n = 3$), or EPP with hyperthermic perfusion ($n = 4$) (44). Intrapleural cisplatin was given at a dose of 100 mg/m^2. There were no operative mortalities. Another small study by Yellin et al. tested the safety of intracavitary hyperthermic cisplatin on 8 patients who underwent EPP and another 18 patients who underwent other procedures for a variety of malignancies. There were no major complications related to the hyperthermic chemotherapy other than empyema (45). A phase I study of intracavitary intraoperative hyperthermic cisplatin with EPP for mesothelioma and amifostine for renal protection was recently completed at the current authors' institution (46). Twenty-nine patients completed the protocol and median survival in resected patients was 20 months. Results of a phase II study of intracavitary hyperthermic cisplatin with sodium thiosulfate with and without amifostine for renal protection were also recently reported by the authors' institution (47). Photodynamic therapy (PDT) was combined with EPP and chemotherapy by Pass et al. who conducted a phase III trial of EPP or P/D, adjuvant cisplatin, interferon-α-2b, and tamoxifen with and without intraoperative PDT. From 1993 to 1996, 48 of 63 patients completed the protocol. Most patients had advanced disease (stage III or IV), and no difference in survival was noted with a median survival of 14 months (48).

VIII. Conclusions

Mesothelioma is a rare disease that challenges physicians in every aspect from diagnosis and staging to treatment. We are still limited by the lack of randomized studies to guide treatment based on stage and subtype of disease. Ideally, each patient should be treated in the setting of a research protocol to enhance overall knowledge of the disease. The lack of consensus and the rarity of the disease make this task quite difficult. The limited data show that patients with epithelial tumors and early-stage disease who undergo aggressive cytoreduction in the setting of a multimodality protocol have a reasonably long-term survival. How to identify these patients preoperatively remains a challenge. Accurate preoperative staging or a prognostic algorithm based on clinical rather than pathologic parameters would greatly assist in this task. Referral to a center of excellence with surgical expertise in EPP or P/D is essential to ensure good postoperative outcomes and reduced operative mortality rates. Finally, the aggressiveness of cytoreduction cannot be further escalated. Rather, enhanced neoadjuvant or adjuvant therapies are needed to improve the local and distant recurrence rates. Improved effectiveness of chemotherapy, radiation, and immunotherapy, as well as methods of delivery for each of these modalities is needed before survival can improve.

Acknowledgment

The authors thank Ann S. Adams for editorial assistance.

References

1. Connelly RR, Spirtas R, Myers MH, et al. Demographic patterns for mesothelioma in the United States. J Natl Cancer Inst 1987; 78:1053–1060.

2. Antman K, Shemin R, Ryan L, et al. Malignant mesothelioma: Prognostic variables in a registry of 180 patients, the Dana-Farber Cancer Institute and Brigham and Women's Hospital experience over two decades, 1965–1985. J Clin Oncol 1988; 6:147–153.

3. Sugarbaker DJ, Garcia JP, Richards WG, et al. Extrapleural pneumonectomy in the multi-modality therapy of malignant pleural mesothelioma. Results in 120 consecutive patients. Ann Surg 1996; 224:288–294.

4. Renshaw AA, Dean BR, Antman KH, et al. The role of cytologic evaluation of pleural fluid in the diagnosis of malignant mesothelioma. Chest 1997; 111:106–109.

5. Dejmek A. Methods to improve the diagnostic accuracy of malignant mesothelioma. Respir Med 1997; 90:191–199.

6. Beauchamp HD, Kundra NK, Aranson R, et al. The role of closed pleural needle biopsy in the diagnosis of malignant mesothelioma of the pleura. Chest 1992; 102:1110–1112.

7. Ho L, Sugarbaker DJ, Skarin AT. Malignant pleural mesothelioma. In: Ettinger DS, ed. Thoracic Oncology. Boston, MA: Kluwer Academic Publishers, 2001:327–373.

8. Boutin C, Rey F. Thoracoscopy in pleural malignant mesothelioma: A prospective study of 188 consecutive patients. Part 1: Diagnosis. Cancer 1993; 72:389–393.

9. Sugarbaker DJ, Flores R, Jacklitsch M, et al. Resection margins, extrapleural nodal status, and cell type determine postoperative long-term survival in trimodality therapy of malignant pleural mesothelioma: Results in extrapleural pneumonectomy for early-stage diffuse malignant pleural mesothelioma 529 183 patients. J Thorac Cardiovasc Surg 1999; 117:54–65.

10. Rusch VW, and the International Mesothelioma Interest Group. A proposed new international TNM staging system for malignant pleural mesothelioma. From the International Mesothelioma Interest Group. Chest 1995; 108:1122–1128.

11. Butchart EG, Ashcroft T, Barnsley WC, et al. Pleuropneumonectomy in the management of diffuse malignant mesothelioma of the pleura: Experience with 29 patients. Thorax 1976; 31:15–24.

12. Boutin C, Rey F, Gouvernet J, et al. Thoracoscopy in pleural malignant mesothelioma: A prospective study of 188 consecutive patients. Part 2: Prognosis and staging. Cancer 1993; 72:394–404.

13. Patz EF Jr, Shaffer K, Piwnica-Worms DR, et al. Malignant pleural mesothelioma: Value of CT and MR imaging in predicting resectability. AJR 1992; 159:961–966.

14. Schneider DB, Clary-Macy C, Challa S, et al. Positron emission tomography with f18-fluorodeoxyglucose in the staging and preoperative evaluation of malignant pleural mesothelioma. J Thorac Cardiovasc Surg 2000; 120:128–133.

15. Benard F, Sterman D, Smith RJ, et al. Prognostic value of FDG PET imaging in malignant pleural mesothelioma. J Nucl Med 1999; 40:1241–1245.

16. Flores RM, Pass HI, Seshan VE, et al. Extrapleural pneumonectomy versus pleurectomy/decortication in the surgical management of malignant pleural mesothelioma: Results in 663 patients. J Thorac Cardiovasc Surg. 2008; 135(3):620–626.

17. Rusch VW. Pleurectomy/decortication in the setting of multimodality treatment for diffuse malignant pleural mesothelioma. Semin Thorac Cardiovasc Surg 1997; 9:367–372.

18. Allen KB, Faber LP, Warren WH. Malignant pleural mesothelioma. Extrapleural pneumonectomy and pleurectomy. Chest Surg Clin North Am 1994; 4:113–126.

19. Brancatisano RP, Joseph MG, McCaughan BC. Pleurectomy for mesothelioma. Med J Aust 1991; 154:455–457.

20. Mychalczak BR, Nori D, Armstrong JG, et al. Results of treatment of malignant pleural mesothelioma with surgery, brachytherapy, and external beam irradiation [Abstract]. Endocurie Hypertherm Oncol 1989; 5:245.

21. Alberts AS, Falkson G, Goedhals I, et al. Malignant pleural mesothelioma: A disease unaffected by current therapeutic maneuvers. J Clin Oncol 1988; 6:527–535.

22. Ruffie R, Feld R, Minkin S, et al. Diffuse malignant mesothelioma of the pleura in Ontario and Quebec: A retrospective study of 332 patients. J Clin Oncol 1989; 7:1157–1168.

23. McCormack PM, Nagasaki F, Hilaris BS, et al. Surgical treatment of pleural mesothelioma. J Thorac Cardiovasc Surg 1982; 84:834–842.

24. Chahinian AP, Pajak TF, Hollan JF, et al. Diffuse malignant mesothelioma. Prospective evaluation of 69 patients. Ann Int Med 1982; 96:746–755.

25. Ball DL, Cruickshank DG. The treatment of malignant mesothelioma of the pleura: Review of a 5-year experience with special reference to radiotherapy. Am J Clin Oncol 1990; 13:4–9.

26. Law MR, Gregor A, Hodson ME, et al. Malignant mesothelioma of the pleura: A study of 52 treated and 64 untreated patience. Thorax 1984; 39:255–259.

27. Wanebo HJ, Martini N, Melamed MR, et al. Pleural mesothelioma. Cancer 1976; 38:2481–2488.

28. Rusch V, Saltz L, Venkatraman E, et al. A phase II trial of pleurectomy/decortication followed by intrapleural and systemic chemotherapy for malignant pleural mesothelioma. J Clin Oncol 1994; 12:1156–1163.

29. Swanson SJ, Grondin SC, Sugarbaker DJ. Technique of pleural pneumonectomy in diffuse mesothelioma. In: Shields TW, LoCicero J III, Ponn RB, eds. General Thoracic Surgery, 5th ed. Philadelphia, PA: Lippincott Williams & Wilkins, 2000:783–790.

30. Worn H. Möglichkeiten und Ergebnisse der chirurgischen Behandlung des malignen Pleuramesotheliomas. Thoraxchir Vask Chir 1974; 22:391–393.

31. DeLaria GA, Jensik R, Faber LP, et al. Surgical management of malignant mesothelioma. Ann Thorac Surg 1978; 26:375–382.

32. DaValle MJ, Faber LP, Kittle CF, et al. Extrapleural pneumonectomy for diffuse malignant mesothelioma. Ann Thorac Surg 1986; 42:612–618.

33. Rusch VW, Piantadosi S, Holmes EC. The role of extrapleural pneumonectomy in malignant pleural mesothelioma. A Lung Cancer Study Group trial. J Thorac Cardiovasc Surg 1991; 102:1–9.

34. Sugarbaker DJ, Heher EC, Lee TH, et al. Extrapleural pneumonectomy, chemotherapy, and radiotherapy in the treatment of diffuse malignant pleural mesothelioma. J Thorac Cardiovasc Surg 1991; 102:10–14.

35. Baldini EH, Recht A, Strauss GM, et al. Patterns of failure after trimodality therapy for malignant pleural mesothelioma. Ann Thorac Surg 1997; 63:334–338.

36. Sugarbaker DJ, Mentzer SJ, DeCamp M, et al. Extrapleural pneumonectomy in the setting of a multimodality approach to malignant mesothelioma. Chest 1993; 103(4 Suppl.):377S–381S.

37. Grondin SC, Sugarbaker DJ. Malignant mesothelioma of the pleural space. Oncology (Huntingt) 1999; 13:919–926.

38. Zellos L, Jaklitsch MT, Bueno R, et al. Treatment of malignant mesothelioma: Extrapleural pneumonectomy with intraoperative chemotherapy. Oper Tech Thorac Cardiovasc Surg: A Comp Atlas 2006; 11(1):45–56.

39. Vogelzang NJ, Rusthoven JJ, Symanowski J, et al. Phase III study of pemetrexed in combination with cisplatin versus cisplatin alone in patients with malignant pleural mesothelioma. J Clin Oncol 2003; 21(14):2636–2644.

40. Rusch VW, Rosenzweig K, Venkatraman E, et al. A phase II trial of surgical resection and adjuvant high-dose hemithoracic radiation for malignant pleural mesothelioma. J Thorac Cardiovasc Surg 2001; 122:788–795.

41. Allen AM, Czerminska M, Jänne PA, et al. Fatal pneumonitis associated with intensity-modulated radiation therapy for mesothelioma. Int J Radiat Oncol Biol Phys 2006; 65(3):640–645.

42. Rice TW, Adelstein DJ, Kirby TJ, et al. Aggressive multimodality therapy for malignant pleural mesothelioma. Ann Thorac Surg 1994; 58:24–29.
43. Stehlin JS Jr. Hyperthermic perfusion for melanoma of the extremities: Experience with 165 patients, 1967 to 1979. Ann N Y Acad Sci 1980; 335:352–355.
44. Ratto GB, Civalleri D, Esposito M, et al. Pleural space perfusion with cisplatin in the multimodality treatment of malignant mesothelioma: A feasibility and pharmacokinetic study. J Thorac Cardiovasc Surg 1999; 117:759–765.
45. Yellin A, Simansky DA, Paley M, et al. Hyperthermic pleural perfusion with cisplatin: Early clinical experience. Cancer 2001; 92(8):2197–2203.
46. Zellos L, Richards W, Capalbo L, et al. A phase I study of extrapleural pneumonectomy and intracavitary intraoperative hyperthermic cisplatin with amifostine cytoprotection for malignant pleural mesothelioma. J Thorac Cardiovasc Surg 2009; 137:453–458.
47. Tilleman T, Richards W, Zellos L, et al. Phase II trial of extrapleural pneumonectomy with intraoperative intrathoracic/intraperitoneal heated cisplatin for malignant pleural mesothelioma. American Association for Thoracic Surgery, Abstract, 88th Annual Meeting, May 10–14, 2008, San Diego, California, USA.
48. Pass HI, Temeck BK, Kranda K, et al. Phase III randomized trial of surgery with or without intraoperative photodynamic therapy and postoperative immunotherapy for malignant pleural mesothelioma. An extrapleural pneumonectomy for early-stage diffuse malignant pleural mesothelioma 531. Surg Oncol 1997; 48:628–633.
49. Weder W, Kestenholz P, Taverna C, et al. Neoadjuvant chemotherapy followed by extrapleural pneumonectomy in malignant pleural mesothelioma. J Clin Oncl 2004; 22:3451–3457.
50. Weder W, Stahel RA, Bernhard J, et al. Multicenter trial of neo-adjuvant chemotherapy followed by extrapleural pneumonectomy in malignant pleural mesothelioma. Ann Oncol 2007; 18:1196–1202.
51. Krug LM, Pass HI, Rusch VW, et al. Multicenter Phase I trial of neoadjuvant pemetrexed plus cisplatin followed by extrapleural pneumonectomy and radiation for malignant pleural mesothelioma. J Clin Oncol 2009; 27:3007–3013.
52. David J. Sugarbaker, Boston, MA. July, 2009. Personal communication.

29
Benign Asbestos–Related Pleural Disease

E. BRIGITTE GOTTSCHALL and LEE S. NEWMAN
National Jewish Health and University of Colorado Denver, and Colorado School of Public Health and School of Medicine, Denver, Colorado, U.S.A.

I. Introduction

Asbestos has attracted attention for centuries, first because of its valuable physical properties, but sadly for the last 50 to 80 years, mostly because of its multiple and varied pulmonary health effects ranging from simple pleural plaques to extensive pleural and parenchymal fibrosis to malignancy. The benign pleural manifestations, including circumscribed pleural plaques, benign pleural effusions, diffuse pleural thickening, and rounded atelectasis, are the focus of this chapter. Mesothelioma is discussed elsewhere in this volume.

II. History

Characteristics that made the industrial use of asbestos popular include insulation against heat, cold, and noise, incombustibility, great tensile strength, flexibility, and weavability, and resistance to corrosion by acids and alkalis. Archeological studies reveal that asbestos fibers were integrated in Finnish pottery as far back as 2500 B.C. Plutarch (ca. 45–124 A.D.) wrote of asbestos wicks for oil lamps. Charlemagne (742–814 A.D.) surprised guests by cleansing asbestos napkins and tablecloths in fire. Asbestos was used in body armor in the 15th century. Gloves, socks, and handbags were made with asbestos in the 18th century. Commercial use of asbestos began in earnest with the Industrial Revolution at the end of the 19th century and peaked after World War II. Over 3000 commercial applications for asbestos were known in 1973 when the first ban against an asbestos product, asbestos spray-on insulation was enacted by the U.S. Environmental Protection Agency. Further, asbestos product bans and tighter asbestos exposure regulations have followed in North America, the European Union, Japan, and Australia. Regrettably, extensive asbestos usage continues in the developing world, making another epidemic of asbestos-related lung disease in the workplaces of these countries almost inevitable. The pleural and parenchymal consequences of asbestos exposure are for the most part incurable. Thus, primary prevention, especially the elimination of asbestos use, holds the key to control of the epidemic.

III. Pathogenesis

Asbestos is the name given to a group of fibrous hydrated magnesium silicates that occur naturally in the environment. Two major geological types of asbestos exist. *Serpentine* fibers are wavy and pliable and readily degrade into finer particles. Chrysotile, the only serpentine fiber, accounts for nearly 95% of commercially used asbestos worldwide. *Amphibole* fibers are needle-shaped and straight and prove to be more resistant to biological degradation. Several amphibole fibers are known, namely, crocidolite, amosite, anthophyllite, tremolite, and actinolite. While crocidolite, amosite, and anthophyllite have been used commercially in small quantities, tremolite and actinolite are mostly found as contaminants of other minerals such as chrysotile, vermiculite, and talc. The mechanism by which asbestos fibers induce pleural and parenchymal disease is not completely understood; however, various pieces of this puzzle have been solved.

Fiber size has been clearly established as a deciding factor of pathogenicity. Stanton et al. in animal studies demonstrated the importance of fiber length in relation to neoplasia (1). Rats exposed to different length asbestos fibers were most likely to develop mesothelioma after the administration of fibers greater than 8 μm long and less than 0.25 μm wide. These findings were further corroborated in animal studies conducted by Pott (2).

Fibrogenicity is also linked to asbestos fiber length. King (3) exposed rabbits to different length asbestos fibers and later examined them for the development of pulmonary fibrosis. Significantly, more fibrosis was produced by long (15 μm) fibers than by short (2.5 μm) ones. Other investigators subsequently confirmed these results (4,5).

The pathogenic importance of fiber size relates, in part, to how different length fibers are lodged in the lung tissue, processed once inhaled, and translocated to the pleura. Short fibers are often phagocytosed and moved from the lung via alveolar clearance mechanisms into the gastrointestinal tract, the hilar lymph nodes, or the pleural space (6). Macrophages are unable to fully engulf the longer fibers, triggering a complex cascade of events, including the release of oxygen radicals, cytokines, chemokines, and growth factors (7). In vitro studies have also demonstrated that long fibers interfere with the cell cytoskeleton, damage chromosomes, and interfere with the mitotic spindle during mitosis (8,9).

While fiber dimension is integral to asbestos pathogenicity, the chemical composition of a fiber plays an important role as well. Fiber composition contributes to fiber durability. When immersed into liquid environment, chrysotile fibers quickly lose their magnesium content leaving behind only a silicon shell. In tissue, they readily separate into their individual fibrils. Consequently, chrysotile is removed from lung tissue much more rapidly than are amphibole fibers. This is an important phenomenon to remember when drawing conclusions regarding pathogenicity of different fiber types based on fiber counts measured in human lung tissue many years after exposure has ceased.

The surface charge of fibers varies. While crocidolite has a negative surface charge, chrysotile is positively charged, resulting in the adsorption of and interaction with different biological materials in the target organ (10).

In summary, the toxicity of asbestos appears intricately related to its morphology and physicochemical properties, but the complete cycle of the events that leads to such varied pulmonary manifestations remains patchy.

IV. Pleural Plaques

A. Epidemiology

The epidemiological evidence for a connection between asbestos exposure and the occurrence of pleural plaques is compelling. The prevalence of pleural plaques is dependent on the population studied. Most estimates of prevalence are based on radiological surveys. The highest attack rates for pleural thickening are found in villages in Turkey and Greece where outcrops contaminated with naturally occurring asbestiform fibers, namely, tremolite, actinolite, or erionite, are used to prepare a whitewash or stucco applied to the inside and outside of dwellings. By the age of 70, 69% of the population of a Turkish village showed evidence of pleural thickening on chest X-ray (11). In Finland, Kiviluoto showed that the vast majority of Finns with bilateral pleural plaques lived in the vicinity of open anthophyllite asbestos pits (12). It is possible that these high rates of pleural thickening in these environmentally exposed populations can be explained by a fiber gradient, with anthophyllite and tremolite showing the strongest association with pleural plaques.

In occupational cohorts with known asbestos exposure, the prevalence of pleural thickening varies widely, ranging from 7.6% in asbestos miners and millers (13) to 58% in insulators (14,15). The large variation in the incidence and prevalence reported in these cohorts can be explained in part by differences in mean age, length of time since first exposure (latency), and dose of exposure among the cohorts studied. The influence of these factors on the prevalence of pleural abnormalities was elegantly confirmed in a recent study by Rohs and colleagues (16) Workers exposed to asbestos contaminated Libby vermiculite ore at an industrial site were first examined in 1980 (17). Among 513 workers, 2.2% showed radiographic evidence of primarily pleural changes consistent with asbestos effects. When 280 of these workers were re-evaluated 25 years later, 28.7% had asbestos-related pleural changes. A significant dose–response of pleural changes with cumulative fiber exposure was evident. A surprising number of workers showed pleural abnormalities. Nearly 14% of those with what would be considered a low-dose cumulative exposure (between 0.25 and 0.74 fibers/cc-years) had pleural disease.

Rogan et al. estimated that 3.9% of the U.S. population aged 35 to 74 years is afflicted with pleural thickening due to occupational asbestos exposure. They based their estimates on chest X-ray data from the National Health and Nutrition Examination Survey (NHANES) II (1976–1980) (18). This prevalence is approximately twice that estimated from NHANES I data (1971–1975) (19). Hillerdal (20) also reported an increase in pleural thickening from 0.2% in 1965 to 2.7% in 1985 in Uppsala county residents over the age of 40 years.

Epidemiological studies may either over- or underestimate the true incidence of pleural plaques when based on radiographs. Recently, increased body mass index (BMI > 30 kg/m^2) was shown to correlate with a greater prevalence of circumscribed pleural thickening on chest radiograph in former crocidolite miners in Wittenoom, Australia (21). This was especially true for thin (<10 mm) shadows covering 25% to 50% of the lateral chest wall. Whether this is due to extra pleural fat or other causes is not clear at this time. However, the finding is of interest in view of the continuing increase in prevalence of obesity among the U.S. population. That chest radiographs can underestimate the presence of pleural plaques has long been known based on autopsy (22–24) and computed tomography (CT) studies (25–27).

Pleural plaques are the most common manifestation of asbestos exposure. When bilateral and partially calcified, they are virtually pathognomonic of past asbestos exposure. The plaques develop slowly over time, with an average latency period from first exposure to radiographically identifiable plaque of 20 to 30 years (28,29). They are not affected by smoking (30). Pleural plaques are associated with lower lung fiber counts than asbestosis (31,32). No threshold exposure has been identified for the occurrence of pleural plaques. While asbestosis has been associated with cumulative, continuous exposures, pleural disease occurs at proportionally higher rates in individuals who have had intermittent exposures (14). Nishimura and Broaddus (33) speculated that intermittent exposures may allow more time for fiber clearance from the lung and for greater accumulation of fibers in the pleura.

Pleural plaques are not known to transform into mesothelioma. However, Hillerdal reported an increased risk for mesothelioma in those with pleural plaques on chest X-ray (34). In a necropsy-based study, Bianchi et al. demonstrated that the presence of plaques >4 cm was a risk indicator for the development of mesothelioma (35). Whether radiographic evidence of pleural plaques is associated with an increased risk of developing lung cancer is controversial. The issue has been addressed in a number of studies of varying design and in reviews without a definitive conclusion (22–24,36–44). Plaques are not causative in the development of lung cancer, but are thought to serve as a surrogate of the magnitude of asbestos exposure. However, temporality of the exposure may play a role in addition to dose, as mentioned earlier for pleural plaques and asbestosis. Any lung cancer in an asbestos-exposed individual should be very closely examined as an asbestos-related lung cancer whether pleural plaques are present or not.

B. Pathogenesis

Inhalation of asbestos fibers results in a spectrum of thoracic manifestations unparalleled by most other toxins. For unknown reasons, the pleura is a major target. The mechanism by which asbestos fibers produce the pleural disorders discussed below is not known for certain, but increasingly sophisticated theories have been proposed. In 1960, Kiviluoto (12) suggested that asbestos fibers poking out of the visceral pleura scratch the parietal pleura during respiration and thus induce an inflammatory reaction in the parietal pleura that eventually leads to pleural thickening. This theory has since been discarded.

Hillerdal (45) in 1980 published a report in which he suggested that some asbestos fibers that have reached the visceral pleura penetrate the pleural space and are swept up by the lymphatic flow and transported to the parietal pleura. As they pass through the parietal pleura, some fibers will actually remain inside macrophages and initiate an inflammatory response that in time leads to pleural thickening. More recently, Boutin et al. (46) published an elegant study adding to our knowledge of how pleural plaques may form. He and his coworkers obtained parietal pleura and lung biospy specimens during thoracoscopy in asbestos-exposed individuals. In the parietal pleura, they secured samples from anthracotic "black spots" and from adjacent normal pleura. Black spots are thought to be a part of the lymphatic system in the pleura and correspond to Kapmeier's foci or "milky spots," which are collections of immune cells surrounding lymphatic stomata (46,47). Transmission electron microscopy (TEM) revealed high concentrations of asbestos fibers in the "black spots" and almost none in the normal pleura. In some cases, higher concentrations of fibers were found in the anthracotic areas of the pleura than in the lung tissue. One-fifth of the fibers recovered from the "black spots" were >5 μm long. This study suggests that the distribution of asbestos fibers throughout the parietal pleura is heterogeneous and could explain the uneven distribution of circumscribed parietal pleural plaques.

Analysis of pleural plaques has identified mainly short, fine asbestos fibers <2 μm long. Animal studies have confirmed that fibers travel into the pleura after tracheal instillation (48,49). Pathology shows that asbestos fibers are embedded (50,51) in the pleura, and in vitro studies of disease mechanism have shown that mesothelial cells exposed to asbestos fibers promote inflammatory events leading to fibrosis (7,52–55).

C. Clinical Presentation

Macroscopically, pleural plaques are discrete, raised, irregularly shaped, shiny lesions of the parietal pleura, with no associated pleural adhesions. Microscopically, on their surface is a normal appearing layer of mesothelial cells. Beneath the mesothelium is fairly acellular, dense, collagenous tissue arranged in a coarse basket weave pattern. Many submicroscopic fibers are visible in these plaques when examined by electron microscopy (56). Plaques are most often found on the posterior and lateral wall of the lower half of the thoracic cage, where they follow the course of the ribs (Fig. 1). They can also form on the domes of the diaphragm, on the mediastinal pleura (especially overlying the heart) (Fig. 2), and rarely on the pericardium itself. They spare the lung apices and costophrenic angles. As Nishimura and Broaddus (33) point out, the intriguing aspect of this distribution is that it corresponds with the distribution of the lymphatic system involved in the clearance of particles from the pleural space. This assumes that asbestos fibers can travel against the normal direction of the lymph flow, as has been reported for coal dust particles (57). Asbestos-related pleural plaques are most often bilateral and symmetrical. If unilateral, most of them seem to form in the left hemithorax based on chest X-ray (58,59). However, a recent CT study did not corroborate this left-sided predominance (60).

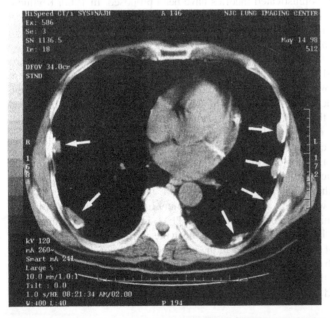

Figure 1   Chest CT with multiple large, localized, partially calcified pleural plaques (*white arrows*) in classic bilateral distribution along the posterior and posterolateral parietal pleura.

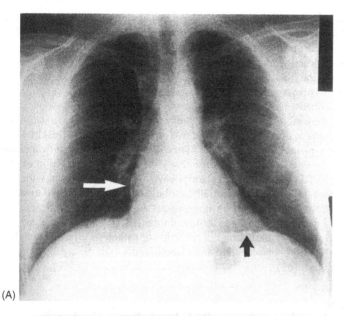

(A)

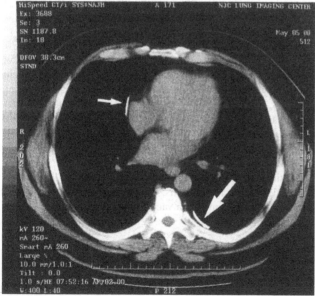

(B)

Figure 2   A former insulator with pleural plaques in multiple locations. (**A**) The chest radiograph shows a thin calcified plaque along the right heart border (*white arrow*) and overlying the dome of the left diaphragm (*black arrow*). (**B**) The chest CT also shows the delicate pleural plaque in the mediastinal pleura overlying the heart (*small white arrow*), but the plaque in the right paraspinous region on chest CT (*large white arrow*) was not visible on chest X-ray.

Chest CT scan has proven to be more sensitive than chest radiography for detecting pleural plaques and for discriminating between pleural fibrosis and extrapleural fat (25–27,61). Gevenois et al. (26) performed a conventional and high-resolution CT (HRCT) scan on 159 asbestos-exposed workers with normal chest radiographs. Of these workers, 37.1% demonstrated pleural thickening on CT scan. Conventional CT proved superior to HRCT in detecting these plaques.

Simple circumscribed asbestos-related pleural plaques usually do not produce clinical symptoms. Often they are discovered incidentally during the clinical evaluation of unrelated health problems or during participation in a screening program. Despite their subclinical presentation, pleural plaques are associated with statistically significant pulmonary function abnormalities (62). Most consistently they lead to a reduction of the forced vital capacity (FVC) (15,63). Pleural plaques have also been associated with airflow limitation (64–68). While this can be partially attributed to the prevalence of tobacco use in asbestos-exposed cohorts, reports in nonsmokers (66) suggest an independent asbestos-related mechanism responsible for airflow limitation. The most plausible scenario is that physiological airflow limitation is a reflection of pathologically apparent, but radiographically occult peribronchiolar fibrosing alveolitis, the early tissue response to inhalation of asbestos fibers (69).

D. Treatment

No specific treatment is needed for circumscribed pleural plaques. However, since they are a marker of exposure and as such are associated with the risk of developing asbestosis and malignancy, regular follow-up of affected individuals is prudent. Recently, much attention has focused on low-dose spiral CT as a lung cancer–screening tool (70,71) by persistently poor five-year survival rates. An expert panel met in 2001 to review the advances in radiology and screening of asbestos-related disease (72). They concluded that data available do not justify broad-based lung cancer screening in asbestos-exposed cohorts. Additionally, the U.S. Preventive Task Force in 2004 recommended neither for nor against using chest CT-scan to screen for lung cancer (73) Asbestos-exposed workers are a well-defined high-risk group in which CT-screening could have great potential. However, for now, the decision to screen with low-dose spiral CT must be made on a case-by-case basis, until further studies are completed.

Regular follow-up visits also offer opportunities to emphasize the importance of smoking cessation and to assist with achieving this, if necessary, and to assure updated immunization records especially for the influenza vaccine and Pneumovax.

V. Diffuse Pleural Thickening

A. Epidemiology

Diffuse pleural thickening has been recognized only recently as a distinct asbestos-related entity. For many years, it was considered to be a part of the spectrum of parenchymal asbestosis (50). On the other hand, it was often not clearly distinguished from circumscribed parietal pleural plaques. It is often touted as the sequel of an asbestos-related benign pleural effusion (74–77). Diffuse pleural thickening is not as specific for asbestos exposure as bilateral partially calcified pleural plaques are, since it has also been associated with other disorders, including parapneumonic exudative effusions, hemothorax, collagen vascular disease, drug exposure, especially bromocriptine (78), and Dressler's syndrome. The incidence of diffuse pleural thickening is thought to be significantly lower than that of pleural plaques. This is supported by a study conducted by Hillerdal (79), who followed 891 cases with pleural thickening due to asbestos exposure and observed that 84 individuals (approximately 10%) developed diffuse pleural thickening over time. Schwartz et al. examined the chest radiographs of 1211 sheet-metal workers and concluded that 260 (21.5%) had developed circumscribed pleural plaques, while again a smaller proportion, only 74 (6.1%), suffered from visceral pleural fibrosis. McLoud et al. (77) could not confirm a significantly lower incidence of diffuse pleural thickening compared to circumscribed pleural thickening when they reviewed chest radiographs of 1373 asbestos-exposed individuals. They found that 10% of the cohort had diffuse pleural thickening and only 16.5% had circumscribed pleural thickening. Some of these differences likely relate to how diffuse pleural thickening is defined by the different investigators or related to the type of asbestos fiber. de Klerk et al. studied workers exposed to crocidolite and found more diffuse pleural thickening than plaques (80).

Diffuse pleural thickening incidence increases with time since first exposure. It is associated with asbestos fiber burden levels that are intermediate between those of levels associated with pleural plaques and those of asbestosis (81–84).

B. Pathogenesis

In contrast to circumscribed pleural plaques, diffuse pleural thickening affects the visceral pleura and typically covers a much larger surface area (Fig. 3). It initially forms in the posterior and posterolateral portions of the lower visceral pleura. With time, it evolves and extends into the costophrenic angles and apices. Diffuse pleural thickening is usually bilateral, but can occur unilaterally. Adhesions between the two pleural sheaths are common. Microscopically, the visceral pleura is replaced by a layer of dense collagenous tissue with a basket weave pattern reminiscent of that found in parietal pleural plaques. Asbestos fibers and bodies can be recovered from the pleuroparenchymal tissue, especially in the vicinity of the pleural thickening (33).

The pathogenesis of diffuse pleural thickening is not precisely known. However, passage of asbestos fibers into the pleural space via lymphatics with a subsequent inflammatory response is also thought to play a role in diffuse pleural thickening. It is not known why some individuals develop circumscribed plaque while others develop diffuse pleural thickening.

C. Clinical Presentation

In contrast to simple parietal plaques, diffuse pleural thickening is often associated with respiratory symptoms. Dyspnea on exertion represents the most common complaint. In a study by Yates et al., 61 out of 64 asbestos-exposed workers with diffuse pleural thickening complained of breathlessness with exertion (85). Occasionally, pleuritic chest pain occurs, most likely due to pleural adhesions in those with diffuse pleural thickening (85,86). Sometimes the pain mimics angina (87).

The physical examination in patients with diffuse pleural thickening can reveal reduced chest expansion, dullness to percussion when the pleural peel has reached significant thickness, and sometimes crackles on auscultation due to concomitant

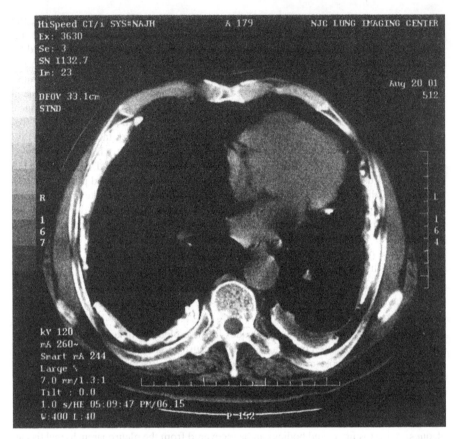

Figure 3 Chest CT depicting extensively calcified thick pleural rind extending around most of the circumference of the lung typical of diffuse pleural thickening.

parenchymal fibrosis. al Jarad and colleagues noted that crackles could be heard in the absence of CT evidence of asbestosis in up to 40% of subjects with diffuse pleural thickening (88).

The radiological features of asbestos-related diffuse pleural thickening have recently been reviewed (83,89). The diagnosis of diffuse pleural thickening on chest radiograph relies on the obliteration of one or both costophrenic angles (78). Based on CT scan, Lynch et al. defined diffuse pleural thickening as a "continuous sheet of pleural thickening more than 5 cm wide, more than 8 cm in craniocaudal extent, and more than 3 mm thick" (90). CT scan often detects fibrous strands, or "crow's feet," extending from the thickened pleura into the lung parenchyma. High-resolution CT scan is superior to chest radiograph in demonstrating the extent of the pleural process. It allows much better visualization of the often-involved paraspinous regions of the pleura that are otherwise obscured by mediastinal structures on chest radiographs. CT scan is also superior in distinguishing between pleural thickening and extrapleural fat.

Several studies have shown that diffuse pleural thickening impairs lung function. The most consistent findings are a decrease in FVC, total lung capacity (TLC), diffusing capacity (DLCO), and exercise tolerance (85,91). In the study by Yates et al. (85) of 64 patients with diffuse pleural thickening, FEV_1 was reduced to 62% and FVC to 77% of predicted. TLC was 71% and DLCO 74% of predicted. Similar results were reported by Kee et al. who studied 53 asbestos-exposed individuals exposed in shipyards or in the construction trades. In this study, the FVC was reduced to 68% of predicted, with a mean DLCO of 72% of predicted (92). Neither study reported DLCO corrected for lung volume, which in the absence of concomitant asbestosis would be expected to be normal.

Interestingly, a1 Jarad et al. showed in 20 patients that severity of disease by CT and chest radiograph scores correlated well with the extent of their pulmonary impairment (93). Schwartz et al. also demonstrated in 60 sheet-metal workers with asbestos-related pleural fibrosis that the greater the volume of pleural fibrosis derived from a three-dimensional reconstructed thoracic HRCT image, the lower the total lung capacity (94).

D. Treatment

Treatment options for those with diffuse pleural thickening and pulmonary impairment are very limited. Attempts have been made at freeing the lung with decortication, but results have been disappointing (79,95). Supportive treatment is often the best option available. Intercurrent respiratory infections should be treated aggressively. Oxygen therapy is necessary for those with hypoxemia at rest or with exertion. The importance of smoking cessation should be stressed. Immunizations are warranted.

VI. Benign Asbestos Pleural Effusion

A. Epidemiology

The epidemiology of asbestos-related benign pleural effusions mirrors that of asbestosis and the other forms of asbestos-related lung and pleural disease. Risk is associated with the same forms of inhaled asbestos that have been linked to asbestosis, asbestos-related lung cancer, mesothelioma, and other pleural disorders. Described in the 1960s (96–102), the so-called benign pleural effusion may in fact portend development of other forms of asbestos-related disease, including pleural fibrosis and possibly mesothelioma (74). In one of the largest studies of prevalence and incidence, Epler and colleagues observed 34 effusions among 1135 workers exposed in a variety of industries, including shipyards, fireproofing product manufacture, and paper mills. The prevalence was dose-related, ranging from 0.2% for peripherally exposed individuals to 7% among those with most severe exposure. It is the most common asbestos-related condition in the first 20 years after exposure, with incidence of 9.2 effusions per 1000 person-years for those exposed at the highest levels and 0.7 effusions per 1000 person-years for those with the least exposure. The effusions can occur as soon as five years after first exposure and have almost always occurred within the first 20 years, although studies differ in their estimates of latency, ranging from a mean of 12 to 30 years. In the Epler study, pleural effusions were five times more likely to occur in asbestos-exposed individuals compared with a nonexposed control group, including effusions related to mesothelioma and lung cancer (74). In light of the rarity of benign pleural effusions in the general population, asbestos exposure should be considered whenever an unexplained exudative effusion is detected. The studies of prevalence and incidence may, in fact, have underestimated the true frequency of asbestos effusions, since many may remain subclinical, preceding development of pleural fibrosis (79).

B. Pathogenesis

The true pathophysiology of asbestos pleural effusions is unknown. As discussed above, animal and human studies have shown that asbestos fibers can migrate to the peripheral lung parenchyma and can be demonstrated in the pleural effusions of asbestos-exposed workers (103–106). These data suggest transpleural seeding of fibers in the parietal pleura (107). Alternatively, in light of the role of lymphatic drainage of asbestos fibers (108), the asbestos fibers might also gain access to the pleura by retrograde lymphatic drainage (57,109). Once in the pleural space, the fibers themselves induce an inflammatory response that results in fluid exudation and clinically obvious effusions. For example, instillation of crocidolite into the pleural space promotes neutrophil chemotaxis (99). Influx of neutrophils and macrophages in the pleural space may help promote resolution of the inflammatory response to asbestos fibers, but also may contribute to pleural fibrosis (110). This low-grade pleural fibrotic reaction is hypothesized to result in altered lymphatic clearance or increased permeability of the parietal pleural. As has been described in the lung parenchyma itself, the pleural inflammatory reaction involves a cascade of inflammatory events involving both neutrophils and macrophages and the release of neutrophil chemotactic factors, oxygen free radicals, leukotrienes, cytokines, and growth factors (7,52,111). Inflammatory changes in both the parietal and visceral pleura are observed. It is noteworthy that pleural fluid eosinophilia has also been described in approximately one-fourth of patients with asbestos pleural effusions, although the role these cells may play in pathogenesis remains open to speculation. The pleural pathology seen in individuals with these effusions is typical of other acute exudative pleural responses, with biopsies demonstrating nonspecific inflammation and fibrosis in those with effusions.

C. Clinical Presentation

Benign asbestos pleural effusion is a diagnosis of exclusion. Benign asbestos effusions are defined as effusions occurring in individuals who have pleural effusion with no other known causes and who have been directly or indirectly exposed to asbestos (74). The effusion is typically exudative and may be hemorrhagic. It is important to exclude other important causes, including infection, malignancy, and pulmonary embolism. This typically requires observation over the course of two to three years. One-half to two-thirds are asymptomatic (74,112), detected as an incidental finding on chest radiograph or thoracic computed tomography. Notably, however, such effusions can be associated with significant pleuritic pain, with or without fever. Of those who present clinically with these effusions, approximately 17% to 50% report pleurisy. Other symptoms include cough and dyspnea. The effusions may be detected in the presence or absence of other findings of asbestos-related disorders such as asbestosis or diffuse pleural thickening. Pleural plaques, especially with calcification, are infrequently seen in concert with asbestos pleural effusions, probably because the effusions occur so much earlier in the course of disease. In approximately 20% of cases, severe diffuse pleural thickening will ensue. While this condition can spontaneously resolve in some cases, it should be considered a chronic condition, prone to recurrences and subsequent diffuse pleural thickening. The typical case will last for approximately one year, spontaneously clear, but then recur in approximately one-third of individuals. The extent of pleural thickening often increases with each episode of effusion (76). Approximately 5% of patients with benign asbestos effusions will later develop malignant mesothelioma, necessitating careful clinical follow-up (101).

Cases are usually first suspected when a unilateral or, less commonly, bilateral pleural effusion is detected on chest radiograph. In one major series, 11% were large (>500 mL) effusions. Confirmation of this diagnosis is customarily made by thoracocentesis, which reveals a typical exudative effusion profile, with elevated total protein, elevated total protein pleural:serum ratio, elevated total lactate dehydrogenase (LDH), pleural LDH:serum LDH ratio, normal glucose level, with elevated while cell count consisting principally of neutrophils, macrophages, and sometimes eosinophils (in one-fourth of cases). Two-thirds will contain mesothelial cells. As discussed above, the effusion is commonly hemorrhagic, even in the absence of malignancy. Nonetheless, when hemorrhagic effusions are detected, additional testing and careful clinical monitoring to rule out malignant mesothelioma or lung cancer should be considered. It is important to recognize that hemorrhagic effusions in asbestos workers do not necessarily implicate mesothelioma.

D. Treatment

There is no known treatment for asbestos pleural effusion that will alter the clinical course of this disorder. When effusions are large and associated with dyspnea, thoracocentesis may help relieve shortness of breath. Anti-inflammatory medications may be prescribed for acute pleurisy symptoms. Diligent follow-up of these cases is important because of the small but significant risk of subsequent mesothelioma. Thoracoscopic pleural biopsy may be warranted in some cases to help clarify whether areas of pleural thickening are due to diffuse pleural fibrosis or malignancy. However, most cases may be followed clinically for signs of improvement, without invasive studies beyond the initial thoracocentesis.

VII. Rounded Atelectasis

A. Epidemiology

Rounded atelectasis is one of the most unusual but distinctive pleural sequelae of asbestos exposure. While uncommon, it is important to recognize because it can mimic lung tumors (113) and provoke unnecessary medical and surgical interventions. The invagination of pleura with associated peripheral lobar collapse was first described in the French literature (114) in relation to infection and complications of therapeutic pneumothorax. Later, Blesovsky (115) made the link between "folded lung" and asbestos exposure when he observed this condition in a pipe fitter, a ship's engineer, and a laborer in a sugar refinery—all of whom had exposures to asbestos and pleural plaques. While rounded atelectasis has been reported as a consequence of pulmonary infarction, Dressler's syndrome, and tuberculous effusion, asbestos is now recognized as the leading cause. Multiple published case series describe the condition and support its association with asbestos exposure, but do not provide good estimates of prevalence and incidence (113,115–124). By inference, rounded atelectasis must be a relatively late and rare event following asbestos exposure, given that Epler and colleagues reported no case in their review of 1135 asbestos workers' chest X-rays (74). Hillerdal estimated a yearly incidence of 5 to 15 cases per 100,000 in men older than age 40 in Sweden, although this denominator was not adjusted for history of asbestos exposure (118).

B. Pathogenesis

The pathogenesis of rounded atelectasis remains speculative. Hanke and Kretzschmar (125) suggested that the condition starts with a pleural effusion that allows infolding of a portion of the lung and the formation of a cleft around an atelectatic segment of lung. Schneider et al. and others (119,121) have questioned this hypothesis because of the rarity with which pleural effusions are seen in cases of rounded atelectasis. However, the process is initiated, the consequence is an infolding of the visceral pleura and of lung tissue subjacent to an area of pleural plaque or pleural thickening. The asbestos-induced pleural plaque itself probably contributes to the invagination of the visceral pleura. At time of thoracotomy, Blesovsky described a thick membrane covering the involved lung segment. Some cases had evidence of adhesions from the lung to the diaphragm with hyalinized plaques on the diaphragm. In another surgical series, predominantly visceral pleural thickening was observed in association with a pleuroparenchymal mass, as well as hyaline plaques on the parietal pleura (120). Histologically, the visceral and parietal pleura show fibrosis with clusters of reactive mesothelial cells and nonspecific inflammatory changes, as well as laminated areas of collapsed pulmonary tissue. Some cases show evidence of interstitial pulmonary fibrosis with lymphocytic infiltration consistent with asbestosis, although in most cases the lung tissue itself appears collapsed but histologically normal (115,120).

C. Clinical Presentation

Patients with rounded atelectasis are often asymptomatic. Occasionally, they may present with cough and either pleuritic or nonpleuritic chest pain. Most commonly, this condition is detected incidentally when a chest radiograph is obtained for purposes of screening for asbestos-related lung disease. The symptoms have been reported to resolve following decortication (120), although such surgical intervention is rarely warranted. Rounded atelectasis is a benign condition that can occur unilaterally or bilaterally, usually in the lower lobes.

On chest radiograph, rounded atelectasis is not necessarily round, but is a pleural-based curvilinear shadow most commonly seen along the posterior surface of the lower lobe, less frequently in the middle lobe or lingula (113,115–121,125). It may have sharp or irregular borders, blurring mostly where the pleura intercalates with blood vessels and bronchi. Entrapment of adjacent lung may create a sweeping, "comet-tail" pattern as the segment of lung becomes compressed into the lung. These findings may be evident on chest radiograph, but usually a CT scan will be needed to provide greater confidence. Signs of lung collapse, such as diaphragmatic elevation, retraction of the fissure, or displaced hilum, are uncommon because rounded atelectasis rarely involves more than a few segments of a single lobe. Other disorders that may be confused with rounded atelectasis on chest radiograph include arteriovenous malformation, loculated effusion or empyema, mesothelioma, metastatic disease, and fibrinous pleurisy.

Rounded atelectasis is best defined by thoracic CT scan (Fig. 4) (117,121). Chronic pleural thickening will be seen adjacent to the curvilinear or oval mass. It can be shown to connect to the pleura. The degree of pleural thickening is the greatest adjacent to

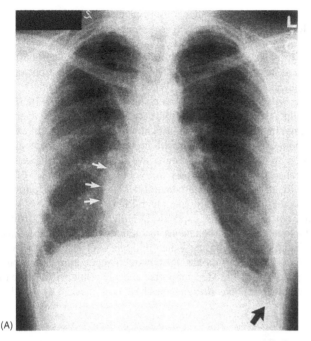

(A)

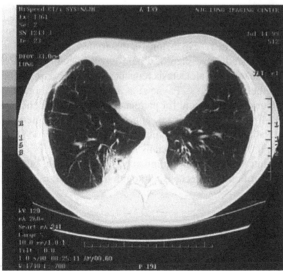

(B)

Figure 4 In a patient with past tremolite exposure, diffuse pleural thickening with rounded atelectasis has developed over time. (**A**) On the chest radiograph, unilateral obliteration of the left costophrenic angle (*black arrow*) can be seen, which is typical for diffuse pleural thickening. In addition, this radiograph depicts a right-sided mass (*white arrows*) located medially and at the level of the heart. (**B**) Computed tomography demonstrates bilateral pleural-based masses associated with pleural thickening. The right-sided mass has a "comet-tail" that is pathognomonic for rounded atelectasis.

the curvilinear mass, even in individuals who show diffuse pleural thickening or pleural plaques elsewhere in the chest.

The findings on CT scan are so characteristic that patients rarely require any form of invasive procedure to make the diagnosis. As discussed above, when the typical "comet sign" is observed, the only major consideration is to have ruled out other known causes of rounded atelectasis (117,121,126). When followed longitudinally, the CT scan and chest radiograph will show no or very slow change over time (118,119,121). Hillerdal performed follow-up assessments in 61 of 64 patients (118), with an average observation period of six years. In this group, 55% had a known history of asbestos exposure. In the observation period, 24 remained stable with no other changes except slight worsening of pleural plaques. In 12 individuals, progressive diffuse pleural thickening and parenchymal changes consistent with asbestosis were observed over the next 2 to 15 years. Two of these individuals developed contralateral benign pleural effusions. An additional 23 patients developed bilateral progressive pleural fibrosis. The patients with rounded atelectasis who did not have asbestos exposure in Hillerdal's cohort remained stable over time, except for one case of spontaneous resolution. Notably, nine of the individuals—all of whom had asbestos exposure—died during the observation period: three from asbestosis and two due to pneumonia. Postobstructive pneumonia and pulmonary thrombosis in entrapped vessels have been reported and can result in death due to rounded atelectasis (127). On rare occasions malignancies have been masked by rounded atelectasis (128).

D. Treatment

There is no specific treatment for rounded atelectasis. In surgical series reported by Blesovsky (115) and later by Payne and colleagues (120), the surgeons were able to release the entrapped lung, resulting in re-expansion of the folded lung segment. In some individuals who had experienced chest pain, the pain resolved with this surgical intervention. In some instances, the rounded atelectasis reoccurred despite stripping of the lung from the pleura. Based on their experience, Payne et al. recommended thoracotomy with removal of the visceral pleura as a treatment for patients with intractable chest pain. However, when the typical CT findings are observed, unnecessary surgical intervention can be avoided in most cases. Patients should be monitored periodically for the stability of the lesion on chest radiograph or CT scan. Clinicians must remain alert for evidence of postobstructive pneumonia, intercurrent lung malignancy, mesothelioma, pulmonary thromboses, or hematoma due to rounded atelectasis, although these are all rare events.

References

1. Stanton MF, Layard M, Tegeris A, et al. Relation of particle dimension to carcinogenicity in amphibole asbestoses and other fibrous minerals. J Natl Cancer Inst 1981; 67(5):965–975.
2. Pott F. Some aspects on the doseometry of the carcinogenic potency of asbestos and other fibrous dusts. Staub Reinhold Luft 1978; 38:486.
3. King EJ. Effect of asbestos and asbestos and aluminium on the lungs of rabbits. Thorax 1946; 1:118.
4. Scymczykiewicz K, Wiecek E. The effect of fibrous and amorphous asbestos on the collagen content in the lungs of guinea pigs. Proceedings of the 13th International Conference of Occupational Hygiene, New York, 1960.

5. Klosterkotter W. Experimentelle Untersuchungen über die Bedeutung der Faserlange für die Asbest-fibrose sowie Untersuchungen über die Beeinflussung der Fibrose durch Polyvinylpyridin-n-oxid. Biologische Wirkungen des Asbestos, 1968:47.

6. Hillerdal G. Nonmalignant pleural disease related to asbestos exposure. Clin Chest Med 1985; 6(1):141–152.

7. Robledo R, Mossman B. Cellular and molecular mechanisms of asbestos-induced fibrosis. J Cell Physiol 1999; 180(2):158–166.

8. Jensen CG, Jensen LC, Reider CL, et al. Long crocidolite asbestos fibers cause polyploidy by sterically blocking cytokinesis. Carcinogenesis 1996; 17(9):2013–2021.

9. Yegles M, Saint-Etienne L, Renier A, et al. Induction of metaphase and anaphase/telophase abnormalities by asbestos fibers in rat pleural mesothelial cells in vitro. Am J Respir Cell Mol Biol 1993; 9(2):186–191.

10. Desai R, Richards RJ. The adsorption of biological macromolecules by mineral dusts. Environ Res 1978; 16(1–3):449–464.

11. Yazicioglu S, Ilçayto R, Balci K, et al. Pleural calcification, pleural mesotheliomas, and bronchial cancers caused by tremolite dust. Thorax 1980; 35(8):564–569.

12. Kiviluoto R. Pleural calcification as a roentgenologic sign of non-occupational endemic anthophyllite-asbestosis. Acta Radiol Suppl 1960; 194:1–67.

13. Irwig LM, du Toit RS, Sluis-Cremer GK, et al. Risk of asbestosis in crocidolite and amosite mines in South Africa. Ann N Y Acad Sci 1979; 330:35–52.

14. Becklake MR. Asbestos and other fiber-related diseases of the lungs and pleura. Distribution and determinants in exposed populations. Chest 1991; 100(1):248–254.

15. Bourbeau J, Ernest P, Chrome J, et al. The relationship between respiratory impairment and asbestos-related pleural abnormality in an active work force. Am Rev Respir Dis 1990; 142(4):837–842.

16. Rohs AM, Lockey JE, Dunning KK, et al. Low-level fiber-induced radiographic changes caused by Libby vermiculite: A 25-year follow-up study. Am J Respir Crit Care Med 2008; 177(6):630–637.

17. Lockey JE, Brooks SM, Jarabek AM, et al. Pulmonary changes after exposure to vermiculite contaminated with fibrous tremolite. Am Rev Respir Dis 1984; 129(6):952–958.

18. Rogan WJ, Ragan NB, Dinse GE. X-ray evidence of increased asbestos exposure in the US population from NHANES I and NHANES II, 1973–1978. National Health Examination Survey. Cancer Causes Control 2000; 11(5):441–449.

19. Rogan WJ, Gladen BC, Ragan NB, et al. US prevalence of occupational pleural thickening. A look at chest X-rays from the first National Health and Nutrition Examination Survey. Am J Epidemiol 1987; 126(5):893–900.

20. Hillerdal G. Pleural plaques in the general population. Ann N Y Acad Sci 1991; 643:430–437.

21. Lee YC, Runnion CK, Pang SC, et al. Increased body mass index is related to apparent circumscribed pleural thickening on plain chest radiographs. Am J Ind Med 2001; 39(1):112–116.

22. Edge JR. Incidence of bronchial carcinoma in shipyard workers with pleural plaques. Ann N Y Acad Sci 1979; 330:289–294.

23. Fletcher DE. A mortality study of shipyard workers with pleural plaques. Br J Ind Med 1972; 29(2):142–145.

24. Kiviluoto R, Meurman LO, Hakama M. Pleural plaques and neoplasia in Finland. Ann N Y Acad Sci 1979; 330:31–33.

25. Friedman AC, Fiel SB, Fisher MS, et al. Asbestos-related pleural disease and asbestosis: A comparison of CT and chest radiography. AJR Am J Roentgenol 1988; 150(2):269–275.

26. Gevenois PA, De Vuyst P, Dedeire S, et al. Conventional and high-resolution CT in asymptomatic asbestos-exposed workers. Acta Radiol 1994; 35(3):226–229.

27. Katz D, Kreel L. Computed tomography in pulmonary asbestosis. Clin Radiol 1979; 30(2):207–213.

28. Becklake MR, Case BW. Fiber burden and asbestos-related lung disease: Determinants of dose–response relationships. Am J Respir Crit Care Med 1994; 150(6 Pt 1):1488–1492.

29. Hillerdal G. Pleural plaques in a health survey material. Frequency, development and exposure to asbestos. Scand J Respir Dis 1978; 59(5):257–263.

30. Yano E, Tanaka K, Funaki M, et al. Effect of smoking on pleural thickening in asbestos workers. Br J Ind Med 1993; 50(10):898–901.

31. Roggli VL, Pratt PC, Brody AR. Asbestos content of lung tissue in asbestos associated diseases: A study of 110 cases. Br J Ind Med 1986; 43(1):18–28.

32. Stephens M, Gibbs AR, Pooley FD, et al. Asbestos induced diffuse pleural fibrosis: Pathology and mineralogy. Thorax 1987; 42(8):583–588.

33. Nishimura SL, Broaddus VC. Asbestos-induced pleural disease. Clin Chest Med 1998; 19(2):311–329.

34. Hillerdal G. Pleural plaques and risk for bronchial carcinoma and mesothelioma. A prospective study. Chest 1994; 105(1):144–150.

35. Bianchi C, Giarelli L, Grandi G, et al. Latency periods in asbestos-related mesothelioma of the pleura. Eur J Cancer Prev 1997; 6(2):162–166.

36. Harber P, Mohsenifar Z, Oren A, et al. Pleural plaques and asbestos-associated malignancy. J Occup Med 1987; 29:641–644.

37. Hillerdal G. Pleural plaques and risk for cancer in the County of Uppsala. Eur J Respir Dis Suppl 1980; 107:111–117.

38. Hillerdal G, Henderson DW. Asbestos, asbestosis, pleural plaques and lung cancer. Scand J Work Environ Health 1997; 23(2):93–103.

39. Mollo F, Andrion A, Colombo A, et al. Pleural plaques and risk of cancer in Turin, northwestern Italy. An autopsy study. Cancer 1984; 54(7):1418–1422.

40. Nurminen M, Tossavainen A. Is there an association between pleural plaques and lung cancer without asbestosis? Scand J Work Environ Health 1994; 20(1):62–64.

41. Partanen T, Nurminen M, Zitting A, et al. Localized pleural plaques and lung cancer. Am J Ind Med 1992; 22(2):185–192.

42. Thiringer G, Blornqvist N, Brolin I, et al. Pleural plaques in chest x-rays of lung cancer patients and matched controls (preliminary results). Eur J Respir Dis Suppl 1980; 107:119–122.

43. Wain SL, Roggli VL, Foster WL Jr. Parietal pleural plaques, asbestos bodies, and neoplasia. A clinical, pathologic, and roentgenographic correlation of 25 consecutive cases. Chest 1984; 86(5):707–713.

44. Weiss W. Asbestos-related pleural plaques and lung cancer. Chest 1993; 103(6):1854–1859.

45. Hillerdal G. The pathogenesis of pleural plaques and pulmonary asbestosis: Possibilities and impossibilities. Eur J Respir Dis 1980; 61(3):129–138.

46. Boutin C, Dumortier P, Rey F, et al. Black spots concentrate oncogenic asbestos fibers in the parietal pleura. Thoracoscopic and mineralogic study. Am J Respir Crit Care Med 1996; 153(1):444–449.

47. Wang NS. Anatomy of the pleura. Clin Chest Med 1998; 19(2):229–240.

48. Sahn SA, Antony VB. Pathogenesis of pleural plaques. Relationship of early cellular response and pathology. Am Rev Respir Dis 1984; 130(5):884–887.

49. Viallat JR, Raybuad F, Passarel M, et al. Pleural migration of chrysotile fibers after intratracheal injection in rats. Arch Environ Health 1986; 41(5):282–286.

50. Becklake MR. Asbestos-related diseases of the lung and other organs: Their epidemiology and implications for clinical practice. Am Rev Respir Dis 1976; 114(1):187–227.

51. Dodson RF, Williams MG Jr, Corn CJ, et al. Asbestos content of lung tissue, lymph nodes, and pleural plaques from former shipyard workers. Am Rev Respir Dis 1990; 142(4):843–847.

52. Choe N, Tanaka S, Xia W, et al. Pleural macrophage recruitment and activation in asbestos-induced pleural injury. Environ Health Perspect 1997; 105(Suppl. 5):1257–1260.

53. Kinnula VL. Oxidant and antioxidant mechanisms of lung disease caused by asbestos fibres. Eur Respir J 1999; 14(3):706–716.

54. Kuwahara M, Kagan E. The mesothelial cell and its role in asbestos-induced pleural injury. Int J Exp Pathol 1995; 76(3):163–170.

55. Kuwahara M, Verma K, Ando T, et al. Asbestos exposure stimulates pleural mesothelial cells to secrete the fibroblast chemoattractant, fibronectin. Am J Respir Cell Mol Biol 1994; 10(2):167–176.

56. Herbert A. Pathogenesis of pleurisy, pleural fibrosis, and mesothelial proliferation. Thorax 1986; 41(3):176–189.

57. Taskinen E, Ahlamn K, Wukeri M. A current hypothesis of the lymphatic transport of inspired dust to the parietal pleura. Chest 1973; 64(2):193–196.

58. Hu H, Beckett L, Kelsey K, et al. The left-sided predominance of asbestos-related pleural disease. Am Rev Respir Dis 1993; 148(4 Pt 1):981–984.

59. Withers BF, Ducatman AM, Yang WN. Roentgenographic evidence for predominant left-sided location of unilateral pleural plaques. Chest 1989; 95(6):1262–1264.

60. Gallego JC. Absence of left-sided predominance in asbestos-related pleural plaques: A CT study. Chest 1998; 113(4):1034–1036.

61. Gamsu G, Aberle DR, Lynch D. Computed tomography in the diagnosis of asbestos-related thoracic disease. J Thorac Imaging 1989; 4(1):61–67.

62. Diagnosis and initial management of nonmalignant diseases related to asbestos. Am J Respir Crit Care Med 2004; 170(6):691–715.

63. Oliver LC, Eisen EA, Greene R, et al. Asbestos-related pleural plaques and lung function. Am J Ind Med 1988; 14(6):649–656.

64. Hedenstierna G, Alexandersson R, Kolmodin-Hedman B, et al. Pleural plaques and lung function in construction workers exposed to asbestos. Eur J Respir Dis 1981; 62(2):111–122.

65. Hjortsberg U, Orbaek P, Aborelius M Jr, et al. Railroad workers with pleural plaques: I. Spirometric and nitrogen washout investigation on smoking and nonsmoking asbestos-exposed workers. Am J Ind Med 1988; 14(6):635–641.

66. Kilburn KH, Warshaw R. Pulmonary functional impairment associated with pleural asbestos disease. Circumscribed and diffuse thickening. Chest 1990; 98(4):965–972.

67. Kilburn KH, Warshaw RH. Abnormal pulmonary function associated with diaphragmatic pleural plaques due to exposure to asbestos. Br J Ind Med 1990; 47(9):611–614.

68. Kilburn KH, Warshaw RH. Abnormal lung function associated with asbestos disease of the pleura, the lung, and both: A comparative analysis. Thorax 1991; 46(1):33–38.

69. Brody AR. The early pathogenesis of asbestos-induced lung disease. Scan Electron Microsc 1984; (Pt 1):167–171.

70. Bach PB, Jett JR, Pastorino U, et al. Computed tomography screening and lung cancer outcomes. JAMA 2007; 297(9):953–961.

71. Markowitz AJ, McPhee SJ. Amyotrophic lateral sclerosis: "Prepare for the worst and hope for the best" (corrected). JAMA 2007; 298(10):1208.

72. Tossavainen A. International expert meeting on new advances in the radiology and screening of asbestos-related diseases. Scand J Work Environ Health 2000; 26(5):449–454.

73. Humphrey LL, Teutsch S, Johnson M. Lung cancer screening with sputum cytologic examination, chest radiography, and computed tomography: An update for the U.S. Preventive Services Task Force. Ann Intern Med 2004; 140(9):740–753.

74. Epler GR, McLoud TC, Gaensler EA. Prevalence and incidence of benign asbestos pleural effusion in a working population. JAMA 1982; 247(5):617–622.

75. Fridriksson HV, Hendenström H, Hillerdal G, et al. Increased lung stiffness of persons with pleural plaques. Eur J Respir Dis 1981; 62(6):412–424.

76. Lilis R, Lerman Y, Selikoff IJ. Symptomatic benign pleural effusions among asbestos insulation workers: Residual radiographic abnormalities. Br J Ind Med 1988; 45(7):443–449.
77. McLoud TC, Woods BO, Carrington CB, et al. Diffuse pleural thickening in an asbestos-exposed population: Prevalence and causes. AJR Am J Roentgenol 1985; 144(1):9–18.
78. Hillerdal G, Lee J, Blomkvist A, et al. Pleural disease during treatment with bromocriptine in patients previously exposed to asbestos. Eur Respir J 1997; 10(12):2711–2715.
79. Hillerdal G. Non-malignant asbestos pleural disease. Thorax 1981; 36(9):669–675.
80. de Klerk NH, Cookson WO, Musk AW, et al. Natural history of pleural thickening after exposure to crocidolite. Br J Ind Med 1989; 46(7):461–417.
81. Gibbs AR, Pooley FD. Analysis and interpretation of inorganic mineral particles in "lung" tissues. Thorax 1996; 51(3):327–334.
82. Gibbs AR, Stephens M, Griffiths DM, et al. Fibre distribution in the lungs and pleura of subjects with asbestos related diffuse pleural fibrosis. Br J Ind Med 1991; 48(11):762–770.
83. Rudd RM. New developments in asbestos-related pleural disease. Thorax 1996; 51(2):210–216.
84. Voisin C, Fisekci F, Voisin-Saltiel S, et al. Asbestos-related rounded atelectasis. Radiologic and mineralogic data in 23 cases. Chest 1995; 107(2):477–481.
85. Yates DH, Browne K, Stidolph PN, et al. Asbestos-related bilateral diffuse pleural thickening: Natural history of radiographic and lung function abnormalities. Am J Respir Crit Care Med 1996; 153(1):301–306.
86. Miller A. Chronic pleuritic pain in four patients with asbestos induced pleural fibrosis. Br J Ind Med 1990; 47(3):147–153.
87. Mukherjee S, de Klerk N, Palmer LJ, et al. Chest pain in asbestos-exposed individuals with benign pleural and parenchymal disease. Am J Respir Crit Care Med 2000; 162(5):1807–1811.
88. al Jarad N, Davies SW, Logan-Sinclair R, et al. Lung crackle characteristics in patients with asbestosis, asbestos-related pleural disease and left ventricular failure using a time-expanded waveform analysis—A comparative study. Respir Med 1994; 88(1):37–46.
89. Peacock C, Copley SJ, Hansell DM. Asbestos-related benign pleural disease. Clin Radiol 2000; 55(6):422–432.
90. Lynch DA, Gamsu G, Aberle DR. Conventional and high resolution computed tomography in the diagnosis of asbestos-related diseases. Radiographics 1989; 9(3):523–551.
91. Shih JF, Wilson JS, Broderick A, et al. Asbestos-induced pleural fibrosis and impaired exercise physiology. Chest 1994; 105(5):1370–1376.
92. Kee ST, Gamsu G, Blanc P. Causes of pulmonary impairment in asbestos-exposed individuals with diffuse pleural thickening. Am J Respir Crit Care Med 1996; 154(3 Pt 1):789–793.
93. al Jarad N, Poulakis N, Pearson MC, et al. Assessment of asbestos-induced pleural disease by computed tomography—Correlation with chest radiograph and lung function. Respir Med 1991; 85(3):203–208.
94. Schwartz DA, Galvin JR, Yagla SJ, et al. Restrictive lung function and asbestos-induced pleural fibrosis. A quantitative approach. J Clin Invest 1993; 91(6):2685–2692.
95. Wright PH, Hanson A, Kreel L, et al. Respiratory function changes after asbestos pleurisy. Thorax 1980; 35(1):31–36.
96. Collins TF. Pleural reaction associated with asbestos exposure. Br J Radiol 1968; 41(489):655–661.
97. Eisenstadt HB. Pleural asbestosis. Am Pract Dig Treat 1962; 13:573–578.
98. Eisenstadt HB. Benign asbestos pleurisy. JAMA 1965; 192:419–421.
99. Gaensler EA, Kaplan AI. Asbestos pleural effusion. Ann Intern Med 1971; 74(2):178–191.
100. Elder J. A study of 16 cases of pleurisy with effusions in ex-miners from Wittenoom Gorge. Aust NZ J Med 1972; 2:328–329.

101. Mattson SB, Ringqvist T. Pleural plaques and exposure to asbestos. A clinical material from a Swedish lung clinic. Scand J Respir Dis Suppl 1970; 75:1–41.
102. Sluis-Cremer GK, Webster I. Acute pleurisy in asbestos exposed persons. Environ Res 1972; 5(4):380–392.
103. Bignon J, Jaurand M, Sebastien P, et al. Interaction of pleural tissue and cells with mineral fibers. Diseases of the Pleural. New York, New York: Masson, 1983:198–207.
104. Morgan A, Evans J, Holmes A. Deposition and clearance of inhaled fibrous materials in the rat: Studies using radioactive tracer techniques. In: Walton W, ed. Inhaled Particles, Vol. IV. Oxford, U.K.: Pergamon Press, 1977:259–274.
105. Sebastien P, Fondimare A, Bignon J, et al. Topographic distribution of asbestos fibres in human lung in relation to occupational and non-occupational exposure. Inhaled Part 1975; 4(Pt 2):435–446.
106. Sebastien P, Janson X, Gaudichet A, et al. Asbestos retention in human respiratory tissues: Comparative measurements in lung parenchyma and in parietal pleura. IARC Sci Publ 1980; (30):237–246.
107. Wang NS. The preformed stomas connecting the pleural cavity and the lymphatics in the parietal pleura. Am Rev Respir Dis 1975; 111(1):12–20.
108. Bignon J, Sebastien P, Gaudichet A. Measurement of Asbestos Retention in the Human Respiratory System Related to Health Effects. Gaithersburg, MD: National Bureau of Standards (Special Publication), 1978:95–119.
109. Suzuki Y, Kohyama N. Translocation of inhaled asbestos fibers from the lung to other tissues. Am J Ind Med 1991; 19(6):701–704.
110. Schwartz DA. New developments in asbestos-induced pleural disease. Chest 1991; 99(1):191–198.
111. Rom WN, Travis WD, Brody AR. Cellular and molecular basis of the asbestos-related diseases. Am Rev Respir Dis 1991; 143(2):408–422.
112. Martensson G, Hagberg S, Pettersson K, et al. Asbestos pleural effusion: A clinical entity. Thorax 1987; 42(9):646–651.
113. Mintzer RA, Cugell DW. The association of asbestos-induced pleural disease and rounded atelectasis. Chest 1982; 81(4):457–460.
114. Roche G, Parent J, Daumet P. Subdivided atelectasis of the lower lobe and the middle lobe during therapeutic pneumothorax. Rev Tuberc 1956; 20(1–2):87–94.
115. Blesovsky A. The folded lung. Br J Dis Chest 1966; 60(1):19–22.
116. Dernevik L, Gatzinsky P. Pathogenesis of shrinking pleuritis with atelectasis—"Rounded atelectasis". Eur J Respir Dis 1987; 71(4):244–249.
117. Doyle TC, Lawler GA. CT features of rounded atelectasis of the lung. AJR Am J Roentgenol 1984; 143(2):225–228.
118. Hillerdal G. Rounded atelectasis. Clinical experience with 74 patients. Chest 1989; 95(4):836–841.
119. Mintzer RA, Gore RM, Vogelzang RL, et al. Rounded atelectasis and its association with asbestos-induced pleural disease. Radiology 1981; 139(3):567–570.
120. Payne CR, Jaques P, Kerr IH. Lung folding simulating peripheral pulmonary neoplasm (Blesovsky's syndrome). Thorax 1980; 35(12):936–940.
121. Schneider HJ, Felson B, Gonzalez LL. Rounded atelectasis. AJR Am J Roentgenol 1980; 134(2):225–232.
122. Stark P. Round atelectasis: Another pulmonary pseudotumor. Am Rev Respir Dis 1982; 125(2):248–250.
123. Szydlowski GW, Cohn HE, Steiner RM, et al. Rounded atelectasis: A pulmonary pseudotumor. Ann Thorac Surg 1992; 53(5): 817–821.
124. Hanke R. Rundatelektasen (Kugel- und Walzenatelektasen): ein Beitrag zur. Differential Diagnose intrapulmonaler Rundherde. ROEFO 1971; 114:164–183.

125. Hanke R, Kretzschmar R. Round atelectasis. Semin Roentgenol 1980; 15(2):174–182.
126. McHugh K, Blaquiere RM. CT features of rounded atelectasis. AJR Am J Roentgenol 1989;
      153(2):257–260.
127. Chen CH, Newman L. Rounded atelectasis complicated by obstructive pneumonia and pul-
      monary arterial thrombosis. Chest 1990; 98(5):1283–1285.
128. Greyson-Fleg RT. Lung biopsy in rounded atelectasis. AJR Am J Roentgenol 1985;
      144(6):1316–1317.

30
Pleural Manifestations of Interstitial Lung Disease

ROBERT P. BAUGHMAN
University of Cincinnati, Cincinnati, Ohio, U.S.A.

I. Introduction

There are a wide variety of interstitial lung diseases (ILD) including occupational interstitial diseases, infectious, collagen vascular, and unknown category. The collagen vascular
diseases, especially systemic lupus erythematosus (SLE), often include pleural disease and
will be discussed elsewhere in this book. Occupational lung diseases, such as asbestos-
related pleural disease, will not be discussed in this chapter. We will concentrate on
pleural diseases related to idiopathic diseases, such as sarcoidosis and Langerhans' cell
histiocytosis (LCH).

With a few exceptions such as asbestosis and SLE, pleural disease is usually a
rare manifestation of an ILD. Pleural manifestations of ILD could include pleural effusions, chylothorax, hemothorax, pleural thickening, pneumothorax, and pleural nodules
or plaques. High-resolution computed tomography (HRCT) is a commonly used method
to evaluate most ILD. This technique may detect subtle pleural manifestations not appreciated on plain chest roentgenogram. For example, subpleural nodules are commonly
seen on HRCT of patients with sarcoidosis (1), but pleural disease is rarely seen with
conventional roentgenograms for sarcoidosis (2,3). Subpleural nodules on HRCT suggest
sarcoidosis rather than other ILD (1). We will discuss the most commonly encountered
pleural manifestations, with a particular emphasis on pleural effusions.

The most common reason for pleural effusion in a patient with ILD is some other
process. Table 1 lists some of the commonly encountered secondary causes of pleural
disease. Congestive heart failure may be related to the underlying disease. An example
is sarcoidosis in which some patients may have a cardiomyopathy due to direct heart
involvement (4). The mean age of patients with idiopathic pulmonary fibrosis (IPF) in
most of the series is more than 60 years (5). Coexisting coronary artery disease may be
encountered, and patients may thus have congestive heart failure. In addition to congestive
heart failure, IPF patients appear to be at increased risk for pulmonary emboli (6). This is
in part due to the pulmonary hypertension the patients may develop, as well as the more
sedentary lifestyle they adapt as a result of their severe dyspnea. Pulmonary hypertension
is also a consequence of advance sarcoidosis (7,8). The use of immunosuppressive therapy
of treatment of sarcoidosis and IPF is common (5,9). This is often a prolonged therapy,
and the patient is at risk for acquiring an opportunistic infection either directly in the
pleura or as a parapneumonic infection (10). Drug-induced pleural effusion may also
be encountered (11). Among these is the docetaxel-associated effusion in patients being
treated for lymphangitic spread of their breast cancer (12).

Table 1 Secondary Causes of Pleural Effusion in Interstitial Lung Diseases

Cause of effusion	Common associations	Comments
Congestive heart failure	Sarcoidosis with cardiac involvement idiopathic pulmonary fibrosis (IPF)	Coexisting coronary artery disease may lead to CHF. Echocardiogram useful to assess left ventricular performance
Parapneumonic effusion	IPF on immunosuppression	Patients receiving chemotherapy may develop complicated pneumonic process
Pulmonary embolism	IPF	Increased risk for patients with cor pulmonale
Malignancy	IPF	Need to differentiate from lymphangitic spread as cause of interstitial lung disease
Drug induced	IPF Lymphangitic spread from cancer	Drug-induced lupus Docetaxel-associated effusion

Some patients with ILD are at increased risk for malignancy. The increased risk of malignancy for patients with IPF was recognized by Turner-Warwick et al. (13). Subsequent studies have confirmed an increased risk for malignancy in these patients (14–16). These are mostly lung cancers (16), usually adenocarcinomas, and they have a peripheral distribution.

In patients with known IPF, the presence of a new pleural effusion should be evaluated. A secondary cause may be identified. In some cases, the secondary cause may be more treatable than the underlying IPF. Treatment of the secondary cause may lead to improvement of symptoms.

II. New Onset of ILD and Pleural Effusion

For many ILD, the mode of onset is gradual. This is particularly true for IPF (5). Detailed questioning of a patient with ILD should be performed to determine if there has been a gradual onset of symptoms over weeks to months. The abrupt onset of pulmonary symptoms and a chest roentgenogram showing both ILD and pleural disease is unusual. It may represent an acute exacerbation of IPF (17). Specific criteria for this diagnosis have been proposed (18). The evaluation of acute decompensation requires excluding infection and malignancy.

In patients with acute ILD and pleural effusion, infection is a major possibility. This includes bacterial pneumonias, such as *Legionella* and even *Streptococcus pneumoniae*. Viral pneumonia can also present this way. Opportunistic infections such as fungi and tuberculosis can cause both effusions and ILD. *Pneumocystis jiroveci* rarely causes pleural fluid, but it can cause pneumothoraces (19). Most infections are suggested on the basis of clinical grounds. The diagnosis of infection-associated pleural effusions is discussed elsewhere in this book.

Malignancy represents another group presenting with acute ILD with pleural effusions. With the exception of a mesothelioma, the presence of malignant cells in the pleural space implies metastases. An interstitial process in the lung can be seen with bronchioloalveolar cell carcinoma (20,21) or with a "pseudolymphoma" due to B-cell proliferation on the MALT tissue (22). Rarely will either of these processes lead to pleural disease. On the other hand, lymphangitic spread of tumor can lead to an interstitial pattern (23,24). Common malignancies causing lymphangitic spread are lung and breast. In one study of patients with lymphangitic breast cancer, pleural effusion preceded or coexisted with the lymphangitic spread in two-thirds of the cases (25). The HRCT scan can be highly suggestive of lymphangitic spread (24). Figure 1 shows a patient with both lymphangitic spread and pleural metastases due to breast cancer. Both bronchoscopy and thoracocentesis were diagnostic in this case.

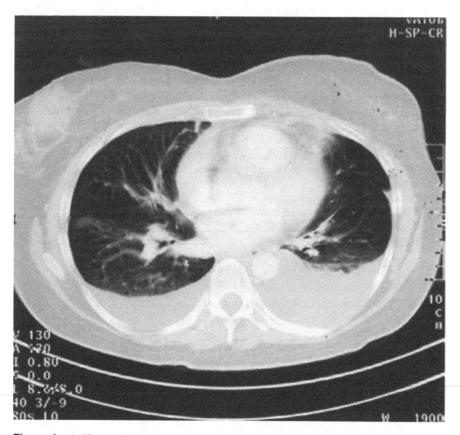

Figure 1 A 47-year-old female with a history of breast cancer who presents with increasing shortness of breath. Chest CT scan demonstrates both ILD and bilateral effusions. Samples obtained by bronchoalveolar lavage and thoracocentesis were both positive for adenocarcinoma consistent with metastatic breast cancer.

III. Chronic ILD of Unknown Cause

When a patient first presents with ILD, the clinician may not be able to determine whether the disease is chronic or not. Therefore, some of the diseases that we classify here may have been present for some time but present as acute disease. Time often clarifies whether a particular disease is chronic or not.

A. Sarcoidosis

Sarcoidosis is a disease characterized by noncaseating granulomas in various organs of the body (26). Traditionally, pleural involvement in sarcoidosis was felt to occur in about 1% to 3% of cases (3,27,28). The use of HRCT has pointed out that subpleural nodules can be seen in sarcoidosis, as well as other ILD such as pneumoconiosis and lymphangitic spread (1). The subpleural nodules have been seen in at least half of the patients reported (1,29). Patients with necrotizing sarcoidosis often have pleural effusions (30). In one series of patients with necrotizing sarcoidosis, pleural involvement was found on CT scan in 6 of 7 cases (31).

In a pair of reviews summarizing the literature of pleural sarcoidosis, Soskel and Sharma have made several observations based on the reported cases (3,27). Figure 2 demonstrates the type of pleural involvement one can see, as well as the underlying lung disease. In this figure, we use Scadding's classification of sarcoidosis lung involvement: Stage 0 is no thoracic disease, Stage 1 is hilar and mediastinal adenopathy alone, Stage 2 is adenopathy plus ILD, Stage 3 is ILD alone, and Stage 4 is fibrotic lung disease (32). Although pleural disease can be seen with any stage of the disease, patients tended to have more advanced disease when they had pleural involvement, although effusions can be found in patients with limited parenchymal lung disease (33). Figure 3 is an example of a patient with pleural disease due to sarcoidosis with Stage 3—parenchymal involvement without adenopathy.

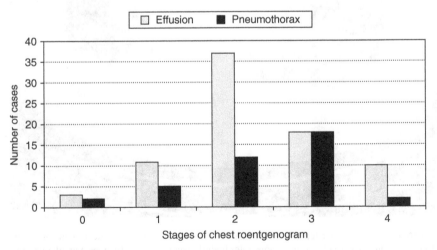

Figure 2 Number of cases of pleural effusion and pneumothorax versus Scadding chest roentgenogram stage (32) in patients with sarcoidosis. *Sources*: Adapted from Refs. 3, 27.

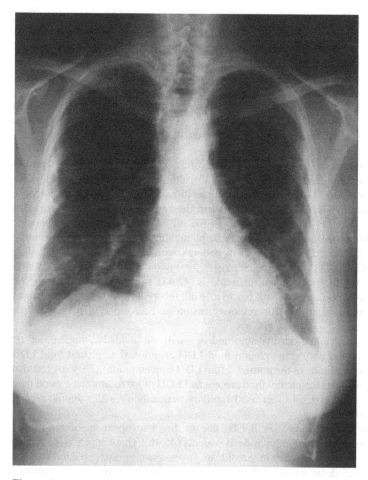

Figure 3 A 51-year-old woman who presented with diffuse lung and pleural disease. Open-lung biopsy demonstrated granulomas in both lung and pleural space, consistent with sarcoidosis.

The incidence of clinically significant pleural effusion for sarcoidosis patients was less than 3% in one prospective study of 181 sarcoidosis patients (33). Two of the cases were left side; three were bilateral. Of the five cases, two were due to congestive heart failure. There seemed to be an association with stage 2 disease by chest roentgenogram stage.

CT scanning may detect pleural disease more frequently. In a study of 61 consecutive sarcoidosis patients undergoing CT scan at one institution (2), 40% had evidence of pleural disease by CT scan, compared to only 11% by conventional chest roentgenogram. Of the 25 cases detected by CT, 20 were pleural thickening and only 5 were effusions. The presence of pleural disease was associated with parenchymal fibrosis and reduced lung volumes on pulmonary function tests.

The reported average age for patients with pleural effusion was found to be 40 years (27). This is not different from the average age found in other large series of sarcoidosis patients (34). The effusions seem to be more common on the right, but are often bilateral (33). Despite the apparently higher prevalence of sarcoidosis in women (34), the number of cases of effusions are often reported as frequently in men as women. It remains to be seen if gender has any affect on pleural involvement in large prospective studies. The pleural effusions are usually described as small to moderate in size. There have been reports of massive effusions (27,35,36). These cases often require chest tube drainage and may require systemic therapy for the sarcoidosis. Pleural fluid has also been reported with pericardial effusion (37).

If the sarcoidosis is the direct cause of the effusion, the fluid is characteristically exudative with a predominance of lymphocytes (33), although increased eosinophils have been occasionally noted (27,38). As in other areas in which there is active sarcoidosis, such as in the bronchoalveolar lavage (BAL) and the cerebral spinal fluid, there is an increase in the CD4:CD8 lymphocyte ratio in the effusion (39,40). This lymphocyte subpopulation found in pleural fluid may indicate pleural histological involvement similar to the lymphocytosis seen in BAL fluid in patients with alveolitis (41). The finding of an increased CD4:CD8 ratio is characteristic for sarcoidosis, but can be seen with other granulomatous diseases, such as tuberculosis (42,43). In patients with lymphocytic effusion of unknown etiology, one still has to rule out tuberculosis and fungal infections even if granulomas are identified. Tuberculous effusion has been reported in a sarcoidosis patient (44).

Huggins et al. pointed out that the fluid is usually in exudative range based on the protein content and not on the pleural fluid LDH criterion (i.e., pleural fluid LDH compared to the upper limits of the normal serum LDH concentration). They suggest that the dysynchrony between the pleural fluid protein and LDH ratios means that pleural fluid in sarcoidosis patients is due to increased capillary permeability with minimal pleural space inflammation (33).

In addition, the effusion may not be due to direct involvement of the pleura. Chylothorax has been reported in sarcoidosis patients (45,46). These appear to be related to mediastinal adenopathy common in sarcoidosis. In one case, a massive pleural effusion associated with sarcoidosis was secondary to brachiocephalic vein obstruction by matted sarcoidosis infiltration in mediastinal lymph nodes (47). Another cause of the pleural effusion is hemothorax, which is rare (27,48).

The prevalence of pneumothorax in sarcoid patients appears to be less than 5% (27), however, it can lead to significant respiratory distress (49). The proposed mechanism of pneumothorax development is unclear, but at least two conditions have been associated with pneumothorax. The first is related to the subpleural necrotizing granulomas mentioned earlier. In some cases, recurrent pneumothoraces was related to the presence of necrotizing granuloma in resected pleural samples (50,51). Another mechanism is the cystic changes commonly found in patients with advanced pulmonary sarcoidosis (Fig. 4). However, patients with advanced fibrotic disease often have associated pleural reaction, as seen in Figure 4. There may be a lower risk for pneumothorax than those seen in other cystic ILD. It is unclear whether systemic treatment will decrease the recurrence of spontaneous lung collapse. Most of the cases require systemic therapy for the treatment of their underlying lung disease. Many cases of pneumothorax from sarcoidosis respond to chest tube alone (27,52). Surgery is usually only necessary when the underlying diagnosis

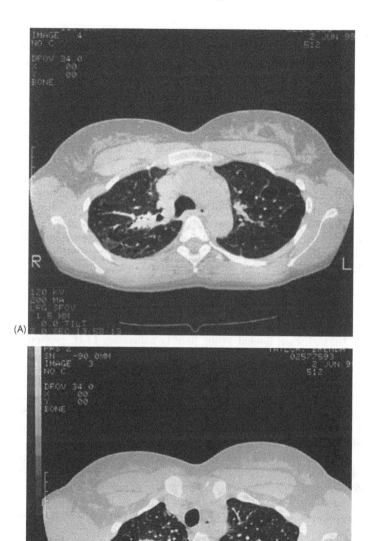

Figure 4 Patient with a 12-year history of sarcoidosis presented with chest pain and hemoptysis. Multiple cystic changes in upper lobe, including mycetoma and pleural reaction on right. Culture of bronchial washings grew *Aspergillus niger*.

is unclear, but has been reported in patients who presented with bilateral pneumothoraces (53). This is different from other ILD, where surgery is often required to assure adequate sclerosis (27). This may be related to the high frequency of granulomatous inflammation present in the pleura, leading to an inflammatory reaction and sclerosis with chest tube drainage.

As illustrated by Figure 4, aspergillomas and locally invasive *Aspergillus* can occur in sarcoidosis (54,55). A pleural reaction is often associated with an aspergilloma (56). Although surgery is done in patients with recurrent pneumothoraces (57), most patients are managed medically. Itraconazole, an azole agent with high activity against *Aspergillus*, has been used with success in some cases (58–60), but not always found useful (61). Voriconazole has been used successfully in one case of itraconazole resistant *Aspergillus fumigatus* causing an aspergilloma (62). The inflammatory reaction to an aspergilloma can contribute to the hemoptysis as well as bronchospasm, and some patients with symptomatic aspergillomas have been treated successfully with corticosteroids (63,64). Current treatment by our group consists of prolonged use of itraconazole and an anti-inflammatory agent such as corticosteroids or methotrexate. Others prefer percutaneous instillation of amphotericin B when possible (60).

B. Langerhans' Cell Histiocytosis

LCH is a spectrum of diseases characterized by Langerhans' cells infiltrating various organs of the body (65). Disease limited to the lung is pulmonary LCH, previously known as eosinophilic granuloma (EG) (66–69). Pulmonary LCH is a smoking-related ILD (70), but systemic LCH can present with pneumothoraces in early childhood (71,72). Pleural manifestations of the disease include pleural effusion, pneumothorax, and pleural thickening (68). The pleural thickening is thought to be the result of a pneumothorax. Spontaneous pneumothorax has long been recognized as an initial presentation of this disorder as well as longstanding disease, with the incidence reported between 4% and 25% (66,69,73–75). Bilateral pneumothoraces in LCH have also been reported. Because of this association, pulmonary LCH should be considered in any young adult smoker who develops a pneumothorax (69). The pathogenesis of spontaneous pneumothorax in LCH may be related to rupturing of subpleural blebs and cysts (69,73). Figure 5 is an example of the honeycombing that can be seen in this condition. In that case, there is associated ground glass from respiratory bronchiolitis, another smoking related ILD (76), that coexisted in this patient. In some cases, end-stage honeycombing may be the cause of the pneumothorax (77).

In a retrospective review of 102 cases of pulmonary LCH seen at one institution (78), 16 (16%) had pneumothorax. Of the 37 total episodes of pneumothoraces (1–5 episodes per patient), 10 patients had more than one episode, often of the opposite side. However, management with observation alone was associated with a recurrence rate for pneumothoraces of 58% to the ipsilateral side compared to 0% after surgical management with pleurodesis. Others have reported that surgical intervention with sclerosis is often required (79,80). Unfortunately reports of recurrent pneumothorax have been noted even following pleurodesis (79).

There is no specific therapy for LCH itself. The discontinuation of smoking is associated with remission in some cases (81,82), while those who continue to smoke may go on to respiratory failure from the disease. Recurrence of LCH into donor lung of

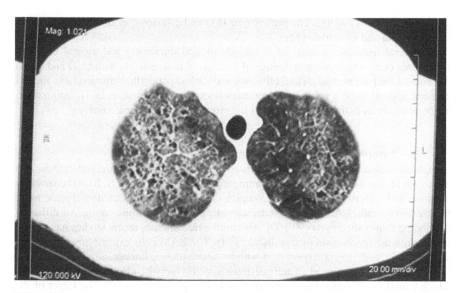

Figure 5 A 48-year-old Caucasian female with history of increasing dyspnea. Patient was a heavy smoker. CT scan revealed diffuse cystic changes as well as ground glass changes.

lung-transplanted patients has been reported in two patients who resumed smoking after transplant (83). The presence of pneumothoraces does not seem to change the overall mortality from pulmonary LCH (78).

Pleural effusions have also been reported in LCH (84,85); however, this is a much less-common manifestation, and the size of the effusion is usually small. In a patient with cystic ILD, the presence of pleural effusion is more characteristic for Erdheim–Chester disease (ECD), sarcoidosis, or lymphangioleiomyomatosis. For those with cystic disease, one also has to consider Birt–Hogg–Dube (BHD) syndrome, a rare inherited genodermatosis characterized by distinctive cutaneous lesions, an increased risk of renal and colonic neoplasia, and the development of pleuropulmonary blebs and cysts but not effusion (86). In a patient with LCH, the presence of a moderate to large effusion should raise the concern of a secondary cause of the effusion, such as malignancy.

C. Erdheim–Chester Disease

ECD is a rare multisystem non-LCH disorder of unknown etiology that occurs in adults. Manifestations include ILD, bone pain, xanthelasma, exophthalmos, and diabetes insipidus. About one-third of patients have pulmonary involvement (87,88). ECD does not have defined criteria and therefore can be difficult to distinguish from LCH, and there has been one report of both occurring in the same patient (89). One difference is the distribution of histiocytic cells in the lung. In ECD, the histiocytes accumulate in the perilymphangitic and subpleural areas. In LCH, histiocytes accumulate in peribronchial distribution (87). Immunohistochemistry identifying the Langerhans' cells (which are CD1 a positive) is also useful, since there are no Langerhans' cells in the ECD lesions (89). The clinical course of the disease is variable, but pulmonary fibrosis is often reported as a cause of death (90,91). The presence of ILD and effusion can also be mistaken for mesothelioma and asbestosis (92).

Pleural manifestations of ECD include pleural thickening and pleural effusion. Wittenberg et al. reviewed the radiological findings of nine patients with ECD and found that four of the patients had pleural effusions and six had pericardial effusion (93). Pleural effusion appears to be a much more common finding in ECD than in LCH. Information is not available as to the characteristic of the effusion or the possible etiology.

D. Lymphangioleiomyomatosis

Lymphangioleiomyomatosis (LAM), formerly known as lymphangiomyomyotosis, is a multisystem disease primarily seen in premenopausal females (94–97). It can be sporadic or associated with tuberous sclerosis complex (TSC) (98), with pulmonary disease more common in sporadic LAM (99). The characteristic pulmonary manifestations are diffusely distributed thin-walled cysts (99,100). Although a rare disease, recent studies have given insight into the mechanism of this disease (94). The LAM cells express smooth muscle actin, desmin, and vimentin consistent with a smooth muscle lineage, although also have features that are not typical of normal muscle cells, namely, electron-dense granules, which contain melanoma-related proteins including glycoprotein 100 (the target of the antibody human melanoma black (HMB)45) and tyrosinase (101), angiotensin-1 converting enzyme (102), and receptors for estrogen and progesterone (103). The abnormal cells appear to be smooth muscle cells which are under some level of estrogen control (94). The close association between tuberous sclerosis and LAM has been supported by the finding of pulmonary LAM in a man with tuberous sclerosis (104). Furthermore, mutations in the tuberous sclerosis complex gene TSC2 have been found in sporadic cases of LAM (105).

Spontaneous pneumothorax is a common presentation in patients with LAM (106,107). The LAM registry examined the completed questionnaires of 395 patients (108). Two-thirds of the patient reported at least one pneumothorax during their lifetime, and over 75% of these had subsequent pneumothoraces. The pneumothoraces can be bilateral (108,109). Patients often require pleurodesis or pleurectomy for management of pneumothoraces (94,107). In one retrospective study, the outcome of 301 initial pneumothoraces, half were treated with either simple aspiration or tube thoracostomy, while the rest were managed surgically or with chemical pleurodesis. Recurrence occurred in 66% of the conservative treatment group, but only 27% of the chemical (27%) and 32% of the surgical (32%) pleurodesis ($p < 0.01$ for both compared to that of conservative treatment) (108).

The mechanism of pneumothorax in LAM is again the rupture of subpleural cavities. In LAM, the appearance of subpleural cystic and micronodular hyperplasia is fairly characteristic (Fig. 6). CT scan is therefore useful for suggesting LAM as the cause of spontaneous pneumothorax. Spontaneous pneumothorax was the initial presentation of 86% of LAM patients in one series (96). CT can also be used to screen for LAM in at risk groups, such as those with tuberous sclerosis (98,105).

Chylothorax is seen in approximately 20% of patients with LAM (106,107, 109,110). One large series found that 8 of 79 (10%) of LAM patients eventually developed chylous effusions (110). Of the eight cases, two were had bilateral effusions and three each had fluid on right or left. Chylous effusion may be the presenting symptom of the

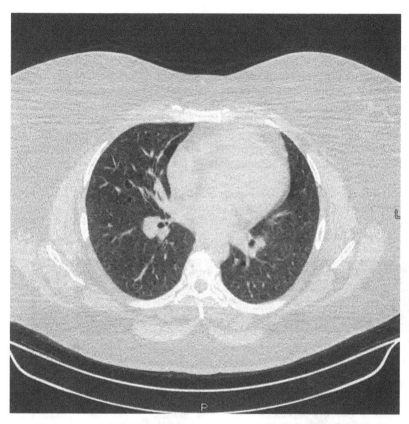

Figure 6 A 37-year-old Caucasian female presented with a spontaneous pneumothorax. No specific cause was identified. One year later, she presented with increasing dyspnea and chest pain. CT scan showed multiple thin walled cysts. Subsequent open-lung biopsy confirmed the diagnosis of lymphangiomyomatosis (LAM).

disease (111). The proposed mechanism is lymphatic obstruction by the LAM cells, and the diagnosis of LAM can be confirmed by cytologic or immunologic examination of the fluid (112,113). More than half of the patients with chylous effusions required pleurodesis or pleurectomy for treatment (94,110). There has been a report of percutaneous catheterization and subsequent embolization to successfully treat chylothorax due to LAM and other conditions (114). A pleurovenous shunt has also been successfully used to control a refractory chylothorax in a LAM patient (115). Chylothorax has also been reported in a male patient with tuberous sclerosis (116).

LAM is usually a disease of women, although it has very rarely been reported in men in association with tuberous sclerosis (104,116). There is a single case report of spontaneous LAM in a male (117). For years, it has been appreciated that LAM progresses in premenopausal women and especially during pregnancy (97,109). Antiestrogen regimens have been used with limited success in patients with LAM (118–120).

One difficulty is the relatively small number of cases and the unpredictable progression of the disease (118,120). However, estrogen alone is not the cause of LAM. Up to 10% of female patients with LAM were diagnosed postmenopause (97). For end-stage disease, lung transplantation has been a successful in some patients (121). A recent study of sirolimus for tuberous sclerosis found that the pulmonary LAM responded in some cases to this therapy (97). A randomized trial of sirolimus for LAM is underway. Doxycycline, a matrix metalloproteinase inhibitor, may also have a role in treating LAM (122).

Benign metastasizing lymphangiomyomatosis (LAM) is another interstitial process that affects the lungs in premenopausal females. It can lead to interstitial changes, parenchymal nodules, and recurrent pneumothorax (Fig. 7) (123–125). Although the clinical features of the patient are similar to those of LAM, there are not as many cystic changes on CT scan as are seen with LAM, and it is felt to represent a slow-growing variant of leiomyosarcoma (126). The lesions are clearly hormone sensitive and respond to anti-estrogen regimens (123,127,128).

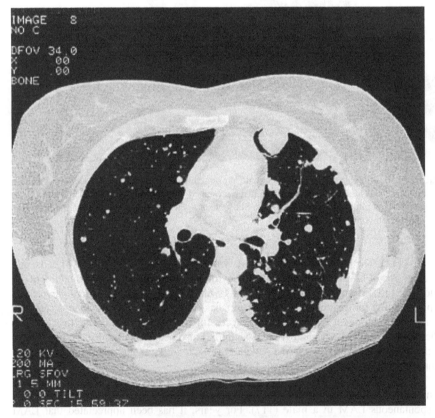

Figure 7 A 30-year-old woman with history of recurrent pneumothoraces. Lung biopsy at time of open pleural sclerosis demonstrated benign metastasizing lymphangiomyomatosis.

E. Churg–Strauss Syndrome

Churg–Strauss syndrome (CSS) is a systemic disease that occurs in patients with a history of asthma or allergies. The syndrome is characterized by vasculitis, extravascular granulomas, eosinophilia, and fever (129–131). The most common pulmonary manifestations of CSS are fleeting infiltrates; however, patients may also develop diffuse reticulonodular opacities and interlobular septal thickening (132–135). Pleural manifestations can include pleural thickening and pleural effusion in about a quarter of patients (134,136). The pleural effusions of CSS are exudative, with a large number of eosinophils and a low glucose (137,138). One patient also was noted to have vasculitis of the pleura on open-lung biopsy (134), another to have necrotizing granulomas (137). The effusion may occur initially or may occur when the disease relapses, as shown in Figure 8. The disease has been associated with the use of antileukotriene therapy (139,140) and the risk of CSS is estimated to be 4.5 times higher in asthmatics on this class of medications (141). However, it is not clear whether these drugs simply unmask an underlying vasculitis when corticosteroids are withdrawn in the chronic asthmatic (141). CSS can occur in patients not receiving those drugs (142). Therapy is usually corticosteroids, but occasionally cytotoxic agents are used (129,130,143).

F. Amyloidosis

Amyloidosis is a disease characterized by the deposition of abnormal protein in the extracellular tissues (144). The amyloid protein characteristically exhibits apple-green birefringence under polarized microscopy and takes up Congo red stain. Typically, it is categorized as primary or secondary. Secondary amyloid is often associated with neoplastic and chronic inflammatory conditions such as rheumatoid arthritis and bronchiectasis. Most often the disease affects multiple organs, but single organ involvement has been described.

Pulmonary amyloid can be isolated or can be a part of systemic amyloid involvement. Autopsy studies have shown that pulmonary involvement is common in primary systemic amyloidosis but not in secondary amyloidosis (145,146). In a Mayo Clinic review of 55 patients with pulmonary amyloid, ILD with or without pleural effusion was common for systemic amyloid but rare for secondary amyloid (147). Others have confirmed this observation (148).

The pleural effusion of amyloidosis can be either transudate or exudate (107–109). Transudative effusions may be secondary to congestive heart failure from cardiac involvement of amyloidosis. The exudative effusions in amyloid have yet to be explained. Nodularity along the pleura has been seen at thoracoscopy in patients with amyloid (110), with direct pleural involvement documented on biopsy (107,108,110). The pleural biopsy may be positive even if the fluid is a transudate (107). Pleural involvement does not always mean systemic amyloidosis (111).

In a detailed retrospective study of persistent pleural effusions in primary systemic amyloid, Berk et al. examined the role of cardiac dysfunction and nephritic syndrome as possible causes of the pleural effusion (149). Of the 636 amyloid patients followed in their clinic, 35 (6%) had persistent large effusions. One-third of the effusions were exudates, using standard criteria. Cadiomyopathy was often identified by echo in these patients, with 81% having right-ventricle abnormalities. When compared to a group of patients with cardiac sarcoidosis and no effusion, there was no difference in either right- or left-side

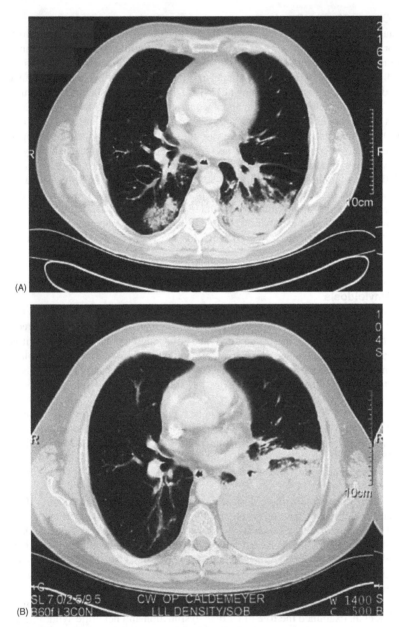

Figure 8 A 50-year-old male asthmatic with 3-month history of cough and shortness of breath noted to have multiple pulmonary infiltrates and peripheral blood eosinophilia. (**A**) Multiple infiltrates prior to open lung biopsy of the right lung lesions. Patient was found to have Churg–Strauss and was treated with corticosteroids. Six months later patient was down to low-dose corticosteroids when he developed worsening dyspnea. (**B**) New left pleural effusion and improvement of parenchymal disease. Examination of left pleural fluid demonstrated 50% eosinophils. The patient improved with increased dosage of corticosteroids.

dysfunction. Normal pulmonary capillary wedge pressure was found in 41% of the patients who had persistent effusions. The authors could not find a role for nephritic syndrome as a cause of most effusions. In fact, the authors identified 14 of the amyloid patients with serum albumin less than 2 g/dL and found that none had effusions. Hypothyroidism was identified in about 20% of the patients with amyloid, and there was no relation to the effusion. In all six cases in which pleural biopsies were performed, amyloid tissue was identified. The authors concluded that pleural effusions due to amyloid were often related to amyloid deposits in the pleural space.

The outcome of untreated pleural effusions from amyloid is poor (149). However, reports indicate that these patients can be treated with sclerosis (149,150).

Pleural thickening without effusion has also been described as a radiological manifestation. Adams et al. described two patients who presented with dyspnea and had diffuse pleural thickening on imaging and who were thought to have mesothelioma. After surgical decortication, the diagnosis of amyloid was made by special stains of the pleura (151).

G. Idiopathic Pulmonary Fibrosis

The ILD have been reclassified based on clinical status and pathological changes (5). A major task for the clinician is to differentiate between nonspecific ILD and usual interstitial pneumonitis (UIP) (152). The term UIP refers to the pathological changes seen. Patients with consistent clinical features and a lung biopsy showing UIP are felt to have IPF (5).

Pneumothorax is the most common pleural disease reported in IPF. In a study of 82 patients with pulmonary fibrosis, 3 (3.6%) of the 46 patients who meet the current criteria for IPF had a spontaneous pneumothorax (153). In addition, the authors found that these patients did not respond well to suction drainage and often required thoracotomy, bleb resection, and pleurectomy. In a retrospective study of the CT scans of 78 patients with UIP, 11% had extra-alveolar air, with 5 having a pneumothorax and 4 having a pneumomediastinum (154). Figure 9 shows a patient who originally presented with a spontaneous pneumothorax and was diagnosed as having UIP at the time of his open sclerosis. As shown in the figure, the probable mechanism of the pneumothorax is rupture of the subpleural honeycombing characteristic of IPF (155). Pneumothorax can be a reason for clinical deterioration and even death in patients with IPF (6).

Pleural thickening is also commonly seen with the subpleural honeycombing characteristic of IPF (156). In a study comparing the HRCT findings of IPF to collagen vascular disease–associated pulmonary fibrosis (CVD-PF), pleural thickening was the most distinguishing feature. Of those studied, 97% of patients with IPF had pleural thickening compared to 33% of the CVD-PF patients. Pleural effusion was seen in only 6% of the IPF patients, but in 26% of the CVD-PF patients (157).

IV. Clinical Evaluation of Pleural Disease in ILD

In evaluating the patient with an interstitial lung process and pleural disease, one needs to first decide whether there is a possible association between the two processes. In a patient with known ILD who has developed a new pleural effusion, one has to consider secondary causes of the pleural effusion, such as congestive heart failure or infection. Workup of these pleural effusions would be similar to what one would do for a patient with a clear chest roentgenogram and a new pleural effusion.

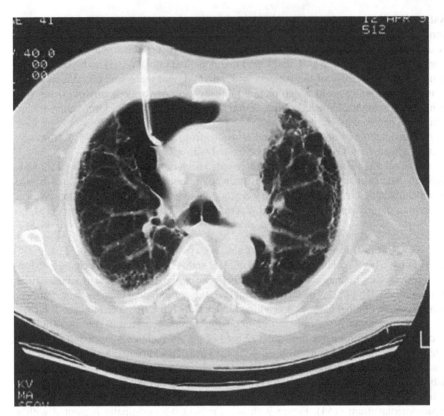

Figure 9 A 70-year-old male who presented with dyspnea and chest pain. Chest CT scan demonstrates pneumothorax as well as subpleural honeycombing consistent with idiopathic pulmonary fibrosis. Open-lung biopsy obtained at time of pleural sclerosis demonstrated usual interstitial pneumonitis.

In the patient who presents symptomatically with new effusion and ILD, one has to consider infection and congestive failure, since these are the most common and treatable conditions. In most cases, these diseases are easily determined based on the clinical evaluation of the patient. Malignancy can be a bit more obscure, but should always be considered as the cause of ILD and pleural effusion.

In the patient with a chronic interstitial lung infiltrate and pleural disease, the pattern of pleural disease may help to determine the underlying process. Table 2 summarizes the relative frequency of pleural effusion and pneumothorax for several ILD. Patients with cystic ILD such as LAM, LCH, and some with sarcoidosis can develop pneumothorax. The presence of a pleural effusion is more frequent in ECD, CSS, LAM; is unusual in sarcoidosis (33); and is extremely rare in LCH. The effusion in CSS usually contains a large number of eosinophils (138). The effusion associated with LAM is often chylous (107,110). In a patient with amyloidosis, the presence of a pleural effusion implies systemic amyloidosis (147).

Table 2 Summary of Pleural Manifestations of Interstitial Lung Diseases

ILD	Pleural effusion	Pneumothorax	Other pleural manifestations
Sarcoidosis	+1[a]	+1	Pleural thickening, nodules, lymphocytic effusion with increased CD4:CD8 ratio
Langerhans cell histiocytosis	Rare	+2	Pleural thickening
Lymphangioleiomyomatosis	+2	+3	Chylothorax common
Erdheim–Chester	+3	Rare	Pleural thickening
Churg–Strauss syndrome	+2	ND	Eosinophilic pleural effusion
Amyloidosis	+2	Rare	Effusion implies systemic amyloidosis
Idiopathic pulmonary fibrosis	Rare	+1	Pleural thickening on HRCT >90% of cases

ND: not described.
[a]Relative score of patients reported to have pleural manifestation: +3 = >40%; +2 = 10–30%; +1 = 1–10%; rare = <1%.

The use of HRCT as part of the routine evaluation of ILD has led to recognition of pleural disease not appreciated on routine chest roentgenogram. This includes the high incidence of subpleural nodules seen in patients with sarcoidosis (1) and the pleural thickening seen with IPF (157). As more attention is placed on pleural disease, more of these correlations will be made.

References

1. Remy-Jardin M, Beuscart R, Sault MC, et al. Subpleural micronodules in diffuse infiltrative lung diseases: Evaluation with thin-section CT scans. Radiology 1990; 177(1):133–139.
2. Szwarcberg JB, Glajchen N, Teirstein AS. Pleural involvement in chronic sarcoidosis detected by thoracic CT scanning. Sarcoidosis Vasc Diffuse Lung Dis 2005; 22(1):58–62.
3. Soskel NT, Sharma OP. Pleural involvement in sarcoidosis. Curr Opin Pulm Med 2000; 6(5):455–468.
4. Deng JC, Baughman RP, Lynch JPI. Cardiac involvement in sarcoidosis. Sem Resp Crit Care Med 2002; 23:513–528.
5. American Thoracic Society/European Respiratory Society International Multidisciplinary Consensus Classification of the Idiopathic Interstitial Pneumonias. Am J Respir Crit Care Med 2002; 165:277–304.
6. Panos RJ, Morrenson R, Niccoli SA, et al. Clinical deterioration in patients with idiopathic pulmonary fibrosis. Causes and assessment. Am J Med 1990; 88:396–404.
7. Baughman RP, Engel PJ, Meyer CA, et al. Pulmonary hypertension in sarcoidosis. Sarcoidosis Vasc Diffuse Lung Dis 2006; 23:108–116.
8. Sulica R, Teirstein AS, Kakarla S, et al. Distinctive clinical, radiographic, and functional characteristics of patients with sarcoidosis-related pulmonary hypertension. Chest 2005; 128(3):1483–1489.
9. Baughman RP, Lower EE. Novel therapies for sarcoidosis. Semin Respir Crit Care Med 2007; 28(1):128–133.
10. Baughman RP, Lower EE. Fungal infections as a complication of therapy for sarcoidosis. QJM 2005; 98:451–456.

11. Antony VB. Drug-induced pleural disease. Clin Chest Med 1998; 19(2):331–340.

12. Shapiro JD, Millward MJ, Rischin D, et al. Activity and toxicity of docetaxel (Taxotere) in women with previously treated metastatic breast cancer. Aus N Z J Med 1997; 27(Feb): 40–44.

13. Turner-Warwick M, Lebowitz M, Burrows B, et al. Cryptogenic fibrosing alveolitis and lung cancer. Thorax 1980; 35:496–499.

14. Lee HJ, Im JG, Ahn JM, et al. Lung cancer in patients with idiopathic pulmonary fibrosis: CT findings. J Comput Assist Tomogr 1996; 20(6):979–982.

15. Mizushima Y, Kobayashi M. Clinical characteristics of synchronous multiple lung cancer associated with idiopathic pulmonary fibrosis. A review of Japanese cases. Chest 1995; 108(5):1272–1277.

16. Le JI, Gribbin J, West J, et al. The incidence of cancer in patients with idiopathic pulmonary fibrosis and sarcoidosis in the UK. Respir Med 2007; 101(12):2534–2540.

17. Kim DS, Park JH, Park BK, et al. Acute exacerbation of idiopathic pulmonary fibrosis: Frequency and clinical features. Eur Respir J 2006; 27(1):143–150.

18. Collard HR, Moore BB, Flaherty KR, et al. Acute exacerbations of idiopathic pulmonary fibrosis. Am J Respir Crit Care Med 2007; 176(7):636–643.

19. Sepkowitz KA, Telzak EE, Gold JW, et al. Pneumothorax in aids. Ann Intern Med 1991; 114(6):455–459.

20. Adler B, Padley S, Miller RR, et al. High-resolution CT of bronchioloalveolar carcinoma. AJR Am J Roentgenol 1992; 159(2):275–277.

21. Greco RJ, Steiner RM, Goldman S, et al. Bronchoalveolar cell carcinoma of the lung. Ann Thorac Sur 1986; 41(Jun):652–656.

22. Mcculloch GL, Sinnatamby R, Stewart S, et al. High-resolution computed tomographic appearance of maltoma of the lung. Eur Radiol 1998; 8:1669–1673.

23. Honda O, Johkoh T, Ichikado K, et al. Comparison of high resolution CT findings of sarcoidosis, lymphoma, and lymphangitic carcinoma: Is there any difference of involved interstitium? J Comput Assist Tomogr 1999; 23(3):374–379.

24. Johkoh T, Ikezoe J, Tomiyama N, et al. CT findings in lymphangitic carcinomatosis of the lung: Correlation with histologic findings and pulmonary function tests. AJR Am J Roentgenol 1992; 158(6):1217–1222.

25. Lower EE, Baughman RP. Pulmonary lymphangitic metastasis from breast cancer. Lymphocytic alveolitis is associated with favorable prognosis. Chest 1992; 102(4):1113–1117.

26. Hunninghake GW, Costabel U, Ando M, et al. ATS/ERS/WASOG statement on sarcoidosis. American Thoracic Society/European Respiratory Society/World Association of Sarcoidosis and Other Granulomatous Disorders. Sarcoidosis Vasc Diffuse Lung Dis 1999; 16(Sep):149–173.

27. Soskel NT, Sharma OP. Pleural involvement in sarcoidosis: Case presentation and detailed review of the literature. Semin Resp Med 1992; 13:492–514.

28. Blackmon GM, Raghu G. Pulmonary sarcoidosis: A mimic of respiratory infection. Semin Respir Infect 1995; 10(3):176–186.

29. Nishimura K, Itoh H, Kitaichi M, et al. Pulmonary sarcoidosis: Correlation of CT and histopathologic findings. Radiology 1993; 189(1):105–109.

30. Harada T, Amano T, Takahashi A, et al. Necrotizing sarcoid granulomatosis presenting with elevated serum soluble interleukin-2 receptor levels. Respiration 2002; 69(5):468–470.

31. Chittock DR, Joseph MG, Paterson NA, et al. Necrotizing sarcoid granulomatosis with pleural involvement. Clinical and radiographic features. Chest 1994; 106(3):672–676.

32. Scadding JG. Prognosis of intrathoracic sarcoidosis in England. Br Med J 1961; 4:1165–1172.

33. Huggins JT, Doelken P, Sahn SA, et al. Pleural effusions in a series of 181 outpatients with sarcoidosis. Chest 2006; 129(6):1599–1604.

34. Baughman RP, Teirstein AS, Judson MA, et al. Clinical characteristics of patients in a case control study of sarcoidosis. Am J Respir Crit Care Med 2001; 164:1885–1889.
35. Carter AB, Hunninghake GW. Massive pleural effusion in diffuse granulomatous disease. Chest 1997; 112(1):284–288.
36. Claiborne RA, Kerby GR. Pleural sarcoidosis with massive effusion and lung entrapment. Kans Med 1990; 91(4):103–105.
37. Navaneethan SD, Venkatesh S, Shrivastava R, et al. Recurrent pleural and pericardial effusions due to sarcoidosis. Plos Med 2005; 2(3):E63.
38. Vafiadis E, Sidiropoulou MS, Voutsas V, et al. Eosinophilic pleural effusion, peripheral eosinophilia, pleural thickening, and hepatosplenomegaly in sarcoidosis. South Med J 2005; 98(12):1218–1222.
39. Groman GS, Castele RJ, Altose MD, et al. Lymphocyte subpopulations in sarcoid pleural effusions. Ann Intern Med 1984; 100:76.
40. Flammang D, Ortho MP, Cadranel J, et al. Pleural, alveolar and blood T-lymphocyte subsets in pleuropulmonary sarcoidosis. Chest 1990; 98(3):782–783.
41. Hunninghake GW, Crystal RG. Pulmonary sarcoidosis: A disorder mediated by excess helper T-lymphocyte activity at sites of disease activity. N Engl J Med 1981; 305: 429–432.
42. Hoheisel GB, Tabak L, Teschler H, et al. Bronchoalveolar lavage cytology and immuno-cytology in pulmonary tuberculosis. Am J Respir Crit Care Med 1994; 149(2 Pt 1):460–463.
43. Baughman RP. Sarcoidosis. Usual and unusual manifestations. Chest 1988; 94:165–170.
44. Yanardag H, Gunes Y. Occurrence of pleural effusion due to tuberculosis in patients with sarcoidosis. Indian J Chest Dis Allied Sci 2005; 47(1):9–11.
45. Parker JM, Torrington KG, Phillips YY. Sarcoidosis complicated by chylothorax. South Med J 1994; 87(8):860–862.
46. Jarman PR, Whyte MK, Sabroe I, et al. Sarcoidosis presenting with chylothorax. Thorax 1995; 50(12):1324–1325.
47. Javaheri S, Hales CA. Sarcoidosis: A cause of innominate vein obstruction and massive pleural effusion. Lung 1980; 157(2):81–85.
48. Watarai M, Yazawa M, Yamanda K, et al. Pulmonary sarcoidosis with associated bloody pleurisy. Intern Med 2002; 41(11):1021–1023.
49. Darquennes K, Van Den BM, Van Swieten HA, et al. A rare cause of spontaneous pneumoth-orax after lifesaving pneumonectomy in a patient with sarcoidosis. Sarcoidosis Vasc Diffuse Lung Dis 2007; 24(1):77–78.
50. Froudarakis ME, Bouros D, Voloudaki A, et al. Pneumothorax as a first manifestation of sarcoidosis. Chest 1997; 112(1):278–280.
51. Lake KB, Sharma OP, Vandyke JJ. Pneumothorax in sarcoidosis. Rev Interam Radiol 1978; 3(1):33–36.
52. Omori H, Asahi H, Irinoda T, et al. Pneumothorax as a presenting manifestation of early sarcoidosis. Jpn J Thorac Cardiovasc Surg 2004; 52(1):33–35.
53. Ayed AK. Bilateral video-assisted thoracoscopic surgery for bilateral spontaneous pneumoth-orax. Chest 2002; 122(6):2234–2237.
54. Wollschlager C, Khan F. Aspergillomas complicating sarcoidosis. A prospective study in 100 patients. Chest 1984; 86(4):585–588.
55. Waldhorn RE, Tsou E, Kerwin DM. Invasive pulmonary aspergillosis associated with aspergilloma in sarcoidosis. South Med J 1983; 76(2):251–253.
56. Franquet T, Muller NL, Gimenez A, et al. Spectrum of pulmonary aspergillosis: Histologic, clinical, and radiologic findings. Radiographics 2001; 21(4):825–837.
57. Wex P, Utta E, Drozdz W. Surgical treatment of pulmonary and pleuro-pulmonary aspergillus disease. Thorac Cardiovasc Surg 1993; 41(1):64–70.

58. Kawana A, Yamauchi Y, Kudo K. Anti-fungal chemotherapy for symptomatic pulmonary aspergilloma. Jpn J Infect Dis 2000; 53(1):29–30.
59. Stevens DA, Kan VL, Judson MA, et al. Practice guidelines for diseases caused by aspergillus. Infectious Diseases Society of America. Clin Infect Dis 2000; 30(4):696–709.
60. Judson MA, Stevens DA. The treatment of pulmonary aspergilloma. Curr Opin Investig Drugs 2001; 2(10):1375–1377.
61. Kawamura S, Maesaki S, Tomono K, et al. Clinical evaluation of 61 patients with pulmonary aspergilloma. Intern Med 2000; 39(3):209–212.
62. Dannaoui E, Garcia-Hermoso D, Naccache JM, et al. Use of voriconazole in a patient with aspergilloma caused by an itraconazole-resistant strain of *Aspergillus fumigatus*. J Med Microbiol 2006; 55(Pt 10):1457–1459.
63. Rosenberg IL, Greenberger PA. Allergic bronchopulmonary aspergillosis and aspergilloma. Long-term follow-up without enlargement of a large multiloculated cavity. Chest 1984; 85(Jan):123–125.
64. Ein ME, Wallace RJ, Williams TJ. Allergic bronchopulmonary aspergillosis-like syndrome consequent to aspergilloma. Am Rev Respir Dis 1979; 119(May):811–820.
65. Lieberman PH, Jones CR, Steinman RM, et al. Langerhans cell (eosinophilic) granulomatosis. A clinicopathologic study encompassing 50 years. Am J Surg Path 1996; 20(May): 519–552.
66. Hoffman L, Cohn JE. Respiratory abnormalities in eosinophilic granuloma of the lung. N Engl J Med 1962; 267:577–589.
67. Tazi A, Soler P, Hance AJ. Adult pulmonary Langerhans' cell histiocytosis. Thorax 2000; 55(May):405–416.
68. Friedman PJ, Liebow AA, Sokoloff J. Eosinophilic granuloma of lung. Clinical aspects of primary histiocytosis in the adult. Medicine 1981; 60(Nov):385–396.
69. Colby TV, Lombard C. Histiocytosis X in the lung. Human Pathology 1983; 14(Oct):847–856.
70. Hance AJ, Basset F, Saumon G, et al. Smoking and interstitial lung disease. The effect of cigarette smoking on the incidence of pulmonary histiocytosis X and sarcoidosis. Ann N Y Acad Sci 1986; 465:643–656.
71. Alavi S, Ashena Z, Paydar A, et al. Langerhans cell histiocytosis manifesting as recurrent simultaneous bilateral spontaneous pneumothorax in early infancy. Pediatr Int 2007; 49(6):1020–1022.
72. Braier J, Latella A, Balancini B, et al. Isolated pulmonary Langerhans cell histiocytosis presenting with recurrent pneumothorax. Pediatr Blood Cancer 2007; 48(2):241–244.
73. Travis WD, Borok Z, Roum JH, et al. Pulmonary Langerhans cell granulomatosis (histiocytosis X). A clinicopathologic study of 48 cases. Am J Surg Pathol 1993; 17(10):971–986.
74. Minghini A, Trogdon SD. Recurrent spontaneous pneumothorax in pulmonary histiocytosis X. Am Surg 1998; 64(11):1040–1042.
75. Watanabe R, Tatsumi K, Hashimoto S, et al. Clinico-epidemiological features of pulmonary histiocytosis X. Intern Med 2001; 40(10):998–1003.
76. Hidalgo A, Franquet T, Gimenez A, et al. Smoking-related interstitial lung diseases: Radiologic–pathologic correlation. Eur Radiol 2006; 16(11):2463–2470.
77. Gore RM, Port RB, Fry WJ. Spontaneous pneumothorax in a patient with honeycomb lung. Chest 1981; 80(2):215–216.
78. Mendez JL, Nadrous HF, Vassallo R, et al. Pneumothorax in pulmonary Langerhans cell histiocytosis. Chest 2004; 125(3):1028–1032.
79. Roland AS. Recurrent spontaneous pneumothorax. N Engl J Med 1964; 270(73):73–77.
80. Gelfand ET, Sheiner NM. Pneumothorax in pulmonary eosinophilic granuloma. Can Med Assoc J 1974; 110(8):937.
81. Von Essen S, West W, Sitorius M, et al. Complete resolution of roentgenographic changes in a patient with pulmonary histiocytosis X. Chest 1990; 98(3):765–767.

82. Negrin-Dastis S, Butenda D, Dorzee J, et al. Complete disappearance of lung abnormalities on high-resolution computed tomography: A case of histiocytosis X. Can Respir J 2007; 14(4):235–237.
83. Etienne B, Bertocchi M, Gamondes JP, et al. Relapsing pulmonary Langerhans cell histiocytosis after lung transplantation. Am J Respir Crit Care Med 1998; 157(1):288–291.
84. Pappas CA, Rheinlander HF, Stadecker MJ. Pleural effusion as a complication of solitary eosinophilic granuloma of the rib. Hum Pathol 1980; 11(6):675–677.
85. Nagaoka S, Maruyama R, Koike M, et al. Cytology of Langerhans cell histiocytosis in effusions: A case report. Acta Cytol 1996; 40(3):563–566.
86. Butnor KJ, Guinee DG Jr. Pleuropulmonary pathology of Birt—Hogg–Dube syndrome. Am J Surg Pathol 2006; 30(3):395–399.
87. Shamburek RD, Brewer HJ, Gochuico BR. Erdheim–Chester disease: A rare multisystem histiocytic disorder associated with interstitial lung disease. Am J Med Sci 2001; 321(Jan): 66–75.
88. Allen TC, Chevez-Barrios P, Shetlar DJ, et al. Pulmonary and ophthalmic involvement with Erdheim–Chester disease: A case report and review of the literature. Arch Pathol Lab Med 2004; 128(12):1428–1431.
89. Kambouchner M, Colby TV, Domenge C, et al. Erdheim–Chester disease with prominent pulmonary involvement associated with eosinophilic granuloma of mandibular bone. Histopathology 1997; 30(4):353–358.
90. Egan AJ, Boardman LA, Tazelaar HD, et al. Erdheim–Chester disease: Clinical, radiologic, and histopathologic findings in five patients with interstitial lung disease. Am J Surg Pathol 1999; 23(1):17–26.
91. Veyssier-Belot C, Cacoub P, Caparros-Lefebvre D, et al. Erdheim–Chester disease. Clinical and radiologic characteristics of 59 cases. Medicine 1996; 75(May):157–169.
92. Saboerali MD, Koolen MG, Noorduyn LA, et al. Pleural thickening in a construction worker: It is not always mesothelioma. Neth J Med 2006; 64(3):88–90.
93. Wittenberg KH, Swensen SJ, Myers JL. Pulmonary involvement with Erdheim–Chester disease: Radiographic and CT findings. AJR Am J Roentgenol 2000; 174(5):1327–1331.
94. Johnson SR. Lymphangioleiomyomatosis. Eur Respir J 2006; 27(5):1056–1065.
95. Mccormack FX. Lymphangioleiomyomatosis: A clinical update. Chest 2008; 133(2):507–516.
96. Ryu JH, Moss J, Beck GJ, et al. The NHLBI lymphangioleiomyomatosis registry: Characteristics of 230 patients at enrollment. Am J Respir Crit Care Med 2006; 173(1):105–111.
97. Urban T, Lazor R, Lacronique J, et al. Pulmonary lymphangioleiomyomatosis. A study of 69 patients. Groupe D'etudes Et De Recherche Sur Les Maladies "Orphelines" Pulmonaires (Germ"O"P). Medicine (Baltimore) 1999; 78(5):321–337.
98. Moss J, Avila NA, Barnes PM, et al. Prevalence and clinical characteristics of lymphangioleiomyomatosis (LAM) in patients with tuberous sclerosis complex. Am J Respir Crit Care Med 2001; 164(4):669–671.
99. Avila NA, Dwyer AJ, Rabel A, et al. Sporadic lymphangioleiomyomatosis and tuberous sclerosis complex with lymphangioleiomyomatosis: Comparison of CT features. Radiology 2007; 242(1):277–285.
100. Pallisa E, Sanz P, Roman A, et al. Lymphangioleiomyomatosis: Pulmonary and abdominal findings with pathologic correlation. Radiographics 2002; 22 Spec No. S185–S198:S185–S198.
101. Matsumoto Y, Horiba K, Usuki J, et al. Markers of cell proliferation and expression of melanosomal antigen in lymphangioleiomyomatosis. Am J Respir Cell Mol Biol 1999; 21(3):327–336.
102. Valencia JC, Pacheco-Rodriguez G, Carmona AK, et al. Tissue-specific renin–angiotensin system in pulmonary lymphangioleiomyomatosis. Am J Respir Cell Mol Biol 2006; 35(1):40–47.

103. Matsui K, Takeda K, Yu ZX, et al. Downregulation of estrogen and progesterone receptors in the abnormal smooth muscle cells in pulmonary lymphangioleiomyomatosis following therapy. An Immunohistochemical Study. Am J Respir Crit Care Med 2000; 161(3 Pt 1):1002–1009.

104. Miyake M, Tateishi U, Maeda T, et al. Pulmonary lymphangioleiomyomatosis in a male patient with tuberous sclerosis complex. Radiat Med 2005; 23(7):525–527.

105. Franz DN, Brody A, Meyer C, et al. Mutational and radiographic analysis of pulmonary disease consistent with lymphangioleiomyomatosis and micronodular pneumocyte hyperplasia in women with tuberous sclerosis. Am J Respir Crit Care Med 2001; 164(4):661–668.

106. Chu SC, Horiba K, Usuki J, et al. Comprehensive evaluation of 35 patients with lymphangioleiomyomatosis. Chest 1999; 115(4):1041–1052.

107. Almoosa KF, Mccormack FX, Sahn SA. Pleural disease in lymphangioleiomyomatosis. Clin Chest Med 2006; 27(2):355–368.

108. Almoosa KF, Ryu JH, Mendez J, et al. Management of pneumothorax in lymphangioleiomyomatosis: Effects on recurrence and lung transplantation complications. Chest 2006; 129(5):1274–1281.

109. Johnson SR, Whale CI, Hubbard RB, et al. Survival and disease progression in UK patients with lymphangioleiomyomatosis. Thorax 2004; 59(9):800–803

110. Ryu JH, Doerr CH, Fisher SD, et al. Chylothorax in lymphangioleiomyomatosis. Chest 2003; 123(2):623–627.

111. Chuang ML, Tsai YH, Pang LC. Early chylopneumothorax in a patient with pulmonary lymphangioleiomyomatosis. J Formos Med Assoc 1993; 92(3):278–282.

112. Tynski Z, Eisenberg R. Cytologic findings of lymphangioleiomyomatosis in pleural effusion: A case report. Acta Cytol 2007; 51(4):578–580.

113. Hirama M, Atsuta R, Mitani K, et al. Lymphangioleiomyomatosis diagnosed by immunocytochemical and genetic analysis of lymphangioleiomyomatosis cell clusters found in chylous pleural effusion. Intern Med 2007; 46(18):1593–1596.

114. Cope C, Kaiser LR. Management of unremitting chylothorax by percutaneous embolization and blockage of retroperitoneal lymphatic vessels in 42 patients. J Vasc Interv Radiol 2002; 13(11):1139–1148.

115. Fremont RD, Milstone AP, Light RW, et al. Chylothoraces after lung transplantation for lymphangioleiomyomatosis: Review of the literature and utilization of a pleurovenous shunt. J Heart Lung Transplant 2007; 26(9):953–955.

116. Foresti V, Casati O, Zubani R, et al. Chylous pleural effusion in tuberous sclerosis. Respiration 1990; 57(6):398–401.

117. Sandrini A, Krishnan A, Yates DH. S-LAM in a man: The first case report. Am J Respir Crit Care Med 2008; 177(3):356.

118. Taveira-Dasilva AM, Stylianou MP, Hedin CJ, et al. Decline in lung function in patients with lymphangioleiomyomatosis treated with or without progesterone. Chest 2004; 126(6):1867–1874.

119. Eliasson AH, Phillips YY, Tenholder MF. Treatment of lymphangioleiomyomatosis. A meta-analysis. Chest 1989; 96(6):1352–1355.

120. Seyama K, Kira S, Takahashi H, et al. Longitudinal follow-up study of 11 patients with pulmonary lymphangioleiomyomatosis: Diverse clinical courses of lam allow some patients to be treated without anti-hormone therapy. Respirology 2001; 6(4):331–340.

121. Boehler A, Speich R, Russi EW, et al. Lung transplantation for lymphangioleiomyomatosis. N Engl J Med 1996; 335(17):1275–1280.

122. Glassberg MK, Elliot SJ, Fritz J, et al. Activation of the estrogen receptor contributes to the progression of pulmonary lymphangioleiomyomatosis via MMP-induced cell invasiveness. J Clin Endocrinol Metab 2008; 93:1625–1633.

123. Banner AS, Carrington CB, Emory WB, et al. Efficacy of oophorectomy in lymphangioleiomyomatosis and benign metastasizing leiomyoma. N Engl J Med 1981; 305(4):204–209.

124. Abramson S, Gilkeson RC, Goldstein JD, et al. Benign metastasizing leiomyoma: Clinical, imaging, and pathologic correlation. AJR Am J Roentgenol 2001; 176(6):1409–1413.

125. Shin MS, Fulmer JD, Ho KJ. Unusual computed tomographic manifestations of benign metastasizing leiomyomas as cavitary nodular lesions or interstitial lung disease. Clin Imaging 1996; 20(1):45–49.

126. Kayser K, Zink S, Schneider T, et al. Benign metastasizing leiomyoma of the uterus: Documentation of clinical, immunohistochemical and lectin-histochemical data of ten cases. Virchows Arch 2000; 437(3):284–292.

127. Wentling GK, Sevin BU, Geiger XJ, et al. Benign metastasizing leiomyoma responsive to megestrol: Case report and review of the literature. Int J Gynecol Cancer 2005; 15(6):1213–1217.

128. Rivera JA, Christopoulos S, Small D, et al. Hormonal manipulation of benign metastasizing leiomyomas: Report of two cases and review of the literature. J Clin Endocrinol Metab 2004; 89(7):3183–3188.

129. Solans R, Bosch JA, Perez-Bocanegra C, et al. Churg–Strauss syndrome: Outcome and long-term follow-up of 32 patients. Rheumatology (Oxford) 2001; 40(7):763–771.

130. Guillevin L, Cohen P, Gayraud M, et al. Churg–Strauss syndrome. Clinical study and long-term follow-up of 96 patients. Medicine (Baltimore) 1999; 78(1):26–37.

131. Jeong YJ, Kim KI, Seo IJ, et al. Eosinophilic lung diseases: A clinical, radiologic, and pathologic overview. Radiographics 2007; 27(3):617–637.

132. Kim YK, Lee KS, Chung MP, et al. Pulmonary involvement in Churgs-Strauss syndrome: An analysis of CT, clinical, and pathologic findings. Eur Radiol 2007; 17(12):3157–3165.

133. Silva CI, Muller NL, Fujimoto K, et al. Churg–Strauss syndrome: High resolution CT and pathologic findings. J Thorac Imaging 2005; 20(2):74–80.

134. Choi YH, Im JG, Han BK, et al. Thoracic manifestation of Churg–Strauss syndrome: Radiologic and clinical findings. Chest 2000; 117(1):117–124.

135. Worthy SA, Muller NL, Hansell DM, et al. Churg–Strauss syndrome: The spectrum of pulmonary CT findings in 17 patients. AJR Am J Roentgenol 1998; 170(2):297–300.

136. Lanham JG, Elkon KB, Pusey CD, et al. Systemic vasculitis with asthma and eosinophilia: A clinical approach to the Churg–Strauss syndrome. Medicine 1984; 63(Mar):65–81.

137. Hirasaki S, Kamei T, Iwasaki Y, et al. Churg–Strauss syndrome with pleural involvement. Intern Med 2000; 39(11):976–978.

138. Erzurum SC, Underwood GA, Hamilos DL, et al. Pleural effusion in Churg–Strauss syndrome. Chest 1989; 95(Jun):1357–1359.

139. Wechsler ME, Finn D, Gunawardena D, et al. Churg–Strauss syndrome in patients receiving montelukast as treatment for asthma. Chest 2000; 117(3):708–713.

140. Guilpain P, Viallard JF, Lagarde P, et al. Churg–Strauss syndrome in two patients receiving montelukast. Rheumatology (Oxford) 2002; 41(5):535–539.

141. Hauser T, Mahr A, Metzler C, et al. The leukotriene-receptor antagonist montelukast and the risk of Churg–Strauss syndrome: A Case-Crossover Study. Thorax 2008; 63:677–682.

142. Bili A, Condemi JJ, Bottone SM, et al. Seven cases of complete and incomplete forms of Churg–Strauss syndrome not related to leukotriene receptor antagonists. J Allergy Clin Immunol 1999; 104(5):1060–1065.

143. Ribi C, Cohen P, Pagnoux C, et al. Treatment of Churg–Strauss syndrome without poor-prognosis factors: A multicenter, prospective, randomized, open-label study of seventy-two patients. Arthritis Rheum 2008; 58(2):586–594.

144. Westermark P. The pathogenesis of amyloidosis: Understanding general principles. Am J Pathol 1998; 152(May):1125–1127.

145. Celli BR, Rubinow A, Cohen AS, et al. Patterns of pulmonary involvement in systemic amyloidosis. Chest 1978; 74(Nov):543–547.
146. Smith RR, Hutchins GM, Moore GW, et al. Type and distribution of pulmonary parenchymal and vascular amyloid. Correlation with cardiac amyloid. Am J Med 1979; 66(Jan):96–104.
147. Utz JP, Swensen SJ, Gertz MA. Pulmonary amyloidosis. The mayo clinic experience from 1980 to 1993. Ann Intern Med 1996; 124(4):407–413.
148. Xu L, Cai BQ, Zhong X, et al. Respiratory manifestations in amyloidosis. Chin Med J (Engl) 2005; 118(24):2027–2033.
149. Berk JL, Keane J, Seldin DC, et al. Persistent pleural effusions in primary systemic amyloidosis: Etiology and prognosis. Chest 2003; 124(3):969–977.
150. Ikeda S, Takabayashi Y, Maejima Y, et al. Nodular lung disease with five year survival and unilateral pleural effusion in AL amyloidosis. Amyloid 1999; 6(4):292–296.
151. Adams AL, Castro CY, Singh SP, et al. Pleural amyloidosis mimicking mesothelioma: A clinicopathologic study of two cases. Ann Diagn Pathol 2001; 5:229–232.
152. Katzenstein AL, Fiorelli RF. Nonspecific interstitial pneumonia/fibrosis. Histologic features and clinical significance. Am J Surg Pathol 1994; 18(2):136–147.
153. Picado C, Gomez DA, Xaubet A, et al. Spontaneous pneumothorax in cryptogenic fibrosing alveolitis. Respiration 1985; 48(1):77–80.
154. Franquet T, Gimenez A, Torrubia S, et al. Spontaneous pneumothorax and pneumomediastinum in IPF. Eur Radiol 2000; 10(1):108–113.
155. Hunninghake GW, Zimmerman MB, Schwartz DA, et al. Utility of a lung biopsy for the diagnosis of idiopathic pulmonary fibrosis. Am J Resp Crit Care Med 2001; 164:193–196.
156. Nishimura K, Kitaichi M, Izumi T, et al. Usual interstitial pneumonia: Histologic correlation with high-resolution CT. Radiology 1992; 182(2):337–342.
157. Lim MK, Im JG, Ahn JM, et al. Idiopathic pulmonary fibrosis vs. Pulmonary involvement of collagen vascular disease: HRCT findings. J Korean Med Sci 1997; 12(6):492–498.

31
Immunological Diseases of the Pleura

KATERINA M. ANTONIOU
Department of Thoracic Medicine Medical School, University of Crete, Heraklion, Crete, Greece

DEMOSTHENES BOUROS
Democritus University of Thrace Medical School, and University Hospital of Alexandroupolis, Alexandroupolis, Greece

ATHOL U. WELLS
Royal Brompton Hospital, London, U.K.

I. Introduction

The systemic autoimmune diseases are a heterogeneous group of inflammatory disorders that can affect the pleura with various frequencies either as single presenting feature or as part of multisystem involvement. Pleural disease in connective tissue disease occurs most frequently in rheumatoid arthritis (RA) and systemic lupus erythematosus (SLE), but there is a considerable variation in the reported prevalence, natural history, and treated course of pleural involvement in both diseases. The definition of pleural disease in other connective tissue disorders is necessarily imprecise. Many of the systemic diseases covered in this chapter are, themselves, rare, and pleural involvement is infrequent; thus, the spectrum of pleural disease is not captured in the medical literature to two standard deviations of disease behavior. It is foolhardy to attempt to generalize from single case reports or retrospective data from very small series.

There are other problems that apply equally to RA, SLE, and other connective tissue diseases. The prevalence and severity of an individual pulmonary feature is likely to be critically dependent upon the nature of the population studied. Potentially important selection biases include evaluation of patients at the onset of disease (following which clinical features may evolve significantly) and presentation to a subspecialty respiratory unit (leading to the selection of patients with particularly vexing pulmonary complications). Furthermore, as clinical experience of unusual diseases accumulates, patients with milder disease are increasingly recognized, especially if ancillary diagnostic tests are developed. A good example of this phenomenon is the widespread determination of serum antineutrophil cytoplasmic antibody levels, leading to a lower diagnostic threshold for Wegener's granulomatosis (WG) in patients with mild or even subclinical disease and a corresponding change in the reported clinical spectrum of disease. In pleural disease, this problem is exacerbated by increasingly sophisticated imaging techniques, allowing the detection of previously unsuspected small effusions of doubtful clinical significance. Plainly, the apparent prevalence of pleural disease will depend utterly upon whether patients are investigated for symptomatic pleural disease, screened radiographically, or undergo computed tomography (CT) by protocol.

Concurrent pathological processes also complicate the definition of pleural disease in connective tissue disorders. Pleural abnormalities may result from renal or cardiac disease, pulmonary emboli, and, especially, pneumonia or empyema, both of which tend to be more prevalent in connective tissue disease. Thus, in many cases, apparent pleural involvement does not, in fact, represent active autoimmune pleuritis, and it becomes increasingly difficult to interpret the significance of occasional case reports of pleural involvement in diseases other than SLE or RA. A further problem is the existence of overlap autoimmune syndromes. For example, pleural disease in patients with apparently isolated systemic sclerosis (SSc) or polymyositis/dermatomyositis (PM/DM) may, in fact, represent incipient overlap with RA or SLE, and the clinical heterogeneity of Churg–Strauss syndrome (CSS) and Wegener's granulomatosus (WG) is notorious.

Finally, treatment is largely anecdotal, with no controlled data, even in cohorts of patients with RA or SLE. This reflects the fact that pleural involvement is often clinically trivial and does not require treatment, a fact not always captured in statements of prevalence.

In this chapter, pleural disease in RA and SLE is covered in greater detail, and the reported experience of pleural disease is summarized briefly in other connective tissue diseases.

II. Rheumatoid Arthritis

Pleural disease (pleuritis, with or without pleural effusion) is the most common intrathoracic manifestation of RA. It usually affects middle-aged men and is characterized by a low pleural fluid glucose level.

A. Incidence

Pleural involvement in RA, first reported in the mid-19th century (1), is found at autopsy in approximately 50% of patients (2). However, only 20% of RA patients experience pleuritic pain at some stage, and many pleural effusions are found incidentally on chest radiography, with overt clinical evidence of pleural disease in less than 5% patients (3–5). In a study of 516 patients with RA, only 17 (3.3%) had pleural effusions, with the prevalence higher in males (7.9%) than in females (1.6%) (3). By contrast, in a controlled study of 309 RA patients, chest radiographic evidence of preexisting pleural disease was seen in 24% of males and 16% of females (compared to 16% and 8% of controlled subjects) (6). Pleuritic pain is also more prevalent in male patients (3,6). Middle-aged men with high rheumatoid factor (RF) titers are mainly affected (7). A genetic predisposition of rheumatoid pleurisy has also been reported with a high prevalence of HLA-B8 and Dw3 associated with rheumatoid pleural effusion (8).

B. Histological Features

Thickening of visceral and parietal pleura is prominent in rheumatoid pleural effusion. The most consistent finding is the replacement of the normal mesothelial cell covering by a pseudo-stratified layer of epithelioid cells, with focal multinucleated giant cells (which differ from foreign body giant cells), regular small papillae containing branching capillaries, and occasional cholesterol clefts (9–11). However, granulomas or necrotic tissue is not routinely found in pleural thoracoscope-guided biopsies (9–11). Typical rheumatoid nodules are an occasional finding (11). These findings are pathognomonic for rheumatoid pleuritis, but histological appearances are nonspecific in many cases and needle biopsy specimens generally show nonspecific evidence of chronic pleuritis (12).

C. Clinical Manifestations

Most patients are asymptomatic, but breathlessness may result from pulmonary compression in large effusions. Fever, cough, and pleuritic pain are occasional complaints (13), and respiratory failure has been precipitated by a large effusion in a patient with preexisting chronic obstructive pulmonary disease (14). Ninety-two (81%) out of 113 patients with rheumatoid pleural effusions, reported before 1968, were male, and the average age of onset was 51 years (range 35–69 years) (3). Rheumatoid effusions are associated with subcutaneous nodules in over 50% patients (3,12,13) and usually develop after the onset of joint manifestations; in only 6% do effusions precede arthritis and in 11%, pleural and systemic disease present concurrently. Pleural effusions are a late manifestation (i.e., developing 10 or more years after the onset of systemic disease) in 20% (3). The presence of pleural disease has not been linked to more severe systemic disease, although associated with a higher prevalence of cardiac and ocular lesions (3).

D. Radiographic Imaging

On chest radiography, effusions are bilateral in 25% (3), with no predilection for either side (12). Effusions are usually small or moderate, but are occasionally massive (14,15), and may be transient, chronic, or recurrent (16). Up to 30% of patients have simultaneous parenchymal lesions (interstitial lung disease or necrobiotic nodules) (3,16), and concurrent pneumothoraces occur in approximately 5% (17). The existence of fluid in the pleural cavity may be confirmed by other techniques such as ultrasound and computed tomography (CT) (18).

E. Diagnosis

The diagnosis of a rheumatoid pleural effusion is made by the exclusion of other causes, although male gender, age in excess of 50, long-standing arthritis, and the presence of subcutaneous nodules all increase the diagnostic likelihood. Effusions are exudative and characterized by high titers of RF, low glucose levels, low pH, and high lactate dehydrogenase (LDH) levels.

F. Differential Diagnosis

In patients with coexisting arthritis and pleural effusions, the major differential diagnosis is SLE. Lupoid effusions are distinguished from rheumatoid effusions by absent or low (1:40) titers of RF, glucose concentrations in excess of 80 mg/dL, lactic dehydrogenase levels of 500 IU/L or less, and pH >7.35.

Rheumatoid pleural effusions are seldom a prolonged source of diagnostic uncertainty. In a study of 40 consecutive patients with exudative pleural effusions, undiagnosed after exhaustive evaluation and followed, on average, for five years, no underlying cause was identified in 32 (80%) cases , but RA was eventually diagnosed in only one case (19).

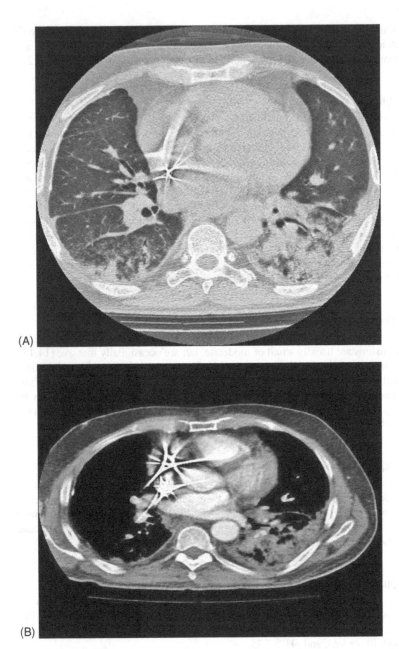

(A)

(B)

Figure 1 Computed tomography of the thorax in a patient with diffuse systemic sclerosis without contrast enhancement showing bilateral parenchymal consolidation and small left pleural effusion (**A**), and the same patient with contrast enhancement showing the left pleural effusion (**B**). (From: Bouros D, et al. Respiration 2008; 75:361–371)

G. Fluid Analysis

The fluid is exudative and nonodorous and may be cloudy, greenish-yellow, or opalescent (9). Glucose levels exceed 3 g/100 mL in 20% to 30% patients, but normal glucose concentrations reduce the likelihood of rheumatoid pleural disease (12). The latter rarely occurs in acute or recent rheumatoid pleurisy. Glucose levels are lower in long-standing rheumatoid effusions.

Other biochemical findings include pH <7.2, LDH levels more than twice the upper limit of the normal serum value, low complement and immune complexes levels, and RF titers (>1:320) that exceed serum titers (13). Further reduction in the value of pH raises the possibility of a concomitant infection.

Whole complement activity and C3, C4 levels are lower in RA pleural fluid than in nonrheumatoid effusions (20). The complement cascade is activated through both classic and alternative pathways in rheumatic pleurisy; in one study, determination of SC5b-9 and C4 d/C4 content in pleural fluid most accurately distinguished between rheumatic, tuberculous, and malignant effusions (21).

As in empyema and tuberculous effusions, the activity of adenosine deaminase (ADA) in rheumatoid effusions is higher in pleural fluid than in serum, indicating local synthesis of ADA by cells within the pleural cavity in RA (22).

H. Fluid Cytology

Cytological examination may disclose a characteristic triad of giant multinucleated macrophages, elongated macrophages, and a background of granular debris (8,16). One or more of these features was present in 24 patients with RA pleuritis (granular necrotic material, $n = 23$; multinucleated giant macrophages, $n = 17$; elongated macrophages, $n = 15$), but in none of 10,000 nonrheumatoid effusions (23). "RA cells" ("ragocytes" with characteristic inclusion bodies, representing phagocytic vacuoles or phagosomes, larger than lysosomes seen in granular leukocytes) are not only sometimes present (24), but may also be seen in tuberculous effusions and empyema (16), and have no diagnostic value (23,25).

I. Glucose

Pleural fluid glucose concentrations of 25 mg/100 mL or less, despite normal serum glucose concentrations, are virtually diagnostic of RA in the absence of bacteria and acid-fast bacilli (26). In a study of 76 rheumatoid effusions, pleural glucose levels were less than 20 mg/dL in 63%, and less than 50 mg/dL in 83% (12). The mechanism for low pleural glucose levels in RA is unknown. The administration of glucose increases serum but not pleural glucose concentrations (5,26). However, pleural glucose is not utilized rapidly; the addition of glucose to pleural fluid in vitro is not associated with significant cellular glucose utilization (5). It has been suggested that the rheumatoid inflammatory process may influence the activity of enzymes contributing to cellular membrane carbohydrate transport (26) or produces substances interfering with glucose entry into pleural fluid (5).

J. Cholesterol

High concentrations of total lipids and cholesterol have been observed in some rheumatoid effusions (5,11,12), and cholesterol crystal formation, an occasional finding, may give

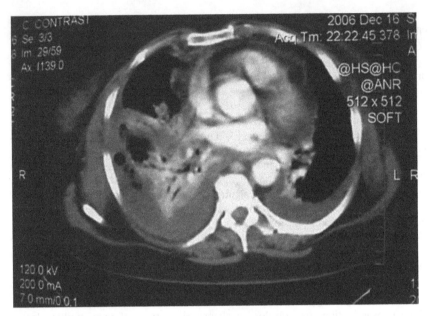

Figure 2 Computed tomography of the thorax in a patient with rheumatoid arthritis showing bilateral pleural effusion. The right pleural effusion was an empyema treated with large bore chest tube drainage and intrapleural instillation of fibrinolytics. The left one was a parapneumonic pleural effusion treated by complete evacuation by thoracocentesis. (From: Bouros D, et al. Respiration 2008; 75:361–371)

rise to an "opalescent sheen" (12). Chronicity or high cellularity is probably necessary for the development of a high pleural fluid lipid or cholesterol content (unless the effusion is a true chylothorax) (5,12).

K. Infection

Empyema may complicate rheumatoid pleural disease, but the reported prevalence is highly variable. Five out of 10 patients with RA pleural effusions observed during a five-year period developed empyema and these patients made up 16% of all adult cases with empyema at that institution (27). By contrast, only 1 out of 19 patients with pleural effusions in RA had empyema (3). In a study of 67 patients with nontuberculous empyema, three were associated with RA (28). It appears that empyema in RA may not only be associated with nodular pleuropulmonary disease and the formation of pyopneumothoraces, but may also occur in the absence of other pleuropulmonary complications of RA. Middle-aged males seem to be particularly susceptible (28). Possible causative factors include corticosteroid therapy, a rheumatoid susceptibility to infection, preexisting chronic bronchopulmonary infection, preexisting rheumatoid effusions, altered biochemical characteristics of pleural fluid, and the formation of bronchopleural fistulas through necrotic rheumatoid nodules (27). A number of recent reports (29–31) have evaluated clinical utility of several biomarkers, sometimes in combination with noninvasive imaging procedures (31), in order to differentiate infectious from noninfectious pleural effusions (29–31). However, their applicability is still under investigation (32).

L. Pneumothorax

This rare complication of RA, thought to occur in approximately 5% of patients with rheumatoid lung (33) and found on chest radiography in 6% of patients with rheumatoid effusions (28), may be bilateral (17) or recurrent (34). The pleural fluid cholesterol content is often increased (11). Pneumothoraces are thought to result from perforation of cavitating rheumatoid nodules into the pleural space, creating continuous leakage. Prolonged chest tube drainage or surgical intervention may be required (35). A triad of rheumatoid lung disease, pneumothorax, and peripheral eosinophilia has been described (36,37).

M. Biopsy

Pleural biopsy is not recommended routinely in RA patients with pleural effusion. Needle biopsy of the pleura has proved disappointing—in most cases, nonspecific granulomatous or fibrotic changes are reported (3,38). On rare occasions pleural rheumatoid nodules are demonstrated, which are diagnostic (38,39).

Thoracoscopy sometimes offers an invaluable supplement to other laboratory data in the evaluation of suspected rheumatoid effusions (7,39,40). The thoracoscopic granular appearance of the parietal pleura and the histopathological changes in tissue gained from thoracoscopic biopsies are often diagnostic (9).

N. Treatment

There is little reported information on the efficacy of therapy in rheumatoid pleural disease. Most effusions are asymptomatic and do not require specific treatment. Initial treatment of pleuritic with nonsteroidal anti-inflammatory agents may suffice. Some patients respond to corticosteroids (3,11,16,41), but others do not (2,42,43), and effusions may recur despite maintenance steroid therapy. Repeated aspirations have been used to control effusions. Occasionally, persistent symptomatic effusions or pleural thickening necessitate decortication (44–46).

Intrapleural installation of corticosteroids has been attempted. In two patients with large persistent, asymptomatic pleural effusions, intrapleural injection was ineffective (42), but a further patient has responded to an injection of 10 mg of depomethylprednisolone (47). However, the role of repeated corticosteroid injections into the pleural space is under investigation.

Decortication should be considered in patients with symptomatic pleural thickening. The significance of pleural thickening can be estimated by serial pleural pressure measurements during therapeutic thoracocentesis; a rapid drop in pleural pressure is noted, which denotes trapping of the lung by thickened pleura (48). However, decortication may be technically difficult in rheumatoid pleural disease (46).

O. Long-Term Outcome

Rheumatoid effusions resolve within four weeks in 50% patients and within four months in two-third of patients (3), but persist for years in approximately 20% (2).

III. Systemic Lupus Erythematosus

A. Incidence

Pleural effusions are common in SLE and are included in the American Rheumatism Association diagnostic criteria for SLE (49). Approximately 30% to 50% of patients develop a pleural effusion during the course of their illness (2,50–53). Pleural abnormalities are found at autopsy in 40% to 93% of cases (54–60), but represent secondary cardiopulmonary complications of SLE, such as heart failure, infection, and pulmonary emboli, rather than lupus pleuritis, in some cases (56). Pleural effusions are variably reported to be more prevalent in females (50) and males (58), with no clear evidence overall of a major association with gender. Pleuritic pain was reported in 60 out of 138 patients in one series, with 14 experiencing repeated episodes (59), and a chest radiographic study disclosed a prevalence of pleural effusion of approximately 35% of patients (60). However, the exact prevalence is difficult to determine, because many patients with transient pleural disease are asymptomatic and may not come to medical attention. Moreover, the clinical features of SLE, including the frequency of pleural disease, vary significantly between ethnic groups (61–66).

B. Histology

Little has been written about the histological features of pleural disease in SLE, perhaps because findings at autopsy represent the end result of multiple episodes, with fibrotic ablation of preceding lesions (60). In an autopsy study of 54 patients, acute fibrinous pleuritis was present in 40%. In 33% of cases, there was evidence of previous inflammation, as shown by pleural fibrosis. Hematoxylin bodies, considered diagnostic by some, were infrequent (67).

C. Clinical Manifestations

Pleuritic pain is the most frequent pleural symptom in SLE, occurring in most patients with lupus pleuritis, although dyspnea and cough are also common (51). Pleuritic pain is often distressing and may be prolonged (59), occasionally necessitating pleurectomy after failure of conservative treatment (68). Frequent findings on examination include fever, pleural rub, and tachycardia (51). Lupus pleuritis is the first manifestation of SLE in only 5% to 10%, but is an early feature in 25% to 30%, usually preceded by arthralgia, and is sometimes associated with pneumonitis and pericarditis (60). Other patients present with painless pleural effusions (69). The prevalence of pleural disease at presentation not only increases in the elderly (sixth decade or later) (70), but pleural involvement is also frequent in children (63,71), and fatal lupus pleuritis has occurred during pregnancy (64). Pleuritis is also a frequent feature of drug-induced lupus syndromes (not covered in this chapter). Finally, pleural effusions may represent complications of SLE (rather than representing primary disease activity), including lupus nephritis, uremia, pneumonia, pulmonary emboli, congestive heart failure, empyema, and other disorders.

D. Radiographic Imaging

On chest radiography, pleural effusions are generally small, but are occasionally massive (72–78). Effusions are bilateral in about 50% of patients, with no major predilection for the right or left side (2), and serial chest radiographs often disclose a change in side (59).

Although pleural involvement was invariably associated with pneumonitis in one study (59), pleural abnormalities are more prevalent than radiographic evidence of interstitial lung disease in other reports (53,60). Other chest radiographic findings include nonspecific alveolar infiltrates, atelectasis, and cardiomegaly, representing cardiomyopathy or pericardial effusions (51,78).

E. Diagnosis

SLE pleuritis should be considered in any patient with an exudative pleural effusion of unknown etiology (60). The diagnosis is often obvious in patients with overt SLE, but in patients with pleuritis in association with nonspecific arthritis, the major differential diagnosis is rheumatoid pleural disease. Laboratory data distinguishing between rheumatoid and lupus pleuritis (51) are covered in the section on rheumatoid arthritis. Measurement of lactic acid has been proposed as a rapid tool to distinguish between bacterial pleural inflammation and other causes of exudative effusions (79), but the measurement of ADA isoenzymes does not enhance the overall diagnostic value of ADA activity in pleural effusions (80).

F. Pleural Fluid Analysis

The pleural fluid is usually exudative, yellow, or serosanguineous (51,60), with rare reports of hemothorax (78,81), and tends to be neutrophilic in patients with pleurisy, but lymphocytic in chronic effusions (51,52). A pleural fluid eosinophilia is generally considered to rule out underlying SLE (82) but has been reported in a single SLE patient (83). Generally, the pH is higher than 7.20, glucose concentrations are slightly decreased (51,84), although usually higher than 60 mg/dL, and LDH levels are lower than 500 IU (51). However, occasional exceptions exist to all three observations (51,52). The clinical features of pleural disease are not linked to pleural pH and glucose levels (52).

As in RA, reductions in pleural fluid complement levels have been observed (3,49–51,85,86), possibly reflecting complement conversion by immune complexes (20,51,52,85,86). Immune complex deposition may engender pleural effusions by increasing capillary permeability (87). Low titer RF positivity is an occasional finding in a lupoid effusion (51). Elevated CA-125 levels have been reported in the pleural fluid of a number of connective tissue diseases, including SLE (88,89); elevated serum CA-125 levels are an indicator of pleural disease in connective tissue disease.

In patients with nondiagnostic serum antinuclear antibody (ANA), RF, anti-DNA antibody, and hemolytic complement levels, the measurement of corresponding pleural levels is diagnostically valueless (90). Similarly, serum antinuclear and associated antibody positivity is not diagnostically useful, although there is a weak association in SLE between anti-RNP positivity and pleuritis (91,92).

G. Pleural Fluid Antinuclear Antibodies

Pleural fluid ANA titers >1:60 and pleural fluid-to-serum ANA ratios >1 are suggestive but not diagnostic of SLE pleuritis; high pleural fluid titers (up to 1:640) are seen occasionally in patients with nonlupoid exudative effusions (93). Most patients with SLE also have higher ANA titers for ssDNA, dsDNA, smooth muscle, and ribonucleoprotein (93,94), although demonstrable pleural fluid ANA are occasionally absent (95). Pleural fluid ANA titer levels may be useful in distinguishing between lupus pleuritis and other causes of pleural disease in SLE patients, in which ANA titers tend to be low or absent (96).

H. Fluid Lupus Cells

Lupus erythematosus (LE) cells are found occasionally in serous effusions in SLE (51,97–103) and may appear at the onset or later in the disease course (104). LE cells also occur in drug-induced lupus pleuritis (97,98). Some have regarded the presence of LE cells in serous effusions as virtually diagnostic of SLE (97–100), although LE cells are occasionally present in malignant pleural effusions (105), rheumatoid joint effusions (106), and have also been reported in pleural fluid, without clinical evidence of SLE (104). However, LE cells are not found in the pleural fluid of all patients with lupoid pleuritis (96) and are usually associated with the presence of serum LE cells; thus, the added value of pleural fluid LE cell positivity is questionable (96). Moreover, the detection of LE cells is not technically straightforward , and may be subjected to significant observer variation (99). Thus, the diagnostic identification of LE cells has largely fallen out of favor.

I. Biopsy

In pleural biopsy specimens from three patients with drug-induced lupus pleural effusions (107) and autopsy pleural specimens from patients with SLE (108), a specific immunoflu-orescent pattern has been observed, characterized by diffused and speckled staining of cell nuclei with anti-immunoglobulin G, anti-IgM, or anti-C3 (107).

Thoracoscopy reveals nodules on the visceral pleura and immunofluorescence of biopsy samples of these nodules demonstrated immunoglobulin deposits (109).

J. Pneumothorax

Pneumothoraces and pneumohemothoraces have been described in adults with SLE (81,110).

K. Treatment

Pleuritic pain in SLE may respond to nonsteroidal anti-inflammatory agents and almost always responds strikingly to corticosteroid therapy, although high doses may be needed for severe pleuritis or large effusions (111). In refractory cases, immunosuppressive agents such as azathioprine and hydroxychloroquine are sometimes but not always efficacious (74,112,113), and monthly cyclosporin courses have been used, with a good outcome (113). Recurrent pleural effusions usually respond to tetracycline (114,115) or talc (74) pleurodesis.

L. Prognosis

Asymptomatic lupoid effusions require no treatment, usually resolve spontaneously (53), and have no known prognostic significance. However, pleuritic pain appears to be an adverse prognostic marker (60,116,117), with a mean survival of less than four years in affected cases in one study (60).

IV. Systemic Sclerosis

Pleural effusions have been reported in both diffused (88,118,119) and limited (120) scleroderma, but are rare. In a formal evaluation of the prevalence of serositis in SSc, none of 37 patients (including 19 with limited SSc) had a pleural effusion, and on review of medical records, pleural effusions were identified in only 4 (7%) out of 58 other SSc patients (121). By contrast, pericardial effusions were present in 17% (121). The very low prevalence of pleural effusions in SSc makes the association uncertain, as a proportion of patients with SSc eventually develop SLE overlap. Thus, an evolving overlap syndrome might give rise to pleural involvement in some patients, including the recently reported case of an 88-year-old woman with SSc and a pleural effusion, eventually diagnosed as an SSc/SLE overlap (122).

In two cases, pleural effusions in SSc have been associated with elevated serum and pleural fluid CA-125 levels (88,118), which were seen to decrease with resolution of the effusion in one case (88). CA-125 levels are usually normal in collagen vascular disease, in the absence of pleural involvement (88), and, thus, it has been suggested that CA-125 levels might reflect the activity of serositis (118).

Pleural fluids in patients with autoimmune diseases are mostly dominated by monocytes and lymphocytes but very rarely contain increased eosinophils. However, it has been recently reported case of a 55-year-old male with Progressive systemic sclerosis-polymyositis overlap syndrome and eosinophilic pleural effusion (123). After the administration of corticosteroid, the pleural effusion decreased promptly, with normalization of serum creatine phosphokinase and C-reactive protein concentrations.

V. Polymyositis/Dermatomyositis

PM/DM are grouped disorders, categorized under the idiopathic inflammatory myopathies and characterized by symmetrical proximal muscle weakness, elevated serum levels of skeletal muscle enzymes, electrophysiological changes consistent with myopathy, and evidence of nonsuppurative inflammation in skeletal muscle tissue (123,124). Dermatomyositis consists of all the manifestations of polymyositis with additional cutaneous features.

Although pleuritic pain is occasionally reported (125–127), overt clinical or radiographic evidence of pleural disease is exceedingly rare. None of the 65 patients with polymyositis ($n = 24$) or dermatomyositis ($n = 41$) had pleural effusions clinically or at autopsy, although histological evidence of fibrinous pleuritis was seen occasionally (125). Two patients with massive pleural effusions have been described, both presenting with marked pyrexia and a good response to corticosteroid therapy (128). Although cardiomyopathy and hypothyroidism might have contributed to pleural fluid accumulation in one case, no confounding features were present in the second patient, a 34-year-old man with dermatomyositis and coexisting interstitial lung disease. It has been recently reported case of anti-Jo-1 syndrome (a rare autoimmune condition that may manifest with various forms of interstitial lung disease), which presented unusually with multiple pulmonary nodules, mimicking carcinoma (129). The patient subsequently developed pleural and pericardial effusions, myopathy, and "mechanic's hand," with similar lesions on the feet. Initially, the patient responded well to immunosuppression but has subsequently progressed to pulmonary fibrosis.

VI. Sjögren's Syndrome

Sjögren's syndrome (SS) is a chronic inflammatory disease characterized by dryness of the mouth (xerostomia), eyes (keratoconjunctivitis sicca), and other mucous membranes (2). SS may be primary or secondary (when associated with RA, SLE, PM/DM, or SSc). Respiratory involvement in primary SS is often clinically mild, although severe symptoms occasionally arise from desiccation of the tracheobronchial tree or lymphocytic infiltration of the lung parenchyma (130). Pleurisy, with or without a pleural effusion, is exceedingly rare in primary SS, but sometimes occurs in secondary SS with accompanying RA or SLE, in keeping with the high prevalence of pleural involvement in those disorders (131).

Overall, pleural effusions have been reported in none of 62 patients with SS (132); in none of 36 patients with primary SS (133); in only 5 out of 349 patients with SS, including 2 with primary SS (134); and in none of 40 patients with primary SS or 26 with secondary SS (135). Pleuritic pain was confined to patients with secondary SS and a control cohort with RA (135).

In a handful of reported pleural effusions associated with primary SS, disease is more often bilateral (131,136,137), but may be unilateral (138), and the fluid is lymphocytic and exudative, with normal glucose levels and pH, and low ADA levels (137–140). Studies of serum and pleural fluid in one patient disclosed rheumatoid factor and anti-SS-A antibody, immune complexes, and activation of complement, all localized to pleural fluid (131). Analysis of pleural fluid T-cell receptor β-chain variable (V β) regions revealed overexpression of V β gene products, including V β 2 and V β 13, previously shown to be overrepresented in salivary glands of SS patients (131). In two instances, pleural effusions associated with primary SS have regressed with corticosteroid therapy (136,137), or improved spontaneously until complete resolution (140).

Pleural involvement in patients with primary SS is so rare that there remains a concern that the pleural effusions described may actually be due to coexisting conditions. A coexisting autoimmune disease such as SLE or RA should first be considered. There have only been nine previous reports of primary SS complicated by pleural effusion (132,137–141).

VII. Ankylosing Spondylitis

Ankylosing spondylitis (AS) is an inflammatory disease involving entheses and joints, especially those in and around the spine, and resulting in chest wall pain, diminished chest wall movement, and a dorsal stoop. Pleural involvement is most frequently associated with apical fibrobullous lung disease, found in a small proportion of AS patients. The initial, mainly fibrotic changes become fibrobullous as the condition progresses, with evolution to prominent cavitation being an occasional feature. Cavities developing within apical fibrotic tissue in AS have a particular predilection for mycobacterial or fungal colonization, especially *Aspergillus fumigatus*, isolated in up to 60% of AS patients with apical cavitation (142). Infection of a cavity may lead to underlying pleural thickening or even empyema.

Other forms of pleural disease in AS are exceedingly rare (143), consisting of a handful of cases with pleural effusions (144–146). In population studies, pleural disease has been identified in 2 out of 53 patients (one tuberculous, one nontuberculous effusion) (147), 2 out of 255 patients (idiopathic bilateral pleural calcification) (148), and 1 out of 200 patients (unexplained pleural thickening) (149). These findings are difficult to interpret, as they might have represented the pleural sequelae of tuberculous or nontuberculous infection, rather than a direct complication of AS. A chest radiographic study of 2080 patients with AS disclosed nonapical pleural disease in 10 patients, which did not differ significantly in prevalence from control subjects and included three transient pleural exudates with normal pleural fluid glucose concentrations and one patient with empyema (150). Recently, a case of pleural and pericardial effusions complicating AS without parenchymal involvement has been reported (151). Patient showed good response to oral corticosteroids with complete resolution of pleural fluid.

VIII. Mixed Connective Tissue Disease

The term mixed connective tissue disease (MCTD), or Sharp's syndrome (152), applies to patients exhibiting a mixture of clinical features of SLE, SSc, and PM/DM, in association with high titers of a circulating ANA, with specificity for a nuclear ribonucleoprotein antigen (snRNP) (153). Pleuropulmonary manifestations, reported to occur in 20% to 80% of patients, include interstitial pneumonitis and fibrosis (20–65%), and pulmonary hypertension (10–45%) (154). Pleural effusions develop during the course of the illness in 50% (154) and pleuritic chest pain is reported in approximately 40% (155). However, despite a high overall prevalence of inflammatory pleural disease, often associated with pericarditis, pleural involvement is seldom an initial manifestation of disease (unlike SLE) (156). In the few reported cases of MCTD in which pleural involvement is the cardinal presenting feature, pleural effusions are sometimes but not always associated with pericarditis (152,156) and may be bilateral (157) or unilateral (158). In general, pleural effusions are small and resolve spontaneously (154).

IX. Eosinophilia–Myalgia Syndrome

Eosinophilia–myalgia syndrome (EMS), a recently defined disorder reaching epidemic proportions in 1989 (159,160), is almost always associated with ingestion of manufactured tryptophan, although occasional idiopathic cases occur (161). Diagnostic criteria are debilitating myalgia and an absolute blood eosinophil count >1.0 (10 × 9) cells/L. The syndrome usually affects Caucasian women older than 35, and clinical data suggest a multisystem disorder, with frequent arthralgia, rash, peripheral edema, elevated aldolase level, and deranged liver function tests. Neuropathy or neuritis occurs in 25% (159) and occasionally ends in paralysis or death. Cough or dyspnea is present in 60%, although less than 10% have pleural effusions on chest radiography (159).

Although the exact pathogenesis of the syndrome remains uncertain (162), cessation of tryptophan ingestion, with or without the addition of corticosteroids, may lead to a rapid complete response, although recovery is often incomplete or prolonged (160) and several deaths have occurred (159,163). Following withdrawal of commercially available preparations of tryptophan, the incidence of EMS has fallen dramatically (159).

Pleural effusions have been reported on chest radiography in 12% out of 178 cases (159) and in 6 out of 18 patients (160). Effusions are usually bilateral and the fluid is sterile and exudative (161,164).

Pleural involvement is not necessarily clinically significant and has no documented therapeutic or prognostic implication. It has been recently described case of a 61-year-old female admitted with acute respiratory failure after using L-tryptophan, hydroxytryptophan, and other drugs (165). The patient presented eosinophilia, together with elevated eosinophil counts in the bronchoalveolar lavage and pleural effusion. After discontinuation of the drugs previously used, corticosteroids were administered, resulting in clinical and radiological improvement within just a few days.

X. Angio-Immunoblastic Lymphadenopathy

Angio-immunoblastic lymphadenopathy (AIL), a disease of unknown etiology and pathogenesis, has variable features of hyperimmunity and immune deficiency. It often resembles Hodgkin's disease (166,167), presenting with fever, true drenching sweats, weight loss, and, often, a rash, generalized lymphadenopathy, and hepatosplenomegaly. Polyclonal hypergammaglobulinemia is usual and hemolytic anemia is frequent (2,166). AIL is uncommon, with 200 cases being reported (167) in the six years following the initial definition of the disease in 1973 (166). The diagnosis is made by histological examination of an enlarged lymph node. The course of the disease is usually progressive, with a median survival of 15 months in 18 fatal cases out of 32 studied in one series (166). Treatments have included prednisone and cyclophosphamide (167), but survival beyond two years is exceedingly rare, and failure to achieve complete remission is associated with a mortality at one year in 90% cases. More intensive chemotherapy is usually unsuccessful and very hazardous, as the risk of severe infection is high.

Histologically, AIL is characterized by a morphological triad: proliferation of arborizing small vessels, prominent immunoblastic proliferation, and amorphous acidophilic interstitial material, with benign appearances (2,166). Progression of disease is thought to represent a nonneoplastic hyperimmune proliferation of B lymphocytes, possibly related to a lack of suppressor T lymphocytes (167,168). Transformations to immunoblastic lymphoma (167) and immunoblastic sarcoma (166) have been reported.

Pleural effusions occur in AIL in at least 10% of cases, with a higher prevalence in some reports. In a Japanese series, pleural effusions were found in 50%, including all five index cases and 8 out of 21 patients previously reported in the Japanese literature (169). In a study of 10 patients, five where found to have a pleural effusion eventually associated with ascites and pedal edema (167). Surprisingly, the characteristics of the pleural fluid (including fundamental features such as protein content) are not well described.

XI. Churg–Strauss Syndrome

Churg–Strauss syndrome (CSS) is characterized by asthma, hypereosinophilia, and necrotizing systemic vasculitis with extravascular eosinophil granulomas. Diagnosis requires satisfaction of at least four American College of Rheumatology criteria: asthma, hypereosinophilia >1500/mm^3 or >10%, paranasal sinusitis, pulmonary infiltration, histological evidence of vasculitis, and mononeuritis multiplex; asthma is the most prevalent clinical manifestation at presentation (170). Although not included in formal diagnostic criteria, weight loss, fever, myalgia, skin involvement, arthralgia, and gastrointestinal involvement are also common (170). The most common thin-section CT findings include bilateral ground glass attenuation, airspace consolidation (predominantly subpleural and surrounded by ground glass attenuation), centrilobular nodules (mostly within ground glass attenuation) bronchial wall thickening, and increased vessel caliber (171).

CSS is often difficult to diagnose, due to striking variations in clinical behavior between patients, and a high frequency of clinical and histological features that overlap with other granulomatous, vasculitic, and eosinophilic disorders (172). "Typical" histological features (necrotizing vasculitis, eosinophilic tissue infiltration, extravascular granulomas) are not consistently captured at biopsy. The significance of an association between leukotriene receptor antagonist administration and CSS remains uncertain (173–177).

Corticosteroid therapy, with or without an immunosuppressive agent (usually cyclophosphamide during initial treatment) results in remission in 90%, although 25% of patients relapse (170); plasma exchange is sometimes warranted in refractory disease. The long-term prognosis is good, although low-dose oral steroid therapy is usually required for asthma for many years, even when clinical evidence of vasculitis regresses rapidly (170).

Although pleural involvement is generally regarded as rare, as shown in a long-term follow-up study of 96 patients (170), a review of the English literature before 1984 disclosed a prevalence of pleural effusions of 30% in 61 patients with documented chest radiograph (172). In a more recent study of nine patients with CSS, pleural effusions were detected in two (as well as two pericardial effusions) (171). In one case with diagnostic features at lung biopsy, thoracocentesis yielded an acidotic exudative effusion with low glucose, low C3, eosinophilia, and a markedly increased RF (178), and in a second case, histological features diagnostic of CSS were present on pleural biopsy (179). Thus, pleural involvement is an occasional feature of CSS.

XII. Wegener's Granulomatosis

Wegener's granulomatosis (WG) is a disease of unknown etiology, characterized histologically by necrotizing granulomatous angiitis. The nose, lungs, and kidneys are classical sites of involvement on which a clinical diagnosis was based historically, but the disease can affect almost all other organ systems (180). Based on a series of 77 patients, pulmonary symptoms (cough, mild dyspnea, hemoptysis, chest pain) occur in more than 95% patients (181). However, reported cohorts vary greatly due to selection bias and a major increase in the detection of subclinical disease with characterization of serological features. Most patients with WG have serum antineutrophil cytoplasmic antibodies, with granular immunofluorescence staining in the cytoplasm (c-ANCA) (182); the measurement of c-ANCA titers is now widespread in suspected autoimmune disease, and less severe WG is increasingly diagnosed.

Characteristic imaging features include nodules and pulmonary infiltrates (181), but chest radiographic appearances often understate the extent of pulmonary involvement and CT is sometimes invaluable (183), especially when it discloses previously undetected cavitation within opacities (181). The course of WG has been dramatically improved by daily treatment with cyclophosphamide and glucocorticoids. Nonetheless, relapses are common (184).

Based upon the studies of small groups of patients, minor pleural involvement is not infrequent. In studies of small groups of patients, effusions were present on chest radiography in 6 out of 11, 4 out of 11, 4 out of 77, and 4 out of 18 cases (181,185–187). Pleural thickening is occasionally evident on chest radiography (187) or CT (188), and pneumothorax has been reported (189). Pleural aspiration has shown an exudative neutrophilic content, with protein levels 38 to 57 g/L in 4 out of 77 cases with an effusion (181).

Pleural effusions in WG are seldom clinically important and generally resolve spontaneously, or regress with the introduction of corticosteroid and/or immunosuppressive treatment.

XIII. Miscellaneous Diseases

Pleural effusions occasionally accompany other connective tissue diseases, including polyarteritis nodosa (190), temporal arteritis (191), giant cell arteritis (192,193), Kawasaki disease (194), Adamantiades–Behcet syndrome (195), human adjuvant disease (196), and adult-onset Still's disease (AOSD) (197–199). The major difficulty in characterizing pleural involvement in these disorders is the paucity of cases of diseases that are, themselves, rare. Thus, steroid-responsive exudative effusions have been reported in temporal arteritis in a handful of cases, but little more is known about this complication (191,200,201). In giant cell arteritis, pulmonary involvement is similarly rare and consists of interstitial infiltration, pulmonary nodules, pulmonary artery vasculitis, granuloma formation, and, in a few cases (192,193), pleural effusions (202–205).

Pleuropulmonary complications are more prevalent in Kawasaki disease. In a series of 129 patients, chest radiographic abnormalities were identified in 15%, invariably within 10 days of the onset, and included reticulonodular patterns, peribronchial cuffing, atelectasis, and air trapping—pleural effusions were found in only 3% of the population (194). The pathological basis of radiographic abnormalities remains uncertain in the absence of histological evaluation, but heart failure was not implicated, and it appears likely that the abnormalities represented lower respiratory tract inflammation and/or pulmonary arteritis, both features of Kawasaki disease (194).

Human adjuvant disease is a connective tissue disease occurring after cosmetic surgery with silicone injections or implants. There is a single report of a chylous effusion developing in association with a lupus-like syndrome, after mammary augmentation with silicone gel-filled prostheses (196).

AOSD is a rare splenic disorder of unknown cause, which may involve other organs, including the liver, kidney, bone marrow, and, less frequently, the lungs. Pulmonary involvement usually consists of pleural effusion or transient pulmonary infiltrates; life-threatening progression to the acute respiratory distress syndrome has been reported. High-dose corticosteroid therapy tends to be used as first-line treatment of pulmonary complications, although responses have also been achieved with cyclophosphamide, azathioprine, and intravenous immunoglobulin (199).

References

1. Fuller HM. On Rheumatism, Rheumatic Gout and Sciatica: Their Pathology, Symptoms and Treatment. New York, NY: S.S. and W. Wood, 1854.
2. Hunninghake GW, Fauci AS. Pulmonary involvement in the collagen vascular diseases. Am Rev Respir Dis 1979; 119:471–503.
3. Walker WC, Wright V. Pulmonary lesions and rheumatoid arthritis. Medicine (Baltimore) 1968; 47:501–520.
4. Hyland RH, Gordon DA, Broder I, et al. A systematic controlled study of pulmonary abnormalities in rheumatoid arthritis. J Rheumatol 1983; 10:395–405.
5. Dodson WH, Hollingsworth JW. Pleural effusion in rheumatoid arthritis. Impaired transport of glucose. N Engl J Med 1966; 275:1337–1342.

6. Jurik AG, Davidsen D, Graudal H. Prevalence of pulmonary involvement in rheumatoid arthritis and its relationship to some characteristics of the patients. A radiological and clinical study. Scand J Rheumatol 1982; 11:217–224.

7. Balbir-Gurman A, Yigla M, Nahir AM, et al. Rheumatoid pleural effusion. Semin Arthritis Rheum 2006; 35:368–378.

8. Hakala M, Tiilikainen A, Hameenkorpi R, et al. Rheumatoid arthritis with pleural effusion includes a subgroup with autoimmune features and HLA-B8, Dw3 association. Scand J Rheumatol 1986; 15:290–296.

9. Faurschou P, Francis D, Faarup P. Thoracoscopic, histological, and clinical findings in nine case of rheumatoid pleural effusion. Thorax 1985; 40:371–375.

10. Aru A, Engel U, Francis D. Characteristic and specific histological findings in rheumatoid pleurisy. Acta Pathol Microbiol Immunol Scand A 1986; 94:57–62.

11. Ferguson GC. Cholesterol pleural effusion in rheumatoid lung disease. Thorax 1966; 21: 577–582.

12. Lillington GA, Carr DT, Mayne GJ. Rheumatoid pleurisy with pleural effusion. Arch Intern Med 1971; 128:764–768.

13. Halla JT, Schronhenloher RE, Volanakis JE. Immune complexes and other laboratory features of pleural effusions. Ann Intern Med 1980; 92:748–752.

14. Pritikin JD, Jensen WA, Yenokida GG, et al. Respiratory failure due to a massive rheumatoid pleural effusion. J Rheumatol 1990; 17:673–675.

15. Brennan SR, Daly JJ. Large pleural effusions in rheumatoid arthritis. Br J Dis Chest 1979; 73:133–140.

16. Joseph J, Sahn SA. Connective tissue diseases and the pleura. Chest 1993; 104:262–270.

17. Ayzenberg O, Reiff DB, Levin L. Bilateral pneumothoraces and pleural effusions complicating rheumatoid lung disease. Thorax 1983; 38:159–160.

18. Brown KK. Rheumatoid lung disease. Proc Am Thorac Soc 2007; 4:443–448.

19. Ferrer JS, Munoz XG, Orriols RM, et al. Evolution of idiopathic pleural effusion: A prospective, long-term follow-up study. Chest 1996; 109:1508–1513.

20. Hunder GG, McDuffie FC, Hepper NG. Pleural fluid complement in systemic lupus erythematosus and rheumatoid arthritis. Ann Intern Med 1972; 76:357–363.

21. Salomaa ER, Viander M, Saaresranta T, et al. Complement components and their activation products in pleural fluid. Chest 1998; 114:723–730.

22. Pettersson T, Ojala K, Weber TH. Adenosine deaminase in the diagnosis of pleural effusions. Acta Med Scand 1984; 215:299–304.

23. Naylor B. The pathognomonic cytologic picture of rheumatoid pleuritis. Acta Cytol 1990; 34:465–473.

24. Sahn SA. Immunologic diseases of the pleura. Clin Chest Med 1985; 6:103–112.

25. Faurschou P. Decreased glucose in RA-cell-positive pleural effusion: Correlation of pleural glucose, lactic dehydrogenase and protein concentration to the presence of RA-cells. Eur J Respir Dis 1984; 65:272–277.

26. Carr DT, McGuckin WF. Pleural fluid glucose. Am Rev Respir Dis 1968; 97:302–305.

27. Jones FL, Blodget RC. Empyema in rheumatoid pleuropulmonary disease. Ann Intern Med 1971; 74:665–671.

28. Dieppe PA. Empyema in rheumatoid arthritis. Ann Rheum Dis 1975; 34:181–185.

29. Alegre J, Surinach JM, Varela E, et al. Diagnostic accuracy of pleural fluid polymorphonuclear elastase in the differentiation between pyogenic bacterial infectious and non-infectious pleural effusions. Respiration 2000; 67:426–432.

30. Alemán C, Alegre J, Segura RM, et al. Polymorphonuclear elastase in the early diagnosis of complicated pyogenic pleural effusions. Respiration 2003; 70:462–467.

31. Alemán C, Alegre J, Andreu J, et al. Accuracy of chest sonography and polymorphonuclear elastase in the assessment of bacterial pleural effusion. Eur J Intern Med 2004; 15:89–92.

32. Bouros D, Panagou P. Pleural fluid polymorphonuclear elastase: Cui bono? Respiration 2003; 70:453–454.
33. Martel W, Abell MR, Mikkelsen WM, et al. Pulmonary and pleural lesions in rheumatoid disease. Radiology 1968; 90:641–653.
34. Adelman HM, Dupont EL, Flannery MT, et al. Case report: Recurrent pneumothorax in a patient with rheumatoid arthritis. Am J Med Sci 1994; 308:171–172.
35. Sharma SS, Reynolds PM. Broncho-pleural fistula complicating rheumatoid lung disease. Postgrad Med J 1982; 58:187–189.
36. Portner MM, Gracie WAJ. Rheumatoid lung disease with cavitary nodules, pneumothorax and eosinophilia. N Engl J Med 1966; 275:697–700.
37. Crisp AJ, Armstrong RD, Grahame R, et al. Rheumatoid lung disease, pneumothorax, and eosinophilia. Ann Rheum Dis 1982; 41:137–140.
38. Anonymous. Pleural effusion in rheumatoid arthritis (editorials). Lancet 1972; 1:480–481.
39. Faurschou P. Rheumatoid pleuritis and thoracoscopy. Scand J Respir Dis 1974; 55: 277–283.
40. Faurschou P. Thoracoscopy in rheumatoid pleural effusion. Pneumologic 1989; 43:69–71.
41. Ward R. Pleural effusion and rheumatoid disease. Lancet 1961; 2:1336.
42. Russell ML, Gladman DD, Mintz S. Rheumatoid pleural effusion: Lack of response to intrapleural corticosteroid. J Rheumatol 1986; 13:412–415.
43. Emerson RA. Pleural effusion complicating rheumatoid arthritis. Br Med J 1956; 1:428.
44. Walker WC, Wright W. Rheumatoid pleuritis. Ann Rheum Dis 1967; 26:467.
45. Brunk JR, Drash EC, Swineford O. Rheumatoid pleuritis successfully treated with decortication. Am J Med 1966; 251:545.
46. Yarbrough JW, Sealy WC, Miller JA. Thoracic surgical problems associated with rheumatoid arthritis. J Thorac Cardiovasc Surg 1975; 69:347–354.
47. Chapman PT, O' Donnell JL, Moller PW. Rheumatoid pleural effusion: Response to intrapleural corticosteroid. Rheumatology 1992; 19:478–480.
48. Light RW, Jenkinson SG, Minh VD, et al. Observations on pleural pressures as fluid is withdrawn during thoracentesis. Am Rev Respir Dis 1980; 121:799–804.
49. Cohen AS, Reynolds WE, Franklin EC. Preliminary criteria for the classification of systemic lupus erythematosus. Bull Rheum Dis 1971; 21:643–648.
50. Pines A, Kaplinsky N, Olchovsky D, et al. Pleuro-pulmonary manifestations of systemic lupus erythematosus: Clinical features of its subgroups. Prognostic and therapeutic implications. Chest 1985; 88:129–135.
51. Halla JT, Schrohenloher RE, Volanakis JE. Immune complexes and other laboratory features of pleural effusions: A comparison of rheumatoid arthritis, systemic lupus erythematosus, and other diseases. Ann Intern Med 1980; 92:748–752.
52. Good JT Jr, King TE, Antony VB, et al. Lupus pleuritis. Clinical features and pleural fluid characteristics with special reference to pleural fluid antinuclear antibodies. Chest 1983; 84:714–718.
53. Alarcon-Segovia D, Alarcon DG. Pleuro-pulmonary manifestations of systemic lupus erythematosus. Dis Chest 1961; 39:7–17.
54. Ropes MW. Systemic Lupus Erythematosus. Cambridge, MA: Harvard University Press, 1976.
55. Miller LR, Greenberg SD, McLarty JW. Lupus lung. Chest 1985; 88:265–269.
56. Haupt HM, Moore GW, Hutchins GM. The lung in systemic lupus erythematosus. Analysis of the pathologic changes in 120 patients. Am J Med 1981; 71:791–798.
57. Gross M, Esterly JR, Earle RH. Pulmonary alterations in systemic lupus erythematosus. Am Rev Respir Dis 1972; 105:572–577.
58. Miller MH, Urowitz MB, Gladman DD, et al. Systemic lupus erythematosus in males. Medicine (Baltimore) 1983; 62:327–334.

59. Harvey AM, Shulman LE, Tumulty PA, et al. Systemic lupus erythematosus: A review of the literature and clinical analysis of 138 cases. Medicine 1954; 33:291–437.
60. Winslow WA, Ploss LN, Loitman B. Pleuritis in systemic lupus erythematosus: Its importance as an early manifestation in diagnosis. Ann Intern Med 1958; 49:70–88.
61. Segasothy M, Phillips PA. Systemic lupus erythematosus in Aborigines and Caucasians in central Australia: A comparative study. Lupus 2001; 10:439–444.
62. Camilleri F, Mallia C. Male SLE patients in Malta. Adv Exp Med Biol 1999; 455: 173–179.
63. Molina JF, Molina J, Garcia C, et al. Ethnic differences in the clinical expression of systemic lupus erythematosus: A comparative study between African-Americans and Latin Americans. Lupus 1997; 6:63–67.
64. Chang CC, Shih TY, Chu SJ, et al. Lupus in Chinese male: A retrospective study of 61 patients. Chung Hua I Hsueh Tsa Chih (Taipei) 1995; 55:143–150.
65. Costallat LT, Coimbra AM. Systemic lupus erythematosus in 18 Brazilian males: Clinical and laboratory analysis. Clin Rheumatol 1993; 12:522–525.
66. Al Rawi Z Al, Shaarbaf H Al, Raheem E, et al. Clinical features of early cases of systemic lupus erythematosus in Iraqui patients. Br J Rheumatol 1983; 22:165–171.
67. Gueft B, Laufer A. Futher cytochemical studies in systemic lupus erythematosus. Arch Pathol 1954; 57:201.
68. Bell R, Lawrence DS. Chronic pleurisy in systemic lupus erythematosus treated with pleurectomy. Br J Dis Chest 1979; 73:314–316.
69. Wang DY, Chang DB, Kuo SH, et al. Systemic lupus erythematosus presenting as pleural effusion: Report of a case. J Formos Med Assoc 1995; 94:746–749.
70. Baker SB, Rovira JR, Campion EW, et al. Late onset systemic lupus erythematosus. Am J Med 1979; 66:727–732.
71. Chantarojanasiri T, Sittirath A, Preutthipan A, et al. Pulmonary involvement in childhood systemic lupus erythematosus. J Med Assoc Thai 1999; 82(Suppl. 1):S144–S148.
72. Bouros D, Panagou P, Papandreou L, et al. Massive bilateral pleural effusion as the only first presentation of systemic lupus erythematosus. Respiration 1992; 59:173–175.
73. Elborn JS, Conn P, Roberts SD. Refractory massive pleural effusion in systemic lupus erythematosus treated by pleurectomy. Ann Rheum Dis 1987; 46:77–80.
74. Kaine JL. Refractory massive pleural effusion in systemic lupus erythematosus treated with talc poudrage. Ann Rheum Dis 1985; 44:61–64.
75. Bulgrin JG, Dubois EL, Jacobson G. Chest roentgenographic changes in systemic lupus erythematosus. Radiology 1960; 74:42.
76. Taylor TL, Ostrum H. The roentgen evaluation of systemic lupus erythematosus. Am J Roentgenol 1959; 82:95.
77. Mathlouthi A, Ben M'rad S, Merai S, et al. Massive pleural effusion in systemic lupus erythematosus: Thoracoscopic and immunohistological findings. Monaldi Arch Chest Dis 1998; 53:34–36.
78. Mulkey D, Hudson L. Massive spontaneous unilateral hemothorax in systemic lupus erythematosus. Am J Med 1974; 56:570.
79. Brook I. Measurement of lactic acid in pleural fluid. Respiration 1980; 40:344–348.
80. Carstens ME, Burgess LJ, Maritz FJ, et al. Isoenzymes of adenosine deaminase in pleural effusions: A diagnostic tool? Int J Tuberc Lung Dis 1998; 2:831–835.
81. Passero FC, Myers AR. Hemopneumothorax in systemic lupus erythematosus. J Rheumatol 1980; 7:183–186.
82. Lakhotia M, Mehta SR, Mathur D, et al. Diagnostic significance of pleural fluid eosinophilia during initial thoracocentesis. Indian J Chest Dis Allied Sci 1989; 31:259–264.
83. Wysenbeek AJ, Pick AI, Sella A, et al. Eosinophilic pleural effusion with high anti-DNA activity as a manifestation of systemic lupus erythematosus. Postgrad Med J 1980; 56:57–58.

84. Carr DT, Lillington GA, Mayne JG. Pleural-fluid glucose in systemic lupus erythematosus. Mayo Clin Proc 1970; 45:409–412.
85. Hunder GG, McDuffie FC, Huston KA, et al. Pleural fluid complement, complement conversion, and immune complexes in immunologic and nonimmunologic diseases. J Lab Clin Med 1977; 90:971–980.
86. Glovsky MM, Louie JS, Pitts WH Jr, et al. Reduction of pleural fluid complement activity in patients with systemic lupus erythematosus and rheumatoid arthritis. Clin Immunol Immunopathol 1976; 6:31–41.
87. Andrews BS, Arora NS, Shadforth MF, et al. The role of immune complexes in the pathogenesis of pleural effusions. Am Rev Respir Dis 1981; 124:115–120.
88. Kimura K, Ezoe K, Yokozeki H, et al. Elevated serum CA125 in progressive systemic sclerosis with pleural effusion. J Dermatol 1995; 22:28–31.
89. Yucel AE, Calguneri M, Ruacan S. False positive pleural biopsy and high CA125 levels in serum and pleural effusion in systemic lupus erythematosus. Clin Rheumatol 1996; 15: 295–297.
90. Small P, Frank H, Kreisman H, et al. An immunological evaluation of pleural effusions in systemic lupus erythematosus. Ann Allergy 1982; 49:101–103.
91. Swaak AJ, Huysen V, Nossent JC, et al. Antinuclear antibody profiles in relation to specific disease manifestations of systemic lupus erythematosus. Clin Rheumatol 1990; 9:82–94.
92. Camilleri F, Mallia C. RNP positivity in Maltese SLE patients. Adv Exp Med Biol 1999; 455:161–166.
93. Khare V, Baethge B, Lang S, et al. Antinuclear antibodies in pleural fluid. Chest 1994; 106:866–871.
94. Riska H, Fyhrquist F, Selander RK, et al. Systemic lupus erythematosus and DNA antibodies in pleural effusions. Scand J Rheumatol 1978; 7:159–160.
95. Ferreiro JE, Reiter WM, Saldana MJ. Systemic lupus erythematosus presenting as chronic serositis with no demonstrable antinuclear antibodies. Am J Med 1984; 76:1100–1105.
96. Wang DY, Yang PC, Yu WL, et al. Comparison of different diagnostic methods for lupus pleuritis and pericarditis: A prospective three-year study. J Formos Med Assoc 2000; 99: 375–380.
97. Carel RS, Shapiro MS, Cordoba O, et al. LE cells in pleural fluid. Arthritis Rheum 1979; 22:936–937.
98. Keshgegian AA. Lupus erythematosus cells in pleural fluid. Am J Clin Pathol 1978; 69: 570–571.
99. Naylor B. Cytological aspects of pleural, peritoneal and pericardial fluids from patients with systemic lupus erythematosus. Cytopathology 1992; 3:1–8.
100. Yoshiyuki OR, Shioya S, Handa K, et al. Lupus erythematosus cells in pleural fluid cytologic diagnosis in two patients. Acta Cytol 1977; 21:215–217.
101. Reda MG, Baigelman W. Pleural effusion in systemic lupus erythematosus. Acta Cytol 1980; 24:553–557.
102. Makashir R, Jayaram G. Lupus erythematosus cells in pleural fluid. Diagn Cytopathol 1988; 4:273–274.
103. Sethi S, Pooley RJ, Yu GH. Lupus erythematosus (LE) cells in pleural fluid: Initial diagnosis of systemic lupus erythematosus by cytologic examination. Cytopathology 1996; 7:292– 294.
104. Chao TY, Huang SH, Chu CC. Lupus erythematosus cells in pleural effusions: Diagnostic of systemic lupus erythematosus? Acta Cytol 1997; 41:1231–1233.
105. Greis M, Atay Z. Zytomorphologische Begleitreaction bei malignen Pleuraerguessen. Pneumonologie 1990; 44(Suppl.):262–264.
106. Hunder GG, Pierre RV. In vivo LE cell phenomenon. Arthritis Rheum 1970; 13:570–571.
107. Chandrasekhar AJ, Robinson J, Barr L. Antibody deposition in the pleura: A finding in drug-induced lupus. J Allergy Clin Immunol 1978; 61:399–402.

108. Pertschuk LP, Moccia LF, Rosen Y, et al. Acute pulmonary complications in systemic lupus erythematosus. Immunofluorescence and light microscopic study. Am J Clin Pathol 1977; 68:553–557.

109. Keane MP, Lynch JP III. Pleuropulmonary manifestations of systemic lupus erythematosus. Thorax 2000; 55:159–166.

110. Jay MS, Jerath R, Van Derzalm T, et al. Pneumothorax in an adolescent with fulminant systemic lupus erythematosus. J Adolesc Health Care 1984; 5:142–144.

111. Brasington RD, Furst DE. Pulmonary disease in systemic lupus erythematosus. Clin Exp Rheumatol 1985; 3:269–276.

112. Ben Chetrit E, Putterman C, Naparstek Y. Lupus refractory pleural effusion: Transient response to intravenous immunoglobulins. J Rheumatol 1991; 18:1635–1637.

113. Sherer Y, Langevitz P, Levy Y, et al. Treatment of chronic bilateral pleural effusions with intravenous immunoglobulin and cyclosporin. Lupus 1999; 8:324–327.

114. McKnight KM, Adair NE, Agudelo CA. Successful use of tetracycline pleurodesis to treat massive pleural effusion secondary to systemic lupus erythematosus. Arthritis Rheum 1991; 34:1483–1484.

115. Gilleece MH, Evans CC, Bucknall RC. Steroid resistant pleural effusion in systemic lupus erythematosus treated with tetracycline pleurodesis. Ann Rheum Dis 1988; 47:1031–1032.

116. Cook RJ, Gladman DD, Pericak D, et al. Prediction of short term mortality in systemic lupus erythematosus with time dependent measures of disease activity. J Rheumatol 2000; 27:1892–1895.

117. Cervera R, Khamashta MA, Font J, et al. Morbidity and mortality in systemic lupus erythematosus during a 5-year period. A multicenter prospective study of 1000 patients. European Working Party on Systemic Lupus Erythematosus. Medicine (Baltimore) 1999; 78: 167– 175.

118. Funauchi M, Ikoma S, Yu H, et al. A case of progressive systemic sclerosis complicated by massive pleural effusion with elevated CA125. Lupus 2000; 9:382–385.

119. Hiramatsu K, Takeda N, Okumura S, et al. Progressive systemic sclerosis associated with massive pleural and pericardial effusion in a 90-year-old woman. Nippon Ronen Igakkai Zasshi 1996; 33:535–539.

120. Lee YH, Ji JD, Shim JJ, et al. Exudative pleural effusion and pleural leukocytoclastic vasculitis in limited scleroderma. J Rheumatol 1998; 25:1006–1008.

121. Thompson AE, Pope JE. A study of the frequency of pericardial and pleural effusions in scleroderma. Br J Rheumatol 1998; 37:1320–1323.

122. Takeda N, Teramoto S, Ihn H, et al. A case of very late onset overlap syndrome of systemic sclerosis and systemic lupus erythematosus. Nippon Ronen Igakkai Zasshi 2000; 37:74–79.

123. Maeshima E, Nishimoto T, Yamashita M, et al. Progressive systemic sclerosis-polymyositis overlap syndrome with eosinophilic pleural effusion. Rheumatol Int 2003; 23:252–254.

124. Pearson CM, Bohan A. The spectrum of polymyositis and dermatomyositis. Med Clin North Am 1977; 61:439–457.

125. Kagen LJ. Polymyositis/dermatomyositis. In: McCarthy DJ, Koopman WJ, eds. Arthritis and Related Conditions. Philadelphia, PA: Lee and Febiger, 1993:1225.

126. Lakhanpal S, Lie JT, Conn DL, et al. Pulmonary disease in polymyositis/ dermatomyositis: A clinicopathological analysis of 65 autopsy cases. Ann Rheum Dis 1987; 46:23–29.

127. Ozawa Y, Kurosaka D, Hashimoto N. An autopsy case of dermatomyositis with rapidly progressive interstitial pneumonia. Nihon Rinsho Meneki Gakkai Kaishi 1995; 18:552–558.

128. Schwarz MI, Matthay RA, Sahn SA, et al. Interstitial lung disease in polymyositis and dermatomyositis: Analysis of six cases and review of the literature. Medicine (Baltimore) 1976; 55:89–104.

129. Miyata M, Fukaya E, Takagi T, et al. Two patients with polymyositis or dermatomyositis complicated with massive pleural effusion. Intern Med 1998; 37:1058–1063.

130. Mogulkoc N, Kabasakal Y, Ekren PK, et al. An unusual presentation of anti-Jo-1 syndrome, mimicking lung metastases, with massive pleural and pericardial effusions. J Clin Rheumatol 2006; 12:90–92.

131. Constantopoulos SH, Tsianos EV, Moutsopoulos HM. Pulmonary and gastrointestinal manifestations of Sjögren's syndrome. Rheum Dis Clin North Am 1992; 18:617–635.

132. Kawamata K, Haraoka H, Hirohata S, et al. Pleurisy in primary Sjögren's syndrome: T cell receptor beta-chain variable region gene bias and local autoantibody production in the pleural effusion. Clin Exp Rheumatol 1997; 15:193–196.

133. Bloch KJ, Buchanan WW, Wohl MJ, et al. Sjögren's syndrome. A clinical, pathological, and serological study of sixty-two cases. Medicine (Baltimore) 1992; 71:386–401.

134. Constantopoulos SH, Papadimitriou CS, Moutsopoulos HM. Respiratory manifestations in primary Sjögren's syndrome. A clinical, functional, and histologic study. Chest 1985; 88: 226–229.

135. Strimlan CV, Rosenow EC III, Divertie MB, et al. Pulmonary manifestations of Sjögren's syndrome. Chest 1976; 70:354–361.

136. Papathanasiou MP, Constantopoulos SH, Tsampoulas C, et al. Reappraisal of respiratory abnormalities in primary and secondary Sjögren's syndrome. A controlled study. Chest 1986; 90:370–374.

137. Kashiwabara K, Kishi K, Narushima K, et al. Primary Sjögren's syndrome accompanied by pleural effusion. Nihon Kyobu Shikkan Gakkai Zasshi 1995; 33:1325–1329.

138. Tanaka A, Tohda Y, Fukuoka M, et al. A case of Sjögren's syndrome with pleural effusion. Nihon Kokyuki Gakkai Zasshi 2000; 38:628–631.

139. Ogihara T, Nakatani A, Ito H, et al. Sjögren's syndrome with pleural effusion. Intern Med 1995; 34:811–814.

140. Alvarez-Sala R, Sanchez-Toril F, Garcia-Martinez J, et al. Primary Sjögren syndrome and pleural effusion. Chest 1989; 96:1440–1441.

141. Teshigawara K, Kakizaki S, Horiya M, et al. Primary Sjogren's syndrome complicated by bilateral pleural effusion. Respirology 2008; 13:155–158.

142. Davies D. Ankylosing spondylitis and lung fibrosis. Q J Med 1972; 41:395–417.

143. Haslock I. Ankylosing spondylitis. Baillieres Clin Rheumatol 1993; 7:99–115.

144. Tanaka H, Itoh E, Shibusa T, et al. Pleural effusion in ankylosing spondylitis: Successful treatment with intra-pleural steroid administration. Respir Med 1995; 89:509–511.

145. Dudley-Hart F, Bogdanovich A, Nichol WD. The thorax in ankylosing spondilitis. Ann Rheum Dis 1950; 9:116–131.

146. Kinnear WJ, Shneerson JM. Acute pleural effusions in inactive ankylosing spondylitis. Thorax 1985; 40:150–151.

147. Zorab PA. The lungs in ankylosing spondylitis. Q J Med 1962; 31:267–280.

148. Crompton GK, Cameron SJ, Langlands AO. Pulmonary fibrosis, pulmonary tuberculosis and ankylosing spondylitis. Br J Dis Chest 1974; 68:51–56.

149. Spencer DG, Park WM, Dick HM, et al. Radiological manifestations in 200 patients with ankylosing spondylitis: Correlation with clinical features and HLA B27. J Rheumatol 1979; 6:305–315.

150. Rosenow E, Strimlan CV, Muhm JR, et al. Pleuropulmonary manifestations of ankylosing spondylitis. Mayo Clin Proc 1977; 52:641–649.

151. Erkan L, Uzun O, Findik S, et al. Isolated pleural and pericardial effusion in a patient with ankylosing spondylitis. Respir Med 2007; 101:356–358.

152. Richard P, Sabouret P, Vayre F, et al. Pleuropericarditis complicated of tamponade disclosing mixed connective tissue disease. Remission with non-steroidal anti-inflammatory agents. Apropos of a case. Ann Cardiol Angeiol (Paris) 1996; 45:513–515.

153. Prakash UB. Lungs in mixed connective tissue disease. J Thorac Imaging 1992; 7:55–61.

154. Prakash UB. Respiratory complications in mixed connective tissue disease. Clin Chest Med 1998; 19:733–746, ix.

155. Sullivan WD, Hurst DJ, Harmon CE, et al. A prospective evaluation emphasizing pulmonary involvement in patients with mixed connective tissue disease. Medicine (Baltimore) 1984; 63:92–107.

156. Beier JM, Nielsen HL, Nielsen D. Pleuritis-pericarditis—An unusual initial manifestation of mixed connective tissue disease. Eur Heart J 1992; 13:859–861.

157. Hoogsteden HC, van Dongen JJ, van der Kwast TH, et al. Bilateral exudative pleuritis, an unusual pulmonary onset of mixed connective tissue disease. Respiration 1985; 48:164–167.

158. Ilan Y, Ben Yehuda A, Okon E, et al. Mixed connective tissue disease presenting as a left sided pleural effusion. Ann Rheum Dis 1992; 51:1157–1158.

159. Swygert LA, Maes EF, Sewell LE, et al. Eosinophilia–myalgia syndrome. Results of national surveillance. JAMA 1990; 264:1698–1703.

160. Martin RW, Duffy J, Engel AG, et al. The clinical spectrum of the eosinophilia–myalgia syndrome associated with L-tryptophan ingestion. Clinical features in 20 patients and aspects of pathophysiology. Ann Intern Med 1990; 113:124–134.

161. Killen JW, Swift GL, White RJ. Eosinophilic fasciitis with pulmonary and pleural involvement. Postgrad Med J 2000; 76:36–37.

162. Strumpf IJ, Drucker RD, Anders KH, et al. Acute eosinophilic pulmonary disease associated with the ingestion of L-tryptophan-containing products. Chest 1991; 99:8–13.

163. Andre M, Canon JL, Levecque P, et al. Eosinophilia–myalgia syndrome associated with L-tryptophan. A case report with pulmonary manifestations and review of the literature. Acta Clin Belg 1991; 46:178–182.

164. Williamson MR, Eidson M, Rosenberg RD, et al. Eosinophilia–myalgia syndrome: Findings on chest radiographs in 18 patients. Radiology 1991; 180:849–852.

165. Grangeia Tde A, Schweller M, Paschoal IA, et al. Acute respiratory failure as a manifestation of eosinophilia–myalgia syndrome associated with L-tryptophan intake. J Bras Pneumol 2007; 33:747–751.

166. Lukes RJ, Tindle BH. Immunoblastic lymphadenopathy. A hyperimmune entity resembling Hodgkin's disease. N Engl J Med 1975; 292:1–8.

167. Cullen MH, Stansfeld AG, Oliver RT, et al. Angio-immunoblastic lymphadenopathy: Report of ten cases and review of the literature. Q J Med 1979; 48:151–177.

168. Shaw RA, Schonfeld SA, Whitcomb ME. A perplexing case of hilar adenopathy. Clinical conference in pulmonary disease from the Ohio State University College of Medicine. Chest 1981; 80:736–740.

169. Sugiyama H, Kotajima F, Kamimura M, et al. Pulmonary involvement in immunoblastic lymphadenopathy: Case reports and review of literature published in Japan. Nihon Kyobu Shikkan Gakkai Zasshi 1995; 33:1276–1282.

170. Guillevin L, Cohen P, Gayraud M, et al. Churg–Strauss syndrome. Clinical study and long-term follow-up of 96 patients. Medicine (Baltimore) 1999; 78:26–37.

171. Choi YH, Im JG, Han BK, et al. Thoracic manifestation of Churg–Strauss syndrome: Radiologic and clinical findings. Chest 2000; 117:117–124.

172. Lanham JG, Elkon KB, Pusey CD, et al. Systemic vasculitis with asthma and eosinophilia: A clinical approach to the Churg–Strauss syndrome. Medicine (Baltimore) 1984; 63: 65–81.

173. Ben Noun L. Drug-induced respiratory disorders: Incidence, prevention and management. Drug Saf 2000; 23:143–164.

174. Wechsler ME, Garpestad E, Flier SR, et al. Pulmonary infiltrates, eosinophilia, and cardiomyopathy following corticosteroid withdrawal in patients with asthma receiving zafirlukast. JAMA 1998; 279:455–457.

175. Wechsler ME, Pauwels R, Drazen JM. Leukotriene modifiers and Churg–Strauss syndrome: Adverse effect or response to corticosteroid withdrawal? Drug Saf 1999; 21:241–251.

176. Wechsler ME, Drazen JM. Zafirlukast and Churg–Strauss syndrome. Chest 1999; 116: 266–267.

177. Wechsler ME, Finn D, Gunawardena D, et al. Churg–Strauss syndrome in patients receiving montelukast as treatment for asthma. Chest 2000; 117:708–713.

178. Erzurum SC, Underwood GA, Hamilos DL, et al. Pleural effusion in Churg–Strauss syndrome. Chest 1989; 95:1357–1359.

179. Hirasaki S, Kamei T, Iwasaki Y, et al. Churg–Strauss syndrome with pleural involvement. Intern Med 2000; 39:976–978.

180. Bambery P, Sakhuja V, Behera D, et al. Pleural effusions in Wegener's granulomatosis: Report of five patients and a brief review of the literature. Scand J Rheumatol 1991; 20: 445–447.

181. Cordier JF, Valeyre D, Guillevin L, et al. Pulmonary Wegener's granulomatosis. A clinical and imaging study of 77 cases. Chest 1990; 97:906–912.

182. Homer RJ. Antineutrophil cytoplasmic antibodies as markers for systemic autoimmune disease. Clin Chest Med 1998; 19:627–639, viii.

183. Papiris SA, Manoussakis MN, Drosos AA, et al. Imaging of thoracic Wegener's granulomatosis: The computed tomographic appearance. Am J Med 1992; 93:529–536.

184. Hoffman GS, Kerr GS, Leavitt RY, et al. Wegener granulomatosis: An analysis of 158 patients. Ann Intern Med 1992; 116:488–498.

185. Gonzalez L, Van Ordstr HS. Wegener's granulomatosis. Review of 11 cases. Radiology 1973; 107:295–300.

186. Bambery P, Katariya S, Sakhuja V, et al. Wegener's granulomatosis in north India. Radiologic manifestations in eleven patients. Acta Radiol 1988; 29:11–13.

187. Fauci AS, Wolff SM. Wegener's granulomatosis: Studies in eighteen patients and a review of the literature. Medicine (Baltimore) 1973; 73:315–324.

188. Weir IH, Muller NL, Chiles C, et al. Wegener's granulomatosis: Findings from computed tomography of the chest in 10 patients. Can Assoc Radiol J 1992; 43:31–34.

189. Jaspan T, Davison AM, Walker WC. Spontaneous pneumothorax in Wegener's granulomatosis. Thorax 1982; 37:774–775.

190. Bosch X, Ramirez J. Bilateral lung images and respiratory insufficiency in an 86-year-old man with polyarteritis nodosa. Med Clin (Barc) 1999; 113:189–197.

191. Turiaf J, Valere PE, Gubler MC. Recurrent pleurisy during temporal arteritis. Poumon Coeur 1967; 23:633–652.

192. Ramos A, Laguna P, Cuervas V. Pleural effusion in giant cell arteritis. Ann Intern Med 1992; 116:957.

193. Gur H, Ehrenfeld M, Izsak E. Pleural effusion as a presenting manifestation of giant cell arteritis. Clin Rheumatol 1996; 15:200–203.

194. Umezawa T, Saji T, Matsuo N, et al. Chest x-ray findings in the acute phase of Kawasaki disease. Pediatr Radiol 1989; 20:48–51.

195. Tunaci A, Berkmen YM, Gokmen E. Thoracic involvement in Behcet's disease: Pathologic, clinical, and imaging features. AJR Am J Roentgenol 1995; 164:51–56.

196. Walsh FW, Solomon DA, Espinoza LR, et al. Human adjuvant disease. A new cause of chylous effusions. Arch Intern Med 1989; 149:1194–1196.

197. Pasteur M, Laroche C, Keogan M. Pleuropericardial effusion in a 50 year old woman. Pleuropericardial effusion caused by adult inset Still's disease. Postgrad Med J 2001; 77: 346–355, 357.

198. Nishio J, Koike R, Iizuka H, et al. A refractory case of adult-onset Still's disease. Nihon Rinsho Meneki Gakkai Kaishi 1997; 20:191–198.

199. Cheema GS, Quismorio FP Jr. Pulmonary involvement in adult-onset Still's disease. Curr Opin Pulm Med 1999; 5:305–309.

200. Romero S, Vela P, Padilla I, et al. Pleural effusion as manifestation of temporal arteritis. Thorax 1992; 47:398–399.

201. Garcia-Alfranca F, Solans R, Simeon C, et al. Pleural effusion as a form of presentation of temporal arteritis. Br J Rheumatol 1998; 37:802–803.

202. Gedalia A, Molina JF, Molina J, et al. Childhoodonset systemic lupus erythematosus: A comparative study of African Americans and Latin Americans. J Natl Med Assoc 1999; 91:497–501.

203. Nadorra RL, Landing BH. Pulmonary lesions in childhood onset systemic lupus erythematosus: Analysis of 26 cases, and summary of literature. Pediatr Pathol 1987; 7:1–18.

204. Katz VL, Kuller JA, McCoy MC, et al. Fatal lupus pleuritis presenting in pregnancy. A case report. J Reprod Med 1996; 41:537–540.

205. Gould DM, Dayes ML. Roentgenologic findings in systemic lupus erythematosus. J Chronic Dis 1955; 2:136–145.

32
Pleural Effusions in Blood Diseases

DESPINA S. KYRIAKOU
University of Thessaly Medical School, University Hospital of Larissa, Larissa, Thessaly, Greece

MICHAEL G. ALEXANDRAKIS
University of Crete Medical School, University Hospital of Heraklion, Heraklion, Crete, Greece

DEMOSTHENES BOUROS
Democritus University of Thrace Medical School, University Hospital of Alexandroupolis, Alexandroupolis, Greece

Pleural effusions can be present in nearly all hematological diseases at presentation or during the clinical course of the disease. The disease itself, drug toxicity, radiotherapy underlying infections, secondary malignancies, autoimmune phenomena, extramedullary hemopoiesis, and other complications may contribute to effusion development (1–71). Non-Hodgkin's lymphomas most commonly are complicated with effusions, especially when mediastinal involvement is present (1,2,65,70,72). The second most common condition is bone marrow transplantation, while pleural effusions rarely accompany the remaining hematological diseases (73).

Applications of Light's criteria for differentiation between exudate and transudate as well as examination of the cells in the fluid by light microscopy, flow cytometry, and gene rearrangement studies are methods to detect malignant involvement of the pleural fluid (3–5). It has been proved that examination of the cytocentrifuge specimens by hematology laboratory is highly sensitive and superior for detection of malignancies than cytopathology (1,16,66,74).

The treatment of pleural effusions depends on the etiology. Disease improvement is accompanied by disappearance of the effusion (75) caused by the disease itself. Recurrent resistant effusions may need intrapleural infusions of cytotoxic drugs (i.e., methotrexate), pleurodesis (i.e., talc), or local treatment with biological drugs, that is, bortezomib or rituximab (33,35,74–78). In cases where the effusion is due to complications such as infection, cardiac failure, etc., treatment of the underlying cause also improves the effusion in most cases.

I. Non-Hodgkin's Lymphomas and Hodgkin's Disease

Pleural effusion in lymphomas is usually observed in advanced disease, and in the majority of reported patients, it is present at diagnosis (4,6,9,10,14,65,70,79–81). The presence of effusion may adversely affect the prognosis of the disease in most cases (1,10,14,79). Pleural effusions occur in up to 20% to 30% of patients with non-Hodgkin's lymphomas (NHL) and Hodgkin's disease (1,71). On the other hand, up to 10% of malignant pleural effusions are due to NHL (2). T-cell lymphomas, especially the lymphoblastic type, most frequently involve the serous fluids (65). Primary mediastinal lymphoma is often accompanied by unilateral or bilateral effusion, especially if there is bulky disease (65). In childhood, mediastinal lymphomas are primarily of the lymphoblastic type and are accompanied usually by pleural effusions. Among patients with lymphomatous pleural effusion, diffuse large B-cell lymphomas is the most frequent type (up to 58%), while about 7% are of the small lymphocytic type (69,81) Low-grade lymphomas such as small lymphocytic lymphoma in stage III and IV are most often associated with pleural effusions due to disease infiltration of the pleura (65,67,70,71,74,75,82). Mucosa-associated lymphoid tissue (MALT) lymphoma of the pleura is a rare type of lymphoma that presents with pleural effusion (83). Other types of primary pleural NHL are very rare (70) and the majority of information in the literature is based on minor observational studies or case reports (1–105).

In the majority of cases the pleural effusion is due to infiltration of the pleura, is an exudate (15–18), and appears serous or serosanguineous on aspiration. It may be unilateral or bilateral and as a rule it causes symptoms such as dyspnea, cough, and chest pain. In 12% of cases the effusion is chylous (1,69,75). Transudative or exudative reactive pleural effusions have also been reported to accompany lung involvement in lymphomas (5,9,13,24–28). In rare cases, especially in advanced stages of low-grade lymphomas with multiple organ infiltration, the pleural effusion is a transudate due to venous compression, cardiac or renal failure, and hypoalbuminemia (23). A case of urinothorax due to ureter obstruction has been reported (64). In Hodgkin's disease, pleural effusion is rarely attributed to infiltration and is most commonly due to other causes (19,20,29). Infections (especially tuberculosis), central lymphatic obstruction, pleural damage due to previous irradiation or chemotherapy, and infiltration by other neoplasms should also be considered in the differential diagnosis (19–23,66,68,105).

Lymphomatous involvement of pleura is often characterized by the presence of clonal lymphocytes in the effusion with the same phenotype as in the affected lymph nodes (2,3,16,18,20,30–32). Thoracocentesis results in a positive cytological diagnosis in 60% to 90% of patients with NHL and pleural involvement. The diagnostic yield may be further increased by thoracoscopy (15–17,33–35,74). In the cases of reactive pleural effusions, lymphocytes are small, mature, polyclonal, and predominantly of the T-cell subset (16,28,36,37). Difficulties in distinguishing morphologically neoplastic from reactive lymphocytes arise often in cytopathological specimens, especially in small lymphocytic/lymphoblastic lymphomas (16). Hematological examination of cytocentrifuge specimens after May–Grunwald/Giemsa staining is highly sensitive to diagnose lymphoma and is superior to cytology (74,75,79,82,84). In addition, flow cytometry, immunocytochemistry, Ig, and TCR rearrangements, as well as oncogene expression studies and cytogenetics, are useful tools for typing and differentiation of lymphoid cells in pleural fluid (15,16,33,38–42,83,106). Combined morphology and immunophenotyping has sensitivity and specificity up to 100% and gives a quick diagnosis as well as information about classification, grade of malignancy, and the presence of viral nucleic acids (65).

Hodgkin's disease rarely affects the pleura and almost in any case it is due to advanced local disease. Pleural damage by radiation or development of schwannoma secondary to radiotherapy has been described (71,105). In addition, treatment-related other secondary neoplasms may develop in the pleura. However, the primary mechanism of pleural effusion in Hodgkin's disease is thoracic duct obstruction and impaired lymphatic drainage (65).

MALT lymphoma of the pleura is rare. Usually, it is disseminated within the lung affecting pleura simultaneously. It is characterized by macrophages within the lymphomatous tissue and most frequently belongs to the low-grade type. It mostly affects gastrointestinal tract but it may develop anywhere in mucosa-associated lymphoid tissue. The diagnosis is made by thoracoscopy and pleural biopsy. Pleural effusion is a common feature if pleura is infiltrated and the fluid usually contains lymphomatous cells of the small cell type. In the differential diagnosis, mesothelioma is the most common feature. The prognosis is very good (9,74,83,106,107–110).

Primary effusion lymphoma (PEL) is a unique clinicopathological entity initially observed in HIV-positive patients when the CD4+ cells are less than 100 to 200/μL. It is recently individualized from the remaining NHL (WHO classification). It accounts for 1% to 2% of NHL in these patients (26,43–51,111–114) and develops mainly in males, homosexuals, and in advanced stages of HIV disease. Occasionally, it appears in other immunosuppressed patients (post-transplantation) (99,100,111,112). PEL has also been reported in childhood (30,44). This lymphoma is of B-cell origin, belongs to the high grade of malignancy group, and is associated with human herpesvirus-8 (HHV-8) (also termed Kaposi sarcoma-HHV) infection. It preferentially grows in liquid phase in serous body cavities (51–57). Very rarely lymphoid masses are detected in these patients. In 50% of cases, coinfection with Epstein–Barr virus (EBV) exists (48,52–54,58,96,113,114). Cases of T-cell or NK-cell phenotypes have been reported but expression of activation markers (CD30, CD38, HLADR) is almost universal (7,38,40,45,46,48,50,61,65). DNA analysis revealed immunoglobulin-heavy chain (IgH) or TCR rearrangements inserted HHV-8 sequences as well as EBV DNA sequences in many cases. In some cases, the malignant cells are HIV+/HSV8+/EBV− in HIV+/HHV8+/EBV+ patients (52,54,60,87,93). In almost all cases, the cells of PEL express CD138/syndecan-1 antigen, suggesting a possible role of this molecule in the serosal preference of these cells (59,90).

Kaposi's sarcoma and multicentric Castelman's disease patients may develop body cavity effusions that either fulfill the criteria of HHV-8–positive PEL or may represent an HHV-8–associated nonneoplastic process (46). In the latter cases, effusions are rich in monocytes/macrophages and in some cases harbor B-cell monoclonal proliferation. These observations support the hypothesis of multistage PEL development and the fact that a prelymphomatous effusion may precede overt body cavity lymphoma. Recently, a tumorous PEL, solid variant of PEL HHV-8 related, has been described in HIV patients with higher levels of CD4+ cells. The strong association to HHV-8 has led to the introduction of antiviral treatment in patients with PEL with improved results.

Pyothorax-associated lymphoma (PAL), develops in the pleural cavity after long-standing pyothorax (62,115), is of exclusively B-cell origin and is strongly associated with EBV infection. HHV-8 is not an obligate pathogen in PAL, as it is not detected in all cases (62). PAL should be defined as a malignant lymphoma developing in chronic inflammation.

II. Acute Leukemias

Pleural effusions are common finding at autopsy in patients with acute leukemia (63). In most cases, microscopic infiltration of the pleura is observed. As these patients die mostly because of infection or hemorrhage, in almost all cases the pleural effusion is hemorrhagic or empyema (63,69). During the course of the disease, pleural effusions are rare events and in most cases reflect underlying infections, hypoalbuminaemia, cardiac or liver failure (69,116–119).

Effusions due to detectable leukemic infiltration in living patients are very rare and only case reports are found in the literature (120–122). Most cases represent acute lymphoblastic leukemia especially of the T-cell type. Involvement of the pleura is more frequent in childhood (123–125). Cases with pleural involvement at presentation are extremely rare and the same is true for extramedullar leukemic development in pleura as the only site (122,126–138). In contrast, extramedular disease in unusual sites such as pleura, are being recognized with increased frequency as long-term survival is improved in these patients (136–140). Granulocytic sarcoma is a solid tumor of myeloid origin and is the solid variant of acute myelogenous leukemia. Development of granulocytic sarcoma in the pleura has been described (129,132,141–143).

Adult T-cell leukemia-lymphoma is a distinct lymphoid malignancy presenting with four types: smoldering, chronic, lymphoma, and acute. In the stage of acute and lymphoma type, pleural (and/or ascitic) effusion may be present (144). In rare cases this disease may be localized to the pleura and/or peritoneum without involvement of other sites. Diagnosis is established by detection of specific surface markers for T lymphocytes and the determination of HTLV-1 viral DNA sequences in mononuclear cells of the effusion (142,144,145).

Unusual cases of hairy cell leukemia and plasma cell leukemia may present with pleural effusions with typical leukemic cells in the pleural fluid (146,147).

In all the above situations, the possibility of other causes for the pleural effusion should be excluded. Infections (bacterial or viral), solid tumors (most commonly adenocarcinoma), and complications of therapy should also be kept in mind when dealing with pleural effusions in leukemic patients. In addition, reactive pleural effusions may also be seen in lung diseases of various etiologies in these patients (121,144). Immunocytochemistry, flow cytometry, electron microscopy, and PCR applied to cytology specimens can contribute to the differential diagnosis, and the findings sometimes need to be confirmed by pleuroscopy and surgical biopsy (121,142,144,148). Cytological examination of pleural effusions has a higher yield in leukemia-lymphoma compared to solid tumors (16). This is explained by the tendency of leukemic blasts to infiltrate tissues and pass through serosal membranes easily due to the lack of adhesion molecules, while cells of most solid tumors usually cluster due to the presence of specialized adhesion mechanisms.

The development of pleural effusion in acute leukemia is rare and its prognostic significance is obscure. Some investigators have found that the presence of a pleural effusion at diagnosis in acute leukemia does not affect the rate of remission and survival. However, others report a worse prognosis, especially in plasmacytic and hairy cell leukemias (146,147).

A pleural effusion in patients with acute leukemias usually disappears quickly after induction chemotherapy if the patient achieves complete remission and may reappear at relapse. If the patients do not achieve remission, they may present with respiratory failure, due to fluid accumulation, necessitating local treatment of the pleural disease. This treatment involves intrapleural chemotherapy, pleurodesis, or frequent drainage (30,149,150).

III. Bone Marrow Transplantation

Pleural effusions are relatively common complications in bone marrow transplantation and result mainly from infections or tumor relapse (152). In the remaining patients with pleural effusion after bone marrow transplantation, acute or chronic graft-versus-host disease (GVHD) is the most common cause (152–154). In these cases, CD8+/HLADR+ lymphocytes with CD57 expression predominate in the fluid (80). Other causes include regimens with high-dose cytotoxic drugs or total body irradiation, post-transplant veno-occlusive disease (VOD), and capillary-leakage syndrome (155–159).

A distinguishable entity called posttransplantation lymphoproliferative disorder has been associated with the reactivation of EBV or cytomegalovirus (CMV) infection. This condition is accompanied by pleural effusion and sometimes by CD4+ lymphocyte expansion. It is a serious and sometimes fatal complication in these patients, who usually are resistant to immunosuppressive therapy (153).

Capillary-leakage syndrome occurs frequently after bone marrow transplantation in addition to GVHD and infections. The underlying pathophysiology is poorly understood, but the clinical manifestations of excessive weight gain, ascites, and edema associated with kidney and liver abnormalities suggest tissue injury in multiple organs. About 50% of allogeneic or autologous transplant recipients develop noncardiogenic pulmonary edema with or without pleural effusions; half of them are accompanied by hepatic dysfunction or renal dysfunction or central nervous system abnormalities. These observations suggest that circulating leukocytes may play a role in the development of the syndrome (156,157).

Hepatic VOD following bone marrow transplantation is associated with high-dose combination cytoreductive therapy during conditioning. Experimental models have suggested that drug-induced injury to hepatic sinusoidal endothelial cells is involved in the pathogenesis. About 50% of patients with VOD develop pleural fluid. VOD nearly always resolves after treatment (158).

IV. Myelodysplastic Syndromes

Pleural effusions in myelodysplastic syndromes (MDS) are rare and, as in most hemopoietic diseases, is a consequence of infection. Rarely, pleural infiltration with the malignant clone is observed, especially during transformation to acute leukemia. Immune disorders are observed in MDS patients with increased frequency but are rarely accompanied by pleural effusion. These cases display systemic vasculitis or eosinophilic infiltration of the lung as the underlying cause (133,160,161).

V. Chronic Leukemias

In chronic leukemias, the incidence of effusions, although rare, is higher than in acute leukemias (147,162–176). In chronic lymphocytic leukemia (CLL), the most common cause of pleural effusion is pleural infiltration. These infiltrations may predispose to the transformation to more aggressive lymphoid neoplasms such as Richter's syndrome and prolymphocytic transformation (165). In CLL the fluid may be hemorrhagic or not and contains numerous lymphocytes identical to those in the blood and bone marrow.

Lymphocytic pleural effusions, cytologically indistinguishable from those in CLL, are well recognized in tuberculous and other nonneoplastic conditions (22,169). Small lymphocytic infiltrations of the pleura are difficult to evaluate histopathologically. Usually, involvement of the pleura in B-CLL may lead to increased proportion of B cells in the pleural effusion with light-chain class restriction and monoclonal IgG heavy-chain rearrangements (170). In most reactive pleural effusions, T cells predominate and a small proportion of polyclonal B cells may be found. A high proportion of T cells, with monoclonal TCR rearrangements, may be found in T-cell neoplasms. Although some investigators suggest that the study of clonality and immunocytochemistry could provide a definite diagnosis, there are case reports where neoplastic infiltration by B-CLL leads to a reactive pleural effusion with predominant polyclonal T cells (168,170).

It is difficult to elucidate the precise pathophysiology of effusion development in each case. Increased lymphatic permeability associated with an active inflammatory-type response, pleural lymphatic obstruction, or more central mediastinal nodal involvement resulting in lymphatic obstruction or obstruction of the thoracic duct with chylothoraces and changes induced by other therapies may be possible mechanisms of effusion development. In cases with reactive effusions, cytotoxic T cells predominate, suggesting a possible antitumor effect of these cells (163,164,167,168).

In chronic myelocytic leukemia (CML) and chronic myelomonocytic leukemia (CMML), the most common cause of pleural effusions is extramedullary hemopoiesis, although pleura is the most uncommon site of extramedullary hemopoiesis in these patients (171–176). Hemopoiesis resembles that of the bone marrow. All the three hemopoietic lineages are present, and the degree of maturation is similar to that of the bone marrow. In Philadelphia-positive cases, the Philadelphia chromosome is detected in the pleural granulocytic cells by conventional cytogenetics and FISH method (66,101). In some cases, the extramedullary hemopoiesis consists of normal hemopoietic tissue only. In some other cases, pleural effusion is due to CML development in the pleura. In the latter case, the predominant cells are mature and immature granulocytes, monocytes, and variable numbers of blasts. The leukemic population is accompanied by variable numbers of reactive lymphocytes, macrophages, and activated mesothelial cells. The differential diagnosis usually presents difficulties, especially when the proportion of blasts is low. The fluid is usually hemorrhagic. Leukocyte alkaline phosphatase, known to be low in CML granulocytes in peripheral blood, has been reported to be normal in leukemic granulocytes of pleural effusions in the same patients. Pleural infiltration in CML and CMML sometimes appears shortly before transformation to acute leukemia, and in these cases the pleural effusion contains a greater proportion of myeloblasts (66,99).

In some cases, the development of pleural effusions is difficult to explain. Patients with CML and CMML may develop pleural fluid during uncontrolled leukocytosis. These effusions may develop without clinical evidence of extramedullary hemopoiesis or leukemic infiltration and are very responsive to conventional chemotherapy (172). Possible obstruction of pleural capillaries or infiltration of interstitial tissue by leukemic cells, increased capillary permeability due to cytokine production, and other nonspecific mechanisms may be responsible for the development of pleural effusions in these patients (172).

In other myeloproliferative disorders (myelofibrosis, polycythemia), the most common cause of pleuritis, other than infection, is extramedullary hemopoiesis and infiltration at the stage of leukemic transformation (171).

Rare conditions, belonging to chronic hematopoietic neoplasms, may be associated with serosal effusions including pleural effusions. Such conditions include systemic mastocytosis, chronic eosinophilic leukemia, and chronic granulocytic leukemia. The effusions in these patients are due to infiltration of the pleura with malignant cells or are reactive with predominantly macrophages, mesothelial cells, and T lymphocytes (141,177,178).

VI. Pleural Effusions Related to the Treatment of Hematological Malignancies

All-trans-retinoic acid (ATRA) is a differentiation agent that can induce complete remission in acute promyelocytic leukemia (APL). Unfortunately, about 50% of patients treated with ATRA may develop a life-threatening complication of uncertain pathogenesis (179). The main clinical signs are respiratory distress, fever, pulmonary infiltrates, weight gain, pleural effusion, renal failure, pericardial effusion, cardiac failure, edema, thromboembolic events, and hypotension. Some patients require mechanical ventilation or dialysis. The lung disease has been ascribed to infiltration of the parenchyma with leukemic or maturing myeloid cells to pulmonary capillaritis and pleuritis. The incidence of death in ATRA syndrome is 1.2% of the total APL patients treated with ATRA, but its occurrence has been associated with shorter remission duration and overall survival. The development of pleural effusion in most cases is of undetermined etiology. Pleural infiltration or pleural inflammation is sometimes the case (179–184).

Other chemotherapeutic regimens have been reported to induce pleural effusion in leukemia patients. High-dose regimens of cytosino-arabinoside, cyclophosphamide, and busulfan and other megatherapies have been reported to be associated with pleural effusions of undetermined pathophysiology. Irradiation of the mediastinum or the total body irradiation that is applied for conditioning in bone marrow transplantation is associated with pleural damage that may lead to pleural effusion (155,185). In addition, pleural effusions have rarely been reported after administration of GM-CSF and high-dose antiglobulin therapy (186,187).

Tyrosine kinase antagonists (biological drugs widely used for the treatment of chronic myelogenous leukemia, bcr/abl+), that is, imatinib, nilotinib, dasatinib, etc., present as a common adverse event edema and effusions. Pleural effusions with various amount of liquid appear in 0.01% to 18% of patients treated with bcr/abl inhibitors. The reason is that these drugs inhibit other tyrosine kinases in a nonspecific way (188,189). Imatinib present this adverse event more often while newer more targeted TKIs like nilotinib and dasatinib present this effect rarely.

VII. Multiple Myeloma

Pleural effusions in multiple myeloma may be due to nephrotic syndrome, pulmonary embolism, congestive heart failure, second neoplasms, and infiltration by the myeloma cells. In a large series of 958 multiple myeloma patients (190), 58 developed pleural effusions of various etiologies. In only six of them was the effusion attributed to infiltration by the myeloma. In other reports, the incidence of myelomatous pleural effusions is estimated to be <1% (191). Almost the whole remaining literature consists of case reports of various types of multiple myelomas or plasmatocytomas infiltrating the pleura. IgA multiple myeloma is responsible for 80% of the cases of multiple myeloma pleural effusions in the literature (192–197).

In most cases, the effusion contains numerous plasma cells secreting monoclonal immunoglobulin (M-component). M-component is identified in the cell-free effusion and is identical to that identified in the serum of the patients. Plasma cells in the effusion are also identical, in morphology and kinetics, to those of the bone marrow of the patients. In rare cases of nonsecreting myeloma, M-component is not found in the effusion. In these cases, the differentiation from lymphomas and undifferentiated carcinomas is usually easy, based on cell morphology and immunocytochemistry. In light-chain myeloma, immunoelectrophoresis of the pleural fluid reveals light chains. Immunocytochemistry and molecular biology may also be helpful (191–197).

A well-recognized complication of multiple myeloma is amyloidosis. Amyloidosis may also present as a complication of other chronic diseases or as the primary type. In exceptional cases, where amyloidosis involves the pleura, an effusion may develop with transudative or exudative features without any characteristic cell type. Diagnosis is made by pleuroscopy and pleural biopsy (198,199).

Waldenström's macroglobulinemia is a rare disorder with lymphoplasmacytic monoclonal proliferation and a high amount of monoclonal IgM immunoglobulin. In rare cases of pleural involvement, lymphoid and plasmatocytoid cells are found in the effusion and monoclonal IgM immunoglobulin in the cell free pleural fluid (200–201).

VIII. Thalassemias

Thalassemia major is characterized by severe anemia that needs to be treated with regular transfusions (202). In homozygous β-thalassemia, anemia develops at about the sixth month after birth because until then fetal hemoglobin (Hb F) effectively replaces hemoglobin A (Hb A). In homozygous α-thalassemia (with four genes affected), severe anemia is obvious at 16 weeks gestational age leading to hydrops fetalis and intrauterine death in most cases. In less severe cases, with nonzero homozygous α-thalassemia, the fetus may develop hydrops with bilateral pleural and ascitic effusions and grow further until birth. Today, with prenatal diagnosis of thalassemia in areas with high prevalence of the disease, cases with hydrops fetalis due to thalassemia are very rarely seen. In hemoglobinopathy H, a variety of α-thalassemia with three a-genes affected, the symptoms of anemia are obvious at birth (202). In β-thalassemia major, chronic anemia, and iron overload lead to cardiovascular damage and insufficiency. In addition, viral infections (HCV, HBV), together with iron overload, may lead to liver insufficiency. Heart and liver insufficiency with hypoalbuminemia are the most common causes of transudative effusions in these patients. Other possible cause of effusions in these patients are venous compression by extramedullary hemopoiesis in the mediastinum, extramedullary hemopoietic tumors in the lung with parapneumonic transudates, and direct infiltration of the pleura by hemopoietic masses producing exudates with erythropoietic precursors in the fluid (202–209). Some microorganisms grow preferentially in iron-rich environments producing infections in these patients at a higher frequency. Effusions may develop during the course of these infections (203,210).

Sickle cell disease is a common disorder in special communities. Sickle cell crisis, a predominant feature of this disease, may be accompanied by pleural effusion because of pulmonary infarction and/or subsequent infections (210–213).

IX. Anemias and Coagulation Disorders

In severe anemias (like megaloblastic anemia or aplastic anemia), cardiac failure is a cause of pleural effusion. Infections are also a common cause of effusions in many anemias, such as Fanconi's anemia, hereditary spherocytosis, other red cell membrane disorders, aplastic anemia, autoimmune anemias treated with corticosteroids, etc. In these cases,

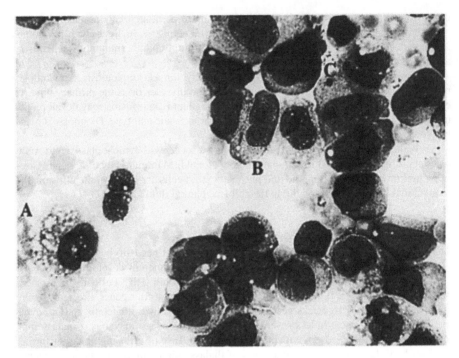

Figure 1 A case of acute nonlymphocytic leukemia. This 60-year-old man presented with chest pain and pleural effusion and no other finding. The effusion contained numerous myeloblasts with Auer bodies and Auer rods. Peroxidase staining was positive. Bone marrow aspiration revealed 60% infiltration with myeloblasts, while the peripheral blood did not contain immature granulocytes. The effusion disappeared after chemotherapy and reappeared at relapse. (**A**) Pleural macrophages, (**B**) blast cell with Auer rods, and (**C**) blast cell with Auer body.

treatment of the underlying cause leads to improvement of the effusion. Pleural effusions in coagulation disorders are almost always due to hemothorax (214–216).

References

1. Elis A, Blickstein D, Mulchanov I, et al. Pleural effusion in patients with non-Hodgkin's lymphoma: A case control study. Cancer 1998; 83:1607–1611.
2. Johnston WW. The malignant pleural effusion. A review of cytopathologic diagnosis of 584 specimens from 472 consecutive patients. Cancer 1985; 56:905–909.
3. Yasuda H, Nakao M, Kanemasa H, et al. T-cell lymphoma presenting with pericardial and pleural effusion as the initial and primary lesion: Cytogenetic and molecular evidence. Intern Med 1996; 35:150–154.
4. Raina V, Boyd G, Soukop M. Longstanding pleural effusion in an elderly man due to non-Hodgkin's lymphoma (multilobulated nuclear cell type). Aust NZ J Med 1990; 20:826–827.
5. Mizuki M, Ueda S, Tagawa S, et al. Natural killer-cell derived large granular lymphocyte lymphoma of lung developed in a patient with hypersensitivity to mosquito bites and reactivated Epstein–Barr virus infection. Am J Hematol 1998; 59:309–315.

6. Suster S, Moran CA. Pleomorphic large cell lymphoma of the mediastinum. Am J Surg Pathol 1996; 20:224–232.

7. Dunphy CH, Collins B, Ramos R, et al. Secondary pleural involvement by an AIDS related anaplastic large cell (CD30+) lymphoma simulating metastatic adenocarcinoma. Diagn Cytopathol 1998; 18:113–117.

8. Patriarcha F, Ermacora A, Skert C. Pleural involvement in a case of monocytoid B-cell lymphoma. Haematologica 1999; 84:949–950.

9. Kodama K, Yokose T, Takahashi K, et al. Low-grade B-cell lymphoma of mucosa-associated lymphoid tissue in the lung: A report of a case with pleural dissemination. Lung Cancer 1999; 24:175–178.

10. Siegert W, Nerl C, Agthe A, et al. Angioimmunoblastic lymphadenopathy (AILD)-type-T cell lymphoma: Prognostic impact of clinical observations and laboratory findings at presentation. The Kiel Lymphoma Study Group. Ann Oncol 1995; 6:659–664.

11. Shepherd SF, A'Hern RP, Pinkerton CR. Childhood T-cell lymphoblastic lymphoma. Does early resolution of mediastinal mass predict for final outcome? The United Kingdom Children's Cancer Study Group (UKCCSG). Br J Cancer 1995; 72:752–756.

12. Naschitz JE, Lazarow N, Yeshurun D. Unilateral chest wall edema with associated pleural effusion: unusual sign of primary retroperitoneal lymphoma. Lymphology 1984; 17: 34–36.

13. Berkman N, Breuer R, Kramer MR, et al. Pulmonary involvement in lymphoma. Leuk Lymphoma 1996; 20:237–299.

14. Snalund JT, Crist WM, Abromowitch M, et al. Pleural effusion is associated with a poor outcome in stage III small non-cleaved cell lymphoma. Leukemia 1991; 5:71–74.

15. Moriki T, Wada M, Takahashi T, et al. Pleural effusion cytology in a case of cytophagic histiocytic panniculitis (subcutaneous panniculitic T-cell lymphoma). A case report. Acta Cytol 2000; 44:1040–1044.

16. Bangerter M, Hildebrand A, Griesshammer M. Combined cytomorphologic and immunophenotypic analysis in the diagnostic workup of lymphomatous effusions. Acta Cytol 2001; 45:307–312.

17. Gulzman J, Bross KJ, Costabel U. Malignant lymphoma in pleural effusions: An immunohistochemical cell surface analysis. Diagn Cytopathol 1991; 7:113–118.

18. Chagnaud BE, Bonsack TA, Kozakewich HP, et al. Pleural effusions in lymphoblastic lymphoma: A diagnostic alternative. J Pediatr Surg 1998; 33:1355–1357.

19. Rondriguez-Garcia JL, Frail G, Moreno MA, et al. Recurrent massive pleural effusion as a late complication of radiotherapy in Hodgkin's disease. Chest 1991; 100:1165–1166.

20. Bishop PC, Elwood PC. Images in clinical medicine. Chylous effusion in Hodgkin's disease. N Engl J Med 1998; 339:1515.

21. Van Renterghem DM, Pauwels RA. Chylothorax and pleural effusions as a late complications of thoracic irradiation. Chest 1995; 108:884–886.

22. Valdes L, Alvarez D, Valle JM, et al. The etiology of pleural effusions in an area with high incidence of tuberculosis. Chest 1996; 109:158–162.

23. Sakemi T, Uchida M, Ikeda Y, et al. Acute renal failure and nephrotic syndrome in a patient with T-cell lymphoma. Nephron 1996; 72:326–327.

24. Collins J, Muller NL, Leung AN, et al. Epstein–Barr-virus associated lymphoproliferative disease of the lung: CT and histological findings. Radiology 1998; 208:749–759.

25. Ooi GC, Chim CS, Lie AK, et al. Computed tomography features of primary pulmonary non-Hodgkin's lymphoma. Clin Radiol 1999; 54:438–443.

26. Ray P, Antoine M, Mary-Krause M, et al. AIDS-related primary pulmonary lymphoma. Am J Respir Crit Care Med 1998; 158:1221–1229.

27. Bazot M, Cadranel J, Benayoun S, et al. Primary pulmonary AIDS-related lymphoma: Radiographic and CT findings. Chest 1999; 11:1282–1286.

28. Aquino SL, Chen MY, Kuo WT, et al. The CT appearance of pleural and extrapleural disease in lymphoma. Clin Radiol 1999; 54:647–650.

29. Moritani T, Aihara T, Oguma E, et al. Spectrum of Epstein–Barr virus infection in Japanese children. A pictorial essay. Clin Imaging 2001; 25:1–8.

30. Das DK, Chowdhury V, Kishore B, et al. CD-30 (Ki-1)-positive anaplastic large cell lymphoma in a pleural effusion. Case report with diagnosis by cytomorphologic and immunocytochemical studies. Acta Cytol 1999; 43:498–502.

31. Bangerter M, Hildebrand A, Griesshammer M. Immunophenotypic analysis of simultaneous specimens from different sites of the same patient with malignant lymphoma. Cytopathology 2001; 12:168–176.

32. Ohori NP, Whisnant RE, Nalesnik MA, et al. Primary pleural effusion post-transplant lymphoproliferative disorder: Distinction from secondary involvement and effusion lymphoma. Diagn Cytopathol 2001; 25:50–53.

33. Pietsch JB, Whitlock JA, Ford C, et al. Management of pleural effusions in children with malignant lymphoma. J Pediatr Surg 1999; 34:635–638.

34. Sahn SA. Malignancy metastatic to the pleura. Clin Chest Med 1998; 19:351–361.

35. Alifano M, Guggino G, Gentile M, et al. Management of concurrent pleural effusion in patients with lymphoma: Thoracoscopy a useful tool in diagnosis and treatment. Monaldi Arch Chest Dis 1997; 52:330–334.

36. Laurini JA, Garcia A, Elsner B, et al. Relation between natural killer cells and neoplastic cells in serious fluids. Diagn Cytopathol; 22:347–350.

37. Green LK, Griffin J. Increased natural killer cells in fluids. A new, sensitive means of detecting carcinoma. Acta Cytol 1996; 40:1240–1245.

38. Matolsky A, Nador RG, Cesarman E, et al. Immunoglobulin VH gene mutational analysis suggests that primary effusion lymphomas derive from different stages of B cell maturation. Am J Pathol 1998; 153:1609–1614.

39. Gaidano G, Carbone A, Dalla-Favera R. Pathogenesis of AIDS-related lymphomas: Molecular and histogenetic heterogeneity. Am J Pathol 1998; 152:623–630.

40. Falzetti D, Crescenzi B, Matteuci C, et al. Genomic instability and recurrent breakpoints are main cytogenetic findings in Hodgkin's disease. Haematologica 1999; 84:298–305.

41. Drexler HG, Uphoff CC, Gaidano G, et al. Lymphoma cell lines: In vitro models for the study of HHV-8(+) primary effusion lymphomas (body cavity based lymphomas). Leukemia 1998; 12:1507–1517.

42. Peterson IM, Raible M. Malignant pleural effusion in Hodgkin's lymphoma. Report of a case with immunoperoxidase studies. Acta Cytol 1991; 35:300–305.

43. Afessa B. Pleural effusions and pneumothoraces in AIDS. Curr Opin Pulm Med 2001; 7: 202–209.

44. Karadeniz C, Guven MA, Ruacan S, et al. Primary pleural lymphoma: An unusual presentation of childhood non-Hodgkin lymphoma. Pediatr Hematol Oncol 2000; 17:695–699.

45. Iwahashi M, Iida S, Sako S, et al. Primary effusion lymphoma with B-cell phenotype. Am J Hematol 2000; 64:317–318.

46. Casado Farinas I, Alonso Martin MJ, Gomez Aguado F, et al. Primary effusion lymphoma associated with type-8 human herpes virus infection. Ann Med Intern 2000; 17: 366–368.

47. Ferrozi F, Tognini G, Mulonzia NW, et al. Primary effusion lymphomas in AIDS: CT findings in two cases. Eur Radiol 2001; 11:623–625.

48. Ascoli V, Siriani MC, Mezzaroma I, et al. Human herpesvirus-8 in lymphomatous and nonlymphomatous body cavity effusions developing in Kaposi's sarcoma and multicentric Castelman's disease. Ann Diagn Pathol 1999; 3:357–363.

49. Ibrahimbacha A, Farah M, Saluza J. An HIV-infected patient with pleural effusion. Chest 1999; 116:1113–1115.

50. Nador RG, Cesarman E, Chadburn A, et al. Primary effusion lymphoma: A distinct clinicopathologic entity associated with Kaposi's sarcoma-associated herpes virus. Blood 1996; 88:645–656.

51. Light RW, Hamm H. Pleural disease and acquired immune deficiency syndrome. Eur Respir J 1997; 10:2638–2643.

52. Ascoli V, Mastroianni CM, Galati V, et al. Primary effusion lymphoma containing human herpesvirus 8 DNA in two AIDS patients with Kaposi's sarcoma. Haematologica 1998; 83:8–12.

53. Beck JM. Pleural disease in patients with acquired immune deficiency syndrome. Clin Chest Med 1998; 19:341–349.

54. Lacost V, Judde JG, Bestett G, et al. Virological and molecular characterization of a new B lymphoid cell line, established from an AIDS patient with primary effusion lymphoma, harboring both KSHV/HHV8 and EBV viruses. Leuk Lymphoma 2000; 38:401–409.

55. Perez MT, Cabanello-Inchausti B, Viamonte M Jr, et al. Pleural body cavity based lymphoma. Ann Diagn Pathol 1998; 2:127–134.

56. Vince A, Begovac J, Kessler H, et al. AIDS-related body cavity-based lymphoma. A case report. Acta Cytol 2001; 45:420–424.

57. Lankester KJ, Lishman S, Ayliffe U, et al. Primary effusion lymphoma and Kaposi's sarcoma in an HIV-infected man. Int J STD AIDS 1998; 9:616–618.

58. Arvanitakis L, Mesri EA, Nador RG, et al. Establishment and characterization of a primary effusion (body cavity based) lymphoma cell line (BC-3) harboring Kaposi's sarcoma-associated herpes virus (KSHV/HHV-8) in the absence of Epstein–Barr virus. Blood 1996; 88:2648–2654.

59. Kuwabara H, Nagai M, Shibanushi T, et al. CD138-positive and Kaposi's sarcoma-associated herpesvirus (KSHV)-negative B-cell lymphoma with serosal spreading of the body cavity and lymphadenopathy: An autopsy case. Human Pathol 2000; 31:1171–1175.

60. Carbone A, Cilia AM, Gloghini A, et al. Establishment of HHV-8-positive and HHV-8-negative lymphoma cell lines from primary lymphomatous effusions. Int J Cancer 1997; 73:562–569.

61. Hocqueloux L, Agbalika F, Oksenhendler E, et al. Long-term remission of an AIDS-related primary effusion lymphoma with antiviral therapy. AIDS 2001; 26(15):280–282.

62. O'Donovan M, Silva I, Uhlam V, et al. Expression profile of human herpesvirus 8 (HHV-8) in pyothorax associated lymphoma and in effusion lymphoma. Mol Pathol 2001; 54:80–85.

63. Suminoe A, Matsuzaki A, Koga Y, et al. Human herpesvirus 6 (HHV-6)-associated pleurisy after unrelated cord blood transplantation in children with chemotherapy-resistant malignant Lymphoma. J Pediatr Hematol Oncol 2007; 29(10):709–712.

64. Karkoulias K, Sampsonas F, Kaparianos A, et al. Urinothorax: An unexpected cause of pleural effusion in a patient with non-Hodgkin lymphoma. Eur Rev Med Pharmacol Sci 2007; 11(6):373–374.

65. Das DK. Serous effusions in malignant lymphomas: A review. Diagn Cytopathol 2006; 34(5): 335–347.

66. Awasthi A, Gupta N, Srinivasan R, et al. Cytopathological spectrum of unusual malignant pleural effusions at a tertiary care centre in north India. Cytopathology 2007; 18(1):28–32.

67. Griffo S, Gravino E, Luciano A, et al. The treatment by V.A.T.S. and M.A.C. of secondary neoplastic pleural effusion in the old patient (>70 years). Acta Biomed 2005; 76(Suppl. 1): 72–75.

68. Vafiadis E, Sidiropoulou MS, Voutsas V, et al. Eosinophilic pleural effusion, peripheral eosinophilia, pleural thickening, and hepatosplenomegaly in sarcoidosis. South Med J 2005; 98(12):1218–1222.

69. Fujisawa S, Tanioka F, Matsuoka T, et al. CD5+ diffuse large B-cell lymphoma with c-myc/IgH rearrangement presenting as primary effusion lymphoma. Int J Hematol 2005; 81(4):315–318.

70. Steiropoulos P, Kouliatsis G, Karpathiou G, et al. Rare cases of primary pleural Hodgkin and non-Hodgkin lymphomas. Respiration 2009; 77(4):459–463.

71. Choi W, Park YH, Paik KH, et al. Peripheral T-cell lymphoma-unspecified (PTCL-U) presenting with hypereosinophilic syndrome and pleural effusions. Korean J Intern Med 2006; 21(1): 57–61.

72. Chang CJ, Cheng JH, Lin MS, et al. Eosinophilic pleural effusion as the first presentation of angioimmunoblastic T cell lymphoma. J Formos Med Assoc 2007; 106(2):156–160.

73. Alexandrakis MG, Passam FH, Kyriakou DS, et al. Pleural effusions in hematologic malignancies. Chest 2004; 125:1546–55 and Chest 2005; 127:1866.

74. Kawahara K, Sasada S, Nagano T, et al. Pleural MALT lymphoma diagnosed on thoracoscopic resection under local anesthesia using an insulation-tipped diathermic knife. Pathol Int 2008; 58(4):253–256.

75. Heffner JE. Diagnosis and management of malignant pleural effusions. Respirology 2008; 13(1):5–20.

76. Kolschmann S, Ballin A, Gillissen A. Clinical efficacy and safety of thoracoscopic talc pleurodesis in malignant pleural effusions. Chest 2005; 128(3):1431–1435.

77. McConkey D, Nawrocki ST, Andtbacka R. Velcade displays promising activity in primary effusion lymphoma cells. Cancer Biol Ther 2005; 4(4):491–492.

78. Lim ST, Rubin N, Said J, et al. Primary effusion lymphoma: Successful treatment with highly active antiretroviral therapy and rituximab. Ann Hematol 2005; 84(8):551–552.

79. Bielsa S, Salud A, Martínez M, et al. Prognostic significance of pleural fluid data in patients with malignant effusion. Eur J Intern Med 2008; 19(5):334–339.

80. Hosoki K, Okada S, Ichinohasama R, et al. Angioimmunoblastic T-cell lymphoma developed with lymphocytic pleural effusion. Intern Med 2007; 46(11):739–742.

81. Vega F, Padula A, Valbuena JR, et al. Lymphoma involving the pleura. A clinicopathologic study of 34 cases diagnosed by pleural biopsy. Arch Pathol Lab Med 2006; 130:1497–1502.

82. Chang H, Sun CF. Detection of B cell lymphoma involvement in T cell-rich serous fluid by immunoglobulin gene rearrangement: A report of 2 cases. Acta Cytol 2008; 52:231–234.

83. Mitchell A, Meunier C, Ouellette D, et al. Extranodal marginal zone lymphoma of mucosa-associated lymphoid tissue with initial presentation in the pleura. Chest 2006; 129:791–794.

84. Anand M, Sharma S, Kumar R, et al. Diagnostic considerations in prolymphocytes in pleural fluid: A case report. Acta Cytol 2008; 52:251–254.

85. Vignes S, Bellanger J. Primary intestinal lymphangiectasia (Waldmann's disease). Orphanet J Rare Dis 2008; 3:5.

86. DeMonaco NA, Jacobs SA. Serum sickness in a patient with follicular lymphoma after rituximab and radioimmunotherapy with ibritumomab tiuxetan. Clin Nucl Med 2007; 32: 933–934.

87. Carbone A, Gloghini A. KSHV/HHV8-associated lymphomas. Br J Haematol 2008; 140: 13–24.

88. Marcelin AG, Motol J, Guihot A, et al. Relationship between the quantity of Kaposi sarcoma-associated herpesvirus (KSHV) in peripheral blood and effusion fluid samples and KSHV-associated disease. J Infect Dis 2007; 196:1163–1166.

89. Mocanu L, Cîmpean AM, Raica M. Expression of cytokeratin MNF116 and vimentin in pleural serous effusions. Rom J Morphol Embryol 2007; 48:291–294.

90. Wies E, Mori Y, Hahn A, et al. The viral interferon-regulatory factor-3 is required for the survival of KSHV-infected primary effusion lymphoma cells. Blood 2008; 111:320–327.

91. Dhingra KK, Singhal N, Nigam S, et al. Unsuspected multiples myeloma presenting as bilateral pleural effusion—A cytological diagnosis. Cytojournal 2007; 4:17.

92. Boulanger E, Meignin V, Afonso PV, et al. Extracavitary tumor after primary effusion lymphoma: Relapse or second distinct lymphoma? Haematologica 2007; 92:1275–1276.

93. Dargent JL, Kains JP, Verhest A. Primary effusion lymphoma presenting as Richter's syndrome. Cytopathology 2007; 18:319–321.

94. Brimo F, Michel RP, Khetani K, et al. Primary effusion lymphoma: A series of 4 cases and review of the literature with emphasis on cytomorphologic and immunocytochemical differential diagnosis. Cancer 2007; 111:224–233.
95. Chen YB, Rahemtullah A, Hochberg E. Primary effusion lymphoma. Oncologist 2007; 12:569–576.
96. Xu D, Coleman T, Zhang J, et al. Epstein–Barr virus inhibits Kaposi's sarcoma-associated herpesvirus lytic replication in primary effusion lymphomas. J Virol 2007; 81:6068–6078.
97. Licci S, Narciso P, Morelli L, et al. Primary effusion lymphoma in pleural and pericardial cavities with multiple solid nodal and extra-nodal involvement in a human immunodeficiency virus-positive patient. Leuk Lymphoma 2007; 48:209–211.
98. Shirokov D, Kadyrova E, Anokhina M, et al. A case of HHV-8-associated HIV-negative primary effusion lymphoma in Moscow. Med Virol 2007; 79:270–277.
99. Kobayashi Y, Kamitsuji Y, Kuroda J, et al. Comparison of human herpes virus 8 related primary effusion lymphoma with human herpes virus 8 unrelated primary effusion lymphoma-like lymphoma on the basis of HIV: Report of 2 cases and review of 212 cases in the literature. Acta Haematol 2007; 117(3):132–144.
100. Carbone A, Gloghini A. HHV-8-associated lymphoma: State-of-the-art review. Acta Haematol 2007; 117(3):129–131.
101. Ishii Y, Shoji N, Kimura Y, et al. Prominent pleural effusion possibly due to imatinib mesylate in adult Philadelphia chromosome-positive acute lymphoblastic leukemia. Intern Med 2006; 45(5): 339–340.
102. Youngster I, Vaisben E, Cohen H, et al. An unusual cause of pleural effusion. Age Ageing 2006; 35(1):94–96.
103. Asuquo BJ, Gould GA. Recurrent chylothorax in a patient with non-Hodgkins lymphoma: Case report. East Afr Med J 2004; 81(4):215–217.
104. Perlman S, Ben-Arie A, Feldberg E, et al. Non-Hodgkin's lymphoma presenting as advanced ovarian cancer—A case report and review of literature. Int J Gynecol Cancer 2005; 15(3): 554–557.
105. Morbidini-Gaffney S. Alpert TE, Hatoum GF. Benign pleural schwanoma secondary to radiotherapy for Hodgkin disease. Am J Clin Oncol 2005; 28:640–641.
106. Mihaescu A, Gebhard S, Chubert P, et al. Application of molecular diagnosis of lymphoid-rich effusions: Study of 95 cases with concomitant immunophenotyping. Diagn Cytopathol 2002; 27:90–95.
107. Natsag J, Tomiyama N, Inoue A, et al. Pulmonary mucosa-associated lymphoid tissue type lymphoma with increased accumulation of fluorine 18-fluorodeoxyglucose on positron emission tomography. J Comput Assist Tomogr 2005; 29:640–643.
108. Nicholson AG. Lymphocytic interstitial pneumonia and other lymphoproliferative disorders in the lung. Semin Respir Crit Care Med 2001; 22(4):409–422.
109. Valdez R, Finn WG, Ross CW, et al. Waldenström macroglobulinemia caused by extranodal marginal zone B-cell lymphoma: A report of six cases. Am J Clin Pathol 2002; 117(3): 495–496.
110. Dolz Aspas R, Toyas Miazza C, Ruiz Ruiz F, et al. Fluctuant pulmonary nodules as presentation of a MALT lymphoma. Ann Med Intern 2003; 20(11):582–584.
111. Rodriguez Salazar MJ, Raya Sanchez JM, Rodriguez Sanchez R, et al. HIV-associated primary body-cavity-based lymphoma: Clinico-biologic features in three patients diagnosed at the same institution. Ann Med Intern 2004; 21:175–178.
112. HisamotoA, Yamane H, Hiraki A, et al. Human herpes virus-8 negative primary effusion lymphoma in a patient with common variable immunodeficiency. Leuk Lymph 2003; 44: 2019–2022.
113. Inoue Y, Tsukasaki K, Nagai K, et al. Durable remmision by sobuzoxane in HIV-seronegative patient with human herpesvirus 8-negative primary effusion lymphoma. Int J Hematol 2004; 79:271–275.

114. Gomyo H, Kajimoto K, Maeda A, et al. t(14;18)(q32;q21)-bearing pleural MALT lymphoma with IgM paraproteinemia: Value of detection of specific cytogenetic abnormalities in the differential diagnosis of MALT lymphoma and lymphoplasmacytic lymphoma. Hematology 2007; 12:315–318.

115. Nakatsuka S, Yao M, Hoshida Y, et al. Pyothorax associated lymphoma: A review of 106 cases. J Clin Oncol 2002; 20:4255–4260.

116. Zhang SF, Guo BY, Wang HL. Clinicopathologic changes in leukemic lung lesions. Zhonghua Nei Ke Za Zhi 1994; 33:99–102.

117. Czader M, Ali SZ. Flow cytometry as an adjunct to cytomorphologic analysis of serous effusions. Diagn Cytopathol 2003; 29(2):74–78.

118. Miyake F, Yoshikawa T, Fujita A, et al. Pneumonia with marked pleural effusion caused by Aspergillus infection. Pediatr Infect Dis J 2006; 25(2):186–187.

119. Collet G, Marty P, Le Fichoux Y, et al. Pleural effusion as the first manifestation of pulmonary toxoplasmosis in a bone marrow transplant recipient. Acta Cytol 2004; 48(1): 114–116.

120. Mori M, Imamura Y, Maegawa H, et al. Cytology of pleural effusion associated with disseminated infection caused by varicella-zoster virus in an immunocompromised patient. A case report. Acta Cytol 2003; 47(3):480–484.

121. Mufti GJ, Oscier DG, Hamblin TJ, et al. Serous effusions in monocytic leukemias. Br J Hematol 1984; 58:547–552.

122. Mitchel CD, Gordon I, Chessells JM. Clinical, haematological, and radiological features in T-cell lymphoblastic malignancy in childhood. Clin Radiol 1986; 37:257–261.

123. Rege K, Powles C, Norton J, et al. An unusual presentation of acute myeloid leukemia with pericardial and pleural effusions due to granulocytic sarcoma. Leuk Lymphoma 1993; 11:305–307.

124. Karimi M, Eshghi P. Unusual lymphoblastic leukemia/lymphoma in Eastern Iran. Indian J Pediatr 2006; 73(7):619–622.

125. Fujisawa S, Tanioka F, Matsuoka T, et al. CD7/CD19 double-positive T-cell acute lymphoblastic leukemia. Int J Hematol 2006; 83(4):324–327.

126. Okada F, Ando Y, Kondo Y, et al. Thoracic CT findings of adult T-cell leukemia or lymphoma. AJR Am J Roentgenol 2004; 182(3):761–767.

127. Stafford CM, Herndier B, Yi ES, et al. Granulocytic sarcoma of the tracheobronchial tree: Bronchoscopic and pathologic correlation Respiration 2004; 71(5):529–532.

128. Fatih T, Selim Y, Mesut A, et al. An unusual cause of unilateral pleural effusion in the setting of aortic stenosis: Acute myeloid leukemia. Intern Med 2007; 46(6):325–327.

129. Farray D, Al-Masri H, Hattersley E, et al. Megakaryoblastic leukemia with involvement of the pleural fluid. Am J Hematol 2005; 79(3):238–239.

130. Dettrick AJ, Robertson T, Morris KL. Diagnosis of granulocytic sarcoma on pleural effusion cytology: Report of a case. Diagn Cytopathol 2004; 31(2):126–128.

131. Azoulay E, Fieux F, Moreau D, et al. Acute monocytic leukemia presenting as acute respiratory failure. Am J Respir Crit Care Med 2003; 167:1329–1333.

132. Uchida A, Miyata A, Ikeda Y, et al. Myeloid/natural killer cell precursor acute leukemia initiated with pleural effusion. Nippon Naika Gakkai Zasshi 2002; 91:2463–2465.

133. Mital OP, Sacham AS, Singh RP, et al. Acute myelogenous leukemia presenting as massive pleural effusion. Indian J Chest Dis 1975; 17:179–181.

134. Hicsönmez G, Cetin M, Yenicesu I, et al. Evaluation of children with myelodysplastic syndrome: Importance of extramedullary disease as a presenting symptom. Leuk Lymphoma 2001; 42(4):665–674.

135. Au WY, Shek TW, Gascoyne RD, et al. Leukemic infiltration of an adenocarcinoma effusion. Br J Haematol 2001; 112(2):257.

136. Saha PK, Agrawal BV, Mishra SK, et al. Pleuropericardial effusion: A presenting manifestation of acute myeloblastic leukemia. Indian Heart J 1977; 29:165–169.

137. Nasilowska-Adamska B, Majewski M, Seferynska I, et al. Predictive value of RT-PCR PML-RARA transcript monitoring for extramedullary relapse of acute promyelocytic leukemia in the pleura, heart and pericardium after allogeneic SCT. Ann Transplant 2007; 12(3):33–38.
138. Nadrous HF, Krowka MJ, McClure RF, et al. Agnogenic myeloid metaplasia with pleural extramedullary leukemic transformation. Leuk Lymphoma 2004; 45:815–818.
139. Disel U, Yavuz S, Paydas S, et al. Extramedullary relapse in the pleura in acute promyelocytic leukemia. Leuk Lymphoma 2003; 44(1):189–191.
140. Park J, Park SY, Cho HI, et al. Isolated extramedullary relapse in the pleural fluid of a patient with acute myeloid leukemia following allogeneic BMT. Bone Marrow Transplant 2002; 30(1):57–59.
141. Dix DB, Anderson RA, McFadden DE, et al. Pleural relapse during hemopoietic remission in childhood acute lymphoblastic leukemia. J Pediatr Hematol Oncol 1997; 19:470–472.
142. Yam LT. Granulocytic sarcoma with pleural involvement. Identification of neoplastic cells with cytometry. Acta Cytol 1985; 29:63–66.
143. Scmetzer HM, Williams W, Gerhartz HH. Detection of acute myeloid leukemia cells in complete remission and in extramedullary sites by clonal analysis. Acta Haematol 1996; 96:83–87.
144. Gutweiler JR, Labelle J, Suh MY, et al. A familial case of pleuropulmonary blastoma. Eur J Pediatr Surg 2008; 18:192–194.
145. Shimoyama M. Diagnostic criteria and classification of clinical subtypes of adult T-cell leukemia-lymphoma. A report from the Lymphoma Study Group (1984–87). Br J Haematol 1991; 79:428–437.
146. Takasugi JE, Godwin JD, Marglin SI, et al. Intrathoracic granulocytic sarcomas. J Thor Imaging 1996; 11:223–230.
147. Fukushima Y, Miyakumi T, Yoshida K, et al. Pleural effusion in a case of plasma cell leukemia after undergoing simple total hysterectomy for uterine cervical carcinoma. Review of multiple myeloma and plasma cell leukemia effusion in Japan. Rinsko Ketsueki 1987; 28:1424–1429.
148. Bouronchle BA. Unusual presentations and complications of hairy cell leukemia. Leukemia 1987; 1:288–293.
149. Bass J, White DA. Thoracentesis in patients with hematologic malignancy: Yield and safety. Chest 2005; 127:2101–2105.
150. Aasebo U, Norum J, Sager G, et al. Intrapleurally instilled mitoxanthrone in metastatic pleural effusions: A phase II study. J Chemother 1997; 9:106–111.
151. Bronner GM, Baas P, Beijnen JH. Pleurodesis in malignant pleural effusion. Ned Tijdschr Geneeskd 1997; 141:1810–1814.
152. Ueda T, Manabe A, Kikuchi A, et al. Massive pericardial and pleural effusion with anasarca following allogeneic bone marrow transplantation. Int J Hematol 2000; 71:394–397.
153. Lechapt-zalcman E, Rieux C, Cordonnier C, et al. Post-transplantation lymphoproliferative disorder mimicking nonspecific lymphocytic pleural effusion in a bone marrow transplant recipient. A case report. Acta Cytol 1999; 43:239–242.
154. Hashino S, Mori A, Kobayashi S, et al. Proliferation of CD4+ lymphocytes in a patient with chronic graft-versus-host disease after allogeneic bone marrow transplantation. Int J Hematol 2000; 71:389–393.
155. Seber A, Khan SP, Kersey JH. Unexplained effusions: association with allogeneic bone marrow transplantation and acute or chronic graft-versus-host disease. Bone Marrow Transplant 1996; 17:207–211.
156. Schaap N, Raymakers R, Schattenberg A, et al. Massive pleural effusion attributed to high-dose cyclophosphamide during conditioning for BMT. Bone Marrow Transplant 1996; 18:247–248.
157. Cahill RA, Spitzer TR, Mazumder A. Marrow engraftment and clinical manifestations of capillary leak syndrome. Bone Marrow Transplant 1996; 18:177–184.

158. Oeda E, Shinohara K, Kamei S, et al. Capillary leak syndrome likely the result of granulocyte colony stimulating factor after high-dose chemotherapy. Intern Med 1994; 33:115–119.

159. Ozkaynak MF, Weinberg K, Kohn D, et al. Hepatic veno-occlusive disease post-bone marrow transplantation in children conditioned with busulphan and cyclophosphamide: Incidence risk factors, and clinical outcome. Bone Marrow Transplant 1991; 7:467–474.

160. Veys PA, McAvinchery R, Rothman MT, et al. Pericardial effusion following conditioning for bone marrow transplantation in acute leukemia. Bone Marrow Transplant 1987; 2: 213–216.

161. Hicsonmez G, Tuncer AM, Sayli T, et al. High dose methylprednisolone, low-dose cytosine arabinoside, and mitoxanthrone in children with myelodysplastic syndromes. Hematol Pathol 1995; 9:185–193.

162. Matsushima T, Murakami H, Kim K, et al. Steroid-responsive pulmonary disorders associated with myelodysplastic syndromes with der(1q; 7p) chromosomal abnormality. Am J Hematol 1995; 50:110–115.

163. Bourantas KL, Tsiara S, Panteli A, et al. Pleural effusion in chronic myelomonocytic leukemia. Acta Hematolol 1998; 99:34–37.

164. Sivakumaran M, Qureshi H, Chapman CS. Chylous effusions in CLL. Leuk Lymphoma 1995; 18:365–366.

165. Andrieu V, Encaoua R, Carbon C, et al. Leukemic pleural effusion in B-cell prolymphocytic leukemia. Hematol Cell Ther 1998; 40:275–278.

166. Shimoni A, Shvidel L, Shtalrid M, et al. Prolymphocytic transformation of B-chronic lymphocytic leukemia presenting as malignant ascites and pleural effusion. Am J Hematol 1998; 59:316–318.

167. Jacobson RJ, Jacobson HJ, Derman DP. Leukemic involvement of the pleura. A case report. S Afr Med J 1977; 52:938–940.

168. Horn KD, Penchansky L. Chylous pleural effusions simulating leukemic infiltrate associated with thoracoabdominal disease and surgery in infants. Am J Clin Pathol 1999; 111:99–104.

169. Ben-Gherit E, Assaf Y, Shnar E. Predominant T-cells in pleural effusion of a patient with B-cell CLL. Acta Hematol 1985; 73:101–103.

170. Cooper C, Watts EJ, Smith AG. *Salmonella septicemia* and pleural effusion as presenting features of hairy cell leukemia. Br J Clin Pract 1987; 41:670–671.

171. Miyahara M, Shimamoto Y, Sano M, et al. Immunoglobulin gene rearrangement in T-cell-rich reactive pleural effusion of a patient with B-cell chronic lymphocytic leukemia. Acta Haematol 1996; 96:41–44.

172. Chubachi A, Wakui H, Miura I, et al. Extramedullary megacaryoblastic tumors following an indolent phase of myelofibrosis. Leuk Lymphoma 1995; 17:351–354.

173. Hicsonmez G, Cetin M, Tunc B, et al. Dramatic resolution of pleural effusion in children with chronic myelomonocytic leukemia following short-course high-dose methylprednisolone. Leuk Lymphoma 1998; 29:617–623.

174. Bourantas KL, Repousis P, Tsiara S, et al. Chronic myelogenous leukemia terminating in acute megakaryoblasting leukemia. Case report. J Exp Clin Cancer Res 1998; 17:234–235.

175. Lancon JP, Charve P, Favre JP, et al. Pleural myeloid metaplasia revealing chronic myelogenous leukemia. Crit Care Med 1986; 14:834–835.

176. Mohapatra MK, Das SP, Mohanty NC, et al. Hemopericardium with cardiac tamponade and pleural effusion in chronic myeloid leukemia. Indian Heart J 2000; 52:209–211.

177. De Renzo A, Micera V, Vaglio S, et al. Induction of alkaline phosphatase activity in chronic myeloid leukemia cells: In vitro studies and speculative hypothesis. Am J Hematol 1990; 35:278–280.

178. Petit A, Pulik M, Gaulier A, et al. Systemic mastocytosis associated with chronic myelomonocytic leukemia: Clinical features and response to interferon alpha therapy. J Am Acad Dermatol 1995; 32:850–853.

179. Farrell SA, Warda LJ, LaFlair P, et al. Adams–Oliver syndrome: A case with juvenile chronic myelogenous leukemia and chylothorax. Am J Med Genet 1993; 47:1175–1179.
180. Davis BA, Cervi P, Amin Z, et al. Retinoic acid syndrome: Pulmonary computed tomography (CT) findings. Leuk Lymphoma 1996; 23:113–117.
181. Schaap N, Raymakers R, Schattenberg A, et al. Massive pleural effusion attributed to high dose cyclophosphamide during conditioning for BMT. Bone Marrow Transplant 1996; 18: 247–248.
182. Camacho LH, Soignet SL, Chanel S, et al. Leukocytosis and the retinoic acid syndrome in patients with acute promyelocytic leukemia treated with arsenic trioxide. J Clin Oncol 2000; 18:2620–2625.
183. Tallman MS, Andersen JW, Schiffer CA, et al. Clinical description of 44 patients with acute promyelocytic leukemia who developed retinoic acid syndrome. Blood 2000; 95:90–95.
184. Nicolls MR, Terada LS, Tuder RM, et al. Diffuse alveolar hemorrhage with underlying pulmonary capillaritis in the retinoic acid syndrome. Am J Respir Crit Care Med 1998; 158:1302–1305.
185. De Botton S, Dombret H, Sanz M, et al. Incidence, clinical features, and outcome of all trans-retinoic acid syndrome in 413 cases of newly diagnosed acute promyelocytic leukemia. The European APL Group. Blood 1998; 92:2712–2718.
186. Woods T, Vidarson B, Mosher D, et al. Transient effusive constrictive pericarditis due to chemotherapy. Clin Cardiol 1999; 22:316–318.
187. Sebach J, Speich R, Fehr J, et al. GM-CSF induced acute eosinophilic pneumonia. Br J Haematol 1995; 90:963–965.
188. Bolanos-Meade J, Keung YK, Cobos E. Recurrent lymphocytic pleural effusion after intravenous immunoglobulin. Am J Hematol 1999; 60:248–249.
189. Kantarjan H, Giles F, Gattermann N, et al. Nilotinib (AMN 107), a highily selective BCR-ABL tyrosine kinase inhibitor, is effective in patients with Philadelphia chromosome-positive chronic myelogenous leukemia in chronic phase following imatinib resistance and intolerance. Blood 2007; 110:3540–3546.
190. Quintás-Cardama A, Kantarjian H, O'Brien S, et al. Pleural effusions in patients with CML treated with dasatinib after imatinib failure. J Clin Oncol 2007; 25:3908–3914.
191. Kintzer JS, Rosenow EC, Kyle RA. Thoracic and pulmonary abnormalities in a multiple myeloma. A review of 958 cases. Arch Intern Med 1978; 138:727–730.
192. Elloumi M, Frikha M, Masmoudi H, et al. Plasmocytic pleural effusion disclosing multiple myeloma. Rev Mol Respir 2000; 17:495–497.
193. Rodriguez JN, Pereira A, Martinez JC, et al. Pleural effusion in multiple myeloma. Chest 1994; 105:622–624.
194. Pacheco A, Perpina A, Eschribano L, et al. Pleural effusion as the first sign of extramedullary plasmatocytoma. Chest 1992; 102:296–297.
195. Palmer HE, Wilson CS, Bardales RH. Cytology and flow cytometry of malignant effusions of multiple myeloma. Diagn Cytopathol 2000; 22:147–151.
196. Manley R, Monteath J, Patton WN. Coincidental presentation of IgA lambda multiple myeloma and pleural involvement with IgM kappa non-Hodgkin's lymphoma. Clin Lab Haematol 1999; 21:61–63.
197. Nagai K, Ando K, Yoshida H, et al. Response of the extramedullary lung plasmatocytoma with pleural effusion to chemotherapy. Ann Hematol 1997; 74:279–281.
198. Meoli A, Willsie S, Fiorella R. Myelomatous pleural effusion. South Med J 1997; 90:65–68.
199. Maeno T, Sando Y, Tsukagoshi M, et al. Pleural amyloidosis in a patient with intractable pleural effusion and multiple myeloma. Respirology 2000; 5:79–80.
200. Knapp MJ, Roggli VL, Kim J, et al. Pleural amyloidosis. Arch Pathol Lab 1988; 112:57–60.
201. Stevenet P, Stevenet A, Helias A, et al. Pleural manifestations of secondary monoclonal dysproteinemia (apropos of 4 cases). Poumon Coeur 1977; 33:143–148.

202. Weatherall DJ, Higgs DR, Bunch C, et al. Hemoglobin H disease and mental retardation: A new syndrome or a remarkable coincidence? N Engl J Med 1981; 305:607–612.

203. Srair HA, Owa JA, Aman HA, et al. Acute chest syndrome in children with sickle cell disease. Indian J Pediatr 1995; 62(2):201–205.

204. Ibabao J, Kassapidis S, Demetis S. et al. Bilateral pleural effusions in a beta-thalassemia intermediate patient with posterior mediastinal extramedullary hemopoietic masses. Hemoglobin 1999; 23:249–253.

205. Urbaniak-Kujda D, Cielinska S, Kapelko-Slowik K, et al. Disseminated nocardiosis as a complication of Evans' syndrome. Ann Hematol 1999; 78:385–387.

206. Peng MJ, Kuo HT, Chang MC. A case of intrathoracic extramedullary hematopoiesis with massive pleural effusion: Successful pleurodesis with intrapleural minocycline. J Formos Med Assoc 1994; 93:445–447.

207. Longaker MT, Laberge JM, Dansereau J, et al. Primary fetal hydrothorax: Natural history and management. J Pediatr Surg 1989; 24:573–576.

208. Smoleniec J, James D. Predictive value of pleural effusions in fetal hydrops. Fetal Diagn Ther 1995; 10:95–100.

209. Ries M, Beinder E, Gruner C, et al. Rapid development of hydrops fetalis in the donor twin following death of the recipient twin in twin-twin transfusion syndrome. J Perinat Med 1999; 27:68–73.

210. Tongsong T, Wanapirak C, Srisomboon J, et al. Antenatal sonographic features of 100 alpha-thalassemia hydrops fetalis fetusis. J Clin Ultrasound 1996; 24:73–77.

211. Becton DL, Friedman HS, Kurtzberg J, et al. Severe mycoplasma pneumonia in three sisters with sickle cell disease. Pediatr Hematol Oncol 1986; 3:259–265.

212. Oestreich AE. Pleural effusions in sickle cell disease. J Natl Med Assoc 1977; 69:579–580.

213. Dekker A, Graham T, Bupp PA. The occurrence of sickle cells in pleural fluid: Report of a patient with sickle cell disease. Acta Cytol 1975; 19:251–254.

214. Butterfield JH, Schwenk NM, Colville DS, et al. Severe generalized reactions to ibuprofen: Report of a case. J Rheumatol 1986; 13:649–650.

215. Clark JH, Fitzgerald JG. Hemorrhagic complications of Henoch-Schonlein syndrome. J Pediatr Gastroenterol Nutr 1985; 4:311–315.

216. Oppermann HC, Wille L. Hemothorax in the newborn. Pediatr Radiol 1980; 9:129–134.

33
Pleural Effusions in HIV

KRISTINA CROTHERS
University of Washington School of Medicine, Seattle, Washington, U.S.A.

LAURENCE HUANG
University of California, San Francisco, California, U.S.A.

I. Introduction

The approach to the evaluation of a pleural effusion in a human immunodeficiency virus (HIV)–infected patient begins with a differential diagnosis that includes all of the causes of both exudative and transudative pleural effusions found in non–HIV-infected individuals. As in all patients, helpful details in investigating the etiology of a pleural effusion can be obtained from presenting complaints and physical examination findings. In particular, duration of illness, symptoms, and the presence of other medical problems can provide significant clues as to the underlying process. For example, a pleural effusion in the setting of the acute onset of fever, cough, and purulent sputum points toward a bacterial parapneumonic process, whereas increasing dyspnea and cough in a patient with cutaneous Kaposi's sarcoma (KS) suggest pleuropulmonary KS. As in non–HIV-infected individuals, evaluation of concomitant radiographic abnormalities and sampling of pleural fluid are crucial diagnostic steps.

The likelihood of different diagnoses is also influenced by a patient's CD4+ T-cell count, the underlying HIV risk factors of the patient, and the prevalence of different diseases in the community. Certain diagnoses are more common in specific populations, such as parapneumonic effusion in injection drug users (IDU) and KS in men who have sex with men (MSM). In areas endemic for *Mycobacterium tuberculosis*, tuberculosis is the most common cause of pleural effusion. An additional consideration is the use of highly active antiretroviral therapy (HAART). Worsening of new pleural effusion, such as in an HIV-infected patient with tuberculosis who initiates treatment with HAART, may also be due to immune reconstitution inflammatory syndrome (IRIS). Therefore, consideration of community, HIV disease state, use of HAART, and risk factors for HIV infection, as well as clinical presentation and concomitant chest radiographic abnormalities are all integral factors in evaluating the etiology of a pleural effusion in an HIV-infected patient.

This chapter will provide an overview of the epidemiology of pleural effusions in hospitalized HIV-infected patients, general diagnostic procedures, and patient outcomes. Individual causes of exudative pleural effusions, namely, infectious and malignant causes will then be discussed in more detail, followed by a review of transudative effusions in HIV-infected patients. Features characteristic of pleural effusions in HIV-infected patients that may be distinct from features seen in HIV-negative patients will be emphasized.

II. Epidemiology of Pleural Effusion in Hospitalized HIV-Infected Patients

In retrospective studies, the prevalence of pleural effusion in hospitalized HIV patients has ranged widely, from 1.7% to 27% of all HIV admissions (1–5). Infections tend to be the most common cause, with the majority being parapneumonic in origin. The next two most common causes of pleural effusion are tuberculosis and malignancy, specifically KS (Table 1) (1–9). Other less frequently reported causes of effusion in these studies of hospitalized HIV patients are processes that can be seen in HIV-negative patients as well, including exudative effusions related to pancreatitis or other intra-abdominal processes, pulmonary embolism, or trauma. Transudative effusions related to congestive heart failure, renal failure, or liver disease also occur.

The etiology of pleural effusion varies depending on a number of factors including the patient population studied and their HIV risk factors. In a study by Afessa, IDUs were more likely to present with pleural effusion (1). While 21% of patients with a history of IDU had pleural effusions, only 7% of heterosexual patients ($p = 0.0001$) and 10% of MSM ($p = 0.0097$) had pleural effusion (1). Among HIV-infected IDUs, the most likely cause of a pleural effusion is infections, given the increased risk for bacterial pneumonia in this population, especially if CD4+ T-cell counts are below 200 cells/μL (10,11). In a retrospective study from Spain, records of 86 hospitalized HIV-infected patients with

Table 1 Reported Causes of Pleural Effusion in Hospitalized HIV-Infected Patients

	References								
	(1)	(4)	(7)	(8)	(2)	(3)	(5)	(6)	(9)
No. of Patients (N)	160	58	30	86	28	30	59	75	91
Incidence per # HIV admits (%)	14.6	5.6	NS	NS	7.2	1.7	26.6	NS	NS
Infectious (%)	42	55	70	88	71	60	66	35	95
Parapneumonic (%)	31	28	47	69	32	33	30	11	4
Empyema (%)	1	–				7	3		
M. tuberculosis (%)	6	14	3	17	21	20	9	12	90
P. jirovecii (%)	3	10	–	2	7	–	15	1	–
Noninfectious (%)	38	45	30	6	29	27	31	47	6
Malignancy (%)	6	40	30	1	25	10	2	47	4
KS (%)	1	33	10	–	7	7	2	43	3
Lymphoma (%)	1	7	17	1	14	–	–	3	1
Lung cancer (%)	3	–	3	–	3	3	–	1	–
CHF (%)	3	2	–	1	3	–	5	–	–
Renal insufficiency (%)	9	–	–	1	–	10	2	–	–
Liver failure (%)	3	–	–	2	–	–	–	–	–
Hypoalbuminemia (%)	8	–	–	–	–	–	19	–	–
Other[a] (%)	9	3	–	–	–	7	5	–	1
Unknown etiology (%)	21	–	–	6	–	10	3	19	–

NS: not stated.
[a] Other causes include pulmonary embolism, pancreatitis, pericarditis, thoracic surgery, chest trauma, atelectasis, ARDS, and subcapsular splenic hematoma.

a pleural effusion were reviewed (8). Ninety-four percent of the patients were IDUs and 54% had AIDS. Overall, 88% of effusions were attributed to infectious causes, and 69% were parapneumonic. In another study from England, 58 consecutive HIV-infected admissions with pleural effusion were prospectively evaluated (4). In this study, 3.4% of patients were IDUs and 69% were MSM. In contrast to the prior study, only 55% of all effusions were attributed to infectious causes, and 28% were parapneumonic. Given the low percentage of IDUs and the high percentage of patients who were MSM, it is not surprising that more effusions proved to be due to KS than to pneumonia in this cohort, illustrating the importance of patient population and specific HIV risk factors in influencing disease presentation.

The etiology of a pleural effusion will also vary with geography and prevalence of disease in the community. In areas with a high rate of tuberculosis, a greater proportion of HIV-infected patients will present with pleural effusion due to tuberculosis. In an investigation of 127 cases of undiagnosed pleural effusion in patients in Rwanda, 86% of effusions were due to *M. tuberculosis*; 83% of these patients who underwent testing were HIV seropositive, indicating a strong association between HIV and tuberculous pleurisy in Africa (9). Other etiologies such as parapneumonic effusion and KS were much less frequent in this population. In contrast, in reports from the United States, at most 20% of effusions in HIV-infected patients were due to *M. tuberculosis* (Table 1) (3).

In addition, the degree of immunosuppression will impact the etiology of a pleural effusion, as the incidence of opportunistic infections and other processes such as AIDS-related lymphoma increases as the CD4+ T-cell count decreases. Whether patients with a lower CD4+ T-cell count are more likely to have a pleural effusion as a complication of underlying disease is unclear. The majority of patients included in the epidemiologic studies described carried a diagnosis of AIDS. In an earlier study, Joseph et al. found that HIV-infected patients with pleural effusion had significantly lower CD4+ T-cell counts than patients without effusion (72 ± 12 cells/μL vs. 274 ± 26 cells/μL; $p < 0.001$) (5). However, a later study by Afessa found that HIV-infected patients with pleural effusion had marginally higher CD4+ T-cell counts (152 ± 186 cells/μL vs. 147 ± 218 cells/μL; $p = 0.0382$) (1).

Finally, the percentages reported in these studies may not be representative of the entire HIV-infected population, because all of these studies have included only hospitalized patients. Therefore, the incidence of effusions secondary to infectious processes may be overestimated in these series, as these patients may be more likely to be hospitalized. Effusions related to malignancy, heart failure, or other less acute processes might be underestimated in these series. These effusions may go unnoticed until the size or other systemic complications cause symptoms, or they may be managed on an outpatient basis.

III. Outcome of HIV-Infected Patients with Pleural Effusion

HIV-infected patients may have a worse outcome if a pleural effusion is present. In the observational study by Afessa, HIV-infected patients with pleural effusion had significantly higher APACHE (acute physiology and chronic health evaluation) II predicted mortality rates than HIV-infected patients without pleural effusion (29% vs. 23%; $p = 0.0001$) (1). The length of hospitalization was on median one day longer (7.6 ± 8.2 days vs. 6.4 ± 6.4 days; $p = 0.0064$), and the in-hospital mortality rate was significantly higher in those with pleural effusion than without (10.0% vs. 5.4%; $p = 0.0407$). However, the presence of pleural effusion was not found to be independently associated with increased mortality [odds ratio (OR) 1.5, 95% confidence interval (CI) 0.8–2.8] (1), suggesting that a pleural effusion may instead be a marker for the severity of underlying disease.

Among HIV-infected patients with community-acquired bacterial pneumonia, the presence of pleural effusion may portend a poor prognosis. In one study from Spain, mortality was significantly increased among HIV-infected patients with community-acquired bacterial pneumonia who had radiologic progression of pneumonia within 48 hours of admission. The presence of pleural effusion on initial chest radiograph was highly associated with radiographic progression (OR, 4.39; 95% CI, 2.09–9.18) on multivariate analysis.

When comparing HIV-infected to HIV-uninfected patients with parapneumonic effusions from bacterial pneumonia or tuberculosis, studies do not suggest a significant difference in morbidity or mortality between those with and without HIV infection (8,12). Specifically, there have been no differences in residual fibrosis, time to resolution of the effusion, or in overall mortality in HIV-infected compared to HIV-uninfected patients with parapneumonic effusions from bacterial pneumonia or tuberculosis.

IV. Diagnostic Evaluation of the HIV-Infected Patient with Pleural Effusion

Evaluation of the HIV-infected patient with a pleural effusion includes routine history, physical examination, and radiographic studies as in the HIV-negative individual. In particular, important clues can be obtained from the presence of bilateral versus unilateral effusions and from concomitant pulmonary abnormalities detected on chest imaging. The presence of bilateral versus unilateral effusions can be suggestive of different diagnoses: bilateral effusions are more commonly seen in KS, lymphoma, and congestive heart failure than are unilateral effusions (4). Unilateral effusions are more likely to be of parapneumonic (4) or tuberculous origin (13,14). The size of a pleural effusion has not generally been helpful in ascertaining its etiology (1,4,5,7,8).

In addition, underlying pulmonary parenchymal and mediastinal abnormalities can provide diagnostic clues. Bilateral pleural effusions with ill-defined peribronchovascular nodules and septal thickening suggest KS (15). Concomitant hilar adenopathy can also be seen with KS (4). A unilateral effusion with focal air space consolidation suggests parapneumonic effusion, while a unilateral effusion with miliary nodules and/or mediastinal lymphadenopathy suggests tuberculosis (4).

Pleural fluid should be sampled promptly, analyzed for cell differential, protein, lactate dehydrogenase (LDH), and glucose, and sent for detailed microbiological analysis. In addition to routine smears and cultures for bacteria, mycobacteria, and fungi, a Wright Giemsa stain can detect fungal elements. Cytological analysis for malignancy should always be performed. Closed pleural biopsy can be particularly useful in the evaluation of tuberculosis as well as lymphoma in HIV-infected patients (13,16). Thoracoscopic evaluation with biopsy can be performed in the evaluation of an undiagnosed effusion and can be particularly useful if confirmation of KS is required (17). Further procedures to consider in working up the undiagnosed pleural effusion include flow cytometry and measurement of pleural fluid adenosine deaminase (ADA) and cryptococcal antigen—these can be suggestive of the diagnoses of malignancy, tuberculosis, and cryptococcus, respectively (18,19).

V. Infectious Causes of Pleural Effusion in HIV-Infected Patients

A. Parapneumonic Effusions

Among the infectious causes of exudative effusions, parapneumonic effusions account for the majority of pleural effusions in HIV-infected hospitalized patients (1,4,8). Pleural effusions are reported in approximately 40% to 50% of HIV-infected patients admitted with bacterial pneumonia (1,20). The high frequency of parapneumonic effusions is not surprising, given the increased susceptibility to bacterial pneumonia (10,11,21) and the high rate of bacteremia in HIV-infected populations with community-acquired pneumonia (CAP), particularly if CD4+ T-cell counts are below 200 cells/μL (22,23). Compared to HIV-negative patients, HIV-infected patients are more likely to have complications from community-acquired bacterial pneumonia, including a greater risk of parapneumonic effusion in one study (24). Out of 137 patients with CAP, 21% of HIV-infected patients had parapneumonic effusions compared to 13% of HIV-negative patients ($p < 0.05$), and 71% of HIV-infected patients required chest tube drainage compared to 44% of HIV-negative patients. Blood cultures and pleural fluid cultures were more likely to be positive in the HIV-infected population (24).

Of microbiological causes, *Staphylococcus aureus* is the most frequently reported cause of parapneumonic effusion in a number of retrospective studies (Table 2) (4,7,8). Seen particularly in HIV-infected IDU, *S. aureus* pneumonia is often complicated by pleural effusions in HIV-infected patients. In one study, nearly one-third of the cases were associated with pleural effusion (25). Pleural effusion due to *S. aureus* infection can be related to CAP, as well as to septic embolism from infectious endocarditis. *S. aureus* infection can result in uncomplicated parapneumonic effusion as well as empyema (8,24–26).

Another very common cause of pneumonia in HIV-infected patients (21,23,27–29), *Streptococcus pneumoniae* is likewise one of the most common causes of parapneumonic pleural effusion (Table 2) (7,8). Although the rate of pneumococcal bacteremia may be up to 100 times greater in HIV-infected patients compared to age-matched HIV-negative patients (29), increased rates of empyema in HIV-infected patients have not been reported (24,29). However, individual cases of more unusual and aggressive manifestations of pneumococcal infection in the pleural space have been reported in patients with HIV infection, including recurrent exudative pleural effusions and pyopneumothorax (30).

Numerous other bacteria have been documented to cause pleural effusion in HIV-infected individuals, including *Staphylococcus epidermidis* and gram negative organisms such as *Pseudomonas aeruginosa* and *Escherichia coli* (5,7,8). *P. aeruginosa* has been reported particularly in IDU and in those with more advanced immunosuppression from HIV (8,31). Although a common cause of pneumonia in HIV-infected patients (27,28), *Haemophilus influenzae* has been infrequently reported as a cause of pleural effusion (4). More unusual organisms can also infect the pleural space, such as *Campylobacter jejuni*, *Salmonella* species, *Nocardia* species, and, rarely, *Rhodococcus equi* (32–35). Pulmonary nocardiosis in HIV-infected patients has been associated with pleural effusion in 10% to 33% of cases, most commonly as a unilateral effusion associated with

Table 2 Reported Infectious Causes of Pleural Effusion in HIV-Infected Hospitalized Patients

	References			
	(4)	(7)	(8)	(5)
Infectious effusions	32/58 (55%)	21/30 (70%)	76/86 (88%)	39/59 (66%)
Presumed bacterial	12 (38%)	6 (29%)	16 (21%)	6 (15%)
S. aureus	2 (6%)	4 (19%)	26 (34%)	1 (3%)
S. pneumoniae		4 (19%)	5 (7%)	8 (21%)
S. epidermidis			4 (5%)	
H. influenzae	1 (3%)			
K. pneumoniae			1 (1%)	
L. pneumophila				1 (3%)
M. pneumoniae				1 (3%)
P. aeruginosa	1 (3%)		6 (8%)	
E. coli				2 (5%)
Enterobacter sp.				1 (3%)
C. jejuni			1 (1%)	
Gram negative bacilli		3 (14%)		
Nocardia sp.		1 (5%)		2 (5%)
M. tuberculosis	8 (25%)	1 (5%)	15 (17%)	5 (13%)
M. avium		2 (10%)		1 (3%)
P. jirovecii	6 (19%)		2 (3%)	9 (23%)
Aspergillus sp.	1 (3%)[a]			
Cryptococcus neoformans	1 (3%)			2 (5%)
Leishmania	1 (3%)[a]			

[a]One patient had both *Aspergillus* and *Leishmania*.

underlying parenchymal abnormalities such as consolidation, mass-like or cavitary lesions (33,36). *Nocardia* empyema requiring tube thoracostomy for drainage has also been described (33).

HIV-infected patients may be more likely to develop complicated parapneumonic pleural effusions than HIV-negative patients. In the study by Gil Suay et al. comparing HIV-infected to HIV-negative patients with CAP and parapneumonic effusion, the HIV-infected patients were more likely to have a complicated clinical course and to develop complicated parapneumonic effusions (24). The HIV-infected patients were younger and were also found to have a significantly longer duration of symptoms prior to admission and a higher fever on admission. Although no differences were observed in pleural fluid pH, protein, LDH, or absolute number of cells, patients with HIV had significantly lower levels of pleural fluid glucose and were more likely to require chest tube drainage. Furthermore, the duration of fever and of intravenous antibiotic treatment and the number of antibiotics were all higher in the HIV-infected group. These findings may be related to the increased frequency of *S. aureus* parapneumonic effusions observed in this study, which included a high proportion of IDU, and the increased complications typically observed with this organism (24). No increase in the number of cases of empyema was reported, however, and no difference in mortality was demonstrated. In another study, no significant difference was detected in the outcome of HIV-infected and HIV-negative patients with either complicated or uncomplicated parapneumonic effusions (8).

Management of parapneumonic effusion in an HIV-infected patient should be the same as in immunocompetent individuals (17). If the patient is an IDU, choice of empiric antibiotics should include coverage for *S. aureus* given the high percentage of parapneumonic effusions in these patients. Empiric coverage for methicillin-resistant *S. aureus* may be warranted depending on local resistance patterns. Antipseudomonal coverage should also be considered, particularly in the more severely immunosuppressed patients. Sampling of pleural fluid is integral in deciding therapy. Given the increased potential for complicated parapneumonic effusions, tube thoracostomy and surgical interventions for drainage may be indicated (37). In cases of empyema not resolving with chest tube drainage, early thoracoscopy for pleural debridement has been advocated (38). In patients with thoracic empyema and CD4+ T-cell counts below 200 cells/μL, additional percutaneous drainage and prolonged tube thoracostomy may be required (39).

B. Mycobacterial Pleural Effusions

Mycobacterium tuberculosis

Mycobacterium tuberculosis is a frequent cause of pleural effusion in HIV. The prevalence of tuberculous pleural effusion varies according to the background rate of tuberculosis in the population reported. *M. tuberculosis* accounts for between 3% and 21% of pleural effusions in HIV-infected hospitalized patients in the United States and Europe (Table 1) (1–8). In contrast, up to 90% of effusions in HIV-infected patients were caused by tuberculosis in Kigali, Rwanda, an area endemic for tuberculosis (9).

Tuberculous pleural effusion tends to occur more commonly in patients with HIV infection, despite substantial overlap in the frequency of disease reported in HIV-infected and HIV-negative populations. Of patients with TB, 8% to 43% of cases in HIV-infected patients have been reported to present with pleural effusion (14,40–44), compared to approximately 4% to 20% of cases in HIV-negative patients in studies from the United States, Europe, and Africa (14,40–43,45). In a review comparing 963 HIV-infected adults to 1000 HIV-negative adults in sub-Saharan Africa, significantly more HIV-infected compared to HIV-negative patients presented with pleural effusion on chest X-ray (16% vs. 6.8%; $p = 0.001$) (42). These results are consistent with the findings in other studies of tuberculosis in South Africa (41,43) and Rwanda (40).

Clinical presentation is similar, although compared to HIV-negative patients, HIV-infected patients with TB pleural effusion were noted to be younger in one study from New York City—this may potentially reflect more cases of primary infection as opposed to reactivation tuberculosis (13). HIV-infected patients have also been reported to present with more prolonged symptoms such as dyspnea, fever, nights sweats, and fatigue (46,47). On radiograph, pleural effusions associated with tuberculosis are usually unilateral and are frequently associated with underlying parenchymal abnormalities (13,40–43). However, pleural effusion may also be the only finding (13). As in HIV-negative patients, 5% to 10% of HIV-infected patients may present with bilateral pleural effusions (13,14,46).

The CD4+ T-cell count influences the presentation of tuberculosis in HIV-infected patients. Although features such as mediastinal adenopathy are more common in patients with CD4+ T-cell counts below 200 cells/μL, manifestations such as cavitary lesions and pleural effusions tend to be more common in patients with higher CD4+ T-cell

Table 3 Relationship Between Degree of Immunosuppression and Presence of Tuberculous Pleural Effusion in HIV-Infected Patients

	Cases with pleural effusion		
References	CD4+ T-cells ≤200 (AIDS)	CD4+ T-cells >200 (no-AIDS)	*p*-value
(40)	15/35 (42%)	6/13 (46%)	0.83
(48)	6/58 (10%)	8/30 (27%)	0.05
(44)	7/98 (7%)	3/30 (10%)	0.70

counts (44,48,49). Although in one study by Jones et al., a higher percentage of patients with CD4+ T-cell counts above 200 cells/μL had pleural effusions, this has not been a consistent finding in other studies (Table 3) (40,44,48). As tuberculous pleuritis is postulated to represent a delayed-type hypersensitivity reaction, with immune response mediated by CD4+ T-cells in the pleural fluid, an increased number of effusions could be explained in patients with higher CD4+ T-cell counts (13,48).

As in the non–HIV-infected patient, a unilateral exudative effusion with lymphocyte predominance and an elevated protein should prompt consideration of tuberculosis. No significant differences between pleural fluid cell differential, protein concentration, or glucose levels have been found between HIV-seropositive and HIV-seronegative individuals with pleural tuberculosis (46). Although usually scarce in tuberculous pleural effusions, an elevated mesothelial cell count can be an unreliable predictor in HIV-infected patients, as increased mesothelial cells have been reported in a small number of cases in HIV-infected patients with effusions due to tuberculosis (50).

If routine cultures are nondiagnostic, a pleural biopsy should be strongly considered. Pleural fluid smears, culture, and pleural biopsy specimens may have a higher yield in HIV-infected patients related to an increased burden of microorganisms in the pleural space (13), although this has not been consistently demonstrated. In one study, pleural biopsy specimens were significantly more likely to be AFB smear-positive in HIV-infected patients compared to HIV-negative patients with pleural tuberculosis (69% vs. 21%; $p < 0.01$) (13), although in other reports no significant differences in the microbiological yield of pleural specimens could be demonstrated (Table 4) (35,46). The percentage of positive results varies greatly between the studies, as it does for HIV-negative patients, related to factors such as amount of fluid sampled, culture techniques, and number of biopsy specimens (51).

Used less commonly in the United States, additional pleural fluid assays to aid in the diagnosis of tuberculosis in immunocompetent patients include measurements of ADA, interferon-gamma (IFN-γ), and lysozyme, and polymerase chain reaction (PCR) to detect *M. tuberculosis*. The role of these studies in HIV-infected patients requires further evaluation (52). ADA is an enzyme that is found in highest concentrations in stimulated T lymphocytes, with elevated levels observed in tuberculous pleural effusions as well as in empyema. It has been shown to have a sensitivity ranging from 90% to 100%, and a specificity of 85% to 100% in immunocompetent patients (45,53,54). In prior studies of HIV patients, ADA had a lower sensitivity due to increased false-negative results (55). However, in an analysis that included the largest number of HIV-infected patients with pleural tuberculosis reported thus far (37 patients), the ADA values did not differ

Table 4 Percent of Cases with Positive Microbiologic Results on Pleural Specimens in Tuberculosis According to HIV Status

	Pleural fluid		Pleural biopsy		
References	Smear (%)	Culture (%)	Histology (%)	Smear (%)	Culture (%)
(9)					
$(N = 90)^a$	1	46	52	NS	50
(13)					
HIV+ ($N = 43$)	15	91	88	69[b]	47[c]
HIV− ($N = 27$)	8	78	71	21	86
(35)					
HIV+ ($N = 22$)	NS	13.6	68.2	NS	18.2
HIV− ($N = 30$)	NS	6.7	53.3	NS	10
(14)					
HIV+ ($N = 22$)	6	64	78	44	40
HIV−[d]		53			

NS: not stated.

[a]Results for HIV+ and HIV− patients combined; HIV positivity rate 83% in the total of 110 patients with pleural TB.

[b]$p < 0.01$ compared to HIV-negative.

[c]$p < 0.05$ compared to HIV-negative.

[d]Rate of pleural fluid AFB culture was taken from control cases seen in HIV-negative patients within the same state during the study period.

significantly from HIV-negative patients, suggesting that it may be equally sensitive in HIV patients (56).

IFN-γ has also been investigated as a potential diagnostic marker for tuberculous pleural effusion. A lymphokine produced by T lymphocytes in response to antigen stimulation, IFN-γ levels increase in tuberculous pleuritis. High sensitivity and specificity of up to 99% and 98%, respectively, have been reported (54). The sensitivity did not differ significantly when compared between 9 HIV-infected and 41 HIV-negative patients. Although the level of IFN-γ tended to be lower in HIV-infected patients, it remained well above the cut-off point of 3.7 U/mL (54). In another study, IFN-γ levels were significantly higher in serum ($p = 0.02$) and pleural fluid ($p = 0.004$) in HIV-infected compared to HIV-uninfected persons (57). Interestingly, PCR has been reported to have a much lower sensitivity of 42% but a high specificity of 99%, with no significant difference in sensitivity reported in the small number of HIV-infected and HIV-negative patients in which it was studied (58).

HIV-infected patients with pleural tuberculosis can be treated with a standard six-month antituberculous regimen, substituting rifabutin for rifampin if patients are on protease inhibitors or certain non-nucleoside reverse-transcriptase inhibitors. Provided appropriate clinical response, prolonged treatment for pleural disease is unnecessary (59). Corticosteroids have been used as adjunctive therapy for pleural tuberculosis. In one randomized, double-blind, placebo-controlled study of 197 HIV-infected persons with pleural tuberculosis, there was no significant survival benefit for those who received prednisolone (60). A Cochrane review of corticosteroids for tuberculous pleurisy analyzed results from six trials and a total of 633 subjects (HIV-uninfected and HIV-infected) (61). The authors concluded that data were insufficient to support evidence-based recommendations for the use of adjunctive corticosteroids in persons with tuberculous pleurisy.

Nontuberculous Mycobacteria

Large pleural effusions due to nontuberculous mycobacteria (NTM) are uncommon in HIV-infected as well as in HIV-negative patients. Although *Mycobacterium avium* complex is the most frequent cause of nontuberculous disease (62) and is often disseminated in AIDS patients, pleural involvement is a rare feature (63). *Mycobacterium kansasii* and *Mycobacterium xenopi* are associated with pleural effusions in only 8% to 18% of cases (64–66), with no significant differences reported between the proportion of cases with pleural involvement in AIDS versus non-AIDS patients (67). Pulmonary disease caused by atypical mycobacteria usually occurs in HIV-infected patients with advanced immunosuppression, often with CD4+ T-cell counts averaging 50 cells/μL (62,66,67). Unlike *M. tuberculosis*, the NTM are unlikely to cause large effusions or isolated pleurisy. This may be related to the often profound immunosuppression of patients with these pathogens, as other features like cavitation that are usually associated with higher CD4+ T-cell counts in patients with *M. tuberculosis* infection are also seen less frequently (66,68,69).

C. Fungal Pleural Effusions

Numerous cases of fungal pleural effusion in HIV-infected patients have been reported. Now classified as a fungus, *Pneumocystis jirovecii* is a frequent cause of opportunistic pneumonia in HIV-infected patients but is not typically associated with pleural effusion. Despite this, a number of cases of pleural effusion have been attributed to *Pneumocystis* pneumonia (PCP) on retrospective review (Table 1) (1,2,4–6). In the study by Joseph et al., 15% of pleural effusions were attributed to PCP (5). However, as no cytological stains were done on pleural fluid specimens to confirm the presence of cysts or trophic forms of *P. jirovecii*, this may be an overestimation. Rather, the presence of pleural effusion in a patient with PCP may be due to a second infection or underlying illness, or may be related to factors associated with the pneumonic process that affect the intrapleural pressure, lymphatic clearance, and permeability of the microcirculation (5).

Rare individual cases that document *P. jirovecii* by cytological examination in the pleural space have been reported (70–72). Of note, all of these cases have been associated with aerosolized pentamidine use, frequently in combination with a pneumothorax, raising the possibility that pleural pneumocystis may be an anatomical extension of subpleural infection that erodes into the pleural space (70).

Another fungus not infrequently reported to cause pleural effusions in HIV-infected patients is *Cryptococcus neoformans* (18,73–77). Pleural effusions in cryptococcal disease are more common in HIV-infected than in non–HIV-infected individuals (78). Reported in association with 5% to 20% of cases of cryptococcal pneumonia (73,74), pleural effusion due to *Cryptococcus* has also preceded disseminated disease and has been seen in the absence of concomitant pulmonary parenchymal disease (18,75–77,79). Methods for diagnosis include fungal smear and culture, as well as closed pleural biopsy and assay for cryptococcal antigen in the pleural fluid (18,76).

In rare cases, disseminated histoplasmosis has been associated with pleural effusion in HIV-infected patients, with microbiological confirmation on thoracentesis as well as a pleural biopsy specimen (80,81). Pleural effusion is an uncommon finding in coccidioidomycosis (82,83) and invasive pulmonary aspergillosis (2,4,84).

D. Other Infectious Causes of Pleural Effusion

Parasitic causes of pleural effusion in HIV-infected patients include invasive amebiasis (85), as well as *Leishmania* (4,6,86). Consideration of these more unusual infections would depend upon the patient's presentation, exposures, and travel history. For example, the cases of amebiasis were reported from an endemic area in Taiwan and were seen in association with liver abscesses. Although a rare disease, pulmonary toxoplasmosis can be associated with pleural effusion in 7% of cases (87).

VI. Malignant Pleural Effusions in HIV-Infected Patients

Malignant pleural effusions in HIV-infected patients can result from tumors that are seen in HIV-negative patients as well as those that are particular to an HIV-infected population. Among the most prevalent AIDS-associated malignancies in HIV patients, KS and non–Hodgkin's lymphoma (NHL) are the most common causes of malignant effusion in HIV-infected patients (88). Bronchogenic carcinoma accounts for approximately 3% of effusions in HIV-infected hospitalized patients (1–3,6,7). Metastatic cancer and rare diseases, as in a case report of a malignant mesothelioma in the absence of asbestos exposure, can also be encountered in the AIDS patient (89). Certain malignant effusions, such as primary effusion lymphoma (PEL) and KS, are seen primarily in those with HIV infection. The characteristics of three causes of malignant pleural effusion particular to AIDS patients are discussed in more detail later.

A. Kaposi's Sarcoma

KS is a mesenchymal tumor involving the blood and lymphatic vessels and can manifest in several different populations, including endemic African KS, classic KS, and KS associated with immunosuppression. Here, we focus on KS-associated with HIV infection, which is seen predominantly in MSM (90). KS was estimated to occur in approximately 10% of AIDS patients prior to the HAART era (91), but the incidence has decreased significantly among populations receiving HAART (90). Pulmonary involvement is evident in 6% to 49% of patients with known mucocutaneous KS, with a higher prevalence of 47% to 75% noted in autopsy series (91). Although uncommon, pulmonary disease can also be seen in up to 15% of patients in the absence of mucocutaneous lesions (92).

Pleural involvement in KS is a frequent complication, with effusions present in approximately 50% of cases (4,91–93). Correspondingly, KS has been the most common malignant effusion in HIV patients, accounting for up to 43% of effusions in HIV-infected patients who present with pleural effusion. However, the reported frequency varies depending on the patient population studied (Table 1) (1–4,6,7).

The most common clinical symptoms of pulmonary KS are dyspnea, nonproductive cough, and fever (92,94). Patients with pulmonary KS typically have advanced HIV, with CD4+ T-cell counts below 150 cells/μL in most series (91), although KS can occur with normal CD4+ T-cell counts as well (95). Pleural fluid is commonly a serosanguineous or bloody exudate with a mononuclear cell predominance (94), although serosanguineous transudates can be found (91,93). Pleural effusion due to KS can present as a chylothorax, presumably related to lymphatic obstruction of the thoracic duct (93,94,96).

The pleural effusions related to KS are bilateral in 65% to 76% of cases (4,15,93). Most effusions are small to moderate in size and, if bilateral, tend to be symmetrical (15). Pleural effusions are reported nearly exclusively in patients with parenchymal lung involvement related to KS (92,97). In the series by O'Brien and Cohn, 3 out of 13 cases of pleuropulmonary KS were reported as having pleural involvement alone on the basis of chest X-ray findings (94), although a CT scan may have detected parenchymal involvement in these patients.

Human-herpes virus 8 (HHV-8) appears to play a central role in pathogenesis of KS, as it is identified in tissues of patients with AIDS-associated KS as well as endemic, classic, and transplant-associated KS (95). The role of HIV infection in the development of KS is unclear, but studies suggest that AIDS-associated KS has a more aggressive clinical course than other types of KS (95). Ongoing work seeks to elucidate disease pathogenesis, and to clarify the controversy whether KS is a true malignancy or a polyclonal, inflammatory response to viral infection (95).

Diagnosis of pleural effusions related to KS can be problematic, as pleural fluid cytology is either negative or reveals only reactive or atypical cells (94,98). Pleural biopsies likewise are usually negative, as KS is confined to the visceral pleura (91,94). Other diagnostic procedures include thoracoscopic evaluation with visualization or biopsy of lesions on the visceral pleura (17). HHV-8 can be identified by molecular techniques including PCR from involved tissue and also from peripheral blood in patients with active KS (99). While the clinical applications and performance of PCR and other approaches to isolate HHV-8 in pleural fluid, serum, or other tissues have not been studied extensively (17), molecular diagnosis represents a promising approach (91). In current practice, the attribution of a pleural effusion to KS is largely based on the combination of clinical presentation, physical examination, and radiographic findings. Although infectious causes should always be considered, the findings of pleural effusion in association with typical parenchymal abnormalities, namely, ill-defined peribronchovascular nodules, perihilar infiltrates, and septal thickening, are suggestive of KS (15,93,100).

Treatment options include chemotherapy, radiation therapy, and HAART. Tumors have been reported to shrink as patients experience an immunological and virological response to HAART (91). Historically, in the pre-HAART era, prognosis has been poor, with median survival ranging between 4 and 12 months in patients with pulmonary KS. Survival appears to be improved, however, in reports of patients treated with HAART (91), although no curative therapy for KS currently exists (90). Other agents to consider include interferon-alpha and chemotherapeutic agents such as doxorubicin, bleomycin, and vinca alkaloids in patients with more advanced disease (90). Recurrent pleural effusions can be problematic and may require repeated drainage; although sclerotherapy is usually ineffective, pleurodesis and pleuroperitoneal shunts are alternative options (88,101).

Immune reconstitution inflammatory syndrome (IRIS) has been reported in patients with KS who are initiated on HAART, within a period varying from one week to several months following initiation of therapy (102,103). Pulmonary manifestations of IRIS related to KS include progression of underlying pulmonary abnormalities, including worsening or new pleural effusion and lymphadenopathy. Although the number of cases reported is small, IRIS with pulmonary involvement from KS has been fatal in some patients and chemotherapy may be considered on an individual basis after a thorough diagnostic evaluation for concurrent infection has been undertaken (103).

B. Non–Hodgkin's Lymphoma

Non–Hodgkin's lymphoma (NHL) is the second most common malignancy in HIV-infected patients (104), which occurs in 2% to 5% of HIV-infected patients (98). Most of these tumors are of B-cell origin and can be classified into one of three histological subtypes: large-cell immunoblastic, small noncleaved cell or Burkitt's, and diffuse large cell (105). Frequently NHL is a disseminated disease with extranodal spread at the time of diagnosis. Pulmonary involvement occurs in 5% to 31% of patients with AIDS-related NHL based on clinical grounds (16,106,107), although a significantly higher proportion have pulmonary involvement documented on autopsy (16).

Pleural effusions are common in AIDS-related NHL. In a retrospective review of 38 cases of pulmonary involvement in NHL in AIDS patients, pleural effusions were detected on chest X-ray in 44%, and in 68% of patients by CT scan (16). In patients with HIV who present with pleural effusion, NHL accounts for approximately 1% to 17% of the cases (Table 1) (1,2,4,6–8). NHL is distinct from AIDS-related primary pulmonary lymphoma, also typically a B-cell tumor, which excludes patients with pleural effusion and includes only those patients with pulmonary parenchymal involvement in the absence of thoracic lymphadenopathy or extrathoracic spread (108,109).

As in many pulmonary illnesses, common presenting features are nonspecific and include dyspnea and cough (16). Most patients have advanced HIV infection, with median CD4+ T-cell counts below 100 cells/μL (16). Pleural fluid is exudative, often with very high levels of LDH (16). Thoracocentesis and pleural biopsy are useful diagnostic steps. The yield of pleural cytology is significantly higher in HIV-associated pulmonary lymphoma as opposed to HIV-negative cases (7). In one report, as few as 11% of cases in HIV-negative individuals had positive results on fluid cytology, with only a 16% yield on closed pleural biopsy (110). In contrast, up to 45% to 75% of cases in HIV-infected individuals had positive results on pleural fluid cytology (16,106), with a 100% yield on closed pleural biopsy specimens reported (16). Flow cytometry of pleural fluid can also be used for diagnosis (19).

Pleural effusions tend to be bilateral in 41% to 55% of cases, with more bilateral effusions detected on CT scan as opposed to chest X-ray (16,106). Associated parenchymal radiographic findings consist primarily of nodules, lobar consolidation, masses, and hilar or mediastinal lymphadenopathy (16,107). Rare prior cases of primary pleural involvement in the absence of detectable systemic lymphadenopathy or parenchymal involvement have been reported as a manifestation of AIDS-associated NHL (106,111). These cases may actually represent PEL, a subset of AIDS-associated NHL, which is discussed further below.

AIDS-related NHLs are generally aggressive tumors with a poor prognosis; median survival has historically been approximately 4 to 10 months prior to HAART (98,112). Although previous studies have indicated that intensive chemotherapy was associated with increased deaths due to infection (98), current studies suggest that combining HAART with more intensive chemotherapy can improve disease-free survival in these patients (112). Pulmonary involvement is treated as a part of systemic disease.

C. Primary Effusion Lymphoma

A subset of NHL, PEL or body-cavity-based lymphomas are tumors that grow exclusively in the pleural, pericardial, or peritoneal cavities as lymphomatous effusions (113). A rare disease, PEL represents approximately 0.13% to 3% of all AIDS-related NHL (114,115). These tumors are found nearly exclusively in HIV-infected patients (116) who are MSM and typically of white race (115,117,118). HIV infection is usually advanced; in one study, peripheral CD4+ T-cell counts averaged 200 cells/μL (115). PEL may occur more commonly in patients with a prior history of KS (115).

Pleural effusions due to PEL can be unilateral or bilateral; by definition, no pulmonary parenchymal or nodal disease is evident (116,118). Pleural disease can include diffuse thickening of the parietal pleura, but no plaque-like or nodular thickening is demonstrable on CT scan (116). Pleural fluid cytology is positive, consistent with the liquid-phase growth pattern of these tumors (116).

Although immunophenotypically indeterminate, PEL tumors are of B-cell genotype with high-grade morphologic features and clonal rearrangements of the immunoglobulin gene (113). HHV-8 is found in all cases of PEL (113,116–118). Detection of HHV-8–associated latent protein within the nuclei of malignant cells by immunohistochemical methods is important in establishing the diagnosis of PEL (119). In addition, Epstein Barr virus (EBV) is demonstrated in nearly all of the AIDS-associated PEL tumors as well, although its role in tumor development and progression is unclear (119).

Prognosis is poor, with median survival on the order of three to six months (113,118–120). Treatment options include HAART and systemic chemotherapy, often with agents known to have activity against intermediate and high-grade NHL. Case reports have suggested a possible role for intrapleural injections with the antiviral drug cidofovir (119).

VII. Causes of Transudative Effusions in HIV-Infected Patients

Most transudative effusions in HIV-infected patients are a result of the same conditions as are seen in HIV-negative individuals, namely, congestive heart failure (CHF), renal insufficiency, and liver disease (Table 1). Treatment consists of management of the underlying medical conditions, as in HIV-negative patients. Whether HIV-infected patients are more likely to develop effusions related to these disease processes has not been studied.

A significant number of transudative effusions in hospitalized HIV-infected patients have been attributed to hypoalbuminemia. In one study, nearly 20% of effusions were attributed to hypoalbuminemia, which was defined as a serum albumin concentration <1.8 g/dL with no other identifiable cause for the effusion (5). The majority of these effusions were classified as small. Whether hypoalbuminemia alone is sufficient to cause a clinically significant pleural effusion, however, is unclear. Rather, hypoalbuminemia is likely to act in concert with another pathological cause in contribution to the formation of an effusion (121). In agreement with this, two studies have reported a significantly decreased serum albumin among hospitalized HIV-infected patients with pleural effusion when compared to HIV-infected patients without pleural effusion (1,5).

VIII. Conclusion

The causes of pleural effusion in HIV-infected patients are diverse. Etiologies to consider include all the causes of transudative and exudative effusions that can be seen in

HIV-uninfected patients. Certain infectious etiologies such as parapneumonic effusions and tuberculosis are encountered very commonly in the HIV-infected patient as well as in the HIV-negative patient. Other etiologies such as KS or PEL will be encountered nearly exclusively in the HIV-infected patient. In addition to routine history and physical examination, key features to be considered include degree of immunosuppression, HIV risk factors and behaviors, regional variability in disease prevalence, and concomitant radiographic abnormalities. Diagnostic evaluation and management choices are generally the same as in HIV-negative individuals.

References

1. Afessa B. Pleural effusion and pneumothorax in hospitalized patients with HIV infection: The Pulmonary Complications, ICU support, and Prognostic Factors of Hospitalized Patients with HIV (PIP) Study. Chest 2000; 117(4):1031–1037.
2. Armbruster C, Schalleschak J, Vetter N, et al. Pleural effusions in human immunodeficiency virus-infected patients. Correlation with concomitant pulmonary diseases. Acta Cytol 1995; 39(4):698–700.
3. Lababidi HMS, Gupta K, Newman T, et al. A retropective analysis of pleural effusion in human immunodeficiency virus infected patients. Chest 1994; 106(2):86S.
4. Miller RF, Howling SJ, Reid AJ, et al. Pleural effusions in patients with AIDS. Sex Transm Infect 2000; 76(2):122–125.
5. Joseph J, Strange C, Sahn SA. Pleural effusions in hospitalized patients with AIDS. Ann Intern Med 1993; 118(11):856–859.
6. Cadranel JL, Chouaid C, Denis M, et al. Causes of pleural effusion in 75 HIV-infected patients. Chest 1993; 104(2):655.
7. Soubani AO, Michelson MK, Karnik A. Pleural fluid findings in patients with the acquired immunodeficiency syndrome: Correlation with concomitant pulmonary disease. South Med J 1999; 92(4):400–403.
8. Trejo O, Giron JA, Perez-Guzman E, et al. Pleural effusion in patients infected with the human immunodeficiency virus. Eur J Clin Microbiol Infect Dis 1997; 16(11):807–815.
9. Batungwanayo J, Taelman H, Allen S, et al. Pleural effusion, tuberculosis and HIV-1 infection in Kigali, Rwanda. AIDS 1993; 7(1):73–79.
10. Hirschtick RE, Glassroth J, Jordan MC, et al. Bacterial pneumonia in persons infected with the human immunodeficiency virus. Pulmonary Complications of HIV Infection Study Group. N Engl J Med 1995; 333(13):845–851.
11. Wallace JM, Hansen NI, Lavange L, et al. Respiratory disease trends in the Pulmonary Complications of HIV Infection Study cohort. Pulmonary Complications of HIV Infection Study Group. Am J Respir Crit Care Med 1997; 155(1):72–80.
12. Cohen M, Sahn SA. Resolution of pleural effusions. Chest 2001; 119(5):1547–1562.
13. Relkin F, Aranda CP, Garay SM, et al. Pleural tuberculosis and HIV infection. Chest 1994; 105(5):1338–1341.
14. Frye MD, Pozsik CJ, Sahn SA. Tuberculous pleurisy is more common in AIDS than in non-AIDS patients with tuberculosis. Chest 1997; 112(2):393–397.
15. Gruden JF, Huang L, Webb WR, et al. AIDS-related Kaposi sarcoma of the lung: Radiographic findings and staging system with bronchoscopic correlation. Radiology 1995; 195(2): 545–552.
16. Eisner MD, Kaplan LD, Herndier B, et al. The pulmonary manifestations of AIDS-related non-Hodgkin's lymphoma. Chest 1996; 110(3):729–736.
17. Beck JM. Pleural disease in patients with acquired immune deficiency syndrome. Clin Chest Med 1998; 19(2):341–349.

18. de Lalla F, Vaglia A, Franzetti M, et al. Cryptococcal pleural effusion as first indicator of AIDS: A case report. Infection 1993; 21(3):192.

19. Lee AM, Katner HP. AIDS-related lymphoma diagnosed by flow cytometry of a pleural effusion. South Med J 1991; 84(10):1278–1279.

20. Cordero E, Pachon J, Rivero A, et al. Community-acquired bacterial pneumonia in human immunodeficiency virus-infected patients: Validation of severity criteria. The Grupo Andaluz para el Estudio de las Enfermedades Infecciosas. Am J Respir Crit Care Med 2000; 162(6):2063–2068.

21. Selwyn PA, Feingold AR, Hartel D, et al. Increased risk of bacterial pneumonia in HIV-infected intravenous drug users without AIDS. AIDS 1988; 2(4):267–272.

22. Clavo-Sanchez AJ, Giron-Gonzalez JA, Lopez-Prieto D, et al. Influence of CD4+ status on the invasiveness of pneumococcal pneumonia in HIV patients. Eur J Clin Microbiol Infect Dis 1996; 15(12):959–960.

23. Falco V, Fernandez de Sevilla T, Alegre J, et al. Bacterial pneumonia in HIV-infected patients: A prospective study of 68 episodes. Eur Respir J 1994; 7(2):235–239.

24. Gil Suay V, Cordero PJ, Martinez E, et al. Parapneumonic effusions secondary to community-acquired bacterial pneumonia in human immunodeficiency virus-infected patients. Eur Respir J 1995; 8(11):1934–1939.

25. Tumbarello M, Tacconelli E, Lucia MB, et al. Predictors of *Staphylococcus aureus* pneumonia associated with human immunodeficiency virus infection. Respir Med 1996; 90(9):531–537.

26. Hernandez Borge J, Alfageme Michavila I, Munoz Mendez J, et al. Thoracic empyema in HIV-infected patients: Microbiology, management, and outcome. Chest 1998; 113(3):732–738.

27. Mundy LM, Auwaerter PG, Oldach D, et al. Community-acquired pneumonia: Impact of immune status. Am J Respir Crit Care Med 1995; 152(4 Pt 1):1309–1315.

28. Burack JH, Hahn JA, Saint-Maurice D, et al. Microbiology of community-acquired bacterial pneumonia in persons with and at risk for human immunodeficiency virus type 1 infection. Implications for rational empiric antibiotic therapy. Arch Intern Med 1994; 154(22):2589–2596.

29. Janoff EN, Breiman RF, Daley CL, et al. Pneumococcal disease during HIV infection. Epidemiologic, clinical, and immunologic perspectives. Ann Intern Med 1992; 117(4):314–324.

30. Rodriguez Barradas MC, Musher DM, Hamill RJ, et al. Unusual manifestations of pneumococcal infection in human immunodeficiency virus-infected individuals: The past revisited. Clin Infect Dis 1992; 14(1):192–199.

31. Kielhofner M, Atmar RL, Hamill RJ, et al. Life-threatening *Pseudomonas aeruginosa* infections in patients with human immunodeficiency virus infection. Clin Infect Dis 1992; 14(2):403–411.

32. Wolday D, Seyoum B. Pleural empyema due to *Salmonella paratyphi* in a patient with AIDS. Trop Med Int Health 1997; 2(12):1140–1142.

33. Uttamchandani RB, Daikos GL, Reyes RR, et al. Nocardiosis in 30 patients with advanced human immunodeficiency virus infection: Clinical features and outcome. Clin Infect Dis 1994; 18(3):348–353.

34. Calore EE, Vazquez CR, Perez NM, et al. Empyema with malakoplakic-like lesions by *Rhodococcus equi* as a presentation of HIV infection. Pathologica 1995; 87(5):525–527.

35. Owino EA, McLigeyo SO, Gathua SN, et al. Prevalence of human immunodeficiency virus infection: Its impact on the diagnostic yields in exudative pleural effusions at the kenyatta national hospital, Nairobi. East Afr Med J 1996; 73(9):575–578.

36. Kramer MR, Uttamchandani RB. The radiographic appearance of pulmonary nocardiosis associated with AIDS. Chest 1990; 98(2):382–385.

37. Feins RH. The role of thoracoscopy in the AIDS/immunocompromised patient. Ann Thorac Surg 1993; 56(3):649–650.

38. Flum DR, Steinberg SD, Bernik TR, et al. Thoracoscopy in acquired immunodeficiency syndrome. J Thorac Cardiovasc Surg 1997; 114(3):361–366.
39. Khwaja S, Rosenbaum DH, Paul MC, et al. Surgical treatment of thoracic empyema in HIV-infected patients: Severity and treatment modality is associated with CD4 count status. Chest 2005; 128(1):246–249.
40. Batungwanayo J, Taelman H, Dhote R, et al. Pulmonary tuberculosis in Kigali, Rwanda. Impact of human immunodeficiency virus infection on clinical and radiographic presentation. Am Rev Respir Dis 1992; 146(1):53–56.
41. Saks AM, Posner R. Tuberculosis in HIV positive patients in South Africa: A comparative radiological study with HIV negative patients. Clin Radiol 1992; 46(6):387–390.
42. Tshibwabwa-Tumba E, Mwinga A, Pobee JO, et al. Radiological features of pulmonary tuberculosis in 963 HIV-infected adults at three Central African Hospitals. Clin Radiol 1997; 52(11):837–841.
43. Lawn SD, Evans AJ, Sedgwick PM, et al. Pulmonary tuberculosis: Radiological features in West Africans coinfected with HIV. Br J Radiol 1999; 72(856):339–344.
44. Perlman DC, el-Sadr WM, Nelson ET, et al. Variation of chest radiographic patterns in pulmonary tuberculosis by degree of human immunodeficiency virus-related immunosuppression. The Terry Beirn Community Programs for Clinical Research on AIDS (CPCRA). The AIDS Clinical Trials Group (ACTG). Clin Infect Dis 1997; 25(2):242–246.
45. Valdes L, San Jose E, Alvarez D, et al. Diagnosis of tuberculous pleurisy using the biologic parameters adenosine deaminase, lysozyme, and interferon gamma. Chest 1993; 103(2): 458–465.
46. Richter C, Perenboom R, Mtoni I, et al. Clinical features of HIV-seropositive and HIV-seronegative patients with tuberculous pleural effusion in Dar es Salaam, Tanzania. Chest 1994; 106(5):1471–1475.
47. Luzze H, Elliott AM, Joloba ML, et al. Evaluation of suspected tuberculous pleurisy: Clinical and diagnostic findings in HIV-1-positive and HIV-negative adults in Uganda. Int J Tuberc Lung Dis 2001; 5(8):746–753.
48. Jones BE, Young SM, Antoniskis D, et al. Relationship of the manifestations of tuberculosis to CD4 cell counts in patients with human immunodeficiency virus infection. Am Rev Respir Dis 1993; 148(5):1292–1297.
49. Post FA, Wood R, Pillay GP. Pulmonary tuberculosis in HIV infection: Radiographic appearance is related to CD4+ T-lymphocyte count. Tuber Lung Dis 1995; 76(6):518–521.
50. Jones D, Lieb T, Narita M, et al. Mesothelial cells in tuberculous pleural effusions of HIV-infected patients. Chest 2000; 117(1):289–291.
51. Morehead RS. Tuberculosis of the pleura. South Med J 1998; 91(7):630–636.
52. Gopi A, Madhavan SM, Sharma SK, et al. Diagnosis and treatment of tuberculous pleural effusion in 2006. Chest 2007; 131(3):880–889.
53. Roth BJ. Searching for tuberculosis in the pleural space. Chest 1999; 116(1):3–5.
54. Villena V, Navarro-Gonzalvez JA, Garcia-Benayas C, et al. Rapid automated determination of adenosine deaminase and lysozyme for differentiating tuberculous and nontuberculous pleural effusions. Clin Chem 1996; 42(2):218–221.
55. Hsu WH, Chiang CD, Huang PL. Diagnostic value of pleural adenosine deaminase in tuberculous effusions of immunocompromised hosts. J Formos Med Assoc 1993; 92(7): 668–670.
56. Riantawan P, Chaowalit P, Wongsangiem M, et al. Diagnostic value of pleural fluid adenosine deaminase in tuberculous pleuritis with reference to HIV coinfection and a Bayesian analysis. Chest 1999; 116(1):97–103.
57. Hodsdon WS, Luzze H, Hurst TJ, et al. HIV-1-related pleural tuberculosis: Elevated production of IFN-gamma, but failure of immunity to *Mycobacterium tuberculosis*. AIDS 2001; 15(4):467–475.

58. Villena V, Rebollo MJ, Aguado JM, et al. Polymerase chain reaction for the diagnosis of pleural tuberculosis in immunocompromised and immunocompetent patients. Clin Infect Dis 1998; 26(1):212–214.

59. Small PM, Fujiwara PI. Management of tuberculosis in the United States. N Engl J Med 2001; 345(3):189–200.

60. Elliott AM, Luzze H, Quigley MA, et al. A randomized, double-blind, placebo-controlled trial of the use of prednisolone as an adjunct to treatment in HIV-1-associated pleural tuberculosis. J Infect Dis 2004; 190(5):869–878.

61. Engel ME, Matchaba PT, Volmink J. Corticosteroids for tuberculous pleurisy. Cochrane Database Syst Rev 2007; (4): CD001876.

62. Chin DP, Hopewell PC. Mycobacterial complications of HIV infection. Clin Chest Med 1996; 17(4):697–711.

63. Rigsby MO, Curtis AM. Pulmonary disease from nontuberculous mycobacteria in patients with human immunodeficiency virus. Chest 1994; 106(3):913–919.

64. Bankier AA, Stauffer F, Fleischmann D, et al. Radiographic findings in patients with acquired immunodeficiency syndrome, pulmonary infection, and microbiologic evidence of *Mycobacterium xenopi*. J Thorac Imaging 1998; 13(4):282–288.

65. Fishman JE, Schwartz DS, Sais GJ. *Mycobacterium kansasii* pulmonary infection in patients with AIDS: Spectrum of chest radiographic findings. Radiology 1997; 204(1): 171–175.

66. Campo RE, Campo CE. *Mycobacterium kansasii* disease in patients infected with human immunodeficiency virus. Clin Infect Dis 1997; 24(6):1233–1238.

67. El-Solh AA, Nopper J, Abdul-Khoudoud MR, et al. Clinical and radiographic manifestations of uncommon pulmonary nontuberculous mycobacterial disease in AIDS patients. Chest 1998; 114(1):138–145.

68. Juffermans NP, Verbon A, Danner SA, et al. *Mycobacterium xenopi* in HIV-infected patients: An emerging pathogen. AIDS 1998; 12(13):1661–1666.

69. Laissy JP, Cadi M, Cinqualbre A, et al. *Mycobacterium tuberculosis* versus nontuberculous mycobacterial infection of the lung in AIDS patients: CT and HRCT patterns. J Comput Assist Tomogr 1997; 21(2):312–317.

70. Horowitz ML, Schiff M, Samuels J, et al. Pneumocystis carinii pleural effusion. Pathogenesis and pleural fluid analysis. Am Rev Respir Dis 1993; 148(1):232–234.

71. Jayes RL, Kamerow HN, Hasselquist SM, et al. Disseminated pneumocystosis presenting as a pleural effusion. Chest 1993; 103(1):306–308.

72. Schaumberg TH, Schnapp LM, Taylor KG, et al. Diagnosis of *Pneumocystis carinii* infection in HIV-seropositive patients by identification of *P. carinii* in pleural fluid. Chest 1993; 103(6):1890–1891.

73. Batungwanayo J, Taelman H, Bogaerts J, et al. Pulmonary cryptococcosis associated with HIV-1 infection in Rwanda: A retrospective study of 37 cases. AIDS 1994; 8(9): 1271–1276.

74. Friedman EP, Miller RF, Severn A, et al. Cryptococcal pneumonia in patients with the acquired immunodeficiency syndrome. Clin Radiol 1995; 50(11):756–760.

75. Grum EE, Schwab R, Margolis ML. Cryptococcal pleural effusion preceding cryptococcal meningitis in AIDS. Am J Med Sci 1991; 301(5):329–330.

76. Katz AS, Niesenbaum L, Mass B. Pleural effusion as the initial manifestation of disseminated cryptococcosis in acquired immune deficiency syndrome. Diagnosis by pleural biopsy. Chest 1989; 96(2):440–441.

77. Newman TG, Soni A, Acaron S, et al. Pleural cryptococcosis in the acquired immune deficiency syndrome. Chest 1987; 91(3):459–461.

78. Fungal infection in HIV-infected persons. American Thoracic Society. Am J Respir Crit Care Med 1995; 152(2):816–822.

79. Miller WT Jr, Edelman JM, Miller WT. Cryptococcal pulmonary infection in patients with AIDS: Radiographic appearance. Radiology 1990; 175(3):725–728.

80. Ankobiah WA, Vaidya K, Powell S, et al. Disseminated histoplasmosis in AIDS. Clinicopathologic features in seven patients from a non-endemic area. N Y State J Med 1990; 90(5):234–238.

81. Marshall BC, Cox JK Jr, Carroll KC, et al. Histoplasmosis as a cause of pleural effusion in the acquired immunodeficiency syndrome. Am J Med Sci 1990; 300(2):98–101.

82. Fish DG, Ampel NM, Galgiani JN, et al. Coccidioidomycosis during human immunodeficiency virus infection. A review of 77 patients. Medicine (Baltimore) 1990; 69(6):384–391.

83. Singh VR, Smith DK, Lawerence J, et al. Coccidioidomycosis in patients infected with human immunodeficiency virus: Review of 91 cases at a single institution. Clin Infect Dis 1996; 23(3):563–568.

84. Staples CA, Kang EY, Wright JL, et al. Invasive pulmonary aspergillosis in AIDS: Radiographic, CT, and pathologic findings. Radiology 1995; 196(2):409–414.

85. Hung CC, Chen PJ, Hsieh SM, et al. Invasive amoebiasis: An emerging parasitic disease in patients infected with HIV in an area endemic for amoebic infection. AIDS 1999; 13(17): 2421–2428.

86. Chenoweth CE, Singal S, Pearson RD, et al. Acquired immunodeficiency syndrome-related visceral leishmaniasis presenting in a pleural effusion. Chest 1993; 103(2):648–649.

87. Rabaud C, May T, Lucet JC, et al. Pulmonary toxoplasmosis in patients infected with human immunodeficiency virus: A French National Survey. Clin Infect Dis 1996; 23(6):1249–1254.

88. Afessa B. Pleural effusions and pneumothoraces in AIDS. Curr Opin Pulm Med 2001; 7(4):202–209.

89. Behling CA, Wolf PL, Haghighi P. AIDS and malignant mesothelioma—Is there a connection? Chest 1993; 103(4):1268–1269.

90. Hengge UR, Ruzicka T, Tyring SK, et al. Update on Kaposi's sarcoma and other HHV8 associated diseases. Part 1: Epidemiology, environmental predispositions, clinical manifestations, and therapy. Lancet Infect Dis 2002; 2(5):281–292.

91. Aboulafia DM. The epidemiologic, pathologic, and clinical features of AIDS-associated pulmonary Kaposi's sarcoma. Chest 2000; 117(4):1128–1145.

92. Huang L, Schnapp LM, Gruden JF, et al. Presentation of AIDS-related pulmonary Kaposi's sarcoma diagnosed by bronchoscopy. Am J Respir Crit Care Med 1996; 153(4 Pt 1): 1385–1390.

93. Khalil AM, Carette MF, Cadranel JL, et al. Intrathoracic Kaposi's sarcoma. CT findings. Chest 1995; 108(6):1622–1626.

94. O'Brien RF, Cohn DL. Serosanguineous pleural effusions in AIDS-associated Kaposi's sarcoma. Chest 1989; 96(3):460–466.

95. Hengge UR, Ruzicka T, Tyring SK, et al. Update on Kaposi's sarcoma and other HHV8 associated diseases. Part 2: Pathogenesis, Castleman's disease, and pleural effusion lymphoma. Lancet Infect Dis 2002; 2(6):344–352.

96. Judson MA, Postic B. Chylothorax in a patient with AIDS and Kaposi's sarcoma. South Med J 1990; 83(3):322–324.

97. Sivit CJ, Schwartz AM, Rockoff SD. Kaposi's sarcoma of the lung in AIDS: Radiologic–pathologic analysis. AJR Am J Roentgenol 1987; 148(1):25–28.

98. White DA. Pulmonary complications of HIV-associated malignancies. Clin Chest Med 1996; 17(4):755–761.

99. Marcelin AG, Motol J, Guihot A, et al. Relationship between the quantity of Kaposi sarcoma-associated herpesvirus (KSHV) in peripheral blood and effusion fluid samples and KSHV-associated disease. J Infect Dis 2007; 196(8):1163–1166.

100. Padley SP, King LJ. Computed tomography of the thorax in HIV disease. Eur Radiol 1999; 9(8):1556–1569.

101. Rubio ER, Chang EE, Kovitz KL. Thoracoscopic management of pleural effusions in Kaposi's sarcoma: A rapid and effective alternative for diagnosis and treatment. South Med J 2002; 95(8):919–921.
102. Connick E, Kane MA, White IE, et al. Immune reconstitution inflammatory syndrome associated with Kaposi sarcoma during potent antiretroviral therapy. Clin Infect Dis 2004; 39(12):1852–1855.
103. Godoy MC, Rouse H, Brown JA, et al. Imaging features of pulmonary Kaposi sarcoma-associated immune reconstitution syndrome. AJR Am J Roentgenol 2007; 189(4):956–965.
104. Powles T, Matthews G, Bower M. AIDS related systemic non-Hodgkin's lymphoma. Sex Transm Infect 2000; 76(5):335–341.
105. Sandler AS, Kaplan L. AIDS lymphoma. Curr Opin Oncol 1996; 8(5):377–385.
106. Sider L, Weiss AJ, Smith MD, et al. Varied appearance of AIDS-related lymphoma in the chest. Radiology 1989; 171(3):629–632.
107. Blunt DM, Padley SP. Radiographic manifestations of AIDS related lymphoma in the thorax. Clin Radiol 1995; 50(9):607–612.
108. Bazot M, Cadranel J, Khalil A, et al. Computed tomographic diagnosis of bronchogenic carcinoma in HIV-infected patients. Lung Cancer 2000; 28(3):203–209.
109. Ray P, Antoine M, Mary-Krause M, et al. AIDS-related primary pulmonary lymphoma. Am J Respir Crit Care Med 1998; 158(4):1221–1229.
110. Celikoglu F, Teirstein AS, Krellenstein DJ, et al. Pleural effusion in non-Hodgkin's lymphoma. Chest 1992; 101(5):1357–1360.
111. Alonso-Villaverde C, Hernandez Flix S, Tomas Mas R, et al. Pleural involvement as a manifestation of AIDS-associated lymphoma. AJR Am J Roentgenol 1994; 163(4):993–994.
112. Tirelli U, Spina M, Gaidano G, et al. Epidemiological, biological and clinical features of HIV-related lymphomas in the era of highly active antiretroviral therapy. AIDS 2000; 14(12): 1675–1688.
113. Cesarman E, Chang Y, Moore PS, et al. Kaposi's sarcoma-associated herpesvirus-like DNA sequences in AIDS-related body-cavity-based lymphomas. N Engl J Med 1995; 332(18):1186–1191.
114. Ibrahimbacha A, Farah M, Saluja J. An HIV-infected patient with pleural effusion. Chest 1999; 116(4):1113–1115.
115. Mbulaiteye SM, Biggar RJ, Goedert JJ, et al. Pleural and peritoneal lymphoma among people with AIDS in the United States. J Acquir Immune Defic Syndr 2002; 29(4):418–421.
116. Morassut S, Vaccher E, Balestreri L, et al. HIV-associated human herpesvirus 8-positive primary lymphomatous effusions: Radiologic findings in six patients. Radiology 1997; 205(2):459–463.
117. Nador RG, Cesarman E, Chadburn A, et al. Primary effusion lymphoma: A distinct clinico-pathologic entity associated with the Kaposi's sarcoma-associated herpes virus. Blood 1996; 88(2):645–656.
118. Ansari MQ, Dawson DB, Nador R, et al. Primary body cavity-based AIDS-related lymphomas. Am J Clin Pathol 1996; 105(2):221–229.
119. Chen YB, Rahemtullah A, Hochberg E. Primary effusion lymphoma. Oncologist 2007; 12(5):569–576.
120. Boulanger E, Gerard L, Gabarre J, et al. Prognostic factors and outcome of human herpesvirus 8-associated primary effusion lymphoma in patients with AIDS. J Clin Oncol 2005; 23(19):4372–4380.
121. Eid AA, Keddissi JI, Kinasewitz GT. Hypoalbuminemia as a cause of pleural effusions. Chest 1999; 115(4):1066–1069.

34
Pleural Effusions in Cardiac Disease

JOHN F. MURRAY
University of California, San Francisco, California, U.S.A.

I. Introduction

Today, life expectancy is increasing in all countries of the world except those that are extremely poor. This means, of course, that more and more people are living longer and longer and will suffer from classic old-age–related medical complications: heart disease, cancer, COPD, and Alzheimer's, and other neurodegenerative diseases. More heart disease means more heart failure with accompanying pleural effusions, the accumulation of transudative liquid in, often, both pleural spaces. Most patients with cardiogenic pleural effusions have congestive failure from some variety of left-sided heart disease; less commonly, pericardial disease or various types of cardiac injury, including heart surgery, may be associated with pleural effusion. Patients with heart disease may also develop pleural effusions of noncardiac origin, especially those caused by pulmonary emboli and bacterial pneumonia. The diagnosis of cardiac-related pleural effusions is ordinarily straightforward, and treatment is focused on the underlying heart disease; sometimes, though, as pointed out in this chapter, variations on the familiar clinical themes may confuse and complicate matters for both patients and physicians.

A. Prevalence

Cardiac disease has been recognized as one of the three most important causes of pleural effusion in virtually all large series of cases reported during the last 50 years; whether cardiac disease tops the ranking or follows malignancy and/or tuberculosis depends on the location and type of institution in which the survey was carried out. In industrialized countries, heart disease usually leads to the list of causes. In the United States, for example, according to Light (1), congestive heart failure will account for 500,000 of the 1,337,000 estimated annual cases of pleural effusion of various types. In some referral institutions, however, malignancies predominate (2), and it must be remembered that tuberculosis remains the most common cause of pleural effusion in countries with a high prevalence of that disease (3).

The frequency of hydrothorax in patients with cardiac disease, as might be expected, depends on two factors: the presence and severity of associated heart failure, and the sensitivity of the method used to detect whether or not effusion is present. These two factors account for the considerable variation in prevalence rates that are found in published reports. For example, using the radiological techniques available in 1941, Bedford and Lovibond (4) found pleural effusions in 39% of 356 patients with overt congestive failure; in 1963, Logue and coworkers (5) conducted a careful radiological study, which included tomography in an unspecified number and reported a prevalence of pleural effusion of 58% in 114 patients with a diagnosis of pulmonary edema; finally, using modern techniques of computed tomography, Kataoka (6) identified pleural effusion(s) in 87% of 60 patients with congestive heart failure. Among 71 patients awaiting cardiac transplantation, however, who were selected by their physicians to have computed tomography, the prevalence of pleural effusion was only 44% (7). In two studies of patients with heart disease hospitalized in intensive care units, the prevalence of pleural effusions detected by sonography was nearly the same, 51% (8) and 56% (9).

II. Pathogenesis

The mechanisms that underlie the formation of the characteristic transudative pleural effusions that are found in patients with congestive heart failure are now reasonably well understood. The small amount of liquid that is normally present in the pleural spaces of healthy humans originates from branches of the systemic circulation that perfuse the parietal pleura, the delicate membrane that lines the outer surface of both pleural cavities; once formed from the capillaries and other tiny blood vessels (collectively known as "microvessels"), the low-protein ultrafiltrate traverses the parietal surface membrane into the pleural spaces; ordinarily, none of the liquid arises from the lungs and enters the pleural spaces through the visceral pleura; by contrast, some liquid (as yet an unknown proportion) is believed to be removed through the visceral pleural (10). Another important pathway—especially for particles, cells, protein, and excess liquid (when present)—is through lymphatic channels that drain both pleural spaces through stomata, microscopic openings that are present only on the parietal pleura (11).

The liquid that collects in the pleural spaces of patients with congestive heart failure comes from within the lungs, and its formation is governed by the hydrostatic and oncotic forces that affect filtration across the microvessels of the pulmonary circulation. Once left ventricular filling pressure is increased, pulmonary capillary hydrostatic pressure rises correspondingly and liquid filtration increases in the lungs. But pleural effusion occurs late in the evolution of the underlying heart disease, well after the onset of congestive failure. In a study of hospitalized patients with congestive heart failure, mean pulmonary arterial wedge pressure was 24 ± 1 mm Hg in the 19 patients with sonographically detectable pleural effusions compared with 17 ± 2 mm Hg in the 18 patients without effusions ($p < 0.01$) (8).

Several inherent safety factors serve to protect the lungs by preventing the development of pulmonary edema, thereby preserving gas exchange. But when these mechanisms are overwhelmed, liquid begins to accumulate, first in the large peribronchovascular interstitial space and last in the alveoli (12). No one knows exactly when along the continuum of worsening edema the liquid begins to spill over into the pleural spaces. Judging from experiments in which the lungs were made progressively edematous, it took time for the lungs to start to leak (13)—presumably, this means that the peribronchovascular interstitium has to be at least partially filled with liquid before it seeps from the subpleural interstitial space into the pleural spaces owing to the prevailing pressure gradient across the visceral pleura (14).

Cardiogenic pleural effusions, therefore, represent pulmonary edema that has leaked across the visceral pleura, an obvious way to rid the lungs of liquid that would otherwise accumulate within them; in other words, the development of pleural effusions retards the onset of alveolar flooding and helps to preserve gas exchange. The amount of edema that flows into the pleural space is substantial. In one experimental preparation, 25% of the total amount of pulmonary edema that formed could be recovered from the pleural spaces (13).

The concentration of protein in pleural liquid sampled from patients with heart failure is low, but not as low as is presumed to exist in the small amount of liquid of systemic origin that is normally present in the pleural spaces of healthy persons. (No satisfactory measurements have been made in healthy humans, but there is no reason to believe that the value would differ greatly from the low value found in sheep.) Measurements in experimental animals showed that the protein concentrations in pulmonary edema liquid within the lungs, liquid in the pleural space, and liquid in the lymphatics that drain the lungs were identical (13). These results corroborate the belief that pleural effusions in patients with congestive heart failure are formed by movement of pulmonary edema from the lungs into the pleural spaces, and also explain why the ratio of the concentration of protein in the hydrothorax to that in the plasma is also low and (usually) satisfies one of Light's criteria of a transudate (15).

Although the routes of formation of pleural liquid in healthy subjects and in patients with congestive heart failure differ, the routes of spontaneous clearance appear to be the same—largely, by bulk flow via lymphatic channels that drain the parietal pleura. (The effect of treatment with diuretics on clearance and protein concentration is considered later.) In theory, then, an increase in pressure in the systemic veins into which lymphatic channels drain might serve to decrease lymph flow, this, in turn, would augment the rate of pleural effusion accumulation by retarding the rate of its clearance. Studies in experimental animals, however, are not clear-cut. Mellins and coworkers (16) were able to produce large pleural effusions by raising systemic venous pressure and lowering plasma oncotic pressure; in contrast, in the experiments of Broaddus et al. (13), an artificial hydrothorax was absorbed even when superior vena caval pressure was elevated. From a clinical point of view, it seems likely that an increase in systemic venous pressure, a common occurrence in congestive heart failure, which by itself is insufficient to cause effusions, will slow the removal of liquid leaking from the lungs into the pleural spaces, thereby contributing to the *formation* of cardiogenic pleural effusions as well as to their *duration*.

III. Congestive Heart Failure

A. Characteristics

For the reasons just discussed, the majority of patients with cardiogenic pleural effusions have congestive heart failure from left ventricular dysfunction, which may be predominantly systolic, diastolic, or mixed. The greater importance of left-sided heart disease compared with the right-sided in the origin of pleural effusions derived from a pair of crucial clinical studies in which intracardiac pressures were measured and the presence or absence of hydrothorax was documented by ultrasonography—left-sided disease was essential and right-sided disease was unimportant (8,17). The most common causes of cardiac hydrothorax in industrialized countries are ischemic heart disease from coronary artery atherosclerosis or hypertension, cardiomyopathy of any etiology, and acquired mitral or aortic valve disease.

Table 1   Radiographic Studies of Laterality of Pleural Effusions in Patients (Pts) with Congestive Heart Failure

References	Method	No. of patients	Location		
			Right	Left	Bilateral
(4)	Standard	136	68	42	26
(18)	Standard	52	20	4	28
(19)	Standard	54	18	17	19
(20)	Standard	70	13	6	51
(21)	Standard	120	18	15	87
(6)	CT	52	5	2	45
(7)	CT	31	7	8	16
Total		515	149	94	272
Percent		100	29	18	53

CT: computed tomography.

There is an oft-repeated clinical maxim dating from the 19th century that says that pleural effusions in congestive heart failure are right-sided or bilateral with right-sided predominance. This led to the belief that a unilateral left hydrothorax in a patient with congestive failure was presumed to be unrelated to heart disease and required special workup. That this is clearly not so can be seen in the results presented in Table 1, which show the findings from seven studies that used chest radiography or computed tomography to detect and localize pleural effusions in patients with congestive heart failure. Slightly more half of all effusions were bilateral, and an additional 29% were confined to the right pleural space. But solitary left hydrothorax was not uncommon and accounted for 18% of the total.

There is no satisfactory explanation for a large localized effusion in either pleural space in the face of left-sided heart disease with pulmonary vascular congestion. Regardless of its origin, an increase in pulmonary capillary pressure should increase liquid filtration equally in both lungs. Obliterative pleuritis and regional differences in intrapulmonary vascular pressures or lymph flows may occasionally influence laterality, but are inadequate causes overall. It has been speculated that cardiogenic effusions may be unilateral in mild congestive heart failure and become bilateral as failure worsens (4). But a more likely explanation relates to the accuracy of the method used to define whether or not an effusion is present. Table 1 shows that when computed tomography is employed, a much higher number of identifiable effusions proves to be bilateral than when less-sensitive standard radiographic techniques are used.

We would expect, therefore, that postmortem examination of patients who died with or of congestive heart failure should demonstrate a preponderance of bilateral hydrothorax—as expected, 290 such patients autopsied at the Mayo Clinic showed that the great majority, 88%, had bilateral pleural effusions larger than 250 mL (22). Of additional interest was the observation that the average quantity of liquid found in the right hemithorax (1084 mL) exceeded that in the left hemithorax (913 mL) by about 16%. In 1935, Dock (23) described the anatomical and hydrostatic forces controlling blood flow from the pulmonary venous bed to the left ventricle that he believed strongly favored the predominance of right over left hydrothorax. Broaddus (24), however, has proposed that the difference may well be explained by the simple facts that the volume, visceral pleural surface area, and leakage rates from the right lung are greater than those from the left lung.

B. Diagnosis

In most patients, the diagnosis of cardiogenic hydrothorax is obvious because the effusion(s) are but one manifestation of the familiar constellation of clinical and radiographic findings that typify the presence of congestive failure in a patient with known left-sided heart disease. Other associated features are cardiac enlargement, arrhythmias, an S-3 gallop, systolic or diastolic murmurs, basilar crackles, venous engorgement, hepatic tenderness, and edema of the lower extremities. It is important to remember that pleural effusions, a sign of left ventricular dysfunction, may develop in the absence of peripheral edema and other signs of right-sided heart disease; this clinical event usually occurs in new-onset left ventricular failure, which most commonly accompanies myocardial infarction. Conversely, pure right-sided heart failure (e.g., from cor pulmonale or pulmonary hypertension) should not be accepted as a sole cause of cardiogenic pleural effusion(s).

Physical examination is not a sensitive way of detecting pleural effusion unless it is large. Most effusions are discovered by standard posteroanterior and lateral radiographic examination, which may be taken as part of a routine checkup or for evaluation of worsening symptoms. Even with high-quality films, pleural liquid collections are likely to be missed unless they are larger than 300 mL—lateral decubitus projections should detect 100 mL or more of liquid (25). The results of a recent study that used thoracic computed tomography as the gold standard for identifying pleural effusions in patients with congestive heart failure indicated that routine radiography missed about 60% of the effusions found by the more sensitive method (26). Portable anteroposterior radiographs, which are often taken with patients in the supine position in intensive care units, are considerably worse, such films cannot be relied on to detect even moderate-sized pleural effusions.

Ultrasonography is clearly superior to standard radiography, particularly for the identification of small pleural effusions, and can be used at the bedside of seriously ill patients, including those in intensive care units. Ultrasonography, because of its relatively low cost, ready availability, and accuracy, would appear to be the method of choice for detecting pleural effusions, if clinically indicated, in patients whose standard films are negative or who cannot be taken to the radiology department. Most of the time, however, it is not necessary to determine if small effusions are present or not because the information does not affect how the patient is treated.

The great majority of cardiogenic hydrothoraces do not need to be verified by thoracocentesis, provided they occur in an appropriate clinical setting. In patients with known or obvious cardiac disease, the presence of unilateral or bilateral pleural effusions can be regarded as one of the associated findings of overt congestive heart failure, which should be evident. Thoracocentesis is seldom indicated, except for the occasional need to relieve breathlessness from a massive liquid collection; other reasons for tapping the chest relate to the importance of finding a noncardiogenic cause for an effusion that requires specific treatment, especially pulmonary embolism and infection.

Classically, cardiogenic pleural effusions are transudates and, as recently documented, have similar biochemical and cellular findings on each side (27). But owing to the efficacy of modern diuretic treatment of congestive heart failure, the typically low protein concentration and, less commonly, the low lactate dehydrogenase (LDH) concentration, may rise to levels found in exudates. In untreated cardiogenic effusions that resolve spontaneously by bulk flow, the concentrations of protein, LDH, and other constituents remain constant. In contrast, in patients treated with diuretics, water is removed at a faster rate than protein, which causes the pleural–serum concentration ratio of protein in the remaining liquid to increase, sometimes to levels that mimic those of an exudate (28). LDH may also rise higher than expected owing to the added influence of cell lysis and trauma from multiple thoracocenteses. This effect may be accompanied by a reduction in serum LDH from the diuresis-induced relief of hepatic congestion that follows improvement of the underlying heart failure; the increase in pleural liquid and the decrease in serum LDH concentrations may occasionally cause the pleural–serum ratio to rise to levels consistent with an exudate. To circumvent the problem of misclassification by Light's criteria, several authors have proposed that when evaluating a hydrothorax in a patient with congestive heart failure, especially after diuresis has begun, if the protein and/or LDH concentration ratios are slightly in the exudative range, one should examine the pleural–serum albumin difference—if the difference is greater than 1.2 g/dL, the effusion is most likely a transudate of cardiac origin (28–29).

Another way of verifying the presence of congestive heart failure or a cardiac hydrothorax is by finding an elevated level of N-terminal probrain natriuretic peptide (NT-proBNP) in serum or, if thoracocentesis is performed, in pleural liquid (30). Measurements of NT-proBNP proved better than the pleural–serum albumin gradient at identifying patients with cardiogenic pleural effusions erroneously classified as exudates according to Light's algorithm (31).

C. Treatment

Therapy of cardiogenic hydrothorax should be directed at the underlying heart disease. Essential elements of treatment include arrhythmia control, preload and afterload reduction, diuresis, sodium restriction, and inotropic agents. Pleural effusions generally respond to these measures, although there may be a lag between improvement in cardiac function and clearing of the chest radiograph. The key feature is that the effusions diminish rather than increase in volume.

Congestive heart failure is apt to wax and wane in severity, and with these changes pleural effusions often worsen and remit. When respiratory function is compromised by a large hydrothorax, thoracocentesis is warranted to improve breathlessness and gas exchange. The role of sclerotherapy in patients with persistent or recurrent symptomatic hydrothorax—despite maximum medical therapy—is controversial. According to one review of the subject, 12 patients have been treated by pleurodesis, with a successful outcome in 10 of them (32). This fits with the observation that successful pleurodesis following talc instillation for recurrent malignant effusions is associated with the presence of (at least some) normal mesothelial lining capable of releasing basic fibroblast growth factor and other fibrogenic substances (33). It should be remembered, though, that the development of pleural effusions in congestive heart failure serves to reduce the accumulation of liquid within the lungs—pleurodesis should worsen pulmonary edema in the affected lung but have no effect on the opposite side.

IV. Pericarditis

Hydrothorax has long been associated with both acute and chronic (constrictive) pericarditis. Owing to the infrequency of the two conditions, however, it remains impossible to make firm statements about the prevalence of associated pleural effusions, their location, and the composition of the liquid.

A. Acute Pericarditis

Weiss and Spodick (34) reviewed the charts and radiographs of 133 consecutively discharged patients with any form of pericardial disease, of these, 35 (26%) had pleural effusion(s). Among the 21 patients with evidence of acute pericarditis (etiology not specified), 15 had only left-sided pleural effusions; 3 had bilateral effusions, left larger than right; and 3 had bilateral effusions of equal size. No patient had either an isolated right-sided effusion or bilateral effusions that were predominately right-sided. Unfortunately, no thoracocenteses were performed.

Our experience at San Francisco General Hospital agrees with that of Weiss and Spodick about the frequency of left-only or left-sided predominance of bilateral pleural effusions, usually small, in patients with acute idiopathic, presumably viral, pericarditis. Thoracocenteses in a few patients revealed exudative, usually lymphocytic liquid that was similar to the liquid obtained from within the pericardium. We have assumed the mechanism of pleural liquid formation to be direct extension of the inflammatory process from within the pericardium to the contiguous pleural membrane(s).

The presence of a small left-sided or bilateral pleural effusion in a patient with acute pericarditis usually poses no diagnostic difficulty. The clinical manifestations are dominated by fever and sharp retrosternal pain, which, typically, is worse when supine and relieved by sitting forward; the diagnosis is strengthened by hearing a pericardial friction rub and/or by finding characteristic electrocardiographic changes. Pericardiocentesis is only indicated if echocardiography reveals tamponade, which is unusual, or in suspected purulent or malignant involvement. Thoracocentesis is seldom warranted unless the pleural collection is huge or does not subside as the pericardial disease resolves.

Treatment is directed at the pericardial disease if a specific cause can be identified, which is seldom the case. Symptomatic treatment with anti-inflammatory agents such as aspirin is generally effective; a three-month course of colchicine improves the outcome and is now widely used; corticosteroids increase the risk of recurrence and are best avoided (35).

B. Chronic (Constrictive) Pericarditis

Pleural effusion is said to be common in patients with chronic constrictive pericarditis, but data are scant. To date, the largest series of 35 surgically proven cases was reported by Plumb and coworkers (36) in which 21 (60%) had pleural effusion(s), which were bilateral in 12 patients and right-sided in 9—unilateral left-sided effusion was never observed. Tomaselli and colleagues (37) also found a 60% prevalence of hydrothorax in 30 patients with constrictive pericarditis of several different causes. The size was not specified, but in 12 patients the effusions were bilateral and symmetrical; in the remaining 6 patients, 3 had right-sided involvement and 3 left-sided. Thus, the left-sided predominance noted in acute pericarditis clearly does not obtain in chronic (constrictive) pericarditis.

There are a few reports of thoracocentesis findings. Of the four patients studied by Tomaselli and colleagues (37), three had exudates and one a transudate, presumably related to contiguous inflammation and congestive failure, respectively, although the precise mechanisms were not specified.

Tuberculous pericarditis, once the chief cause of constrictive pericarditis, has been replaced by mediastinal radiation, idiopathic involvement, and the after-effects of cardiac surgery. Restrictive cardiomyopathy can also cause systemic venous congestion and needs to be differentiated. Doppler echocardiography, Doppler tissue imaging, magnetic resonance imaging, and cardiac catheterization are all useful (35). Good results may follow pericardiectomy, but these results vary.

V. Postcardiac Injury Syndrome

In 1956, Dressler (38) reported 10 cases of a postmyocardial infarction syndrome, which was characterized by fever, pericarditis, pleurisy, and pneumonitis, a constellation of findings that had been previously recognized after mitral valve commissurotomy (39). As the indications for and use of open-heart surgery proliferated during the 1960s and thereafter, the onset of fever, pericarditis, and pleural effusion within a few weeks, occasionally months, of the operation was called the postpericardiotomy syndrome, a serious complication that has led to bypass graft closure and fatal cardiac tamponade (40). Similar sequelae have been reported following blunt chest trauma, percutaneous left ventricular puncture, implantation of a pacemaker, and radio frequency ablation for cardiac arrhythmias. Owing to the similarities in clinical manifestations and, presumably, in etiology, these disorders are now known collectively as the postcardiac injury syndrome (41), the prevalence of which varies with the type of injury to the heart. (Some authors, though, refer to the postpericardiotomy syndrome and the two terms appear interchangeable.) Following open-heart surgery the syndrome occurs in 10% to 50% of patients (40). The incidence, however, is much lower following myocardial infarction and, in recent years the syndrome is believed to have virtually disappeared (42).

Patients with the postcardiac injury syndrome usually complain of precordial pain and nearly always have fever and evidence of pericarditis (audible friction rub and/or typical echocardiographic or electrocardiographic abnormalities); pleural effusion is common but not invariable; pneumonitis is less frequent. In Dressler's original series, 6 of 10 patients (60%) with the syndrome following myocardial infarction had pleural effusions (38); of 38 postoperative surgical patients analyzed by Kaminsky and coworkers (43), 68% had pleural effusions. The hydrothorax is left-sided in the majority of patients and bilateral in the remainder, isolated right-sided involvement is rare. The exudative liquid is bloody in 30% of the cases. Either monocytes or polymorphonuclear cells may predominate. The etiology of the postcardiac injury syndrome remains mysterious, but is speculated to be an autoimmune process related to the presence of antimyocardial antibodies, which target antigens exposed by damage to heart muscle (44); such antibodies have also been identified in the pleural liquid of one afflicted patient (45).

The onset of fever with symptoms of pericarditis in association with pleural effusion and sometimes pneumonitis a week or two after some sort of cardiac trauma, most frequently open-heart surgery, is now so common and easy to recognize that the diagnosis should present no problem. Symptomatic treatment with anti-inflammatory agents is generally effective, although recurrences may occur. Prophylactic use of corticosteroids has not prevented the syndrome from occurring (44), but owing to the success of colchicine in treating acute pericarditis (see above), a placebo-controlled, multicenter trial of colchicine for the primary prevention of the postpericardiotomy syndrome has been planned and should be underway (46).

VI. Coronary Artery Revascularization

Constant improvements and favorable results from percutaneous coronary intervention (PCI) served to slow down the decades-long relentless steady increase in the number of coronary artery bypass graft (CABG) operations performed each year, but specific indications for one procedure or the other seem to be emerging from the many studies that have been carried out to date (47). This means hundreds of thousands of CABG operations in industrialized countries during coming years and, given the substantial incidence of pleural effusions related to the procedure (see below), myocardial revascularization surgery has moved up to fifth on the list of frequent causes of hydrothorax in industrialized countries—after congestive heart failure, pneumonia, malignancy, and pulmonary embolism (48).

The spectrum of pleural effusions after CABG surgery has been thoroughly reviewed by Heidecker and Sahn (49), who have classified them according to their time of onset after the operation—an abbreviated and modified version of their classification is shown in Table 2.

A. Immediate (During the First Week Following CABG)

Pleural effusions during the immediate postoperative period following CABG surgery are extremely common: from 41% to 87% (49). The majority of these are small, left-sided, and related to pain from the median sternotomy, chest tube placement, and impaired movement of the left hemidiaphragm, which is probably related in part to intraoperative left phrenic nerve injury. Collectively, these transient insults compel patients to breathe rapidly and

Table 2 Timetable of Common Causes of Pleural Effusions After Coronary Artery Bypass Graft Surgery

Immediate (during the first week)
  Atelectasis
  Internal mammary artery graft
  Congestive heart failure
Early (during the first 2 mo)
  Postcardiac injury syndrome
  Resolving hemothorax
Late (2–12 mo later)
  Postcardiac injury syndrome
  Lymphocytic effusion of unknown etiology
  Lung entrapment
  Constrictive pericarditis
  Congestive heart failure

shallowly, which often leads to radiographically detectable bibasilar atelectasis and small bilateral or left-sided pleural effusions. Prevention and therapy are directed at minimizing atelectasis by controlling pain and encouraging deep breathing. These types of effusions usually resolve spontaneously within two weeks.

Pleural effusion(s) in the immediate postoperative period may also follow CABGs that involve internal mammary artery grafting, which often injures the neighboring parietal pleura. Most of these effusions are generally small and occur on the side from which the internal mammary artery was harvested; large effusions, however, may occur with a reported incidence of from 0.5% to 8.5% after CABG surgery (49).

Patients who require surgical revascularization may already have sustained myocardial damage from the effects of their diseased coronary arteries. Congestive heart failure with bilateral transudative pleural effusions may supervene from the added surgical effects of a "stunned" myocardium, vigorous intraoperative liquid administration, or the development of perioperative myocardial ischemia. Such effusions are usually small and respond to diuretics.

B. Early (During the First Two Months Following CABG)

The pleural effusions attributable to the direct effects of CABG surgery are evident during the first few days following the operation, tend to be small, predominate in the left pleural space, and resolve quickly. But that is not the end of the story. In a retrospective study by Light and coworkers (50), of 3707 patients who had had CABG procedures, "large" effusions (greater than 25% of a hemithorax) were found in 29 (0.78%) of the patients. Causes were identified in 10 patients (congestive heart failure, $n = 7$; pericarditis, $n = 2$; and pulmonary embolism, $n = 1$), the remaining 19 patients with significant hydrothorax of unknown etiology were subdivided into two groups depending on the gross appearance of the liquid—bloody and nonbloody.

The bloody effusions reached their maximum size early (12.6 days), had high LDH values, contained mesothelial cells, monocytes, and (less frequently) eosinophils, and were relatively easy to control with one to three therapeutic thoracocenteses. By contrast, the nonbloody effusions developed much later (48.8 days) had lower values of LDH, contained chiefly small lymphocytes, and were much more difficult to manage clinically. In a later prospective, follow-up of 312 patients after CABG surgery, 62.4% had radiographically detectable pleural effusions, most of which were small and predominantly left-sided—nearly 10% had large effusions (48).

A reasonable conclusion is that large bloody effusions represent slowly evolving hemothoraces resulting from the CABG surgery itself, whereas, as emphasized by Heidecker and Sahn (49), the nonbloody effusions may represent manifestations of the postcardiac injury syndrome. Full-blown postcardiac injury syndrome, as described in an earlier section, includes pericarditis, which is generally considered a sine qua non for the diagnosis, as well as fever, dyspnea, and radiographically discernable pleural effusion(s) and pneumonitis; moreover, the onset typically occurs about three weeks after surgery. Not all cases of nonbloody post-CABG pleural effusions have had the usual accompanying features of the syndrome, nor did all have antimyocardial antibodies, when these were looked for. But the best explanation remains that some sort of limited (or forme fruste) of the postcardiac injury syndrome plays a role in the development of pleural effusions during the first few months after CABG.

C. Late (2–12 Months Later)

Three months after CABG surgery on 200 patients, 20% had pleural effusions (51), the possible causes of which are listed in Table 2. The postcardiac injury syndrome and lymphocytic effusions, which may be a manifestation of evolving cardiac injury, are common occurrences. These are important because of the intensive treatment required to deal with dyspnea, persistence and/or recurrences, and pleural thickening with entrapment of the lung: therapeutic options include anti-inflammatory agents, multiple thoracenteses, tube thoracostomy, pleural sclerosis, and pleurectomy (49).

Constrictive pericarditis (see earlier description) is an uncommon late manifestation of CABG surgery, with a reported incidence ranging from 0.2% (52) to 2.3% (53). And as would be expected, underlying myocardial damage in patients with coronary artery disease severe enough to warrant CABG, may worsen in the months following surgery, and cause congestive heart failure with pleural effusions. In this instance, measurement of NT-proBNP should help in the differential diagnosis (30).

VII. Other Causes

Most pleural effusions in patients with heart disease are related to one of the cardiac abnormalities just described. But patients with heart disease also have an increased susceptibility to certain other—noncardiogenic—causes of pleural effusion.

A. Pulmonary Embolism

Patients hospitalized for congestive heart failure or acute myocardial infarction are at increased risk of developing and dying from pulmonary embolism (54), which is often associated with pleural effusion. Patients with cardiac disease who undergo surgical procedures on their hearts—such as CABG, valve replacement, and even pacemaker implantation—or elsewhere in the body are considered at high risk for pulmonary embolism.

B. Pneumonia

Community-acquired pneumonia occurs with increased frequency in patients with advanced heart disease. In a review of 300 consecutive patients hospitalized for congestive heart failure, over half had some form of respiratory infection, chiefly acute bronchitis and pneumonia; in most cases, the infection was the precipitating cause of admission (55). In another study, heart disease was the most frequent underlying condition associated with hospitalization for community-acquired pneumonia, exceeding even the contribution of alcoholism, chronic lung disease, and diabetes mellitus as risk factors (56). Confusion may occur because pneumonia is often complicated by a parapneumonic effusion or empyema, which may be mistaken for a cardiogenic hydrothorax.

C. Antiarrhythmia Agents

Two drugs used to treat arrhythmias in patients with heart disease are known to induce pleural effusions. Amiodarone causes multiorgan toxicity of which fibrosing interstitial pneumonitis is the most serious and sometimes fatal, although uncommon, pleural effusions coexisting with parenchymal involvement have also been reported (57). Similarly, procainamide can cause pleural effusions as part of a drug-induced lupus reaction (58).

VIII. Summary

Hydrothorax from congestive heart failure, the most common cause of pleural effusion in the industrialized countries of the world, is usually easily diagnosed by the presence of many clinical and radiographic features of underlying cardiac dysfunction. Cardiogenic effusions are caused by leakage of pulmonary edema liquid from the lungs into the pleural spaces. Acute and chronic pericarditis, injury to the myocardium and pericardium, especially by CABG and other cardiac operations, are also frequently complicated by the development of pleural effusions. The mechanisms of liquid formation in these disorders remain obscure: possibilities include contiguous spread of cardiac inflammation to the neighboring pleural surfaces, surgical trauma, and immune dysfunction.

References

1. Light RW. Pleural Diseases, 5th ed. Philadelphia, PA: Lippincott Williams & Wilkins, 2007: 111.
2. Storey DD, Dines DE, Loles DT. Pleural effusion: A diagnostic dilemma. JAMA 1976; 236:2183–2186.
3. Valdes L, Alvarez D, Valle JM, et al. The etiology of pleural effusions in an area with high incidence of tuberculosis. Chest 1996; 109:158–162.
4. Bedford DE, Lovibond JL. Hydrothorax in heart failure. Br Heart J 1941; 3:93–111.
5. Logue RB, Rogers JV, Gay BB. Subtle roentgenographic signs of left heart failure. Am Heart J 1963; 65:464–473.
6. Kataoka H. Pericardial and pleural effusions in decompensated chronic heart failure. Am Heart J 2000; 139:918–923.
7. Lewin S, Goldberg L, Dec GW. The spectrum of pulmonary abnormalities on computed chest tomographic imaging in patients with advanced heart failure. Am J Cardiol 2000; 86: 98–100.
8. Wiener-Kronish JP, Matthay MA, Callen PW, et al. Relationship of pleural effusions to pulmonary hemodynamics in patients with heart failure. Am Rev Respir Dis 1985; 132:1253–1256.
9. Mattison LE, Coppage L, Alderman DF, et al. Pleural effusions in the medical ICU. Prevalence, causes, and clinical implications. Chest 1997; 111:1018–1023.
10. Zoochi L. Physiology and pathophysiology of pleural fluid turnover. Eur Respir J 2002; 20:1545–1558.
11. Staub NC, Wiener-Kronish JP, Albertine KH. Transport through the pleura. Physiology of normal liquid and solute exchange in the pleural space. In: Chrétien J, Bignon J, Hirsh A, eds. The Pleura in Health and Disease. New York, NY: Marcel Dekker Inc., 1985: 169–193.
12. Staub NC. Pathophysiology of pulmonary edema. In: Staub NC, Taylor AE, eds. Edema. New York, NY: Raven Press, 1984:719–746.
13. Broaddus VC, Wiener-Kronish JP, Staub NC. Clearance of lung edema into the pleural space of volume-loaded, anesthetized sheep. J Appl Physiol 1990; 68:2623–2630.
14. Bhattacharya J, Gropper MA, Staub NC. Interstitial fluid pressure gradient measured by micropuncture in excised dog lung. J Appl Physiol 1984; 56:271–277.
15. Light RW, MacGregor MI, Luchsinger PC, et al. Pleural effusions: The diagnostic separation of transudates and exudates. Ann Intern Med 1972; 77:507–513.
16. Mellins RB, Levine DR, Fishman AP. Effect of systemic and pulmonary venous hypertension on pleural and pericardial fluid accumulation. J Appl Physiol 1970; 29:564–569.
17. Wiener-Kronish JP, Goldstein R, Matthay RA, et al. Lack of association of pleural effusion with chronic pulmonary arterial and right atrial hypertension. Chest 1987; 92:967–970.
18. McPeak EM, Levine SA. The preponderance of right hydrothorax in congestive heart failure. Ann Intern Med 1946; 25:916–927.

19. Peterman TA, Brothers SK. Pleural effusion in congestive heart failure and in pericardial disease. N Engl J Med 1983; 309:313.
20. Weiss JM, Spodick DH. Laterality of pleural effusions in chronic congestive heart failure. Am J Cardiol 1984; 53:951.
21. Woodring JH. Distribution of pleural effusion in congestive heart failure: What is atypical? South Med J 2006; 98:518–523.
22. Race GA, Scheifley CH, Edwards JE. Hydrothorax in congestive heart failure. Am J Med 1957; 22:83–89.
23. Dock W. The anatomical and hydrostatic basis of orthopnea and of right hydrothorax in cardiac failure. Am Heart J 1935; 10:1047–1055.
24. Broaddus VC. Transudative pleural effusions. In: Loddenkemper R, Antony VB, eds. Pleural Disease. Eur Respir Monog 2002; 22:157–176.
25. Paré JA, Fraser RG. Synopsis of Diseases of the Chest. Philadelphia, PA: W. B. Saunders, 1983:104.
26. Kataoka H, Takada S. The role of thoracic ultrasonography for evaluation of patients with decompensated chronic heart failure. J Am Coll Cardiol 2000; 35:1638–1646.
27. Kalomendidis I, Rodriguez M, Barnette R, et al. Patient with bilateral pleural effusion. Are the findings the same in each fluid? Chest 2003; 124:167–176.
28. Broaddus VC. Diuresis and transudative effusions—Changing the rules of the game. Am J Med 2001; 110:732–735.
29. Burgess LJ, Maritz FJ, Taljaard JJF. Comparative analysis of the biochemical parameters used to distinguish between pleural transudates and exudates. Chest 1995; 1604–1609.
30. Kolditz M, Halank M, Schiemanck CS, et al. High diagnostic accuracy of NT-proBNP for cardiac origin of pleural effusions. Eur Respir J 2006; 28:144–150.
31. Porcel JM, Chorda J, Cao G, et al. Comparing serum and pleural fluid pro-brain natriuretic peptide (NT-proBNP) levels with pleural-to-serum albumin gradient for the identification of cardiac effusions misclassified by Light's criteria. Respirology 2007; 12:654–659.
32. Glazer M, Berkman N, Lafair JS, et al. Successful talc slurry pleurodesis in patients with nonmalignant pleural effusion. Report of 16 cases and review of the literature. Chest 2000; 117:1404–1409.
33. Sudduth CD, Sahn SA. Pleurodesis for nonmalignant pleural effusions. Recommendations. Chest 1992; 102:1855–1860.
34. Weiss JM, Spodick DH. Association of left pleural effusion with pericardial disease. N Engl J Med 1983; 308:696–697.
35. Little WC, Freeman GL. Pericardial disease. Circulation 2006; 113:1622–1632.
36. Plumb GE, Bruwer AJ, Clagett OT. Chronic constrictive pericarditis: Roentgenologic findings in 35 surgically proven cases. Mayo Clin Proc 1957; 32:555–566.
37. Tomaselli G, Gamsu G, Stulbarg JS. Constrictive pericarditis presenting as pleural effusion of unknown origin. Arch Intern Med 1989; 149:201–203.
38. Dressler W. A post-myocardial-infarction syndrome. Preliminary report of a complication resembling idiopathic, recurrent, benign pericarditis. JAMA 1956; 160:1379–1383.
39. Janton DH, Glover RP, O'Neil TJE, et al. Results of the surgical treatment of mitral stenosis. Circulation 1952; 6:321–333.
40. Miller RH, Horneffer PJ, Gardner TJ, et al. The epidemiology of the postpericardiotomy syndrome: A common complication of surgery. Am Heart J 1988; 116:1323–1329.
41. Khan AH. The postcardiac injury syndromes. Clin Cardiol 1992; 15:67–72.
42. Spodick DH. Decreased recognition of the post-myocardial infarction (Dressler) syndrome in the postinfarct setting. Does it masquerade as "idiopathic pericarditis" following silent infarcts? Chest 2004; 126:1410–1411.
43. Kaminsky ME, Rodan BA, Chen JTT, et al. Postpericardiotomy syndrome. AJR 1982; 138:503–508.

44. Wessman DE, Stafford CM. The postcardiac injury syndrome: Case report and review of the literature. South Med J 2006; 99:309–314.

45. Kim S, Sahn SA. Postcardiac injury syndrome. An immunologic pleural fluid analysis. Chest 1996; 109:570–572.

46. Imazio M, Cecchi E, Demichelis B, et al. COPPS investigators. Rational and design of the COPPS trial: A randomized, placebo-controlled, multicentre study of the use of colchicine for the primary prevention of postpericardiotomy syndrome. J Cardiovasc Med (Hagerstown) 2007; 8:1044–1048.

47. Carrozza JP. Drug-eluting stents—Pushing the envelope beyond the labels? N Engl J Med 2008; 358:405–407.

48. Light RW, Rogers JT, Moyers JP, et al. Prevalence and clinical course of pleural effusion at 30 days after coronary artery and cardiac surgery. Am J Respir Crit Care Med 2002; 166: 1567–1571.

49. Heidecker J, Sahn SA. The spectrum of pleural effusions after coronary artery bypass grafting surgery. Clin Chest Med 2006; 27:267–283.

50. Light RW, Rogers JT, Cheng D-C, et al. Large pleural effusions occurring after coronary artery bypass grafting. Ann Intern Med 1999; 130:891–896.

51. Aarnio P, Kettunen S, Harjula A. Pleural and pulmonary complications after bilateral internal mammary artery grafting. Scand J Thorac Cardiovasc Surg 1991; 25:175–178.

52. Fowler NO. Constrictive pericarditis: Its history and current status. Clin Cardiol 1995; 18: 341–350.

53. Matsuyama K, Matsumoto M, Sugita T, et al. Clinical characteristics of patients with constrictive pericarditis after coronary bypass surgery. Jpn Circ J 2001; 65:480–482.

54. Darze ES, Latado AL, Guimarães AG, et al. Acute pulmonary embolism is an independent predictor of adverse events in severe decompensated heart failure patients. Chest 2007; 131:1838–1843.

55. Flint FJ. The factor of infection in heart failure. Br Med J 1954; 2:1018–1022.

56. Sullivan RJ Jr, Dowdle WR, Marine WM, et al. Adult pneumonia in a general hospital. Etiology and host risk factors. Arch Intern Med 1972; 129:935–942.

57. Mittal SR, Maheshwari M. Amiodarone-induced exudative pleural effusions—A case report and review of the literature. Indian Heart J 2006; 58:352–355.

58. Smith PR, Nacht RI. Drug-induced lupus pleuritis mimicking pleural space infection. Chest 1992; 101:268–269.

35
Pleural Effusions in Pregnancy and Gynecological Diseases

KATERINA M. ANTONIOU and NIKOLAOS M. SIAFAKAS
Department of Thoracic Medicine Medical School, University of Crete, Heraklion, Crete, Greece

DEMOSTHENES BOUROS
Democritus University of Thrace Medical School, and University Hospital of Alexandroupolis, Alexandroupolis, Greece

I. Introduction

Pulmonary effusion (PE) has been reported to accompany several gynecological conditions, mostly as a clinical feature of a systemic abnormality or seldom as an isolated extragynecological sign of a heterogeneous group of disorders (Table 1). The PEs related to pregnancy are rare in overall incidence, although they remain as a particularly devastating problem affecting not only the health of a young and presumably previously healthy and productive member of society, but also very often the life of the fetus or newborn infant. Pregnant women may potentially be at risk for misdiagnosis of pleural disease. The main reason for this is the obscure clinical features masked by the main event of pregnancy. The classical approach to differential diagnosis of PE can be missed if women avoid essential diagnostic techniques (e.g., chest X-ray) out of concern for the health of the fetus. However, the serious consequences of certain pleural diseases for maternal and fetal well-being require effective management of these unusual complications.

In this chapter, we will discuss PE associated with special gynecological diseases or with the intrapartum and postpartum periods either resulting from a primary pleural disease or representing an important clinical manifestation of a pregnancy-related systemic or pulmonary abnormality (Table 1). Secondary PE due to specific disorders, for example, tuberculous PE, will be discussed within the framework of the particularity of coexistence with pregnancy.

II. Pleural Effusion in Gynecology

A. Ovarian Hyperstimulation Syndrome

Pharmacological ovarian stimulation, a well-established therapeutic procedure in the field of infertility, has been widely used in the last decade (1). This treatment modality consists of ovulation induction with human chorionic gonadotropin (hCG) alone or in combination with clomiphene. It has become the gold standard method since the introduction of in vitro fertilization. One of the most common complications of this treatment is the development of the ovarian hyperstimulation syndrome (OHSS), defined as the shift of serum from the

Table 1 PE in Gynecology and Obstetrics

Related to gynecological conditions
Ovarian hyperstimulation syndrome (OHSS)
Meigs' syndrome
Endometriosis
Related to obstetrics and pregnancy
Benign postpartum effusion
Antiphospholipase antibody-related PE
Choriocarcinoma
Chylothorax
Associated with lymphangiomyomatosis
Traumatic
Other
Hemothorax related to neurofibromatosis
Ruptured diaphragm
Hominis empyema
Urinothorax
Specific
Tuberculosis pleural effusion
Parapneumonic pleural effusion

intravascular space to the third space, and mainly to the abdominal cavity that occurs when the ovaries become enlarged due to follicular stimulation. It is characterized by ovarian enlargement, ascites, pleural effusion, hypovolemia, hemoconcentration, oliguria, and rarely thromboembolism. Its incidence is 0.1% to 4% of ovulation induction treatments (1), but the low incidence is increasing worldwide through the expansion of infertility treatments (1,2). The syndrome can fall into four clinical stages of increasing severity: (1) mild, with abdominal distension and discomfort; (2) moderate, with ascites on ultrasound examination; (3) severe, with ascites clinically apparent with or without another effusion (pleural, rarely pericardial), and a hemoconcentration [hematocrit >45% and white blood cell (WBC) count >15,000 cells/mL]; and (4) critical, with, in addition to the above signs, hypovolemic shock, an acute renal and respiratory cells per milliliter failure, a marked hemoconcentration (hematocrit >55% and WBC count >25,000), and thrombotic disorders (3). It can be extremely severe, with a morbidity reaching 5% of in vitro fertilizations (1).

The pathophysiology of the syndrome is not completely understood, and no specific therapy or prevention is available. This syndrome represents an overexpression of the normal ovulatory process described in normal pregnancy. It is thought that certain systemic and ovarian biosynthetic cytokines and vasoactive and angiogenic factors that are produced in excess during induction of ovulation, initiate the cascade of events that leads to OHSS.

The mechanisms underlying the clinical manifestations of OHSS involve an increased permeability of the ovarian capillaries and other mesothelial vessels triggered by the release of vasoactive substances of the ovaries under hCG stimulation (4). Although other mechanisms, such as increased peripheral arteriolar dilatation (5), have been proposed as causes of the hemodynamic alterations seen in OHSS, there is now a general consensus that women with ovaries primed with follicle stimulating hormone/luteinizing hormone (FSH/LH) and subsequently exposed to hCG develop a clinical picture in which the ultimate pathophysiological step is increased vascular permeability (VP) (6). As hCG has no direct vasoactive properties (7), investigations have aimed to detect the vasoactive substance responsible for this condition. Information gathered over the last decade has pointed to vascular endothelial growth factor (VEGF) as being crucial to the development of OHSS syndrome. Studies in rodents and humans have shown that levels of ovarian VEGF and VEGFR-2 mRNA levels and VP are already increased by stimulation with gonadotrophins, which precedes hCG administration. The administration of hCG pushes all of these parameters to their maximum. A linear correlation is found between increased expression of VEGF/VEGFR-2 mRNAs and enhanced VP, with both peaking 48 hours after injection of hCG (8). It has been demonstrated that the ovary is the main source of VEGF and other cytokines produced in hyperstimulation, and that increased capillary permeability and ascites are phenomena predominantly related to the ovaries (8).

The origin of pleural effusion is believed to be secondary to fluid shift from abdominal ascites. In patients with bilateral effusions, the probable mechanism that has been suggested is capillary leak into the pleural space itself. In the particular cases of isolated pleural effusions, the pathogenesis is more complex, with the unilaterally increased permeability remaining unexplained. The pleural effusions with OHSS are usually right-sided. In the series of 33 patients with pleural effusion reported by Abramov et al. (9), 17 (52%) effusions were right-sided, 9 (27%) were bilateral, and 7 (21%) were left-sided. Two recently reported studies included a total of seven cases of isolated pleural effusions with OHSS, six of which were unilaterally right-sided (10,11). Some authors suggest that this preferential location might be explained by a capillary leak and exudation into the pleural space due to the decreased right lymphatic drainage as compared to the left side (10). In addition, ascitic-related pleural effusions are also predominant in the right side because of the transfer through diaphragmatic defect or hiatus (12). The pleural fluid in patients with OHSS is an exudate. In the case-series of Abramov et al. (13), the mean pleural fluid protein was 4.1 g/dL, whereas the mean plasma protein was 4.4 g/dL.

The unpredictable individual responses to ovulation inducers make the prevention of OHSS very difficult. The following risk factors have been identified: age <35 years, presence of a polycystic ovarian disease prior to stimulation, a number of follicles >10, estradiol plasma concentration >2000 pg/mL, and an ongoing active pregnancy (10). Several recent studies reported the possible prognostic importance of serial cytokines as markers of this syndrome. Chen and colleagues have reported that the levels of VEGF and IL-6 in ascites dropped significantly during the course of OHSS, and levels of VEGF were significantly correlated with levels of IL-1β, IL-8, and TNF-α, as well as progesterone concentrations, hematocrit, and WBC counts (14). A similar study suggests that follicular fluid IL-6 concentrations at the time of oocyte retrieval and serum IL-8 concentrations on the day of embryo transfer may serve as early predictors of this syndrome (15).

Patients with OHSS initially develop abdominal discomfort and distension, followed by nausea, vomiting, and diarrhea. As the syndrome worsens, the patients develop evidence of ascites and then hydrothorax or breathing difficulties. In the most severe stages, the patient develops increased blood viscosity owing to hemoconcentration, coagulation abnormalities, and diminished renal function (13,16). Respiratory symptoms develop 7 to 14 days after the hCG injection (16,17). The OHSS as a complication of hormonal treatment is usually mild in degree. In cases of increased risk, the patients' monitoring should be very cautious, with repeated ultrasonographic examinations and plasma hormonal determinations. The severity of OHSS varies with the delay between the onset of symptoms and the stimulation: within three to seven days of hCG administration, it is often moderate to severe, while a later onset (12–17 days) often signals a more severe clinical form (11). The treatment is mainly supportive (bed rest and avoidance of further hormonal treatment), and the symptoms usually resolve spontaneously. Hemoconcentration should be treated with intravenous fluids to avoid acute renal failure. Some approaches for preventing OHSS, which are based on its pathophysiology, are now applied. Studies show a reduced incidence of OHSS when rLH or a gonadorelin-releasing hormone (GnRH) analog is used to trigger the final steps of oocyte maturation. Prophylactic administration of CB2, a dopamine agonist, is associated with a significant reduction in the incidence of symptoms and signs of moderate/severe OHSS. This drug inhibits VEGFR-2 phosphorylation and signaling. A specific treatment is, therefore, available. Larger trials are necessary for confirming its efficacy and safety (8).

Large pleural effusions with respiratory discomfort should be treated by intercostal drainage. In conclusion, chest physicians should be more aware of this syndrome in order to ensure a better and minimally invasive management of these potentially pregnant women. The OHSS has to be considered in the differential diagnosis of pleural effusion in young women undergoing ovulation induction for in vitro fertilization, because of its increasing prevalence (13).

B. Endometriosis

Although endometriosis is generally confined to the pelvis, it may occur at remote sites with unusual manifestations. Thoracic endometriosis is a relatively rare condition, with a varying clinical presentation and is usually diagnosed from a history of recurrent chest pain with or without hemoptysis termed as catamenial hemoptysis. This monthly presentation coincides with the menstrual cycle, with the pain occurring at the time of menstruation. The most common presentation of the disease is right-sided pneumothorax (18). Hemothorax, recurrent hemoptysis, chest pain, and asymptomatic pulmonary nodules occur less commonly (19–21).

Ectopic endometrium in distant sites from the pelvis is well described. It causes symptoms relative to the site where the bleeding occurs. Rare examples include pulmonary endometriosis and endometriosis associated with ascites. Muneyyirci-Delale et al. (22) presented 4 cases, reviewed the literature of 23 additional cases, and found that 8 (30%) out of the 27 patients also presented with pleural effusion. Bhojawala et al. (23) published 12 cases of both bloodstained ascites and pleural effusion with endometriosis since the first report by Meigs (24). The ascitic and/or pleural fluid are described as a bloodstained or chocolate-colored fluid (23). The etiology of thoracic endometriosis remains speculative, with two possible theories having been suggested. The first of these is a vascular theory whereby endometrial cells are transported via the venous system to the right side of the heart and thereafter via the pulmonary artery to peripheral sites of the lungs. Ascites may result from rupture of endometriosis or chocolate cysts leading to peritoneal irritation (25), or it may occur in a similar way to that in Meigs' syndrome (26,27). Recurrent hemorrhagic ascites secondary to endometriosis is an unusual occurrence, more than 50 cases have been reported since 1954 (27,28). However, evidence in human and non-human primates suggests a genetic basis for endometriosis (29). The pleural effusion generally occurs on the right [although Yu and Grimes reported bilateral pleural effusions (30)] and is thought to be due to ascitic fluid gaining entrance to the pleural cavity through the diaphragm.

The treatment of massive ascites, pleural effusion, and endometriosis is difficult. The medical treatment of this syndrome is temporary and merely confirms the fact that the hypoestrogenic state is the desired curative course. The use of the hypothalamus-derived GnRH agonists in the treatment of endometriosis would seem to be extremely helpful in establishing a course of therapy, aiming to suppress the hypophyseal–gonadal axis, so as to ensure a regression of the endometrial implants. If medical treatment fails, surgical resection of the endometriomas is suggested, although relapse rate may be high (31). A case report by Shek et al. recommended a GnRH analog agonist (nafarelin acetate) administered through nasal route and thoracocentesis as the initial treatment for endometriosis-related ascites and/or pleural effusion (32). Out of the 31 patients reviewed by Muneyyirci-Delale et al., only three were managed without laparotomy (22). Total abdominal hysterectomy and bilateral salpingo-oophorectomy are the most commonly performed procedures (22). At operation, endometriosis usually involved surrounding structures such as the fallopian tubes, ovaries, appendix, sigmoid colon, and omentum (22).

C. Meigs' Syndrome

In 1937, Meigs and Cass (33) reported the clinical picture of ovarian fibroma associated with ascites and pleural effusion in seven patients. Thereafter, the syndrome was referred to as Meigs' syndrome (24). Meigs proposed that the true Meigs' syndrome be limited to benign and solid ovarian tumors (fibroma, thecoma, and granulose cell tumor) (24). In contrast, pseudo-Meigs' syndrome is a condition characterized by nonmalignant ascites and/or pleural effusion due to pelvic tumors other than solid benign ovarian tumors (e.g., other benign cysts of the ovary, leiomyomas of the uterus, and teratomas) (34,35). Meigs still prefers to reserve his name for only those cases in which the primary neoplasm is a benign solid ovarian tumor (24). Light classifies any patient with a pelvic neoplasm associated with ascites and pleural effusion, in whom surgical removal of the tumor results in permanent disappearance of the ascites and pleural effusion, as having Meigs' syndrome (36).

Fibromas are associated with ascites in approximately 10% to 15% of all cases. Ascites probably occurs by means of a transudative mechanism through the tumor surface that exceeds the peritoneum's capacity to reabsorb the fluid (37). Other possible mechanisms include obstruction of peritoneal lymphatics by tumor or increased permeability of the neovasculature with protein leakage. The plausible theory is that the pressure on the lymphatic vessels in the tumor itself causes the escape of fluid through the surface lymphatics, which are situated just beneath the single-layered cuboid epithelium covering the tumor. CA-125 has been demonstrated to be elevated in benign conditions, such as pelvic-inflammatory disease, endometriosis, uterine leiomyoma, and early pregnancy (37). There are several reports of Meigs' syndrome with elevated CA-125 levels. All these cases prove that elevated CA-125 levels are common in patients with this syndrome (37,38). Results of immunoperoxidase stains suggest that serum elevation of CA-125 antigen is caused by mesothelial expression of the antigen rather than by the fibroma (37). A recent report found differences in changes in VEGF levels in pleural effusion and ascites after removal of ovarian tumor complicated by Meigs' syndrome. Postoperative VEGF levels decreased in the patient's pleural fluid but not in the peritoneal fluid. Although the mechanism of this phenomenon is clear thus far, the possibility of differences in kinetics of fluid in the peritoneal and pleural cavity has been shown. This finding may provide a clue that the mechanism of the development of the pleural effusion and ascites in Meigs' syndrome may differ (39). The findings of a recent report suggest the involvement of vasoactive growth factors such as fibroblast growth factor and VEGF and of the inflammatory cytokine IL-6 in the pathogenesis of Meigs' syndrome (5). All the three factors possess potent VP-enhancing properties, and all have been associated with capillary leakage and with the formation of ascites and pleural effusion in other gynecological abnormalities such as the OHSS (8).

Patients with Meigs' syndrome usually have a chronic illness characterized by weight loss, pleural effusion, ascites, and a pelvic mass (24). The pleural effusion is right-sided in about 70% of the patients, left-sided in 10%, and bilateral in 20% (40). The only symptom referable to the pleural effusion is shortness of breath. The ascites may not be evident on physical examination. The pleural fluid is usually an exudate. Most pleural fluids secondary to Meigs' syndrome have a protein level above 3.0 g/dL (12). The pleural fluid has usually low WBC (fewer than $1000/mm^3$) and is occasionally bloody (41). The diagnosis of Meigs' syndrome should be considered in all women who have pelvic masses, ascites, and pleural effusions. Laparotomy is required for the correct diagnosis of ovarian tumors since peritoneal cytology, tumor markers, and other indicators of malignant pathology may be misleading. The diagnosis is confirmed when the ascites and the pleural effusion resolve postoperatively and do not reoccur. Postoperatively, the pleural fluid disappears rapidly and is usually completely gone within two weeks (42).

III.   Pregnancy-Related Pleural Effusion

A.   Benign Postpartum PE

Asymptomatic PE presented in the immediate postpartum period is a benign condition that is not clinically significant but should be included in the differential diagnosis of diseases occurring in the postpartum period. Benign PE may develop in the immediate postpartum period within a week after delivery. Hessen reported the first prospective clinical study of the presentation of PE in 23% of a group of 92 women 7 to 12 days after a normal delivery (43). Another 14% of the population under study had radiographic findings compatible with a probable PE. In the study of Hessen, a control group of 300 healthy individuals, including 163 nonpregnant women and 137 men, underwent a similar radiographic evaluation. Radiographic findings of a small effusion were identified in 12 (4%) subjects and a probable small effusion in 18 (6%). In the above study, no information is reported on the cardiorespiratory status of the studied patients. Subsequently, several investigators examined, either prospectively or retrospectively, women with uncomplicated labor and delivery. Hughson et al. (44) studied retrospectively 112 women who had delivered vaginally and had posteroanterior and lateral chest X-ray within 24 hours of delivery. Two independent radiologists reviewed the radiographs using a scoring system that reflected the degree of costophrenic angle blunting. None of the patients had evidence of cardiorespiratory disease. The authors reported moderate-sized PE in 4% of the patients and small in 46%, which were bilateral in 75% (44). Based on this observation, the same group conducted a prospective study wherein 30 similar patients were evaluated using the same methodology. PE was reported in 20 (67%) and in 11 (36%) it was bilateral. Both retrospective and prospective studies of Hughson and colleagues (44) reported that the presence of the PE was not correlated with any of the clinical features they analyzed including age, weight gain during pregnancy, hematocrit, serum protein, existence of preeclampsia, duration and difficulty of labor, use of intravenous fluids, or administration of oxytocin. The presence of postpartum PE was also not correlated with a major obstetric complication or with an adverse fetal outcome.

In another study, Stark and Pollack (45) reviewed chest radiographs of 45 women within 48 hours of labor and delivery. Forty-four of the 45 patients had radiographic evidence of small PE. However, the case-series design (women were evaluated for fever or respiratory symptoms) and the high proportion of delivery by cesarean section are particular biases not allowing acceptance of the high incidence of the postpartum PE reported in this study (45).

The plain chest radiographs without decubitus views have a low sensitivity and specificity for the detection of PE (46). In contrast, thoracic ultrasonographic scans provide a sensitive and specific method for the detection of PEs in very low volumes—3 to 5 mL (46–48). Thus, Udeshi and colleagues examined women postpartum for the presence of PE using thoracic ultrasonography (49). Out of the 50 patients studied, all examined within 48 hours of labor and delivery, 29 had delivered by the vaginal route and the other 21 underwent a cesarean section. Only 1 out of the 50 patients evaluated had ultrasonic evidence of PE. Since this patient had experienced severe preeclampsia complicated by pulmonary edema, the authors concluded that PEs rarely occur after an uncomplicated vaginal or cesarean delivery (49). In contrast to the above report, Gourgoulianis et al. (50) in a case-control study examined 31 postpartum women delivered vaginally and normally, and 22 healthy nonpregnant women as control group with thoracic ultrasonography. They reported ultrasonic evidence of PE in 7 out of the 31 (23%) patients and in none of the 22 healthy controls (50). The authors concluded that the physiological conditions of pregnancy, labor, and normal delivery could promote transudation of fluid into the pleural space because of the increased hydrostatic pressure in the systemic circulation and the decreased colloid osmotic pressure. Moreover, the repeated Valsalva maneuvers of parturition may further promote pleural effusion through an increase of intrathoracic pressure and an impairment of the lymphatic drainage of the pleural space.

In a subsequent study, Wallis et al. (51) designed a case-series study aiming to determine the incidence of the postpartum PE in patients with moderate to severe preeclampsia. Nine (26.5%) out of the 34 individuals had ultrasonic findings of PE. There was no difference in the severity of the preeclampsia, radiographic appearance of pulmonary edema, or the amount of intravenous fluids between those with and without PE. However, the investigators reported a 10-fold higher incidence of perinatal fetal mortality in women who experienced a postpartum PE (51).

Since thoracic ultrasonography is more sensitive than chest radiography (46,47), it is likely that the true incidence of postpartum PE related to normal labor and delivery is closer to the case-series and case-control studies (49–51) that have used ultrasound evaluation. Postpartum small size, asymptomatic PE is not clinically significant but should be included in the differential diagnosis of the pleural diseases occurring in the postpartum period. However, moderate-to-large effusions, particularly if accompanied by signs and symptoms of a complicated disease, should be evaluated and managed as pleural effusions similar to other clinical settings.

B. Antiphospholipid Antibody–Related PE

In addition to the "normal" phenomenon of the benign postpartum pleural effusion, which usually occurs immediately after labor and delivery, there have been two studies (52,53) reporting a systemic disease with pulmonary effusion and pulmonary infiltrates a few weeks after delivery. In the first study, Kochenour et al. (52) presented a series of three women with antiphospholipid antibodies (aPL) and a postpartum syndrome of pleuropulmonary disease, fever, and cardiac manifestations. Each patient had either lupus anticoagulant or anticardiolipin antibodies or both. However, none of the patients had antinuclear antibodies or fulfills the criteria for the diagnosis of systemic lupus erythematosus (52). Two out of the three patients experienced thromboembolic episodes. Based on the association between aPL and fetal loss, fetal growth retardation, and preeclampsia, investigators suggested that patients with aPL are at risk for a serious autoimmune postpartum syndrome. The second report is a case report of a patient at 29 weeks' gestation who had elevated blood pressure, proteinuria, and early intrauterine growth retardation (53). Studies were positive for the presence of both lupus anticoagulant and anticardiolipin antibodies. After delivery, chest pain and a pleural effusion developed as further manifestations of the patient's autoimmune disease. In addition to the known association between antiphospholipid syndrome and instances of fetal death (54,55), the above studies (52,53) demonstrate another important relationship between these immunological markers and serious pleuropulmonary and cardiac disorders in the postpartum period. The authors propose that aPL syndrome be considered if patients experience serious pleuropulmonary or/and cardiac disease in the first month after delivery (52). On the other hand, pregnant women with positive aPL may benefit from immunosuppressive therapy and prophylactic anticoagulation to prevent life-threatening thromboembolic disease (52,53). More recently, a randomized study has been conducted to compare the two most efficacious therapeutic regimens, intravenous immunoglobulin (IVIG) and anticoagulation with low molecular weight (LMW) heparin and low-dose aspirin, in women with recurrent pregnancy loss associated with aPL (56). The women treated with LMW heparin and low-dose aspirin had a higher rate of live births (84%) than those treated with IVIG (57%). Treatment with LMW heparin and low-dose aspirin should be considered as the standard therapy for recurrent pregnancy loss due to aPL (56).

C. Choriocarcinoma

Choriocarcinoma is a form of gestational trophoblastic disease (GTD), a heterogeneous group of interrelated lesions that may occur after any gestational experience (e.g., abortion, ectopic, or term pregnancy). The pathogenesis is unique because the maternal tumor arises from fetal, not maternal, tissue. It is commonly metastatic to several organs such as lung, brain, liver, pelvis, vagina, spleen, intestine, and kidney (57). Pulmonary metastatic GTD poses problems in diagnosis and management and has a poorer prognosis than the nonmetastatic variant. The overall survival rate at two years after diagnosis in the series of Kumar et al. (57) was 65%. Pleural effusion may occur mostly as a consequence of a metastatic disease to the pleura or to the neighboring subpleural lung parenchyma. Rarely, the vascular dissemination of the trophoblastic tissue undergoes pulmonary infarction secondary to tumor emboli presenting as pleural effusion.

In many patients of the case-series study of Kumar et al. (57), the pulmonary lesions were asymptomatic. However, patients may present with the following signs and symptoms (57,58):

Dyspnea secondary to tumor emboli and pulmonary infarction,
Cough and hemoptysis due to bronchial or parenchymal lesions,
Persistent gradually worsening dyspnea secondary to lung parenchyma metastases, and
Pleuritic pain as a result of pleural metastatic disease.

Most patients with choriocarcinoma and pulmonary lesion have an antecedent molar pregnancy, although an associated choriocarcinomatous lesion in the uterus is absent in the majority of them (57). Fewer than 5% of patients have other gestational experience such as abortion, ectopic, immediate-term or term pregnancy. However, a higher mortality has been observed when the antecedent pregnancy ended at term (57,58). Choriocarcinomatous pleural effusion may be due to the metastatic pleural disease or to the pulmonary tumor embolism and is usually hemorrhagic. The pleural involvement frequently causes large hemothorax (pleural fluid/blood hematocrit >50%) (59,60) leading to severe dyspnea and respiratory failure. In addition, gestational trophoblastic neoplasms can present as pulmonary nodules without significant disease of the reproductive organs. This entity must be considered in the differential diagnosis in any female of reproductive age who presents with multiple pulmonary nodules. Thoracotomy has a limited role in the initial evaluation of patients with this disease. However, it may be needed in patients who have evidence of persistent pulmonary disease, despite appropriate therapy (61).

Since the clinical presentation of the metastatic choriocarcinoma in pleura and lungs is the same as in pulmonary embolism, these two entities should be carefully sorted out, taking into account that metastatic choriocarcinoma treated wrongly with anticoagulants may lead to fatal spontaneous hemorrhage from the brain. Several management options are available for patients who are symptomatic and require some form of therapy, such as chest tube drainage, outpatient thoracocentesis for recurrent effusions to prevent respiratory stress, and the development of fibrothorax and trapped lung.

D. Chylothorax

Associated with Lymphangiomyomatosis

Pulmonary lymphangiomyomatosis (LAM) is a rare idiopathic lung disease that afflicts women of childbearing age (62–64). It is characterized pathologically by the proliferation of atypical pulmonary interstitial smooth muscle in the pulmonary blood vessels, airways, and lymphatic channels, and by cysts formation (64). Pulmonary LAM presents almost exclusively in premenopausal women (64,65). More than 70% of the patients are between 20 and 40 years of age at the onset of the disease. Only 6% are more than 50 years of age at presentation, many of them associated with hormone replacement therapy (65). The disease causes dyspnea, pneumothorax, chylous pleural effusion, hemoptysis, and eventually respiratory failure. At presentation, most of the patients have airflow obstruction, relatively normal lung volumes, and a low diffusing capacity of the lung (ILCO) (64,65).

Extrapulmonary manifestations include abdominal and pelvic masses occurring along axial lymphatics (now termed lymphangioleiomyoma), chylous ascites, and in more than 80% renal angiomyolipomas (66). The pathogenesis of LAM is unknown, but data are accumulating that suggest a role for abnormalities in proteins involved in the synthesis of catecholamines (62,67). It is likely that estrogen plays a central role in disease progression, since the disease does not present prior to menarche and only rarely after menopause (64). Estrogen and progesterone receptors have been demonstrated in biopsy tissue (68,69). Furthermore, the disease is known to accelerate during pregnancy (70–75), and there is some evidence that women with LAM are less likely to become pregnant (65). Out of the 50 cases of the study of Johnson and Tattersfield (65), 28 had been pregnant and 27 had had children. Seven out of the 50 developed their first symptom of LAM when pregnant or postpartum ($n = 4$). Out of the seven patients, one pregnancy was uncomplicated and one was terminated. The other five patients had complications during pregnancy, while two developed a chylous pleural effusion and three experienced one or more pneumothoraces. The overall incidence of complications was 11 times higher during pregnancy than at other times (65). In the same study, the two patients with chylous pleural effusion (one bilateral and one unilateral) were treated initially by aspiration and intercostal drainage. One woman with unilateral effusion needed further procedures including thoracotomy, thoracic duct ligation, and pleurectomy (65). On the basis of observations that women with LAM present an increased incidence of complications during pregnancy, patients should be aware of this before conception.

Traumatic

Chylothorax nonassociated with LAM has been rarely reported in pregnancy (76,77). It can be classified as traumatic etiology because the condition seems to be a consequence after a prolonged difficult vaginal delivery with the obstructed expiratory effort of the Valsalva maneuver transmitting high intrathoracic pressures to thoracic structures. This mechanism causes main lymphatic duct rupture and chylothorax. Difficult childbirth has been reported as an unusual etiology for the formation of chylothorax. Doctors should take into account this diagnosis when lymphoma, LAM, malignancies, and miscellaneous other causes of chylothorax are not evident. The management of this condition is the same as with any other traumatic chylothorax (78).

E. Other

Neurofibromatosis-Related Hemothorax

Massive spontaneous intrathoracic hemorrhage related to neurofibromatosis has been reported in two cases during the first week after delivery (79). Neurofibromatosis is an idiopathic disease characterized by abnormal proliferation of fibrous tissue in the skin and viscera. Effects of pregnancy on the clinical course of neurofibromatosis are known to include worsening of cutaneous lesions, increased incidence of hypertension, and renal artery rupture. Vessel wall rupture in areas of vascular neurofibromatous infiltration is the possible mechanism of hemorrhagic pleural effusion.

Ruptured Diaphragm

Prolonged and tiring vaginal delivery generates high intrathoracic and intra-abdominal pressures with rapid acceleration and deceleration during the effort to utilize the Valsalva maneuvers. This delivery mechanism may cause rupture of the diaphragm, a rare but serious complication of pregnancy commonly associated with hemorrhagic pleural effusion (80–84). Onset of the rupture usually presents with acute abdominal pain with varying degree of dyspnea nausea and emesis because of the herniated bowel (80,81). In the case of a strangulated herniated bowel, serious manifestations may occur such as cyanosis and shock (80). Chest roentgenography and computed tomography revealed bowel in the left hemithorax, compatible with a left-sided diaphragmatic rupture. Delayed rupture of diaphragm not related with labor but associated with intrauterine pregnancy has seldom been reported (85,86). In one case report, this delayed ruptured diaphragm presented as pleural empyema (87). Surgical therapy is the cornerstone of management, particularly when a diaphragmatic defect is symptomatic. The route of delivery may be individualized for patients with diaphragmatic repairs in whom there has been sufficient time for healing (84).

Mycoplasma hominis *Empyema*

Mycoplasma hominis frequently colonizes the genital tract, but is rarely isolated from the respiratory tract (88). The significance of *M. hominis* in respiratory infections must be interpreted with caution. *M. hominis* has been isolated from respiratory secretions in 1% to 3% of healthy persons, 8% of patients with chronic respiratory complaints, and 14% of persons engaging in orogenital sex (89). Thus, *M. hominis* is probably rarely capable of causing lower respiratory tract infection. Dissemination of *M. hominis* has been documented in women with a febrile illness after delivery (88). Occasional reports exist in which *M. hominis* has been isolated from pure culture from empyema fluid (90,91). Intrathoracic infection with *M. hominis* has been reported to cause complicated pleural empyema in two case reports. The first involved a postpartum 16-year-old patient (92) with complicated pleural empyema, and the second was the case of a 32-year-old woman in her 29th week of pregnancy with persistent pleural effusion (93).

Urinothorax

Relaxation of ureteral smooth muscle induced by hormones producing ureteral atony and pressure on the ureters by the gravid uterus may result in mild-to-moderate dilatation of the collecting systems of the kidney (94). This functional hydronephrosis, which tends to be more prominent on the right, is not usually associated with renal dysfunction (94). However, moderate or severe hydronephrosis is a well-recognized complication in the previously pregnant women (94,95). The degree of obstruction is rarely sufficient to cause acute renal failure due to ureteral obstruction by the gravid uterus (96). In some cases, the normalization of renal function in the lateral recumbent position relieves pressure on the ureters by the uterus, and its recurrence when supine confirms the diagnosis. Occasionally, pyelonephritis coexists with pregnancy because of a moderate-to-severe ureteral obstruction (97). Acute oliguric renal failure associated with bacterial pyelonephritis is a rarely recognized clinical entity in pregnancy (98).

Pleural effusion related either to functional hydronephrosis and/or pyelonephritis has been reported during pregnancy (94,96,99,100). In some reports patients presented with large pleural effusion and renal failure (96,99). In most cases, the pleural fluid is transudate. In some case reports, the transudative pleural effusion may represent urinothoraces (101). The diagnosis of urinothorax is confirmed by demonstrating a pleural fluid-to-serum creatinine ratio of greater than 1 (102).

F. Pleural Effusion of Specific Etiology

When a pleural effusion of specific etiology such as tuberculous or parapneumonic is diagnosed in coexistence with pregnancy, a number of challenging clinical problems should promptly managed. The complete review of these conditions is discussed elsewhere in this book. Here, we will focus on available important clinical evidence of management of tuberculosis (TB) and infectious pleural effusions relevant for the maternal and infant well-being.

Tuberculous Pleural Effusion

The prevalence of TB, especially extrapulmonary tuberculosis, is increasing worldwide (103). Despite the fact that extrapulmonary tuberculosis does not affect the course of pregnancy, labor, or the perinatal outcome, a higher rate of antenatal maternal hospitalization along with low Apgar scores and low birth weight in infants has been reported (103). Diagnosis of pleural TB remains a challenge. Among nonconventional tests, ADA and IFN-γ have the best sensitivity and specificity, but they are biomarkers of the inflammatory process in the pleural space and do not confirm the etiologic agent (104). Nucleic acid amplification tests (NAATs) and serology are promising but require further development to improve sensitivity (104). The clinical manifestations of tuberculous pleural effusion in the pregnant woman are not different from those in nonpregnant individuals, and the same is true concerning the treatment modalities. Thus, the treatment rationale in established TB pleural effusion is recommended in pregnancy, although it is not verified in this group of women (105). None of the first-line drugs has been shown to be teratogenic (106). Streptomycin should be avoided, as it may be ototoxic (106). In the United States, caution is recommended regarding the use of pyrazinamide. The American Thoracic Society guidelines state that pyrazinamide should be avoided in pregnancy but can be given after the first trimester (105). In summary, isoniazid in combination with ethambutol and rifampicin is recommended for a pregnant woman with TB (107). If a fourth drug is warranted, then pyrazinamide could be added after the third trimester. Routine therapeutic abortion is not medically indicated for a pregnant woman who is taking first-line antituberculous drugs (105). Pregnant women with suspected TB pleural effusion should be targeted for tuberculin skin testing (108). There are some cases when the pregnant women have positive tuberculin test but the pleural effusion finally is diagnosed as of a different cause than TB. In this case, the patient is diagnosed as having latent tuberculosis infection (108).

Parapneumonic Pleural Effusion

An important predisposing factor to the development of severe pneumonic infections and parapneumonic pleural effusion or empyema during pregnancy is the altering of the maternal immune system. Whereas the clinical features of bacterial pneumonia during pregnancy are not dramatically different from those seen in the nonpregnant patient, complications are more frequently reported, reflecting a possible delay of recognition of pneumonia. Madinger et al. reported a case-series study of 25 patients in whom diagnoses of bacterial pneumonia were initially overlooked in five cases. This delay was possibly related to the increased incidence of serious complications, including empyema, in nearly half of all the patients in this series (109).

A detailed discussion of the clinical manifestations and the diagnosis of parapneumonic pleural effusion or empyema are beyond the scope of this review (see other chapters). Generally, the presentation and diagnosis of parapneumonic effusion or empyema do not differ between nonpregnant and pregnant patients, although the physiological changes of pregnancy make it difficult for the pregnant woman to tolerate a large parapneumonic effusion. The management of parapneumonic effusion or empyema in pregnant women is similar to nonpregnant, taking into account the basic recommendations regarding the use of antibiotic therapy in pregnancy (110,111). Chest tube for evacuation of large or complicated parapneumonic effusions is not contraindicated. Intrapleural instillation of fibrinolytic agents has been shown in a number of studies to be an effective and safe mode of treatment in complicated parapneumonic effusions and empyema, minimizing the need for surgical intervention (112). However, fibrinolysis in the management of complicated multiloculated empyemas is generally not recommended in pregnancy because of limited experience (112–115).

References

1. Golan A, Ron-el R, Herman A, et al. Ovarian hyperstimulation syndrome: An update review. Obstet Gynecol Surv 1989; 44:430–440.
2. Schenker JG, Ezra Y. Complications of assisted reproductive techniques. Fertil Steril 1994; 61:411–422.
3. Navot D, Bergh PA, Laufer N. Ovarian hyperstimulation syndrome in novel reproductive technologies: Prevention and treatment. Fertil Steril 1992; 58:249–261.
4. Varma TR, Patel RH. Ovarian hyperstimulation syndrome. A case history and review. Acta Obstet Gynecol Scand 1988; 67:579–584.
5. Balasch J, Fabregues F, Arroyo V. Peripheral arterial vasodilation hypothesis: A new insight into the pathogenesis of ovarian hyperstimulation syndrome. Hum Reprod 1998; 13: 2718–2730.
6. Vlahos NF, Gregoriou O. Prevention and management of ovarian hyperstimulation syndrome. Ann N Y Acad Sci 2006; 1092:247–264.
7. Gómez R, Simon C, Remohi J, et al. Vascular endothelial growth factor receptor-2 activation induces vascular permeability in hyperstimulated rats, and this effect is prevented by receptor blockade. Endocrinology 2002; 143:4339–4348.
8. Soares SR, Gómez R, Simón C, et al. Targeting the vascular endothelial growth factor system to prevent ovarian hyperstimulation syndrome. Hum Reprod Update. April 2, 2008 [Epub ahead of print].
9. Abramov Y, Barak V, Nisman B, et al. Vascular endothelial growth factor plasma levels correlate to the clinical picture in severe ovarian hyperstimulation syndrome. Fertil Steril 1997; 67:261–265.
10. Man A, Schwarz Y, Greif J. Pleural effusion as a presenting symptom of ovarian hyperstimulation syndrome. Eur Respir J 1997; 10:2425–2426.
11. Roden S, Juvin K, Homasson JP, et al. An uncommon etiology of isolated pleural effusion. The ovarian hyperstimulation syndrome. Chest 2000; 118:256–258.
12. Light RW. Pleural diseases. Dis Mon 1992; 38:261–331.
13. Abramov Y, Elchalal U, Schenker JG. Febrile morbidity in severe and critical ovarian hyperstimulation syndrome: A multicentre study. Hum Reprod 1998; 13:3128–3131.
14. Chen CD, Wu MY, Chen HF, et al. Prognostic importance of serial cytokine changes in ascites and pleural effusion in women with severe ovarian hyperstimulation syndrome. Fertil Steril 1999; 72:286–292.
15. Chen CD, Chen HF, Lu HF, et al. Value of serum and follicular fluid cytokine profile in the prediction of moderate to severe ovarian hyperstimulation syndrome. Hum Reprod 2000; 15:1037–1042.

16. Levin MF, Kaplan BR, Hutton LC. Thoracic manifestations of ovarian hyperstimulation syndrome. Can Assoc Radiol J 1995; 46:23–26.
17. Gregory WT, Patton PE. Isolated pleural effusion in severe ovarian hyperstimulation: A case report. Am J Obstet Gynecol 1999; 180:1468–1471.
18. Carter EJ, Ettensohn DB. Catamenial pneumothorax. Chest 1990; 98:713–716.
19. Wilkins SB, Bell-Thomson J, Tyras DH. Hemothorax associated with endometriosis. J Thorac Cardiovasc Surg 1985; 89:636–638.
20. Elliot DL, Barker AF, Dixon LM. Catamenial hemoptysis. New methods of diagnosis and therapy. Chest 1985; 87:687–688.
21. Horsfield K. Catamenial pleural pain. Eur Respir J 1989; 2:1013–1014.
22. Muneyyirci-Delale O, Neil G, Serur E, et al. Endometriosis with massive ascites. Gynecol Oncol 1998; 69:42–46.
23. Bhojawala J, Heller DS, Cracchiolo B, et al. Endometriosis presenting as bloody pleural effusion and ascites-report of a case and review of the literature. Arch Gynecol Obstet 2000; 264:39–41.
24. Meigs JV. Fibroma of the ovary with ascites and hydrothorax. Meigs' syndrome. Am J Obstet Gynecol 1954; 67:962–987.
25. Joseph J, Sahn SA. Thoracic endometriosis syndrome: New observations from an analysis of 110 cases. Am J Med 1996; 100:164–170.
26. Chervenak FA, Greenlee RM, Lewenstein L, et al. Massive ascites associated with endometriosis. Obstet Gynecol 1981; 57:379–381.
27. Ekoukou D, Guilherme R, Desligneres S, et al. Endometriosis with massive hemorrhagic ascites: A case report and review of the literature. J Gynecol Obstet Biol Reprod (Paris) 2005; 34:351–359.
28. Palayekar M, Jenci J, Carlson JA Jr. Recurrent hemorrhagic ascites: A rare presentation of endometriosis. Obstet Gynecol 2007; 110:521–522.
29. Kennedy S. Is there a genetic basis to endometriosis? Semin Reprod Endocrinol 1997; 15:309–318.
30. Yu J, Grimes DA. Ascites and pleural effusions associated with endometriosis. Obstet Gynecol 1991; 78:533–534.
31. Augoulea A, Lambrinoudaki I, Christodoulakos G. Thoracic endometriosis syndrome. Respiration 2008; 75:113–119 [Epub June 28, 2007.
32. Shek Y, De Lia JE, Pattillo RA. Endometriosis with a pleural effusion and ascites. Report of a case treated with nafarelin acetate. J Reprod Med 1995; 40:540–542.
33. Meigs JV, Cass JW. Fibroma of the ovary with ascites and hydrothorax. Am J Obstet Gynecol 1937; 33:249–267.
34. Chen FC, Fink RL, Jolly H. Meigs' syndrome in association with a locally invasive adeno-carcinoma of the fallopian tube. Aust N Z J Surg 1995; 65:761–762.
35. Ryan RJ. Pseudo-Meigs syndrome. Associated with metastatic cancer of ovary. N Y State J Med 1972; 72:727–730.
36. Light RW. Diagnostic principles in pleural disease. Eur Respir J 1997; 10:476–481.
37. Abad A, Cazorla E, Ruiz F, et al. Meigs' syndrome with elevated CA125: Case report and review of the literature. Eur J Obstet Gynecol Reprod Biol 1999; 82:97–99.
38. Kurai M, Shiozawa T, Noguchi H, et al. Leiomyoma of the ovary presenting with Meigs' syndrome. J Obstet Gynaecol Res 2005; 31:257–262.
39. Ishiko O, Yoshida H, Sumi T, et al. Vascular endothelial growth factor levels in pleural and peritoneal fluid in Meigs' syndrome. Eur J Obstet Gynecol Reprod Biol 2001; 98:129–130.
40. Majzlin G, Stevens FL. Meigs' syndrome: Case report and review of literature. J Int Coll Surg 1964; 42:625–630.
41. Neustadt JE, Levy RC. Hemorrhagic pleural effusion in Meigs' syndrome. JAMA 1968; 204:81–82.

42. Jimerson SD. Pseudo-Meigs' syndrome. An unusual case with analysis of the effusions. Obstet Gynecol 1973; 42:535–537.
43. Hessen I. Roentgen examination of pleural fluid. Acta Radiol 1951; 86:62–64.
44. Hughson WG, Friedman PJ, Feigin DS, et al. Postpartum pleural effusion: A common radiologic finding. Ann Intern Med 1982; 97:856–858.
45. Stark P, Pollack MS. Pleural effusions in the postpartum period. Radiologe 1986; 26:471–473.
46. Eibenberger KL, Dock WI, Ammann ME, et al. Quantification of pleural effusions: Sonography versus radiography. Radiology 1994; 191:681–684.
47. Lipscomb DJ, Flower CD, Hadfield JW. Ultrasound of the pleura: An assessment of its clinical value. Clin Radiol 1981; 32:289–290.
48. Matalon TA, Neiman HL, Mintzer RA. Noncardiac chest sonography. The state of the art. Chest 1983; 83:675–678.
49. Udeshi UL, McHugo JM, Crawford JS. Postpartum pleural effusion. Br J Obstet Gynaecol 1988; 95:894–897.
50. Gourgoulianis KI, Karantanas AH, Molyvdas PA. Peripartum pleural effusion. Chest 1997; 111:1467–1468.
51. Wallis MG, McHugo JM, Carruthers DA, et al. The prevalence of pleural effusions in pre-eclampsia: An ultrasound study. Br J Obstet Gynaecol 1989; 96:431–433.
52. Kochenour NK, Branch DW, Rote NS, et al. A new postpartum syndrome associated with antiphospholipid antibodies. Obstet Gynecol 1987; 69:460–468.
53. Ayres MA, Sulak PJ. Pregnancy complicated by antiphospholipid antibodies. South Med J 1991; 84:266–269.
54. Backos M, Rai R, Baxter N, et al. Pregnancy complications in women with recurrent miscarriage associated with antiphospholipid antibodies treated with low dose aspirin and heparin. Br J Obstet Gynaecol 1999; 106:102–107.
55. Caruso A, De Carolis S, Di Simone N. Antiphospholipid antibodies in obstetrics: New complexities and sites of action. Hum Reprod Update 1999; 5:267–276.
56. Triolo G, Ferrante A, Ciccia F, et al. Randomized study of subcutaneous low molecular weight heparin plus aspirin versus intravenous immunoglobulin in the treatment of recurrent fetal loss associated with antiphospholipid antibodies. Arthritis Rheum 2003; 48: 728–731.
57. Kumar J, Ilancheran A, Ratnam SS. Pulmonary metastases in gestational trophoblastic disease: A review of 97 cases. Br J Obstet Gynaecol 1988; 95:70–74.
58. Libshitz HI, Baber CE, Hammond CB. The pulmonary metastases of choriocarcinoma. Obstet Gynecol 1977; 49:412–416.
59. Johnson TR Jr, Comstock CH, Anderson DG. Benign gestational trophoblastic disease metastatic to pleura: Unusual cause of hemothorax. Obstet Gynecol 1979; 53:509–511.
60. Sudduth CD, Strange C, Campbell BA, et al. Metastatic choriocarcinoma of the lung presenting as hemothorax. Chest 1991; 99:527–528.
61. McNair OM Jr, Polk OD Jr. Pulmonary disease in gestational trophoblastic neoplasms. J Natl Med Assoc 1992; 84:713–7166.
62. Kalassian KG, Doyle R, Kao P, et al. Lymphangioleiomyomatosis: New insights. Am J Respir Crit Care Med 1997; 155:1183–1186.
63. Sullivan EJ. Lymphangioleiomyomatosis: A review. Chest 1998; 114:1689–1703.
64. NHLBI Workshop Summary. Report of workshop on lymphangioleiomyomatosis. National Heart, Lung, and Blood Institute. Am J Respir Crit Care Med 1999; 159:679–683.
65. Johnson SR, Tattersfield AE. Clinical experience of lymphangioleiomyomatosis in the UK. Thorax 2000; 55:1052–1057.
66. Urban T, Lazor R, Lacronique J. Pulmonary lymphangioleiomyomatosis. A study of 69 patients. Groupe d'Etudes et de Recherche sur les Maladies "Orphelines" Pulmonaires (GERM "O" P). Medicine (Baltimore) 1999; 78:321–337.

67. Beck GJ, Sullivan EJ, Stoller JK, et al. Lymphangioleiomyomatosis: New insights. Am J Respir Crit Care Med 1997; 156:670.
68. Berger U, Khaghani A, Pomerance A, et al. Pulmonary lymphangioleiomyomatosis and steroid receptors. An immunocytochemical study. Am J Clin Pathol 1990; 93:609–614.
69. Ohori NP, Yousem SA, Sonmez-Alpan E, et al. Estrogen and progesterone receptors in lymphangioleiomyomatosis, epithelioid hemangioendothelioma, and sclerosing hemangioma of the lung. Am J Clin Pathol 1991; 96:529–535.
70. Brunelli A, Catalini G, Fianchini A. Pregnancy exacerbating unsuspected mediastinal lymphangioleiomyomatosis and chylothorax. Int J Gynaecol Obstet 1996; 52: 289–290.
71. Hughes E, Hodder RV. Pulmonary lymphangiomyomatosis complicating pregnancy. A case report. J Reprod Med 1987; 32:553–557.
72. Lieberman J, Agliozzo CM. Intrapleural nitrogen mustard for treating chylous effusion of pulmonary lymphangioleiomyomatosis. Cancer 1974; 33:1505–1511.
73. Monteforte WJ Jr, Kohnen PW. Angiomyolipomas in a case of lymphangiomyomatosis syndrome: Relationships to tuberous sclerosis. Cancer 1974; 34:317–321.
74. Silverstein EF, Ellis K, Wolff M, et al. Pulmonary lymphangiomyomatosis. Am J Roentgenol Radium Ther Nucl Med 1974; 120:832–850.
75. Yockey CC, Riepe RE, Ryan K. Pulmonary lymphangioleiomyomatosis complicated by pregnancy. Kans Med 1986; 87:277–278, 293.
76. Cammarata SK, Brush RE, Hyzy RC Jr. Chylothorax after childbirth. Chest 1991; 99: 1539–1540.
77. Tornling G, Axelsson G, Peterffy A. Chylothorax as a complication after delivery. Acta Obstet Gynecol Scand 1987; 66:381–382.
78. Valentine VG, Raffin TA. The management of chylothorax. Chest 1992; 102:586–591.
79. Brady DB, Bolan JC. Neurofibromatosis and spontaneous hemothorax in pregnancy: Two case reports. Obstet Gynecol 1984; 63:35S–38S.
80. Bernhardt LC, Lawton BR. Pregnancy complicated by traumatic rupture of the diaphragm. Am J Surg 1966; 112:918–922.
81. Diddle AW, Tidrick RT. Diaphragmatic hernia associated with pregnancy. Am J Obstet Gynecol 1941; 41:317–318.
82. Wolfe CA, Peterson MW. An unusual cause of massive pleural effusion in pregnancy. Thorax 1988; 43:484–485.
83. Rajapaksa DS. Traumatic diaphragmatic hernia in pregnancy. Ceylon Med J 1986; 31: 153–155.
84. Flick RP, Bofill JA, King JC. Pregnancy complicated by traumatic diaphragmatic rupture. A case report. J Reprod Med 1999; 44:127–130.
85. Dudley AG, Teaford H, Gatewood TS Jr. Delayed traumatic rupture of the diaphragm in pregnancy. Obstet Gynecol 1979; 53:25S–27S.
86. Henzler M, Martin ML, Young J. Delayed diagnosis of traumatic diaphragmatic hernia during pregnancy. Ann Emerg Med 1988; 17:350–353.
87. Goldstein AI, Gazzaniga AB, Ackerman ES, et al. Strangulated diaphragmatic hernia in pregnancy presenting as an empyema. J Reprod Med 1972; 9:135–139.
88. Platt R, Lin JS, Warren JW, et al. Infection with *Mycoplasma hominis* in postpartum fever. Lancet 1980; 2:1217–1221.
89. Mufson MA. *Mycoplasma hominis*: A review of its role as a respiratory tract pathogen of humans. Sex Transm Dis 1983; 10:335–340.
90. Vogel U, Luneberg E, Kuse ER, et al. Extragenital *Mycoplasma hominis* infection in two liver transplant recipients. Clin Infect Dis 1997; 24:512–513.
91. Madoff S, Hooper DC. Nongenitourinary infections caused by *Mycoplasma hominis* in adults. Rev Infect Dis 1988; 10:602–613.

92. Word BM, Baldridge A. *Mycoplasma hominis* pneumonia and pleural effusion in a postpartum adolescent. Pediatr Infect Dis J 1990; 9:295–296.

93. Fabbri J, Tamm M, Frei R, et al. *Mycoplasma hominis* empyema following pleuropneumonia in late pregnancy. Schweiz Med Wochenschr 1993; 123:2244–2246.

94. Fried AM. Hydronephrosis of pregnancy: Ultrasonographic study and classification of asymptomatic women. Am J Obstet Gynecol 1979; 135:1066–1070.

95. Brandes JC, Fritsche C. Obstructive acute renal failure by a gravid uterus: A case report and review. Am J Kidney Dis 1991; 18:398–401.

96. Weiss Z, Shalev E, Zuckerman H, et al. Obstructive renal failure and pleural effusion caused by the gravid uterus. Acta Obstet Gynecol Scand 1986; 65:187–189.

97. Heffner JE, Sahn SA. Pleural disease in pregnancy. Clin Chest Med 1992; 13:667–678.

98. Thompson C, Verani R, Evanoff G, et al. Suppurative bacterial pyelonephritis as a cause of acute renal failure. Am J Kidney Dis 1986; 8:271–273.

99. Corriere JN Jr, Miller WT, Murphy JJ. Hydronephrosis as a cause of pleural effusion. Radiology 1968; 90:79–84.

100. Carey MP, Ihle BU, Woodward CS, et al. Ureteric obstruction by the gravid uterus. Aust N Z J Obstet Gynaecol 1989; 29:308–313.

101. Kamble RT, Bhat SP, Joshi JM. Urinothorax: A case report. Indian J Chest Dis Allied Sci 2000; 42:189–190.

102. Sahn SA. The diagnostic value of pleural fluid analysis. Semin Respir Crit Care Med 1995; 1:269–276.

103. Jana N, Vasishta K, Saha SC, et al. Obstetrical outcomes among women with extrapulmonary tuberculosis. N Engl J Med 1999; 341:645–649.

104. Trajman A, Pai M, Dheda K, et al. Novel tests for diagnosing tuberculous pleural effusion: What works and what does not? Eur Respir J. 2008; 31:1098–1106.

105. Diagnostic standards and classification of tuberculosis in adults and children. Am J Respir Crit Care Med 2000; 161:1376–1395.

106. BTS-guidelines. Chemotherapy and management of tuberculosis in the United Kingdom: Recommendations 1998. Joint Tuberculosis Committee of the British Thoracic Society. Thorax 1998; 53:536–548.

107. Snider DE Jr, Layde PM, Johnson MW, et al. Treatment of tuberculosis during pregnancy. Am Rev Respir Dis 1980; 122:65–79.

108. ATS/CDC statement. Targeted tuberculin testing and treatment of latent tuberculosis infection. Am J Respir Crit Care Med 2000; 161:S221–S247.

109. Madinger NE, Greenspoon JS, Ellrodt AG. Pneumonia during pregnancy: Has modern technology improved maternal and fetal outcome? Am J Obstet Gynecol 1989; 161:657–662.

110. Montella KR. Pulmonary pharmacology in pregnancy. Clin Chest Med 1992; 13:587–595.

111. Rubin P. Fortnightly review: Drug treatment during pregnancy. BMJ 1998; 317:1503–1506.

112. Bouros D, Schiza S, Siafakas N. Fibrinolytics in the treatment of parapneumonic effusions. Monaldi Arch Chest Dis 1999; 54:258–263.

113. Bouros D, Schiza S, Siafakas N. Utility of fibrinolytic agents for draining intrapleural infections. Semin Respir Infect 1999; 14:39–47.

114. Bouros D, Schiza S, Tzanakis N, et al. Intrapleural urokinase versus normal saline in the treatment of complicated parapneumonic effusions and empyema. A randomized, double-blind study. Am J Respir Crit Care Med 1999; 159:37–42.

115. Bouros D, Tzouvelekis A, Antoniou KM, et al. Intrapleural fibrinolytic therapy for pleural infection. Pulm Pharmacol Ther 2007; 20:616–626.

36
Pleural Effusions in the Intensive Care Unit

IOANNIS PNEUMATIKOS
Critical Care Department, University Hospital of Alexandroupolis, Democritus University Thrace, Alexandroupolis, Greece

CHARIS ROUSSOS
Critical Care Department, Evangelismos Hospital, National and Capodistrian University of Athens, Athens, Greece

I. Introduction

Pleural effusion (PE) is defined as the excessive accumulation of fluid in the pleural space indicating an imbalance between pleural fluid formation and removal. PEs are rarely a manifestation of primary pleural disease. They usually reflect a pulmonary or extrapulmonary disorder (1). Accordingly, the clinical importance of PEs arises primarily from what they really represent (infection, malignancy, heart failure, pulmonary embolism, hemothorax, or other) and secondarily from their impact on respiratory physiology.

The incidence of PEs in the intensive care unit (ICU) seems to be common and varies with screening methods, from approximately 8% for physical examination to more than 60% for routine lung ultrasound (LUS) (2). Patients in ICU may develop PEs for two reasons: as a consequence of their primary disease or as a result of several supportive and therapeutic interventions. Critically ill patients are prone to some individual conditions predisposing to the development of PEs. For example, they are frequently intubated and mechanically ventilated requiring analgesia, sedation, or paralysis. Accordingly, they are at risk for developing atelectasis and ventilator-associated pneumonia (VAP) often associated with PEs. Moreover, many ICU patients who present with hypotension and hemodynamic instability are treated with aggressive hydration, leading to fluid overload thus promoting interstitial edema formation and pleural transudation. Apart from traumatic effusions and empyema, most PEs are free effusions and are associated with atelectasis, heart failure, fluid overload, hypo-albuminemia, or abdominal diseases.

II. Pathophysiology

The pleura space lies between the inner surface of chest wall (parietal pleura) and the surface of the lungs (visceral pleura). This space is normally filled with a very small amount of colorless alkaline fluid, which serves as a coupling system. In normal conditions, fluid enters the pleural space from the capillaries in the parietal pleura and is removed via the lymphatics situated in the parietal pleura. Fluid can also enter the pleural space from the interstitial spaces of the lung via the visceral pleura or from the peritoneal cavity via small holes in the diaphragm. Pleural fluid turnover is estimated to be ~ 0.15 mL/(kg $\cdot$ h). The lymphatics have the capacity to absorb 20 times more fluid than is normally formed.

The total absorbing capacity of the parietal pleural is of the order of 30 mL/hr of fluid, equivalent to 700 mL/day (3). Accordingly, a PE may occur when excessive formation of fluid can overwhelm these efficient absorptive mechanisms or when there is decreased fluid absorption by the lymphatics.

PEs are traditionally classified as either transudates or exudates (4). A transudative PE develops when *the systemic factors* influencing the formation or absorption of pleural fluid are altered. Examples of conditions producing transudative PE are left ventricular failure, pulmonary embolism, and cirrhosis. In contrast, an exudative PE develops when *local factors* influencing the formation and absorption of pleural fluid are altered. Examples of conditions producing exudative PEs are bacterial or viral pneumonia, malignancy, and pulmonary embolism.

III. Etiology

Only three studies have prospectively referred to the frequency and etiology of PEs in the ICU (1,2,5) (Table 1).

Fartoukh et al. found that of 1351 patients admitted to three medical intensive care units (MICUs) during a period of one year, 113 patients had physical and radiographic evidence of PE yielding an annual incidence of 8.4% (1). Routine thoracocentesis was

Table 1 Causes of Pleural Effusions in Intensive Care Unit Patients

	ICU patients			Non-ICU patients	
Causes of pleural effusions	Mattison et al. (2), $N = 62$	Fartoukh et al. (1), $N = 113$	Chih-Yen et al. (5), $N = 94^a$	Light (4), $N = 150$	Heffner et al. (65), $N = 1754$
Congestive heart failure	22 (35.5%)	28 (24.8%)	9 (10%)	39 (26%)	330 (18.8%)
Atelectasis	14 (23%)	2 (1.7%)	-	-	-
Cirrhosis	5 (8%)	6 (5.3%)	2 (2.1%)	5 (3.3%)	49 (2.8%)
Hypoalbuminemia	5 (8%)	-	7 (7.4%)	-	28 (1.6%)
Nephrotic syndrome	-	1 (0.8%)	-	3 (2%)	39 (2.2%)
Parapneumonic effusions	7 (11%)	29 (25.6%)	36 (38.3%)	26 (17.3%)	244 (13.4%)
Pulmonary embolism	-	5 (4.4%)	-	5 (3.3%)	47 (2.7%)
Empyema	1 (2%)	12 (10.6%)	15 (16%)	/	-
Malignancies	2 (3%)	11 (9.7%)	1 (1%)	43 (28.7%)	569 (32.4%)
Tuberculosis	-	2 (1.7%)	-	14 (9.3%)	306 (17.4%)
Pancreatitis	1 (2%)	2 (1.7%)	2 (2%)	6 (4%)	11 (0.6%)
Postsurgical effusions	-	-	1 (1%)	-	-
Collagen vascular disease	-	-	1 (1%)	-	29 (1.6)
Uremic pleurisy	1 (2)%	-	-	-	-
Hemothorax	-	4 (3.4%)	-	2 (1.3%)	
Trauma	-	-	-	-	15 (0.8%)
Sepsis	-	-	10 (10.6%)	-	-
Other	1 (2%)	-	-	7 (4.7%)	87 (4.5%)
Unknown	3 (5%)	6 (5.3%)	8 (9%)	-	-

[a]Febrile patients with PEs admitted to ICU in 1-year study.

performed in 82 patients. Twenty (24.4%) patients had a transudate, 35 (42.7%) patients had an infectious exudate, and 27 (32.9%) patients had a noninfectious exudate. In three patients, no cause was found.

The prevalence and causes of PEs in patients admitted to a MICU are also prospectively studied by Mattison et al. using chest X-rays (CXRs) reviewed daily and LUS performed within 10 hours of their latest chest radiograph. In 100 consecutive admissions to the MICU with stays greater than 24 hours, the prevalence of PEs was 62%, with 41% being present on admission (2). Most PEs were small, and two-thirds were due to noninfectious causes, namely, heart failure 22 (35%) of 62, and atelectasis 14 (23%) of 62; when compared with patients who never had effusions during their MICU stay, patients with PEs had statistically significant lower serum albumin concentration, higher acute physiology and chronic health evaluation II (APACHE II) scores during the initial 24 hours of MICU stay, longer MICU stays, and longer mechanical ventilation days. No patient died as a direct result of his or her PE.

In another prospective study, all consecutive patients admitted to an MICU with fever $>38°C$ for >8 hours were screened prospectively for physical and radiographic evidence of PE (5). During the one-year study period, 1640 patients were admitted to the MICU, of these, 94 were febrile patients with simultaneously PEs proven by CXRs and LUS. Routine thoracocentesis and pleural fluid cultures were performed in all patients under portable LUS guidance. In all, 58 (62%) patients had infectious exudates, 28 (30%) patients had transudates, and 8 (8%) patients had noninfectious exudates.

IV. Imaging

A. Chest Radiograph

In the upright patient, a PE can be diagnosed with adequate sensitivity with the help of a standard postero-anterior (PA) CXR: blunting of the costophrenic angle usually occurs in the presence of approximately 200 mL of pleural fluid, although the plain film can be normal with up to 500 mL fluid (6,7). Lateral decubitus films are occasionally useful as free fluid gravitates to the most dependent part of the chest wall (8). As the effusion size increases the characteristic meniscus becomes apparent (9). Complete opacification of the hemithorax with contralateral mediastinal shift occurs with massive PEs although no mediastinal shift occurs if there is associated pulmonary collapse or mediastinal fixation (10). Large PEs can also invert the ipsilateral hemidiaphragm, particularly on the left, as the liver splints the right hemidiaphragm. Complicated parapneumonic effusions (PPEs) and empyemas can appear as simple PEs on CXR, but are more often seen in association with consolidation. They are commonly unilateral, and, if bilateral, the infected side is usually larger. A PE can become loculated as it evolves, causing irregular lentiform fluid collections. Loculated or subpulmonic PEs may be difficult to diagnose on a standard PA CXR. Hemidiaphragm elevation and/or lateral displacement of the diaphragm apex are the main signs of a subpulmonic PE.

In the ICUs, bedside CXRs are frequently obtained on a daily basis as a complement to the physical examination (11). They are readily available, easy and quick to perform, and much less expensive than any other imaging modality. Nearly all CXRs taken in the ICU are obtained with patients lying in a semirecumbent position (SCXR). However, despite great improvement in quality some technical and diagnostic limitations

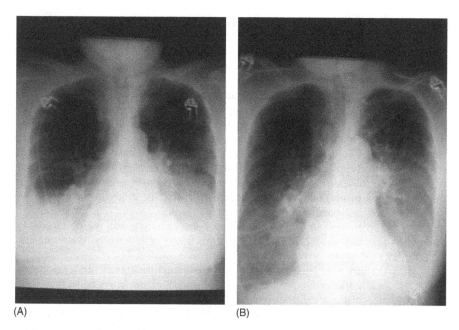

(A)   (B)

Figure 1   Chest radiograph of a critically ill patient with bilateral pleural effusion—(**A**) in semire-cumbent position: blunting of the costophrenic angle and the characteristic meniscus becomes apparent, and (**B**) in supine position: increased homogeneous density over the lower and middle lung fields of both hemithoraces that does not obliterate normal bronchovascular markings.

remain (12): First, during the acquisition procedure, the patient and the thorax often move, decreasing the spatial resolution of the radiological image. Second, the film cassette is placed posterior to the thorax. Third, the X-ray beam originates anterior, at a shorter distance than recommended and quite often not tangentially to the diaphragmatic dome, thereby making difficult the correct interpretation of the silhouette sign. These technical difficulties often result to incorrect assessment of several pulmonary disorders such as a PE.

The most common radiographic finding of a PE in a SCXR is increased homogeneous density over the lower lung field that does not obliterate normal bronchovascular markings, does not show air bronchogram, and does not show hilar or mediastinal displacement until the effusion is massive (Fig. 1). Other common signs are blunted of costofrenic angle and loss of hemidiaphragm silluette (13,14). Apical pleural capping is a sign usually indicating large PEs. A normal SCXR does not exclude the presence of a PE. The overall accuracy of a SCXR for detecting a PE with reference to decubitus view has been estimated to be 0.67 to 0.95. A more recent study using the LUS as gold standard estimated the accuracy of SCXR to 82% (13).

B. Lung Ultrasound
LUS was demonstrated to detect PEs a long time ago (15–17). However, it has taken quite some time for LUS to gain acceptance for the bedside diagnosis of PEs in the ICUs.

LUS shows better sensitivity and reliability for diagnosis of PEs than bedside SCXR (18–20). It rules out other etiologies such as atelectasis, consolidation, mass, or an elevated hemidiaphragm, takes less time than SCXR and can be repeated serially at the bedside. The skills required to detect PEs are easy to acquire, as suggested by several publications (15,17,18).

Briefly, with the patient lying in supine position, a PE should be sought on a longitudinal view using a short probe directly applied to the chest wall. The probe must be oriented upward and downward, laterally and medially, and then anteriorly and posteriorly in order to obtain a complete anatomic assessment of the area. A PE is described as an anechoic or hypoechoic layer between two pleural layers. The lung behind a PE appears either aerated or consolidated in the case of large PEs. If no PE is visible, this means absent or minimal PE. Assessment of a PE requires attention to spleen or liver and diaphragm, especially when pleural puncture is considered. PEs can be easily distinguished from spleen and liver by visualization of the so-called "sinusoid sign." The "sinusoid sign" indicates the centrifugal shifting of the lung towards the chest wall during inspiration. This sign is mandatory as it confirms PE with a specificity of 97% when the gold standard is the withdrawal of pleural fluid (21).

LUS evaluation of PEs in mechanically ventilated patients is very important in two ways: first, it allows the quantification of pleural fluid and hence helps in deciding whether thoracocentesis should be performed in high-risk patients (17,22–24); and, second it provides visual guidance for thoracocentesis (21,23,24). In the supine position, an inter-pleural distance at the lung base, defined as the distance between the lung and the posterior chest wall ≥50 mm is highly predictive of a PE ≥500 mL (18,24). Another important contribution of LUS is to provide noninvasive information about the nature (transudate or exudates) of a PE. Transudates are always anechoic. In contrast, a liquid with mobile particles or septa is suggestive of exudate, hemothorax or purulent pleurisy and should be analyzed (Fig. 2) (25).

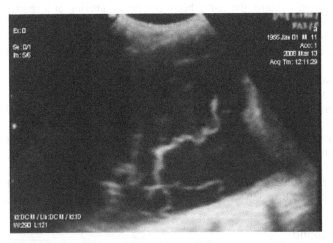

Figure 2 Lung ultrasound in an ICU patient showing a parapneumonic pleural effusion. Note the floating strands and septa within the complex septated effusion.

C. Computerized Tomography (CT) Scan

CT scan is the most accurate examination for detecting and characterizing PEs and it has made a major impact on their diagnosis and management. CT scan has the advantage over LUS in that it can evaluate the pleural surface better, and it is ideal to evaluate the lung parenchyma and tracheobronchial tree (26). For the most accurate assessment of the pleural surface, chest CT scan should be performed with IV contrast (Fig. 3). Although moving a critically ill patient for a CT scan has potential risks, the diagnostic advantage can be justified in the stable patient when the clinical course is not compatible with the proposed diagnosis suggested by the portable CXR. In selected patients with multiple trauma, chest CT scan often provides additional diagnostic information and positively affects patients management and outcome (27,28).

In simple uncomplicated PEs the CT scan shows crescent-shaped opacities in the posterior and basal portions of the hemithorax. Although thoracocentesis and analysis of the pleural fluid are the mainstay in identifying the etiology of a PE, CT often can suggest the diagnosis. For example, empyemas often have a characteristic appearance on CT scan; when IV contrast is used, an empyema classically will show enhancement of both the parietal and visceral pleural surfaces, a picture that is known as the "split pleura" sign (29).

V. Pleural Fluid Examination

In evaluating PEs, clinicians perform thoracocentesis and pleural fluid examination. Pleural fluid analysis is useful in establishing the etiology of a PE (Table 2). With a presumptive clinical diagnosis in concert and with a good working knowledge of pleural fluid analysis, a definitive or confident clinical diagnosis can be expected in up to 95% of patients (30).

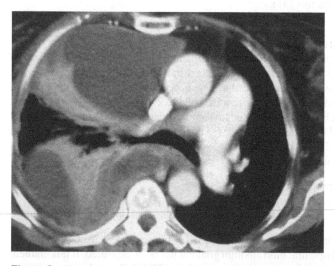

Figure 3 Contrast-enhanced CT scan of the chest at the level of the conus of the pulmonary artery showing a massive loculated parapneumonic PE on the right hemithorax displacing the mediastinum to the left.

Table 2 Pleural Fluid Analysis for Differential Diagnosis

All pleural effusions	Exudates	Other tests
Protein	Gram stain/culture	Glucose
LDH	Acid fast stain/culture	Amylase
pH	Fungal stain/culture	Adenosine deaminase
Cell count	Cytologic examination	Antinuclear antibody titer
Cholesterol		Triglycerids

The selection of the tests depends on clinical condition.

A. Observation

The color, characteristics, and odor of the pleural fluid may either be diagnostic or help narrow the differential diagnosis (30). Although an exudate cannot be definitely excluded, a clear, straw-colored fluid usually suggests a transudate. Sanguineous fluid (hematocrit <1%) is not helpful diagnostically. However, when the fluid is grossly bloody and trauma is absent, the differential diagnosis should include malignancy, post–cardiac injury syndrome or pulmonary infarction. A hemothorax is most commonly due to blunt or penetrating chest trauma but may also occur with invasive procedures. If pus is aspirated, an empyema is established. Pus is determined by its gross appearance, which is a thick, viscous, yellow-white, opaque fluid. If the pus has a putrid odor, an anaerobic infection is confirmed. A white or milky pleural fluid suggests either a chylothorax or a cholesterol effusion, although an empyema may simulate this appearance. Finally, if a central venous catheter has migrated extravascularly into the mediastinum with subsequent rupture of the mediastinal parietal pleura, the pleural fluid will be similar to the infusate. This is especially characteristic in patients receiving total parenteral nutrition and is more likely to occur in left-sided catheters (31).

B. Light's Criteria

After obtaining a sample of pleural fluid the clinician should determine whether the effusion is a transudate or exudate. If the fluid is a transudate, the possible causes are relatively few and further diagnostic procedures are not necessary. In contrast, if the fluid is an exudate, further diagnostic tests are required (Table 2).

According to Light's criteria, transudative and exudative PEs are differentiated by comparing protein and lactate dehydrogenase (LDH) concentrations in the pleural fluid to those in the blood (32). Exudative PEs meet at least one of the following criteria, whereas transudative PEs meet none:

1. Pleural fluid protein/serum protein >0.5
2. Pleural fluid LDH/serum LDH >0.6.
3. Pleural fluid LDH more than two-thirds of the normal upper limit for serum.

Light's criteria may label approximately 25% of transudates as exudates. In these conditions, the serum-to-pleural fluid albumin gradient has been measured. If this gradient is greater than 1.2 g/dL, then the patient has a transudative PE (4). Recently, a combination of PE cholesterol concentration (criterion for exudates: PE-CHOL >60 mg/dL) and PE lactate dehydrogenase LDH activity (criterion for exudates: PE-LDH >280 UI/L) seems to have at least the same or highest discriminatory potential than Light's criteria and the added advantage that no patient plasma is needed for correct classification (33,34).

C. pH

The pH of normal pleural fluid is approximately 7.62 owing to active transport of HCO_3^- into the pleural space. A low pH is seen in inflammatory and infiltrative disorders such as infected parapneumonic effusions, empyema, malignancies, collagen vascular disease, and oesophageal rupture. Urinothorax is the only transudative effusion that can be present with a low pleural fluid pH (35). A parapneumonic pleural fluid with pH <7.2 is an indication for pleural drainage (32).

D. Glucose

The glucose concentration in transudates and in most exudates is similar to that in the serum as glucose is of low molecular weight and moves from blood to pleural fluid by simple diffusion across the endothelial and mesothelial membranes. Diseases with low pleural fluid pH may also have a low pleural fluid glucose concentration, defined as <60 mg/dL or a pleural fluid/serum glucose ratio of <0.5 (36).

E. Amylase

An elevated pleural fluid amylase (>upper limit of normal for serum) indicates that the PE is caused by pancreatic disease, oesophageal rupture, or pleural malignancy. The clinical setting usually separates these entities, and determination of the pleural fluid amylase isoenzyme pattern can differentiate malignancy from pancreatic disease.

F. Other Laboratory Tests

Other tests that routinely should be obtained on exudative pleural fluids are Gram stain and cultures, cell counts and differential, cytology, and a marker for tuberculous pleuritis. The diagnosis of tuberculous pleuritis is strongly suggested by a pleural fluid adenosine deaminase level above 50 IU/L (30).

VI. Management of PEs in the ICU

A. Diagnostic Thoracocentesis

When a PE has been recognized in an ICU patient, a question is usually asked: Is it necessary to perform a diagnostic thoracocentesis in an attempt to establish the cause? PEs usually require diagnostic thoracocentesis when the fluid is suspected infected, or suspected blood, and when large enough to cause ventilatory compromise (37). Exceptions might be patients with secure clinical diagnosis and only a small amount of pleural fluid as in atelectasis or patients with uncomplicated congestive heart failure (20). Observation may be warranted in these situations but thoracocentesis should be performed if there are adverse changes.

Until the coming of LUS, diagnostic or therapeutic thoracocentesis in critically ill patients was classically performed through a posterolateral approach with the head of the bed elevated as close to 90° angle as possible. In this position, thoracocentesis was approached along the posterior axillary line. Nevertheless, in patient receiving mechanical ventilation, it may be hazardous to attempt a blind thoracocentesis for a suspected PE, especially if the effusion is small or if the patient is on a high level of positive end-expiratory pressure (21). Under such circumstances, the potential risk for pneumothorax or other complications is high. Specially designed thoracocentesis trays are now available with a spring-loaded, blunt-tip needle that avoids puncture of the lung (38).

Nowadays, the value of LUS not only for a simple thoracocentesis but also for drainage of a PE is well recognized (39). LUS is especially valuable in guiding drainage of loculated or very small effusions. Although LUS-guided thoracocentesis becomes a routine procedure, strict criteria are mandatory: briefly, with the patient adequately positioned on his back or in supine position, one must check for an inspiratory distance of at least 15 mm with the effusion visible at the adjacent upper and lower intercostals spaces. The operator must also check for the absence of interposition of lung, heart, liver, or spleen during the respiratory cycle to avoid puncture of such organs that can potentially cause catastrophic complications (24). The "sinusoid sign" has the advantage of being clearly correlated with a low viscosity of the pleural fluid thus allowing the insertion of a fine needle with minimal trauma. Once an optimal and safe position for thoracocentesis has been determined, the skin should be marked and disinfected and the patient should remain in the exact same position in which the LUS was performed. Optimally, the puncture should be done within seconds to minutes of the marking. Lichtenstein et al. evaluated the feasibility and safety of LUS-aided thoracocentesis in 40 patients receiving mechanical ventilation (21). No complications occurred in the 45 LUS-aided thoracenteses, all performed by intensive care physicians. Similar results have been obtained in a more recent comparable study by Mayo et al. with the pneumothorax to occur only in 3 of 232 cases (40).

B. Therapeutic Thoracocentesis

The main indications of therapeutic thoracocentesis in a critically ill patient are to drainage empyema or hemothorax, and to improve ventilatory compromise in cases of massive effusions. Small PEs do not usually require therapeutic thoracocentesis and typically will resolve with conservative management. However, in critically ill patients with acute respiratory failure, catheter drainage of even a small PE can improve oxygenation significantly (41,42).

The technique of therapeutic thoracocentesis is essentially the same as for diagnostic thoracocentesis except that a blunt-tip needle or a plastic catheter rather than a sharp-tip needle should be used. This reduces the risk of pneumothorax, which may occur as fluid is removed and the lung expands toward the chest wall.

The use of small-bore pig-tail catheters placed under radiographic guidance offers a reliable treatment of uncomplicated PEs and is a safe and less invasive alternative to tube thoracostomy (43,44). Moreover, a central venous catheter inserted using a Seldinger technique may be efficacious, well tolerated, and with minimal complications in draining uncomplicated large PEs (45).

Because LUS do not permit a detailed assessment of the pleural process or evaluate the lung parenchyma or airways, CT is increasingly used in the management of complex PEs. Using CT guidance, it is relatively easy to place drainage catheters in specific loculations regardless of size and location. CT fluoroscopy allows real-time continuous monitoring of catheter placement, increasing the success of the procedure and further reducing complications (40). Recently, the development of portable CT has offered the potential to obviate patient transport and its attendant shortcomings (46,47). Although the experience is still limited, portable CT provides the opportunity for bedside drainage procedures (46).

VII. Empyema

Empyema is defined as "pus" in the pleural space or as a PE with microorganisms detected by Gram stain. Empyema may be parapneumonic or nonparapneumonic in origin, and infected pleural fluid may be free or loculated (48) (Table 3). Empyema is a rare diagnosis in the ICU because most patients have usually received antibiotics (that easily penetrate pleural space) for pneumonia, thus preventing the progression of the pleural space infection (49). Nevertheless, empyema becomes more likely if the suspect fluid collection is adjacent to pneumonia. Because of the diagnostic limitations of portable CXRs in ICU, the diagnosis of a pleural empyema can be missed. Although decubitus views and LUS enchance the likelihood of finding the effusion, CT is the definite way to confirm a free or loculated fluid collection, especially if small or loculated (Fig. 2). For febrile and franky septic patients, especially those with an underlying pneumonia, the search for an empyema is reasonable.

Apart from antibiotic therapy, treatment of patients with pleural empyema consists mainly of thorough drainage of the infected pleural fluid by prompt insertion of thoracostomy tube(s) of sufficient caliber. CT guidance can be invaluable in guiding the placement of several drainage catheters. Failure to resolve the acute phase satisfactorily can require an open thoracotomy and pleural stripping or decortications. Video-assisted thoracic surgery (VATS) may be more effective than chest-tube drainage and less invasive than open thoracotomy. This technique plays a bridging role between medical and surgical management and assumed a great importance during the last decade (50,51). Intrapleural fibrinolytic drugs administration (52–55) may probably be useful in patients who are poor surgical candidates or for health care settings in which surgical interventions are unavailable (56).

Table 3 Etiology of Empyema Thoracis in the ICU

Parapneumonic empyemas	Nonparapneumonic empyemas
Pneumonia	Abdominal sepsis
Lung abscess	Abdominal trauma
Bronchiectasis	Chest trauma
	Esophageal perforation
	Mediastinitis
	Postthoracocentesis
	Postthoracostomy
	Postthoracotomy

VIII. Hemothorax

Hemothorax (HE) is defined as a bloody PE in which the pleural fluid hematocrit is at least 50% that of the peripheral blood (4). According to its cause, HE can be divided into two major categories: (*i*) traumatic and (*ii*) nontraumatic or spontaneous hemothorax. Thoracic injury is the most common cause of hemothorax encountered in ICU and should be suspected in any patient with blunt or penetrating chest trauma. If a PE is found on the admitting CXR, thoracocentesis should be performed immediately and the hematocrit should be measured on the fluid. The HE may not be recognized on the initial CXR or LUS. Thus, patients with severe chest trauma should have follow up CXRs three to six hours after the accident (57). Most patients with traumatic HE can be managed with chest tube drainage and do not require thoracotomy. However, exploratory thoracotomy should be strongly considered when more than 2 L of blood is evacuated initially from the chest or if bleeding continues at a rate exceeding 100 mL/hr. Video-thoracoscopy may replace thoracotomy in selected patients and seems to be safe and effective in the treatment of HE. To avoid prolonged operations, conversions to thoracotomy and complications, it should be performed as soon as possible (58). Video-thoracoscopy must also be considered as the procedure of choice for the treatment of retained posttraumatic HE (drainage of clotted hemothorax) in order to avoid late complications such as fibrothorax, empyema, and trapped lung (59).

Other causes of HE in ICU patients include invasive procedures such as placement of central venous catheters, thoracocentesis, percutaneous aspiration or biopsy (60), and pulmonary infarction, malignancy or ruptured aortic aneurysm. HE is also a rare complication of anticoagulation (61).

IX. Chylothorax

Chylothorax is the accumulation of chyle in the pleural space and is caused by disruption of the thoracic duct or its collaterals (4,62). Chylothorax occurs infrequently in the ICU, and, when it occurs, it is almost always traumatic. Among traumatic chylothoraces, iatrogenic causes constitute the majority. Thoracic surgery constitutes the majority of iatrogenic causes (63). Chylothorax is suspsected when the pleural fluid has a distinctive milky, white appearance. The presence of chylomicrons and a triglyceride level >110 mg/dL in the aspirated pleural fluid confirms the diagnosis of chylothorax. Intercostal tube drainage is the initial step in large chylothoraces that cause respiratory distress. During the period of excessive chyle leak, patients almost always require total parenteral nutrition to avoid or reverse hypovolaemia, immunosuppression, and protein and electrolyte deficiencies. Aggressive surgical therapy is recommended for posttraumatic or postsurgical chylothorax. The surgical intervention of choice in thoracic duct injury is thoracic, abdominal, or cervical ligation of the thoracic duct (63). Thoracoscopic ligation of thoracic duct has also been well described (64).

X. Conclusions

PEs are common in the ICU patients but they can easily go unrecognized due to technical and diagnostic limitations of supine portable CXRs. They are usually small, uncomplicated and postoperative and resolve with conservative management. However, if infection is considered a thoracocentesis should be done without delay. The diagnosis of PEs in ICU patients has been revolutionized with the advent of LUS. LUS shows better diagnostic sensitivity and reliability than bedside CXR, and is especially valuable for thoracocentesis in ventilated patients. CT has major advantages over LUS in the area of image-guided thoracocentesis and should be preferred for drainage of loculated PEs. Although routine thoracocentesis has been proved, a simple and safe means of improving the diagnosis and treatment of PEs in ICU patients the impact of this intervention on the prognosis is unknown.

References

1. Fartoukh M, Azoulay E, Galliot R, et al. Clinically documented pleural effusions in medical ICU patients: How useful is routine thoracentesis? Chest 2002; 121:178–184.
2. Mattison LE, Coppage L, Alderman DF, et al. Pleural effusions in the medical ICU: Prevalence, causes, and clinical implications. Chest 1997; 111:1018–1023.
3. Miserocchi G. Physiology and pathophysiology of pleural fluid turnover. Eur Respir J 1997; 10:219–225.
4. Light RW. Pleural Diseases, 7th ed. Philadelphia, PA: Lippincott Williams & Wilkins, 2007.
5. Chih-Yen Tu, Wu-Huei Hsu, Te-Chun Hsia,et al. Pleural effusions in febrile medical ICU patients. Chest 2004; 126:1274–1280.
6. Woodring GH. Recognition of pleural effusion on supine radiographs: How much fluid is requires? AJR 1984; 142:59.
7. Blackmore CC, Black WC, Dallas RV, et al. Pleural fluid volume estimation: A chest radiograph prediction rule. Acad Radiol 1996; 3:103–109.
8. Kocijancic I, Vidmar K, Ivanovi-Herceg Z. Chest sonography versus lateral decubitus radiography in the diagnosis of small pleural effusions. J Clin Ultrasound 2003; 31:69–74.
9. Henschke CI, Davis SD, Romano PM, et al. Pleural effusions: Pathogenesis, radiologic evaluation, and therapy. J Thorac Imaging 1989; 4:49–60.
10. Liberson M. Diagnostic significance of the mediastinal profile in massive unilateral pleural effusions. Am Rev Respir Dis 1963; 88:176–180.
11. Graat ME, Hendrikse KA, Spronk PE, et al. Chest radiography practice in critically ill patients: A postal survey in the Netherlands. BMC Med Imaging 2006; 6:8.
12. Bouhemad B, Zhang M, Rouby JJ. Clinical review: Bedside lung ultrasound in critical care practice. Critical Care 2007; 11:205.
13. Emamian SA, Kaasbol MA, Olsen JF, et al. Accuracy of the diagnosis of pleural effusion on supine chest X-ray. Eur Radiol 1997; 7(1):57–60.
14. Ruskin JA, Gurney JW, Thorsen MK, et al. Detection of pleural effusions on supine chest radiographs AJR Am J Roentgenol 1987; 148(4):681–683.
15. Joyner CR, Herman RJ, Reid JM. Reflected ultrasound in the detection and localization of pleural effusions. JAMA 1967; 200:399–402.
16. Freimanis AS. Ultrasound and thoracentesis. JAMA 1977; 238:1631.
17. Gryminski J, Krakowka P, Lypacewicz G. The diagnosis of pleural effusion by ultrasonic and radiologic techniques. Chest 1976; 70:33–37.
18. Eibenberger KL, Dock WI, Ammann ME, et al. Quantification of pleural effusions: Sonography versus radiography. Radiology 1994; 191:681–684.
19. Coppage L, Jolles H, Henry DA. Imaging of the chest in the intensive care setting. In: Shoemaker WC, Ayres SM, Grenvik A, Holbrook PR, eds. Textbook of Critical Care. Philadelphia, PA: Saunders, 1995:332–347.
20. Sahn SA. Pleural disease in the critically ill patients. In: Irvin RS, Cerra FB, Rippe MJ, eds. Intensive Care Medicine, 4th ed. Philadelphia, PA: Lippincott Williams & Wilkins, 1999:710–727.

21. Lichtenstein D, Hulot JS, Rabiller A, et al. Feasibility and safety of ultrasound-aided thoracentesis in mechanically ventilated patients. Intensive Care Med 1999; 25:955–958.

22. Roch A, Bojan M, Michelet P, et al. Usefulness of ultrasonography in predicting pleural effusions > 500 mL in patients receiving mechanical ventilation. Chest 2005; 127: 224–232.

23. Vignon P, Chastagner C, Berkane V,et al. Quantitative assessment of pleural effusion in critically ill patients by means of ultrasonography. Crit Care Med 2005; 33:1757–1763.

24. Balik M, Plasil P, Waldauf P, et al. Ultrasound estimation of volume of pleural fluid in mechanically ventilated patients. Intensive Care Med 2006; 32:318–321.

25. Yang PC, Luh KT, Chang DB, et al. Value of sonography in determining the nature of pleural effusion: Analysis of 320 cases. Am J Roentgenol 1992; 159:29–33.

26. Rubinowits A, Siegel M, Tocino I. Thoracic Imaging in the ICU. Crit Care Clinics 2007; 23:539–573.

27. Mirvis SE, Tobin CD, Kostrubiak I, et al. Thoracic CT in detecting occult disease in critically ill patients. AJR 1987; 148:685.

28. Peruzzi W, Garner W, Bools J, et al. Portable chest roentgenography and computed tomography in critically ill patients. Chest 1988; 93:722.

29. Stark DD, Federle MP, Goodman PC,et al. Differentiating lung abscess and empyema: Radiography and computed tomography. AJR Am J Roentgenol 1983; 141:163–167.

30. Sahn SA. The value of pleural fluid analysis. Am J Med Sci 2008; 335(1):7–15.

31. Walshe C, Phelan D, Bourke J, et al. Vascular erosion by central venous catheters used for total parenteral nutrition. Intensive Care Med 2007; 33(3):534–537.

32. Light RW, MacGregor MI, Luschsinger PC, et al. Pleural effusions: The diagnostic separation of transudates and exudates. Ann Intern Med 1972; 62:57–63.

33. Romero S, Martinez A, Hernandez L, et al. Light's criteria revisited: Consistency and comparison with new proposed alternative criteria for separating pleural transudates from exudates. Respiration 2000; 67(1):18–23.

34. Leers MP, Kleinveld HA, Scharnhorst V. Differentiating transudative from exudative pleural effusion: should we measure effusion cholesterol dehydrogenase? Clin Chem Lab Med 2007; 45(10):1332–1338.

35. Miller KS, Wooten S, Sahn SA. Urinothorax: A cause of low pH transudative pleural effusions. Am J Med 1988; 85(3):448–449.

36. Sahn SA. Pathogenesis and clinical features of diseases associated with a low pleural fluid glucose. In: Chretien J, Bignon J, Hirsch A, eds. The Pleural in Health and Disease. New York, NY: Marcel Dekker, 1985:267–285.

37. Myers DL. Pleural disease. In: Civetta JM, Taylor RW, Kirby RR, eds. Critical Care. Philadelphia, PA: Lippincott, 1988:1133–1142.

38. Grodzin CJ, Balk RA. Indwelling small pleural catheter needle thoracocentesis in the management of large pleural effusions. Chest 1997; 11:981.

39. Beaulieu Y, Marik PE. Bedside ultrasonography in the ICU. Chest 2005; 128:1766–1781.

40. Mayo PH, Goltz HR, Tafreshi M, et al. Safety of ultrasound guided thoracentesis in patients receiving mechanical ventilation. Chest 2004; 125:1059–1062.

41. Trotman-Dickenson B. Radiology in the intensive care unit (Part 2). J Intensive Car Med 2003; 18(5):239–252.

42. Talmor M, Hydo L, Gershenwald JG, et al. Beneficial effects of chest tube drainage of pleural effusion in acute respiratory failure refractory to positive end-expiratory pressure ventilation. Surgery 1998; 123(2):137–143.

43. Colice GL, Rubins JB. Practical management of pleural effusions. When and how should fluid accumulation be drained? Postgrad Med 1999; 105:67–77.

44. Grodzin CJ, Balk RA. Indwelling small pleural catheter needle thoracocentesis in the management of large pleural effusions. Chest 1997; 111:981–988.

45. Singh K, Loo S, Bellomo R. Pleural drainage using central venous catheters. Crit Care 2003; 7(6):R191–R194.

46. White CS, Meyer CA, Wu J, et al. Portable CT: Assessing thoracic disease in the intensive care unit. Am J Radiol 1999; 173:1351–1356.

47. Teichgraber UKM, Pinkerneele J, et al. Portable computed tomography performed on the intensive care unit. Intensive Care Med 2003; 29:491–495.

48. Papiris S, Roussos Ch. Pleural effusions in the intensive care unit. In: Bouros D, ed. Pleural Diseases, 1st ed. New York, NY: Marcel Dekker, 2004:741–765.

49. Strange C. Pleural complications in the intensive care unit. Clin Chest Med 1999; 20:317–327.

50. Bouros D, Antoniou KM, Chalkiadakis G, et al. The role of video-assisted thoracoscopic surgery in the treatment of parapneumonic empyema after the failure of fibrinolytics. Surg Endosc 2002; 16151–16154.

51. Luh SP, Chou MC, Wang LS, et al. Video-assisted thoracoscopic surgery in the treatment of complicated parapneumonic effusions or empyemas: Outcome of 234 patients. Chest 2005; 127:1427–1432.

52. Bouros D, Schiza S, Patsourakis G, et al. Intrapleural streptokinase versus urokinase in the treatment of complicated parapneumonic effusions: A prospective, double-blind study. Am J Respir Crit Care Med 1997; 155:291–295.

53. Bouros D, Schiza S, Tzanakis N, et al. Intrapleural urokinase versus normal saline in the treatment of complicated parapneumonic effusions and empyema: A randomized, double-blind study. Am J Respir Crit Care Med 1999; 159:37–42.

54. Diacon AH, Theron J, Schuurmans MM, et al. Intrapleural streptokinase for empyema and complicated parapneumonic effusions. Am J Respir Crit Care Med 2004; 170:49–53.

55. Maskell NA, Davies CWH, Nunn AJ, et al. U.K. controlled trial of intrapleural streptokinase for pleural infection. N Engl J Med 2005; 352:865–874.

56. Heffner JE. Multicenter trials of treatment for empyema—After all these years. N Engl J Med 2005; 352:926–928.

57. Yeam I, Sassoon C. Hemotorax and chylothorax. Curr Opin Pulm Med 1997; 3:310–314.

58. Ambrogi MC, Lucchi M, Dini P, et al. Videothoracoscopy for evaluation and treatment of hemothorax. J Cardiovasc Surg (Torino) 2002; 43(1):109–112.

59. Morales Uribe CH, Villegas Lanau MI, Petro Sánchez RD. Best timing for thoracoscopic evacuation of retained post-traumatic hemothorax. Surg Endosc 2008; 22(1):91–95.

60. Hsu WH, Chiang CD, Hsu JY, et al. Ultrasound guided fine-needle aspiration biopsy of lung cancer. J Clin Ultrasound 1996; 24:225–233.

61. Mrug M, Mishra PV, Lusane HC, et al. Hemothorax and retroperitoneal hematoma after anticoagulation with enoxaparin. South Med J 2002; 95(8):936–938.

62. Nair SK, Petko M, Hayward MP. Aetiology and management of chylothorax in adults. Eur J Cardiothorac Surg 2007; 32(2):362–369.

63. Merrigan B, Winter D, O'Sullivan G. Chylothorax. Br J Surg 1997; 84:15–20.

64. Janssen J, Joosten J, Postmus P. Thoracoscopic treatment of postoperative chylothorax after coronary artery bypass surgery. Thorax 1994; 49:12.

65. Heffner JE, Highland K, Brown LK. A meta-analysis derivation of continuous likelihood ratios for diagnosing pleural fluid exudates. Am J Respir Crit Care Med 2003; 167(12):1591–1599.

37
Pleural Effusions in Gastrointestinal Tract Diseases

EPAMINONDAS N. KOSMAS
3rd Department of Pulmonary Medicine, Chest Diseases Hospital "Sotiria",
Voula, Athens, Greece

VLASIS S. POLYCHRONOPOULOS
3rd Chest Department, Sismanogleion General Hospital, Athens, Greece

I. General Considerations

Diseases of the gastrointestinal (GI) tract are sometimes associated with pleural effusion causing either transudative or exudative pleural effusions. Transudative pleural effusions occur when the systemic factors influencing the formation and absorption of pleural fluid are altered so that pleural fluid accumulates. In the majority of the cases, the transudative pleural effusion is related causally to cirrhosis and ascites. Exudative pleural effusions related to GI diseases, are usually secondary to acute or chronic diseases and conditions affecting pancreas, liver and biliary tract, esophagus, hernias or they represent a complication of abdominal surgery. A particular category of exudative pleural effusions is the metastatic invasion of the pleura by abdominal neoplasms. Table 1 shows GI diseases associated with transudative, exudative, and malignant pleural effusions.

Since the etiology of pleural effusion is very often a challenge to diagnose, the clinician must always have in mind the possibility of an underlying abdominal disease in any pleural effusion of undetermined origin.

II. Transudative Pleural Effusion

A. Hepatic Hydrothorax

A transudative pleural effusion may occur occasionally as a complication of hepatic cirrhosis and, in this case, it is called hepatic hydrothorax. Pleural effusions secondary to hepatic cirrhosis are rare (5–6%) and usually occur when ascitic fluid is present (1). Several studies with large series of cirrhotic patients have confirmed the coexistence of ascitic and pleural fluid (2,3). In a proportion of patients, the ascites is not clinically evident, however, the presence of ascitic fluid can almost always be detected with ultrasonography (4).

Pleural effusion in patients with cirrhosis and ascites are usually right-sided (67%), but may also be left-sided (16%) or bilateral (16%) (1–3).

Pathogenesis and Pathophysiology

Patients with advanced cirrhosis and portal hypertension often show an abnormal extracellular fluid volume regulation, which results in the accumulation of fluid, as ascites, pleural

Table 1 Gastrointestinal Tract Diseases Associated
with Pleural Effusions

Transudative
  Hepatic hydrothorax (cirrhosis, ascites)
  Hepatic chylothorax
  Retroperitoneal fibrosis
Exudative
  Acute pancreatitis
  Pancreatic abscess
  Pancreatic pseudocyst (chronic pancreatic effusion)
  Pancreatic ascites
  Subphrenic abscess
  Intrahepatic abscess
  Parasitic liver abscess (amebiasis, echinococcosis)
  Intrasplenic abscess
  Esophageal rupture
  Diaphragmatic hernia
  Biliary tract disorders
  After abdominal surgery
  After endoscopic variceal sclerotherapy
  After liver transplantation
Malignant
  Stomach
  Colon
  Pancreas
  Liver
  Cholangiocarcinoma

---

effusion or edema. This abnormality in volume regulation is associated with significant changes in the splachnic and renal circulation that induce sodium and water retention (5). Plasma oncotic pressure is low in patients with cirrhosis, mainly due to hypoalbuminemia, and one might hypothesize that this is the principal pathophysiologic mechanism of pleural fluid accumulation. It has been reported that in experimental animals the induction of decreased plasma oncotic pressure results to the accumulation of pleural fluid. However, this mechanism is not considered anymore as the predominant cause of pleural effusion in cirrhotic patients with ascites. The accumulation of fluid into the pleural space appears to be caused by transfer of the ascitic fluid from the peritoneal cavity to the pleural cavity.

It is a subject for discussion whether this transfer of fluid from the peritoneal to the pleural cavity is either direct through diaphragmatic pores/defects or a transfer through the diaphragmatic lymphatic system. Johnston and Loo (2) have shown that after the intraperitoneal injection of India ink, cells in the pleural fluid contained many carbon particles, whereas carbon particles were not detected in peripheral blood cells. Furthermore, when they injected intravenously radiolabeled albumin, they first detected albumin in the ascitic fluid, and then in the pleural fluid. When they injected the labeled protein intraperitoneally, the concentration of protein was greater in the pleural fluid than that in the plasma; when the same material was injected intrapleurally, the radiolabeled albumin was detected in plasma before it appeared in ascitic fluid. The authors concluded that the pleural effusion in cirrhotic patients with ascites originates from the passage of ascitic fluid from the peritoneal to the pleural cavity through the lymphatic vessels of the diaphragm. However, this conclusion seems to be wrong, since, two decades later, Datta et al. (6) reported completely different findings. They observed that when labeled human protein was injected intraperitoneally in patients with ascites and pleural effusion, the protein was picked up by the lymphatic system in the diaphragm, and then it moved across the mediastinal lymphatic channels towards the subclavian vein and therefore protein did not enter the pleural cavity.

On the other hand, when Lieberman et al. (3) induced pneumoperitoneum by introducing 0.5 to 1.0 L of air into the peritoneal cavity of five patients with cirrhosis, ascites, and pleural effusion, they observed in all patients, the development of hydropneumothorax during the first 48 hours after the introduction of air. Moreover, when they performed thoracoscopy in their patients, they saw air bubbles coming through diaphragm, probably through, otherwise undetected, diaphragmatic defects. At postmortem examination, diaphragmatic defects were demonstrated in two of their patients. Later, Mouroux et al. (7) visualized the diaphragmatic defects in the diaphragm during thoracoscopy. Hence, these investigators, along with the data studied, disputed the diaphragmatic lymphatic system to be the channel through which fluid passes from the peritoneal to the pleural cavity. In a recent study, Huang et al. (8) studied 11 patients with hepatic hydrothorax via thoracoscopy. They classified their morphologic findings into four types: type I, no obvious defect (1 patient); type II, blebs lying on the diaphragm (4 patients); type III, diaphragmatic fenestrations (8 patients); and type IV, multiple diaphragmatic gaps (1 patient). All these data support the hypothesis that the pleural effusion arises from the passive movement of fluid from peritoneal to pleural space through defects or pores in the diaphragm. The role of these defects in the pathogenesis of hepatic hydrothorax provides a satisfactory explanation to why hydrothorax is much more common on the right side than on the left side. It is thought that cirrhosis-related pleural transudate is more common on the right hemithorax because the right hemidiaphragm is more likely to have embryologic developmental defects (9). Recent scintigraphic studies (10–13) with intraperitoneal injection of technetium-99m (Tc-99m) sulfur colloid have verified the above theory by providing evidence of a one-way flow of fluid from the peritoneal to pleural cavity, even in the rare cases of hepatic hydrothorax without ascitic fluid (14–16).

The pathophysiologic basis of this theory relies on the increased intra-abdominal pressure caused by the presence of ascitic fluid. The increased intra-abdominal pressure poses a stretch pressure on the diaphragm, thus causing microscopic defects or magnifying preexisting defects. In addition, the increased intra-abdominal pressure acts as the driving pressure, which leads to the one-way transfer of fluid from the peritoneal to the pleural cavity through these diaphragmatic defects. The possibility that in some patients the transfer of ascitic fluid across the diaphragm by the lymphatic vessels may be important in the production of pleural fluid cannot be excluded. However, the dominant mechanism is the direct movement of the fluid through diaphragmatic defects or pores (1). Another observation supporting this mechanism is that when chest tubes were placed in order to relieve dyspnea from large pleural effusions, the amount of ascitic fluid was rapidly decreased (within minutes).

Clinical Manifestations

The clinical picture of patients with hepatic hydrothorax is the one of the cirrhotic patient with ascites. In case of a large effusion, the patient may be dyspneic. It has to be noted that the amount of pleural fluid is usually large and may occupy the entire hemithorax, and this is probably because the transfer of the fluid from the abdomen to the pleural space is continued, until the equilibration of both pressures, pleural and peritoneal. Light et al. have measured the pleural pressures in patients with pleural effusions secondary to ascites, and they found them to be higher than in patients with transudative pleural effusions of other etiology (17). As noted above, hepatic hydrothorax is much more common on the right side and only rare cases may be on the left side or bilateral.

Diagnosis

The diagnosis of hepatic hydrothorax is usually easy and is based on thoracocentesis and abdominal paracentesis. Both fluids are transudates and although the pleural fluid protein tends to be higher than the ascitic fluid protein level, it is still below 3.0 g/dL, pleural fluid lactate dehydrogenase (LDH) is also low. Occasionally, the fluid is bloodtinged or even bloody and such a finding is not excluding the diagnosis since the patient may have a poor coagulation profile due to cirrhosis. The differential cell count may be variable with predominance of either polymorphonuclear cells or lymphocytes.

In one series of 60 patients with cirrhosis and pleural effusion (18), a diagnosis other than hepatic hydrothorax was established in 30% of patients and this alternate diagnosis was much more common when the effusion was left-sided or when there was no ascites. Alternative diagnoses included spontaneous bacterial pleuritis, tuberculosis, adenocarcinoma, parapneumonic effusion, and undiagnosed exudates. Pleural effusion related to pancreatic ascites will be excluded by the measurement of amylase levels, while cytologic examination of both fluids should be always performed in order to rule out malignant disease.

As mentioned above, when hepatic hydrothorax is suspected in a patient with a large pleural effusion and cirrhosis but without clinically evident ascites, an abdominal ultrasonography should be performed in order to reveal the presence of ascitic fluid (4). Intraperitoneal spraying of indocyanine green or intraperitoneal injection of Tc-99m and subsequent radionuclide scintigraphy of peritoneal and pleural cavities may facilitate diagnosis in cases of a nondiagnostic ultrasonography and may help with respect to treatment decision (14–16).

In patients with cirrhosis, ascites, and pleural effusion, it is important to be aware of the possibility of pleural infection, which is analogous to bacterial peritonitis that may complicate the clinical course in these patients. Xiol et al. (19) reported on 24 episodes of spontaneous bacterial empyema in 16 (13%) out of 120 patients admitted with a diagnosis of hepatic hydrothorax. In 14 of the 24 cases of bacterial pleuritis, there was a concomitant spontaneous bacterial peritonitis. The term bacterial pleuritis is preferable than the term bacterial empyema, since in most of the cases the pleural fluid was not frank pus. Patients with spontaneous bacterial pleuritis tend to have worse liver disease. Diagnosis of bacterial pleuritis in a patient with cirrhosis and ascites is established when pneumonia is excluded, when there is a positive culture of the pleural fluid along with a neutrophil count >250 cells/mm^3, or even a negative culture along with a neutrophil count >500 cells/mm^3. Pathogenic agents usually include *Escherichia coli*, *Enterococcus* species, *Streptococcus* species, and *Streptococcus pneumoniae* (19). The treatment of bacterial pleuritis is an appropriate antibiotic according to bacterial susceptibility; placement of chest tubes is not indicated.

Treatment

The treatment of hepatic hydrothorax should be directed toward the therapeutic measures for the ascites, since hydrothorax originates from the transfer of ascitic fluid into the pleural cavity. The patient should be started on a low-salt diet and should be given diuretics, with the more appropriate combination being furosemide (40–160 mg daily) and spironolactone (100–400 mg daily) (20). Therapeutic thoracocenteses are of temporary benefit since the pleural fluid usually re-accumulates rapidly.

Although the majority of patients respond well to salt restriction and the administration of diuretics, some patients remain dyspneic due to the persistence of large pleural effusion and ascites. In these patients, liver transplantation or alternatively implantation of a transjugular intrahepatic portal systemic shunt (TIPS) should be considered. Many recent studies (10,21–25) addressed the issue of the beneficial effects of TIPS in patients with refractory hepatic hydrothorax. All studies proved the effectiveness and safety of the procedure, documenting a significant advantage with respect to treatment and survival rates in those patients assigned to TIPS as compared to those assigned to serial thoracocenteses.

Another alternative treatment option is videothoracoscopy with an attempt to close the diaphragmatic defects and to perform pleurodesis. Aerosolized talc pleurodesis at the time of thoracoscopy has been proven effective in controlling recurrence of the pleural effusion (26). Mouroux et al. (27) reported their results in 8 patients; diaphragmatic defects were found and closed in 6 out of the 8 patients, while talc pleurodesis was performed in all patients. In all patients, the combination was proved effective. In a more recent study (28) of 18 patients who were subjected to thoracoscopy combined with talc insufflation, the results are not so encouraging in comparison with the results of the Mouroux study. In a minority of patients (28%), the diaphragmatic defects were detected and closed while the whole procedure was successful only in 48% of patients. However, videothoracoscopy remains an acceptable alternative method when neither liver transplantation nor TIPS are available or feasible. It has to be mentioned herein that using talc for pleurodesis has been associated recently with the development of acute respiratory distress in approximately 5% of patients with a mortality rate of about 1%.

A successful surgical repair of hepatic hydrothorax in the absence of ascites has been reported recently (29). The method consists of induction of pneumoperitoneum in order to identify possible defects in the diaphragm and of direct suture of the defect.

B.   Pleural Effusion as a Complication of Percutaneous Transhepatic Coronary Vein Occlusion

Patients with bleeding esophageal varices are sometimes managed by injecting Gelfoam or other materials transhepatically into the coronary vein in an attempt for the injected material to lodge in the esophageal veins and stop the bleeding (30). It has been noticed that, sometimes, pleural fluid rapidly accumulates after this procedure in patients with ascites. According to Light (1), the pleural effusion arises from the iatrogenic diaphragmatic defect, which allows the ascitic fluid to flow into the pleural space. Pleural effusions may also appear by the same mechanism after percutaneous transhepatic cholangiography.

C. Cirrhotic Chylothorax

Chylothorax is a rare and apparently underestimated manifestation of cirrhosis, resulting from transdiaphragmatic passage of chylous ascites. In one series of 809 patients, 24 patients had pleural effusions being chylothoraces. Five of these patients (20%) were found to have liver cirrhosis (31).

Cirrhotic chylous effusions were transudates with distinct biochemical fluid characteristics (significantly lower protein, LDH, and cholesterol levels as compared to chylous effusions resulting from other causes).

D. Retroperitoneal Fibrosis

Reports from Japan have identified cases of retroperitoneal fibrosis associated with transudative pleural effusions (32,33). Retroperitoneal fibrosis is considered to be an extremely rare cause of pleural effusion, and the possible pathophysiologic mechanism appears to be the extrahepatic portal vein obstruction.

III. Exudative Pleural Effusion

As mentioned above, exudative pleural effusions may arise as a manifestation during the clinical course of various GI diseases, acute or chronic, affecting pancreas, liver, biliary tract, esophagus, hernias, intra-abdominal abscesses or as a complication of various surgical and other invasive procedures (Table 1).

A. Pancreatic Diseases

Four different nonmalignant pancreatic diseases are associated with an exudative pleural effusion: acute pancreatitis, pancreatic abscess, chronic pancreatitis with pseudocyst, and pancreatic ascites.

Acute Pancreatitis

In older times, it was thought that the incidence of pleural effusion with acute pancreatitis was low, ranging from 3% to 17%. The introduction of computed tomography (CT scan) in everyday clinical practice revealed that many cases of acute pancreatitis may be associated with the presence of a pleural effusion, with usually minimal findings on chest X-ray, given that the amount of pleural fluid is usually small. Lankisch et al., in a series of 133 consecutive patients admitted in hospital due to acute pancreatitis, reported that about 50% of them had a pleural effusion on CT scan during the first three days from admission (34). The effusion is usually bilateral (77%), while occasionally it is left-sided (16%) or right-sided (8%). In the vast majority of the patients, pleural cavity contains a small amount of fluid. In one report from Italy in which 539 patients where included (35), pleural effusion was present in 77 (14%) patients had a pleural effusion (44% bilateral, 32% left-sided, and 24% right-sided). Maringhini et al. (36) have also reported a 20% incidence of pleural effusion among patients with acute pancreatitis.

The presence of pleural effusion, in patients with acute pancreatitis, has been correlated with a more severe clinical course and poor outcome of the pancreatic disease. Heller et al. (37) studied 116 patients with mild pancreatitis and 19 patients with severe pancreatitis. The incidence of pleural effusion was much higher in the group of severe pancreatitis compared to that in the group of patients with mild pancreatitis

(84% vs. 8.6%, respectively). Similarly, Talamini et al. (35) studied 539 patients and found that the presence of a pleural effusion, along with serum creatinine, within the first 24 hours from admission, were correlated with mortality risk, with a diagnosis of necrotizing pancreatitis and with risk of developing infected necrosis. In another series of 100 patients (36), it has been documented that the presence of ascitic and pleural fluids was accurate independent predictors of severity in acute pancreatitis.

The pathophysiologic mechanism of exudative pleural effusion during the clinical course of acute pancreatitis seems to be the transdiaphragmatic transfer, via the diaphragmatic lymphatic vessels, of the exudative fluid produced from the acute inflammation of both pancreas and diaphragm (38). This pancreatic exudate enters the lymphatic vessels on the peritoneal side of the diaphragm toward the pleural side of the diaphragm. The increased content of the fluid in pancreatic enzymes contributes to the formation of pleural effusion by increasing the permeability of lymphatic vessels resulting in the leakage of the fluid into the pleural cavity, and by obstructing the pleural lymphatics and decreasing the pleural lymphatic flow (39). It has to be mentioned that the diaphragm itself may be inflamed from the adjacent acute pancreatic inflammation and this is because of the proximity between pancreas tail and the diaphragm.

The clinical presentation of patients with acute pancreatitis and pleural effusion is usually dominated by the abdominal symptoms, including pain, nausea, and vomiting. Occasionally, patients report symptoms indicative of respiratory disease, such as pleuritic chest pain and/or dyspnea. The chest radiography may reveal a small or moderate pleural effusion, elevation of the diaphragm and, sometimes basilar infiltrates (30). In addition, on ultrasound or fluoroscopy, the diaphragm is sluggish or even immobile.

Differential diagnosis consists of pneumonia or pulmonary embolism, complicated by pleural effusion. The diagnosis is usually established by demonstrating a high serum amylase or lipase level in a patient with abdominal pain, nausea, or vomiting. When the diagnosis of acute pancreatitis is confirmed and the pleural effusion is asymptomatic and of small or moderate size, thoracocentesis should not be performed. Thoracocentesis, diagnostic or therapeutic, should be restricted only for patient's relief from dyspnea due to a large effusion and in order to rule out empyema in a persistently febrile patient.

Pleural fluid is an exudate, with high protein and LDH levels, and occasionally is serosanguineous or even bloody. Glucose level is similar to that of the blood and polymorphonuclear leukocytes predominate with respect to the differential white blood cell (WBC) count. The fluid WBC usually vary from 1000 to 50,000 cells/mm^3. Pleural fluid amylase in patients with acute pancreatitis and pleural effusion is usually higher than serum amylase and remains elevated for a longer period in comparison with the serum amylase (30,39,40). The pleural fluid amylase level in patients with acute pancreatitis tends to be lower than that in patients with chronic pancreatic disease. Fluid levels of phospholipase A2 are also high in patients with acute pancreatitis (41), while the fluid levels of trypsinogen-activation peptide are low (42).

In the vast majority of patients with acute pancreatitis and a small- or moderate-size effusion, there is not any indication for any additional treatment beyond the treatment of acute pancreatitis. Therapeutic thoracocentesis and pleural fluid drainage are indicated only for relief in large effusions causing dyspnea or for empyema drainage due to superinfection. The pleural effusion usually resolves spontaneously as the acute pancreatitis subsides. In case of nonresolving effusion within two to three weeks, one must consider the possibility of a pancreatic abscess or pseudocyst (30). A beneficial effect of oral administration of high-dose octreotide has been reported (43).

Pancreatic Abscess

Pancreatic abscess usually follows an episode of acute pancreatitis. In most of the cases, acute pancreatitis responds to therapy within 10 to 14 days. When the clinical course of acute pancreatitis is not favorable and 10 to 21 days after the initiation of medical treatment although an with an initial response was observed, and the patient becomes febrile with recurrence of abdominal pain and peripheral blood leukocytosis, the formation of a pancreatic abscess must be suspected (44). Pancreatic abscess must be suspected also if the patient is diagnosed as pancreatitis, but he doesn't improve, even if he is on the appropriate treatment. Whenever there is a suspicion of a pancreatic abscess development, abdominal ultrasonography and CT scanning must be performed without any delay. It is very important to mention that the mortality rate in not-drained pancreatic abscesses is very high ($\approx$100%); therefore, the need of immediate diagnostic confirmation and surgical drainage is essential and urgent (39,44).

Pleural effusion is a frequent finding in patients with pancreatic abscess. Miller et al. (44), in their series of 63 patients with pancreatic abscess, have reported an incidence rate of 38% with respect to the presence of a pleural effusion. Pleural fluid amylase level is high, however, there is lack of data concerning pleural fluid characteristics in patients with pancreatic abscess (30).

Pancreatic Pseudocyst and Chronic Pancreatic Pleural Effusion

A pancreatic pseudocyst (a term implying that this is not a cyst with true walls) represents a collection of fluid and debris with a high content in pancreatic enzymes, which is usually situated near or within the pancreas. The walls consist of granulation tissue without an epithelial lining (30). Approximately 10% of patients with acute pancreatitis have a clinically significant pseudocyst. Pancreatic pseudocysts rarely (5%) are followed with a pleural effusion (45). According to Rockey and Cello in their review on pancreatic pseudocysts (45), pleural effusions are relatively uncommon.

The primary mechanism for the development of pleural effusion in patients with a chronic pseudocyst is the formation of a pancreatic-pleural fistula between the pancreas and the pleural space (30,45). Once fluid enters the pleural cavity, the pancreatic-pleural fistula is likely to result in a massive effusion. A secondary mechanism is the passage of the pseudocyst fluid into the mediastinum through the esophageal or aortic hiatus. This passage may result either to the formation of a mediastinal pseudocyst or to the decompression into one or both pleural spaces (30,46–49) or to an enzymic mediastinitis (50). An extremely rare complication of a pancreatic pseudocyst is the formation of a pancreatic-bronchial fistula (51).

Most patients with chronic pancreatic pleural effusion are men. In about 90% of male patients, the pancreatic disease is a result of alcoholism. General symptoms, such as malaise, fatigue, and weight loss, and respiratory symptoms, such as chest pain and dyspnea, usually dominate the clinical picture in these patients (45,50,52). Uchiyama et al. (52), in one series of 113 patients, reported that the main complaints were dyspnea (42%) and chest pain (29%), while the frequency of upper abdominal pain was impressively low (23%) for a disease affecting the upper abdomen. The lack of abdominal symptoms may be attributed to the fact that the pancreatic-pleural fistula decompresses the pseudocyst.

The effusion, as mentioned above, is usually large or even massive, occupying the entire hemithorax. It is usually affecting the left hemithorax, but occasionally is right-sided (20%) or bilateral (15%) (45,52). It is important to notice that the diagnosis of chronic pancreatic pleural effusion is frequently missed, because of the lack of typical abdominal symptoms and the absence of prior pancreatic disease.

The diagnosis should be suspected in any case of a patient who looks chronically ill and who has a large or even massive pleural effusion, particularly left-sided. A good proportion of the patients have a history of prior pancreatic disease or abdominal trauma (30). However, many patients have no such history. The more useful laboratory test for establishing the diagnosis is the measurement of pleural fluid amylase. Pleural fluid amylase levels are markedly elevated (usually >1000 U/L), whereas the serum amylase may be normal or mildly elevated (30). It has to be mentioned here that the specificity of high amylase in pleural fluid is not 100%, therefore, one must think of the other causes of high amylase levels in the fluid, such as malignant pleural effusions or esophageal diseases (40,53). Measurement of amylase isoenzymes on pleural fluid appears to be helpful in the differential diagnosis between malignant and pancreatic effusion, because with malignant effusions, the amylase is of the salivary type than of the pancreatic type (54). Peripheral blood eosinophilia (>500 cells/mm^3) was found in 21 (17%) patients in one series of 122 cases with chronic pancreatitis (55). Eosinophilia frequently developed in association with severe damage to neighboring organs (pleural effusion, pericarditis, ascites), as well as in association with pancreatic pseudocyst (55).

CT scanning of the chest and abdomen usually establishes the diagnosis, revealing both the pancreatic pseudocyst and the pancreatic-pleural fistula (30,49–51,56). Endoscopic retrograde cholangiopancreatography (ERCP) plays an important role in the evaluation and management of patients with that kind of fistula. The greatest utility for ERCP is to define preoperatively the precise anatomic relationship between the fistula and the adjacent structures, such as the pancreas, the diaphragm, and the pleura (30,49–51,56).

The initial treatment of patients with a pancreatic pseudocyst and a pleural effusion is usually nonsurgical. It has to be noted that therapeutic thoracocentesis is not helpful since the fluid has the tendency to re-accumulate rapidly (52). The concept of the conservative treatment is to reduce pancreatic secretions in order to achieve regression of the pseudocyst and functional closure of the fistula (57). The insertion of a nasogastric tube is required in all patients and intravenous hyperalimentation is given. The administration of somatostatin or octreotide, a synthetic analogue of somatostatin, has shown benefit in some patients (58,59). It is known that somatostatin exerts an inhibitory action on pancreatic exocrine secretion (45). It has been shown that somatostatin decreases the output from an external pancreatic fistula by more than 80% (30). Some authors recommend serial thoracocenteses and subsequent tube thoracostomy if the effusion recurs, but there is no evidence that such procedure is beneficial (30). If the above conservative treatment fails, the treatment of choice is surgical.

Surgical intervention should be considered whenever the patient remains symptomatic and the pleural effusion persists or continues to accumulate, after two weeks of treatment. Approximately 50% of patients, and particularly those with more severe pancreatic disease, require surgery (30). The preoperative assessment consists of ERCP and abdominal CT scan, which are helpful in planning the appropriate surgical procedure. Recently, some patients have been successfully treated by placing stents in the pancreatic duct at the time the ERCP is performed (60,61). Depending on the location of the pseudocyst within pancreas and of the duct with the leak, different procedures are available, such as distal pancreatectomy, direct anastomosis between the leak and a jejunal loop or internal drainage of the cyst into the stomach or into a jejunal loop (30,62–64). In an attempt to avoid the surgical procedure, some investigators have tried to drain the pseudocyst percutaneously under CT guidance (65,66). A catheter is inserted through the anterior abdominal wall and the stomach towards the pseudocyst cavity and it accomplishes drainage from the cyst into the stomach. Maintenance of this drainage for 15 to 20 days is thought to create a fistulous tract between the pseudocyst and the stomach. Lang et al. have reported a success rate of 77% in their series of 26 patients (66). However, there are not many available data in the literature regarding the percutaneous drainage. In addition, Brelvi et al. (67) introduced nasopancreatic drainage, a novel approach for treating internal pancreatic fistulas and pseudocysts. It seems that this method did not gain popularity as of yet.

The prognosis of these patients is usually favorable. The mortality rate in a series of 96 patients was approximately 5% (44). Patients who died as a direct result of the pancreatic disease were managed conservatively and died of sepsis. In patients with chronic pleural effusions secondary to pancreatic pseudocystic disease, pleural thickening is a probable complication and decortication may be needed. Sometimes, the pleural thickening resolves gradually over months and a watchful waiting is necessary prior to decide a decortication. Clinicians must be aware of unusual manifestations of pancreatic pseudocysts, such as mediastinal extension of the pseudocyst, obstructive jaundice, intraperitoneal rupture, pancreatic ascites, pancreaticobronchial fistula, and massive hemorrhage due to the development of a false aneurysm in a branch of the celiac axis in the wall of the pseudocyst, as they require different surgical management (64). One very uncommon complication of pancreatic pleural effusion is the development of a bronchopleural fistula. In this situation, chest tube should be inserted immediately to drain the pleural space and to protect the lung from the fluid, which has a high enzymatic content (39).

Pancreatic Ascites

Development of pancreatic ascites is attributed to leakage of fluid from a pseudocyst directly into the peritoneal cavity via an internal pancreatic fistula, and is characterized by high amylase and protein levels (68). Some of these patients happen to have a defect in their diaphragm and they subsequently develop large pleural effusion, as a result of the flow of fluid from the peritoneal cavity in the same way that pleural effusion develops secondary to cirrhotic ascites. Approximately 20% of patients with pancreatic ascites have a pleural effusion (68). Over one-half of the patients had no history of inflammatory pancreatic disease (69). However, a history of chronic alcoholism is associated with the syndrome of pancreatic ascites (70,71). Most patients with pancreatic ascites and pleural effusion are initially thought to have cirrhotic ascites. The diagnosis is easily established if amylase levels are measured in both peritoneal and pleural fluids.

Common symptoms of this syndrome are intermittent abdominal pain, nausea, vomiting, and considerable weight loss, which occurs despite fluid retention (70). Patients complain of dyspnea whenever the pleural effusion is large. The diagnosis of pancreatic ascites is made if amylase and protein levels of the peritoneal and pleural fluid are high (68,69). Serum amylase is usually, but not always, elevated (69). Hypoalbuminemia is common as well (70). The internal pancreatic fistula is successfully demonstrated in most instances by ERCP (69).

The treatment of pancreatic ascites is the same as for pancreatic pseudocyst and chronic pancreatic pleural effusion, except serial abdominal paracenteses rather than serial therapeutic thoracocenteses are performed. Initial treatment is nonoperative (nasogastric suction, hyperalimentation, administration of somatostatin or octreotide), with a success rate of 32% to 48% (69,71–73). In an attempt to determine risk factors for failure of conservative treatment, Parekh and Segal studied 23 patients with pancreatic ascites or effusion (72). They observed that serum sodium and albumin levels were significantly lower and the ratio of fluid total protein-to-serum total protein was significantly higher in the group that failed to heal in response to conventional medical therapy. In addition, they found that the patients with severe pancreatitis did not respond to the nonsurgical treatment, implying that patients with advanced pancreatic disease should be selected for early surgery (72).

When nonoperative medical therapy fails, then surgery is performed to drain or to resect the internal fistula (73), with an overall success rate of 82% (69). In a series of 49 patients (73), conservative treatment was successful in 18 patients, while the remaining 31 patients were assigned to surgical treatment. The different surgical procedures were the internal pancreatic drainage, the external pancreatic drainage, and the distal pancreatectomy with fistula resection. It seems that internal pancreatic drainage was the ideal surgical treatment for patients with pancreatic ascites and/or pleural effusion that did not respond to medical treatment (73). An alternative choice is the endoscopic placement of a stent across the pancreatic duct disruption (74).

B. Subphrenic Abscess

Subphrenic abscess continues to be a significant clinical problem despite the development of potent antibiotics. Approximately 80% of subphrenic abscesses result from abdominal surgical procedures, such as splenectomy, gastrectomy, exploratory laparotomy, laparoscopic cholecystectomy, etc. (75–77). Splenectomy, as gastrectomy, is likely to be complicated by a left subphrenic abscess. On the other hand, only 1% of intra-abdominal operations are complicated by a subphrenic abscess. Sanders states that in a total of 1566 operations, only 15 patients presented a postoperative subphrenic abscess (76). The time interval between the surgical procedure and the development of a subphrenic abscess usually lies to one to three weeks but can be as long as five to six months. Rarely, a subphrenic abscess may develop without any surgical procedure in the abdomen, as a result of gastric, appendiceal or duodenal perforation, diverticulitis, cholecystitis, pancreatitis or trauma (78). In such patients, the diagnosis may be easily missed because of the atypical clinical picture. In a series of 22 patients with antecedent abdominal operations, the diagnosis was established before the patient's death in only 41% (78).

Subphrenic abscesses are discussed in this chapter because a pleural effusion is a common manifestation, occurring in about 60% to 80% of patients with a subphrenic abscess, and is usually small to moderate in size, although sometimes may be large enough to occupy a large part of the hemithorax (76,78,79).

Carter and Brewer proposed as possible pathogenetic mechanism the transfer of abscess material from the subphrenic-inflamed location into the pleural cavity via the diaphragmatic lymphatics (79). However, there is doubt on that theory, as culture of pleural fluid is rarely positive. There is a general belief that the pathogenesis of the subphrenic abscess–induced pleural effusion is probably related to the inflammation of the diaphragm. This inflammation probably increases the permeability of the capillaries in the diaphragmatic pleura and causes the accumulation of pleural fluid (30).

The clinical symptoms and signs of patients with subphrenic abscess and pleural effusion are due to the abdominal and chest disease. As reported in one series of 125 cases, 44% of patients had exclusively chest findings, with the pleuritic chest pain being the dominant symptom (79). Patients may have no abdominal symptoms at the time of presentation. The majority of patients with a postoperative subphrenic abscess have fever, leukocytosis, and abdominal pain or tenderness (78,79), however, not all the patients have characteristic symptoms or localizing signs (30).

The diagnosis of subphrenic abscess should be considered whenever the patient develops a pleural effusion several days or weeks after an abdominal operation or when the patient has an exudative polymorphonuclear effusion of otherwise undetermined cause. Examination of the pleural fluid usually reveals a polymorphonuclear type of exudate. The WBC count of the fluid may approach 30,000 to 50,000 cells/mm^3, but the pH and glucose level remain above 7.20 and 60 mg/dL respectively, and is very uncommon for the pleural fluid to be infected (30). However, there are occasional case reports of empyema formation (77).

Radiographic examination usually reveals the presence of the pleural fluid, and additional radiographic findings include basal pneumonitis, compression atelectasis or elevation of the diaphragm on the affected side. The pathognomonic finding is an air-fluid level below the diaphragm outside the GI tract. The patient must be in upright or lateral decubitus position for the best demonstration (75). Sometimes a displacement of intra-abdominal viscera can be noticed on radiographs. Contrast studies including barium enema are sometimes helpful in demonstrating the extraluminal location of gas leakage or displacement of normal structures. Abdominal CT scan is the best imaging procedure to establish the diagnosis (80). CT scan is more sensitive and has the advantage over other methods (gallium scanning, ultrasonography) of detecting the precise anatomical location and magnitude of the abscess, while ultrasonic examination is technically difficult in the left upper abdominal quadrant because of overlying lung, ribs, and gas in the GI tract. Gallium scans are not always positive when subphrenic abscesses are present with a 36% rate of false-negative findings.

Optimal treatment consists of the administration of broad-spectrum antibiotics and also cover for anaerobic organisms and drainage, either percutaneously under CT guidance or surgically. Because the results with the two procedures seem comparable, it is recommended that percutaneous drainage could be used in most cases, although posterior subphrenic abscesses are best approached surgically. The catheter should be inserted under CT guidance and should be maintained in place for a mean of six days.

Sepsis is the commonest and life-threatening complication of subphrenic abscess. In a series of 125 patients with a subphrenic abscess (79), 23% of the patients had positive blood cultures and in those patients the mortality rate was impressively high, approaching 93%. However, even in nonseptic abscesses, the mortality rate is still high, ranging from 20% to 45% (75,78,79). This unfavorable prognosis is mainly due to delayed diagnosis or even lack of a diagnosis. It is important to consider the possibility of a subphrenic abscess in every patient presenting with exudative pleural effusion containing predominantly polymorphonuclear leukocytes and particularly when this picture follows an abdominal surgical procedure.

C. Intrahepatic Abscess

About 20% of patients with a liver abscess develop pleural effusion, with the same mechanism as the subphrenic abscess (30). Half of these patients have a history of hepatolithiasis or other hepatobiliary disease, while the remaining 50% have no known disease predisposing to the development of a liver abscess (81). There are occasional reports of liver abscesses with right-sided pleural effusions manifested during the clinical course of disseminated infections from various pathogens, such as *Mycobacterium tuberculosis* (82) or *Corynebacterium afermentans lipophilum* (83).

As the mortality rate is quite high, nearly 100%, in patients with untreated intrahepatic abscesses, clinicians should be very careful when evaluating a right-sided exudative pleural effusion with predominance of polymorphonuclear leukocytes (30). In a multivariate analysis of risk factors in 73 patients with pyogenic liver abscess and overall mortality rate 19%, it was revealed that clinical jaundice, pleural effusion, bilobar abscess, profound hypoalbulinemia, hyperbilirubinemia, hypertransaminasemia, elevated serum alkaline phosphatase level and marked leukocytosis, were associated with a higher mortality rate (84).

Most of the patients with pyogenic intrahepatic abscesses have anorexia and fever accompanied by chills, while abdominal pain is common, but frequently not localized to the right upper quadrant. In the majority of cases, there is an enlargement and tenderness of the liver (81).

Laboratory tests may reveal leukocytosis, anemia, and elevated alkaline phosphatase and bilirubin levels. Because none of the above test is invariably present, the diagnosis of pyogenic liver abscess is best established by an abdominal CT scan and alternatively by an abdominal ultrasound study. Abdominal CT scanning may detect abscesses and fluid-filled intrahepatic lesions of small diameter. Because not all the fluid-filled lesions are pyogenic liver abscesses (differential diagnosis includes cysts, hematomas, hemangiomas, amebic abscesses), diagnosis can be established definitely by percutaneous aspiration under CT or ultrasound guidance, provided that ultrasound is not diagnostic.

Treatment consists of the administration of parenteral antibiotics and drainage of the abscess. CT-guided or ultrasound-guided percutaneous needle aspiration is the procedure of choice for draining the abscess (81,85,86). Persistent fever, pain, and tenderness in the right upper quadrant, and leukocytosis are indications for multiple aspirations (86). Laparotomy is indicated either when aspiration has failed or when there are signs of peritonitis and clinical deterioration (81).

D. Parasitic Liver Abscess

Amebic liver abscess is the most common extra-intestinal site of infection by *Endamoeba histolytica*. In turn, pleural-pulmonary amebiasis is the most common complication of amebic liver abscess and usually is attributed to the erosion of the abscess through the diaphragm to involve the pleural space or lung parenchyma (87,88). The mortality rate varies between 2% and 3% (89). There have been efforts to define possible prognostic factors in large series (89,90) in terms of both clinical and laboratory indices. The presence of jaundice, large or multiple abscesses, acute abdomen, liver failure, sepsis, dyspnea, drop of in hematocrit, prothrombin time, albumin, LDH, urea nitrogen, and pleural effusion has been recognized as predictors of severity (89,90).

The significance and severity of a pleural effusion in patients with amebic liver abscesses varies from the mild cases of "sympathetic" transudates to the more severe cases of amebic empyema and formation of hepatobronchial fistula. Transudative "sympathetic" pleural effusions and atelectasis are common accompaniments of liver abscesses and do not indicate extension of disease. Patients with pleural-pulmonary complications have an exudative effusion and present with cough, pleuritic pain, and dyspnea. Empyema due to rupture of the abscess into the pleural cavity presents with sudden respiratory distress, fever, and pain, and has a substantial mortality. In some instances, a hepatobronchial fistula forms and has been associated with spontaneous drainage of the hepatic abscess.

The diagnosis of amebiasis-induced pleural effusion is suggested by the discovery of "chocolate sauce" or "anchovy paste" appearance of the pleural fluid. *E. histolytica* is usually demonstrable in the pleural fluid. Abdominal ultrasonography serves as a useful diagnostic aid (91).

Treatment consists of metronidazole 750 mg per os 3 times a day for 5 to 10 days plus diloxanide furoate 500 mg 3 times a day for 10 days for intraluminal infection. Chloroquine has been used as well (91). Severe cases require, in addition to amebicidal treatment, either percutaneous aspiration or surgical drainage of pus, especially in patients with ruptured abscesses (89). Patients with abscesses that rupture into the thoracic cavity must be treated by either thoracotomy or needle aspiration (89).

The hydatid cysts of *Echinococcus granulosus* form in the liver in 50% to 70% of patients and in the lung in 20% to 30% of patients. Pleural disease develops when either a hepatic or parenchymal lung cyst ruptures into the pleural space (87). The patient develops an acute illness with severe chest pain, dyspnea, and sometimes shock, secondary to severe allergic reactions to parasitic antigens suddenly released. The diagnosis is established by recognition of daughter cysts in the pleural fluid. Optimal treatment is surgical resection to drain the pleural space and removal of the original cyst.

E. Splenic Abscess

Intrasplenic abscess is actually a very unusual clinical entity. There are approximately 20 cases, which have been reported in U.S. hospitals during the period 1950–1990. Most of them presented with an associated left-sided pleural effusion (92,93). Splenic abscess, although a rare clinical entity, may occur de novo in septic ICU patients and is associated with significant mortality. In the majority of the patients, the splenic suppurative disease is caused from primary hematogenous dissemination of infection, such as endocarditis (94). Various pathogens have been identified, such as *Candida albicans, Streptococcus viridans, E. Coli, Citrobacter freundii, Enterobacter, Staphylococcus aureus,* etc. (93,94). Particularly vulnerable population is those patients who suffer from diseases causing splenic abnormalities, such as chronic hemolytic anemia or sickle cell anemia (92). Mortality rate ranges between 40% and 50%.

Fever is usually present, accompanied by chills and vomiting (94). Left upper quadrant tenderness and leukocytosis appear in almost all patients (94). The diagnosis is not easily made since not all patients with a splenic abscess complain of a localized pain or tenderness in the left upper quadrant. The presence of a left-sided pleural effusion with thrombocytosis is a combination of findings that is suggestive of the disease (93).

Unexplained thrombocytosis in a septic patient with persistent left pleural effusion is suggestive of splenic abscess. The diagnosis can be made with an abdominal CT scan or ultrasonography and can be confirmed by fine needle aspiration (94,95).

The treatment of choice consists of splenectomy plus antibiotics (94), while catheter drainage could be considered as an alternative approach (95).

F. Esophageal Rupture

Esophageal perforation is an uncommon clinical emergency in which any delay in diagnosis and treatment may result in mortality rate becoming as high as 100% (96,97). Rupture of esophagus most commonly is a complication of esophagoscopy, particularly when there is an attempt to dilate an esophageal structure or to remove a foreign body (98). Keszler and Buzna, in a series of 108 consecutive patients with esophageal perforation, reported that 67% of the events occurred as a complication of an esophagoscopic procedure (98). However, esophageal perforation is a rare complication of esophagoscopy, as the reported incidence of perforation following an esophagoscopic examination is below 1% (96). Importantly, the endoscopist usually does not realize that the esophagus has been perforated. Less frequent, causes of an esophageal rupture include the insertion of a Blakemore tube for esophageal varices, foreign bodies, chest trauma, chest surgery, gastric intubation, and carcinomas (30,96). Finally, spontaneous rupture of the lower part of esophagus may occur as a complication of vomiting (Boerhaave's syndrome).

Mediastinum is a sterile compartment of the human body and the entrance of oropharyngeal and esophageal contents contaminates this sterile part and produces an acute mediastinitis. When the mediastinal pleura ruptures, a pleural effusion develops, frequently complicated by pneumothorax. Most of the morbidity from esophageal rupture is the result of infection of the mediastinum and pleural space by microorganisms of the oropharyngeal bacterial flora (99).

Clinical manifestations of esophageal rupture depend of the cause of perforation. As mentioned above, in cases of "iatrogenic" perforation, endoscopists usually do not realize the trauma they have caused. Such patients usually report persistent chest or epigastric pain within several hours of the procedure. Patients with spontaneous (non-iatrogenic) rupture of the esophagus, usually have a history of vomiting and chest pain, followed by a sensation of tearing or bursting in the lower part of the chest or the epigastrium. Chest pain is very strong and is often not relieved by opiates. Hematemesis is present frequently and dyspnea may be the main symptom (100). Subcutaneous emphysema is usually a late complication of esophageal rupture (100). Very rarely, the appearance of symptoms is not so dramatic as mentioned above and patients may have only mild distress.

Pleural effusion, often left-sided, is present in about 60% of patients with esophageal rupture while pneumothorax is present in about 25% of them (96). In a retrospective 15-year chart review, chest X-ray was abnormal in all patients, and revealed pleural effusion and/or pneumothorax (101). Diagnosis of esophageal rupture is necessary to be made as soon as possible, because of the high mortality rate (60%). When a patient who appears acutely ill has an exudative left-sided pleural effusion and reports a history of an endoscopic esophageal procedure or vomiting, esophageal cancer, etc., he should be very carefully evaluated for esophageal rupture. Examination of pleural fluid is very helpful because it is characterized by a high amylase level (particularly of the salivary isoenzyme), a low pH, and the presence of squamous epithelial cells and sometimes of ingested food particles.

High amylase levels appear to be the best indication of esophageal rupture (53,100). In the experimental model, the pleural fluid amylase level is elevated within two hours of esophageal rupture. The origin of the amylase is salivary rather than pancreatic because the saliva, with its high amylase content, enters the pleural space through the defect in the esophagus (102). Pleural fluid pH is usually decreased. Dye and Laforet (103) concluded that a pleural fluid pH below 6.0 is highly suggestive of esophageal rupture. Low pH was traditionally attributed to the leakage of acidic gastric content through the esophageal tear towards pleural space. Recent reports from Good et al. demonstrated that leukocyte metabolism may be the major contributing factor to the low pleural fluid pH in these patients (104), since patients with severe pleural infections and an intact esophagus frequently have a pleural pH below 6.0. Squamous epithelial cells are usually found with Wright's stain of pleural fluid of patients with esophageal perforation, since these cells enter the pleural cavity through the esophageal perforation. Eriksen documented the presence of those cells in all of 14 such patients (105). The demonstration of food in the pleural fluid is the pathognomonic finding of esophageal perforation (106). Another characteristic of the pleural fluid from patients with esophageal rupture is that smear and cultures frequently reveal multiple organisms.

Simple chest radiography may be of help, as it reveals the pleural effusion and/or the pneumothorax, and it may reveal a mediastinal widening or the presence of air (pneumomediastinum) within the mediastinal compartments. Contrast radiologic studies of the esophagus establish the diagnosis of esophageal perforation by detecting an esophageal disruption. Hexabrix, a water-soluble agent (320 mg/mL) is preferred from barium, because the latter, once it leaks into the mediastinum or pleural space, produces a marked inflammatory reaction in the pleura. Gastrographin or Hexabrix are not known to produce this reaction, but the former may cause bronchospasm (107). The contrast studies are positive in about 85% of patients but when the perforation is small or has already closed spontaneously, the esophagogram may not be diagnostic. It has been suggested that contrast studies of the esophagus could be performed in the decubitus position when perforation is suspected. A chest CT scan may facilitate the diagnosis if the contrast studies are not helpful. The morphologic alterations seen on chest CT scan that are suggestive of esophageal rupture, include the presence of extraesophageal air, periesophageal fluid, and esophageal wall thickening, while occasionally the site of perforation may be visible.

The treatment for esophageal rupture and pleural effusion or pneumothorax (or pneumomediastinum) is surgical. Mediastinotomy with repair of the esophageal perforation and drainage of the pleural cavity and mediastinum is the surgical procedure of choice. Parenteral antibiotics should be given to treat mediastinitis and pleural infection. It is important to perform the operation the soonest possible, because any delay may increase the mortality rate. If primary repair is not possible because damaged tissue cannot hold the sutures, the patient can be managed with T-tube intubation of the esophageal defect.

G. Abdominal Surgical Procedures

Small pleural effusion is a usual finding following abdominal operations, particularly of the upper abdomen. According to George and Light, about 50% of patients develop small pleural effusions within 48 to 72 hours after the surgical procedure (108). Moreover, Nielsen et al. reported a more frequent incidence (about 70%) of pleural effusion after upper abdominal surgery (109). Pleural effusions are usually related to diaphragmatic irritation or atelectasis.

Since in the majority of cases (80%) the pleural effusion is small, the fluid is detected only in the lateral decubitus position. A larger and usually left-sided effusion may follow splenectomy. Thoracocentesis is performed only when the thickness of the fluid layer is more than 10 mm on decubitus film. In about 80% of cases, the fluid is exudative and without any other characteristic finding. Other causes of postoperative pleural effusion are pulmonary embolism, respiratory infection with parapneumonic effusion, postoperative atelectasis, and subphrenic abscess. The majority of effusions occur within the first 72 hours after the abdominal surgery and resolve spontaneously.

H. Diaphragmatic Hernia

Diaphragmatic hernias can either cause or mimic a pleural effusion. When the hernia is strangulated, a pleural effusion is usually present.

Hernias through the diaphragm should be suspected whenever an apparent pleural effusion has an atypical shape or location. The presence of air in the herniated intestine is the diagnostic clue. The possibility of a strangulated diaphragmatic hernia should always be considered in patients with left pleural effusion and signs of an acute abdominal trauma. At least 90% of these hernias are traumatic and occur in the left side, because the liver protects the right hemidiaphragm (110). Strangulation may occur months or even years after a car accident, which is usually the cause of abdominal trauma.

Pleural fluid, almost always present, is a serosanguineous exudate, with predominantly polymorphonuclear leukocytes. The diagnosis is suggested by the presence of an air-fluid level in the left pleural space. Sometimes contrast imaging studies of the GI tract (i.e., barium enema) are necessary to establish the diagnosis.

The treatment is imperative and consists of immediate surgical operation to prevent gangrene of the strangulated viscera (110).

I. Variceal Sclerotherapy

Endoscopic variceal sclerotherapy is nowadays the main form of treatment for patients who present with hemorrhage from ruptured esophageal varices. The incidence of pleural effusion after the above procedure seems to depend on the sclerosant, which has been used. Saks et al. report pleural effusions in 50% of 38 such patients in which 5% sodium morrhuate was used as a sclerosing agent (111). Similar are the results of Bacon et al. (48% of 65 patients) (112) who used the same sclerosant as in the Saks study. In contrast, Parikh et al. (113), who used absolute alcohol as the sclerosant, reported an incidence of pleural effusion only in 19% of 31 patients. Most of the effusions are small with no predilection for the right or left pleural cavity. Sometimes, bilateral pleural effusions have been observed.

Pathogenesis of the pleural effusion is probably related to the extravasation of the sclerosant into the esophageal mucosa, which results to an intense inflammatory reaction affecting the mediastinum and the pleura (112). Pleural fluid is usually exudative and no treatment is necessary, unless if the fluid persists for more than one to two days, the patient is febrile, and more than 25% of the hemithorax is occupied in chest X-ray. In all these cases, a thoracocentesis is necessary in order to rule out an infection or an esophagopleural fistula, especially if the fluid amylase level is high. Recently, it has been demonstrated that an alternative method, endoscopic ligation of esophageal varices, significantly reduced the adverse effects associated with sclerotherapy, such as pyrexia, retrosternal pain, and pleural effusion (114).

J. Bilious Pleural Effusion

Bilious pleural effusion is a rare complication of biliary tract disorders and occurs only when there is a fistula between the biliary tract and the pleural space. The most common cause is a thoracoabdominal trauma, while less frequent causes include a parasitic (i.e., echinococcus) liver disease, suppurative complications of biliary tract obstruction, postoperative strictures of bile ducts, percutaneous biliary drainage or the stent placement for an obstructed biliary system (115,116). Very rarely, the biliary-pleural fistula is large enough to allow the passage of gallstones into the pleural cavity.

The instillation of bile into the pleural space produces an inflammatory reaction. The diagnosis should be suspected in any patient with an obstructed biliary system who presents a pleural effusion. Interestingly, the pleural fluid does not necessarily appear to be bile. Although the fluid bilirubin level may be lower than that anticipated, the ratio of the pleural fluid-to-serum bilirubin usually is greater than 1.0 in these patients (30).

The optimal treatment is the reestablishment of normal biliary drainage. In most of the cases of bilious pleural effusion, the treatment of choice consists of decortication of pleural space (115). It should be remembered that the incidence of empyema is high in these patients (about 50%), so clinicians should be aware of this complication to treat effectively.

K. Pleural Effusion Following Liver Transplantation

Most of the patients who undergo a liver transplantation, develop a postoperative pleural effusion. The frequency varies from 75% to 95% of patients, according to various studies (117,118). The pleural effusion usually develops within 72 hours of transplantation, usually in right-sided or bilateral; in the last case, the amount of fluid on the right side is greater than that of the left side.

Pleural effusion following liver transplantation may be large and may cause respiratory symptoms. Bilik et al. (119) reported that in 48 children who were recipients of a liver transplant, a large pleural effusion manifested in 23 out of them and required the placement of chest tubes.

The pathogenesis of the liver transplant–induced pleural effusion is unclear as of yet. It has been suggested that the effusion may be due to irritation or injury of the right hemidiaphragm during the operation. The effusion gradually increases during the first 3 postoperative days and then gradually resolves within several weeks to several months. Patients with continuously enlarging effusions should be evaluated for subdiaphragmatic pathology (i.e., hematomas, abscesses, etc.). The pleural effusion can be prevented effectively if a fibrin sealant is sprayed on the undersurface of the diaphragm at the time of transplantation (120).

IV. Metastatic Pleural Effusions

Carcinoma of any organ can metastasize to the pleura. However, carcinomas of the lung, breast, ovary, and lymphomas account for approximately 80% of malignant pleural effusions (121). In approximately 6% to 7% of patients with malignant pleural effusions, the primary site is unknown when the diagnosis of malignant pleural effusion is first established.

Neoplasms of the GI tract are recognized as rare causes of malignant pleural effusions. Carcinoma of the stomach is relatively more common, accounting for 1% to 3% of metastatic effusions, while colon carcinoma and pancreatic carcinoma are even more rare (less than 1% of malignant effusions) (122,123). Malignant effusions due to invasion of pleura from hepatocellular carcinoma (124) or cholangiocarcinoma (125) are extremely rare.

The most common symptoms reported by patients with malignant pleural effusions are dyspnea, chest pain, weight loss, malaise, anorexia, and symptoms attributable to the tumor itself. Chest radiography is essential in revealing the pleural effusion. The size of the effusion usually is large with the fluid occupying the entire hemithorax. Malignant disease is the most common cause of a massive pleural effusion.

The pleural fluid usually is an exudate. Most pleural effusions that meet exudative criteria by LDH level but not by the protein level are malignant pleural effusions. The presence of bloody fluid (red blood cell count >100,000 cells/mm^3) suggests malignant pleural disease. The predominant cells in the pleural fluid differential white cell count of these effusions are lymphocytes in about 45% and other mononuclear cells in about 40%. Pleural fluid eosinophilia is very uncommon.

In most cases, the positive cytologic examination of the fluid establishes the diagnosis. Pleural biopsy has a moderate diagnostic yield ranging from 40% to 74%, which may improve with thoracoscopy or open thoracotomy. However, these diagnostic procedures, if positive, establish the diagnosis of the pleural involvement by an adenocarcinoma, and they are not helpful in indicating the adenocarcinoma primary site. Immunohistochemical staining of the fluid sometimes may be of help, while the measurement of tumor markers in the fluid has no utility. Consequently, when clinicians face the challenge of diagnosing a pleural effusion secondary to adenocarcinoma of unknown primary site, they must perform an abdominal CT scan, contrast radiologic examination of stomach and colon, gastroscopy, and colonoscopy.

Palliative treatment of malignant pleural effusions depending of the site of primary tumor and the symptoms consists of repeated therapeutic thoracocenteses, systemic chemotherapy, placement of chest tubes, chemical pleurodesis with intrapleural injection of a sclerosing agent, pleuroperitoneal shunt, and pleurectomy.

The prognosis in patients with malignant pleural effusions is poor, although it obviously varies according to the histologic features of the tumor. Prognosis is worse if the pleural fluid glucose level is below 60 mg/dL or the pleural fluid pH is less than 7.30 (126). Low fluid glucose level and low fluid pH indicates that the patient has a high tumor burden in his pleural space. In a relatively recent series, the mean survival was five months with GI cancer (126).

References

1. Light RW. Transudative pleural effusions. In: Light RW, ed. Pleural Diseases. Philadelphia, PA: Lippincott Williams & Wilkins, 2007:120–133.
2. Johnston RF, Loo RV. Hepatic hydrothorax: Studies to determine the source of the fluid and report of thirteen cases. Ann Intern Med 1964; 61:385–401.
3. Lieberman FL, Hidemura R, Peters RL, et al. Pathogenesis and treatment of hydrothorax complicating cirrhosis with ascites. Ann Intern Med 1966; 64:341–351.

4. Rubinstein D, McInnes IE, Dudley FJ. Hepatic hydrothorax in the absence of clinical ascites: Diagnosis and management. Gastroenterology 1985; 88:188–191.

5. Cardenas A, Gines P. Pathogenesis and treatment of fluid and electrolyte imbalance in cirrhosis. Semin Nephrol 2001; 21:308–316.

6. Datta N, Mishkin FS, Vasinrapee P, et al. Radionuclide demonstration of peritoneal-pleural communication as a cause for pleural fluid. JAMA 1984; 252:210–217.

7. Mouroux J, Hebuterne X, Perrin C, et al. Treatment of pleural effusion of cirrhotic origin by videothoracoscopy. Br J Surg 1994; 81:546–547.

8. Huang PM, Chang YL, Yang CY. The morphology of diaphragmatic defects in hepatic hydrothorax: Thoracoscopic findings. J Thorac Cardiovasc Surg 2005; 139:141–145.

9. Lazaridis KN, Frank JW, Krowka MJ, et al. Hepatic hydrothorax: Pathogenesis, diagnosis and management. Am J Med 1999; 107:262–267.

10. Degawa M, Hamasaki K, Yano K, et al. Refractory hepatic hydrothorax treated with transjugular intrahepatic portosystemic shunt. J Gastroenterol 1999; 34:128–131.

11. Schuster DM, Mukundan S Jr, Small W, et al. The use of the diagnostic radionuclide ascites scan to facilitate treatment decision for hepatic hydrothorax. Clin Nucl Med 1998; 23:16–18.

12. Mittal BR, Maini A, Das BK. Peritoneopleural communication associated with cirrhotic ascites: Scintigraphic demonstration. Abdom Imaging 1996; 21:69–70.

13. Park CH, Pham CD. Hepatic hydrothorax: Scintigraphic confirmation. Clin Nucl Med 1995; 20:278–280.

14. Kakizaki S, Katakai K, Yoshinaga T, et al. Hepatic hydrothorax in the absence of ascites. Liver 1998; 18:216–220.

15. Daly JJ, Potts JM, Gordon L, et al. Scintigraphic diagnosis of peritoneo-pleural communication in the absence of ascites. Clin Nucl Med 1994; 19:892–894.

16. Benet A, Vidal F, Toda R, et al. Diagnosis of hepatic hydrothorax in the absence of ascites by intraperitoneal injection of 99 m-Tc Fluor colloid. Postgrad Med 1992; 68:153–154.

17. Light RW, Jenkinson SG, Minh V, et al. Observations on pleural pressures as fluid is withdrawn during thoracentesis. Am Rev Respir Dis 1980; 121:799–804.

18. Xiol X, Castellote J, Cortes-Beut R. Usefulness and complications of thoracentesis in cirrhotic patients. Am J Med 2001; 111:67–69.

19. Xiol X, Castellvi JM, Guardiola J, et al. Spontaneous bacterial empyema in cirrhotic patients: A prospective study. Hepatology 1996; 23:719–723.

20. Runyon BA. Care of patients with ascites. N Engl J Med 1994; 330:337–342.

21. Rossle M, Ochs A, Gulberg V, et al. A comparison of paracentesis and transjugular intrahepatic portosystemic shunting in patients with ascites. N Engl J Med 2000; 342:1701–1707.

22. Gordon FD, Anastopoulos HT, Crenshaw W, et al. The successful treatment of symptomatic, refractory hepatic hydrothorax with transjugular intrahepatic portosystemic shunt. Hepatology 1997; 25:1366–1369.

23. Haskal ZJ, Zuckerman J. Resolution of hepatic hydrothorax after TIPS placement. Chest 1994; 106:1293–1295.

24. Strauss RM, Martin LG, Kaufman SL, et al. Transjugular intrahepatic portal systemic shunt for the management of symptomatic cirrhotic hydrothorax. Am J Gastroenterol 1994; 89:1520–1522.

25. Conklin LD, Estrera AL, Weiner MA, et al. Transjugular intrahepatic portosystemic shunt for recurrent hepatic hydrothorax. Ann Thorac Surg 2000; 69:609–611.

26. Vargas FS, Milanez JR, Filomeno LT, et al. Intrapleural talc for the prevention of recurrence in benign or undiagnosed pleural effusions. Chest 1994; 106:1771–1775.

27. Mouroux J, Perrin C, Venissac N, et al. Management of pleural effusion of cirrhotic origin. Chest 1996; 109:1093–1096.

28. Milanez de Campos JR, Filho LO, Werebe EC, et al. Thoracoscopy and talc poudrage in the management of hepatic hydrothorax. Chest 2000; 118:13–17.

29. Yaguchi T, Harada A, Sakakibara T, et al. A successful surgical repair of the hepatic hydrothorax using pneumoperitoneum: Report of a case. Surg Today 1999; 29:795–798.

30. Light RW. Pleural effusion secondary to diseases of the gastrointestinal tract. In: Light RW, ed. Pleural Diseases. Philadelphia, PA: Lippincott Williams & Wilkins, 2007:252–265.

31. Romero S, Martin C, Hernandez L, et al. Chylothorax in cirrhosis of the liver: Analysis of its frequency and clinical characteristics. Chest 1998; 114:154–159.

32. Gatanaga H, Ohnishi S, Miura H, et al. Retroperitoneal fibrosis leading to extrahepatic portal vein obstruction. Intern Med 1994; 33:346–350.

33. Sassa H, Kondo J. Tsuboi H, et al. A case of idiopathic retroperitoneal fibrosis with chronic pericarditis. Intern Med 1992; 31:414–417.

34. Lankisch PG, Droge M, Becher R. Pleural effusions: A new negative prognostic parameter for acute pancreatitis. Am J Gastroenterol 1994; 89:1849–1851.

35. Talamini G, Uomo G, Pezzilli R, et al. Serum creatinine and chest radiographs in the early assessment of acute pancreatitis. Am J Surg 1999; 177:7–14.

36. Maringhini A, Ciambra M, Patti R, et al. Ascites, pleural, and pericardial effusions in acute pancreatitis. A prospective study of incidence, natural history and prognostic role. Dig Dis Sci 1996; 41:848–852.

37. Heller SJ, Noordhoek E, Tenner SM, et al. Pleural effusion as a predictor of severity in acute pancreatitis. Pancreas 1997; 15:222–225.

38. Gumaste V, Singh V, Dave P. Significance of pleural effusion in patients with acute pancreatitis. Am J Gastroenterol 1992; 87:871–874.

39. Kaye MD. Pleuropulmonary complications of pancreatitis. Thorax 1968; 23:297–306.

40. Light RW, Ball WC. Glucose and amylase in pleural effusions. JAMA 1973; 225:257–260.

41. Makela A, Kuusi T, Nuutinen P, et al. Phospholipase A2 activity in body fluids and pancreatic tissue in patients with acute necrotising pancreatitis. Eur J Surg 1999; 165:35–42.

42. Mayer JM, Rau B, Siech M, et al. Local and systemic zymogen activation in human acute pancreatitis. Digestion 2000; 62:164–170.

43. Karakoyunlar O, Sivrel E, Tanir N, et al. High-dose octreotide in the management of acute pancreatitis. Hepatogastroenterology 1999; 46:1968–1972.

44. Miller TA, Lindenauer SM, Frey CF, et al. Proceedings: Pancreatic abscess. Arch Surg 1974; 108:545–551.

45. Rockey DC, Cello JP. Pancreaticopleural fistula. Report of 7 patients and review of the literature. Medicine 1990; 69:332–344.

46. Standaert L, Verstappen G, Malbrain H, et al. Hemorrhagic pleural effusion and mediastinal mass: Presenting symptoms in a child with pseudocyst of the pancreas. J Pediatr Gastroenterol Nutr 1983; 2:329–331.

47. Ahmad N, Auld CD, Lawrence JR, et al. Pancreatic mediastinal pseudocyst: Report of two cases simulating intrathoracic disease. Scott Med J 1991; 36:146–147.

48. Zeilender S, Turner MA, Glauser FL. Mediastinal pseudocyst associated with chronic pleural effusions. Chest 1991; 99:1318–1319.

49. Lee DH, Shin DH, Kim TH, et al. Mediastinal pancreatic pseudocyst with recurrent pleural effusion. Demonstration by endoscopic retrograde cholangiopancreatogram and subsequent computed tomography scan. J Clin Gastroenterol 1992; 14:68–71.

50. Iacono C, Procacci C, Frigo F, et al. Thoracic complications of pancreatitis. Pancreas 1989; 4:228–236.

51. Izbicki JR, Wilker DK, Waldner H, et al. Thoracic manifestations of internal pancreatic fistulas: Report of five cases. Am J Gastroenterol 1989; 84:265–271.

52. Uchiyama T, Suzuki T, Adachi A, et al. Pancreatic pleural effusion: Case report and review of 113 cases in Japan. Am J Gastroenterol 1992; 87:387–391.

53. Branca P, Rodriguez RM, Rogers JT, et al. Routine measurement of pleural fluid amylase is not indicated. Arch Intern Med 2001; 161:228–232.

54. Kramer MR, Saldana MJ, Cepero RJ, et al. High amylase levels in neoplasm-related pleural effusion. Ann Intern Med 1989; 110:567–569.
55. Tokoo M, Oguchi H, Kawa S, et al. Eosinophilia associated with chronic pancreatitis: An analysis of 122 patients with definite chronic pancreatitis. Am J Gastroenterol 1992; 87:455–460.
56. Bronner MH, Marsh WH, Stanley JH. Pancreaticopleural fistula: Demonstration by computed tomography and endoscopic retrograde cholangiopancreatography. J Comput Tomogr 1986; 10:167–170.
57. Closset J, Gelin M. The management of pancreatic ascites and pancreaticopleural effusion. Acta Gastroenterol Belg 2000; 63:269–270.
58. Pederzoli P, Bassi C, Falconi M, et al. Conservative treatment of external pancreatic fistulae with parenteral nutrition along or in combination with continuous intravenous infusion of somatostatin, glucagon or calcitonin. Surg Gynecol Obstet 1986; 163:428–432.
59. Singh P, Holubka J, Patel S. Acute mediastinal pancreatic fluid collection with pericardial and pleural effusion. Complete resolution after treatment with octreotide acetate. Dig Dis Sci 1996; 41:1966–1971.
60. Safadi BY, Marks JM. Pancreatic-pleural fistula: The role of ERCP in diagnosis and treatment. Gastrointest Endosc 2000; 51:213–215.
61. Hastier P, Rouquier P, Buckley M, et al. Endoscopic treatment of wirsungo-cysto-pleural fistula. Eur J Gastroenterol Hepatol 1998; 10:527–529.
62. Kotsis L, Agocs L, Kostic S, et al. Transdiaphragmatic cyst-jejunostomy with Roux-en-Y loop for an exclusively mediastinal pancreatic pseudocyst. Scand J Thorac Cardiovasc Surg 1996; 30:181–183.
63. Tsang TM, Tam PK. Pancreatic pleural effusion: An indication for emergency distal pancreatectomy and Roux-en-Y pancreatico-jejunostomy. J Pediatr Surg 1995; 30:1632–1633.
64. Christensen NM, Demling R, Mathewson C Jr. Unusual manifestations of pancreatic pseudocysts and their surgical management. Am J Surg 1975; 130:199–205.
65. Faling LJ, Gerzof SG, Daly BD, et al. Treatment of chronic pancreatitic pleural effusion by percutaneous catheter drainage of abdominal pseudocyst. Am J Med 1984; 76:329–333.
66. Lang EK, Paolini RM, Pottmeyer A. The efficacy of palliative and definitive percutaneous versus surgical drainage of pacreatic abscesses and pseudocysts. South Med J 1991; 84: 55–64.
67. Brelvi ZS, Jonas ME, Trotman BW, et al. Nasopancreatic drainage: A novel approach for treating internal pancreatic fistulas and pseudocysts. J Assoc Acad Minor Phys 1996; 7:41–46.
68. Lipsett PA, Cameron JL. Internal pancreatic fistula. Am J Surg 1992; 163:216–220.
69. Cameron JL, Kieffer RS, Anderson WJ, et al. Internal pancreatic fistulas: Pancreatic ascites and pleural effusions. Ann Surg 1976; 184:587–593.
70. Hotz J, Goebell H, Herfarth C, et al. Massive pancreatic ascites without carcinoma. Report of three cases. Digestion 1977; 15:200–216.
71. Uchiyama T, Yamamoto T, Mizuta E, et al. Pancreatic ascites—A collected review of 37 cases in Japan. Hepatogastroenterology 1989; 36:244–248.
72. Parekh D, Segal I. Pancreatic ascites and effusion. Risk factors for failure of conservative therapy and the role of octreotide. Arch Surg 1992; 127:707–712.
73. da Cunha JE, Machado M, Bacchela T, et al. Surgical treatment of pancreatic ascites and pancreatic pleural effusion. Hepatogastroenterology 1995; 42:748–751.
74. Kochhar R, Goenka MK, Nagi B, et al. Pancreatic ascites and pleural effusion treated by endoscopic pancreatic stent placement. Indian J Gastroenterol 1995; 14:106–107.
75. Connell TR, Stephens DH, Carlson HC, et al. Upper abdominal abscess: A continuing and deadly problem. Am J Roentgenol 1980; 134:759–765.
76. Sanders RC. Post-operative pleural effusion and subphrenic abscess. Clin Radiol 1970; 21:308–312.

77. Kelty CJ, Thorpe JA. Empyema due to spilled gall stones during laparoscopic cholecystectomy. Eur J Cardiothorac Surg 1998; 13:107–108.

78. Sherman NJ, Davis JR, Jesseph JE. Subphrenic abscess: A continuing hazard. Am J Surg 1969; 117:117–123.

79. Carter R, Brewer LA. Subphrenic abscess: A thoracoabdominal clinical complex. Am J Surg 1964; 108:165–174.

80. Alexander ES, Proto AV, Clark RA. CT differentiation of subphrenic abscess and pleural effusion. Am J Roentgenol 1983; 145:47–51.

81. Chu KM, Fan ST, Lai EC, et al. Pyogenic liver abscess. An audit of experience over the past decade. Arch Surg 1996; 131:148–152.

82. Roy R, Goyal RK, Gupta N. Tuberculous liver abscess. J Assoc Physicians India 2000; 48:241–243.

83. Dykhuisen RS, Douglas G, Weir J, et al. *Corynebacterium afermentans* subsp. Lipophilum: Multiple abscess formation in brain and liver. Scand J Infect Dis 1995; 27:637–639.

84. Lee KT, Sheen PC, Chen JS, et al. Pyogenic liver abscess: Multivariate analysis of risk factors. World J Surg 1991; 15:372–377.

85. Wong KP. Percutaneous drainage of pyogenic liver abscesses. World J Surg 1990; 14:492–497.

86. Baek SY, Lee MG, Cho KS, et al. Therapeutic percutaneous aspiration of hepatic abscesses: Effectiveness in 25 patients. AJR Am J Roentgenol 1993; 160:799–802.

87. Light RW. Pleural diseases. Dis Mon 1992; 28:263–331.

88. Lyche KD, Jensen WA, Kirsch CM, et al. Pleuropulmonary manifestations of hepatic amebiasis. West J Med 1990; 153:275–278.

89. Chuah SK, Chang-Chien CS, Sheen IS, et al. The prognostic factors of severe amebic liver abscess: A retrospective study of 125 cases. Am J Trop Med Hyg 1992; 46:398–402.

90. Munoz LE, Botello MA, Carillo O, et al. Early detection of complications in amebic liver abscess. Arch Med Res 1992; 23:251–253.

91. Tony JC, Martin TK. Profile of amebic liver abscess. Arch Med Res 1992; 23:249–250.

92. Sarr MG, Zuidema GD. Splenic abscess: Presentation, diagnosis and treatment. Surgery 1982; 92:480–485.

93. Ho HS, Wisner DH. Splenic abscess in the intensive care unit. Arch Surg 1993; 128:842–848.

94. Green BT. Splenic abscess: Report of six cases and review of the literature. Am Surg 2001; 67:80–85.

95. Tikkakoski T, Siniluoto T, Paivansalo M, et al. Splenic abscess. Imaging and intervention. Acta Radiol 1992; 33:561–565.

96. Michel L, Grillo HC, Malt RA. Operative and nonoperative management of esophageal perforations. Ann Surg 1981; 194:57–63.

97. Reeder LB, DeFilippi VJ, Ferguson MK. Current results of therapy for esophageal perforation. Am J Surg 1995; 169:615–617.

98. Keszler P, Buzna E. Surgical and conservative management of esophageal perforation. Chest 1981; 80:158–162.

99. Maulitz RM, Good JT Jr, Kaplan RL, et al. The pleuropulmonary consequences of esophageal rupture: An experimental model. Am Rev Respir Dis 1979; 120:363–367.

100. Abbott OA, Mansour KA, Logan WD Jr, et al. Atraumatic so-called "spontaneous" rupture of the esophagus. J Thorac Cardiovasc Surg 1970; 59:67–83.

101. Lemke T, Jagminas L. Spontaneous esophageal rupture: A frequently missed diagnosis. Am Surg 1999; 65:449–452.

102. Sherr HP, Light RW, Merson MH, et al. Origin of pleural fluid amylase in esophageal rupture. Ann Intern Med 1972; 76:985–986.

103. Dye RA, Laforet EG. Esophageal rupture: Diagnosis by pleural fluid pH. Chest 1974; 66:454–456.

104. Good JT Jr, Antony VB, Reller LB, et al. The pathogenesis of the low pleural fluid pH in esophageal rupture. Am Rev Respir Dis 1983; 127:702–704.

105. Eriksen KR. Oesophagopleural fistula diagnosed by microscopic examination of pleural fluid. Acta Chir Scand 1964; 128:771–777.

106. Drury M, Anderson W, Heffner JE. Diagnostic value of pleural fluid cytology in occult Boerhaave's syndrome. Chest 1992; 102:976–978.

107. Ginai AZ. Experimental evaluation of various available contrast agents for use in the gastrointestinal tract in case of suspected leakage: Effects on pleura. Br J Radiol 1986; 59:887–894.

108. Light RW, George RB. Incidence and significance of pleural effusion after abdominal surgery. Chest 1976; 69:621–626.

109. Nielsen PH, Jensen SB, Olsen AD. Postoperative pleural effusion following upper abdominal surgery. Chest 1989; 96:1133–1135.

110. Aronchick JM, Epstein DM, Gefter WB, et al. Chronic traumatic diaphragmatic hernia: The significance of pleural effusion. Radiology 1988; 168:675–678.

111. Saks BJ, Kilby AE, Dietrich PA, et al. Pleural and mediastinal changes following endoscopic injection sclerotherapy of esophageal varices. Radiology 1983; 149:639–642.

112. Bacon BR, Bailey-Newton RS, Connors AF Jr. Pleural effusions after endoscopic variceal sclerotherapy. Gastroenterology 1985; 88:1910–1914.

113. Parikh SS, Amarapurkar DN, Dhawan PS, et al. Development of pleural effusion after sclerotherapy with absolute alcohol. Gastrointest Endovasc 1993; 39:404–405.

114. Tsugawa K, Hashizume M, Migou S, et al. Endoscopic ligation of oesophageal varices compared with injection sclerotherapy in primary biliary cirrhosis. Eur J Gastroenterol 2000; 12(10):1111–1115.

115. Ivatury RR, O'Shea J, Rohman M. Post-traumatic thoracobiliary fistula. J Trauma 1984; 24:438–441.

116. Delco F, Domenigheti G, Kauzlaric D, et al. Spontaneous biliothorax (thoracobilia) following cholecystopleural fistula presenting as an acute respiratory insufficiency. Chest 1994; 106:961–963.

117. Spizarny DL, Gross BH, McLoud T. Enlarging pleural effusion after liver transplantation. J Thorac Imaging 1993; 8:85–87.

118. Afessa B, Gay PC, Plevak DJ, et al. Pulmonary complications of orthotopic liver transplantation. Mayo Clin Proc 1993; 68:427–434.

119. Bilik R, Yellen M, Superina RA. Surgical complications in children after liver transplantation. Pediatr Surg 1992; 27:1371–1375.

120. Uetsuji S, Komada Y, Kwon AH, et al. Prevention of pleural effusion after hepatectomy using fibrin sealant. Int Surg 1994; 79:135–137.

121. Sahn SA. Malignant pleural effusions. In: Fishman AP, ed. Fishman's Pulmonary Diseases and Disorders. New York, NY: McGraw-Hill, 1998:1429–1438.

122. Spriggs AI, Boddington MM. The Cytology of Effusions, 2nd ed. New York, NY: Grune & Stratton, 1968.

123. Anderson CB, Philpott GW, Ferguson TB. The treatment of malignant pleural effusions. Cancer 1974; 33:916–922.

124. Falconieri G, Zanconati F, Colautti I, et al. Effusion cytology of hepatocellular carcinoma. Acta Cytol 1995; 39:893–897.

125. Tamai M, Tanimura H, Yamaue H, et al. Nasobiliary drainage for spontaneous bile peritonitis due to cholangiocarcinoma. Nippon Geka Hokan 1991; 60:195–202.

126. Sanchez-Armengol A, Rodriguez-Panadero F. Survival and talc pleurodesis in metastatic pleural carcinoma, revisited. Report of 125 cases. Chest 1993; 104:1482–1485.

38
Pleural Effusions in Pulmonary Embolism

LUIS PUENTE-MAESTU
Hospital Universitario Gregorio Marañón, Madrid, Spain

VICTORIA VILLENA
Hospital Universitario 12 de Octubre, Madrid, Spain

I. Introduction

Pulmonary embolism (PE) is responsible for approximately 20 deaths per 100,000 inhabitants per year in the United States (1–3). Untreated PE is associated with an overall mortality rate of approximately 30%—although more than half of this is due to underlying conditions like cancer and myocardial infarction (4,5)—which can be decreased between 2% and 8% with the institution of appropriate treatment (6–8).

Most of the deaths due to PE occur within the first few hours of the event (6,9). Although the majority of patients with a PE live beyond these first few hours, it is apparent from long-term studies that, if untreated, recurrent PE, possibly with fatal consequences, is common in this population (7). It is, therefore, imperative that effective therapy be instituted after a thromboembolic event. However, it has been reported that only 30% of patients with PE at autopsy had received the diagnosis before death (10), and it is estimated that 5% of patients undergoing autopsies (11,12) had died of undiagnosed PE. Thus, many deaths can be prevented by a more accurate diagnosis of this condition (2).

Pleural effusion visible in the chest radiography occurs in 10% to 50% of patients with PE (13–21), thus, it may be a clue for PE diagnosis. Furthermore, among the patients of the International Cooperative Pulmonary Embolism Registry (ICOPER), 36% of the 39 patients diagnosed with PE at autopsy who had a chest radiograph had a pleural effusion (20). In studies conducted in Worcester, Massachusetts (2), and Olmsted County, Minnesota (3), the incidence of venous thromboembolism was 1 case per 1000 inhabitants per year. Symptomatic PE occurs in approximately 30% of the patients with deep venous thrombosis, but if one counts the asymptomatic events, some 50% to 60% of the patients with deep venous thrombosis may develop PE (22). From these data and the reported prevalence of pleural effusion around 30% (13–21), a fair amount of pleural effusions can be expected to be due to PE. To give only an example, more pleural effusions should be expected to be due to PE than due to lung cancer (23). In striking contrast with those estimations, most clinicians feel that PE is an infrequent cause of pleural effusion (24). Furthermore, several series studying the prevalence of the different causes of pleural effusions find PE to be an uncommon cause, with figures lower than 6% of the effusions studied, in spite of different epidemiological contexts and durations of collection of the series (25–31). On the one hand, it is likely that in patients diagnosed with PE and associated pleural effusions, the etiology of the effusion would be assumed to be the PE and no further diagnostic workout is performed (and arguably may not be required if the clinical course is favorable); on the other hand, however, it may occur that PE is not often be considered in undiagnosed pleural effusions, that pleural effusions related to PE are attributed to other causes easier to recognize when several concomitant potential causes are present (e.g., heart failure, atelectasis, or infection), or that postmortem diagnoses are not included in these series, which might underestimate the number of cases due to PE. For example, in an autopsy series of 290 patients with congestive heart failure and pleural effusions, 60 (21%) had pulmonary emboli (32). Thus, in every patient with undiagnosed pleural effusion in which pulmonary thromboembolism is clinically probable, the diagnosis of PE should be sought.

II. Mechanisms

In the normal pleural space, there is a steady state in which the rate of the formation of liquid matches the rate of absorption. Therefore, pleural fluid starts to accumulate when either an increase in entry rate or a reduction in exit rate occurs. It is likely that both mechanisms contribute, since the absorbing pleural lymphatics have a large reserve capacity to deal with excess pleural liquid (33) and an isolated decrease in exit rate is unlikely to be the sole cause because the normal entry rate is low. Even if the exit of liquid ceased entirely, accumulation of fluid would take many days to become evident. As an example, at a normal entry rate in the pleural space of 0.01 mL/(kg · hr), only 15 to 20 mL would accumulate per day if the exit were completely shut off (34).

Potential mechanisms operating in PE include:

1. An increase in entry rates of liquid by increase in capillary permeability or by elevated hydrostatic pressures in pulmonary and systemic veins, and perhaps by lowering pleural pressure due to atelectasis.
2. Pulmonary embolism might also decrease exit rates of pleural liquid by increasing the systemic venous pressure (hindering lymphatic drainage) or perhaps by decreasing pleural pressure (hindering lymphatic filling). In one study, though, the calculated lymphatic flow for patients with PE was 0.18 mL/(kg · hr), which is only slightly lower than the maximal exit rate measured for sheep [0.28 mL/ (kg · hr)] (34).

Bynum and Wilson (35) studied the characteristics of pleural fluids associated with PE, and apparently 24% of the effusions were transudates (35). In recent series (21,36), when all three Light's criteria to differentiate exudates from transudates (25) were employed, all the effusions associated with PE fell into the exudate category. The transudative effusions associated with PE described by Bynum and Wilson (35) had a protein ratio higher than what would be expected if the only source of fluid were the ultrafiltration from capillaries of the systemic circulation of the pleural membranes due to increased microvascular pressures. Thus, if they indeed were transudates, most of the liquid must had come from another source, such as the leakage of interstitial fluid of the lung (37).

The most relevant mechanisms by which PE can produce exudates is the increase in the permeability of the capillaries of the lung by ischemia or more probably by release of inflammatory mediators such as vascular endothelial growth factor from the platelets of the thrombi (38). The excess of interstitial fluid so formed will leak into the pleural space throughout the visceral pleura (39). Apparently, visceral pleura capillaries are supplied by bronchial circulation (40), and thus inflammatory mediators released into the pulmonary circulation do not influence them. It is possible, however, that inflammatory mediators released by the ischemia of the adjacent lung could affect visceral pleura capillaries.

As many as 65% of the pleural effusions associated with PE have a blood-tinged appearance (35,36,41). The passing of red cells into the pleural space seems to be related, at least in part, to the existence of an adjacent pulmonary infarction, as indicated by the fact that 88% of the patients with infiltrates suggestive of infarction had bloody effusions (35). However, up to 30% of the pleural effusions associated with PE without apparent pulmonary infiltrates in chest X-ray also were bloody in appearance (35).

III. Clinical Picture

A. Epidemiology and Natural History

The incidence of PE increases with age—for each year increase in age its incidence doubles (2,3,42,43). Three-quarters of the cases of PE occur in people older than 50 years and approximately 90% in those older than 40 years (43). Prospective series find a male predominance in venous thromboembolic episodes (2,3). Interestingly, though, retrospective reports of cases of PE find a slight female predominance (42,43). The available experience regarding pleural effusions associated with PE is limited, but it also appears that effusions due to PE are more frequent in patients older than 40 years and particularly in those older than 50 years (21,27,28). It has to be noted, however, that in this range of ages, the most prevalent cause recognized of exudative and transudative effusions are neoplasms and heart failure, respectively (25–28) (see introduction).

Pleural effusion has been found by chest radiography in 10% to 30% of patients with PE (13–21) and between 40% and 70% when computed tomography is used (13–21). It was seen in 23% of the 2322 patients included in the ICOPER who had chest radiographs (20) and it occurred more often when acute PE followed certain surgical procedures [e.g., general abdominal surgery (33%)] than others [e.g., orthopedic surgery (19%)]. Nevertheless, these differences may reflect the incidence of common radiographic abnormalities after specific surgical procedures, rather than different chest abnormalities caused by PE. The delay between initial presentation and thoracocentesis in the study of Romero et al. (36) was 6.8 ± 5.2 days, and between thoracocentesis and the diagnosis of PE, the delay was 2 ±3 days.

In the absence of complications, pleural effusions tend to reach their maximum size early. In the only study to our knowledge aimed specifically at describing the clinical picture of pleural effusions associated with PE (14), the maximal size had been reached on the first chest radiograph in 57 out of the 62 (92%) pleural effusions attributed to PE, and in only 2 (2%) did its size increase after the third day. In those two cases, other causes (i.e., infection in one and recurrence of the PE in the other) were thought responsible for the late increase in effusion.

The course of resolution of these effusions has not been extensively studied. In the series of Bynum and Wilson (14), although 18 out of 25 (72%) pleural effusions without parenchymal infiltrates resolved in less than seven days, in all 31 patients with associated parenchymal consolidation effusions persisted longer than seven days. This might reflect, at least in part, the larger size at the onset of effusions associated with pulmonary infarctions. No data are reported on the time resolution of the cases that persisted for more than seven days (14). Thus, if an effusion increases after the third day, recurrent PE, hemothorax from anticoagulation, secondary infection, or an alternate diagnosis should be suspected (14,44,45).

Most effusions secondary to PE evolve to complete resolution, however, some can leave minimal sequels. In one study in which 58 angiographically proven pulmonary infarcts in 32 patients were followed by chest radiography, 9 (16%) showed pleural diaphragmatic adhesions and 6 (10%) localized pleural thickening. In all cases, the features had improved when compared with the original abnormality (46).

The two main acute complications of pleural effusions associated with PE are infection (14) and hemothorax (44,45). Both are rare, presenting in less than 1% of the cases (14). The worst, because of its high mortality, is massive hemothorax. Its causes are not clear; it may be spontaneous, secondary to anticoagulation therapy or, likely, to both. The clinical picture consists of a sudden or rapid deterioration of the hemodynamic status of the patient, marked increase in the size of the pleural effusion, which usually fills the whole hemithorax, and secondary deterioration of the respiratory function (44,45). The hematocrit is frequently lower than previous values, although not as much as would be expected by the hemodynamic repercussion (44,45). The pleural fluid is frank blood (44,45). Hematocrit values that equal those of the blood are almost the rule. At autopsy, massive unilateral hemothorax and evidence of parenchymal necrosis are seen (44,45). The term acute rupture of pulmonary infarction has been proposed for those cases in which parenchymal necrosis is evident (45). Acute hemothorax must be distinguished from recurrent embolism and from bleeding from other sources. The evident increase in the effusion on the chest radiography points toward this complication and the analysis of the fluid confirms its bloody nature. The treatment consists of immediate withdrawal of thrombolytic or anticoagulant medication, repositioning of volume with fresh blood, and drainage of the pleural space (44,45). Emergency surgical intervention can be considered, although its utility has not been proven.

Another rare pleural complication after pulmonary infarction is the development of persistent, usually small, left-sided, or bilateral pleural effusions (47,48). The effusions are associated with the classical signs and symptoms of the postcardiac-injury syndrome (49) (i.e., chest pleuritic in nature, fever, leukocytosis, an elevated erythrocyte sedimentation rate, and variable combinations of pulmonary infiltrates and pleural or pericardial effusions). The effusions are hemorrhagic in 70% of cases and frankly bloody in 30% (47,48,50). Patients with postpulmonary-infarction syndrome, typically present symptoms one week or more after a pulmonary infarction (47,48,50). In one report, for example, 65% of affected patients presented within 3 months and 100% within 12 months (51). The response to treatment with glucocorticoids for both postcardiac and postpulmonary syndromes is dramatic (47,48), but it would probably respond to nonsteroidal anti-inflammatory agents as well, since the majority of patients with postcardiac-injury syndrome (in whom glucocorticoids are relatively contraindicated) respond well to nonsteroidal anti-inflamatories (52). The pathogenesis of this postpulmonary-infarction syndrome is unclear, but appears to be an immunological reaction (47).

B. Clinical Manifestations

There is little information on whether patients with PE and pleural effusions present a different clinical picture than patients with PE but without pleural effusion. The available information suggests that chest pain on the side of the effusion is more common when PE has an associated pleural effusion (14,53). In one study of patients without prior cardiopulmonary disease who had a PE diagnosed by arteriography (54), pleural effusion was present in 67 out of 119 (56%) of those patients who reported a syndrome of "pulmonary infarction or hemorrhage" (defined as pleuritic pain or hemoptysis as presentation symptoms). On the other hand, 6 out of 31 (19%) of those reporting isolated dyspnea and none of the 5 (0%) patients with circulatory collapse had pleural effusion (54).

Effusions secondary to PE generally are small and occupy less than one-third of the hemithorax, but they can be of any size (13–21,36). On plain chest radiographs they usually are unilateral, even in the presence of bilateral pulmonary emboli, however, around 15% may show bilateral effusions (21,25–28,36). This proportion may be higher with computed tomography (19). Loculated pleural effusions have been described as a possible radiologic appearance of PE when the diagnosis is delayed for some time (usually more than two weeks) after the symptoms developed (21,55) and may be confounded with empyema (55). Pleural effusion may occur independently in the presence of visible infarction. Pulmonary infiltrates suggestive of pulmonary infarction has been found in 13% to 95% of the cases (14–21,36,54,56). Pooling these series together only around half of the pleural effusions associated with PE showed peripheral infiltrates suggestive of pulmonary infarction (14–21,36,54,56).

To our knowledge, there are no specific data on the frequency of the combination of pleural effusion with other common radiographic signs associated with PE (i.e., cardiac enlargement, elevated hemidiaphragm, enlargement of pulmonary arteries, atelectasis, pulmonary congestion, and oligemia) and their value to lead one to suspect PE in pleural effusions of difficult diagnosis. Using helical computed tomography, no radiological sign, with the exception of wedge-shaped infiltrates, differentiated between effusions due to PE and those due to other causes (19). In one series, the frequency of pulmonary effusions was not different between patients with central and peripheral clots (21).

C. Pleural Fluid Characteristics

The reported characteristics of pleural fluid associated with PE are variable (21,35,36). Among the 26 patients of Bynum and Wilson (35), 24% of effusions were transudates (35). Nevertheless, pleural fluid lactate dehydrogenase (LDH) was not measured in all cases (35). In two recent series (21,36) using all three Light's criteria for differentiating transudate from exudates (which include pleural effusion-to-plasma LDH ratio) (25), all effusions were classified as exudates. Pleural fluid pH has not been reported to be lower than 7.20 (21,36). In the series of Porcel et al. (21), 1 out of 26 subjects in which pleural effusions associated with PE could be analyzed had adenosine deaminase higher than 40 U/L.

A blood-tinged or bloody-appearing fluid has been reported in more than half of the cases (21,35,36,41). The blood cell count is >10,000 cells/mm^3 in 58% to 73% of patients, and it is >100,000 cells/mm^3 in 15% to 18% of patients (35,36).

The white blood cell count ranges from <100 cells/mm^3 to >50,000 cells/mm^3 (21,35,36). A polymorphonuclear leukocyte predominance has been found in 60% of patients (35,36). Nevertheless, more than 80% lymphocytes may be found in 15% of patients (35). Pleural eosinophilia (>10% eosinophils) has also been reported in around 20% of these patients (36,57). In addition, a higher mesothelial cell score in comparison to other effusions has also been found (36). Interestingly, in a small series of loculated pulmonary effusions due to PE, dominance of lymphocytes was found (55). The pleural fluid glucose typically is normal (21,35,36,55).

IV. Diagnosis

The diagnostic value of pleural effusion in patients suspected of having a PE has been analyzed in several studies. Worsley et al. (17) looked at the predictive value of different radiological signs in 1063 patients involved in the Prospective Investigation of Pulmonary Embolism Diagnosis (PIOPED). The population consisted of patients in which PE was clinically suspected. Pleural effusions were noted in 47% of 383 and 39% of 680 patients with and without PE, respectively. Pleural effusion was a poor predictor of PE (17). In a subsample of 500 patients of the Prospective Investigative Study of Acute Pulmonary Embolism Diagnosis (PISA-PED), pleural effusion was seen in 45% of 202 patients with PE and 35% of 298 patients without PE. While the difference was statistically significant, again its specificity was low (58). In a different population of subjects, that is, young patients who presented with acute chest pain, McNeil et al. (53) found that the presence of pleural effusion increased the likelihood of PE.

A few studies have looked at the predictive value for PE of the size of the effusion in patients in which PE had been clinically suspected, but the information produced is contradictory. While Goldberg et al. (59), in a retrospective study, reported that 43% of those patients with large pleural effusions actually had PE versus 28% and 30% of those patients with small pleural effusions and without pleural effusions, respectively, neither Talbot et al. (56) nor Shah et al. (19) (the latter using helical computed tomography) found that the size of the effusion discriminated between patients with and without PE. In the series of Talbot et al. (56), though, small effusions were more frequent in patients with PE than patients without PE. These results are consistent with the general finding that pleural effusions were predominantly small in the majority of the reports of pleural effusion associated with PE (13–22,35,36).

In summary, the characteristics of pleural fluids associated with PE are unspecific in a majority of cases (36). The diagnostic value of the pattern believed to be more specific, that is, a blood-tinged exudate rich in polymorphonuclear leukocytes has not been studied. Pulmonary embolism should be a diagnostic consideration in every patient with an acute, unilateral pleural effusion, particularly if it is an exudate or even in transudates with relatively high levels of proteins (35,36), or if it is associated with acute chest pain of pleuritic characteristics (14,53). Some evidence suggests that pleural effusions due to PE are most frequently small or medium size (13–22,35,36,53–59) and do not enlarge after the third day of presentation (14). PE is seldom the cause of significant bilateral pleural effusions on plain chest radiographs (14,17,21,35,36,53–59), but in one series of bilateral effusions without enlarged cardiac shadow, 10 out of 78 cases (13%) were diagnosed with PE (60). Particular caution is needed with effusions thought to be due to heart failure, since in certain circumstances a significant proportion of them can be due to or may have a concomitant PE (32,60). In a small series, levels of N-terminal pro-brain natriuretic peptide higher than 2220 pg/mL in pleural fluid was able to distinguish between effusions due to congestive heart failure from those due to PE (61). Pleural effusion increases the likelihood of PE in subjects with suspected PE, but the specificity as diagnostic criterion for PE was low (53,56,58).

A. Clinical Probability Assessment

The most commonly reported symptoms, signs, and predisposing conditions found in several large cohorts of subjects diagnosed with PE are described in Table 1 (15,16,58,62–71). However, the frequency of many of these symptoms and signs is similar in patients who are thought to have a PE and those who do not (15,16,58,62–71).

Clinicians appear to be able to assign meaningful probabilities for PE prior to specific tests. In PIOPED, for example, clinical probabilities were rated as low (0–19%), intermediate (20–79%), or high (80–100%). Among patients determined clinically to have a high probability of disease prior to lung scanning, 67% were found to have PE; in contrast, only 9% of those assigned a low probability had it, but intermediate probabilities were assigned in the majority of patients (64%) (63). In another large multicentric trial, the PISA-PED, a standardized diagnostic protocol was used, and a clinical probability of PE was assigned out of three alternatives: very likely (90%), possible (50%), or unlikely (10%). PE was diagnosed in only 9% of the patients with unlikely clinical presentation and in 91% of those in whom the disease was considered likely on clinical grounds. Again, the majority of patients had intermediate probabilities (64). Similar findings were noted in other large prospective studies (65,66). An algorithm (Table 2) on the combination of seven variables containing three blocks of information: (1) key symptoms and signs at presentation, (2) the clinician assessment of the likelihood of an alternative diagnosis,

Table 1 Incidence of Symptoms, Signs, and Predisposing Conditions in Patients with PE

	Incidence (%)
Symptoms	
Dyspnea	75–80
Pleuritic pain	44–74
Fainting or syncope	13–26
Cough	11–53
Hemoptysis (rarely massive)	9–30
Signs	
Tachypnea	70–92
Tachycardia	24–44
Fourth heart sound	24–34
Accentuated pulmonary component of the second heart sound	23–53
Rales	18–51
Signs of lower extremity deep venous thrombosis	17–32
Cyanosis	16–19
Fever	7–43
Preexisting diseases	
Cardiac or pulmonary diseases	33–38
Malignant neoplasm	6–10
Predisposing risk factors	
Immobilization	55–59
Surgery	40
Previous venous disease	34–43
Bone fracture of lower extremities	23

Sources: Adapted from Refs. 15–17, 58, 62–71.

Table 2   Clinical Decision Rule

Clinical decision rule	
Clinical symptoms of DVT (leg swelling, pain with palpation)	3.0
Other diagnosis less likely than pulmonary embolism	3.0
Heart rate >100	1.5
Immobilization (≥3 days) or surgery in the previous 4 wk	1.5
Previous DVT/PE	1.5
Hemoptysis	1.0
Malignancy	1.0
Probability score	
Traditional clinical probability assessment	
High	>6.0
Moderate	2.0–6.0
Low	<2.0
Simplified clinical probability assessment*	
PE likely	>4.0
PE unlikely	≤4.0

*Clinical probability of pulmonary embolism unlikely: 4 or less points; clinical probability of pulmonary embolism likely: more than 4 points.
Source: Adapted from Refs. 67 and 68.

and (3) the presence of risk factors has been proposed to classify patients in three groups (high, moderate, or low) as to pretest probability of PE. This scheme was validated in 1239 patients with suspected PE; PE was ultimately documented in 3% of patients with a low pretest probability, 28% with a moderate pretest probability, and 78% with a high pretest probability (67). Recently (Table 2), a simpler modified classification of risk has been shown to be useful (68).

In summary, only a minority of patients with PE have no important clinical manifestation of the disease. However, no single symptom or sign or combination of them is sufficient to diagnose PE; in spite of their lack of specificity, combinations of symptoms, signs, and epidemiological data allow one to assign meaningful probabilities for pulmonary emboli.

B.   Laboratory Abnormalities

Blood Gas Analysis

Routine laboratory findings including arterial blood gases are nonspecific (15,58,69,70). Arterial blood gases usually reveal hypoxemia, hypocapnia, and respiratory alkalosis, but 10% to 20% of patients with PE may have an arterial oxygen pressure higher than 80 mm Hg (15,58,69). Furthermore, the criterion that is considered most sensitive, the alveolar-arterial gradient for oxygen, is normal (i.e., <15 mm Hg) in 6% to 16% of patients with PE (15,58,69). While arterial blood gases have a limited role in the diagnosis of PE, oxygen saturation can be useful to initially assess the severity (71), besides a sudden deterioration of arterial blood gases in the context of a patient with acute respiratory symptoms (dyspnea, chest pain, fainting, or tachypnea), when both the symptoms and the abnormal alveolar-arterial gradient for oxygen cannot be explained by an alternative cause, especially if accompanied by risk factors for PE, there is a high clinical probability of PE (72).

Natriuretic Peptides and Troponins

Natriuretic peptides are frequently higher in patients with PE than in patients without PE (73) and serum troponins are high in 30% to 50% of the patients with moderate to large PE (74), however, available evidence suggests that they are neither sensitive nor specific enough to be useful diagnostic tests (73,74). Troponin and natriuretic peptides, though, may be valuable prognostic markers (74–76).

C. Electrocardiogram

Electrocardiogram is often abnormal, but the most frequent findings are generally nonspecific ST and T-wave changes, especially in V_1–V_4 leads (77). Other frequent abnormalities are tachycardia and atrial fibrillation (15,43,58,77,78). Seventy percent of patients without preexisting cardiovascular disease in PIOPED presented an abnormal electrocardiogram. The most common abnormalities (49%) were nonspecific ST segment and T-wave changes (16). In the Urokinase Pulmonary Embolism Trial, electrocardiographic abnormalities were demonstrated in 87% of patients with massive or submassive PE. Only 26% had manifestations of right ventricle overload [T-wave inversion in right precordial leads, S1Q3/S1Q3T3, transient right bundle branch block, P-wave "pulmonale," or pseudo-infarction (S1S2S3)] (78). In the PISA-PED, right ventricular overload was seen in 50% of the patients with PE and 12% of the subjects without PE (58). In summary, electrocardiogram often presents unspecific abnormalities, but it can be helpful in the integrative interpretation of pretest probability of PE.

D. Chest Radiography

Only around 10% of chest radiographs were interpreted as normal in a large series of patients with PE (15–17,20,43,56,58). The most frequent changes described in prospective studies are described in Table 3. The most common chest radiographic finding was atelectasis and/or parenchymal areas of increased opacity; however, the prevalence was not significantly different from that in patients without PE (15–17,58). Pleural effusion

Table 3   Chest Radiographic Abnormalities Associated with Acute Pulmonary Embolism

Abnormality	Incidence (%)
Cardiac enlargement	27–61
Pleural effusion	23–45
Elevated hemidiaphragm	20–62
Pulmonary artery enlargement	16–19
Atelectasis	18–32
Infiltrate	12–17
Oligemia	8–45
Pulmonary infarction	5–15
Pulmonary congestion	1–14
Amputation of pulmonary artery	<1–15

Sources: Adapted from Refs. 17, 20, 55, 57.

increases the likelihood of PE in subjects with suspected PE, but the specificity as diagnostic criterion for PE was low (53,56,58). Miniati et al. (58) found that amputation of hilar artery, oligemia, or consolidations compatible with infarction were present in 45%, 36%, and 15% of patients with PE, respectively. These abnormalities occurred only in 1% of patients without PE. They were good predictors of PE when associated with certain symptoms.

Thus, although chest radiographs are essential in the investigation of suspected PE, their main value is to exclude diagnoses that clinically mimic PE. The signs considered more specific are rare in most series, and their predictive value is not proven.

E. D-Dimer

Levels of D-dimer higher than 500 ng/mL are detectable in nearly all patients with PE with accurate assays (79,80). On the other hand, low D-dimer levels have been found in only about 25% of patients without PE (80). It is unlikely that D-dimer assays would be helpful in patients with recent surgery (within three months) or with malignancy, since so a few of these patients have D-dimer levels below 500 ng/mL (80). The use of D-dimer has been extensively studied. This experience suggests that a D-dimer lower than 500 ng/mL measured by quantitative ELISA in patients with a low or moderate pretest probability are associated with a posttest probability of PE below 5%. Quantitative latex D-dimer test and haemagglutination D-dimers had higher rate of false-negative and may be insufficient as a stand-alone test in patient populations with a higher prevalence of PE, thus, they only can exclude PE in patients with a low clinical probability (67,68,70,79–87).

F. Lung Scanning

Three prospective studies, involving a considerable number of patients, on ventilation/perfusion scanning in the diagnosis of PE (63,64,88–92) have established the value of this technique, particularly when combined with clinical probability (Table 2). From the available evidence, it can be concluded that (1) a normal perfusion lung scan virtually excludes the diagnosis of PE; (2) a high-probability lung scan indicates a high likelihood of emboli, particularly in patients with a high clinical suspicion; and (3) the combination of a low-probability scan with a low probability on clinical grounds is associated with less than 4% of false-negatives, most of them with small emboli (63), further testing might not be needed in such patients. Roughly, 70% of patients present with combinations of clinical and lung ventilation/perfusion scan that cannot confirm or exclude the diagnosis of pulmonary emboli with certainty (63,88–92).

Chest radiographs are used to evaluate lung scans for PE. In patients with pleural effusions, the fluid may gravitate to different regions of the pleural space, depending upon the position of patients, and thus apparent defects can be seen in different locations than the effusion in the chest radiograph when each is performed in different positions (93). In addition, pleural effusion may enter the major fissures when the patients lie down. In moderate or large effusions, a therapeutic thoracocentesis before ventilation/perfusion scan has been recommended (93), measuring the pleural fluid pressure in order to aspirate as much fluid as possible (94). Following the criteria of Biello et al. (95) for the interpretation of defects in lung scans corresponding with radiological abnormalities, Goldberg et al. (59) found that 45% of patients with matched ventilation–perfusion defects of the same size as the effusion were angiographically positive for PE. They concluded that

matched ventilation–perfusion scans corresponding to radiologically evident pleural effusions are of intermediate probability for PE. Thus, they did not recommend revision of
the traditional lung interpretative criteria based upon pleural effusions.

G.   Alveolar Dead Space

In 1 trial out of 398 subjects, a combination of the seven-variable clinical model (Table 2),
nonenzyme-linked immunosorbent assay D-dimer test (positive/negative), and alveolar
dead-space fraction ($\leq$0.15, negative; and >0.15, positive) was used. When two of these
three criteria were negative, PE was excluded. This approach was as safe as a standard
strategy of starting with ventilation–perfusion scan (96). While these results need of
confirmation the approach is appealing because in a fairly larger proportion (34% using
the three test vs. 18% only with the clinical probability assessment and the D-dimer) PE
could be discarded at beside.

H.   Venous Studies

Two modalities of noninvasive venous studies have been tested color-flow Doppler
with compression ultrasound and impedance plethysmography. Compared to venography, venous ultrasonography has high sensitivity (89–100%) and specificity (89–100%)
for the detection of a first episode of proximal deep venous thrombosis (97). Impedance
pletismography offers lower sensitivity, similar specificity, is portable, and its cost is
lower in comparison to venous ultrasonography (98). The rationality under the use of
lower extremity venous studies is that if venous thrombosis is detected, the treatment
would be equally anticoagulation and therefore no further testing would be necessary,
particularly in patients with intermediate clinical or scanning probabilities (99–104),
however, less than 30% of PE show venous thrombosis detected by ultrasound and 3% of
false-positives have been reported (105). Complete lower limb venous ultrasonography
examining both the proximal (femoral and popliteal) and distal (calf) veins in this setting
seems to significantly increase this yield (106).

Venous studies have shown to be helpful in the management of PE, but the predictive
value of the studies depends on their completeness and the quality of the operator, thus
they probably should be reserved for centers with experience.

I.   Helical Computed Tomography

Helical computed tomograph pulmonary angiography (CTPA) with intravenous contrast
has gained acceptance for the diagnosis of PE in part due to its availability (107,108).
Potential additional benefits of CTPA are its ability to help in the diagnosis of competing
diseases (19,109) and potentially to image the subdiaphragmatic deep veins (even the legs)
at the same session (110). Different reports have shown specificities generally greater
than 90%, but wide differences in sensitivities (109,111–114). In the largest study to date
(824 patients), the accuracy of CTPA was determined by comparison against a composite
reference standard (114). Sensitivity was 83% and specificity 96%. The addition of
venous-phase imaging further improved the sensitivity (to 90%). As with lung scintigraphy the accuracy was affected by considering clinical pre-test probability. The positive
predictive values were 96%, 92%, and 58%, and the negative predictive values were
96%, 89%, and 60%, respectively, with high, intermediate, or low clinical probabilities.

The variability in sensitivities among studies may be due to differences in patient selection, extent of pulmonary emboli, technology, and readers' experience. Thus, the extrapolation of the operating characteristics of CTPA from published studies to one's local environment must be undertaken with some caution (114). If local experience and technique are of good quality, the main recognized limitation of helical CTPA is its lack of resolution for detecting isolated subsegmental emboli. In a meta-analysis of 23 studies reported on 4657 patients with negative CTPA results, who did not receive anticoagulation, the three-month rate of subsequent venous thromboembolic events was 1.4% and the three-month rate of fatal PE was 0.51% (115), similar to that seen after negative results on conventional pulmonary angiography (10). On the other hand, the three-month rate of subsequent thromboembolic events was 5.3% in subjects with negative CTPA, but with a high clinical probability of PE (115).

Thus, provided that the equipment, methodology and experience of the interpreters of the images are adequate, CTPA is a fairly sensitive and specific procedure. Furthermore, it is safe in most instances to withhold anticoagulation after negative CTPA results. Caution is warranted, however, when there are discrepancies between CTPA results and the clinical probability of PE, and in such instances additional tests are usually necessary.

J. Magnetic Resonance Angiography

Technological advances, including respiratory gating, ultrafast techniques performed during breath holding, and the use of gadolinium, offer promise for an expanded role of magnetic resonance imaging. Preliminary studies show sensitivities between 98% and 70% with high specificity (116–118). Magnetic resonance imaging is also useful for studying the venous systems of the pelvis and lower extremities.

Currently, magnetic resonance does not seem to offer advantages over CTPA and its availability is lower.

K. Pulmonary Angiography

This is the definitive diagnostic technique in PE. A negative pulmonary angiogram seems to exclude clinically relevant PE. Mortality is <0.5% and morbidity about 5%, usually related to catheter insertion or contrast reactions (63,119).

L. Multimodality Algorithms

Two systematic reviews of multimodalty strategies that combined clinical assessment of pretest probability of PE, D-dimer determination and lung scintigraphy with noninvasive tests for lower extremity venous thrombosis and in a few studies CTPA (86,120) concluded that (1) high-probability ventilation–perfusion lung scan or positive venous ultrasonography in patients with a moderate or high pretest probability are associated with a greater than 85% post-test probability of PE; (2) a normal appearance on lung scan, a negative CTPA along with a negative venous ultrasonography and a D-dimer concentration <500 mg/L measured by quantitative ELISA in patients with a low or moderate pretest probability were associated with a posttest probability of PE below 5%; and (3) low-probability ventilation–perfusion lung scan, magnetic resonance angiography, a quantitative latex D-dimer test, and haemagglutination D-dimers had higher false-negative rates and can only exclude PE in patients with a low pretest probability (86,120). None of these algorithms have shown to perform substantially better than the others (86,120). These approaches are only considered appropriate if the patient is stable (i.e., hemodynamically stable and without severe hypoxemia).

Only one large (3306 patients) prospective study has analyzed a simplified algorithm using a modified version of the Well's criteria for clinical pretest probability assessment (Table 2), quantitative ELISA D-dimer, and CTPA (68). In this study, PE was discarded in 1028 subjects by a clinical categorization as "unlikely PE" and low D-dimer and less than 0.5% had thrombombomebolic events during the three months of follow-up. In the rest of the subjects CTPA was performed, resulting negative results in 1436 subjects who were not treated. Less than 1.5% had thromboembolic events and only 0.2% had fatal events (68). This study suggests that when good CTPA is available other image tests might not be necessary, however, the cost-efficiency of this approach has not been established and may vary depending on the availability and quality of other resources such as venous ultrasonography and lung scintigraphy.

V. Conclusion

Pleural effusions due to PE are frequently not recognized as such. Pleural fluid characteristics and radiological characteristics are variable, therefore, PE should be considered in the differential diagnosis of every patient with an acute pleural effusion, particularly if unilateral, medium size and of exudative nature. The decision whether to pursue further diagnostic procedures requires clinical judgment that is guided by the patient's presentation. The presence of thromboembolic risk, pleuritic chest pain, dyspnea, tachypnea, or fainting, the likelihood of alternative diagnosis, and the association to other radiological and electro-cardiographic alterations will allow us to decide on the basis of the clinical probability for PE. PE is very unlike in those not presenting any important clinical manifestation of the disease. If PE is suspected and if the patient is stable, combinations of clinical assessment, D-dimer testing, dead-space assessment, lung scanning, venous ultrasound, or CTPA will confirm or exclude acute pulmonary emboli in most patients. In other cases, pulmonary angiography remains the gold standard for diagnosis.

References

1. Dismuke SE, Wagner EH. Pulmonary embolism as a cause of death. The changing mortality in hospitalized patients. JAMA 1986; 255:2039–2042.
2. Anderson FA Jr, Wheeler HB, Goldberg RJ, et al. A population-based perspective of the hospital incidence and case-fatality rates of deep vein thrombosis and pulmonary embolism: The Worcester DVT Study. Arch Intern Med 1991; 151:933–938.
3. Silverstein MD, Heit JA, Mohr DN, et al. Trends in the incidence of deep venous thrombosis and pulmonary embolism. A 25 yr population based study. Arch Intern Med 1998; 158:585–593.
4. Barritt DW, Jordon SC. Anticoagulant drugs in the treatment of pulmonary embolism: A controlled trial. Lancet 1960; 1:1309–1313.
5. Kanis JA. Heparin in the treatment of pulmonary thromboembolism. Thromb Diath Haemorrh 1974; 32:519–527.
6. Alpert JS, Smith R, Carlson J, et al. Mortality in patients treated for pulmonary embolism. JAMA 1976; 236:1477–1480.

7. Carson JL, Kelley MA, Duff A, et al. The clinical course of pulmonary embolism. N Engl J Med 1992; 326:1240–1245.

8. Douketis JD, Kearon C, Bates S, et al. Risk of fatal pulmonary embolism in patients with treated venous thromboembolism. JAMA 1998; 279:458–462.

9. Donaldson GA, Williams C, Scanell J. A reappraisal of the application of the Trendelenburg operation to massive fatal embolism. N Engl J Med 1963; 268:171–174.

10. Goldhaber SZ, Hennekens CH, Evans DA, et al. Factors associated with correct antemortem diagnosis of major pulmonary embolism. Am J Med 1982; 73:822–826.

11. Morgenthaler TI, Ryu JW. Clinical characteristics of fatal pulmonary embolism in a referral hospital. Mayo Clin Proc 1995; 70:417–424.

12. Stein PD, Henry JW. Prevalence of acute pulmonary embolism among patients in a general hospital and at autopsy. Chest 1995; 108:978–981.

13. Moser KM. Pulmonary embolism. Am Rev Respir Dis 1977; 115:829–852.

14. Bynum LJ, Wilson JE. Radiographic features of pleural effusions in pulmonary embolisms. Am Rev Respir Dis 1978; 117:829–834.

15. Stein PD, Terrin ML, Hales CA, et al. Clinical, laboratory, roentgenographic, and electrocardiographic findings in patients with acute pulmonary embolism and no pre-existing cardiac or pulmonary disease. Chest 1991; 100:598–603.

16. Stein PD, Saltzman HA, Weg JG. Clinical characteristics of patients with acute pulmonary embolism. Am J Cardiol 1991; 68:1723–1724.

17. Worsley DF, Alavi A, Aronchick JM, et al. Chest radiographic findings in patients with acute pulmonary embolism: Observations from the PIOPED study. Radiology 1993; 189: 133–136.

18. Coche EE, Müller NL, Kim K. Acute pulmonary embolism: Ancillary findings at helical CT. Radiology 1998; 207:753–758.

19. Shah AA, Davis SD, Gamsu G, et al. Parenchyma and pleural findings in patients with and without acute pulmonary embolism detected at helical CT. Radiology 1999; 211: 147–153.

20. Elliott CG, Goldhaber SZ, Visani L, et al. Chest radiographs in acute pulmonary embolism. Results from the International Cooperative Pulmonary Embolism Registry. Chest 2000; 118:33–38.

21. Porcel JM, Madroñero AB, Pardina M, et al. Analysis of pleural effusions in acute pulmonary embolism: Radiological and pleural fluid data from 230 patients. Respirology 2007; 12:234–239.

22. Moser KM, Fedullo PF, LitteJohn JK, et al. Frequent asymptomatic pulmonary embolism in patients with deep venous thrombosis. JAMA 1994; 271:223–225.

23. Olsen JH. Epidemiology of lung cancer. In: Spiro SG, ed. Carcinoma of the Lung. Sheffield, U.K.: European Respiratory Journals Ltd., 1995:1–18.

24. Griner PF. Bloody pleural fluid following pulmonary infarction. JAMA 1967; 202:123–125.

25. Light RW, MacGregor MI, Luchsinger PC, et al. Pleural effusions: The diagnostic separation of transudates and exudates. Ann Intern Med 1972; 77:507–613.

26. Storey DD, Dines DE, Coles DT. Pleural effusion: A diagnostic dilemma. JAMA 1976; 236:2183–2186.

27. Marel M, Zrustova M, Stasny B, et al. The incidence of pleural effusion in a well-defined region: Epidemiologic study in central Bohemia. Chest 1993; 104:1486–1489.

28. Valdés L, Alvarez D, Valle JM, et al. The etiology of pleural effusions in an area with high incidence of tuberculosis. Chest 1996; 109:158–162.

29. Preterman TA, Speicher CE. Evaluating pleural effusions: A two stage laboratory approach. JAMA 1984; 252:1051–1053.

30. Mattison LE, Copagge L, Alderman F, et al. Pleural effusion in the medical ICU: Prevalence, causes and clinical implications. Chest 1997; 111:1018–1023.

31.   Villena V, López Encuentra A, Echave-Sustaeta J, et al. Prospective study of 1000 consecutive patients with pleural effusion. Etiology of the effusion and characteristics of the patients. Arch Bronconeumol 2002; 38:21–26.
32.   Race GA, Scheifley CH, Edward JE. Hydrothorax in congestive heart failure. Am J Med 1957; 22:83–89.
33.   Broaddus VC, Wiener-Kronish JP, Berthiaume Y, et al. Removal of pleural liquid and protein by lymphatics in awake sheep. J Appl Physiol 1988; 64:384–390.
34.   Stewart PB. The rate of formation and lymphatic removal of fluid in pleural effusions. J Clin Invest 1963; 42:258–262.
35.   Bynum LJ, Wilson JE II. Characteristics of pleural effusions associated with pulmonary embolism. Arch Intern Med 1976; 136:159–162.
36.   Romero Candeira S, Hernández Blasco L, Soler MJ, et al. Biochemical and cytological characteristics of pleural effusions secondary to pulmonary embolism. Chest 2002; 121:465–469.
37.   Light RW. Diseases of the pleura. Curr Opin Pulm Med 1995; 1:313–317.
38.   Cheng D, Rodriguez RM, Perkett EA, et al. Vascular endothelial growth factor in pleural fluid. Chest 1999; 116:760–765.
39.   Wiener-Kronish JP, Broaddus VC, Albertine KH, et al. Relationship of pleural effusions to increased permeability pulmonary edema in anesthetized sheep. J Clin Invest 1988; 82:1422–1429.
40.   Albertine KH, Wiener-Kronish JP, Roos PJ, et al. Structure, blood supply, and lymphatic vessels of the sheep's visceral pleura. Am J Anat 1982; 165:277–294.
41.   Villena V, López-Encuentra A, García-Luján R, et al. Clinical implications of appearance of pleural fluid at thoracentesis. Chest 2004; 125:156–159.
42.   Stein P, Huang H, Afzal A, et al. Incidence of acute pulmonary embolism in a general hospital. Chest 1999; 116:909–913.
43.   Goldhaber SZ, Visan L, DeRosa M for ICOPER. Acute pulmonary embolism: Clinical outcomes in the International Cooperative Pulmonary Embolism Registry (ICOPER). Lancet 1999; 353:1386–1389.
44.   Simon H, Daggett WM, DeSanctis R. Hemothorax as a complication of anticoagulant therapy in the presence of pulmonary infarction. JAMA 1969; 208:1830–1834.
45.   Wick MR, Ritter JH, Schuller D. Ruptured pulmonary infarction: A rare, fatal complication of thromboembolic disease. Mayo Clin Proc 2000; 75:639–642.
46.   McGoldrick PJ, Rudd TG, Figley MM, et al. What becomes of pulmonary infarcts. AJR 1979; 133:1039–1045.
47.   Sklaroff HJ. The post-pulmonary infarction syndrome. Am Heart J 1979; 98:772–776.
48.   Jerjes-Sanchez C, Ibarra-Perez C, Ramirez-Rivera A, et al. Dressler-like syndrome after pulmonary embolism and infarction. Chest 1987; 92:115–117.
49.   Dressler W. The post-myocardial infarction syndrome: A report of forty-four cases. Arch Intern Med 1959; 103:28.
50.   Stelzner TJ, King TE Jr, Antony VB, et al. The pleuropulmonary manifestations of postcardiac injury syndrome. Chest 1983; 84:383–387.
51.   Welin L, Vedin A, Wilhelmsson C. Characteristics, prevalence, and prognosis of postmyocardial infarction syndrome. Br Heart J 1983; 50:140–145.
52.   Khan AH. The postcardiac injury syndromes. Clin Cardiol 1992; 15:67–72.
53.   McNeil BJ, Hessel SJ, Branch WT. Measures of clinical efficacy: 3, The value of lung scan in the evaluation of lung patients with pleuritic chest pain. J Nucl Med 1976; 17:163–164.
54.   Stein P, Henry JW. Clinical characteristics of patients with acute pulmonary embolism stratified according to their presenting syndromes. Chest 1997; 112:74–79.
55.   Erkan L, Fýndýk S, Uzun O, et al. A new radiologic appearance of pulmonary thromboembolism: Multiloculated pleural effusions. Chest 2004; 126:298–302.

56. Talbot S, Worthington BS, Roebuck EJ. Radiographic signs of pulmonary embolism and pulmonary infarction. Thorax 1973; 28:198–203.
57. Adelman M, Albelda SM, Gottlieb J, et al. Diagnostic utility of pleural fluid eosinophilia. Am J Med 1984; 77:915–920.
58. Miniati M, Predileto R, Formichi B, et al. Accuracy of clinical assessment in the diagnosis of pulmonary embolism. Am J Respir Crit Care Med 1999; 158:864–871.
59. Goldberg SN, Richardson DD, Palmer EL, et al. Pleural effusion and ventilation/perfusion scan interpretation for acute pulmonary embolus. J Nucl Med 1996; 37:1310–1313.
60. Rabin CB, Blackman NS. Bilateral pleural effusions. Its significance in association with a heart of normal size. J Mt Sinai Hosp 1957; 24:45–63.
61. Liao H, Na MJ, Dikensoy O, et al. Diagnostic value of pleural fluid N-terminal pro-brain natriuretic peptide levels in patients with cardiovascular diseases. Respirology 2008; 13:53–57.
62. Bell WR, Simon TL, DeMets DL. The clinical features of submassive and massive pulmonary emboli. Am J Med 1977; 62:355–360.
63. The PIOPED Investigators. Value of the ventilation/perfusion scan in acute pulmonary embolism. Results of the prospective investigation of pulmonary embolism diagnosis (PIOPED). JAMA 1990; 263:2753–2759.
64. Miniati M, Pistolesi M, Marini G, et al. Value of perfusion lung scan in the diagnosis of pulmonary embolism: Results of the Prospective Investigative Study of Acute Pulmonary Embolism Diagnosis (PISA-PED). Am J Respir Crit Care Med 1996; 154:1387–1393.
65. Perrier A, Bounameaux H, Morabia A, et al. A diagnosis of pulmonary embolism by a decision analysis-based strategy including clinical probability, D-dimer levels, and ultrasonography: A management study. Arch Intern Med 1996; 156:531–536.
66. Stein PD, Henry JW, Gottschalk A. The addition of clinical assessment to stratification according to prior cardiopulmonary disease further optimizes the interpretation of ventilation/perfusion lung scans in pulmonary embolism. Chest 1993; 104:1472–1476.
67. Wells PS, Ginsberg JS, Anderson DR, et al. Use of a clinical model for safe management of patients with suspected pulmonary embolism. Ann Intern Med 1998; 129:997–1005.
68. van Belle A, Büller HR, Huisman MV, et al. Christopher Study Investigators. Effectiveness of managing suspected pulmonary embolism using an algorithm combining clinical probability, D-dimer testing, and computed tomography. JAMA 2006; 295:172–179.
69. Rodger MA, Carrier M, Jones GN, et al. Diagnostic value of arterial blood gas measurement in suspected pulmonary embolism. Am J Respir Crit Care Med 2000; 162:2105–2108.
70. Egermayer P, Town GI, Turner JG, et al. Usefulness of D-dimer, blood gas, and respiratory rate measurements for excluding pulmonary embolism. Thorax 1998; 53:830–834.
71. Kline JA, Hernandez-Nino J, Newgard CD, et al. Use of pulse oximetry to predict in-hospital complications in normotensive patients with pulmonary embolism. Am J Med 2003; 115:203–208.
72. Hyers TM. Venous thromboembolism. Am J Respir Crit Care Med 1999; 159:1–14.
73. Kiely DG, Kennedy NS, Pirzada O, et al. Elevated levels of natriuretic peptides in patients with pulmonary thromboembolism. Respir Med 2005; 99:1286–1291.
74. Horlander KT, Leeper KV. Troponin levels as a guide to treatment of pulmonary embolism. Curr Opin Pulm Med 2003; 9:374–377.
75. Kostrubiec M, Pruszczyk P, Bochowicz A, et al. Biomarker-based risk assessment model in acute pulmonary embolism. Eur Heart J 2005; 26:2166–2172.
76. Söhne M, en wolde M, Boomsma F, et al. Brain natriuretic peptide in hemodynamically stable acute pulmonary embolism. J Thromb Haemost 2006; 4:552–556.

77. Ferrari E, Imbert A, Chevalier T, et al. The ECG in pulmonary embolism: Predictive value of negative T waves in precordial leads-80 case reports. Chest 1997; 111:537–543.

78. The Urokinase Pulmonary Embolism Trial: A national cooperative study. Circulation 1973; 47(Suppl. 2):1–108.

79. Goldhaber SZ, Simons GR, Elliott CG, et al. Quantitative plasma D-dimer levels among patients undergoing pulmonary angiography for suspected pulmonary embolism. JAMA 1993; 270:2819–2822.

80. Bounameaux H, de Moerloose P, Perrier A, et al. Plasma measurement of D-dimer as diagnostic aid in suspected venous thromboembolism: An overview. Thromb Haemost 1994; 71:1–6.

81. Bates SM, Grand'Maison A, Johnston M, et al. A latex D-dimer reliably excludes venous thromboembolism. Arch Intern Med 2001; 161:447–453.

82. Ginsberg JS, Wells PS, Kearon C, et al. Sensitivity and specificity of a rapid whole-blood assay for D-dimer in the diagnosis of pulmonary embolism. Ann Intern Med 1998; 129:1006–1011.

83. Oger E, Leroyer C, Bressollette L, et al. Evaluation of a new, rapid and quantitative D-dimer test in patients with suspected pulmonary embolism. Am J Respir Crit Care Med 1998; 158:65–70.

84. Roy PM, Colombet I, Durieux P, et al. Systematic review and meta-analysis of strategies for the diagnosis of suspected pulmonary embolism. BMJ 2005; 331:259.

85. Kruip MJ, Leclercq MG, van der Heul C, et al. Diagnostic strategies for excluding pulmonary embolism in clinical outcome studies. A systematic review. Ann Intern Med 2003; 138:941–951.

86. Lee AY, Julian JA, Levine MN, et al. Clinical utility of a rapid whole-blood D-dimer assay in patients with cancer who present with suspected acute deep venous thrombosis. Ann Intern Med 1999; 131:417–423.

87. Farrell S, Hayes T, Shaw M. A negative SimpliRED D-dimer assay result does not exclude the diagnosis of deep vein thrombosis or pulmonary embolus in emergency department patients. Ann Emerg Med 2000; 35:121–125.

88. Hull RD, Hirsh CJ, Carter CJ, et al. Diagnostic value of ventilation–perfusion lung scanning, in patients with suspected pulmonary embolism. Chest 1985; 88:819–828.

89. Hull RD, Raskob GE. Low-probability lung scan findings: A need for change. Ann Intern Med 1991; 114:142–143.

90. Bone RC. The low-probability scan. A potentially lethal reading. Arch Itern Med 1993; 153:2621–2622.

91. Tapson VF, Carroll BA, Davidson BL, et al. The diagnostic approach to acute venous thromboembolism. Am J Respir Crit Care Med 1999; 160:1043–1066.

92. Stein PD, Gottschalk A. Critical review of ventilation–perfusion scans in acute pulmonary embolism. Prog Cardiovasc Dis 1994; 37:13–24.

93. Light RW. Pleural Diseases. 4th ed. Philadelphia, PA: Lippincott Williams & Wilkins, 2001.

94. Villena V, Lopez-Encuentra A, Pozo F, et al. Measurement of pleural pressure during therapeutic thoracentesis. Am J Respir Crit Care Med 2000; 162:1534–1538.

95. Biello DR, Mattar AG, McKnight RC, et al. Ventilation–perfusion studies in suspected pulmonary embolism. AJR Am J Roentgenol 1979; 133:1033–1037.

96. Rodger MA, Bredeson CN, Jones G, et al. The bedside investigation of pulmonary embolism diagnosis study: A double-blind randomized controlled trial comparing combinations of 3 bedside tests vs. ventilation–perfusion scan for the initial investigation of suspected pulmonary embolism. Arch Intern Med 2006; 166:181–187.

97. Kearon C, Ginsberg JS, Hirsh J. The role of venous ultrasonography in the diagnosis of suspected deep venous thrombosis and pulmonary embolism. Ann Intern Med 1998; 129:1044–1049.

98. Wells PS, Hirsh J, Anderson DR, et al. Comparison of the accuracy of impedance plethys-mography and compression ultrasonography in outpatients with clinically suspected deep venous thrombosis. Thromb Haemost 1995; 74:1423–1427.

99. Stevens SM, Elliott CG, Chan KJ, et al. Withholding anticoagulation after a negative result on duplex ultrasonography for suspected symptomatic deep venous thrombosis. Ann Intern Med 2004 15; 140:985–991.

100. Hull RD, Raskob GE, Ginsberg A, et al. A noninvasive strategy for the treatment of patients with suspected pulmonary embolism. Arch Intern Med 1994; 154:289–297.

101. Wells PS, Ginsberg JS, Anderson DR, et al. Use of a clinical model for safe man-agement of patients with suspected pulmonary embolism. Ann Intern Med 1998; 129: 997–1005.

102. Wells PS, Anderson DR, Rodger M, et al. Derivation of a simple clinical model to cate-gorize patients probability of pulmonary embolism: Increasing the models utility with the SimpliRED D-dimer. Thromb Haemost 2000; 83:416–420.

103. Perrier A, Desmarais S, Miron MJ, et al. Non-invasive diagnosis of venous thromboembolism in outpatients. Lancet 1999; 353:190–195.

104. Musset D, Parent F, Meyer G, et al. Evaluation du Scanner Spiralé dans l'Embolie Pul-monaire study group. Diagnostic strategy for patients with suspected pulmonary embolism: A prospective multicentre outcome study. Lancet 2002; 360:1914–1920.

105. Turkstra F, Kuijer PM, van Beek EJ, et al. Diagnostic utility of ultrasonography of leg veins in patients suspected of having pulmonary embolism. Ann Intern Med 1997; 126: 775–781.

106. Elias A, Colombier D, Victor G, et al. Diagnostic performance of complete lower limb venous ultrasound in patients with clinically suspected acute pulmonary embolism. Thromb Haemost 2004; 91:187–195.

107. Trowbridge RL, Araoz PA, Gotway MB, et al. The effect of helical computed tomography on diagnostic and treatment strategies in patients with suspected pulmonary embolism. Am J Med 2004; 116:84–90.

108. Garg K, Welsh CH, Feyerabend AJ, et al. Pulmonary embolism: Diagnosis with spiral CT and ventilation–perfusion scanning-correlation with pulmonary angiographic results or clinical outcome. Radiology 1998; 208:201–208.

109. Schoepf UJ, Goldhaber SZ, Costello P. Spiral computed tomography for acute pulmonary embolism. Circulation 2004; 109:2160–2167.

110. Loud PA, Katz DS, Klippenstein DL, et al. Combined CT venography and pulmonary angiog-raphy in suspected thromboembolic disease: Diagnostic accuracy for deep venous evaluation. Am J Roentgenol 2000; 174:161–164.

111. Remy-Jardin M, Remy J, Wattinne L, et al. Central pulmonary thromboembolism: Diagnosis with volumetric CT with the single-breath-holding technique comparison with pulmonary angiography. Radiology 1992; 185:381–387.

112. Drucker EA, Rivitz SM, Shepard JA, et al. Acute pulmonary embolism: Assessment of helical CT for diagnosis. Radiology 1998; 209:235–241.

113. Rathbun SW, Raskob GE, Whitsett TL. Sensitivity and specificity of helical computed tomog-raphy in the diagnosis of pulmonary embolism: A systematic review. Ann Intern Med 2000; 132:227–232.

114. Stein PD, Fowler SE, Goodman LR, et al. PIOPED II Investigators. Multidetector computed tomography for acute pulmonary embolism. N Engl J Med 2006; 354:2317–2327.

115. Moores LK, Jackson WL Jr, Shorr AF, et al. Meta-analysis: Outcomes in patients with sus-pected pulmonary embolism managed with computed tomographic pulmonary angiography. Ann Intern Med 2004; 141:866–874.

116. Meaney JF, Weg JG, Chenevert TL, et al. Diagnosis of pulmonary embolism with magnetic resonance angiography. N Engl J Med 1997; 336:1422–1427.

117. Gupta A, Frazer CK, Ferguson JM, et al. Acute pulmonary embolism: Diagnosis with MR angiography. Radiology 1999; 210:353–359.
118. Oudkerk M, van Beek EJ, Wielopolski P, et al. Comparison of contrast-enhanced magnetic resonance angiography and conventional pulmonary angiography for the diagnosis of pulmonary embolism: A prospective study. Lancet 2002; 359:1643–1647.
119. Stein PD, Athanasoulis C, Alavi A, et al. Complications and validity of pulmonary angiography in acute pulmonary embolism. Circulation 1992; 85:462–468.
120. Kruip MJ, Leclercq MG, van der Heul C, et al. Diagnostic strategies for excluding pulmonary embolism in clinical outcome studies. A systematic review. Ann Intern Med 2003; 138:941–951.

39
Pleural Effusions in Children

JOHN N. TSANAKAS and ELPIS HATZIAGOROU
Aristotelian University of Thessaloniki, Hippokration General Hospital, Thessaloniki, Greece

I. Introduction

Pleural effusions (PE) in children are caused by the same factors that cause PE in adults, but they appear with a different incidence, related to age. In the neonate, PE are usually present either as a part of a generalized disease, like *hydrops fetalis* or congenital heart disease, or as an isolated finding, like chylothorax, intrauterine or perinatal infection, transient tachypnea of the newborn, persistent hypertension of the newborn, etc. (1). In older children, the most common cause is bacterial pneumonia, followed by heart failure, rheumatic disorders, and malignancies (2). Tuberculous effusions are also increasing in frequency (3). In this chapter, we will focus on the most common causes of pleurisy in the pediatric population, the diagnostic approach, and management.

Pleural space is the space formed between the parietal and visceral pleurae. It is a continuous compartment, covering the lung as an envelope filled with a relatively acellular fluid (4,5). This pleural fluid is mainly formed by filtration of fluid from subpleural capillaries at a quantity, which is estimated between 0.1 and 0.2 mL/kg under normal conditions. It acts as a lubricant between the two pleural layers, moves actively from the visceral to the parietal pleura, and is drained there by small openings, called stomata (6–9). Stomata communicate with the pulmonary lymphatics, which drain into the mediastinum, then into the thoracic duct, and finally into the venous circulation. Therefore, the pleural fluid quantity is influenced by changes in its production (e.g., increased vascular permeability in pneumonia) or removal (e.g., increased lymphatic pressure in heart failure, mediastinal tumors).

According to its content, the pleural fluid can be classified as transudate, exudate, and empyema. Transudates are noninflamed fluids, which result from an imbalance between hydrostatic and oncotic pressures. They contain little protein and few mononuclear cells, and their concentrations of glucose, pH, and LDH are similar to those in serum (10). Exudates are the result of inflammation of pleura or obstruction of lymphatic flow. Empyemas (Greek εν + πύον = pus within a space) are heavily infected exudates. The distinction between the three categories of pleural fluid is based on certain markers. A practical classification of PE in children is based on the assessment of the pleural fluid (Table 1).

II. Clinical Presentation

The clinical presentation is related to the cause and the size of the effusion. If, for example, the underlying disease is pneumonia, then cough, fever, and malaise, or even lethargy and

Table 1   Classification of Pleural Effusions in Children

Transudate	Exudate
Congestive heart failure	Infection
Nephrotic syndrome	Malignancy
Chylothorax	Hemothorax
Collagen vascular disease	Pancreatitis
Pulmonary emboli	Perforation of esophagus
Hypothyroidism	Pulmonary infarction
Liver cirrhosis	
Iatrogenic	

cyanosis may precede the development of dyspnea (11). Noninfectious diseases like malignancies may not cause any symptoms if the amount of pleural fluid is small. On the other hand, large infusions may cause cough, respiratory distress of various degree, and orthopnea. Pain on inspiration may be the first sign of an effusion, originating from the sensitive innervation of the parietal pleura (12). The pain may be referred to the ipsilateral shoulder or the abdomen (13). In some cases, abdominal symptoms may mimic acute appendicitis and gastroenteritis (14).

Specific signs include asymmetrical movement of the affected side, dullness to percussion, decreased tactile and voice fremitous, diminished breath sounds, and voice egophony above the effusions. Large effusions may cause scoliosis, contralateral cardiac and tracheal displacement, and/or hepatomegaly, signs that are more prominent in young infants and babies (10). However, the younger the child is the more difficult to elicit and relay on the physical findings. This is due to the poor cooperation of the sick infant and the small size of the rib cage, which transmits the auscultatory findings to the unaffected side.

III. Investigation

The clinical suspicion of PE will be confirmed by various image techniques and examination of the pleural fluid. A chest radiograph in the upright position may show blunting of the costophrenic angle if the amount of fluid is more than 100 to 200 mL, depending on the size of the child. A chest film in the supine position may not show any abnormality if the amount of fluid is small or may appear as a "diffuse haziness" in the affected side (15). Lateral decubitus films, taken with the child lying on the affected side, are more sensitive as they can detect the presence of smaller amounts of fluid, but are applicable only in cooperative patients. A sign of fluid loculation is the inability of the liquid to shift from the upright to decubitus position. The amount of fluid adequate for thoracentesis is considered if the fluid layer is at least 10 mm thick in the decubitus film. Large collections may also cause a shift of the mediastinum to the opposite site [Fig. 1(A)].

Ultrasonography is a very helpful method for the detection of the amount of fluid and its composition in the pleural space (16). It can also distinguish pleural thickening or lung abscess from clear fluid (17). Ultrasound can distinguish the serous anechoic fluid, with no evidence of fibrinous organization from the thick purulent fluid–formatting septations (Figs. 1 and 2). Repeated sonographs are also helpful in monitoring the progress of the disease (16).

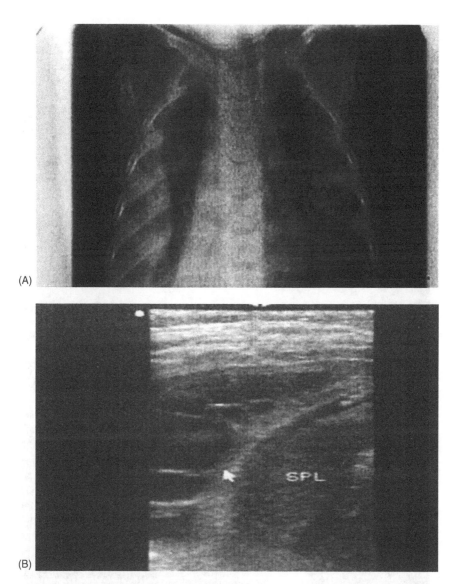

Figure 1 (A) A 2-year-old girl with right-side empyema pushing the trachea to the left. (B) Ultrasonography shows the difference in echogenicity of the pleural fluid, indicating the presence of septated membranes and loculated areas in the pleural space. Tube drainage plus fibrinolysis were successful.

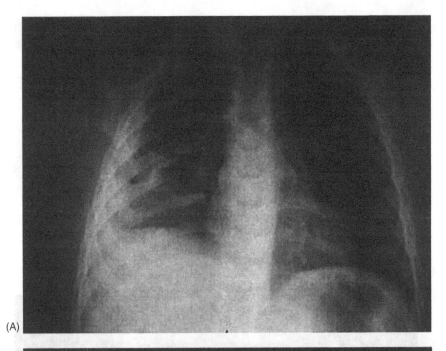

(A)

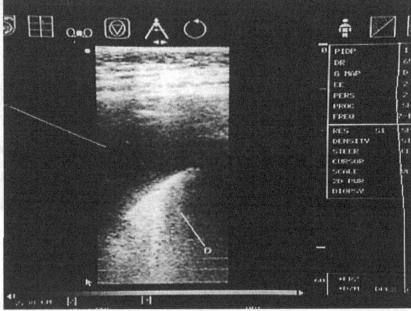

(B)

Figure 2   (A) A 6-year-old boy with right-side pleurisy. (B) Ultrasonography shows the homogeneous echogenicity of the pleural fluid, a sign of uncomplicated effusion. No need for tube drainage or fibrinolysis.

Computed tomography (CT) is helpful for the assessment of atelectasis or probable lung compression. However, being an expensive and time-consuming method, requiring a lot of cooperation, it is not routinely used in children with PE (18). Its application is justified only in selected cases with complicated PE, where there is a need to discriminate abscess formation from empyema, or when an underlying lung disorder is suspected (19).

Thoracocentesis and pleural fluid analysis are necessary investigations for the majority of children with PE, with an exception of minor effusions of obvious cause, like uncomplicated viral infections, congestive heart failure, nephrotic syndrome, and ascites (20). Some investigators advocate thoracocentesis in every child with PE, while others reserve it only to those with a suspicion of an infection (21,22). In our institution, we perform thoracocentesis in all children presenting with PE, excluding those with very little fluid and those who need drainage tubes.

Thoracocentesis is a relatively safe procedure in children, with no absolute contraindications and rare complications, the most common of which is pain at the insertion site. Other complications include iatrogenic pneumothorax, infection, intercostal nerve damage, and puncture of the liver or spleen (23). Ultrasounds help to determine the exact location for thoracocentesis, which is usually 1 to 2 cm below the onset of dullness to percussion (21,24).

The procedure (Table 2) must be followed up carefully under strictly aseptic conditions to avoid contamination of the pleural space. Examination of the pleural fluid is of utmost importance for the majority of PE in children. The gross appearance of the fluid will help to distinguish the milky fluid of chylothorax from the purulent fluid of empyema or from the pale yellow liquid of a transudate or an exudate. Bloody fluid may be due to trauma or malignancy. Further chemical and cellular analyses are necessary to confirm the diagnosis (Table 3).

The diagnostic value of these tests for the differentiation between transudates and exudates is not as strong as it is in adults, and the results should always be interpreted in relation to the clinical findings (25,26). Pleural fluid pH in discriminating transudates

Table 2 Procedure for Thoracentesis

Parental information	Inform the parents and the child (if possible) of the procedure and the need for it.
Sedation	Use chloral hydrate or midazolam to relieve agitation.
Position of patient	Older children may be comfortably seated, leaning forward over a pillow. Young infants and babies must be supine leaning on the affected side, supported by an assistant.
Analgesia	Is achieved with topical application of xylocaine.
Technique	The exact site for thoracentesis will be decided with the aid of ultrasonography, which must be performed immediately before the procedure. The needle is usually inserted at the 7th interspace in the mid-axillary or the posterior axillary line, aiming toward the center of the rib below the interspace. Upon entering the skin, move the needle and the skin up so that the needle passes over the top of the rib and into the pleural space. Aspirate a small amount of fluid and gently remove the needle.

Source: Adapted from Ref. 13.

Table 3 Laboratory Studies for Pleural Fluid Specimens

Chemistry	Glucose, protein, pH, LDH, amylase, cholesterol, triglycerides
Cytology	Total and differential cell count; cytological examination for malignancy
Microbiology	Gram stain, bacterial culture

from exudates and empyemas in children has been proposed by some authors (21) with the additional advantage of rapid diagnosis (27). Pneumococcal antigen detection in pleural fluid specimens from children provides a rapid and sensitive method of diagnosis of pneumococcal empyema, which can be confirmed by specific pneumolysin PCR when culture results are negative. Broad-range 16S rDNA PCR has value in detecting bacterial agents responsible for culture-negative pleural empyema (28).

IV. Diagnostic and Therapeutic Approach

A rational approach to the child with PE is presented in Figure 3.

A. Parapneumonic Effusions

These are by far the most common cause of PE in the pediatric population. They are usually complications of pneumonias and may be caused by viruses like influenza, parainfluenza, adenovirus, and rhinovirus, or by bacteria like *Staphylococcus aureus*, *Streptococcus pneumoniae*, and *Haemophilus influenzae*. Other less common organisms include *Streptococcus pyogenes*, Enterobacteriaceae, anaerobes, *Legionella*, and *Histoplasma*. The incidence of infectious PE in hospitalized children varies between 50% and 78%, with a recent increase in empyemas (29–31). *S. aureus* used to be the predominant causative organism of empyema, but recently has been replaced by *S. pneumoniae*, followed by *H. influenzae* (32). In a number of cases the bacterial pathogen cannot be isolated.

The clinical presentation of parapneumonic effusions varies, with empyema being the worst end. Cough, chest pain, progressive dyspnea, and high fever not responding to antibiotics are highly suggestive of empyema. Examination of the pleural fluid will help to establish the diagnosis. With no proper treatment, the pleural fluid passes within hours from the exudative stage (clear, serous, sterile fluid) to the fibrinopurulent stage (thick pus with fibrin clots, formatting fibrin membranes, with collections of fluid in between), and finally within one to three weeks to the organizational stage (invasion of fibroblasts and formation of a thick nonelastic pleura) (33).

The management of a parapneumonic effusion involves eradication of the causative organism using the proper antibiotics and drainage of the pleural cavity at the earliest possible stage. Effusions, which are enlarging and/or compromising respiratory function, should not be managed by antibiotics alone. Consideration should be given to early active treatment, as conservative treatment results in prolonged duration of illness and hospital stay (34).

The choice of proper antibiotics largely depends on the results of the pleural fluid or blood culture, which are not always positive (14,35). As a first-line combination, the use of a third-generation cephalosporin plus antistaphylococcal β-lactamase–resistant penicillin is recommended in all cases with empyema (32). In cases of resistant streptococci or anaerobic pathogens, clindamycin should be used, while vancomycin should be reserved

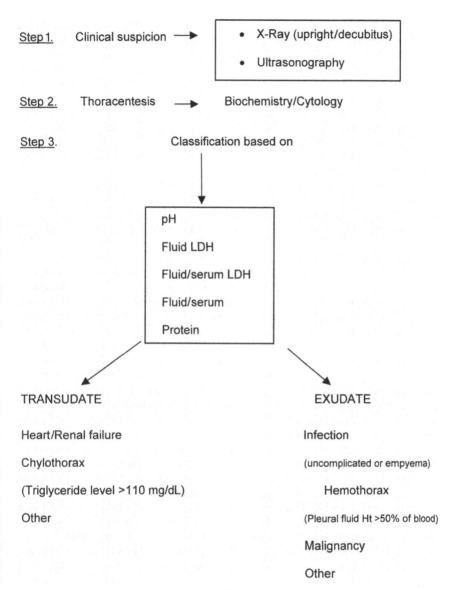

Step 1. Clinical suspicion ⟶ • X-Ray (upright/decubitus)

• Ultrasonography

Step 2. Thoracentesis ⟶ Biochemistry/Cytology

Step 3. Classification based on

pH

Fluid LDH

Fluid/serum LDH

Fluid/serum

Protein

TRANSUDATE

Heart/Renal failure

Chylothorax

(Triglyceride level >110 mg/dL)

Other

EXUDATE

Infection

(uncomplicated or empyema)

Hemothorax

(Pleural fluid Ht >50% of blood)

Malignancy

Other

Figure 3   Steps for the diagnosis of common PE in children.

for the very severe life-threatening cases of methicillin-resistant *S. aureus*. Once the causative organism is identified, the proper antibiotic should replace the empirical regime.

Drainage of the pleural cavity has changed during the last decade from a more conservative policy to an earlier operative treatment (14,35,36). The treatment of choice is related to the phase of the pleural fluid. During the exudative or early fibrinopurulent stage, a tube drainage and fibrinolytics may be effective, whereas at the organizational stage, interventional thoracoscopy or thoracotomy is necessary. The accuracy of ultrasonography in the detection of the location and the quantity and the quality of the pleural fluid has led to a more rational treatment and reduced hospitalization (16). Computed tomography may be helpful, but may not be adequate to differentiate between the fibrinopurulent and organizing phases of empyema (37).

In case of chest drainage, the drain should be removed once there is clinical resolution. A drain that cannot be unblocked should be removed but replaced if significant pleural fluid remains. Since there is no evidence that large bore chest drains confer any advantage, small drains (including pigtail catheters) should be used whenever possible to minimize patient discomfort (34).

Chest physiotherapy is not beneficial and should not be performed in children with empyema, while early mobilization and exercise are strongly recommended (34). It is important that the child be encouraged not to stay immobilized in bed while having the tube, as this may lead to impaired pulmonary toilet and retardation of clearing the pleural space.

The efficacy of fibrinolysis as an adjunct treatment in complicated PE has been well documented in adult studies (38,39), with negligible adverse reactions in the recommended doses (40). Some authors, however, believe that when compared with video-assisted thoracoscopic surgery, fibrinolysis is inferior (41). Intrapleural fibrinolytics shorten hospital stay and are recommended by British Thoracic Society (BTS) for any complicated parapneumonic effusion (thick fluid with loculations) or empyema (overt pus) in children. There have been seven pediatric case series in children reporting a total of 136 cases treated with streptokinase, urokinase, or alteplase (34,42–44). All indicate increased pleural drainage with these agents and overall a successful outcome without surgery in 90% (123) cases. There is no evidence that any of the three fibrinolytics are more effective than the others, but only urokinase has been studied in a randomized controlled trial in children, which is recommended, by the BTS guidelines (34). However, some authors stress the risk of possible anaphylactic reactions by using streptokinase or urokinase. For this reason, urokinase is not any more available in the United States and has been replaced by tissue plasminogen activator. This is a recombinant fibrinolytic agent that is being used by many physicians to facilitate the drainage of loculated PE in children, in the United States (45). Some centers recommend the use of tube placement at an early stage (46), while others advocate early surgical intervention (either thoracotomy or video-assisted thoracoscopic surgery) as a first-line intervention in children with empyema (47–50). Others recommend the use of surgical treatment 10 days after the beginning of medical treatment, providing there is no improvement (50) (Fig. 4). According to BTS guidelines, patients should be considered for surgical treatment if they have persisting sepsis in association with a persistent pleural collection, despite chest tube drainage and antibiotics. Other circumstances where surgery is more likely to be required are complex empyema with significant lung pathology (e.g., delayed presentation with a significant peel and trapped lung), bronchopleural fistula with pyopneumothorax, and secondary empyema (34). We believe that while surgical treatment is the method of choice for selected cases, like complicated empyemas, following necrotizing pneumonitis (51) for the great majority of parapneumonic effusions, tube drainage and fibrinolytics should be the first-line treatment. An algorithm for a rational approach to treatment of parapneumonic effusions is shown in Figure 5.

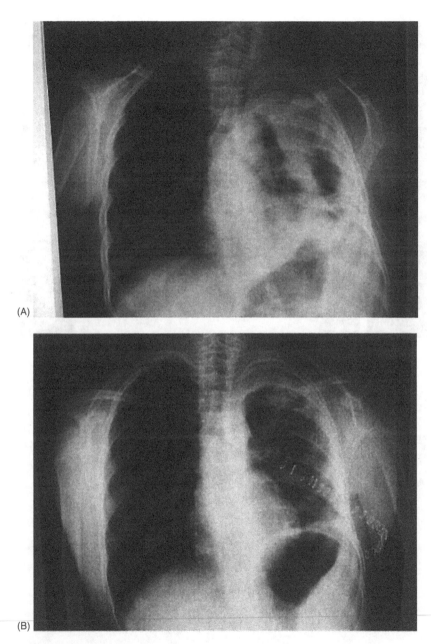

Figure 4 (**A**) An 8-year-old girl with left-sided staphylococcal empyema. Note the displacement of the trachea to the right. Tube drainage and fibrinolytics were tried for 10 days with no definite improvement. Lung decortication was decided upon. (**B**) The same patient immediately after the lung decortication. (*Continued*)

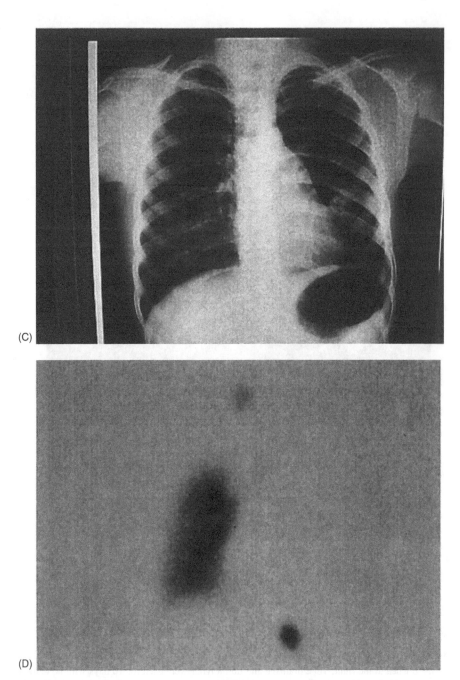

(C)

(D)

Figure 4   (*Continued*) (**C**) The patient 3 months later. (**D**) Ventilation scan before the surgical intervention.

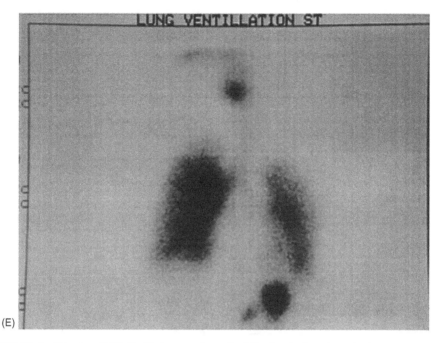

(E)

Figure 4 (*Continued*) (**E**) Ventilation scan 3 months following the lung decortication.

In our institution, we routinely use ultrasonography for the diagnosis and follow-up of all parapneumonic effusions. Diagnostic thoracocentesis is performed in the great majority of children with PE, followed by tube drainage and fibrinolytics in every case with purulent loculated fluid.

Urokinase should be given twice daily for three days (six doses in total) using 40,000 units in 40 mL 0.9% saline for children aged one year or above, and 10,000 units in 10 mL 0.9% saline for children aged under one year (34). Children with coagulation disorders or with hemorrhagic pleural fluid are excluded. Urokinase is injected in the pleural cavity through the drainage tube, which remains clamped for the following four hours. Then the pleural fluid is drained with gentle suction via a negative pressure pump (we apply continuous negative pressure −18 mm Hg for children older than 12 years and −10 mm Hg for the younger ones). The above is repeated for four days, with serial daily sonograms for evaluation. If the condition is not improving after four days, we proceed to open thoracotomy and lung decortication. Out of 68 children with parapneumonic effusions treated in our clinic in the last three years, in 16 cases urokinase was added to treatment, while in 2 cases open thoracotomy was necessary. In contrast to adults, most parapneumonic effusions in children resolve, with no serious complications. A residual pleural thickening with mild abnormalities on lung function, either obstructive or restrictive, has been reported, mainly in younger children (52,53). Mortality rates for complicated empyemas are between 6% and 9%, mainly in young infants less than two years of age. With rational antibiotic therapy and prompt intervention, most children are absolutely well after a period of 3 to 18 months (Fig. 6).

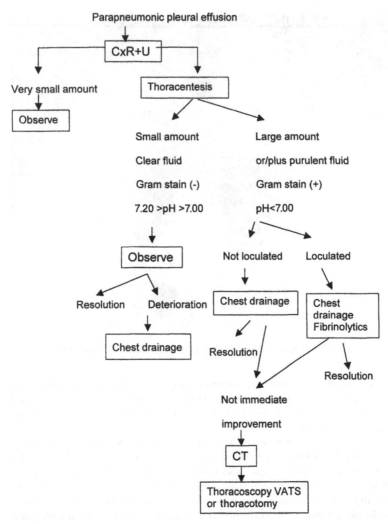

Figure 5   Algorithm for the management of parapneumonic effusions in children. *Abbreviations*: CXR, chest X-ray; US, ultrasonography; CT, computed tomography; VATS, video-assisted thoracoscopic surgery.
Source: Adapted from Refs. 33, 37.

B.   Tuberculous Effusions

Tuberculosis (TB) remains a worldwide disease, increasing recently, especially in Africa, Asia, and urban areas of Europe and North America (54). It is estimated that 450,000 children under the age of 15 years die annually from TB (55). Tuberculous pleurisy is not uncommon in children, particularly in adolescents. It is usually the consequence of subpleural granulomas or hematogenous spread of *Tubercle bacilli*.

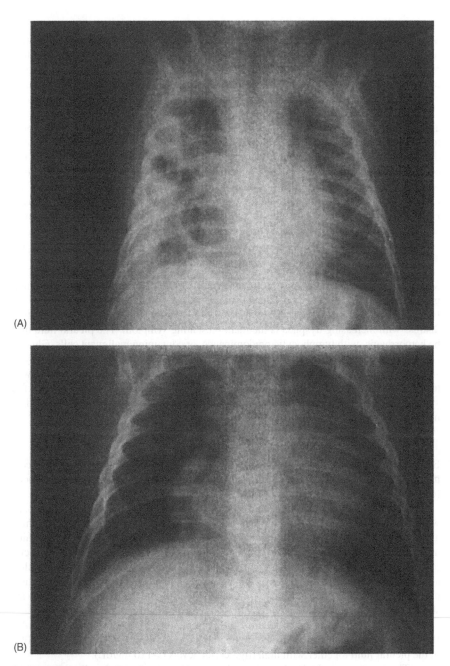

(A)

(B)

Figure 6 (**A**) A 2-month-old boy with multiple bullae formation and pleural effusion due to *Staphylococcus aureus*. Tube drainage and prolonged anti-staphylococcal treatment (4 weeks) were given. (**B**) Complete recovery 3 months later.

The combination of pleural and hilar adenopathy found in the majority of cases is highly suggestive of TB, but in some patients pleurisy is the only presenting manifestation of the disease. TB effusions are usually unilateral, presenting suddenly with fever, chest pain on inspiration, and shortness of breath of various severity, depending on the amount of the accumulated pleural fluid. Tuberculin tests have a high sensitivity and should be used to confirm the diagnosis in all suspicious cases (56). Examination of the fluid shows a lymphocytic predominance, low glucose, and pH between 7.0 and 7.3. *Tubercle bacilli* are found in almost half of the fluid cultures. Presence of TB granulomas is found in 50% to 80% of pleural biopsies (57). However, a biopsy should be performed only in case of diagnostic difficulty. Other specific diagnostic tests like adenosine deaminase activity test or interferon-γ levels have very high sensitivity and specificity, which reaches the level of 95%. They are recommended for routine use in countries with a high incidence of TB (58,59). Most children with TB pleurisy respond excellent to antituberculous treatment. However, adding a course of steroids for two to four weeks causes a dramatic improvement in symptoms in patients with large effusions and shift of the mediastinum (Fig. 7).

C. Malignant Effusions

Malignancies are the third most common cause of PE in children, with lymphomas predominating (Fig. 8). They are usually unilateral, resulting from obstruction of the lymphatics in the lung or from direct invasion of pleura by malignant cells. Respiratory distress with increasing dyspnea is the main presenting symptom. The pleural fluid may be hemorrhagic, with lymphocytic predominance, or containing malignant cells. Glucose and pH are within normal limits (60). Immunochemical stain studies are necessary in some cases for making the diagnosis (61). Malignant effusions generally respond well to chemotherapy and irradiation. Thoracocentesis, though helpful for temporary relief of symptoms, should be carried out with caution, as aggressive removal of the pleural fluid may be followed by reexpansion pulmonary edema (62).

D. Chylothorax

By this term, we mean the accumulation of lymph fluid within the pleural cavity. Accumulation of chylous may appear during the fetal period (congenital) or later in childhood (63).

Congenital chylothorax is the most common cause of pleural effusion in the neonate, with an incidence of 1:10,000 deliveries. Among the most common cause is a congenital abnormality of lymph vessels (lymphangiomatosis or lymphangiectasia) or congenital heart disease. Less common causes are lobar sequestration or mediastinal malignancies (64). Neonates with chylothorax present immediately at birth with difficulty to establish adequate respiration. Resuscitation is cumbersome and sometimes intense effort causes pneumothorax to the neonatal lung. On examination, the trachea and mediastinum are shifted to the contralateral side, with dullness to percussion of the ipsilateral thorax.

Ultrasonography helps to identify the presence of chylothorax even antenatally. However, the diagnosis is established by finding large numbers of lymphocytes (>90%) in the pleural fluid together with high triglyceride levels (>110 mg/dL).

Thoracostomy and tube drainage is the immediate treatment for all neonates with chylothorax to facilitate the expansion of the compressed lung. If the accumulation of chyle persists for long, management of fluids, nutrition, and electrolytes becomes necessary (65).

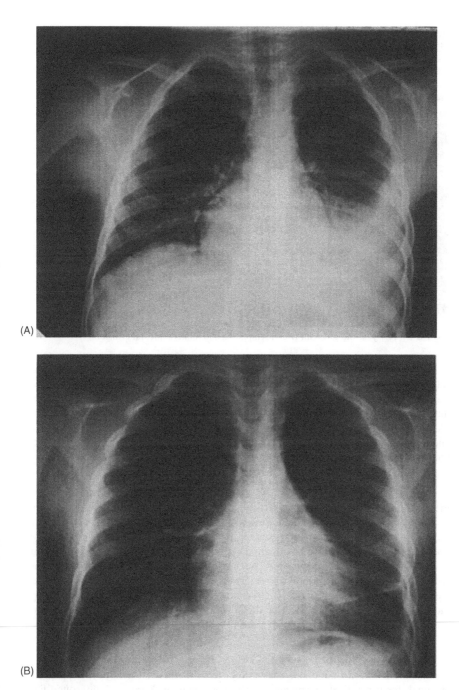

Figure 7 (**A**) A 9-year-old girl with tuberculous pleural effusion with no hilar adenopathy. Note that the findings are not specific. (**B**) The same patient after 3 months of antituberculous treatment. No tube drainage was necessary.

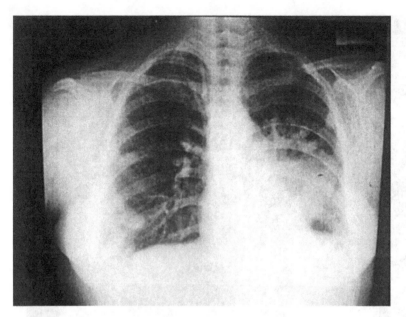

Figure 8 A 4-year-old girl with B-cell lymphoma and bilateral pleural effusion.

Chylothorax beyond the neonatal period is usually a postoperative complication, related to cardiothoracic interventions or central venous catheterizations (66,67). Rarely, it may be the result of obstruction of the thoracic duct by a tumor. The presentation and diagnosis is the same as in congenital chylothorax. Management is a combination of pleural drainage and special diet with medium-chain triglyceride oil, fat-free oral foods, and/or total parenteric nutrition. If the situation is not improving in two to four weeks, then pleurodesis is attempted.

V. Summary

PE in children have similar etiology as in adults, but they appear with a different incidence according to the age of presentation. The most common PE in the pediatric population are those of infectious origin, usually presenting as complications of pneumonias. Fibrinolysis for complicated PE seems to be effective in children, but we are waiting for the results of large studies to confirm this impression. Moreover, though conservative treatment with tube drainage and fibrinolysis remains the first-choice approach for complicated parapneumonic effusions, surgical intervention like video-assisted thoracoscopy or open thoracotomy and lung decortication should not be delayed if there is no immediate improvement.

Acknowledgment

We thank Dr. Maria Badouraki, Senior Register in Pediatric Radiology, Hippokration Hospital, for her critical review and helpful comments on X-ray and ultrasound films, used in the manuscript.

References

1. Greenough A. Pleural effusion. In: Greenough A, Roberton NRC, Milner AD, eds. Neonatal Respiratory Disorders. London: Arnold Publishers, 1996:426–435.
2. Orenstein D. Diseases of the pleura. In: Behram R, Kliegman R, Jenson H, eds. Nelson Textbook of Pediatrics. 16th ed. Philadelphia: W. B. Saunders Co., 2000:1329–1331.
3. Dinwiddie R. Diagnosis and Management of Paediatric Respiratory Disease. 2nd ed. New York: Churchill Livingstone, 1997:121.
4. Albertine KH, Wiener KJ, Bastacky J, et al. No evidence for mesothelial cell contact across the costal pleural space of sheep. J Appl Physiol 1991; 10:123–134.
5. Kobzik L. The lung. In: Cortan R, Kumar V, Collins T, eds. Pathologic Basis of Disease. Philadelphia: W. B. Saunders Co., 1999:749–751.
6. Wang NS. The performed stomas connecting the pleural cavity and the lymphatics in the parietal pleura. Am Rev Respir Dis 1975; 11:12–20.
7. Miserocchi G, Venturoli D, Negrini D, et al. Intrapleural fluid movements described by a porous flow model. J Appl Physiol 1992; 73:2511–2516.
8. Rusch V, Ginsberg R. Chest wall, pleura lung and mediastinum. In: Schwartz S, ed. Principles of Surgery. 7th ed. New York: McGraw-Hill, 1999:669–670.
9. Sahn SA. State of the art: The pleura. Am Rev Respir Dis 1988; 138:184–234.
10. Panitch HB, Papastamelos C, Schidlow V. Abnormalities of the pleural space. In: Taussig LM, Landau LI, eds. Pediatric Respiratory Medicine. St Louis: Mosby, 1999:1178–1196.
11. Maziah W, Choo KE, Ray JG. Empyema thoracis in hospitalized children in Kelantan, Malaysia. J Trop Pediatr 1995; 41:185–188.
12. Givan DC, Eigen H. Common pleural effusions in children. Clin Chest Med 1998; 19:363–371.
13. Zeitlin PL. Pleural effusions and empyema. In: Loughlin GM, Eigen H, eds. Respiratory Disease in Children. Philadelphia: Lippincott Williams & Wilkins, 1994:453–463.
14. Shankar KR, Kenny SE, Okoye BO, et al. Evolving experience in the management of empyema thoracis. Acta Pediatr 2000; 89:417–420.
15. Woodring JH. Recognition of pleural effusions on supine radiographs. How much fluid is required? Am J Roentgenol 1984; 142:59–64.
16. Ramnath RR, Heller RM, Ben-Ami T, et al. Implications of early sonographic evaluation of parapneumonic effusions in children with pneumonia. Pediatrics 1998; 101:68–71.
17. Libscomb DJ, Flower CDR, Hadfield JW. Ultrasound of the pleura: An assessment of its clinical value. Clin Radiol 1981; 32:289–290.
18. Donnelly LF, Klosterman LA. CT appearance of parapneumonic effusions in children: Findings are not specific for empyema. AJR Am J Roentgenol 1997; 169:179–182.
19. Moon WK, Kim WS, Kim IO, et al. Complicated pleural tuberculosis in children: CT evaluation. Pediatr Radiol 1999; 29:153–157.
20. Butani L, Polinsky MS, Kaiser BA, et al. Pleural effusion complicating acute peritoneal dialysis in haemolytic uremic syndrome. Pediatr Nephrol 1998; 12:772–774.
21. Montgomery M. Air and liquid in pleural space. In: Chernick V, Boat T, Kending E, eds. Disorders of the Respiratory Tract in Children. 6th ed. Philadelphia: W. B. Saunders Co., 1998:389–411.
22. Papastamelos C. Pleural effusions. In: Schidlow DV, Smith DS, eds. A Practical Guide to Pediatric Respiratory Disease. Philadelphia: Hanley & Belfus, Inc., 1994:436–445.
23. Haddad G, Palazzo R. Diagnostic approach to respiratory disease. In: Behram R, Kliegman R, Jenson H, eds. Nelson Textbook of Pediatrics. 16th ed. Philadelphia: W. B. Saunders Co., 2000:1257.
24. Ghaye B, Dondelinger RF. Imaging guided thoracic interventions. Eur Respir J 2001; 17:507–528.
25. Alkrinawi S, Chernick V. Pleural fluid in hospitalized pediatric patients. Clin Pediatr 1996; 35:5–9.

26. Heffner JE. Evaluating Diagnostic Tests in the Pleura. Diseases of the Pleura, Clinics in Chest Medicine. Vol. 19. Philadelphia: W. B. Saunders, 1998:277–293.

27. Azoulay E, Farthoukh M, Galliot R, et al. Rapid diagnosis of infectious pleural effusions by use of reagent strips. Clin Infect Dis 2000; 31:914–919.

28. Monnier A, Carbonnelle E, Zahar JR, et al. Microbiological diagnosis of empyema in children: Comparative evaluations by culture, polymerase chain reaction, and pneumococcal antigen detection in pleural fluids. Clin Infect Dis 2006; 42:1135–1140.

29. Hardie W, Bokulic R, Garcia VF, et al. Pneumococcal pleural empyemas in children. Clin Infect Dis 1996; 22:1057–1063.

30. Rees JHM, Spencer DA, Parikh D, et al. Increase in incidence of childhood empyema in West Midlands, U.K. Lancet 1997; 349:342.

31. Alkrinawi S, Chernick V. Pleural infection in children. Semin Respir Infect 1996; 11:148–154.

32. Campbell JD, Nataro JP. Pleural empyema. Pediatr Infect Dis J 1999; 18:725–726.

33. Ham H, Light RW. Parapneumonic effusion and empyema. Eur Respir J 1997; 10:1150–1156.

34. Balfour-Lynn IM, Abrahamson E, Cohen G, Hartley J, King S, Parikh D, Spencer D, Thomson AH, Urquhart D and on behalf of the Paediatric Pleural Diseases Subcommittee of the BTS Standards of Care Committee. BTS Guidelines for the Management of Pleural Infection in Children. Thorax 2005; 60;1–21.

35. Meier AH, Smith B, Raghavan A, et al. Rational treatment of empyema in children. Arch Surg 2000; 135:907–912.

36. Doski J, Lou D, Hicks B, et al. Management of parapneumonic collections in infants and children. J Pediatr Surg 2000; 35:265–270.

37. Cassina PC, Hauser M, Hillejan L, et al. Video-assisted thoracoscopy in the treatment of pleural empyema: Stage-based management and outcome. J Thorac Cardiovasc Surg 1999; 117:234–238.

38. Davies RJ, Traill ZC, Gleeson FV. Randomised controlled trial of intrapleural streptokinase in community acquired pleural infection. Thorax 1997; 52:416–421.

39. Bouros D, Schiza S, Tzanakis N, et al. Intrapleural urokinase versus normal saline in the treatment of complicated parapneumonic effusions and empyema. Am J Respir Crit Care Med 1999; 159:37–42.

40. Davies CW, Lok S, Davies RJO. The systematic fibrinolytic activity of intrapleural streptokinase. Am J Respir Crit Care Med 1998; 157:328–330.

41. Wait M, Sharma S, Hohn J, et al. A Randomized trial of empyema therapy. Chest 1997; 111:1548–1551.

42. Krishnan S, Amin N, Dozor A, et al. Urokinase in the management of complicated parapneumonic effusions in children. Chest 1997; 112:1579–1583.

43. Barbato A, Panizzolo C, Monciotti C, et al. Use of urokinase in childhood pleural empyema. Pediatr Pulmonol 2003; 35:50–55.

44. Wells RG, Havens PL. Intrapleural fibrinolysis for parapneumonic effusion and empyema in children. Radiology 2003; 228:370–378.

45. Beers SL, Abramo TJ. Pleural effusions. Pediatr Emerg Care 2007; 23(5):330–334.

46. Sasse S, Nguyen T, Mulligan M, et al. The effects of early chest tube placement on empyema resolution. Chest 1997; 111:1679–1683.

47. Patton RM, Abrams RS, Gauderer MWL. Is thoracoscopically aided pleural debridement advantageous in children? Am Surg 1999; 65:69–72.

48. Kercher K, Attori R, Hoover D, et al. Thoracoscopic decortication as first-line therapy for pediatric parapneumonic empyema. Chest 2000; 118:24–27.

49. Rescola FJ, West KW, Gingalewski CA, et al. Efficacy of primary and secondary video-assisted thoracic surgery in children. J Pediatr Surg 2000; 35:134–138.

50. Balquet M, Larroquet M, Gruner M. Current surgical treatment for pleural empyema in children. Pediatr Pulmon 1999; 18(Suppl.):109.

51. Wong KS, Chiu CH, Yeow KM, et al. Necrotising pneumonitis in children. Eur J Pediatr 2000; 159:684–688.

52. Redding GJ, Walund LD, Jones JW, et al. Lung function in children following empyema. Am J Dis Child 1990; 144:1337–1342.

53. Hoff SJ, Neblett WW, Heller RM, et al. Postpneumonic empyema in childhood: Selecting appropriate therapy. J Pediatr Surg 1989; 24:659–664.

54. Enarson DA, Ait-Khaled N. Tuberculosis. In: Annesi-Maesano I, Gulsvic A, Viegi G, eds. Respiratory Epidemiology in Europe. European Respiratory Monograph. Sheffield, UK: European Respiratory Society 2000; 67–91.

55. Gremin BJ. Tuberculosis—The resurgence of our most lethal infectious disease—A review. Pediatr Radiol 1995; 25:620–626.

56. Merino JM, Carpintero I, Alvarez T, et al. Tuberculous pleural effusion in children. Chest 1999; 115:26–30.

57. Seibert AF, Haynes J Jr, Middleton R. Tuberculous pleural effusion: Twenty-year experience. Chest 1991; 99:883–886.

58. Burgess LJ, Maritz FJ, Le Roux I, et al. Use of adenosine deaminase as a diagnostic tool for tuberculous pleurisy. Thorax 1995; 50:593–594.

59. Wongtim S, Silachamroon U, Ruxrungtham K, et al. Interferon gamma for diagnosing tuberculous pleural effusions. Thorax 1999; 54:921–924.

60. Strings AI, Van Hegan RI. Cytologic diagnosis of lymphomas of serous effusion. J Clin Pathol 1981; 34:1311–1325.

61. Cohen I, Loberant N, King E, et al. Rhabdomyosarcoma in a child with massive pleural effusion: Cytological diagnosis from pleural fluid. Diagn Cytopathol 1999; 21:125–128.

62. Pietsch JB, Whitlock JA, Ford C, et al. Management of pleural effusions in children with malignant lymphoma. J Pediatr Surg 1999; 34:635–638.

63. Chernick V, Reed MH. Pneumothorax and chylothorax in the neonatal period. J Pediatr 1970; 76:624–632.

64. Hilliard RI, Mckendry JB, Phillips MJ. Congenital abnormalities of the lymphatic system: A new clinical classification. Pediatrics 1990; 86:988–994.

65. Dubin PJ, King IN, Gallagher PG. Congenital chylothorax. Curr Opin Pediatr 2000; 12:505–509.

66. Buttiker V, Fanconi S, Burger R. Chylothorax in children. Guidelines for diagnosis and management. Chest 1999; 116:682–687.

67. Madhavi P, Jameson R, Robinson MJ. Unilateral pleural effusion complicating central venous catheterization. Arch Dis Child Fetal Neonatal Ed 2000; 82:F248–F249.

40
Pneumothorax

CHARLIE STRANGE
Medical University of South Carolina, Charleston, South Carolina, U.S.A.

I. Introduction

Pneumothorax is defined as air in the pleural space. Traumatic pneumothoraces can occur following both blunt and penetrating injuries to the chest, although the most common traumatic pneumothorax occurs following iatrogenic needle puncture of the lung. Spontaneous pneumothoraces are divided into primary and secondary subtypes. Primary spontaneous pneumothorax occurs in the absence of underlying lung disease, while secondary spontaneous pneumothorax occurs with increased frequency compared to the general population associated with most lung diseases.

Spontaneous pneumothorax incidence has been estimated at 13.7/100,000 per year for men and 3.2/100,000 per year for women from data extracted from Olmsted County, Minnesota, where 141 cases were seen from 1950 to 1974 (1). The incidence in females is likely higher today, because chronic obstructive pulmonary disease (COPD) prevalence has risen. Approximately equal numbers of patients will have primary and secondary spontaneous pneumothorax.

This chapter is designed to cover the breadth of literature on pneumothorax while keeping the focus on the clinical presentation of disease, appropriate diagnostic testing, and stratified treatment approaches. Recent consensus studies have provided an approach to disease that will need confirmation of algorithms and objective trials to establish appropriate therapy.

II. Traumatic Pneumothorax

Traumatic pneumothorax from blunt or penetrating injury to the thorax occurs commonly. In one recent series of major trauma cases, pneumothorax was present in approximately 20% of cases and was associated with more clinical instability than cases without pneumothorax (2). Any pneumothorax, regardless of size, should receive a chest tube because the extent of organ injuries is usually incompletely known at the time of presentation. Observation is not recommended for this group of patients, because any hemodynamic instability results in emergent thoracotomy. Therefore any remote chance of tension pneumothorax should be avoided. Although a few chest tubes may be placed for small pneumothoraces that might not progress, the single case with hemodynamic instability from pneumothorax that could have been prevented while cardiac contusions, aortic dissections, and pericardial tamponade remain in the differential diagnosis suggests that an aggressive treatment algorithm is warranted.

III. Iatrogenic Pneumothorax

Iatrogenic pneumothoraces most commonly follow needle punctures of the lung. When needle aspiration cytology of the lung is performed for lung cancer diagnosis, the frequency of pneumothorax is related to the degree of airway obstruction, the depth of needle puncture, needle size, and the number of fissures crossed. Other common causes of iatrogenic pneumothorax include complications of central venous catheter placement (3), tracheostomy (4), thoracentesis bronchoscopy, gastric tube placement (5), and pericardiocentesis. Some pulmonary specialists have advocated letting air into the pleural space during thoracentesis to produce an air contrast evaluation of the pleura to define the extent of lung entrapment (6). Rare cases associated with acupuncture (7) and from self-inflicted needle puncture in Münchausen's syndrome (8) have been reported.

The natural history of iatrogenic pneumothoraces is different than in other forms of pneumothorax because the needle puncture site usually heals within 24 hours. Pneumothorax is radiographically evident within an hour of needle puncture in the majority of cases (9), and onset more than four hours after intervention is rare. Therefore, observation is used more frequently than in other pneumothoraces, and short-term interventions such as small-caliber chest tubes with Heimlich valves have become popular.

IV. Primary Spontaneous Pneumothorax

Approximately half of all pneumothoraces occur in the absence of clinically apparent underlying lung disease. The demographics of this population include disproportionate representation of individuals aged 15 to 30 years, of tall stature, and with thin body habitus (10). This body habitus produces a larger gradient in pleural pressure and greater distending pressure in apical alveoli, which may be important in pneumothorax development.

Some evidence from case reports of siblings with disease suggests that genetic factors may predispose some individuals to develop pneumothorax (11). In most series, more than 90% smoke cigarettes (12). Pneumothorax incidence is related to the number of cigarettes smoked, with relative risk >50 for smokers who consume more than one pack per day (13). Lung function tests after resolution of pneumothorax are usually normal.

In some respects, the primary designation is a misnomer, because high-resolution chest computed tomography (CT) has suggested the presence of subpleural areas of air space enlargement in the majority of these patients (14). These "emphysema-like changes" are commonly bilateral and rarely present in nonsmoking, age-matched controls. Lung density measurements in areas not involved were normal in one study (15). This finding has generated considerable controversy, but no data exist proving that the site of pneumothorax generation is from these lesions. Furthermore, contralateral pneumothorax is no more common in patients who have contralateral emphysema-like changes than in those without contralateral CT abnormalities (16).

Because the frequency of bullae is high, a tendency to stratify patients on the basis of their lung anatomy has become more common. The stratification scheme of Vanderschueren is presented in Table 1. This controversy extends itself into treatment decisions, since staple bullectomy has been recommended for patients with bullae seen on radiograph or CT. It should be noted that no randomized controlled trials of bullectomy versus nonbullectomy pleurodesis have been performed for either primary or secondary spontaneous pneumothorax.

Table 1 Pneumothorax Classification

Stage 1: Anatomically normal lungs
Stage 2: Pleural adhesions
Stage 3: Blebs < 2 cm
Stage 4: Blebs > 2 cm

Source: From Ref. 68.

The physiological factor that induces pneumothorax development is an increased transpleural pressure. Epidemiological trials have demonstrated that atmospheric pressure changes are associated with increased pneumothorax incidence (17–19). Pneumothoraces associated with compressed air diving or skydiving have been described. Patients whose occupation requires contact with swings in barometric pressure should consider pleurodesis.

V. Secondary Spontaneous Pneumothorax

A variety of lung diseases can be complicated by pneumothorax. Although the most common disease in case series is usually chronic obstructive lung disease, the heterogeneity of other diseases makes specific diagnosis a particularly important aspect of pneumothorax management.

Many diseases have established diagnoses at the time of pneumothorax presentation. Cystic fibrosis patients have a 0.6% yearly risk of pneumothorax that is seen in older patients with more advanced lung disease (20). Asthmatic patients have been noted to have significant risks for pneumothorax if mechanically ventilated (21). Increased pneumothorax frequency in idiopathic pulmonary fibrosis (22) generally occurs in established disease with extensive subpleural honeycomb change.

Pneumothorax occurs most commonly in the obstructive lung diseases. Because of expiratory airflow obstruction, the path of least resistance for subpleural air may remain across the visceral pleural surface, perpetuating the air leak. The other factor favoring pneumothorax development in these diseases is that elastin destruction is common in both the airway and visceral pleura.

Although no comprehensive studies of human pleural histology following pneumothorax have been performed, some small case series have suggested that visceral pleural connective tissue is reduced.

Some rare diseases are associated with an increased pneumothorax risk. Birt–Hogg–Dube syndrome is an autosomal dominant disease characterized by large lung cysts and increased risk for renal cell carcinoma (23). Pneumothorax is often the herald symptom in an affected patient (Fig. 1). Pneumothorax has been seen with Marfan syndrome and Ehlers–Danlos syndrome (24).

A particularly morbid form of pneumothorax is seen in the acquired immunodeficiency syndrome (AIDS). When pneumothorax occurs it is usually the consequence of subpleural cysts caused by *Pneumocystis jiroveci*, often being prophylaxed with inhaled pentamidine. Pneumothorax is often protracted, and home chest tubes have been used with frequency in this disorder (25,26). Pneumothorax incidence appears to have lessened with the availability of other systemic therapies for pneumocystis.

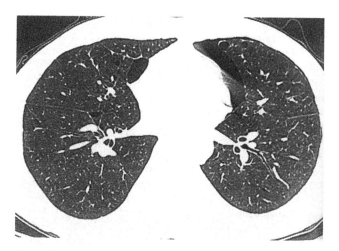

Figure 1 Chest CT scan of a 35-year-old male occasional smoker with Birt–Hogg–Dube syndrome who presented with pneumothorax. The client's father had had five previous pneumothoraces and renal cell carcinoma. Unilateral thoracotomy was performed for definitive recurrence prevention. Note the multiple cysts within the lung and left pneumothorax.

When pneumothorax occurs with an undiagnosed interstitial lung disease seen on radiograph, the possibilities of Langerhans cell granulomatosis (27) and lymphangioleiomyomatosis (28) should be considered. Both these diseases carry a pneumothorax prevalence greater than 15%. CT can help in differential diagnosis. Other interstitial lung diseases that have some component of obstruction also carry increased incidence of pneumothorax. These diseases include sarcoidosis, berylliosis, bronchiolitis obliterans with organizing pneumonia, and Sjögren's bronchiolitis, among others (29).

VI. Persistent Airleak and Bronchopleural Fistula

A pneumothorax in which the lung continues to have a hole through which air travels is designated as having a persistent airleak. The term bronchopleural fistula (BPF) has usually been reserved as a designation for patients on mechanical ventilation with a significant air leak arising from a bronchial source sufficient to impair alveolar ventilation. Unfortunately, the degree of airleak that qualifies as significant is not well defined and is often the subject of controversy. Furthermore, large BPF will sometimes spontaneously heal and transition through a period when the degree of airleak is small. Therefore, most clinicians do not discern a difference between BPF and persistent airleak terminology. Instead, the volume of airleak and its source are important in defining management.

Bronchopleural fistulae are most commonly seen postoperatively following thoracic operations and as complications of acute respiratory distress syndrome (30). Although few randomized trials of therapy have been performed, these patients are often sufficiently ill that elective thoracoscopy for pleural closure is precluded. Nonoperative interventions include optimizing mechanical ventilation to keep airflow across the fistula as low as possible to assist pleural healing. Keeping positive end expiratory pressure as low as possible is usually the best strategy (31). Most recently, endobronchial one-way valves have been developed for patients with refractory persistent airleaks.

The technique of endobronchial therapy for BPF closure requires an assessment of the source of leak. This usually begins with balloon endobronchial occlusion during bronchoscopy to identify the site(s) of leak. Unfortunately, significant collateral ventilation may occur in patients with COPD, forcing endobronchial therapy to target lobar or larger targets. Although some chemical agents that obstruct the airways have been given to decrease airleak, an experience with removable endobronchial one-way valves has emerged as an effective therapy (32–35). These valves are placed in target airways with removal from four to six weeks later once the airleak has spontaneously healed.

Recognizing that significant CO_2 is eliminated by some BPFs (36), aggressive closure of these airleaks is not always indicated. When insufficient alveolar ventilation results despite optimal ventilatory management, options of timed chest tube pressurization can limit the amount of ventilated air traversing the pleura (37,38). Double lumen endotracheal tubes may also be used (39). Of interest is that patients with acute respiratory distress syndrome (ARDS) have no difference in mortality when stratified for the presence or absence of pneumothorax (40).

A. Clinical Presentation

Pleuritic chest pain is the most common symptom at pneumothorax presentation but is present in only 90% of patients (41). The onset of pain can be abrupt or indolent. Radiation to the ipsilateral shoulder is common. Occasionally, patients can feel unusual fluttering sensations within the chest that correspond to Hampton's crunch, an unusual sound heard on physical examination suspected to arise from air escaping from within trapped spaces in the major or minor fissures.

Dyspnea is nearly universal in secondary spontaneous pneumothorax and in COPD is often out of proportion to the size of the pneumothorax (42). Because alveolar ventilation drops as lung volumes are reduced, hypercapnia is common. Hypoxemia results from both ventilation–perfusion mismatch and shunt that can be as large as 20% (43). Presentation to medical care can be at times distant from symptom onset. In some series, more than 50% of patients waited more than 24 hours before emergency room arrival (44). Presentation after lung transplant can be catastrophic since both pleural spaces may communicate (45).

B. Diagnosis

Although CT is the most specific diagnostic modality, the chest radiograph usually demonstrates pleural air. The optimal technique to obtain chest radiography has been the subject of extensive study. Upright radiographs are superior to supine films. Although expiratory films should theoretically increase visceral pleural density and enhance pneumothorax detection, clinical trials have shown no difference between detection rates from radiographs obtained in full inspiration.

Some series have noted that physicians tend to underestimate the size of pneumothorax from chest radiography (46). Current treatment algorithms have therefore attempted to simplify recommendations using the distance from the lung apex to the thoracic apex as a surrogate measure for percentage lung collapse (47). These recommendations have recently been validated with computed tomography (48). Plain radiographs in supine patients in the ICU carry significant risks of missed pneumothorax. In the supine position, two-thirds of pneumothoraces are found in the subpulmonic space or along the mediastinal pleura (49). Although lateral decubitus views can help clarify some cases, CT remains superior if available. The consequences of a missed pneumothorax in the ICU are significant since 50% may advance to tension (49).

Thoracic ultrasound is also a useful test to detect pneumothorax. The test is not sensitive when subcutaneous air is present but is otherwise both sensitive and specific in the hands of a trained operator (50). Lightweight portable ultrasound machines now in common medical use can be used to detect pneumothorax in aerospace medicine and terrestrial trauma patients. The ultrasound experience has shown high levels of sensitivity and specificity for both the presence and enlargement of pneumothorax compared to CT, the gold standard (51).

VII. Tension Pneumothorax

Tension pneumothorax is a condition most often seen in hospitalized patients. Although radiographic signs of a positive intrapleural pressure are often seen in pneumothorax, the definition is usually reserved for those patients with physiological manifestations of tension. Radiographic signs include the deep sulcus sign, mediastinal shift, rib splaying, and diaphragmatic depression. Physiological signs of tension include dyspnea, increased pulsus paradoxus, tachycardia, hypoxemia, and hypotension.

Tension pneumothorax occurs more commonly under positive pressure ventilation. The diagnosis in these patients is often made at bedside before radiographic conformation by the absence of breath sounds and asymmetrical ventilation on chest observation. If the lung is consolidated and therefore unable to collapse, tension physiology can occur with a small or localized pneumothorax (52). A rush of air should accompany the placement of an intravenous catheter through the intercostal space. More formal chest thoracostomy tube placement can be performed electively.

Since tension pneumothorax is frequently catastrophic, any pneumothorax seen in mechanically ventilated patients should receive chest tube drainage (53). It is reassuring to know that properly treated pneumothoraces do not seem to increase mortality in ARDS (40).

VIII. Therapy

Therapy for pneumothorax remains complicated. Any discussion of therapeutic options must include a discussion of recurrence prevention. In the largest prospective clinical trial of pneumothorax therapy, the VA Cooperative Trial randomized 520 patients to pleural tetracycline or placebo (54). The five-year recurrence risk for the placebo patients was 32% for primary spontaneous pneumothorax and 41% for secondary spontaneous disease. The majority of pneumothoraces occurred within the first year after the herald event. Although intrapleural tetracycline decreased the pneumothorax recurrence rate to 25%, commercial unavailability and alternatives such as intrapleural talc make this study of historical importance for the natural history of pneumothorax.

IX. Observation

Observation is the recommended treatment modality for stable patients in the recent American College of Chest Physicians Delphi Consensus Statement of Management of

Table 2 Criteria Necessary for Pneumothorax Observation

Clinical stability
Stable vital signs
Ability to speak in full sentences
Normal oxygenation
Lack of progression
Unchanging pneumothorax size over 4 hours
Access to emergency care
Proximity to emergency care
Sufficient resources to return for worsening

Source: From Ref. 47.

Spontaneous Pneumothorax (47). Some criteria must be met before a pneumothorax can be safely observed (Table 2). The pneumothorax should be small enough so that progression in size can be detected (55). Although judging the size of a pneumothorax from an upright chest radiograph is not very accurate, pneumothoraces that are smaller than 3 cm from the lung apex to the apex of the thoracic cavity can usually be watched safely. The patient should be symptomatically stable. In secondary spontaneous pneumothoraces, this criterion is rarely met because of the underlying cardiopulmonary reserve. Lastly, sufficient resources should be immediately available for lung reexpansion should the patient decompensate. Observation might occur at home if the patient has been watched without pneumothorax progression for at least four hours and the patient has ready access to emergency services for worsening.

Observation allows for intrapleural air to be resorbed through the pleural vasculature. If the patient is on supplemental oxygen at the time of pneumothorax, the pleural air may contain sufficient oxygen for rapid resorption. More commonly, pleural air rich in nitrogen is resorbed at 1.25% of the pleural volume per day, suggesting a usual course of a few weeks for pneumothorax resolution (56). Oxygen speeds pleural nitrogen resorption by increasing the transvascular gradient for nitrogen resorption by at least a factor of four (57,58).

Few clinical series have systematically used observation. In one series of 40 patients in which observation was used for with pneumothorax, 9 of 40 required subsequent chest tube placement. A 32% recurrence rate was recorded with two deaths (59).

X. Aspiration

Small catheter aspiration is a procedure that is often used when lung collapse is large, the onset of symptoms is distant from presentation, and patients are stable. The technique of aspiration involves placement of a small catheter into the pleural space to withdraw air. Serial aliquots of air can be withdrawn by 50 mL syringe until gentle pressure is felt or 3 to 4 L of air has been aspirated. The catheter is withdrawn or a Heimlich valve is attached until a chest radiograph confirms reexpansion. If no subsequent air leak is seen through the Heimlich valve when placed to water seal, a stopcock can close the catheter. Subsequent radiographs in four hours show completely expanded lungs in approximately 65% to 80% of cases.

The advantage of leaving the small-bore catheter in place during the aspiration procedure is to avoid a second intervention should the lung leak be persistent. Conversion to a water-sealed chest tube is as simple as connecting the catheter to a pleural drainage device.

XI. Chest Thoracostomy Tubes

Chest tube placement should be performed for any patient with clinical instability or when a large pneumothorax complicates secondary spontaneous pneumothorax. Chest tube size is usually adequate with thoracostomy tubes >20 French, although the largest BPFs during ARDS have been measured at 16 L/min, a flow that requires tubes of at least 32 French to handle. Chest tubes should be placed on water seal and not suction since airleak cessation occurs more quickly when suction is avoided (60). The exception occurs when the lung is not expanded on water seal alone or when a large air leak (bubbles ≥4/7 on the water seal chamber of most closed system chest drainage devices) is ongoing (60).

Intercostal tube removal remains somewhat controversial, with some physicians believing that tube clamping improves the ability to accurately detect ongoing pleural airleak. What is clear from several studies is that recurrence rates are substantial if chest tubes are pulled immediately after air bubbles stop traversing the water-seal chamber. By waiting an additional 12 to 48 hours, chest tube removal is usually successful (61).

XII. Chest Thoracotomy Tube Pleurodesis

Since pneumothorax recurrence is common, procedures that decrease the risk have been used. It should be noted that a chest tube alone does not alter the recurrence rate of pneumothorax (62). Options for pleurodesis include thoracoscopy, thoracotomy, and application of chemical sclerosing agents through a chest tube (63). The VA Cooperative Study was the first trial to demonstrate the efficacy of intrapleural tetracycline in a prospective, randomized controlled trial. Although pleural tetracycline decreased pneumothorax recurrence, the recurrence rate still remained unacceptably high. Since the removal of tetracycline from the market, doxycycline has been used with similar results. Talc pleurodesis through a chest tube has been performed by mixing 5 g of talc in sterile saline as a slurry. When administered through the chest tube and allowed to dwell in the thorax for two hours, significant amounts of talc are deposited on the pleural surface. Although larger trials of talc slurry pleurodesis have been performed in malignant pleural effusions, the efficacy in preventing pneumothorax recurrence from small case series appears to approach 90% (64). Thoracoscopy that has followed talc slurry pleurodesis failures has noted an asymmetrical talc deposition with most of the substance localized to lung fissures.

XIII. Thoracoscopy and Pleuroscopy

Thoracoscopy for pneumothorax allows inspection of the pleural surface, electrocautery of persistent areas of airleak, application of talc poudrage that dusts the surface of the lung and parietal pleura under visualization, abrasion of one or more pleural surfaces, and resection of bullae. The difficulty in evaluating the efficacy of thoracoscopy for pneumothorax is that different combinations of interventions have been used in different series and no randomized trials have been completed. The most controversial intervention is the issue of whether bullectomy is indicated for patients in whom bullae that exceed 2 cm in greatest diameter are noted on CT scan or at time of thoracoscopy. Although pleurodesis success has been noted to be less when large bullae are seen, longer duration of airleak usually complicates a bullectomy procedure. Furthermore, the success rate of talc poudrage alone appears to be equally effective when compared to bullectomy/abrasion procedures. Other comparisons between talc poudrage and abrasion have suggested that talc is the more successful intervention (65).

Some controversy has developed over the safety of talc administration. Sterile asbestos-free talc is available in multiple formulations in the United States and abroad. Particle size generally remains proprietary information. Although there is good evidence that some talc particles are removed from the pleural space and traverse pleural lymphatics to the mediastinal lymph nodes and to the systemic circulation, no evidence of organ injury has been suggested. The possible exception is a perivascular lymphocytic infiltrate that has been seen in the lung of animal models of intrapleural talc (66). The rare cases of respiratory failure that have been seen after talc administration (discussed in more detail in other chapters) appear more common when large doses of talc are administered. Although no increased incidence of cancer has been seen 30 years after pleural talc administration, some practitioners use these data to suggest that young individuals should avoid talc pleurodesis. The last concern is that the pneumothorax risk factor of cigarette smoking is also a risk factor for lung cancer or lung transplant that may need subsequent chest surgery. Although surgery is not precluded by previous talc, the operations are more difficult and have more associated morbidity.

XIV. Thoracotomy

Some practitioners still suggest that thoracotomy remains the procedure of choice for recurrent pneumothoraces, since recurrence rates remain less than 2% in most case series. Series using thoracoscopy have slightly higher rates of recurrence. The major morbidity of thoracotomy includes a postthoracotomy pain syndrome that usually resolves over time. For patients with bilateral disease, the option of a median sternotomy has been used.

XV. Timing of Interventions

Considerable controversy surrounds the timing of pneumothorax intervention for pleurodesis. In primary spontaneous pneumothorax in which the risk of death is low because the cardiopulmonary reserve is high, pneumothorax has often been viewed as a nuisance disease. Because the recurrence rate is approximately 30%, any intervention to effect pleurodesis will result in unnecessary treatment of 70% of patients. The counterargument is that pneumothorax death is a tragedy in young individuals and is likely underreported. Primary economic analyses suggest that money can be saved by intervening with talc poudrage by thoracoscopy in first presentations of disease (67).

In the ACCP consensus document, pleurodesis was recommended after the first secondary spontaneous pneumothorax and after the second primary spontaneous pneumothorax.

XVI. Future Research

Since little can be done—other than smoking cessation initiatives—as primary prevention, most research will need to focus on the best treatment modalities. Unfortunately, trials performed in the past have been retrospective case series or small nonrandomized prospective trials. The next generation of pneumothorax research will require prospective, randomized clinical trials. The likelihood of such trials being performed is not high since pneumothorax remains a sporadic disease in which therapy must be initiated rather quickly in most cases. No obvious economic incentives are likely to emerge to foster clinical trials in this area.

High on the list of priorities for research is whether bullectomy is needed when thoracoscopy is performed for continuing BPF or for recurrence prevention. The needed trial would require computed tomography to stratify patients and randomize comparable groups to bullectomy with talc poudrage and talc poudrage alone. An issue is whether interventional pulmonologists should be performing therapy in all patients in the absence of bullectomy capabilities.

References

1. Melton LJ III, Hepper NG, Offord KP. Incidence of spontaneous pneumothorax in Olmsted County, Minnesota: 1950 to 1974. Am Rev Respir Dis 1979; 120(6):1379–1382.
2. Di Bartolomeo S, Sanson G, Nardi G, et al. A population-based study on pneumothorax in severely traumatized patients. J Trauma 2001; 51(4):677–682.
3. Eerola R, Kaukinen L, Kaukinen S. Analysis of 13800 subclavian vein catheterizations. Acta Anaesthesiol Scand 1985; 29(2):193–197.
4. Arola MK. Tracheostomy and its complications. A retrospective study of 794 tracheostomized patients. Ann Chir Gynaecol 1981; 70(3), 96–106.
5. Wendell GD, Lenchner GS, Promisloff RA. Pneumothorax complicating small-bore feeding tube placement. Arch Intern Med 1991; 151(3), 599–602.
6. Huggins JT, Sahn SA, Heidecker J, et al. Characteristics of trapped lung: Pleural fluid analysis, manometry, and air-contrast chest CT. Chest 2007; 131(1):206–213.
7. Ernst E, White AR. Prospective studies of the safety of acupuncture: A systematic review. Am J Med 2001; 110(6):481–485.
8. Urschel JD, Miller JD, Bennett WF. Self-inflicted pneumothoraces. Ann Thorac Surg 2001; 72(1):280–281.
9. Dennie CJ, Matzinger FR, Marriner JR, et al. Transthoracic needle biopsy of the lung: Results of early discharge in 506 outpatients. Radiology 2001; 219(1), 247–251.
10. Melton LJ III, Hepper NG, Offord KP. Influence of height on the risk of spontaneous pneumothorax. Mayo Clin Proc 1981; 56(11):678–682.
11. Koivisto PA, Mustonen A. Primary spontaneous pneumothorax in two siblings suggests autosomal recessive inheritance. Chest 2001; 119(5):1610–1612.
12. Light RW. Pleural Diseases. 2nd ed. Philadelphia, PA: Lea & Febiger, 1990.
13. Bense L, Eklund G, Wiman LG. Smoking and the increased risk of contracting spontaneous pneumothorax. Chest 1987; 92(6):1009–1012.
14. Bense L, Lewander R, Eklund G, et al. Nonsmoking, non-alpha 1-antitrypsin deficiency-induced emphysema in nonsmokers with healed spontaneous pneumothorax, identified by computed tomography of the lungs. Chest 1993; 103(2):433–438.
15. van Belle AF, Lamers RJ, ten Velde GP, et al. Diagnostic yield of computed tomography and densitometric measurements of the lung in thoracoscopically-defined idiopathic spontaneous pneumothorax. Respir Med 2001; 95(4):292–296.

16. Schramel FM, Zanen P. Blebs and/or bullae are of no importance and have no predictive value for recurrences in patients with primary spontaneous pneumothorax. Chest 2001; 119(6): 1976–1977.

17. Bense L. Spontaneous pneumothorax related to falls in atmospheric pressure. Eur J Respir Dis 1984; 65(7):544–546.

18. Smit HJ, Deville WL, Schramel FM, et al. Atmospheric pressure changes and outdoor temperature changes in relation to spontaneous pneumothorax. Chest 1999; 116(3):676–681.

19. Scott GC, Berger R, McKean HE. The role of atmospheric pressure variation in the development of spontaneous pneumothoraces. Am Rev Respir Dis 1989; 139(3):659–662.

20. Flume PA, Strange C, Ye X, et al. Pneumothorax in cystic fibrosis. Chest 2005; 128(2): 720–728.

21. Afessa B, Morales I, Cury JD. Clinical course and outcome of patients admitted to an ICU for status asthmaticus. Chest 2001; 120(5):1616–1621.

22. Franquet T, Gimenez A, Torrubia S, et al. Spontaneous pneumothorax and pneumomediastinum in IPF. Eur Radiol 2000; 10(1):108–113.

23. Schmidt LS, Warren MB, Nickerson ML, et al. Birt–Hogg–Dube syndrome, a genodermatosis associated with spontaneous pneumothorax and kidney neoplasia, maps to chromosome 17p11.2. Am J Hum Genet 2001; 69(4):876–882.

24. Yellin A, Shiner RJ, Lieberman Y. Familial multiple bilateral pneumothorax associated with Marfan syndrome. Chest 1991; 100(2):577–578.

25. Afessa B. Pleural effusion and pneumothorax in hospitalized patients with HIV infection: The Pulmonary Complications, ICU support, and Prognostic Factors of Hospitalized Patients with HIV (PIP) Study. Chest 2000; 117(4):1031–1037.

26. Vricella LA, Trachiotis GD. Heimlich valve in the management of pneumothorax in patients with advanced AIDS. Chest 2001; 120(1):15–18.

27. Mendez JL, Nadrous HF, Vassallo R, et al. Pneumothorax in pulmonary Langerhans cell histiocytosis. Chest 2004; 125(3):1028–1032.

28. Almoosa KF, Ryu JH, Mendez J, et al. Management of pneumothorax in lymphangioleiomyomatosis: Effects on recurrence and lung transplantation complications. Chest 2006; 129(5):1274–1281.

29. Wu S, Sagawa M, Suzuki S, et al. Pulmonary fibrosis with intractable pneumothorax: New pulmonary manifestation of relapsing polychondritis. Tohoku J Exp Med 2001; 194(3): 191–195.

30. Gammon RB, Shin MS, Groves RH Jr, et al. Clinical risk factors for pulmonary barotrauma: A multivariate analysis. Am J Respir Crit Care Med 1995; 152(4 Pt 1):1235–1240.

31. Strange C, Jantz M. Pneumothorax. In: Bouros D, ed. The Pleura. Lung Biology in Health and Disease, Vol. 186. New York: Marcel Dekker, 2004:661–676.

32. Fann JI, Berry GJ, Burdon TA. The use of endobronchial valve device to eliminate air leak. Respir Med 2006; 100(8):1402–1406.

33. Ferguson JS, Sprenger K, Van Natta T. Closure of a bronchopleural fistula using bronchoscopic placement of an endobronchial valve designed for the treatment of emphysema. Chest 2006; 129(2):479–481.

34. Mitchell KM, Boley TM, Hazelrigg SR. Endobronchial valves for treatment of bronchopleural fistula. Ann Thorac Surg 2006; 81(3):1129–1131.

35. Toma TP, Kon OM, Oldfield W, et al. Reduction of persistent air leak with endoscopic valve implants. Thorax 2007; 62(9):830–833.

36. Bishop MJ, Benson MS, Pierson DJ. Carbon dioxide excretion via bronchopleural fistulas in adult respiratory distress syndrome. Chest 1987; 91(3):400–402.

37. Blanch PB, Koens JC Jr, Layon AJ. A new device that allows synchronous intermittent inspiratory chest tube occlusion with any mechanical ventilator. Chest 1990; 97(6): 1426–1430.

38. Carvalho P, Thompson WH, Riggs R, et al. Management of bronchopleural fistula with a variable-resistance valve and a single ventilator. Chest 1997; 111(5):1452–1454.
39. Strange C. Double-lumen endotracheal tubes. Clin Chest Med 1991; 12(3):497–506.
40. Weg JG, Anzueto A, Balk RA, et al. The relation of pneumothorax and other air leaks to mortality in the acute respiratory distress syndrome. N Engl J Med 1998; 338(6):341–346.
41. Seremetis MG. The management of spontaneous pneumothorax. Chest 1970; 57(1):65–68.
42. Dines DE, Clagett OT, Payne WS. Spontaneous pneumothorax in emphysema. Mayo Clin Proc 1970; 45(7):481–487.
43. Norris RM, Jones JG, Bishop JM. Respiratory gas exchange in patients with spontaneous pneumothorax. Thorax 1968; 23(4):427–433.
44. O'Hara VS. Spontaneous pneumothorax. Mil Med 1978; 143(1):32–35.
45. Slebos DJ, Elting-Wartan AN, Bakker M, et al. Managing a bilateral pneumothorax in lung transplantation using single chest-tube drainage. J Heart Lung Transplant 2001; 20(7): 796–797.
46. Engdahl O, Toft T, Boe J. Chest radiograph—A poor method for determining the size of a pneumothorax. Chest 1993; 103(1):26–29.
47. Baumann MH, Strange C, Heffner JE, et al. Management of spontaneous pneumothorax: An American College of Chest Physicians Delphi consensus statement. Chest 2001; 119(2): 590–602.
48. Noppen M, Alexander P, Driesen P, et al. Quantification of the size of primary spontaneous pneumothorax: Accuracy of the Light index. Respiration 2001; 68(4):396–399.
49. Tocino IM, Miller MH, Fairfax WR. Distribution of pneumothorax in the supine and semirecumbent critically ill adult. AJR Am J Roentgenol 1985; 144(5):901–905.
50. Dulchavsky SA, Schwarz KL, Kirkpatrick AW, et al. Prospective evaluation of thoracic ultrasound in the detection of pneumothorax. J Trauma 2001; 50(2):201–205.
51. Soldati G, Testa A, Sher S, et al. Occult traumatic pneumothorax: Diagnostic accuracy of lung ultrasonography in the emergency department. Chest 2008; 133(1):204–211.
52. Gobien RP, Reines HD, Schabel SI. Localized tension pneumothorax: Unrecognized form of barotrauma in adult respiratory distress syndrome. Radiology 1982; 142(1):15–19.
53. Chen KY, Jerng JS, Liao WY, et al. Pneumothorax in the ICU: Patient outcomes and prognostic factors. Chest 2002; 122(2):678–683.
54. Light RW, O'Hara VS, Moritz TE, et al. Intrapleural tetracycline for the prevention of recurrent spontaneous pneumothorax. Results of a Department of Veterans Affairs cooperative study. JAMA 1990; 264(17):2224–2230.
55. Wolfman NT, Myers WS, Glauser SJ, et al. Validity of CT classification on management of occult pneumothorax: A prospective study. AJR Am J Roentgenol 1998; 171(5): 1317–1320.
56. Kircher LT Jr, Swartzel RL. Spontaneous pneumothorax and its treatment. J Am Med Assoc 1954: 155(1):24–29.
57. Northfield TC. Oxygen therapy for spontaneous pneumothorax. Br Med J 1971; 4(5779): 86–88.
58. England GJ, Hill RC, Timberlake GA, et al. Resolution of experimental pneumothorax in rabbits by graded oxygen therapy. J Trauma 1998; 45(2):333–334.
59. O'Rourke JP, Yee ES. Civilian spontaneous pneumothorax. Treatment options and long-term results. Chest 1989; 96(6):1302–1306.
60. Cerfolio RJ, Bass C, Katholi CR. Prospective randomized trial compares suction versus water seal for air leaks. Ann Thorac Surg 2001; 71(5):1613–1617.
61. Sharma TN, Agnihotri SP, Jain NK, et al. Intercostal tube thoracostomy in pneumothorax— Factors influencing re-expansion of lung. Indian J Chest Dis Allied Sci 1988; 30(1):32–35.
62. Andrivet P, Djedaini K, Teboul JL, et al. Spontaneous pneumothorax. Comparison of thoracic drainage vs immediate or delayed needle aspiration. Chest 1995; 108(2):335–339.

63. Almind M, Lange P, Viskum K. Spontaneous pneumothorax: Comparison of simple drainage, talc pleurodesis, and tetracycline pleurodesis. Thorax 1989; 44(8):627–630.

64. Kennedy L, Sahn SA. Talc pleurodesis for the treatment of pneumothorax and pleural effusion. Chest 1994; 106(4):1215–1222.

65. Cardillo G, Facciolo F, Regal M, et al. Recurrences following videothoracoscopic treatment of primary spontaneous pneumothorax: The role of redo-videothoracoscopy. Eur J Cardiothorac Surg 2001; 19(4):396–399.

66. Kennedy L, Harley RA, Sahn SA, et al. Talc slurry pleurodesis. Pleural fluid and histologic analysis. Chest 1995; 107(6):1707–1712.

67. Torresini G, Vaccarili M, Divisi D, et al. Is video-assisted thoracic surgery justified at first spontaneous pneumothorax? Eur J Cardiothorac Surg 2001; 20(1):42–45.

68. Vanderschueren RG. Pleural talcage in patients with spontaneous pneumothorax. Poumon Coeur 1981; 37(4):273–276.

41
Hemothorax

PAUL E. VAN SCHIL and PHILIPPE G. JORENS
Antwerp University Hospital, Edegem, Antwerp, Belgium
PATRIQUE SEGERS
Academic Medical Center, Amsterdam, The Netherlands

I. Introduction

Hemothorax is defined as accumulation of a significant amount of blood in the pleural space. By pure visualization of pleural fluid, it is clinically difficult to judge the amount of blood, and usually this is overestimated (1). For a hemothorax, the hematocrit of the pleural fluid should be at least 50% that of the peripheral blood (2). A massive hemothorax is defined as the accumulation of more than 800 mL of blood (3). It should be noted that the pleural space can contain up to 6 L of blood (4). On chest X-ray, the amount is considered significant when there is opacification of either diaphragmatic dome or when the depth of blood on the lateral decubitus film exceeds 2 cm at its deepest point (5). In a prospective study on the value of computed tomography (CT) in blunt chest trauma, hemothorax was defined on CT scan as an intrapleural collection of fluid that is equivalent to blood (30–100 Hounsfield units) with a thickness of more than 10 mm (6). Immediate insertion of a chest drain is the best prophylaxis against pleural space complications (4). The latter, listed in Table 1, result from an inadequately drained hemothorax.

A clotted or retained hemothorax is defined as a persisting or residual bloody effusion obscuring 25% or more of the lung field after three days (5). Empyema is present when there is pus or an infected clot in the pleural cavity. This occurs in 5% to 10% of cases after tube thoracostomy (5,7). The first phase is exudative, followed by the fibrinopurulent stage when there are fibrin deposits with loculation of fluid (8). When this is not adequately treated, a pleural peel develops—the third or organizing phase (9).

A persisting pleural effusion is an exudative pleuritis and occurs in more than 10% of cases after removal of the chest tubes. Such effusions are usually nonbloody, and most resolve spontaneously without pleural space sequelae (1). A thoracocentesis should be performed to rule out infection.

The incidence of fibrothorax is 1% after hemothorax. A dense fibrous peel develops on the lung surface, leading to a trapped lung, inhibiting lung expansion. In such cases decortication is necessary (4).

II. Etiology

Possible causes of hemothorax are listed in Table 2. The blunt or penetrating trauma is most frequently encountered (Fig. 1). Sources of bleeding include the chest wall, lung, diaphragm, blood vessels, and mediastinum. Abdominal causes, such as lacerations of

Table 1   Pleural Space Complications
of Hemothorax

Clotted or retained hemothorax
Empyema
Persisting pleural effusion
Fibrothorax, trapped lung

spleen or liver with an associated diaphragmatic injury, can also give rise to a hemothorax (3). Rib fractures should not be considered to be minor injuries. In a series of 711 patients with rib fractures, a hemo- or pneumothorax was found in 32% of patients, and 26% had a lung contusion (10). Mortality was higher than 10% in this series. In our own series of 187 thoracic-trauma patients, hemothorax was diagnosed in 55 or 29.4% patients (11). Associated injuries were present in 40 (72.7%) patients. Rib fractures were associated with hemothorax in 35.3% of patients, with pneumothorax in 42.1%, and with lung contusion in 60.1% (11).

In the nontraumatic group, pleural tumors and complications of anticoagulant therapy are most frequent (12). A large hemothorax in a patient operated for empyema is shown in Figure 2. Hemothorax may also occur after spontaneous pneumothorax. The incidence ranges from 2.0% to 7.3% (13). Three possible mechanisms exist to explain hemorrhage in hemopneumothorax. First, a torn adhesion between the parietal and visceral pleurae may be the cause. Second, rupture of vascularized bullae or underlying lung parenchyma may represent the bleeding source. Third mechanism is hemorrhage from

Table 2   Causes of Hemothorax

Traumatic
    Blunt trauma
    Penetrating trauma
Iatrogenic
    Puncture of subclavian artery or vein
    Thoracentesis
    Puncture or biopsy of pleural or pulmonary lesions
    Transbronchial biopsy
    Cardiac or thoracic surgery
Nontraumatic
    Pleural tumors (primary—metastatic)
    Complication of anticoagulation therapy
    Bleeding disorder such as hemophilia, thrombocytopenia
    Lung metastases
    Spontaneous pneumothorax
    Rupture of pleural adhesions
    Pleural endometriosis
    Leaking aortic dissection or aneurysm
    Arteriovenous malformations
    Pancreatic pseudocyst
    Neurofibromatosis

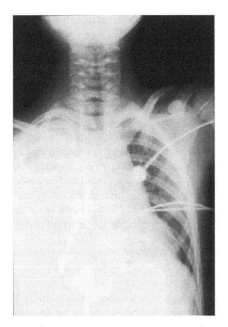

Figure 1   Massive hemothorax in a 10-year-old boy after penetrating injury of the subclavian artery.

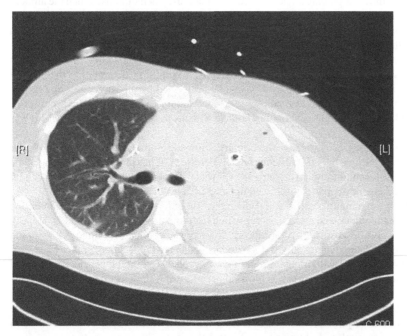

Figure 2   CT scan demonstrating left hemothorax in a patient who underwent thoracotomy for empyema due to iatrogenic esophageal perforation.

torn congenital aberrant vessels branching from the pleural surface and distributed in and around the bulla in the apex of the lung.

In children also, the most common cause of hemothorax is trauma. Other causes include subpleural arteriovenous malformations and malignancy (8).

III. Clinical Presentation

General symptoms depend on the amount of blood in the pleural space and range from minimal to life-threatening shock. Symptoms and signs are those of bleeding and pleuritis. Less than 250 mL of blood in the pleural space gives only a few symptoms. In case of massive hemothorax, patient will present with tachypnea, tachycardia, pallor, hypotension, and cardiovascular collapse (3). On clinical examination, there are diminished or absent breath sounds on the involved side and dullness to percussion. Routine laboratory tests are performed including hemoglobin, hematocrit, and coagulation tests. In case of severe blood loss, enough blood is matched and general resuscitation measures started to correct the hypovolemic shock.

IV. Diagnosis

In every patient with a thoracic trauma a chest radiograph is obtained, preferentially in the upright position. In the supine position, only haziness will be present on the involved side. In a study of 130 patients with blunt chest trauma, a hemothorax was not diagnosed correctly on the initial chest radiograph in 24% of patients (14). In a more upright position, blunting of the costophrenic angle is noted in a small-sized hemothorax. When the amount of blood increases, a dense opacification is found on the affected hemithorax (Figs. 1 and 2) with a possible mediastinal shifting to the contralateral side. In 50% of traumatic cases a pneumothorax is also present. In any case, a follow-up chest radiograph should be taken after 24 hours to judge the specific evolution (12). When no upright chest radiograph can be obtained or in case of doubt, ultrasonography is helpful in determining the amount of blood in the pleural space (15). This can be performed by the surgeon or emergency physician during the initial evaluation of the chest-trauma patient (16). The accuracy of ultrasound examination in penetrating thoracic wounds has been reported to be as high as 97.3% (17).

Chest radiography remains the primary screening study for the assessment of victims of chest trauma, but CT, particularly multidetector CT, has progressively changed the imaging approach to trauma patients (18). Nowadays, CT is readily available especially as many emergency departments are equipped with a CT scanner.

Early after trauma, differential diagnosis should be made between hemothorax, diaphragmatic injury, and atelectasis for which the thoracic CT scanning is most helpful.

However, as cost is a major concern nowadays, the value of routine CT scanning of the chest in hemodynamically stable patients is disputed (17). On the other hand, in a study of 103 patients with blunt chest trauma, thoracic CT scanning provided additional information in 65% of cases (6). CT was especially valid in detecting lung contusions, pneumo-, and hemothorax. The specific findings on CT had direct consequences in early trauma management in 42% of the total study population, mostly regarding chest tube placement and respiratory care. Compared to historical controls, use of CT resulted in less cases of respiratory failure and ARDS, and also in a reduced mortality (6).

So, CT scanning of the chest can be recommended in the initial diagnostic workup in severe chest trauma, except in patients who are hemodynamically unstable or when there is an indication for urgent surgical intervention.

The use of serial chest X-rays to evaluate patients with penetrating thoracic trauma is a common practice. In a recent prospective study evaluating whether a noncontrast chest CT is as reliable as a six-hour chest X-ray for detecting delayed thoracic injuries after penetrating thoracic trauma, 118 patients were included (19). All initial chest X-rays were negative. CT identified six patients with a pneumothorax and one patient with a hemothorax. Two patients required surgical intervention. There were no delayed findings on chest X-ray provided the CT was negative. The use of serial chest X-rays provided no additional information, which was not available on the initial chest CT (19).

In persisting or recurrent pleural effusions for which a precise diagnosis should be obtained, thoracocentesis is indicated with puncture of the pleural fluid, if necessary under ultrasonographic or CT guidance. Hematocrit, glucose, and protein content should be determined and a specimen is also sent for bacteriological examination to rule out empyema. Thoracocentesis should be considered as a diagnostic procedure and is not indicated for treatment of hemothorax (3).

V. Treatment

Depending on the clinical stage of the patient, general measures are taken for resuscitation and to correct hypovolemia. Hemodynamically unstable patients are taken to the operating room at once. Therapeutic options for hemothorax and its complications are listed in Table 3.

A. Tube Thoracostomy

Early drainage of every hemothorax by a chest tube is indicated to obtain a complete lung expansion and to reduce the incidence of empyema and fibrothorax (4). Approximately 85% of all hemothoraces can be treated by a chest drain only (3). A large-bore tube should be inserted in the fifth intercostal space on the midaxillary line and directed posteriorly to the costophrenic angle (Fig. 3). In case of massive bleeding, an autotransfusion device can be used for rapid processing and reinfusion of blood. Tube thoracostomy provides a precise measure of blood loss and its evolution over time (20). By apposing the pleural surfaces, bleeding from the pulmonary parenchyma or pleural lacerations usually stops spontaneously, as a natural tamponade is created (12,20). In an experimental study of massive hemothorax, chest tube clamping did not decrease hemorrhage or mortality and

Table 3 Treatment Options for Hemothorax and
Its Complications

Tube thoracostomy
Fibrinolytic treatment
Thoracoscopy or VATS
Thoracotomy
    Early: massive or persisting blood loss
    Late: clotted hemothorax, empyema, fibrothorax

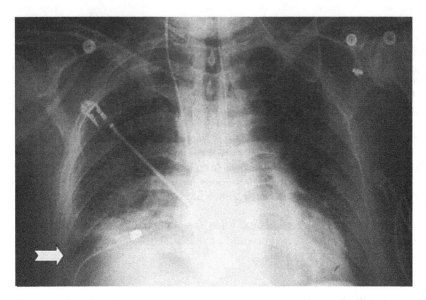

Figure 3   Insertion of a basal chest tube in a patient with hemophilia A who underwent cholecystectomy complicated by right hemothorax.

did not improve hypotension (21). For these reasons, clamping is not recommended in the treatment of a large hemothorax.

By applying suction to the drains, chest tube duration can be decreased, potentially leading to a shorter length of hospital stay (22). When drainage becomes less than 50 mL over six hours, the chest tubes should be removed as they can serve as conduits for pleural infection and subsequent empyema (5). Prophylactic antibiotics are indicated as they reduce the incidence of empyema and pneumonia in patients with chest tubes for traumatic hemopneumothoraces (23–25). However, the precise dosage and optimal duration remain to be determined. Usually, a first-generation cephalosporin is administered for no longer than 24 hours (26).

In one retrospective study of 57 chest drains, the overall complication rate was 30%, but there was only one major complication, a thoracic empyema (27). No insertional complications were encountered. However, in another retrospective study, the overall complication rate was significantly higher for chest tubes inserted on the inpatient ward as compared to the emergency department or operating room (28).

A short-period treatment aiming at removing the chest tube within 24 hours combined with early mobilization was evaluated in 1845 patients, 7.5% of whom had a blunt chest trauma (5). In total, 91% of patients could be treated by tube thoracostomy only, and hospital stay was less than 48 hours in 82% of the patients, a remarkable achievement. General principles of treatment included early mobilization, adequate analgesia, and vigorous physiotherapy. In this study, the failure rate of conservative treatment without chest drain was 26%. Empyema was found to occur more frequently in patients with a significantly longer mean drainage time or an increased volume of blood loss (5).

B. Fibrinolytic Treatment

When a residual clotted hemothorax develops, there is an ongoing controversy whether this should be treated conservatively or more aggressively by thoracotomy or video-assisted thoracic surgery (VATS). Pleural blood can be absorbed spontaneously, but adverse sequelae of an incomplete evacuation may develop (Table 1), favoring a more aggressive approach (16). Intrapleural administration of the fibrinolytic agents streptokinase and urokinase has been reported as an effective nonoperative treatment of residual collections or so-called retained hemothorax. The first use of streptokinase in hemothorax was described in 1949 (29). Thereafter, several authors reported beneficial effects of intrapleural fibrinolytic treatment (30–33). A recent study included patients with an undrained traumatic hemothorax, defined as more than 300 mL of intrathoracic blood estimated by CT scan on the third day after chest tube insertion (34). Out of 203 patients with a traumatic hemothorax, managed by tube thoracostomy, 25 (12.3%) patients developed an undrained hemothorax. Successful resolution was seen in 92% of patients within 3.4 ± 1.4 days of fibrinolytic treatment. No bleeding or other significant complications related to fibrinolytic treatment were recorded (34).

A retrospective study evaluated 65 patients with posttraumatic-retained hemothoraces managed by VATS or intrapleural streptokinase (35). The use of VATS diminished the need for thoracotomy and also shortened hospital stay. However, this was a nonrandomized study and it should be noticed that fibrinolytic treatment is a minimally invasive procedure, which can be applied repeatedly in critically ill patients.

Regarding the specific technique, streptokinase (250,000 IU) or urokinase (100,000 IU) is diluted in 100-mL saline solution and injected through the chest tube which is clamped for four hours. Daily drainage is recorded and the chest tubes are removed when drainage becomes less than 50 mL over 24 hours. Fibrinolytic treatment seems to be most effective for a clotted hemothorax when it is applied within 10 days of injury (Fig. 4). Otherwise, organization of the clot leads to a fibrous peel and fibrothorax, necessitating a decortication by thoracotomy, at least four to five weeks later (12). At the present time, there is no consensus on the duration of fibrinolytic treatment, the amount and frequency of instillation, and the precise assessment of response.

C. Thoracoscopy or VATS

As most patients with a hemothorax can be treated by a thoracic drain, only 10% to 20% need an operative intervention. These represent a high-risk group (3). VATS or thoracoscopy is a less-invasive treatment modality, which can replace thoracotomy in selected cases. Nowadays, in hemodynamically stable patients, diagnostic and therapeutic thoracoscopy plays an important role in the trauma setting. Its use in penetrating chest injuries was first described in 1946 (36). VATS uses minimal incisions, possibly reducing postoperative pain and hospital stay (37,38). A hemodynamically stable patient, presenting with persistent hemorrhage through the chest tube, is a classic indication for early thoracoscopic intervention in trauma. VATS offers a complete visualization of the pleural cavity; blood can be evacuated and the source of bleeding can also be determined (16). Lacerated pulmonary segments can be repaired or resected, and chest-wall bleeding may be clipped, coagulated or sutured. Other current indications for VATS in thoracic trauma are clotted hemothorax early after the injury, evaluation of a persistent air leak, mediastinal injuries, and also inspection of the diaphragm to rule out traumatic rupture (9,17,38–40). Diaphragmatic injuries are difficult to diagnose, as they might be overlooked in

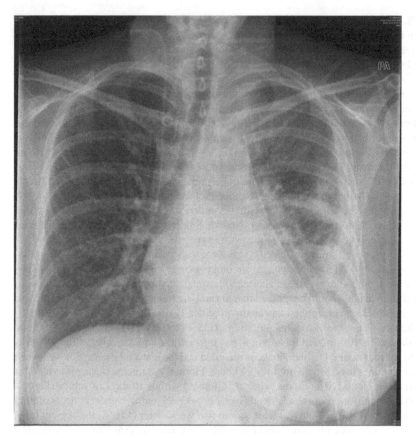

Figure 4   Chest X-ray after fibrinolytic treatment in the patient with hemothorax (Fig. 2) showing almost complete resolution.

conventional trauma imaging without gross herniation of intra-abdominal contents into the thoracic cavity. In some cases, diaphragmatic defects can be closed during thoracoscopy as well (38).

Contraindications for VATS are hemodynamically unstable patients who should proceed immediately to sternotomy or thoracotomy, suspected great vessel or cardiac injury, obliteration of the pleural space, which renders the introduction of the thoracoscope impossible, and inability to tolerate single-lung ventilation (9,39). In this respect, a VATS procedure should be performed within five days of the original injury to avoid developing fibrosis from an organizing bloody effusion.

In a study of 58 patients with residual traumatic hemothorax, chest radiograph taken on the second day after injury was compared to CT scanning of the thorax (7). Chest X-ray was found to be unreliable, with an incorrect interpretation in 48%. In 31% of patients, the treatment decision based on chest X-ray was changed from operative to nonoperative management, or vice versa. In this way, CT scanning adds more diagnostic information and is considered the gold standard on which to base therapeutic decisions. Arbitrarily, a volume of 500 mL of blood is chosen as the cut-off value for performing a thoracoscopic procedure (41). Early thoracoscopic evacuation of retained blood has proven to be safe and effective. In a prospective randomized trial, 39 patients with retained hemothoraces were randomized between a second tube thoracostomy and a VATS procedure (42). In the VATS group duration of tube drainage, total hospital stay and costs were reduced. Although VATS represents a more complex and expensive approach, it may be a more efficient and economical strategy for treatment of traumatic-retained hemothoraces.

Complications occur in less than 10% of VATS procedures, of which atelectasis is the most common (43). Conversion rates of VATS range from 1.7% to 24%; for this reason patients should always be prepared for thoracotomy (39). Also in the management of posttraumatic empyema, VATS has been successfully performed (44), but it should be reserved for early cases before the organizing phase sets in.

D. Thoracotomy

With the advent of fibrinolytic treatment and thoracoscopic procedures, the number of thoracotomies for the management of traumatic hemothorax will probably diminish. No precise criteria for intervention have been established (12). An initial blood loss of more than 1.5 L or a persisting blood loss of more than 250 mL/hr for three consecutive hours is generally regarded as an indication for urgent exploration by sternotomy or thoracotomy, especially in unstable patients (1,3,16). In our series of 55 hemothoraces, an urgent thoracotomy was performed in 6 or 10.9% patients (11).

Although there is a trend towards nonoperative or delayed treatment in patients with aortic rupture and severe associated lesions, suspected aortic injury with a massive left-sided hemothorax is still an indication for urgent left thoracotomy and repair (17). Rare cases of traumatic aortic dissection without complications can be treated conservatively (45). Other indications for immediate thoracotomy are cardiac tamponade, evidence of a major bronchial rupture, sucking chest wounds, and injury of the aortic arch vessels (12,16,26,38). Cardiac injuries are mostly approached by sternotomy.

In case of bleeding from lung parenchyma, selective ligation of bleeding vessels is advocated after placement of long vascular clamps or staplers to the entrance and exit sites of injured lobes. This technique is known as pulmonotomy or pulmonary tractotomy (16,17). A so-called trauma pneumonectomy is performed in cases of massive bleeding by stapling of the pulmonary hilum, but carries a high mortality (46,47).

Emergency room thoracotomy is mainly indicated in penetrating injuries with recent cardiac arrest or massive blood loss, but overall survival rates are less than 10% (17,48). Contraindications are penetrating trauma with no signs of life on the accident scene and blunt trauma without signs of life on arrival in the emergency department.

Late indications for thoracotomy after traumatic injuries include clotted hemothorax, empyema, and fibrothorax. A retained or clotted hemothorax 7 to 10 days after injury is no longer an indication for fibrinolytic treatment or thoracoscopy due to organization of the clot. Open thoracotomy is necessary to open up the different loculations, drain the effusion, and remove the fibrous peel to obtain a complete lung expansion (3). Empyema in the organizing phase should also be treated by thoracotomy to allow full evacuation of all purulent collections and debridement of devitalized tissue (20). In case of fibrothorax or trapped lung, a decortication is performed. Good results have been described even if the fibrothorax has been present for 10 years or more (2,12).

E. Treatment of Nontraumatic Hemothorax

In case of a nontraumatic hemothorax, treatment depends on the underlying disorder. Pulmonary arteriovenous malformations are treated by embolization or surgical resection and ligation (8). Transcatheter arterial coil embolization is also an effective method for the treatment of spontaneous hemothorax after aneurysm rupture in neurofibromatosis (49).

Coagulation disorders are corrected by administration of specific blood products. Anticoagulation is stopped or reduced in case of a significant hemothorax occurring as complication of overzealous anticoagulant therapy.

Diagnosis of pleural tumors and treatment of recurrent pneumothorax and endometriosis can be performed by thoracoscopy (50,51). A leaking aortic aneurysm or dissection is an indication for thoracotomy or sternotomy with repair by an interposition graft (52). Iatrogenic hemothorax requires insertion of a chest drain. Only in cases of massive or persistent bleeding is a thoracotomy indicated for repair of the bleeding vessel or lung lesion.

VI. Conclusion

The most common cause of hemothorax is chest trauma. For precise diagnosis in severe chest injury, CT of the thorax is recommended. Most hemothoraces can be adequately treated by insertion of a chest drain, which provides the best prophylaxis against pleural space complications. Thoracotomy is indicated only in cases of massive or persistent bleeding. A clotted or retained hemothorax early after injury is an indication for fibrinolytic treatment or thoracoscopy. Complete drainage is necessary to avoid late complications such as empyema or fibrothorax. The latter usually necessitates an open thoracotomy for adequate drainage and removal of the fibrous peel.

References

1. Sahn SS. Diseases of the pleura and pleural space. In: Baum GL, Crapo JD, Celli BR, Karlinsky JB, eds. Textbook of Pulmonary Diseases. Philadelphia: Lippincott-Raven, 1998:1483–1498.
2. Light RW. Diseases of the pleura, mediastinum, chest wall and diaphragm. In: George RB, Light RW, Matthay MA, Matthay RA, eds. Chest Medicine. Philadelphia, PA: Lippincott, 2005:415–447.
3. Owens MW, Milligan SA, Eggerstedt JM, et al. Thoracic trauma, surgery and perioperative management. In: George RB, Light RW, Matthay MA, Matthay RA, eds. Chest Medicine. Philadelphia: Lippincott, 2005:564–588.
4. Glinz W. Chest Trauma. Diagnosis and Management. Berlin: Springer-Verlag, 1981.
5. Knottenbelt JD, Van Der Spuy JW. Traumatic hemothorax—Experience of a protocol for rapid turnover in 1,845 cases. S Afr J Surg 1994; 32:5–8.
6. Trupka A, Waydhas C, Hallfeldt KK, et al. Value of thoracic computed tomography in the first assessment of severely injured patients with blunt chest trauma: Results of a prospective study. J Trauma 1997; 43:405–412.
7. Velmahos GC, Demetriades D, Chan L, et al. Predicting the need for thoracoscopic evacuation of residual traumatic hemothorax: Chest radiograph is insufficient. J Trauma 1999; 46:65–70.
8. Zeitlin PL. Pleural effusions and empyema. In: Loughlin GM, Eigen H, eds. Respiratory Disease in Children. Baltimore, MD: Williams & Wilkins, 1994:453–463.
9. Lowdermilk GA, Naunheim KS. Thoracoscopic evaluation and treatment of thoracic trauma. Surg Clin North Am 2000; 80:1535–1542.

10. Ziegler DW, Agarwal NN. The morbidity and mortality of rib fractures. J Trauma 1994; 37:975–979.

11. Segers P, Van Schil P, Jorens PG, et al. Thoracic trauma: An analysis of 187 patients. Acta Chir Belg 2001; 101:277–282.

12. Light RW, Garay Lee YC. Pneumothorax, chylothorax, hemothorax and fibrothorax. In: Murray JF, Nadel JA, eds. Textbook of Respiratory Medicine, Part 3. Philadelphia: W. B. Saunders Company, 2005:1961–1988.

13. Hsu NY, Shih CS, Hsu CP, et al. Spontaneous hemopneumothorax revisited: Clinical approach and systemic review of the literature. Ann Thorac Surg 2005; 80:1859–1863.

14. Drummond DS, Craig RH. Traumatic hemothorax: Complications and management. Am Surg 1967; 33:403–408.

15. McEwan K, Thompson P. Ultrasound to detect haemothorax after chest injury. Emerg Med J 2007; 24:581–582.

16. Graeber GM, Prabhakar G, Shields TW. Blunt and penetrating injuries of the chest wall, pleura, and lungs. In: Shields TW, LoCicero J III, Ponn RB, Rusch VW, eds. General Thoracic Surgery. Philadelphia: Lippincott, 2005:951–971.

17. Feliciano DV, Rozycki GS. Advances in the diagnosis and treatment of thoracic trauma. Surg Clin North Am 1999; 79:1417–1429.

18. Mirvis SE. Imaging of acute thoracic injury: The advent of MDCT screening. Semin Ultrasound CT MR 2005; 26:305–331.

19. Magnotti LJ, Weinberg JA, Schroeppel TJ, et al. Initial chest CT obviates the need for repeat chest radiograph after penetrating thoracic trauma. Am Surg 2007; 73:569–573.

20. Winterbauer RH. Non malignant pleural effusions. In: Fishman AP, ed. Fishman's Pulmonary Diseases and Disorders. New York: McGraw-Hill, 1998:1411–1427.

21. Ali J, Qi W. Effectiveness of chest tube clamping in massive hemothorax. J Trauma 1995; 38:59–63.

22. Davis JW, Mackersie RC, Hoyt DB, et al. Randomized study of algorithms for discontinuing tube thoracostomy drainage. J Am Coll Surg 1994; 179:553–557.

23. Sanabria A, Valdivieso E, Gomez G, et al. Prophylactic antibiotics in chest trauma: A meta-analysis of high-quality studies. World J Surg 2006; 30:1843–1847.

24. Gonzalez RP, Holevar MR. Role of prophylactic antibiotics for tube thoracostomy in chest trauma. Am Surg 1998; 64:617–621.

25. Wilson RF, Nichols RL. The EAST practice management guidelines for prophylactic antibiotic use in tube thoracostomy for traumatic hemopneumothorax: A commentary. J Trauma 2000; 48:758–759.

26. Meyer DM. Hemothorax related to trauma. Thorac Surg Clin 2007; 17:47–55.

27. Bailey RC. Complications of tube thoracostomy in trauma. J Accid Emerg Med 2000; 17:111–114.

28. Chan L, Reilly KM, Henderson C, et al. Complication rates of tube thoracostomy. Am J Emerg Med 1997; 15:368–370.

29. Tillett WS, Sherry S. The effect in patients of streptococcal fibrinolysin (streptokinase) and streptococcal deoxyribonuclease on fibrinous, purulent and sanguineous pleural exudations. J Clin Invest 1949; 23:173–179.

30. Vogelzang RL, Tobin RS, Burstein S, et al. Transcatheter intracavitary fibrinolysis of infected extravascular hematomas. Am J Roentgenol 1987; 148:378–380.

31. Inci I, Ozcelik C, Ulku R, et al. Intrapleural fibrinolytic treatment of traumatic clotted hemothorax. Chest 1998; 114:160–165.

32. Jerjes-Sanchez C, Ramirez-Rivera A, Elizalde JJ, et al. Intrapleural fibrinolysis with streptokinase as an adjunctive treatment in hemothorax and empyema: A multicenter trial. Chest 1996; 109:1514–1519.

33. Moulton JS, Benkert RE, Weisiger KH, et al. Treatment of complicated pleural fluid collections with image-guided drainage and intracavitary urokinase. Chest 1995; 108:1252–1259.

34. Kimbrell BJ, Yamzon J, Petrone P, et al. Intrapleural thrombolysis for the management of undrained traumatic hemothorax: A prospective observational study. J Trauma 2007; 62:1175–1179.

35. Oguzkaya F, Akçali Y, Bilgin M. Videothoracoscopy versus intrapleural streptokinase for management of posttraumatic retained hemothorax: A retrospective analysis of 65 cases. Injury 2005; 36:526–529.

36. Branco JMC. Thoracoscopy as a method of exploration in penetrating injuries of the chest. Dis Chest 1946; 12:330–335.

37. Heniford BT, Carrillo EH, Spain DA, et al. The role of thoracoscopy in the management of retained thoracic collections after trauma. Ann Thorac Surg 1997; 63:940–943.

38. Cetindag IB, Neideen T, Hazelrigg SR. Video-assisted thoracic surgical applications in thoracic trauma. Thorac Surg Clin 2007; 17:73–79.

39. Lang-Lazdunski L, Mouroux J, Pons F, et al. Role of videothoracoscopy in chest trauma. Ann Thorac Surg 1997; 63:327–333.

40. Carrillo EH, Richardson JD. Thoracoscopy in the management of hemothorax and retained blood after trauma. Curr Opin Pulm Med 1998; 4:243–246.

41. Velmahos GC, Demetriades D. Early thoracoscopy for the evacuation of undrained haemothorax. Eur J Surg 1999; 165:924–929.

42. Meyer DM, Jessen ME, Wait MA, et al. Early evacuation of traumatic retained hemothoraces using thoracoscopy: A prospective randomized trial. Ann Thorac Surg 1997; 64:1396–1401.

43. Krasna MJ, Deshmukh S, McLaughlin JS. Complications of thoracoscopy. Ann Thorac Surg 1996; 61:1066–1069.

44. Sosa JL, Pombo H, Puente I, et al. Thoracoscopy in the evaluation and management of thoracic trauma. Int Surg 1998; 83:187–189.

45. Goverde P, Van Schil P, Delrue F, et al. Traumatic type B aortic dissection. Acta Chir Belg 1996; 96:233–236.

46. Wagner JW, Obeid FN, Karmy-Jones RC, et al. Trauma pneumonectomy revisited: The role of simultaneous stapled pneumonectomy. J Trauma 1996; 40:590–594.

47. Baumgartner F, Omari B, Lee J, et al. Survival after trauma pneumonectomy: The pathophysiologic balance of shock resuscitation with right heart failure. Am Surg 1996; 62:967–972.

48. Kaiser LR, DiPierro FW. Thoracic trauma. In: Fishman AP, ed. Fishman's Pulmonary Diseases and Disorders. New York: McGraw-Hill, 1988:1661–1669.

49. Arai K, Sanada J, Kurozumi A, et al. Spontaneous hemothorax in neurofibromatosis treated with percutaneous embolization. Cardiovasc Intervent Radiol 2007; 30:477–479.

50. Van Schil P, Van Meerbeeck J, Vanmaele R, et al. Role of thoracoscopy (VATS) in pleural and pulmonary pathology. Acta Chir Belg 1996; 96:23–27.

51. Van Schil PE, Vercauteren SR, Vermeire PA, et al. Catamenial pneumothorax caused by thoracic endometriosis. Ann Thorac Surg 1996; 62:585–586.

52. Ochsner J, Ancalmo N. Descending thoracic aortic aneurysm. Chest Surg Clin North Am 1992; 2:291–309.

42
Chylothorax and Pseudochylothorax

MICHAEL TOUMBIS
Chest Diseases Hospital of Athens "Sotiria", Athens, Greece

I. Chylothorax

Chylothorax is a rather acute pleural effusion characterized by the presence of chyle into one or both pleural cavities. Due to its high-fat content, the pleural fluid is usually milky. Analysis of the pleural fluid reveals high levels of triglycerides and chylomicrons. Before considering the aetiopathogenic, clinical, biochemical, and therapeutic features of chylothorax, essential data concerning the anatomy of thoracic duct and the physiology of chyle will be briefly mentioned.

A. Anatomy of the Thoracic Duct

The thoracic duct extends from the abdomen to the root of the neck, varying in length from 37 to 45 cm. It originates from the cisterna chyli at the level of L-2 vertebra, and ascents into the thorax through the aortic hiatus to the right of the midline. At the level of T-5 or T-6 vertebra, it crosses to the left of the spine and continues upward along the lateral aspect of esophagus behind the aorta and the left subclavian artery. It ultimately joins the junction of the left subclavian vein and the left internal jugular vein (1).

Although it is considered as a single structure, thoracic duct is commonly multiple in part of its course and may consist of up to eight separate channels with extensive lymphatic and venous communications (2). Occasionally, the duct divides into two branches, one in the usual left side and the other in the right side. The right lymphatic duct terminates at the junction of the right subclavian vein and the right internal jugular vein, and drains the right side of the head and neck, right upper limb, right lung, right side of the heart, and the convex surface of liver. The left lymphatic duct drains the remaining parts of the body (3).

This anatomy explains several clinically important issues: (*i*) chylothorax is usually right-sided as the largest part of the thoracic duct is within the right hemithorax; (*ii*) bilateral chylothorax can be formed when the damage of thoracic duct is at the level of midline; (*iii*) left-sided chylothorax tends to occur when the damage of the duct is at the level of aorta; and (*iv*) obstruction of the thoracic duct per se does not result in a chylothorax, because of the duct's extensive lymphatic and venous communications—this means that it can be tied off therapeutically without adverse consequences (4).

B. Physiology of Chyle

The thoracic duct normally transports 1500 to 2500 mL of chyle daily, derived from the gastrointestinal tract (60%), the liver (35%), and the skeletal tissue (15%) (5). Basal lymph flow is about 30 mL/(kg · day). It drops to 10 mL/(kg · day) during starvation. The ingestion of a fatty meal increases the flow of lymph in the thoracic duct by a factor of 2 to 10 for several hours. The ingestion of water also increases the flow of chyle, whereas the ingestion of proteins or carbohydrates has little effect (6).

Conventional dietary lipids consist mainly of long-chain triglyceride containing predominantly fatty acids of chain length ≥16. The ingested short-chain fatty acids are transported directly by the portal system. About 60% to 70% of ingested dietary lipids pass through the lymphatic system, mainly as chylomicrons, at a concentration of 5 to 30 g/L (6). By the time they reach the thoracic duct, chylomicrons are 80% to 95% triglycerides. Once they are in circulation, hydrolysis of the triglycerides rapidly degrades them to cholesterol-rich particles.

Chylomicrons and lipoproteins are molecular complexes of lipids and proteins that transport the water-insoluble lipids in a water-compatible colloidal form. Therefore, triglycerides, cholesterol, fat-soluble vitamins (A, D, E, and K), and antibodies are found in chyle (6). The protein content of chyle varies between 2 and 3 g/dL, with an albumin-to-globulin ratio of approximately 3:1. The electrolyte composition is similar to that of serum. Lymphocytes constitute 95% of the chyle cellular component. Some 90% of them are T lymphocytes (400–6000/mm³). Erythrocytes are also present, numbering between 50 and 600/mm³ (1).

C. Etiology

Chylothorax may be classified according to etiology as traumatic, nontraumatic, congenital, and idiopathic (Table 1).

The incidence of traumatic chylothoraces is approximately 25% and is largely iatrogenic in nature (7). Because of its anatomic course, the thoracic duct is vulnerable to traumatic injury during any thoracic surgical procedure and especially during surgery on the thoracic vertebral column, or on the left hemithorax near the hilum. The occurrence of chylothorax has most often been described following esophageal resection, with incidence varying between 0.6% and 4%. Higher incidence is reported for the transhiatal technique than for the thoracic approach (8). The estimated incidence of chylothorax after cardiovascular surgery is 0.25% to 0.50% and the condition is most commonly seen with surgery for Fallot's tetralogy, patent ductus arteriosus, and coarctation of the aorta (9). Chylothorax has also been reported as a complication of thoracoplasty, pneumonectomy, thoracic sympathectomy, mobilization of the left subclavian artery, stellate ganglion blockage, cervical node dissection, radical neck dissection, surgical intervention below the diaphragm, and several therapeutic and diagnostic procedures, like central venous cannulation, translumbar arteriography, and esophageal sclerotherapy (1,3,9,10).

Approximately 20% of cases of traumatic chylothorax are due to noniatrogenic causes. Penetrating injuries to the neck, chest, or abdomen due to gunshot or stab wounds may directly lacerate the thoracic duct or its tributaries. Chylothorax may occur following blunt injury to the clavicle, ribs or vertebrae, and blast and crush injuries (9–11).

Among the nontraumatic causes, the most common is malignancy accounting for more than 50% of cases, with lymphoma being the leading cause (70%). Other malignant causes include primary or metastatic tumors that cause mediastinal mass effect, disrupting or compressing the thoracic duct. Lymphoma or other mediastinal malignancy causing disruption or obstruction of the lower portion of the thoracic duct tends to cause

Table 1 Etiology of Chylothorax

Traumatic
  Iatrogenic trauma
    Cervical, thoracic, abdomen surgery
    Central venous cannulation
    Translumbar arteriography
    Esophageal sclerotherapy
  Noniatrogenic trauma
    Blunt
    Penetrating
Nontraumatic
  Malignant diseases
    Lymphoma
    Metastatic carcinoma
    Kaposi's sarcoma
  Mediastinal tumors
    Teratoma
    Retrosternal goiter
  Infectious diseases
    Tuberculosis, filariasis
  Diseases affecting the lymph vessels
    Lymphangioleiomyomatosis
    Gorham's syndrome
    Thoracic duct cyst
    Yellow nail syndrome, Castleman's disease
  Miscellaneous
    Sarcoidosis, Bechet's syndrome
  Transudative
    Cirrhosis of the liver, heart failure, nephrotic syndrome
Congenital lymphatic malformation
  Thoracic duct atresia
  Lymphatic aplasia, hypoplasia, dysplasia
  Varicose lymphatics, megalolymphatics
  Lymphangioma, lymphangiomatosis
  Intestinal lymphangiectasia; protein-losing enteropathy
Idiopathic

right-sided chylothorax. When the upper half of the thoracic duct is affected, chylothorax is commonly left-sided (12–14).

Intraluminal rapid obstruction of great veins by neoplasmatic cells, infective organisms, and thrombosis may be associated with chylothorax. Chylothorax due to superior vena cava thrombosis is frequently bilateral and often fatal, especially in children. A few cases of chylothorax as late complication of thoracic irradiation have been reported (3,15,16).

Among the diseases that are directly affecting the lymph vessels, lymphangioleiomyomatosis and Gorham's syndrome are most commonly associated with chylothorax. Lymphangioleiomyomatosis is a rare lung disease affecting females and characterized by an abnormal proliferation of smooth muscle–like cells causing progressive obstruction of the airways, lymphatics, and blood vessels. The frequency of chylothorax related to lymphangioleiomyomatosis, appears to be less frequent in recent series than that in some older reports (7–29%) (17,18). Gorham's syndrome characterized by massive osteolysis is a very rare disease and is complicated by chylothorax in 17% cases (19).

Cases of chylothorax with biochemical characteristics of transudate have been reported in patients with nephrotic syndrome, cardiac failure, and cirrhosis with chylous ascites (20–22). Finally, chylothorax is extremely rare complication of most of the remaining nontraumatic diseases listed in Table 1 (1,3,10,14).

Congenital chylothorax occurs spontaneously and is usually detected in infancy. Under this broad etiologic heading, it is possible to include thoracic atresia, lymphatic aplasia, lymphatic hypoplasia, lymphatic dysplasia, varicose lymphatics, lymphangioma, lymphangiomatosis, and lymphangiectasis (3,17,23,24). Congenital lymphatic malformations can be associated to Down syndrome, Noonan syndrome, *hydrops fetalis*, Turner syndrome, and lymphedema (3).

Idiopathic chylothorax is uncommon and comprises cases where no cause has been identified. These cases may be associated with fixation of the thoracic duct by previous infection, trauma or anomaly of the underlying vertebra and sudden overstretching of the fixed duct by strenuous activity (25). A sudden increase in duct pressure from stretching or coughing, especially after a heavy and fatty meal when the duct is engorged, may be a contributory factor (1).

D. Clinical Manifestations

In chylothorax, the clinical manifestations may be mild or severe depending on the amount and rate of chyle loss. Nontraumatic chylothorax usually develops slowly and the clinical picture is that of fatigue, dyspnea on exertion, and heaviness and discomfort in the affected side. Pleuritic chest pain and high fever are rare because chyle is not irritating to the pleural surface.

In traumatic chylothorax, a latent period varying between a few hours and several months, with an average of 7 to 10 days, usually occurs between the trauma and the onset of symptomatic chylothorax (26). The duration of this period is related to the size of the damaged lymphatic vessel, the rate of the leakage of chyle, and the ongoing medical management following the trauma. Dietary restriction or administration of opiates for pain relief prolongs this period (1). It is worthy to mention that in traumatic chylothorax there may be an initial phase of accumulation of chyle within the mediastinum, forming a chyloma, which is usually asymptomatic. With increasing pressure, the mediastinal pleural becomes breached and chyle spills over into the pleural cavity. In this cause, the rapidly developing effusion may produce serious respiratory distress and shock (27).

Many patients with chylothorax present with features of hypovolemia and hypotension from the massive sequestration of fluid in the pleural space. Progressive weakness, emaciation, and general apathy occur in a short period if there is protracted escape of large amounts of chyle. In the neonate, birth asphyxia and respiratory failure are major symptoms of congenital chylothorax, requiring resuscitation and mechanical ventilation (28).

During prolonged chyle drainage, the body's reserves of protein, fat, and electrolytes are depleted. Hyponatremia, acidosis, and hypocalcaemia are the most commonly found consequences (26). Both cell-mediated and humoral immunity are impaired too. Hypoalbuminemia and lymphopenia in conjunction with an impaired immune response, including lowered antibody levels, increase the risk of bacterial and viral sepsis (29).

E. Diagnosis

In chylothorax, the pleural fluid is usually milky or creamy. However, two other types of pleural fluid may appear milky and need to be distinguished: (*i*) Chyliform or pseudochylous pleural effusion in which the milkiness is due to cholesterol and/or lecithin–globulin complexes; the addition of 2 mL of ethyl ether clears the milkiness in chylothorax but not in pseudochylothorax. (*ii*) Empyema in which the milkiness is due to the suspension of leukocytes, which, unlike chylomicrons, settle out on standing or centrifugation (18). It is important to mention that chylous effusions can be bloody, yellow or green turbid, serous or serosanguineous in almost 50% of cases (6).

The diagnosis of chylous effusion is made by analysis of pleural fluid. Triglyceride levels greater than 110 mg/dL are highly suggestive of a chylous effusion (6). Occasionally, high pleural triglyceride levels can be found in patients with chyliform effusions or with hypertriglyceridemia. A pleural fluid-to-serum triglyceride ratio higher than 1.0 excludes patients with triglyceridemia, and pleural fluid-to-serum cholesterol ratio lower than 1.0 excludes chyliform effusions (14).

Pleural fluid triglyceride levels below 50 mg/dL virtually exclude the diagnosis of chylothorax. In patients with triglyceride levels between 50 and 110 mg/dL, or if there is any doubt about the diagnosis, lipoprotein electrophoresis should be performed. The demonstration of chylomicrons by the latter test is considered the gold standard for a biochemical diagnosis of chylothorax.

The administration of cream or other foodstuff of high-fat content is a helpful diagnostic test in clinical settings; it induces a dramatic change in the color, content, and the amount of the pleural fluid. A thoracocentesis performed one hour after the patient ingests butter mixed with lipophilic dye, preferably Drug and Cosmetic Green Number 6, should yield green pleural fluid if a chylothorax is present (27).

On plain radiographs, the changes with chylothorax cannot be distinguished from other effusions. Traumatic damage to the thoracic duct can firstly present as posterior mediastinal mass (30), which after it ruptures into the pleural space is no longer visible radiographically. If an underlying tumor, and lymphoma in particular, is suspected, computed tomography (CT) can be a useful tool.

Lymphangiography provides useful information regarding the site and size of the leak. It may identify complete transection or laceration of the duct and thus may guide management toward a surgical or a conservative approach. It may also demonstrate lymphoma, duck blockage with collaterals and lymphatic malformations, including lymphangiectasia (31). Occasionally and particularly in nontraumatic chylothorax, the site of leakage cannot be localized. In such case, lymphoscitigraphy may be an alternative to lymphangiography (32).

Thoracoscopy can provide useful help in cases in which the cause has not been found by the above methods. It can be used as a diagnostic and therapeutic tool at the same time. Biopsy of the lung, especially of any suspicious part seen at CT, could be performed, since this is the best way to diagnose, for instance, a lymphangioleiomyomatosis (10).

F. Treatment

There are two approaches to the treatment of chylothorax: conservative management and surgical interventions (Table 2). Most agree that either approach must be considered in the light of the specific aetiological type of chylothorax and the patient's general condition.

The initial management of any chylothorax is usually conservative. It involves drainage of the pleural cavity, replacement of fluid and nutritional losses, reduction of the

Table 2 Treatment of Chylothorax

Conservative	Surgical
Drainage	Ligation of the thoracic duct
Replacement of nutritional and fluid losses	Thoracotomy
Reduction of chyle production	VATS
Dietary modifications	Pleuroperitoneal shunt
Somatostatin, octreotide, NO	Pleurectomy
Embolization	
Pleurodesis	
Respiratory care	
Treatment	

chyle production, and respiratory care. This appears to be successful in many cases, and particularly in those characterized by few or no symptoms and small volumes of chyle loss.

Drainage of chylothorax decompresses both the pleural space and the thoracic lymphatics, and re-expands the lung giving a dramatic improvement in symptomatology (33).

In order to avoid hypovolemia and hypotension, the daily fluid lost via the pleural drains should be replaced by at least an equivalent volume of intravenous fluid, preferably in the form of plasma protein fraction or albumin solution.

To minimize thoracic lymphatic flow, and to maintain nutrition, treatment with a medium-chain triglyceride (MCT) diet or total parenteral alimentation has been recommended (34). After large losses or foregut reconstruction surgery, total parenteral nutrition is the preferred method of nutritional support (35).

Several case reports and series have shown that somatostatin and its synthetic analogue octreotide are probably effective and safe in the management of chylothorax. Although their exact mechanism of action is not well defined, they likely induce leak closure by decelerating the lymph flow. The treatment lasts for 1 to 2 weeks. In successful cases, a substantial reduction of lymph drainage is evident within the first few days of treatment (36).

In infants and neonates with congenital chylothorax, supportive mechanical ventilation is usually necessary, even after the chyle has been adequately drained, because of either insufficient lung expansion, persistent fetal circulation, or lung hypoplasia. The addition of positive end–expiratory pressure to mechanical ventilation increases intrathoracic pressure, approximates the two intrapleural surfaces to obliterate the pleural cavity and retard chyle leakage (28).

In some cases, treatment of the underlying disease is very important and sometimes causes resolution of chylothorax. Examples are corticosteroids in sarcoidosis or treatment of heart failure. Furthermore, certain varieties of lymphoma are very responsive to chemotherapy or radiation therapy and these options should be considered after removing pleural fluid to treat symptoms (37).

Chemical pleurodesis has been a successful therapeutic option in many chronic or recurrent pleural effusions. This option is sometimes preferred in terminally ill patients with chylothorax without subjecting them to a thoracotomy, and in patients with persistent chylothorax due to lymphoma, which otherwise respond to chemotherapy or radiation (37).

Although attempts have been successfully made by interventional radiologists to cannulate and embolize the leaking thoracic duct (38), success has been limited and the procedure is not reproducible at many centers.

Aggressive surgical therapy is recommended for posttraumatic or postsurgical chylothorax. Many advocate conservative management for a maximum of 2 weeks in the absence of a strong indication for surgery. The general consensus is that surgical management should be adopted if medical management of chylothorax fails. In general terms, surgical intervention offers better results than that of conservative management when the daily chyle leak exceeds 1.5 L in an adult or >100 mL/kg body weight per day in a child. Surgical intervention is usually indicated when the chyle drainage rate is more than 1 L/day for a period of more than five days (10,39,40).

Thoracic duct ligation has been the most effective operation in the management of chylothorax. It has 90% to 95% success rate with low mortality and morbidity (3,41). In case the site of leakage is not identifiable, a supradiaphragmatic mass ligature of the thoracic duct in the area between the azygos vein and the aorta has been suggested (42).

Pleural decortication and surgical pleurodesis may be indicated when the chylothorax is complicated, loculated, or the site of chyle leak cannot be established.

Video-assisted thoracic surgery (VATS) is becoming more widely used in the treatment of persistent chylothorax, because of easy manageability and low morbidity. VATS-guided procedures include: (*i*) treatment of the identified site of the leakage with suture, clips, and fibrin glue; (*ii*) insufflated talc pleurodesis; (*iii*) repairing of the pleural defect; and (*iv*) placement of pleuroperitoneal shunts. Extensive pleural adhesions can be a serious problem for VATS and may force conversion to an open thoracotomy (43,44).

Pleuroperitoneal shunt has been used with varying success in the management of refractory chylothorax, in both adults and children (45,46). It alleviates the respiratory symptoms of chylothorax without the loss of fluids, electrolytes, nutrients, and lymphocytes associated with the chest tube drainage. It is not recommended in the presence of a markedly elevated right atrial or vena cava pressures, and of simultaneous chylous ascites.

II. Pseudochylothorax

Pseudochylothorax, often synonymously called chyliform or cholesterol pleurisy, is an even more rare lipid pleural effusion than chylothorax. The pleural effusion is characterized by an excessive cholesterol content (>200 mg/dL), and occasionally by the presence of cholesterol crystals, which are thought to be diagnostic.

A. Pathogenesis

The precise pathogenetic mechanism of cholesterol accumulation in the pleural cavity remains obscure. The anatomic substratum of pseudochylothorax is a fibrotic, grossly thickened, and poorly vascularized pleura (47). It has been suggested that because of the above anatomic characteristics, cholesterol diffuses out of the pleural space at an abnormally slow rate, resulting in both the deposition in the pleura tissue and the accumulation of cholesterol in the pleural cavity (48).

The origin of the cholesterol has not been elucidated. It is probably derived from serum lipoproteins. It has been suggested that in acute inflammation, pleural barrier opens to plasma low-density lipoproteins (LDL) that are cholesterol-riched. In more chronic effusions, cholesterol changes its lipoprotein-binding characteristics toward the high-density lipoprotein (HDL) region, possibly due to local metabolism. In protracted chronic pleurisy eventually leading to a chyliform effusion, these blood-derived HDL molecules may progressively be trapped in the pleural space with a further rise in total cholesterol (49).

Factors determining the formation of cholesterol crystals are not clear. It seems to be a natural consequence of the high concentration of cholesterol. Supersaturation results in crystallization of cholesterol in both the fluid and the thick pleura.

B. Etiology

Tuberculosis is by far the most frequent cause of pseudochylothorax. In a recent comprehensive review of 174 published cases of pseudochylothorax, tuberculosis accounted for 54% of all cases (50). Patients who have had therapeutic pneumothorax for tuberculosis seem to be particularly prone to this condition. It has been suggested that tuberculous pseudochylothorax will be extinguished, because of the abandonment of routines like pneumothorax treatment.

Rheumatoid arthritis (RA) is the second leading cause of pseudochylothorax, accounting for 9% of all published cases (50). In recent years, the early diagnosis and precocious and aggressive treatment resulted in substantial decrease of pseudochylothorax associated with RA.

Other reported diseases associated with pseudochylothorax include paragonimiasis, lung cancer, hepatopulmonary echinococcosis, alcoholism, syphilis, diabetes mellitus, Hodgkin disease, heart failure, nephritic syndrome, trauma or hemothorax, Behcet's disease, and coronary artery bypass surgery (47).

C. Clinical Manifestations

Pseudochylothorax tends to develop in patients with long-standing pleural effusions. It has been reported that the average time required for the evolution of a pleural effusion to chyliform effusion is five years or more (48,50). In the majority of reported nontuberculous cases, the time of evolution was less than three years. Pseudochylothorax occurs most commonly in men than in women. Out of 68 patients whose sex was reported, 53 (78%) were men and 15 (22%) were women. The age of the patients ranged from 10 to 81 years (50).

Patients with pseudochylothorax are usually asymptomatic. When symptoms occur, they are related to the underlying disease, or to the impairment of lung function due to the effusion and/or thickened and calcified pleura. The most common symptom is dyspnea.

Complications of an untreated pseudochylothorax include respiratory insufficiency, infections (e.g., tuberculosis, fungal infection, and nonspecific infection) and bronchopulmonary or pleurocutaneous fistulae (47).

D. Diagnosis

The clinical context in which the effusion occurs is so characteristic that pseudochylothorax rarely causes any diagnostic confusion and especially with a true chylothorax. Long-standing pleural effusion with thickened or calcified pleura is the main characteristic.

The gross appearance of the fluid does not allow a specific diagnosis. It is usually thick, and appears milky or turbid. The milkiness is due to cholesterol and/or lecithin–globulin complexes (26). Nevertheless, its appearance may range from the resemblance of soft white cheese to that of motor oil (51). When the fluid is milky or turbid, it should be differentiated from empyema and chylothorax. In empyema, the milkiness disappears with centrifugation. The addition of 2 mL ethyl ether clears the milkiness in chylothorax but not in pseudochylothorax (26).

The diagnosis of chyliform effusion is made by the analysis of pleural fluid. Cholesterol levels in chyliform effusions are variable. They are usually very high, ranging from 150 to 4500 mg/dL (up to 30 g/dL). In clinical routine, cholesterol levels above 200 mg/dL strongly suggest a chyliform effusion (49). Lower levels may be found after repeated aspirations due to a dilution effect.

Many pseudochylous effusions contain cholesterol crystals, which are thought to be diagnostic (48). They seem to be a natural consequence of the high concentration of cholesterol. Their existence gives a distinct, satin-like sheen to the pleural fluid. Microscopically, they present a typical rhomboid configuration. Rarely, high-triglyceride levels (271–458 mg/dL) may be found in chyliform effusions (48,49). In the latter case, the absence of chylomicrons in protein electrophoresis confirms the diagnosis of pseudochylothorax.

Pleural biopsy and histologic examination has a low yield for etiologic diagnosis, and can be associated with complications. In cases of tuberculosis, the yield of this procedure with subsequent culture is not much higher than that of fluid culture alone. Thus, in patients with pseudochylothorax of suspected tuberculous origin, biopsy can be delayed until fluid culture proved negative (50).

Paragonimiasis should be strongly suspected, if blood eosinophilia, pseudochylothorax, and a high level of immunoglobulin E in pleural effusion are detected. Diagnosis can be confirmed by finding the characteristic eggs of paragonimous or by specific ELISA and immunoblot serologic tests (52).

The radiographic features of chyliform effusion, with the exception of a loculated pleural collection or pleural thickening, which may be indicative of the long duration of the lesion, are not different from those of other forms of pleural effusion. Interestingly, the presence of fat–fluid or fat–calcium level at CT seems to be unique finding of chyliform effusion and is most commonly caused by tuberculous empyema (53).

E. Treatment

In most cases of pseudochylothorax, there is a benign course, and it is only if the patient has symptoms or if there has been a significant increase in size that any intervention is needed.

Thoracocentesis is performed to relieve dyspnea, and to prevent the above-mentioned complications. In some patients, the chyliform effusion does not reaccumulate after the initial thoracocentesis. However, repeated aspirations are usually needed, and this procedure may be complicated by empyema or bronchopulmonary or pleurocutaneous fistula. (47).

Decortication should be the last therapeutic step for recurrent and symptomatic patients, provided their clinical condition is improved by the aspirations (47,50).

The management of patients with pseudochylothorax should be directed to the underlying disease too. Specific pharmaceutical treatment should be given in cases with active tuberculosis or paragonimiasis.

References

1. Merrigan BA, Winter DC, O'Sullivan GC. Chylothorax. Br J Surg 1997; 84:15–20.
2. Rosenberg A, Abrams HL. Radiology of the thoracic duct. AJR 1971; 111:807–820.
3. Paes ML, Powell H. Chylothorax: An update. Br J Hosp Med 1994; 51:482–490.
4. Lampson RS. Traumatic chylothorax. A review of the literature and report of a case treated by mediastinal ligation of the thoracic duct. J Thorac Surg 1948; 17:778–791.
5. Yoffey JM, Courtice FC. Lymphatics, Lymph and Lymphoid Tissue. Cambridge, MA: Harvard University Press, 1956.
6. Staats BA, Ellefson RD, Budahn LL, et al. The lipoprotein profile of chylous and nonchylous pleural effusions. Mayo Clin Proc 1980; 55:700–704.
7. Cerfolio RJ, Allen MS, Deschamps C, et al. Postoperative chylothorax. J Thorac Cardiovasc Surg 1996; 112:1361–1366.
8. Bolger C, Walsh TN, Tanner WA, et al. Chylothorax after oesophagectomy. Br J Surg 1991; 78:587–588.
9. Wilson AG. The pleura and pleural disorders. In: Amstrong P, Wilson AG, Dee P, eds. Imaging of Diseases of the Chest. Chicago: Year Book Medical, 1990:627–702.
10. Nair KS, Petko M, Hayward MP. Aetiology and management of chylothorax in adults. Eur J Cardiothoracic Surg 2007; 32:362–369.
11. Fraser RG, Paré JAP, Paré PD, et al. The pleura. In: Fraser RG, Paré JAP, Paré PD, Fraser RS, Generux GP, eds. Diagnosis of Diseases of the Chest, 3rd ed. Philadelphia, PA: W. B. Saunders Company, 1991:2712–2793.
12. Light RW. Chylothorax and pseudochylothorax. In: Light RW, ed. Pleural diseases 3rd ed. Baltimore, MD: Williams & Wilkins, 1995:284–298.
13. Arunabh, Fei AM. Chylothorax: A review. Clin Pulm Med 1997; 4:63–70.
14. Romero S. Nontraumatic chylothorax. Curr Opin Pulm Med 2000; 6:287–291.
15. Kramer SS, Taylor GA, Garfinkel DJ, et al. Lethal chylothoraces due to superior vena caval thrombosis in infants. Am J Radiol 1981; 137:559–563.
16. Van Renterghem DM, Pauwels RA. Chylothorax and pleural effusion as late complications of thoracic irradiation. Chest 1995; 108:886–887.
17. Kitaichi M, Nishimura K, Itoh H, et al. Pulmonary lymphangioleiomatosis: A report of 46 patients including a clinicopathologic study of prognostic factors. Am J Respir Crit Care Med 1995; 151:527–533.
18. Urban T, Lazor R, Lacronique J, Murris M, Labrune S, Valeyere D, Cordier JF, for the Groupe D'Etuties et de Recherche sur les Maladies "orphelines" Pulmonaires. Pulmonary lymphangioleimyomatosis: A study of 69 patients. Medicine 1999; 78:321–337.
19. Tie MLH, Poland GD, Rosenow III EC. Chylothorax in Gorham's syndrome. A common complication of a rare disease. Chest 1994; 105:208–213.
20. Moss R, Hinds S, Fedullo AJ. Chylothorax: A complication of the nephritic syndrome. Am Rev Respir Dis 1989; 140:1436–1437.
21. Romero S, Martin C, Hernandes L, et al. Chylothorax in cirrhosis of the liver: Analysis of its frequency and clinical characteristics. Chest 1998; 114:154–159.
22. Rector WG. Spontaneous chylous ascites of chirrosis. J Clin Gastroenterol 1984; 6: 369–372.
23. Browse NL, Allen DR, Wilson NM. Management of chylothorax. Br J Surg 1997; 84:1711–1716.
24. Levine C. Primary disorders of the lymphatic vessels: A unified concept. Pediatr Surg 1989; 24:233–240.
25. Meade RH. Spontaneous chylothorax. Arch Intern Med 1952; 90:30–36.
26. Sassoon CS, Light RW. Chylothorax and pseudochylothorax. Clin Chest Med 1985; 6: 163–171.
27. Bessone LN, Ferguson TB, Burford TH. Chylothorax. Ann Thorac Surg 1971; 12:527–550.

28. van Straaten HLM, Gerards LJ, Krediet TG. Chylothorax in the neonatal period. Eur J Pediatr 1993; 152:2–5.
29. Machleder HL, Paulus H. Clinical and immunological alterations observed in patients undergoing long-term thoracic duct drainage. Surgery 1978; 84:157–165.
30. Higgins CB, Mulder DG. Mediastinal chyloma. A roentgenographic sign of chylous fistula. JAMA 1970; 211:1188.
31. Ngan H, Fok M, Wong J. The role of lymphography in chylothorax following thoracic surgery. Br J Radiol 1988; 61:1032–1036.
32. Pui MH, Yueh TC. Lymphoscintigraphy in chyluria, chyloperitoneum and chylothorax. J Nucl Med 1998; 39:1292–1296.
33. Kelly RF, Shumway SJ. Conservative management of postoperative chylothorax using somatostatin. Ann Thorac Surg 2000; 69:1944–1945.
34. Jensen GL, Mascioli EA, Meyer LP, et al. Dietary modification of chyle composition in chylothorax. Gastroenterology 1989; 97:761–765.
35. Peterson B, Jacobson BB. Medium chain triglycerides for the treatment of spontaneous neonatal chylothorax. Acta Paediatr Scand 1977; 66:121–125.
36. Kalomenidis I. Octreotide and chylothorax. Curr Opin Pulm Med 2006; 12:264–267.
37. O'Callaghan AM, Mead GM. Chylothorax in lymphoma: Mechanisms and management. Ann Oncol 1995; 6:603–607.
38. Cope C, Salem R, Kaiser LR. Management of chylothorax by percutaneous catheterisation and embolization of the thoracic duct: Prospective trial. J Vasc Interv Radiol 1999; 10:1248–1254.
39. Yeam I, Sassoon C. Hemothorax and chylothorax. Curr Opin Pulm Med 1996; 3:310–314.
40. Selle JG, Snyder WH, Schreiber JT. Chylothorax: Indications for surgery. Ann Surg 1973; 177:245–249.
41. Robinson CLN. The management of chylothorax. Ann Thorac Surg 1985; 39:90–95.
42. Patterson GA, Todd TRJ, Delarue NC, et al. Supradiaphragmatic ligation of the thoracic duct in intractable chylous fistula. Ann Thorac Surg 1981; 32:44–49.
43. Peillon C, D'Hont C, Melki J, et al. Usefulness of video thoracoscopy in the management of spontaneous and postoperation chylothorax. Surg Endosc 1999; 13:1106–1109.
44. Wurnig PN, Hollaus PH, Ohtsuka T, et al. Thoracoscopic direct clipping of the thoracic duct for chylopericardium and chylothorax. Ann Thorac Surg 2000; 1662–1665.
45. Murphy MC, Newman BM, Rodgers BM. Pleuroperitoneal shunts in the management of persistent chylothorax. Ann Thorac Surg 1989; 48:195–200.
46. Engum SA, Rescorla FJ, West KW, et al. The use of pleuroperitoneal shunts in the management of persistent chylothorax in infants. J Pediatr Surg 1999; 34:286–290.
47. Hillerdal G. Chylothorax and pseudochylothorax. Eur Respir J 1997; 10:1157–1162.
48. Coe JE, Aikawa JK. Cholesterol pleural effusion. Arch Intern Med 1961; 108:763–774.
49. Hamm H, Pfalzer B, Fabel H. Lipoprotein analysis in a chyliform pleural effusion: Implications for pathogenesis and diagnosis. Respiration 1991; 58:294–300.
50. Garcia-Zamalloa A, Riuz-Irastorza G, Aguayo FJ, et al. Pseudochylothorax. Report of 2 cases and review of the literature. Medicine (Baltimore) 1999; 78:200–207.
51. Johnson JR, Falk A, Iber C, et al. Paragonimiasis in the United States: A report of nine cases in immigrants. Chest 1982; 82:168–171.
52. Inoue Y, Kawaguchi T, Yoshida A, et al. Paragonimiasis miyazakii associated with bilateral pseudochylothorax. Intern Med 2000; 39:579–582.
53. Song J-W, Im J-G, Goo JM, et al. Pseudochylous pleural effusion with fat-fluid levels: Report of six cases. Radiology 2000; 216:478–480.

43
The Pleural Space and Organ Transplantation

MARC A. JUDSON and STEVEN A. SAHN
Division of Pulmonary, Critical Care, Allergy and Sleep Medicine, Medical University of South Carolina, Charleston, South Carolina, U.S.A.

I. Introduction

The number of living organ transplant recipients has reached a level where subspecialists and generalists are involved in the medical management of these patients. In particular, it has become essential for pulmonologists to have a detailed understanding of pulmonary problems associated with organ transplantation.

This chapter serves as a review of the spectrum of pleural disease as it relates to organ transplantation, both before and after the procedure. Pleural considerations of each organ transplant will be reviewed separately, although many of the infectious complications and posttransplant lymphoproliferative disorders (PTLD) relate to the level and duration of immunosuppression and are not organ-specific. Table 1 lists the pleural diseases posttransplantation that are not related to a specific organ transplant.

II. Bone Marrow Transplantation

A. Evaluation of Pleural Disease Pretransplant

Bone marrow transplantation (BMT) is performed for a variety of diseases including aplastic anemia, thalassemias, immunodeficiency and genetic disorders, leukemias, lymphomas, and solid-organ malignancies (1). Pleural effusions associated with these diseases should be evaluated by thoracocentesis prior to BMT to exclude infection and residual tumor (2).

Pleural effusions are rare at the time of diagnosis in Hodgkin's disease but not uncommon in non–Hodgkin lymphoma. A review of the literature (3) reported that only 1 (0.3%) of 269 patients with Hodgkin disease had a pleural effusion at presentation, whereas the incidence of pleural effusion with untreated non–Hodgkin's lymphoma has been reported to be 12% to 71% (4–7). As Hodgkin disease progresses, the incidence of pleural effusions increases to 30% in some series (8,9) and 30% to 60% at postmortem (10). The postmortem involvement of non–Hodgkin lymphoma appears to be higher still with a reported frequency of 72% in one series (11). Extrapleural involvement with lymphoma may also be seen with displacement or invasion of the extrapleural fat stripe (12).

Pleural effusions associated with Hodgkin lymphoma are usually a consequence of lymphatic or venous obstruction from mediastinal adenopathy (9,13), whereas direct pleural infiltration is the predominant cause in non–Hodgkin lymphoma (3,4). Chylous pleural effusions may result from obstruction of the thoracic duct from tumor (4,14);

Table 1 Pleural Disease After
Transplantation (Not Organ-Specific)

Pleural effusion
Infection
Uncomplicated parapneumonic
Complicated parapneumonic/empyema
PTLD with pleural involvement
Primary effusion lymphoma
Iatrogenic
Central venous line
Pleural effusion
Hemothorax
Chylothorax
Pneumothorax

Abbreviation: PTLD, posttransplant lymphoproliferative disorder.
Source: Adapted from Ref. 2.

this is more common with non–Hodgkin lymphoma than Hodgkin disease (15). Because pleural infiltration is a more common cause of pleural effusion in non–Hodgkin lymphoma than Hodgkin lymphoma, the diagnosis of lymphomatous pleural effusion is more easily established with non–Hodgkin lymphoma. The presence of bloody fluid suggests direct pleural involvement, and a transudate is usually seen early in the course of impaired lymphatic pleural space drainage (3). The nucleated cell count is often low, with a predominance of lymphocytes that may approach 100% (16). The pH and glucose level are usually normal, but they may be low (10). Cytological examination of the pleural fluid and pleural biopsy have a diagnostic yield of 73% to 90% in non–Hodgkin's lymphoma (4,17). The combination of immunophenotypic analysis with cytological examination has increased the sensitivity and specificity to as high as 100% for non–Hodgkin's lymphoma (18), so that thoracocentesis alone is the diagnostic procedure of choice for this malignancy (5,18,19).

Although thoracocentesis needs to be performed in patients with lymphoma prior to BMT to exclude infection (14), the presence of lymphomatous pleural involvement is not an absolute contraindication to BMT (2,20). However, the presence of pleural involvement portends a greater risk of relapse of Hodgkin disease after BMT (21). In a study of 100 consecutive patients with Hodgkin disease receiving autologous BMT, the presence of pleural disease prior to BMT was found to be a poor prognostic factor for disease-free survival. None of the seven patients with pleural disease prior to BMT were free from relapse at three years (21). Bone marrow transplantation has also been successfully performed in patients with non–Hodgkin lymphoma with pleural involvement (22).

Treatment of lymphoma may result in pleural disease. Methotrexate may cause pleurisy (23), pleural effusion (23,24), and pleural thickening (25). In one report, pleurisy occurred in 14 (4%) of 317 patients who received one to several 50-mg intramuscular doses of methotrexate (23). Four (29%) of the 14 patients developed pleural effusions without parenchymal infiltrates. Bleomycin has been reported to cause pleural effusion and pleural thickening (26,27). These pleural complications have always been associated with an interstitial pneumonitis from bleomycin. A case of massive bilateral pleural effusions has been reported that was thought to be an idiosyncratic reaction from high-dose cyclophosphamide (4200 mg intravenously for two consecutive days) with Mesna rescue given as pretreatment prior to BMT (28).

Radiation therapy to the thorax can cause pleural effusions by two mechanisms: (1) radiation pleuritis and (2) systemic venous hypertension, lymphatic obstruction, or constrictive pericarditis from mediastinal fibrosis (3,29–31). Ipsilateral pleural effusions have been reported in 6% of patients with breast carcinoma who received radiation therapy (32), all of whom received 4000 to 6000 rads. These effusions developed between two weeks and six months after completion of radiation therapy, and all the patients had radiation pneumonitis either prior to or simultaneously with the pleural effusion. These effusions lasted a minimum of four months to several years. Over time, the amount of fluid remained constant or decreased slightly, and there was an increase in the degree of adhesions and tendency for loculation.

Pleural effusions may also occur 1–2 or more years after completion of intensive (4000–6000 rads) mediastinal radiation from mediastinal fibrosis that causes constrictive pericarditis, superior vena cava syndrome, or lymphatic obstruction (33). These complications should be considered if other causes of pleural effusion have been excluded and the appropriate time has elapsed between completion of radiation therapy and the development of a pleural effusion.

Postradiation pleural effusion can be successfully treated with talc poudrage or talc slurry (34). Both have a success rate approaching 90% (34).

Chylothorax may be a late complication of thoracic radiation (14). This is caused by radiation-induced fibrosis and occlusion of intrathoracic vessels, and alterations in lymphatic flow that can lead to lymph leakage (35,36). Talc pleurodesis is also effective in this setting (37).

Pleural effusions may develop prior to BMT from fluid overload secondary to intravenous hydration or infusion of blood products. This is probably a common cause of pleural effusion prior to BMT, although to our knowledge the incidence of pleural effusions from fluid overload has not been determined.

Spontaneous pneumothorax may rarely occur in patients with lymphoma (38), usually after thoracic radiation (39,40). It is more common with Hodgkin than non–Hodgkin lymphoma. In one series (39), the incidence of spontaneous pneumothorax in patients with Hodgkin lymphoma who received thoracic radiation was 2.2% (3 out of 138 patients). Most patients received radiation within three years of the pneumothorax and most were younger than 30 years of age (39–42). It has been postulated that pneumothorax develops in these patients from radiation pneumonitis coupled with the presence of subapical blebs that often cause pneumothoraces in tall asthenic individuals (43). Pneumothorax from cytotoxic chemotherapy without radiation occurs much less commonly than from radiation therapy (34,35,44,45). It has been proposed that chemotherapy-induced pneumothorax results from rapid tumor lysis leading to tissue necrosis or from rupture of subpleural-based tumor nodules (43).

B. Evaluation of Pleural Disease Posttransplant

Approximately half of BMT recipients develop a pulmonary complication, and half will die of the complication (46,47). Pleural effusions and other noninfectious pulmonary

Table 2   Pleural Disease After Bone Marrow Transplantation[a]

Pleural effusion
Hepatic veno-occlusive disease
Recurrent tumor
Iatrogenic
Volume overload
GVHD
Pneumothorax from obstructive airway disease (chronic GVHD)

[a]See Table 1 for additional pleural diseases associated with transplantation.
Abbreviation: GVHD, graft-versus-host disease.
Source: Adapted from Ref. 2.

complications have been reported in 10% to 39% of patients following BMT (47–49). Causes of pleural disease after BMT are listed in Table 2.

Noninfectious Causes of Pleural Effusion

We suspect that the most common cause of pleural effusion after BMT is fluid overload because of intravenous over-hydration or the need for blood products. These effusions are usually right-sided or bilateral with more fluid in the right pleural space. Thoracocentesis is not required if a pleural effusion develops in an appropriate temporal relationship to the intravenous administration of a large volume of fluids and/or blood products, and the patient has no clinical evidence of infection (2).

Because BMT recipients frequently require central venous access and invasive procedures, iatrogenic pleural effusions may occur. A chylothorax has been reported in a BMT recipient as a complication of right subclavian vein thrombosis from a central venous catheter insertion (50).

A syndrome of multiorgan failure from a generalized capillary endothelial injury ("capillary leak syndrome") may occur after BMT (51). This syndrome occurs within one week of engraftment and is characterized by fever, rash, hypotension, edema including ascites and pleural effusions (51,52). Renal and hepatic failure are common (52). This syndrome may occur in autologous and allogeneic BMT recipients (52). It has been proposed that the capillary leak may be the result of generalized endothelial damage initiated by chemo/radiotherapy conditioning regimens and enhanced by mediators, proteolytic enzymes, and toxic oxygen metabolites released from leukocytes (14,52–54). It is known that leukocytes of patients recovering from BMT have abnormally high oxidative metabolism and often secrete large quantities of cytokines (55). Although there was a report of 29 BMT recipients who developed this syndrome (52) with associated pleural effusions, the frequency of pleural effusions was not noted and pleural fluid characteristics were not reported.

Hepatic veno-occlusive disease (VOD) is a fibrous obliteration of hepatic venules characterized by jaundice, hepatomegaly and/or right upper quadrant pain, ascites, and/or unexplained weight gain (56). VOD occurs in approximately 20% of allogeneic and 5% to 10% of autologous BMTs in which chemotherapy or radiotherapy is used prior to transplantation (56–59). Pleural effusions have been observed in 50% (7/14) of BMT recipients who developed VOD after transplantation compared to 3% (1/36) of BMT recipients without VOD (iatrogenic pleural effusion) (60). Patients with pleural effusion and VOD had either tachypnea (4/7) or no respiratory signs or symptoms (3/7). It is thought that the pleural fluid probably originates in the peritoneal space because most patients have ascites and none have cardiomegaly (60). The effusions are right-sided or bilateral, with the larger effusion on the right side. VOD usually precedes the development of a pleural effusion by seven days. VOD lasts from postoperative day 13 to day 29, whereas pleural effusions are present from postoperative day 20 through day 27 (60). Both VOD and the pleural effusions resolve without thoracocentesis or tube thoracostomy.

Graft-versus-host disease (GVHD) is a serious complication of allogeneic BMT (61). On occasion, GVHD following BMT is associated with sterile serosal effusions (62,63). In a review of 1905 allogeneic BMT recipients, 15 (0.8%) patients were identified who had effusions in two or more of the following cavities: pleural, peritoneal, and pericardial (48). VOD and iatrogenic causes explained eight of these multiple effusions. The remaining seven "unexplained" multiple effusions were the result of either acute or chronic GVHD. Five out of seven had associated cytomegalovirus (CMV) disease. All the effusions were transudative and developed after engraftment, and in 6 out of 7 cases, the effusions developed within 100 days of BMT. Four of the patients required chest tube drainage. Most effusions resolved within one month, although they were present at death in four patients. An additional case has been reported of a massive pleural and pericardial effusion from chronic GVHD after allogeneic BMT (64). The diagnosis was established by immunophenotypic analysis of pleural fluid lymphocytes.

PTLD may develop early after BMT, and the clinical course is often rapidly progressive with a high mortality (65). The majority of these disorders are of B-cell phenotype and are associated with Epstein–Barr virus (EBV) or CMV infections (66,67). It is thought that an early deficiency in EBV- and CMV-specific cytotoxic T cells may be responsible for this disorder (14,66,67). Isolated ascites may occur in BMT patients developing PTLD (68). A case was reported of isolated pleuroperitoneal effusions from PTLD in a BMT recipient (62). The diagnosis was established by morphological, immunocytological, and molecular studies that demonstrated B-cell origin of the lymphocytes and high titers of EBV.

Isolated pleural effusions may be a manifestation of leukemia relapse after BMT. The diagnosis of pleural relapse can be confirmed by immunophenotyping, cytogenetic, and gene rearrangement studies of pleural lymphocytes obtained by thoracocentesis (69,70).

Infectious Causes of Pleural Effusion

The incidence of pleural effusions of an infectious cause after BMT is unknown. One report (47) identified pleural effusions in 16% out of 57 BMT recipients within the first 100 days after BMT. Five (39%) out of 13 patients with "nonbacterial, nonfungal pneumonia" had pleural effusions, which included pneumonias characterized as "idiopathic," "unknown," and from CMV, mycobacteria, and *Pneumocystis carinii*. One effusion was a *Candida albicans* empyema that required thoracostomy tube drainage. Other cases of pleural effusions from *Nocardia* species, toxoplasmosis, *Candida* species, and other fungi have been reported (71–75). We suspect that bacterial pathogens are responsible for the majority of infectious pleural effusions after BMT despite a lack of evidence in the medical literature.

Pneumothorax

Chronic GVHD after BMT is associated with airflow obstruction. Causes of obstruction include bronchitis, bronchiolitis obliterans, emphysema-like changes, and bronchospasm

(46). Spontaneous pneumothorax and pneumomediastinum have been reported in BMT recipients with obstructive airway disease from chronic GVHD (76–79). The pneumothoraces occur after the lung disease progresses to end-stage.

III. Heart Transplantation

A. Evaluation of Pleural Disease Pretransplant

Pulmonary venous hypertension is the major factor for the development of pleural effusions in congestive heart failure (3,80). Chest radiographs of patients with pleural effusions from congestive heart failure typically show cardiomegaly and bilateral small-to-moderate pleural effusions of relatively equal size, with the right slightly greater than the left. There is usually evidence of pulmonary vascular congestion, and the severity of pulmonary edema usually correlates with the presence of pleural effusions (80). The pleural fluid is transudative with predominantly mesothelial cells and lymphocytes, and it is unusual to observe more than 10% neutrophils. Acute diuretic therapy may cause elevations of pleural fluid total protein and lactate dehydrogenase (LDH) levels as well as pleural fluid-to-serum ratios of total protein and LDH. However, these transudates develop increased protein and LDH concentrations and resemble exudates in only 8% to 37% of cases (81,82).

Pleural effusions have been observed radiographically in 45 (34%) of 132 potential heart transplant recipients (83), but an analysis of these effusions have not been reported. Ettinger and Trulock (84) stated that a thoracocentesis is not mandatory in the pretransplant workup of a patient with congestive heart failure unless the cause of the effusion is unclear or atypical clinical or radiographic features are present. These atypical features include a unilateral effusion, bilateral effusions of disparate size, absence of cardiomegaly, fever, pleuritic chest pain, and an inappropriately low Pao_2 (3). If a thoracocentesis is performed, a transudate usually confirms congestive heart failure as the cause of the effusion. Some heart transplant candidates may have pleural effusions with equivocal or exudative characteristics because of diuretic therapy (see above), but other causes of pleural exudates should be excluded by appropriate tests.

B. Posttransplant Considerations

Causes of pleural disease after heart transplantation are listed in Table 3.

Noninfectious Causes of Pleural Effusion

Pleural effusions occur in as many as 78% of cardiac surgical patients during the immediate postoperative period. The majority are small, bilateral, or left-sided, and are often associated with atelectasis (85). Pleural effusions may result from congestive heart failure, postsurgical hemorrhage, iced saline cardioplegia solution, and entry of blood through unrecognized pleural tears (85–87).

Similar to these results found in general cardiac surgery patients, a retrospective study of 72 heart transplant recipients found that 85% developed a pleural effusion on a chest radiograph or chest CT within one year of surgery (88). Of those with effusions, the majority were similarly bilateral (49/61, 80%) or left-sided (10/72, 14%). The majority were small, occupying less than 25% of the hemithorax and resolved within the first year following transplantation.

Table 3 Pleural Diseases After Heart Transplantation[a]

Pleural effusion
Infection associated with preoperative pulmonary infarction
Parapneumonic effusion (uncomplicated)
Empyema
Cytomegalovirus[b]
Pericarditis
Hemothorax/diagnosis secondary to endomyocardial biopsy
Pneumothorax
Iatrogenic secondary to endomyocardial biopsy

[a]See Table 1 for additional pleural diseases associated with transplantation.
[b]Appears to be more common after heart transplantation than after other solid-organ transplantations.
Source: Adapted from Ref. 2.

These findings are disparate from three other reports where the frequency of pleural effusions after cardiac transplantation were much lower. However, these two studies were all reports of respiratory complications after heart transplantation; and therefore, small clinically insignificant effusions were probably not included. Lenner and colleagues reported the development of pleural effusions as a complication of cardiac transplantation in 6.7% (10/159) recipients (89). In this study, pleural effusions were deemed to be a complication if the effusion occupied more than 25% of a hemithorax, required drainage, or antibiotic therapy. Schulman and coworkers also reported a low frequency of pleural effusion as a respiratory complication (8/94, 9%) after heart transplantation (90). Of the eight effusions reported in this study, two were associated with pericarditis, one was malignant, one was iatrogenic, and four were unexplained. Two of the unexplained effusions resolved spontaneously, and the other two demonstrated nonspecific pleural inflammation at autopsy.

A patient has been reported who underwent cardiac transplantation for sarcoidosis and developed massive pleural and pericardial effusions within two weeks after transplantation (91). The pericardial effusion caused pericardial tamponade that responded to pericardiocentesis but recurred and eventually required a pericardial window. The pleural effusion re-accumulated after thoracocentesis and eventually required chemical pleurodesis. The pleural fluid was exudative and lymphocyte-predominant. The etiologies of the pleural and pericardial effusions were never determined. A heart transplant patient has been described who developed Kaposi's sarcoma one year after transplantation and eight years later developed a pleural effusion from primary-effusion lymphoma (92). This lymphoma as well as Kaposi's sarcoma are caused by human herpes virus 8 (HHV-8) (93). The lymphoma was diagnosed by immunophenotypic, genotypic, and ultrastructural studies of pleural fluid lymphocytes obtained from thoracocentesis.

A chylothorax rarely occurs after heart transplantation. These usually occur one to three weeks after transplantation (94,95). It has been postulated that injury to collateral lymphatics in the anterior mediastinal, thymic, or parasternal areas may cause a chylothorax (94). These collaterals may develop after injury from previous cardiac surgery (94), although this complication has been reported in cardiac transplant recipients who have never had a previous procedure (95). If a chest tube is placed, the chylothorax may pose problems in cyclosporine dosing, as the high hydrophobicity of the drug causes accumulation in the lipid-rich chylous fluid that is eliminated via the chest tube. High oral doses or intravenous cyclosporine may be required in these cases (96).

Infectious Causes of Pleural Effusion

In a review of respiratory complications of 94 consecutive heart transplant recipients (90), empyemas developed in 8 (9%) patients. Bacteria and *Aspergillus* species were the most common pathogens.

The pathogenesis of empyema formation after heart transplantation may involve pulmonary infarction. Pulmonary infarctions often develop in the early postoperative period in heart transplant recipients from inadequate collateral circulation from the pulmonary and bronchial arteries or venous stasis because of heart failure, edema, or infection (97,98). These pulmonary infarcts may become infected from bronchial contamination. The infected infarction may develop into a lung abscess, empyema, and/or bronchopleural fistula (99,100). The infarctions that lead to empyema usually are acute and occur within a week prior to heart transplantation in most cases (99,100). Empyemas after heart transplantation have been reported from *Salmonella enteritidis* (101), *Pseudomonas paucimobilis* (102), *Streptococcus pneumoniae* (103), *Serratia marcescens* (104), *Pseudomonas aeruginosa* (105) (with *Candida* pericarditis), and *Legionella pneumophila* (106) (with bronchopleural fistula). These empyemas usually occur within four months of transplantation. A pleuromediastinal cutaneous fistula is a rare complication of heart transplantation that is associated with pneumothorax and may occur early after the procedure from a sternal wound infection (107).

Pleural effusions associated with CMV pneumonia have been reported in heart transplant recipients (108,109). All these patients eventually had pulmonary infiltrates in addition to the effusions, although in one patient a unilateral effusion preceded bilateral pulmonary infiltrates by 12 days (108). These infections occurred between one and six months after transplantation, which is the period in which CMV pneumonitis frequently develops (110).

Pneumothorax/Hemothorax

Pneumothoraces have occurred in heart transplant recipients as the result of infectious and iatrogenic complications. Pneumothoraces and bronchopleural fistulas have been reported with empyemas in recipients with preoperative pulmonary infarctions (99,100) and in one recipient with a *L. pneumophila* empyema (106).

Hemothorax may occur after endomyocardial biopsy to exclude allograft rejection (111). This is a rare complication that occurred only once (0.2%) in a series of 661 endomyocardial biopsies of heart transplant recipients in one series (112), twice (0.6%) out of 339 procedures in another series (113), and in 2 (0.9%) of 232 patients in a third (the number of biopsies was not reported) (107). A case has been reported of a spontaneous hemothorax two weeks after heart transplantation that was treated by tube thoracostomy with evacuation of a large hematoma (114). Pneumothorax is also rare with endomycardial biopsy after heart transplantation, occurring in 1 (0.3%) out of 338 procedures in one series (113).

C. Donor Considerations

Because a number of heart transplant candidates are critically ill with unstable hemodynamics and a short-life expectancy, attempts have been made to liberalize the donor criteria. One heart transplant group broadened selection criteria for donor hearts to include heart donors with pleural disease (115). Eleven hearts from donors with severe chest trauma, pneumothorax in 5/11 and hemothorax in 8/11, were used for heart transplantation. The one-year actuarial survival of recipients with these allografts was not different from those receiving donor hearts fulfilling standard donor criteria.

IV. Liver Transplantation

A. Evaluation of Pleural Disease Pretransplant

Pleural effusions occur in approximately 5% of patients with cirrhosis in the absence of significant cardiopulmonary disease, and it is referred to as hepatic hydrothorax (116). The fluid is a transudate and most often (70%) right-sided, although it may be bilateral (15%) or unilateral on the left (15%) (117). Hepatic hydrothorax usually occurs with clinical ascites, although it may form in its absence. These effusions are thought to be the result of pleuroperitoneal communications through diaphragmatic defects with the normal fluctuation of intrathoracic pressure with respiration causing unidirectional movement of fluid (118). Thoracocentesis reveals a serous transudate with a low nucleated cell count and a predominance of mononuclear cells, a pH > 7.40, a glucose similar to serum, and a low amylase (3). Pleural fluid and ascitic fluid have similar characteristics, with protein and LDH concentrations tending to be slightly higher in pleural fluid (119).

Exclusion of other intrathoracic causes of pleural fluid accumulation, including infection, thromboembolic disease, and metastatic carcinoma, is important in the pretransplant evaluation process, particularly when exudative or hemorrhagic effusions are identified (120). Therefore, a diagnostic thoracocentesis should be performed in liver transplant candidates with pleural effusions, especially if the effusions are left-sided or associated with fever or pleuritic chest pain.

In a series of liver transplant recipients (121), pleural effusions were found preoperatively in 8 (18%) of 44 patients. Four of the effusions were less than 10% of the hemithorax, whereas four occupied more than 25%. The mean preoperative arterial oxygen tension of patients with pleural effusions was significantly lower than in patients without effusions (75 ± 14 mm Hg vs. 88 ± 12 mm Hg; $p < 0.05$). The total lung capacity was decreased in 4 (50%) of 8 with preoperative pleural effusion compared to 10 (27%) of 36 without effusion. In another series (122), 7 (39%) of 18 liver transplant recipients had pleural effusions at the time of transplantation. Preoperative ascites was more common in those with pleural effusions (5/9, 55%) than in those without ascites (2/9, 22%). Preoperative respiratory complications including pleural effusions have been shown by regression analysis to be a significant risk factor for postoperative respiratory complications after liver transplantation (123).

B. Posttransplant Considerations

Causes of pleural disease after liver transplantation are listed in Table 4.

Pleural Effusions in the Early Postoperative Period

Pleural effusions are common in the immediate postoperative period after liver transplantation (124). Data concerning early postoperative pleural effusions after liver transplantation are shown in Table 5. The incidence of pleural effusions after liver transplantation has been reported to be between 16% and 100% within the first week after the operation

Table 4 Pleural Diseases After Liver Transplantation[a]

Pleural effusion
Transudative effusion (common and early after liver transplantation)[b]
Subphrenic abscess (uncommon)
Parapneumonic effusion
Suprahepatic stenosis of inferior vena cava (rare)
Lymphocele (rare)
Sirolimus toxicity (rare; at present only reported after liver transplantation)

[a]See Table 1 for additional pleural diseases associated with transplantation.
[b]See Table 5.
Source: Adapted from Ref. 2.

(121,123–134). The effusions are usually isolated right effusions or are bilateral and are rarely isolated to the left pleural space (135). Thoracocentesis or tube thoracostomy was required in 0% to 19% of cases for respiratory embarrassment (125,126,129,132). The pleural fluid typically has the characteristics of a transudate (124,125,127). The effusions usually develop and enlarge over the first three days to one week after surgery (126,127,129). Most effusions resolve within two to three weeks, although occasionally they persist for several months (121,126). In one series (126), 7 (70%) of 10 liver transplant recipients whose effusions were increasing more than 72 hours after surgery had subdiaphragmatic disease (three hematomas, one biloma, and three subphrenic abscesses). Other studies (127,129) have reported that the effusions typically enlarge over the first postoperative week before subsiding.

On the basis of these data, we do not believe that routine thoracocentesis is warranted if a pleural effusion develops in the early postoperative period following liver

Table 5 Pleural Effusion Early After Liver Transplantation

n	Incidence of effusion (%)	Postoperative day	Isolated right effusion (%)	Bilateral effusions (%)	Isolated left effusion (%)	References
300	69	NR	NR	NR	NR	(132)
18	72	3	62	38	0	(133)
43	77	7	55	45	0	(127)
42	95	3	NR	NR	NR	(134)
14	86	7	71	29	0	(135)
21	48	NR	NR	NR	NR	(136)
9	100	NR	33	67	0	(137)
16	69	NR	NR	NR	NR	(138)
31	68	NR	NR	NR	NR	(139)
187	37	NR	NR	NR	NR	(140)
44	41	<30	NR	NR	NR	(130)
131	38	NR	66	20	14	(131)
100	23	NR	NR	NR	NR	(129)
70	16	NR	NR	NR	NR	(142)

NR: not reported.

transplantation. However, a thoracocentesis is indicated for left-sided effusions, effusions that continue to enlarge beyond the first postoperative week, effusions that persist more than three weeks after transplantation, fever without an obvious clinical explanation, or the development of pleuritic chest pain.

Postoperative pleural effusions occur in the majority of pediatric liver transplant recipients as they do in adults (136,137). Pleural effusions may cause respiratory compromise more commonly in the pediatric population, as respiratory embarrassment from pleural effusion has been reported in more than 30% of 60 pediatric liver transplant recipients (136). These patients required thoracocentesis or tube thoracostomy. In one study of adults undergoing liver transplantation, only 10% (19/184) developed pleural effusions that required an intervention (135).

Several mechanisms have been proposed to explain the high incidence of pleural effusions in the early postoperative period after liver transplantation. Surgical trauma, injury to the right hemidiaphragm from right upper abdominal dissection and retraction, peri-operative infusion of blood products, residual ascites, hypoalbuminemia, and atelectasis all may contribute to the development of effusions (121,125,132). Operative transection of hepatic lymphatics may also make an important contribution to the development of the effusions. The human liver is connected to the undersurface of the diaphragm by ligaments that contain lymphatics. It has been demonstrated in a swine model (swine and human lymphatics have a similar distribution) (138) that hepatic lymphatics communicate with the visceral pleural lymphatics via the pulmonary ligament (138). When the native liver is removed during liver transplantation, these lymphatics are not ligated but transected. These severed lymphatics connecting the liver to the visceral pleura are then free to deposit lymph. It has been proposed that leakage of lymph from these unattached lymphatics results in the immediate development of ascites and subsequent postoperative right pleural effusions via congenital or acquired diaphragmatic defects (138).

Respiratory compliance may also contribute to the development of pleural effusions after liver transplantation. In one study of 18 liver transplant recipients (122), postoperative respiratory compliance was lower in patients with bilateral effusions than in those with right-sided or no effusions. These authors postulated that the decreased compliance was the result of an increased interstitial volume related to the administration of peri-operative blood products and intravenous fluids.

Infectious Causes of Pleural Effusion

It has been proposed that empyema may occur after liver transplantation by contamination of the postoperative right hydrothorax (139). This is consistent with the observation that a postoperative pleural effusion is a risk factor for pneumonia in liver transplant recipients (125). Patients with empyemas after liver transplantation need aggressive management because immunosuppressive medications inhibit inflammatory and immune mechanisms (139).

To our knowledge, only one study has examined the incidence of pleural infections after liver transplantation (140). Five (8%) of 60 liver transplant recipients developed pleural infections. The responsible pathogens were *Aspergillus* species (two cases), *Escherichia coli*, *Enterobacter/Klebsiella* species, and *Toxoplasma gondii*. Pleural infections were responsible for 4% (5/139) of the infectious complications in these patients. Pleural effusions in liver transplant recipients have also been described with *Nocardia* species, CMV, non-*Aspergillus* fungi, *P. carinii*, histoplasmosis, legionellosis, and *Mycobacterium tuberculosis* (125,141–145).

Noninfectious Pleural Disease

Rarely a pleural effusion will be the primary manifestation of lymphoma related to PTLD after liver transplantation (146–148). These usually occur months to years after transplantation. The diagnosis may sometimes be made by cytological and flow cytometric analysis of pleural fluid (146,148).

Pleural effusion has been reported as a manifestation of sirolimus toxicity (149). Pleural effusions were thought to be related to sirolimus use in 17% (15/91) liver transplant recipients who received the drug (149). Pleural effusions have not been reported with sirolimus after transplantation of other solid organs or with other macrolide immunosuppressants.

A lymphocele is another rare cause of a pleural effusion after liver transplantation (150). These effusions are right-sided and develop several weeks to months after liver transplantation (150). The lymphoceles may be successfully excised at laparoscopy.

Diaphragmatic paralysis after liver transplantation may present with atelectasis, right pleural effusion, and respiratory failure (151). Diaphragmatic plication is usually successful in resolving respiratory failure (151).

A case of a large right pleural effusion has been reported from suprahepatic stenosis of the inferior vena cava four months after liver transplantation in a one-year-old girl (152). It was thought that the effusion was secondary to ascites and hepatic hydrothorax. The patient was successfully treated by percutaneous balloon angioplasty of the stenotic segment.

Because liver transplant recipients often undergo invasive procedures such as central line insertions and liver biopsies, iatrogenic complications such as hemothorax and pneumothorax may rarely occur (153–158).

C. Donor Considerations

The critical shortage of solid organs available for transplantation has prompted an evaluation of grafts previously considered marginal for transplantation (159). Adult-to-adult living-donor liver transplantation (LDLT) developed rapidly in the 1990s and peaked in 2001 accounting for 10% of liver transplantations that year (159). Either a left or right hepatectomy can be performed for transplantation (160). One and three-year survival after LDLT to deceased-donor liver transplantation (DDLT), although the results may not be comparable in that the severity of illness tends to be lower in those selected for LDLT than DDLT (160).

Pleural disease may occur as a complication in donors after LDLT. Table 6 lists the frequency of this complication, which varies from 2% to 37% (160–163). This

Table 6 Pleural Effusion Early After Living-Donor Liver Transplantation

n effusion (%)	Incidence of postoperative	Effusion reported as complication	References
83	37	No	(169)
34	21	Yes	(171)
112	7[a]	Yes	(170)
386	2	Yes	(172)

[a] Includes empyemas.

variability can be accounted by the fact that some studies only accounted for effusions that were classified as complications (161,163) and required an intervention whereas others included all effusions detected radiographically (160). Postoperative pleural effusions and all respiratory complications appear to occur more commonly in donors who undergo a right hepatectomy than a left one (161). Readmission for a pleural effusion after LDLT does not appear to be associated with the size of the liver resection or postoperative albumin changes (162). Postoperative empyemas and iatrogenic pneumothoraces have been reported after LDLT (161).

V. Kidney Transplantation

A. Evaluation of Pleural Effusions Pretransplant

Pleural effusions are found in approximately 20% of patients receiving chronic hemodialysis at the time of hospitalization (164). The majority of these effusions are caused by congestive heart failure, uremic pleurisy, atelectasis, and parapneumonic effusions. Patients with parapneumonic effusions and atelectasis are more likely to have unilateral effusions than patients with heart failure. The presence of chest pain was not more frequent in patients with parapneumonic effusions than other nonheart failure effusions, but it was not more common when compared with patients with heart failure effusions (164).

Uremic pleural effusions are usually associated with a fibrinous pleuritis (165). Pleuritic chest pain and cough are presenting complaints in one-third of cases, but dyspnea is unusual (166). Pleural friction rubs are common (166,167). The chest radiograph usually shows a moderate pleural effusion that may be unilateral or bilateral, although occasionally the effusion is massive (166,168–170). These effusions are usually serosaganuinous to bloody (166,168); however, the fluid may be serous (166,169). The number of nucleated cells tends to be less than 1500/μL and is usually lymphocyte-predominant; however a neutrophil predominance and pleural fluid eosinophilia have been reported (166,168). The pleural effusions typically resolve with continued dialysis over several weeks, but they may recur (166). Fibrothorax requiring decortication may complicate these effusions (169–171). Uremic pleural effusions are diagnosed clinically when other causes of exudates, particularly tuberculosis pleurisy, have been excluded. Rare causes of pleural effusions in patients undergoing dialysis include brachiocephalic vein stenosis and/or clot from a previous dialysis catheter placement (172) and "reflux chylothorax" from a clot originating at the dialysis catheter site propagating to the left subclavian vein and obstructing the thoracic duct (173).

It has been suggested (84) that pre-renal transplant evaluation of pleural effusions should exclude disease entities that may cause significant morbidity, particularly tuberculosis, empyema, pulmonary infarction, and malignancy. If hypervolemia is suspected as the cause of the effusion, aggressive dialysis resulting in negative fluid balance may be attempted in lieu of thoracocentesis; if the effusion resolves, volume overload is confirmed. Otherwise, pleural fluid should be obtained for routine analysis, cytology, and culture. Pleural tissue should be examined histologically as well as cultured to evaluate for tuberculosis.

There is a paucity of literature describing pleural disease in kidney transplant candidates. One study (174) determined that 10% of diabetic and 4.5% of nondiabetic renal transplant candidates ($p > 0.05$) had pleural effusions on their preoperative chest

Table 7   Pleural Disease After Kidney Transplantation[a]

Pleural effusion
Urinothorax
Perirenal lymphocele
Legionella[b]
Nocardia[b]
Other parapneumonic effusions

[a]See Table 1 for additional pleural diseases associated with transplantation.
[b]Appears to be more common after kidney transplantation than after other solid-organ transplants based on frequent case reports.
Source: Adapted from Ref. 2.

radiographs. The outcome of these patients compared to patients without effusions was not addressed. A study of pediatric renal transplantation identified six children with pleural and pericardial effusions prior to transplantation associated with heart failure, ascites, or splenomegaly (175). The outcome of these patients was not different from the general renal transplant population.

B.   Posttransplant Considerations

Causes of pleural disease after kidney transplantation are listed in Table 7.

Noninfectious Causes of Pleural Effusion

Several cases of urinothorax have been reported after renal transplantation (176–179). This complication occurs within three weeks of transplantation (176–179). The effusion is usually ipsilateral to the transplanted kidney (176,177), but not always (179). Typically the urine output decreases and serum creatinine increases in concert with the development of the pleural effusion. The cause of urinothorax in these cases is ureteral obstruction that requires surgical repair. Renal failure, oliguria, and the urinothorax resolve rapidly after surgical repair of the affected ureter. A urinothorax may diagnosed by pleural fluid analysis revealing a pleural fluid-to-serum ratio of creatinine that is greater than 1.0; it is the only cause of a low-pH transudate (180).

Cases of PTLD with pleural involvement have been reported after renal transplantation (181–184). T-cell leukemia, anaplastic large cell lymphoma, large-cell (B-cell) lymphoma, and non–Hodgkin's lymphoma have been reported. These tumors have developed three to eight years after transplantation. The effusions are usually associated with other chest radiographic abnormalities, such as pulmonary nodules or a mediastinal mass. In all cases, the diagnosis of malignancy was made by histological and immunohistochemical analysis of pleural fluid cells obtained by thoracocentesis.

Two cases have been described of renal transplant recipients developing a pleural effusion secondary to a perirenal lymphocele 7 and 10 years after transplantation (185,186). We suspect pleural effusion is a rare complication of perirenal lymphocele, as no effusions were described in five studies reporting a total of 47 perirenal lymphoceles after kidney transplantation (187–191). An exudative effusion with 90% lymphocytes was reported in one patient (185). Refractory ascites and pleural effusions resolved after peritoneovenous shunt placement in one case, whereas in the other case a peritoneovenous shunt was inadequate to drain the rapidly accumulating pleural fluid (186). Removal of the graft and retransplantation was required, although the kidney had been functioning normally.

One case of skin lesions and pleural effusion from Kaposi's sarcoma in a renal transplant recipient has been reported (192). Human herpes virus 8 was identified from polymerase chain reaction of a pleural biopsy specimen. One case has been reported of sarcoidosis presenting as a pleural effusion 17 months after renal transplantation (193). Noncaseating granulomas were identified in both pleural and lung tissue. The patient was receiving tacrolimus but not corticosteroids at presentation, and the effusion resolved when after the patient received 20 mg/day of prednisone.

In a retrospective review of the anesthesia complications of 500 consecutive renal transplants (194), one hemothorax occurred as a complication of central line placement. Another recipient developed an idiopathic postoperative pneumothorax.

Infectious Causes of Pleural Disease

As with other organ transplants, pleural infections after renal transplantation usually relate to the level of immunosuppression and are not specific for kidney transplantation. In a review of 173 kidney transplants recipients (195), pulmonary infections developed in 73 (43%) of 173. Forty-nine (65%) of the infections were caused by bacteria, and 5 (10%) of these were associated with pleural effusions. In a review of 142 renal transplantations in India (196), 27 (19%) of 142 recipients developed pulmonary infection, and bacteria were solely responsible for only 3 (11%) of 27 of these infections. Three (11%) of the 27 had pleural effusions, and all 3 had tuberculosis.

Renal transplantation is a risk factor for *Legionella* pneumonia, and pleural effusions are common (43–90%) in renal transplant recipients who develop *Legionella* pneumonia (197–202). The parapneumonic effusions have been reported to be isolated (203), associated a pulmonary infiltrate (197–201), and initially isolated with subsequent development of an infiltrate (202). The diagnosis of these *Legionella* infections is often made from stains or cultures of pleural fluid (197,198,200,202).

Several cases of *Nocardia* pneumonia with pleural involvement have been reported (196,204–208). Most occurred within the first four months after transplantation or with treatment of graft rejection (204,205,208). Chest radiographs revealed isolated pleural effusions (205) or effusions associated with pulmonary infiltrates (205, 207,208).

Tuberculosis can develop in a renal transplant patient from primary infection, reactivation, or from transplantation of an infected graft (209,210). The frequency of these infections after transplantation varies with the prevalence of tuberculosis infection, as 10 (37%) of 27 of all pulmonary infections were attributable to *M. tuberculosis* in a review of renal transplants performed in India (196) where tuberculosis is endemic. The risk of developing tuberculosis posttransplant seems most closely related to the total corticosteroid dose as opposed to the use of other immunosuppressive therapy (211). Infection with Bacillus Calmette-Guerin is probably very rare, as no cases were reported in a series of 487 renal transplant recipients from South Africa where 21 cases of tuberculosis were reported (210). Tuberculous pleural effusions have been described in some renal transplant recipients (196,209,210,212–216). The diagnostic value for tuberculosis of the adenosine deaminase activity in pleural fluid of a renal transplant patient remains high despite the use of immunosuppressive agents (217).

Pleural effusions have been reported in renal transplant recipients from cryptococcal infections (218,219), pneumocystis pneumonia (220), and *Rhodococcus equi* (221). Empyemas have been reported from staphylococcal (222) and *Salmonella* species (223). Two cases of pneumothorax from necrotizing pulmonary infections after renal transplantation have been reported (224). The responsible pathogens were not clearly elucidated as both patients were concomitantly treated for *Candida* species and aerobic gram negative bacilli that were cultured from sputum.

Clinical data suggest that most parapneumonic effusions in renal transplant recipients do not require pleural space drainage, as in one series only 3 (1%) out of 273 consecutive renal transplants required a surgical procedure to drain the pleural space (225). The procedures used were rib resection, thoracotomy with decortication, and rib resection with decortication.

VI. Lung and Heart–Lung Transplantation

A. Pretransplant Considerations

Preexisting pleural disease was initially thought to be a contraindication to lung transplantation (226). This belief was based on reports of frequent postoperative deaths after heart–lung transplantation that were attributed to pleural hemorrhage from lysis of pleural adhesions (227). Because heart–lung transplantation must be performed with cardiopulmonary bypass that requires anticoagulation, the degree of pleural hemorrhage was probably greater in these series than for patients undergoing single-lung transplantation who rarely require cardiopulmonary bypass unless they have severe pulmonary hypertension (228). Double-lung transplantation is now performed by the sequential single-lung technique where during one operation a single-lung transplantation is performed followed by a contralateral lung transplantation (229). Therefore, cardiopulmonary bypass is now rarely required for double-lung transplantation (230,231). As long as cardiopulmonary bypass can be avoided for lung transplantation, there is only a minimal risk of significant pleural hemorrhage (232). An additional concern is that extensive pleural adhesions may prolong dissection and anesthesia time and may result in severe air leaks that are difficult to control. Although pleural hemorrhage has now become less of a problem after lung transplantation, pleural fibrosis may still increase the risks of the procedure. In one study of 32 cystic fibrosis, patients who received lung transplantation, patients with severe pleural disease detected by CT scanning had significantly longer hospital stay (50.5 days vs. 23.3 days; $p < 0.05$) and required mechanical ventilation longer (9.5 ± 13 days vs. 2 ± 2.3 days; $p = 0.06$) than those with minimal pleural disease (233). Another retrospective study of patients who underwent lung transplantation for lymphangioleiomyomatosis showed that those who had undergone a prior pleurodesis were at higher risk of postoperative pleural-related bleeding (234).

The management of pleural disease in a patient with cystic fibrosis considered for lung transplantation is problematic. Because of their chronic suppurative lung disease and lifelong requirements for immunosuppression after transplantation, recipients with cystic fibrosis require double-lung transplantation (235). More than 3% of patients with cystic fibrosis develop at least one pneumothorax in their lifetime (236). Pneumothorax may be treated by observation, tube thoracostomy with or without pleurodesis, surgical/thoracoscopic resection of blebs with or without talc poudrage, pleural abrasion, and parietal pleurectomy (237). The degree and extent of pleurodesis depends upon the procedure that is used. There has been concern about the effects of pleurodesis on the patient's candidacy for lung transplantation (238). When lung transplantation was in its infancy, it was thought that patients who had undergone a prior pleurodesis or pleurectomy had an unacceptably high rate of postoperative bleeding (239). An informal survey of cystic fibrosis centers found that many patients had been denied transplantation because of undergoing a previous pleural ablation and that most physicians had altered their approach to managing pneumothorax because of transplantation (240). It has been argued that a surgical pleurodesis is preferable to a chemical pleurodesis as there may be fewer diffused adhesions that might complicate the transplant procedure (241). The current consensus is that pleurodesis is not an absolute contraindication to lung transplantation (242). It has been recommended that a pneumothorax in a patient with cystic fibrosis being considered for lung transplantation be treated initially with chest tube drainage and observation for as long as five days (240,241). If the air leak persists for more than five days, it has been suggested that a procedure that minimizes the extent of pleurodesis be attempted, such as thoracotomy or thoracoscopic stapling with apical (limited) talc poudrage. This approach will be successful as 85% of pneumothoraces in cystic fibrosis result from rupture of apical blebs (243). The length of time that the air leak is observed without a surgical procedure should be individualized, as it might be appropriate to wait more than two weeks if the air leak is diminishing. Only if the limited pleurodesis procedure fails should diffuse chemical pleurodesis or extensive parietal pleurectomy be considered. Even if unrestricted chemical pleurodesis or pleurectomy is required, lung transplant is not absolutely contraindicated as several cystic fibrosis patients have undergone successful transplantation after extensive pleural procedures (244). In a study comparing lung transplant patients who had previously undergone intrapleural procedures to 18 matched lung transplant recipients who had not had such procedures, there was no statistically significant difference in operating time, blood loss, transfusion requirements, time intubated, and intensive care unit time (245). There was also no difference in spirometry at 6 months and 12 months after transplantation.

Pleurovenous shunting may be used as an alternative to a surgical procedure to temporize a symptomatic pleural effusion as a bridge to lung transplantation. This approach has been successful with a hepatic hydrothorax prior to liver transplantation and for chylothorax prior lung transplantation for lymphangioleiomyomatosis (246).

B. Early Postoperative Pleural Complications

Pneumothorax, air leak, and pleural effusion are common early postoperative problems after lung transplantation (247). Most air leaks resolve spontaneously within a few days of lung transplantation; however, approximately 10% of lung transplant recipients will have a prolonged air leak lasting at least two weeks after surgery (248). Typically, these air leaks resolve with tube thoracostomy alone and do not require further intervention (248). Pneumothoraces may occasionally be seen in the early postoperative period because of undersized donor lungs (232,249). These are usually small, insignificant, and resolve within days to weeks.

A pneumothorax may also occur from dehiscence of the bronchial anastomosis (232,250). Total dehiscence is rare and is usually life threatening, as it is extremely difficult to control the air leak and re-expand the allograft. Lesser degrees of bronchial dehiscence occasionally occur (232) and are complicated by air leaks that usually heal with conservative management. Occasionally, a pneumothorax will develop in the native lung in the postoperative period after single-lung transplantation (251). These are thought to result from positive pressure mechanical ventilation to the diseased native lung. Pleural effusions are extremely common in the early postoperative period, reaching up to 100% in frequency (247,252). These effusions are usually small to moderate in size and are ipsilateral to the graft (247,253). Rarely they may be massive (253). Most resolve spontaneously within 14 days after transplantation, although rarely they may increase in volume over the first three postoperative weeks (252). There are several explanations for the development of pleural fluid in the early postoperative period. First, alveolar capillaries have increased permeability during the first few days after transplantation because of allograft ischemia, denervation, and subsequent reperfusion (254). Second, lymphatic flow is severely disrupted from transection of lung lymphatics during the operation. Animal studies have demonstrated that allograft lymphatics are reconstituted and become functional two to four weeks after transplantation (255,256), corresponding to the time when pleural effusions resolve after human-lung transplantation. Third, pleural effusions are associated with acute lung rejection (257), an event that occurs once in almost all lung transplant recipients and is most common in the second to sixth week after transplant (258). Even though pleural effusions may occur with acute lung rejection, the sensitivity, specificity, and positive and negative predictive value of a pleural effusion detected on chest CT for the diagnosis of acute lung rejection is poor (Table 8) (259). Although the combined CT findings of volume loss, pleural effusion, and septal thickening is very specific for the diagnosis of acute lung rejection, this is a relatively uncommon occurrence (259). However, because acute lung rejection may be associated with a pleural effusion, we propose that a patient with established acute lung rejection does not require investigation of a small-to-moderate sized pleural effusion unless the pleural effusion fails to decrease within one to two days after treatment for rejection. Fourth, positive fluid balance in the early postoperative period may contribute to the development of pleural effusions, although these effusions often develop while the patient is in extreme negative fluid balance.

Pleural effusions occasionally require drainage if they cause symptoms or remain large so that infection or rejection are possible causes. In one large study of 214 lung transplant recipients, 31 (14%) developed pleural effusions that were thought to require

Table 8 Chest CT Radiographic Findings After Acute Lung Rejection

CT radiographic findings	Sensitivity	Specificity	+Pred value[a]	−Pred value[b]
Pleural effusion	44	50	47	47
Ground glass opacity	44	77	68	55
Volume loss and pleural effusion	25	83	63	50
Volume loss, pleural effusion, and septal thickening[c]	8	100	100	20

$n = 34$, rejection; $n = 30$, control.
[a]Positive predictive value
[b]Negative predictive value
[c]Only 11 of the 64 had this finding.
Source: Adapted from Ref. 259.

drainage (260). They were drained with image-guided small-bore catheters. This technique was successful, but drainage was often prolonged and occasionally required multiple catheter placements.

Living lobar lung transplantation has been developed so that the donor, typically a parent of a recipient with cystic fibrosis, can receive a donor lung lobe that usually "grows" with the child so that the thoracic cavity remains filled (261). In one study of 87 living lobar lung transplantations (262), pleural space problems developed in 24 (35%) and included air leak or bronchopleural fistula for more than seven days, pneumothorax, loculated pleural effusion, and empyema. Empyema was uncommon (2/76, 3%) despite that 87% (76/87) of the recipients had cystic fibrosis.

Chylothorax may occur early after lung transplantation. Usually, this occurs in patient with lymphangioleiomyomatosis (263–266). This most often occurs within the first week to months after lung transplantation (263,265). Treatments for this condition have included pleurovenous shunts (264), diet manipulation including medium-chain triglycerides, thoracic duct ligation, needle aspiration, pleurectomy, and pleurodesis (263,265,266). Chylothoraces have also been reported one to five weeks after heart–lung transplantation for diseases other than lymphangioleiomyomatosis (267). They have been successfully treated with thoracic duct ligation or oral aminocaproic acid in one case (267).

The characteristics of the pleural fluid that occurs immediately after lung transplantation has been described in nine successful single-lung transplant recipients who had no clinical evidence of infection or rejection (268). The effusions were initially bloody, exudative, and neutrophil-predominant. Over the subsequent seven days, the percentage of neutrophils and concentration of LDH and protein decreased, whereas the percentage of macrophages and lymphocytes increased. These initial pleural fluid findings were similar to control patients who had undergone nontransplant cardiothoracic surgery. Daily pleural fluid output gradually decreased except in one patient with the pulmonary re-implantation response (254), a form of noncardiogenic pulmonary edema that occurs within four days of lung transplantation. This patient required re-intubation for respiratory failure, and resolution of his pulmonary edema was paralleled by a decrease in his daily pleural fluid output. We suspect that there was a close correlation between pleural fluid output and lung edema in this patient because of the disruption of lung lymphatics that did not allow for rapid clearance of fluid from the pleural space. Two additional cases have been reported of lung transplantation with graft failure and capillary leak in the immediate postoperative period in which the pleural fluid output was 7 and 10 L/day, respectively (269). Interestingly, both patients had a dramatic decrease in pleural fluid output coupled with marked clinical improvement after administration of Cl-esterase inhibitor that was postulated to reverse the capillary leak.

Hemothorax and empyema may also occur in the early postoperative period after lung transplantation (232,247). These may be associated with airway dehiscence, wound infection, or lysis of pleural adhesions. A multivariate analysis suggested that hemothorax and persistent air leak after lung transplantation were associated with increased postoperative mortality (247). One case of chest tube suction–associated unilateral negative pressure pulmonary edema has been reported two months after lung transplantation (270). Lung transplant recipients may be at higher risk of this complication soon after transplantation because of compromised lymphatic drainage.

An HLA analysis has been done to determine the rate of influx of recipient cells into the pleural space after lung transplantation (271). Donor cells appear to be rapidly cleared from the pleural space, with less than 1% of pleural cells being of donor origin by postoperative day 8.

Pleural fluid analysis has been performed of effusions associated with acute lung rejection (257). The fluid is exudative and often contains more than 90% lymphocytes.

C. Long-Term Postoperative Pleural Complications

In one study of 144 lung transplant recipients (248), pleural complications were found to be less frequent with single-lung transplantation (5/53, 9%) than double-lung transplantation (25/81, 27%) ($p < 0.05$). All but one of the pleural complications after single-lung transplantation were pneumothoraces that persisted more than 14 days. No patient developed an empyema or parapneumonic effusion after single-lung transplantation. In contrast, 11 (12%) of 81 double-lung transplant recipients developed pleural infections: 7 (8%) empyemas, and 4 (5%) parapneumonic effusions; 3 of the empyemas were fatal. Pleural complications were most common in patients with cystic fibrosis (10/29, 34%) and chronic obstructive pulmonary disease (12/47, 26%). Chest CT scan, a more sensitive test to detect pleural disease than clinical findings demonstrated that 86% (50/58) lung transplant recipients has a pleural alteration one year after the procedure (247).

Parapneumonic effusions are common with pneumonia after lung transplantation, having been reported in 33 (73%) of 45 episodes of pneumonia in one series (272). Pleural effusion was equally common when the pathogen was bacterial, fungal, mycobacterial, or viral.

Empyemas occur commonly after lung transplantation. Several cases of *Burkholderia cepacia* empyema and other *Burkholderia* species have been reported after double-lung transplantation for cystic fibrosis (248,273–275); some of these patients developed empyema necessitatis (274). CT evidence of a pleural effusion was found in 73% (33/45) of lung transplant recipients with pneumonia in one series (272). Pathogens causing infected pleural effusions and empyemas after lung and heart–lung transplantation have included *Legionella* species (276), staphylococcal and streptococcal species (277), *P. aeruginosa* (253,272), *Listeria monocytogenes* (278), *M. tuberculosis* (279–281), CMV (272), *Aspergillus* species (272), and *Candida* species (282).

Rarely, a pleural effusion may result from abnormalities of the pulmonary venous anastomosis, such as thrombosis, kinking, or fibrosis. These abnormalities may cause unilateral or bilateral pulmonary edema with pleural effusions and may mimic allograft rejection, opportunistic infection, or congestive heart failure. Although this complication often occurs in the immediate postoperative period, pleural effusions from pulmonary venous abnormalities has been reported more than a year after lung transplantation (283). As with other solid-organ transplants, PTLD may be seen after lung transplantation and is occasionally associated with pleural effusion (284,285).

An iatrogenic pneumothorax may occur secondary to transbronchial biopsy or percutaneous biopsy for surveillance of rejection or pulmonary infection. In a review of 39 lung transplant centers that perform surveillance bronchoscopy for lung rejection, 95% (37/39) reported a pneumothorax rate of less than 5% of the time and 97% (38/39) reported a frequency of chest tube placement less than 5% of the time (286). In a study of review of 320 transbronchial lung biopsies performed for clinically suspected infection of rejection, 8 (2.5%) of 320 developed a pneumothorax (287). A pneumothorax may occur from progressive underlying lung disease in the native lung of a single-lung transplant recipient (vide infra) or superimposed disorders in the allograft, such as invasive fungal disease. Finally, a pneumothorax may occur as the result of recurrence of a disease in the allograft. This may be seen when a patient with lymphangioleiomyomatosis develops recurrent disease (288).

Pleural fibrosis has been found at autopsy in heart–lung transplant recipients (289). Although this has been attributed to the surgical procedure, an animal study revealed that pleural fibrosis developed in recipients who received allografts but not in those who received an autograft (their own heart–lung bloc) (290). This suggests that surgery was not responsible for the fibrosis, and the investigators suspected that its development was related to chronic rejection.

One late-onset chylothorax has been reported four months after heart–lung transplantation (291). It was successfully treated with diet manipulation. A case of mesothelioma post-lung transplantation that presented with a hemorrhagic effusion has been reported (292).

D. Interpleural Communication After Double-Lung and Heart–Lung Transplantation

During the course of a heart–lung transplant, the anterior pleural reflections are severed so that an interpleural communication develops (293–296). Therefore, air or fluid can move between the pleural spaces. Similar interpleural communication has also been observed after heart transplantation and thoracic surgery in patients with previous mediastinotomy (294). Interpleural communication may also occur after bilateral sequential lung transplantation performed through bilateral anterolateral thoracotomies and transverse sternotomy (clamshell) because anterior pleural reflections are also severed with this approach. This phenomenon has been demonstrated to persist for more than two years after heart–lung transplantation (293,294), and it is likely permanent.

Awareness of interpleural communication after heart–lung transplantation is important because pleural disease in these recipients should be managed aggressively. Empyemas need to be aggressively and adequately drained so that the infected pleural contents do not spill into the contralateral pleural space. A tension pneumothorax in such recipients is likely to be bilateral and, hence, life-threatening. Usually, a single thoracostomy tube is adequate for a heart–lung or lung transplant recipient with bilateral pneumothoraces (297,298). However, a case has been reported where a single chest tube failed to adequately drain a bilateral pneumothoraces in a heart–lung transplant recipient, and a contralateral tension pneumothorax developed (299). The transplant had been performed two years previously, and the authors postulated that pleural scar formation had sealed the interpleural communication. Careful radiographic monitoring is therefore recommended when using a single chest tube in this situation. An unusual situation has been reported where a pneumothorax in the native lung of a single-lung transplant recipient failed to resolve because of contralateral stenosis of the airway anastomosis (300). This was successfully treated with placement of a stent in the anastomosis.

E. Pleural Considerations in the Contralateral Lung After Single Lung Transplantation

Pleural complications may develop in the native lung of a single-lung transplant recipient. Pneumothorax is the most common complication, and this is not an unexpected finding in patients with end-stage restrictive or obstructive disease. These secondary spontaneous pneumothoraces rarely resolve permanently with tube thoracostomy (301). Thoracoscopic talc poudrage (302) and thoracoscopic partial pleurectomy (2,303) have both been successful in long term.

Donor Considerations

Because potential lung donors may have undergone significant trauma, it is not uncommon for them to have sustained a pneumothorax. Although pneumothorax was initially a contraindication for lung donation, this criterion has been liberalized (304). It is recommended that the extent of the air leak and area of related lung injury be assessed to determine if the lung should be donated (304).

VII. Summary

Pleural disease has important clinical implications both before and after organ transplantation. Pleural effusions are common in candidates for heart, liver, and kidney transplantation. A thoracocentesis is not mandatory in these patients but should be performed if clinical or radiographic features suggest that the effusion is not the result of organ failure. Posttransplant pleural infections and PTLD relate to the level and duration of immunosuppression and are not organ-specific. Some posttransplant pleural effusions are organ-specific and are described in the text. The treatment of pleural disease in potential lung transplant candidates should minimize the extent of pleurodesis. Pleural effusions are to be expected after lung transplantation. Interpleural communication, an expected finding after heart–lung or double-lung transplantation, has therapeutic implications.

References

1. Armitage JO. Bone marrow transplantation. N Engl J Med 1994; 330(12):827–838.
2. Judson MA, Sahn SA. The pleural space and organ transplantation. Am J Respir Crit Care Med 1996; 153(3):1153–1165.
3. Sahn SA. State of the art. The pleura. Am Rev Respir Dis 1988; 138(1):184–234.
4. Xaubet A, Diumenjo MC, Marin A, et al. Characteristics and prognostic value of pleural effusions in non-Hodgkin's lymphomas. Eur J Respir Dis 1985; 66(2):135–140.
5. Chaignaud BE, Bonsack TA, Kozakewich HP, et al. Pleural effusions in lymphoblastic lymphoma: A diagnostic alternative. J Pediatr Surg 1998; 33(9):1355–1357.
6. Castellino RA, Bellani FF, Gasparini M, et al. Radiographic findings in previously untreated children with non-Hodgkin's lymphoma. Radiology 1975; 117(3 Pt 1):657–663.
7. Berkman N, Breuer R, Kramer MR, et al. Pulmonary involvement in lymphoma. Leuk Lymphoma 1996; 20(3–4):229–237.
8. Fisher AM, Kendall B, Van Leuven BD. Hodgkin's disease: A radiological survey. Clin Radiol. 1962; 13:115–127.
9. Bernardeschi P, Bonechi I, Urbano U. Recurrent pleural effusion as manifesting feature of primitive chest wall Hodgkin's disease. Chest 1988; 94(2):424–426.
10. Wong FM, Grace WJ, Rottino A. Pleural effusions, ascites, pericardial effusions and edema in Hodgkin's disease. Am J Med Sci 1963; 246:678–682.
11. Costa MB, Siqueira SA, Saldiva PH, et al. Histologic patterns of lung infiltration of B-cell, T-cell, and Hodgkin lymphomas. Am J Clin Pathol 2004; 121(5):718–726.
12. Aquino SL, Chen MY, Kuo WT, et al. The CT appearance of pleural and extrapleural disease in lymphoma. Clin Radiol 1999; 54(10):647–650.

13. Au V, Leung AN. Radiologic manifestations of lymphoma in the thorax. AJR Am J Roentgenol 1997; 168(1):93–98.
14. Alexandrakis MG, Passam FH, Kyriakou DS, et al. Pleural effusions in hematologic malignancies. Chest 2004; 125(4):1546–1555.
15. Weick JK, Kiely JM, Harrison EG Jr, et al. Pleural effusion in lymphoma. Cancer 1973; 31(4):848–853.
16. Yam LT. Diagnostic significance of lymphocytes in pleural effusions. Ann Intern Med 1967; 66(5):972–982.
17. Jenkins PF, Ward MJ, Davies P, et al. Non-Hodgkin's lymphoma, chronic lymphatic leukaemia and the lung. Br J Dis Chest 1981; 75(1):22–30.
18. Bangerter M, Hildebrand A, Griesshammer M. Combined cytomorphologic and immunophenotypic analysis in the diagnostic workup of lymphomatous effusions. Acta Cytol 2001; 45(3):307–312.
19. Pietsch JB, Whitlock JA, Ford C, et al. Management of pleural effusions in children with malignant lymphoma. J Pediatr Surg 1999; 34(4):635–638.
20. Grimwade DJ, Chopra R, King A, et al. Detection and significance of pulmonary Hodgkin's disease at autologous bone marrow transplantation. Bone Marrow Transplant 1994; 13(2):173–179.
21. Poen JC, Hoppe RT, Horning SJ. High-dose therapy and autologous bone marrow transplantation for relapsed/refractory Hodgkin's disease: The impact of involved field radiotherapy on patterns of failure and survival. Int J Radiat Oncol Biol Phys 1996; 36(1):3–12.
22. Elis A, Blickstein D, Mulchanov I, et al. Pleural effusion in patients with non-Hodgkin's lymphoma: A case-controlled study. Cancer 1998; 83(8):1607–1611.
23. Walden PA, Mitchell-Weggs PF, Coppin C, et al. Pleurisy and methotrexate treatment. Br Med J 1977; 2(6091):867.
24. Everts CS, Westcott JL, Bragg DG. Methotrexate therapy and pulmonary disease. Radiology 1973; 107(3):539–543.
25. Urban C, Nirenberg A, Caparros B, et al. Chemical pleuritis as the cause of acute chest pain following high-dose methotrexate treatment. Cancer 1983; 51(1):34–37.
26. Pascual RS, Mosher MB, Sikand RS, et al. Effects of bleomycin on pulmonary function in man. Am Rev Respir Dis 1973; 108(2):211–217.
27. Holoye PY, Luna MA, MacKay B, et al. Bleomycin hypersensitivity pneumonitis. Ann Intern Med 1978; 88(1):47–49.
28. Schaap N, Raymakers R, Schattenberg A, et al. Massive pleural effusion attributed to high-dose cyclophosphamide during conditioning for BMT. Bone Marrow Transplant 1996; 18(1):247–248.
29. Kramer G, Gans S, Rijnders A, et al. Long term survival of a patient with malignant pleural mesothelioma as a late complication of radiotherapy for Hodgkin's disease treated with 90 yttrium-silicate. Lung Cancer 2000; 27(3):205–208.
30. Rodriguez-Garcia JL, Fraile G, Moreno MA, et al. Recurrent massive pleural effusion as a late complication of radiotherapy in Hodgkin's disease. Chest 1991; 100(4):1165–1166.
31. Morrone N, Gama e Silva Volpe VL, Dourado AM, et al. Bilateral pleural effusion due to mediastinal fibrosis induced by radiotherapy. Chest 1993; 104(4):1276–1278.
32. Bachman AL, Macken K. Pleural effusions following supervoltage radiation for breast carcinoma. Radiology 1959; 72(5):699–709.
33. Whitcomb ME, Schwarz MI. Pleural effusion complicating intensive mediastinal radiation therapy. Am Rev Respir Dis 1971; 103(1):100–107.
34. Kennedy L, Harley RA, Sahn SA, et al. Talc slurry pleurodesis. Pleural fluid and histologic analysis. Chest 1995; 107(6):1707–1712.
35. Van Renterghem DM, Pauwels RA. Chylothorax and pleural effusion as late complications of thoracic irradiation. Chest 1995; 108(3):886–887.

36. Shalev A, Borer H, Reusser P, et al. Chylothorax as the initial manifestation of malignant Hodgkin lymphoma. Schweiz Rundsch Med Prax 1998; 87(20):690–693.

37. Vargas FS, Milanez JR, Filomeno LT, et al. Intrapleural talc for the prevention of recurrence in benign or undiagnosed pleural effusions. Chest 1994; 106(6):1771–1775.

38. Okam M, Alsolaiman M, Brau A, et al. Spontaneous pneumothorax as the first manifestation of lymphoma: A rare presentation and the importance of diagnostic biopsy. South Med J 2003; 96(1):99–100.

39. Pezner RD, Horak DA, Sayegh HO, et al. Spontaneous pneumothorax in patients irradiated for Hodgkin's disease and other malignant lymphomas. Int J Radiat Oncol Biol Phys 1990; 18(1):193–198.

40. Yellin A, Benfield JR. Pneumothorax associated with lymphoma. Am Rev Respir Dis 1986; 134(3):590–592.

41. Penniment MG, O'Brien PC. Pneumothorax following thoracic radiation therapy for Hodgkin's disease. Thorax 1994; 49(9):936–937.

42. Rowinsky EK, Abeloff MD, Wharam MD. Spontaneous pneumothorax following thoracic irradiation. Chest 1985; 88(5):703–708.

43. Melton LJ III, Hepper NG, Offord KP. Influence of height on the risk of spontaneous pneumothorax. Mayo Clin Proc 1981; 56(11):678–682.

44. Hsu JR, Chang SC, Perng RP. Pneumothorax following cytotoxic chemotherapy in malignant lymphoma. Chest 1990; 98(6):1512–1513.

45. Stein ME, Shklar Z, Drumea K, et al. Chemotherapy-induced spontaneous pneumothorax in a patient with bulky mediastinal lymphoma: A rare oncologic emergency. Oncology 1997; 54(1):15–18.

46. Krowka MJ, Rosenow EC III, Hoagland HC. Pulmonary complications of bone marrow transplantation. Chest 1985; 87(2):237–246.

47. Noble PW. The pulmonary complications of bone marrow transplantation in adults. West J Med 1989; 150(4):443–449.

48. Seber A, Khan SP, Kersey JH. Unexplained effusions: Association with allogeneic bone marrow transplantation and acute or chronic graft-versus-host disease. Bone Marrow Transplant 1996; 17(2):207–211.

49. Schwarer AP, Hughes JM, Trotman-Dickenson B, et al. A chronic pulmonary syndrome associated with graft-versus-host disease after allogeneic marrow transplantation. Transplantation 1992; 54(6):1002–1008.

50. Schiller G. Chylothorax as a complication of central venous catheter-induced superior vena cava thrombosis. Bone Marrow Transplant 1992; 9(4):302.

51. Powles R, Pedrazzini A, Crofts M, et al. Mismatched family bone marrow transplantation. Semin Hematol 1984; 21(3):182–187.

52. Cahill RA, Spitzer TR, Mazumder A. Marrow engraftment and clinical manifestations of capillary leak syndrome. Bone Marrow Transplant 1996; 18(1):177–184.

53. Holler E, Kolb HJ, Moller A, et al. Increased serum levels of tumor necrosis factor alpha precede major complications of bone marrow transplantation. Blood 1990; 75(4):1011–1016.

54. Antin JH, Ferrara JL. Cytokine dysregulation and acute graft-versus-host disease. Blood 1992; 80(12):2964–2968.

55. Leino L, Lilius EM, Nikoskelainen J, et al. Neutrophils are responsible for the reappearance of chemiluminescence after allogeneic bone marrow transplantation. Bone Marrow Transplant 1990; 6(6):391–394.

56. Rollins BJ. Hepatic veno-occlusive disease. Am J Med 1986; 81(2):297–306.

57. Jones RJ, Lee KS, Beschorner WE, et al. Venoocclusive disease of the liver following bone marrow transplantation. Transplantation 1987; 44(6):778–783.

58. Dulley FL, Kanfer EJ, Appelbaum FR, et al. Venocclusive disease of the liver after chemoradiotherapy and autologous bone marrow transplantation. Transplantation 1987; 43(6):870–873.

59. Brugieres L, Hartmann O, Benhamou E, et al. Veno-occlusive disease of the liver following high-dose chemotherapy and autologous bone marrow transplantation in children with solid tumors: Incidence, clinical course and outcome. Bone Marrow Transplant 1988; 3(1):53–58.

60. Ozkaynak MF, Weinberg K, Kohn D, et al. Hepatic veno-occlusive disease post-bone marrow transplantation in children conditioned with busulfan and cyclophosphamide: Incidence, risk factors, and clinical outcome. Bone Marrow Transplant 1991; 7(6):467–474.

61. Weisdorf D, Haake R, Blazar B, et al. Treatment of moderate/severe acute graft-versus-host disease after allogeneic bone marrow transplantation: An analysis of clinical risk features and outcome. Blood 1990; 75(4):1024–1030.

62. Lechapt-Zalcman E, Rieux C, Cordonnier C, et al. Posttransplantation lymphoproliferative disorder mimicking a nonspecific lymphocytic pleural effusion in a bone marrow transplant recipient. A case report. Acta Cytol 1999; 43(2):239–242.

63. Shulman HM, Sullivan KM, Weiden PL, et al. Chronic graft-versus-host syndrome in man. A long-term clinicopathologic study of 20 Seattle patients. Am J Med 1980; 69(2):204–217.

64. Ueda T, Manabe A, Kikuchi A, et al. Massive pericardial and pleural effusion with anasarca following allogeneic bone marrow transplantation. Int J Hematol 2000; 71(4):394–397.

65. Orazi A, Hromas RA, Neiman RS, et al. Posttransplantation lymphoproliferative disorders in bone marrow transplant recipients are aggressive diseases with a high incidence of adverse histologic and immunobiologic features. Am J Clin Pathol 1997; 107(4):419–429.

66. Lucas KG, Small TN, Heller G, et al. The development of cellular immunity to Epstein–Barr virus after allogeneic bone marrow transplantation. Blood 1996; 87(6):2594–2603.

67. Papadopoulos EB, Ladanyi M, Emanuel D, et al. Infusions of donor leukocytes to treat Epstein–Barr virus-associated lymphoproliferative disorders after allogeneic bone marrow transplantation. N Engl J Med 1994; 330(17):1185–1191.

68. Shapiro RS, McClain K, Frizzera G, et al. Epstein–Barr virus associated B cell lymphoproliferative disorders following bone marrow transplantation. Blood 1988; 71(5):1234–1243.

69. Dix DB, Anderson RA, McFadden DE, et al. Pleural relapse during hematopoietic remission in childhood acute lymphoblastic leukemia. J Pediatr Hematol Oncol 1997; 19(5):470–472.

70. Motherby H, Ross B, Kube M, et al. Pleural carcinosis confirmed by adjuvant cytological methods: A case report. Diagn Cytopathol 1998; 19(5):370–374.

71. Couraud S, Houot R, Coudurier M, et al. Nocardial pulmonary infection. Rev Mal Respir 2007; 24(3 Pt 1):353–357.

72. Collet G, Marty P, Le Fichoux Y, et al. Pleural effusion as the first manifestation of pulmonary toxoplasmosis in a bone marrow transplant recipient. Acta Cytol 2004; 48(1):114–116.

73. Dohmen K, Harada M, Ishibashi H, et al. Ultrasonographic studies on abdominal complications in patients receiving marrow-ablative chemotherapy and bone marrow or blood stem cell transplantation. J Clin Ultrasound 1991; 19(6):321–333.

74. Merz WG, Sandford GR. Isolation and characterization of a polyene-resistant variant of *Candida tropicalis*. J Clin Microbiol 1979; 9(6):677–680.

75. Lai CC, Liaw SJ, Hsiao YC, et al. Empyema thoracis due to *Rhizopus oryzae* in an allogenic bone marrow transplant recipient. Med Mycol 2006; 44(1):75–78.

76. Kurzrock R, Zander A, Kanojia M, et al. Obstructive lung disease after allogeneic bone marrow transplantation. Transplantation 1984; 37(2):156–160.

77. Galanis E, Litzow MR, Tefferi A, et al. Spontaneous pneumomediastinum in a patient with bronchiolitis obliterans after bone marrow transplantation. Bone Marrow Transplant 1997; 20(8):695–696.

78. Suzuki T, Saijo Y, Ebina M, et al. Bilateral pneumothoraces with multiple bullae in a patient with asymptomatic bronchiolitis obliterans 10 years after bone marrow transplantation. Bone Marrow Transplant 1999; 23(8):829–831.

79. Cazzadori A, Di Perri G, Bonora S, et al. Fatal pneumothorax complicating BAL in a bone marrow transplant recipient with bronchiolitis obliterans. Chest 1997; 111(5):1468–1469.

80. Wiener-Kronish JP, Matthay MA, Callen PW, et al. Relationship of pleural effusions to pulmonary hemodynamics in patients with congestive heart failure. Am Rev Respir Dis 1985; 132(6):1253–1256.

81. Shinto RA, Light RW. Effects of diuresis on the characteristics of pleural fluid in patients with congestive heart failure. Am J Med 1990; 88(3):230–234.

82. Chakko SC, Caldwell SH, Sforza PP. Treatment of congestive heart failure. Its effect on pleural fluid chemistry. Chest 1989; 95(4):798–802.

83. Wright RS, Levine MS, Bellamy PE, et al. Ventilatory and diffusion abnormalities in potential heart transplant recipients. Chest 1990; 98(4):816–820.

84. Ettinger NA, Trulock EP. Pulmonary considerations of organ transplantation. Part 3. Am Rev Respir Dis 1991; 144(2):433–451.

85. Carter AR, Sostman HD, Curtis AM, et al. Thoracic alterations after cardiac surgery. AJR Am J Roentgenol 1983; 140(3):475–481.

86. Thorsen MK, Goodman LR. Extracardiac complications of cardiac surgery. Semin Roentgenol 1988; 23(1):32–48.

87. Henry DA, Jolles H, Berberich JJ, et al. The post-cardiac surgery chest radiograph: A clinically integrated approach. J Thorac Imaging 1989; 4(3):20–41.

88. Misra H, Dikensoy O, Rodriguez RM, et al. Prevalence of pleural effusions post orthotopic heart transplantation. Respirology 2007; 12(6):887–890.

89. Lenner R, Padilla ML, Teirstein AS, et al. Pulmonary complications in cardiac transplant recipients. Chest 2001; 120(2):508–513.

90. Schulman LL, Smith CR, Drusin R, et al. Respiratory complications of cardiac transplantation. Am J Med Sci 1988; 296(1):1–10.

91. Lee JT, Durzinsky DS, Wilson WR, et al. Pericardial tamponade and massive pleural effusion complicating orthotopic heart transplantation. J Cardiovasc Surg (Torino) 1999; 40(3):377–379.

92. Jones D, Ballestas ME, Kaye KM, et al. Primary-effusion lymphoma and Kaposi's sarcoma in a cardiac-transplant recipient. N Engl J Med 1998; 339(7):444–449.

93. Karcher DS, Alkan S. Human herpesvirus-8-associated body cavity-based lymphoma in human immunodeficiency virus-infected patients: A unique B-cell neoplasm. Hum Pathol 1997; 28(7):801–808.

94. Bowerman RE, Solomon DA, Bognolo D, et al. Chylothorax: Report of a case complicating orthotopic heart transplantation. J Heart Lung Transplant 1993; 12(4):665–668.

95. Conroy JT, Twomey C, Alpern JB. Chylothorax after orthotopic heart transplantation in an adult patient: A case complicated by an episode of rejection. J Heart Lung Transplant 1993; 12(6 Pt 1):1071.

96. Repp R, Scheld HH, Bauer J, et al. Cyclosporine losses by a chylothorax. J Heart Lung Transplant 1992; 11(2 Pt 1):397–398.

97. Parker BM, Smith JR. Pulmonary embolism and infarction; a review of the physiologic consequences of pulmonary arterial obstruction. Am J Med 1958; 24(3):402–427.

98. Murray JR. The pathogenesis, diagnosis, and treatment of pulmonary embolus. Calif Med 1971; 114(6):36–43.

99. Young JN, Yazbeck J, Esposito G, et al. The influence of acute preoperative pulmonary infarction on the results of heart transplantation. J Heart Transplant 1986; 5(1):20–22.

100. Cavarocchi NC, Carp NZ, Mitra A, et al. Successful heart transplantation in recipients with recent preoperative pulmonary emboli. J Heart Transplant 1989; 8(6):494–498.

101. Bieber E, Quinn JP, Venezio FR, et al. *Salmonella* empyema in a heart transplant recipient. J Heart Transplant 1989; 8(3):262–263.

102. Cover TL, Appelbaum PC, Aber RC. *Pseudomonas paucimobilis* empyema after cardiac transplantation. South Med J 1988; 81(6):796–798.

103. Amber IJ, Gilbert EM, Schiffman G, et al. Increased risk of pneumococcal infections in cardiac transplant recipients. Transplantation 1990; 49(1):122–125.

104. DePinto D, Park S, Houck J, et al. Successful treatment of mediastinitis and empyema in a heart transplant patient: One-stage procedure. J Heart Lung Transplant 1993; 12(5):883–884.

105. Canver CC, Patel AK, Kosolcharoen P, et al. Fungal purulent constrictive pericarditis in a heart transplant patient. Ann Thorac Surg 1998; 65(6):1792–1794.

106. Copeland J, Wieden M, Feinberg W, et al. Legionnaires' disease following cardiac transplantation. Chest 1981; 79(6):669–671.

107. Knisely BL, Mastey LA, Collins J, et al. Imaging of cardiac transplantation complications. Radiographics 1999; 19(2):321–339 [discussion 340–341].

108. Rees AP, Meadors M, Ventura HO, et al. Diagnosis of disseminated cytomegalovirus infection and pneumonitis in a heart transplant recipient by skin biopsy: Case report. J Heart Lung Transplant 1991; 10(2):329–332.

109. Schulman LL, Reison DS, Austin JH, et al. Cytomegalovirus pneumonitis after cardiac transplantation. Arch Intern Med 1991; 151(6):1118–1124.

110. Dummer JS, White LT, Ho M, et al. Morbidity of cytomegalovirus infection in recipients of heart or heart–lung transplants who received cyclosporine. J Infect Dis 1985; 152(6):1182–1191.

111. Aarnio P, Harjula A, Heikkila L, et al. Surgery after heart transplantation. Scand J Thorac Cardiovasc Surg 1990; 24(1):21–22.

112. Anastasiou-Nana MI, O'Connell JB, Nanas JN, et al. Relative efficiency and risk of endomyocardial biopsy: Comparisons in heart transplant and nontransplant patients. Cathet Cardiovasc Diagn 1989; 18(1):7–11.

113. Grande AM, Minzioni G, Martinelli L, et al. Echo-controlled endomyocardial biopsy in orthotopic heart transplantation with bicaval anastomosis. G Ital Cardiol 1997; 27(9):877–880.

114. DiSesa VJ, Sloss LJ, Cohn LH. Heart transplantation for intractable prosthetic valve endocarditis. J Heart Transplant 1990; 9(2):142–143.

115. Schuler S, Parnt R, Warnecke H, et al. Extended donor criteria for heart transplantation. J Heart Transplant 1988; 7(5):326–330.

116. Johnston RF, Loo RV. Hepatic hydrothorax; studies to determine the source of the fluid and report of thirteen cases. Ann Intern Med 1964; 61:385–401.

117. Krowka MJ, Cortese DA. Pulmonary aspects of chronic liver disease and liver transplantation. Mayo Clin Proc 1985; 60(6):407–418.

118. Krowka MJ, Cortese DA. Pulmonary aspects of liver disease and liver transplantation. Clin Chest Med 1989; 10(4):593–616.

119. Lieberman FL, Hidemura R, Peters RL, et al. Pathogenesis and treatment of hydrothorax complicating cirrhosis with ascites. Ann Intern Med 1966; 64(2):341–351.

120. Ettinger NA, Trulock EP. Pulmonary considerations of organ transplantation. Part I. Am Rev Respir Dis 1991; 143(6):1386–1405.

121. Afessa B, Gay PC, Plevak DJ, et al. Pulmonary complications of orthotopic liver transplantation. Mayo Clin Proc 1993; 68(5):427–434.

122. Tallgren M, Hockerstedt K, Lindgren L. Respiratory compliance during orthotopic liver transplantation. Acta Anaesthesiol Scand 1996; 40(6):760–764.

123. Hasegawa S, Mori K, Inomata Y, et al. Factors associated with postoperative respiratory complications in pediatric liver transplantation from living-related donors. Transplantation 1996; 62(7):943–947.

124. O'Brien JD, Ettinger NA. Pulmonary complications of liver transplantation. Clin Chest Med 1996; 17(1):99–114.

125. Golfieri R, Giampalma E, Morselli Labate AM, et al. Pulmonary complications of liver transplantation: Radiological appearance and statistical evaluation of risk factors in 300 cases. Eur Radiol 2000; 10(7):1169–1183.

126. Spizarny DL, Gross BH, McLoud T. Enlarging pleural effusion after liver transplantation. J Thorac Imaging 1993; 8(1):85–87.
127. Olutola PS, Hutton L, Wall WJ. Pleural effusion following liver transplantation. Radiology 1985; 157(3):594.
128. Costello P, Williams CR, Jenkins RW, et al. The incidence and implications of chest radiographic abnormalities following orthotopic liver transplantation. Can Assoc Radiol J 1987; 38(2):90–95.
129. Shieh WB, Chen CL, Wang KL. Respiratory changes and pulmonary complications following orthotopic liver transplantation. Transplant Proc 1992; 24(4):1486–1488.
130. Kim ST, Kim SJ, Park KW, et al. Early experience of liver transplantation at Seoul National University Hospital. Transplant Proc 1996; 28(3):1695–1696.
131. Cohen JD, Singer P, Keslin J, et al. Immediate postoperative course and complications of orthotopic liver transplantation: The first 31 adult patients. Transplant Proc 1997; 29(7): 2882.
132. Duran FG, Piqueras B, Romero M, et al. Pulmonary complications following orthotopic liver transplant. Transpl Int 1998; 11(Suppl. 1):S255–S259.
133. Hong SK, Hwang S, Lee SG, et al. Pulmonary complications following adult liver transplantation. Transplant Proc 2006; 38(9):2979–2981.
134. Jiang Y, Lv LZ, Cai QC, et al. Liver transplant for 70 patients with end-stage liver diseases. Hepatobiliary Pancreat Dis Int 2007; 6(1):24–28.
135. Adetiloye VA, John PR. Intervention for pleural effusions and ascites following liver transplantation. Pediatr Radiol 1998; 28(7):539–543.
136. Bilik R, Yellen M, Superina RA. Surgical complications in children after liver transplantation. J Pediatr Surg 1992; 27(11):1371–1375.
137. Moulin D, Clement de Clety S, Reynaert M, et al. Intensive care for children after orthotopic liver transplantation. Intensive Care Med 1989; 15(Suppl. 1):S71–S72.
138. Collins JD, Disher AC, Shaver ML, et al. Imaging the hepatic lymphatics: Experimental studies in swine. J Natl Med Assoc 1993; 85(3):185–191.
139. Robinson LA, Moulton AL, Fleming WH, et al. Intrapleural fibrinolytic treatment of multiloculated thoracic empyemas. Ann Thorac Surg 1994; 57(4):803–813 [discussion 813–814].
140. Schroter GP, Hoelscher M, Putnam CW, et al. Infections complicating orthotopic liver transplantation: A study emphasizing graft-related septicemia. Arch Surg 1976; 111(12):1337–1347.
141. Golfieri R, Giampalma E, Sama C, et al. Pulmonary complications following orthotopic liver transplant: Radiologic patterns and epidemiologic considerations in 100 cases. Rays 1994; 19(3):319–338.
142. Raby N, Forbes G, Williams R. Nocardia infection in patients with liver transplants or chronic liver disease: Radiologic findings. Radiology 1990; 174(3 Pt 1):713–716.
143. Knollmann FD, Maurer J, Bechstein WO, et al. Pulmonary disease in liver transplant recipients. Spectrum of CT features. Acta Radiol 2000; 41(3):230–236.
144. Oh YS, Lisker-Melman M, Korenblat KM, et al. Disseminated histoplasmosis in a liver transplant recipient. Liver Transpl 2006; 12(4):677–681.
145. Codeluppi M, Cocchi S, Guaraldi G, et al. Posttransplant *Mycobacterium tuberculosis* disease following liver transplantation and the need for cautious evaluation of Quantiferon TB GOLD results in the transplant setting: A case report. Transplant Proc 2006; 38(4):1083–1085.
146. Wolford JF, Krause JR. Posttransplant mediastinal Burkitt-like lymphoma. Diagnosis by cytologic and flow cytometric analysis of pleural fluid. Acta Cytol 1990; 34(2):261–264.
147. Hoffmann H, Schlette E, Actor J, et al. Pleural posttransplantation lymphoproliferative disorder following liver transplantation. Arch Pathol Lab Med 2001; 125(3):419–423.
148. Ohori NP, Whisnant RE, Nalesnik MA, et al. Primary pleural effusion posttransplant lymphoproliferative disorder: Distinction from secondary involvement and effusion lymphoma. Diagn Cytopathol 2001; 25(1):50–53.

149. Montalbano M, Neff GW, Yamashiki N, et al. A retrospective review of liver transplant patients treated with sirolimus from a single center: An analysis of sirolimus-related complications. Transplantation 2004; 78(2):264–268.

150. Merenda R, Gerunda GE, Neri D, et al. Laparoscopic surgery after orthotopic liver transplantation. Liver Transpl 2000; 6(1):104–107.

151. Smyrniotis V, Andreani P, Muiesan P, et al. Diaphragmatic nerve palsy in young children following liver transplantation. Successful treatment by plication of the diaphragm. Transpl Int 1998; 11(4):281–283.

152. Zajko AB, Claus D, Clapuyt P, et al. Obstruction to hepatic venous drainage after liver transplantation: Treatment with balloon angioplasty. Radiology 1989; 170(3 Pt 1):763–765.

153. Larson AM, Chan GC, Wartelle CF, et al. Infection complicating percutaneous liver biopsy in liver transplant recipients. Hepatology 1997; 26(6):1406–1409.

154. Lovell M, Baines D. Fatal complication from central venous cannulation in a paediatric liver transplant patient. Paediatr Anaesth 2000; 10(6):661–664.

155. Pirenne J, Aerts R, Yoong K, et al. Liver transplantation for polycystic liver disease. Liver Transpl 2001; 7(3):238–245.

156. Galati JS, Monsour HP, Donovan JP, et al. The nature of complications following liver biopsy in transplant patients with Roux-en-Y choledochojejunostomy. Hepatology 1994; 20(3):651–653.

157. Kalayoglu M, D'Alessandro AM, Knechtle SJ, et al. Preliminary experience with split liver transplantation. J Am Coll Surg 1996; 182(5):381–387.

158. Torgay A, Pirat A, Candan S, et al. Internal jugular versus subclavian vein catheterization for central venous catheterization in orthotopic liver transplantation. Transplant Proc 2005; 37(7):3171–3173.

159. Foster R, Zimmerman M, Trotter JF. Expanding donor options: Marginal, living, and split donors. Clin Liver Dis 2007; 11(2):417–429.

160. Yi NJ, Suh KS, Cho JY, et al. Three-quarters of right liver donors experienced postoperative complications. Liver Transpl 2007; 13(6):797–806.

161. Dondero F, Taille C, Mal H, et al. Respiratory complications: A major concern after right hepatectomy in living liver donors. Transplantation 2006; 81(2):181–186.

162. Schumann R, Bonney I, McDevitt LM, et al. Extent of right hepatectomy determines postoperative donor albumin and bilirubin changes: New insights. Liver Int 2008; 28(1):95–98.

163. Lee SY, Ko GY, Gwon DI, et al. Living donor liver transplantation: Complications in donors and interventional management. Radiology 2004; 230(2):443–449.

164. Jarratt MJ, Sahn SA. Pleural effusions in hospitalized patients receiving long-term hemodialysis. Chest 1995; 108(2):470–474.

165. Hopps HC, Wissler RW. Uremic pneumonitis. Am J Pathol 1955; 31(2):261–273.

166. Berger HW, Rammohan G, Neff MS, et al. Uremic pleural effusion. A study in 14 patients on chronic dialysis. Ann Intern Med 1975; 82(3):362–364.

167. Nidus BD, Matalon R, Cantacuzino D, et al. Uremic pleuritis—A clinicopathological entity. N Engl J Med 1969; 281(5):255–256.

168. Galen MA, Steinberg SM, Lowrie EG, et al. Hemorrhagic pleural effusion in patients undergoing chronic hemodialysis. Ann Intern Med 1975; 82(3):359–361.

169. Rodelas R, Rakowski TA, Argy WP, et al. Fibrosing uremic pleuritis during hemodialysis. JAMA 1980; 243(23):2424–2425.

170. Harnsberger HR, Lee TG, Mukuno DH. Rapid, inexpensive real-time directed thoracentesis. Radiology 1983; 146(2):545–546.

171. Gilbert L, Ribot S, Frankel H, et al. Fibrinous uremic pleuritis: A surgical entity. Chest 1975; 67(1):53–56.

172. Wright RS, Quinones-Baldrich WJ, Anders AJ, et al. Pleural effusion associated with ipsilateral breast and arm edema as a complication of subclavian vein catheterization and arteriovenous fistula formation for hemodialysis. Chest 1994; 106(3):950–952.

173. Van Veldhuizen PJ, Taylor S. Chylothorax: A complication of a left subclavian vein thrombosis. Am J Clin Oncol 1996; 19(2):99–101.

174. Heino A. Operative and postoperative non-surgical complications in diabetic patients undergoing renal transplantation. Scand J Urol Nephrol 1988; 22(1):53–58.

175. Chen Y, Yen TH, Liu KL, et al. Outcome of renal transplantation in children with pericardiopleural effusion. Transplant Proc 2004; 36(7):2032–2033.

176. Kuzbary Y, Lasher JC, Blumhardt R, et al. Renal transplant extravasation of urine through a chest tube: An unusual appearance on radionuclide imaging. Nucl Med Commun 1984; 5(10):655–659.

177. Carcillo J Jr, Salcedo JR. Urinothorax as a manifestation of nondilated obstructive uropathy following renal transplantation. Am J Kidney Dis 1985; 5(3):211–213.

178. Salcedo JR. Urinothorax: Report of 4 cases and review of the literature. J Urol 1986; 135(4):805–808.

179. Kees-Folts D, Cole BR. Ureteral urine leak presenting as a pleural effusion in a renal transplant recipient. Pediatr Nephrol 1998; 12(8):666–667.

180. Miller KS, Wooten S, Sahn SA. Urinothorax: A cause of low pH transudative pleural effusions. Am J Med 1988; 85(3):448–449.

181. Hayashi K, Hoshida Y, Ohnoshi T, et al. Primary pulmonary non-Hodgkin's lymphoma in a Japanese renal transplant recipient. Int J Hematol 1993; 57(3):245–250.

182. Lippman SM, Grogan TM, Carry P, et al. Post-transplantation T cell lymphoblastic lymphoma. Am J Med 1987; 82(4):814–816.

183. Jimenez-Heffernan JA, Viguer JM, Vicandi B, et al. Posttransplant CD30 (Ki-1)-positive anaplastic large cell lymphoma. Report of a case with presentation as a pleural effusion. Acta Cytol 1997; 41(5):1519–1524.

184. Levendoglu-Tugal O, Weiss R, Ozkaynak MF, et al. T-cell acute lymphoblastic leukemia after renal transplantation in childhood. J Pediatr Hematol Oncol 1998; 20(6):548–551.

185. DeCamp MM, Tilney NL. Late development of intractable lymphocele after renal transplantation. Transplant Proc 1988; 20(1):105–109.

186. Sollinger HW, Starling JR, Oberley T, et al. Severe "weeping" kidney disease after transplantation: A case report. Transplant Proc 1983; 15(4):2157–2160.

187. Bear RA, McCallum RW, Cant J, et al. Perirenal lymphocyst formation in renal transplant recipients: Diagnosis and pathogenesis. Urology 1976; 7(6):581–586.

188. Schweizer RT, Cho S, Koutz KS, et al. Lymphoceles following renal transplantation. Arch Surg 1972; 104(1):42–45.

189. Morley P, Barnett E, Bell PR, et al. Ultrasound in the diagnosis of fluid collections following renal transplantation. Clin Radiol 1975; 26(2):199–207.

190. Braun WE, Banowsky LH, Straffon RA, et al. Lymphoceles associated with renal transplantation: Report of fifteen cases and review of the literature. Proc Clin Dial Transplant Forum 1973; 3:185–189.

191. Koehler PR. Injuries and complications of the lymphatic system following renal transplantation. Lymphology 1972; 5(2):61–67.

192. Gomez-Roman JJ, Ocejo-Vinyals JG, Sanchez-Velasco P, et al. Presence of human herpesvirus 8 DNA sequences in renal transplantation-associated pleural Kaposi sarcoma. Arch Pathol Lab Med 1999; 123(12):1269–1273.

193. Schmidt RJ, Bender FH, Chang WW, et al. Sarcoidosis after renal transplantation. Transplantation 1999; 68(9):1420–1423.

194. Heino A, Orko R, Rosenberg PH. Anaesthesiological complications in renal transplantation: A retrospective study of 500 transplantations. Acta Anaesthesiol Scand 1986; 30(7):574–580.

195. Vereerstraeten P, De Koster JP, Vereerstraeten J, et al. Pulmonary infections after kidney transplantation. Proc Eur Dial Transplant Assoc 1975; 11:300–307.

196. Jha R, Narayan G, Jaleel MA, et al. Pulmonary infections after kidney transplantation. J Assoc Physicians India 1999; 47(8):779–783.

197. Thacker WL, Benson RF, Schifman RB, et al. *Legionella tucsonensis* sp. nov. isolated from a renal transplant recipient. J Clin Microbiol 1989; 27(8):1831–1834.

198. McKinney RM, Wilkinson HW, Sommers HM, et al. *Legionella pneumophila* serogroup six: Isolation from cases of legionellosis, identification by immunofluorescence staining, and immunological response to infection. J Clin Microbiol 1980; 12(3):395–401.

199. Bock BV, Kirby BD, Edelstein PH, et al. Legionnaires' disease in renal-transplant recipients. Lancet 1978; 1(8061):410–413.

200. Marshall W, Foster RS Jr, Winn W. Legionnaires' disease in renal transplant patients. Am J Surg 1981; 141(4):423–429.

201. Moore EH, Webb WR, Gamsu G, et al. Legionnaires' disease in the renal transplant patient: Clinical presentation and radiographic progression. Radiology 1984; 153(3):589–593.

202. Foster RS Jr, Winn WC Jr, Marshall W, et al. Legionnaires' disease following renal transplantation. Transplant Proc 1979; 11(1):93–95.

203. Levin AS, Caiaffa Filho HH, Sinto SI, et al. An outbreak of nosocomial Legionnaires' disease in a renal transplant unit in Sao Paulo, Brazil. Legionellosis Study Team. J Hosp Infect 1991; 18(3).243–248.

204. Santamaria Saber LT, Figueiredo JF, Santos SB, et al. Nocardia infection in renal transplant recipient: Diagnostic and therapeutic considerations. Rev Inst Med Trop Sao Paulo 1993; 35(5):417–421.

205. Lovett IS, Houang ET, Burge S, et al. An outbreak of Nocardia asteroides infection in a renal transplant unit. Q J Med 1981; 50(198):123–135.

206. Ochiai T, Amemiya H, Watanabe K, et al. Successful treatment of Nocardia asteroides infection with minocycline in kidney transplant patients. Jpn J Surg 1978; 8(2):138–144.

207. Tzamaloukas AH, Ahlin T, Katzestein D, et al. Association of pulmonary embolism and pulmonary nocardiosis in renal transplant recipients. Transplantation 1982; 33(5):569.

208. Arduino RC, Johnson PC, Miranda AG. Nocardiosis in renal transplant recipients undergoing immunosuppression with cyclosporine. Clin Infect Dis 1993; 16(4):505–512.

209. Lakshiminarayan S, Sahn SA. Tuberculosis in a patient after renal transplantation. Tubercle 1973; 54(1):72–76.

210. Hall CM, Willcox PA, Swanepoel CR, et al. Mycobacterial infection in renal transplant recipients. Chest 1994; 106(2):435–439.

211. Vandermarliere A, Van Audenhove A, Peetermans WE, et al. Mycobacterial infection after renal transplantation in a Western population. Transpl Infect Dis 2003; 5(1):9–15.

212. Wood M, Wallin JD, O'Neill W Jr. Disseminated tuberculosis in a renal transplant recipient: Presentation as an anterior mediastinal mass. South Med J 1983; 76(12):1577–1579.

213. Malhotra KK, Dash SC, Dhawan IK, et al. Tuberculosis and renal transplantation— Observations from an endemic area of tuberculosis. Postgrad Med J 1986; 62(727):359–362.

214. Kaaroud H, Beji S, Boubaker K, et al. Tuberculosis after renal transplantation. Transplant Proc 2007; 39(4):1012–1013.

215. Lattes R, Radisic M, Rial M, et al. Tuberculosis in renal transplant recipients. Transpl Infect Dis 1999; 1(2):98–104.

216. Park YS, Choi JY, Cho CH, et al. Clinical outcomes of tuberculosis in renal transplant recipients. Yonsei Med J 2004; 45(5):865–872.

217. Chung JH, Kim YS, Kim SI, et al. The diagnostic value of the adenosine deaminase activity in the pleural fluid of renal transplant patients with tuberculous pleural effusion. Yonsei Med J 2004; 45(4):661–664.

218. Conces DJ Jr, Vix VA, Tarver RD. Pleural cryptococcosis. J Thorac Imaging 1990; 5(2):84–86.

219. Lye WC, Chin NK, Lee YS. Disseminated cryptococcosis presenting with a pleural effusion in a kidney transplant recipient: Early diagnosis by pleural biopsy and successful treatment with oral fluconazole. Nephron 1993; 65(4):646.

220. Balasubramanian VP, Komorowski RA, Santo Tomas LH. *Pneumocystis carinii* pneumonia with pleural effusion in a non-HIV host. WMJ 2006; 105(1):62–65.

221. Gonzalez-Roncero FM, Gentil MA, Rodriguez-Algarra G, et al. Medical management of pneumonia caused by *Rhodococcus equi* in a renal transplant recipient. Am J Kidney Dis 2002; 39(2):E7.

222. Spencer CD, Crawford GE. Nontoxic staphylococcal pneumonia with empyema in a renal transplant recipient. West J Med 1982; 136(2):147–149.

223. Berk MR, Meyers AM, Cassal W, et al. Non-typhoid salmonella infections after renal transplantation. A serious clinical problem. Nephron 1984; 37(3):186–189.

224. Polga JP, Watnick M, Herman PG. Pneumothorax following lung abscess in the renal transplant patient. J Can Assoc Radiol 1973; 24(2):116–118.

225. Castaneda MA, Garvin PJ. General surgical procedures in renal allograft recipients. Am J Surg 1986; 152(6):717–721.

226. Egan TM, Kaiser LR, Cooper JD. Lung transplantation. Curr Probl Surg 1989; 26(10):673–751.

227. Tazelaar HD, Yousem SA. The pathology of combined heart-lung transplantation: An autopsy study. Hum Pathol 1988; 19(12):1403–1416.

228. Bando K, Keenan RJ, Paradis IL, et al. Impact of pulmonary hypertension on outcome after single-lung transplantation. Ann Thorac Surg 1994; 58(5):1336–1342.

229. Kaiser LR, Pasque MK, Trulock EP, et al. Bilateral sequential lung transplantation: The procedure of choice for double-lung replacement. Ann Thorac Surg 1991; 52(3):438–445 [discussion 445–446].

230. de Hoyos A, Demajo W, Snell G, et al. Preoperative prediction for the use of cardiopulmonary bypass in lung transplantation. J Thorac Cardiovasc Surg 1993; 106(5):787–795 [discussion 795–796].

231. Triantafillou AN, Pasque MK, Huddleston CB, et al. Predictors, frequency, and indications for cardiopulmonary bypass during lung transplantation in adults. Ann Thorac Surg 1994; 57(5):1248–1251.

232. Collins J, Kuhlman JE, Love RB. Acute, life-threatening complications of lung transplantation. Radiographics 1998; 18(1):21–43 [discussion 43–47].

233. Dusmet M, Winton TL, Kesten S, et al. Previous intrapleural procedures do not adversely affect lung transplantation. J Heart Lung Transplant 1996; 15(3):249–254.

234. Almoosa KF, Ryu JH, Mendez J, et al. Management of pneumothorax in lymphangioleiomyomatosis: Effects on recurrence and lung transplantation complications. Chest 2006; 129(5):1274–1281.

235. Shennib H, Adoumie R, Noirclerc M. Current status of lung transplantation for cystic fibrosis. Arch Intern Med 1992; 152(8):1585–1588.

236. Flume PA, Strange C, Ye X, et al. Pneumothorax in cystic fibrosis. Chest 2005; 128(2):720–728.

237. Flume PA. Pneumothorax in cystic fibrosis. Chest 2003; 123(1):217–221.

238. Seddon DJ, Hodson ME. Surgical management of pneumothorax in cystic fibrosis. Thorax 1988; 43(9):739–740.

239. Smyth RL, Higenbottam TW, Scott JP, et al. Transplantation of the lungs. Respir Med 1989; 83(6):459–466.

240. Noyes BE, Orenstein DM. Treatment of pneumothorax in cystic fibrosis in the era of lung transplantation. Chest 1992; 101(5):1187–1188.

241. Noppen M, Dhondt E, Mahler T, et al. Successful management of recurrent pneumothorax in cystic fibrosis by localized apical thoracoscopic talc poudrage. Chest 1994; 106(1):262–264.

242. Schidlow DV, Taussig LM, Knowles MR. Cystic Fibrosis Foundation consensus conference report on pulmonary complications of cystic fibrosis. Pediatr Pulmonol 1993; 15(3):187–198.

243. Rich RH, Warwick WJ, Leonard AS. Open thoracotomy and pleural abrasion in the treatment of spontaneous pneumothorax in cystic fibrosis. J Pediatr Surg 1978; 13(3):237–242.

244. Madden BP, Hodson ME, Yacoub MH, et al. Heart–lung transplantation for cystic fibrosis. BMJ 1992; 304(6830):835–836.

245. Dosanjh A, Jones L, Yuh D, et al. Pleural disease in patients undergoing lung transplantation for cystic fibrosis. Pediatr Transplant 1998; 2(4):283–287.

246. Artemiou O, Marta GM, Klepetko W, et al. Pleurovenous shunting in the treatment of nonmalignant pleural effusion. Ann Thorac Surg 2003; 76(1):231–233.

247. Ferrer J, Roldan J, Roman A, et al. Acute and chronic pleural complications in lung transplantation. J Heart Lung Transplant 2003; 22(11):1217–1225.

248. Herridge MS, de Hoyos AL, Chaparro C, et al. Pleural complications in lung transplant recipients. J Thorac Cardiovasc Surg 1995; 110(1):22–26.

249. Griffith BP, Zenati M. The pulmonary donor. Clin Chest Med 1990; 11(2):217–226.

250. Mills NL, Boyd AD, Gheranpong C. The significance of bronchial circulation in lung transplantation. J Thorac Cardiovasc Surg 1970; 60(6):866–878.

251. Venuta F, Boehler A, Rendina EA, et al. Complications in the native lung after single lung transplantation. Eur J Cardiothorac Surg 1999; 16(1):54–58.

252. Chiles C, Guthaner DF, Jamieson SW, et al. Heart–lung transplantation: The postoperative chest radiograph. Radiology 1985; 154(2):299–304.

253. Raju S, Heath BJ, Warren ET, et al. Single- and double-lung transplantation. Problems and possible solutions. Ann Surg 1990; 211(6):681–691 [discussion 691–693].

254. Todd TR. Early postoperative management following lung transplantation. Clin Chest Med 1990; 11(2):259–267.

255. Ruggiero R, Fietsam R Jr, Thomas GA, et al. Detection of canine allograft lung rejection by pulmonary lymphoscintigraphy. J Thorac Cardiovasc Surg 1994; 108(2):253–258.

256. Winter JB, Groen M, Petersen AH, et al. Reduced antibody responses after immunization in rat lung transplants. Am Rev Respir Dis 1993; 147(3):664–668.

257. Judson MA, Handy JR, Sahn SA. Pleural effusion from acute lung rejection. Chest 1997; 111(4):1128–1130.

258. Trulock EP. Management of lung transplant rejection. Chest 1993; 103(5):1566–1576.

259. Gotway MB, Dawn SK, Sellami D, et al. Acute rejection following lung transplantation: Limitations in accuracy of thin-section CT for diagnosis. Radiology 2001; 221(1):207–212.

260. Marom EM, Palmer SM, Erasmus JJ, et al. Pleural effusions in lung transplant recipients: Image-guided small-bore catheter drainage. Radiology 2003; 228(1):241–245.

261. Date H, Yamane M, Toyooka S, et al. Current status and potential of living-donor lobar lung transplantation. Front Biosci 2008; 13:1433–1439.

262. Backhus LM, Sievers EM, Schenkel FA, et al. Pleural space problems after living lobar transplantation. J Heart Lung Transplant 2005; 24(12):2086–2090.

263. Dauriat G, Brugiere O, Mal H, et al. Refractory chylothorax after lung transplantation for lymphangioleiomyomatosis successfully cured with instillation of povidone. J Thorac Cardiovasc Surg 2003; 126(3):875–877.

264. Fremont RD, Milstone AP, Light RW, et al. Chylothoraces after lung transplantation for lymphangioleiomyomatosis: Review of the literature and utilization of a pleurovenous shunt. J Heart Lung Transplant 2007; 26(9):953–955.

265. Boehler A, Speich R, Russi EW, et al. Lung transplantation for lymphangioleiomyomatosis. N Engl J Med 1996; 335(17):1275–1280.

266. Pechet TT, Meyers BF, Guthrie TJ, et al. Lung transplantation for lymphangioleiomyomatosis. J Heart Lung Transplant 2004; 23(3):301–308.

267. Ziedalski TM, Raffin TA, Sze DY, et al. Chylothorax after heart/lung transplantation. J Heart Lung Transplant 2004; 23(5):627–631.

268. Judson MA, Handy JR, Sahn SA. Pleural effusions following lung transplantation. Time course, characteristics, and clinical implications. Chest 1996; 109(5):1190–1194.

269. Struber M, Hagl C, Hirt SW, et al. C1-esterase inhibitor in graft failure after lung transplantation. Intensive Care Med 1999; 25(11):1315–1318.

270. Memtsoudis SG, Rosenberger P, Sadovnikoff N. Chest tube suction-associated unilateral negative pressure pulmonary edema in a lung transplant patient. Anesth Analg 2005; 101(1):38–40, table of contents.

271. Judson MA, Sahn SA, Hahn AB. Origin of pleural cells after lung transplantation: From donor or recipient? Chest 1997; 112(2):426–429.

272. Collins J, Muller NL, Kazerooni EA, et al. CT findings of pneumonia after lung transplantation. AJR Am J Roentgenol 2000; 175(3):811–818.

273. Snell GI, de Hoyos A, Krajden M, et al. *Pseudomonas cepacia* in lung transplant recipients with cystic fibrosis. Chest 1993; 103(2):466–471.

274. Noyes BE, Michaels MG, Kurland G, et al. *Pseudomonas cepacia* empyema necessitatis after lung transplantation in two patients with cystic fibrosis. Chest 1994; 105(6):1888–1891.

275. Khan SU, Gordon SM, Stillwell PC, et al. Empyema and bloodstream infection caused by *Burkholderia gladioli* in a patient with cystic fibrosis after lung transplantation. Pediatr Infect Dis J 1996; 15(7):637–639.

276. Brooks RG, Hofflin JM, Jamieson SW, et al. Infectious complications in heart–lung transplant recipients. Am J Med 1985; 79(4):412–422.

277. Horvath J, Dummer S, Loyd J, et al. Infection in the transplanted and native lung after single lung transplantation. Chest 1993; 104(3):681–685.

278. Janssens W, Van Raemdonck D, Dupont L, et al. Listeria pleuritis 1 week after lung transplantation. J Heart Lung Transplant 2006; 25(6):734–737.

279. Penketh AR, Higenbottam TW, Hutter J, et al. Clinical experience in the management of pulmonary opportunist infection and rejection in recipients of heart–lung transplants. Thorax 1988; 43(10):762–769.

280. Dromer C, Nashef SA, Velly JF, et al. Tuberculosis in transplanted lungs. J Heart Lung Transplant 1993; 12(6 Pt 1):924–927.

281. Schulman LL, Scully B, McGregor CC, et al. Pulmonary tuberculosis after lung transplantation. Chest 1997; 111(5):1459–1462.

282. Emery RW, Graif JL, Hale K, et al. Treatment of end-stage chronic obstructive pulmonary disease with double lung transplantation. Chest 1991; 99(3):533–537.

283. Liguori C, Schulman LL, Weslow RG, et al. Late pulmonary venous complications after lung transplantation. J Am Soc Echocardiogr 1997; 10(7):763–767.

284. Collins J, Muller NL, Leung AN, et al. Epstein–Barr-virus-associated lymphoproliferative disease of the lung: CT and histologic findings. Radiology 1998; 208(3):749–759.

285. Siegel MJ, Lee EY, Sweet SC, et al. CT of posttransplantation lymphoproliferative disorder in pediatric recipients of lung allograft. AJR Am J Roentgenol 2003; 181(4):1125–1131.

286. Kukafka DS, O'Brien GM, Furukawa S, et al. Surveillance bronchoscopy in lung transplant recipients. Chest 1997; 111(2):377–381.

287. Chan CC, Abi-Saleh WJ, Arroliga AC, et al. Diagnostic yield and therapeutic impact of flexible bronchoscopy in lung transplant recipients. J Heart Lung Transplant 1996; 15(2):196–205.

288. Chen F, Bando T, Fukuse T, et al. Recurrent lymphangioleiomyomatosis after living-donor lobar lung transplantation. Transplant Proc 2006; 38(9):3151–3153.

289. Yousem SA, Burke CM, Billingham ME. Pathologic pulmonary alterations in long-term human heart–lung transplantation. Hum Pathol 1985; 16(9):911–923.

290. Haverich A, Dawkins KD, Baldwin JC, et al. Long-term cardiac and pulmonary histology in primates following combined heart and lung transplantation. Transplantation 1985; 39(4):356–360.

291. Shitrit D, Izbicki G, Starobin D, et al. Late-onset chylothorax after heart-lung transplantation. Ann Thorac Surg 2003; 75(1):285–286.

292. Chhajed PN, Bubendorf L, Hirsch H, et al. Mesothelioma after lung transplantation. Thorax 2006; 61(10):916–917.

293. Engeler CE, Olson PN, Engeler CM, et al. Shifting pneumothorax after heart–lung transplantation. Radiology 1992; 185(3):715–717.

294. Wittich GR, Kusnick CA, Starnes VA, et al. Communication between the two pleural cavities after major cardiothoracic surgery: Relevance to percutaneous intervention. Radiology 1992; 184(2):461–462.

295. Paranjpe DV, Wittich GR, Hamid LW, et al. Frequency and management of pneumothoraces in heart–lung transplant recipients. Radiology 1994; 190(1):255–256.

296. Sacks EM, Unger EC. Heart–lung transplantation: Postoperative pleural effusion. AJR Am J Roentgenol 1990; 154(6):1344–1345.

297. Slebos DJ, Elting-Wartan AN, Bakker M, et al. Managing a bilateral pneumothorax in lung transplantation using single chest-tube drainage. J Heart Lung Transplant 2001; 20(7):796–797.

298. Holland SA, Hutton LC, McKenzie FN. Radiologic findings in heart–lung transplantation: A preliminary experience. Can Assoc Radiol J 1989; 40(2):94–97.

299. Lee YC, McGrath GB, Chin WS, et al. Contralateral tension pneumothorax following unilateral chest tube drainage of bilateral pneumothoraces in a heart–lung transplant patient. Chest 1999; 116(4):1131–1133.

300. Chhajed PN, Malouf MA, Tamm M, et al. Resolution of native lung pneumothorax by insertion of a nitinol stent for bronchostenosis in the transplanted lung. Respirology 2002; 7(4):377–379.

301. Spaggiari L, Rusca M, Carbognani P, et al. Contralateral spontaneous pneumothorax after single lung transplantation for fibrosis. Acta Biomed Ateneo Parmense 1993; 64(1–2):29–31.

302. Venuta F, Rendina EA, de Giacomo T, et al. Thoracoscopic treatment of recurrent contralateral pneumothorax after single lung transplantation. J Heart Lung Transplant 1994; 13(3):555–557.

303. Waller DA, Conacher ID, Dark JH. Videothoracoscopic pleurectomy after contralateral single-lung transplantation. Ann Thorac Surg 1994; 57(4):1021–1023.

304. Shumway SJ, Hertz MI, Petty MG, et al. Liberalization of donor criteria in lung and heart–lung transplantation. Ann Thorac Surg 1994; 57(1):92–95.

44
Pleural Disease as a Complication of Radiotherapy and Radiofrequency Ablation

JOSÉ M. PORCEL
Department of Internal Medicine, Arnau de Vilanova University Hospital, Lleida, Spain

I. Introduction

Radiotherapy (RT) has become a standard treatment option for a wide range of malignancies. Radiation can be considered as packets of energy in the form of photons or particles. Radiation dose is the term that describes the quantity of energy deposited per mass of a tissue, and is frequently expressed using the International System unit *gray* (Gy), which equals 1 J/kg. An older unit of dose is the *rad*, which is equal to 1/100 Gy or 1 cGy (1).

Incidental irradiation of adjacent normal structures is inevitable during RT, resulting in acute and long-term side effects. Early or acute effects typically occur within weeks or a few months after irradiation; an example is radiation pneumonitis. Late effects, on the other hand, occur months to years after irradiation; an example is lung and mediastinal fibrosis. The risk of these complications, particularly high with old suboptimal irradiation techniques, has decreased with the introduction of modern technologies. However, despite the efforts to reduce radiation-induced late toxicity, physicians are still seeing survivors of Hodgkin's disease (HD) who were treated in earlier decades with extended-field RT, presenting with severe organ damage and functional disabilities (2).

From a technological point of view, there are two general types of RT (1): (*i*) brachytherapy, which is usually administered with internal sources and (*ii*) teletherapy, or external-beam therapy, in which high photon energies are delivered with linear accelerators. In the last decade, three-dimensional conformal RT (3DCRT) has become the standard of care for treating tumors amenable to ionizing radiation. A more sophisticated form of RT called intensity-modulated RT (IMRT) is a technique that maximizes the homogeneous delivery of radiation to the planned target while sparing normal tissue. The delivery of IMRT can utilize multileaf collimators or linear accelerators mounted on an industrial robot arm (stereotactic radiosurgery).

On the other hand, radiofrequency ablation (RFA) has evolved as a new technique that can potentially be applied to patients with lung or liver tumors who are not surgical candidates (3). RFA utilizes radio waves that are emitted from a probe implanted within a tumor to generate heat, causing coagulation necrosis of the tumoral tissue. In this chapter, we will review pleural toxicities produced by different modalities of RT and RFA (Table 1).

Table 1 Pleural Toxicities After Radiotherapy and Radiofrequency Ablation

Technique	Pleural involvement
Chest radiotherapy	
Conventional	Frequent: pleural thickening (~20%)
	Infrequent: early and late pleural effusions (0–10%), pneumothorax (0–2%)
	Rare: chylothorax, mesothelioma
Radiosurgery	Pneumothorax (10–30%)
Brachytherapy	Pneumothorax (0–4% by bronchoscopy, up to 30% by CT)
Radiofrequency ablation	
Liver tumors	Infrequent: pleural effusion (<2.5%)
	Rare: hemothorax, pneumothorax
Lung tumors	Pneumothorax (~50%), pleural effusion (~10%)

II. Pleural Involvement Following Chest Radiotherapy

A. Conventional RT

Early Pleural Effusions

RT is an integral component of the locoregional management of breast cancer and early-stage HD, as well as a frequently recommended treatment for advanced lung and esophageal tumors. Radiation pneumonitis is reported in about 10% of patients receiving definitive external-beam RT for lung cancer, but this incidence is lower in HD and breast cancer patients who receive mediastinal irradiation (2%) (4). Radiation damage to the lungs is rarely seen below 20 Gy, whereas it is common in areas receiving 30 to 40 Gy, and almost inevitable over 40 Gy. Radiation pneumonitis usually develops one to three months after completing RT, and presents with dry cough, dyspnea, low-grade fever, and rales. In most cases, these symptoms are mild and resolve spontaneously (5).

Pleural effusions may accompany acute radiation pneumonitis. In old series, between 5% and 10% of patients receiving 40 to 60 Gy to the hemithorax for breast cancer developed pleural effusions attributed to, and within six months of, RT (6,7). Virtually all patients had concomitant radiation pneumonitis. The effusions were small and lasted from four months to several years (6). The pleural fluid associated with radiation pleuritis has not been well characterized, but in two reported cases the fluid was a hemorrhagic exudate with multiple-vacuolated mesothelial cells (8). It should be noted that a history of RT does not affect the cytopathologic interpretation of pleural fluid (9).

The incidence of postradiation pleural effusion has now dramatically decreased. A recent prospective study evaluated the prevalence and grade of pleuropulmonary abnormalities in the chest radiographs of 186 patients with breast cancer, all of whom received postlumpectomy or postmastectomy RT with a total dose of 50 Gy (10). The chest radiographs were normal in 54% at three months, in 61% at six months, and in 84% at one year after RT. Grade 2 pneumonitis (linear streaky), the most common abnormality, was noted in 22.5%, 28%, and 16% of patients at the end of 3, 6, and 12 months, respectively. Abnormalities in the pleura consisted of an elevated diaphragm, a diffuse contour, or adhesions of the diaphragm, and were observed in 17% at three months and in 19% at six months after RT. However, no associated pleural fluid was detected in any plain radiograph. There were only three patients who showed pleural abnormalities without lung changes.

The pathophysiological mechanism of early pleural effusions caused by RT is probably an increase in capillary permeability resulting from damage to the microvasculature and mesothelial cells. Activation of mesothelial cells, recruitment of inflammatory cells into the pleural space, and a disordered fibrin turnover will ultimately lead to pleural fibrosis.

Late Pleural Effusions

In addition to the moderate and often asymptomatic effusions that can accompany radiation pneumonitis during the first months after completing RT, pleural effusions may also occur as a late complication of mediastinal radiation. Extended-field radiation of the mediastinum (i.e., radiation to the areas of disease and surrounding lymph nodes), once responsible for much of the late toxicities seen in patients with HD, is now considered an outdated treatment and has been substituted for involved-field radiation (i.e., only to known areas of disease).

In a series of 68 inoperable patients with stage I non–small-cell lung cancer that received hypofractioned RT (mean total dose of 37.5 Gy), 2 (3%) developed a benign pleural effusion as a late side effect (11). The combination of two series of patients (for a total of 112), who achieved a complete response after definitive chemoradiotherapy (total radiation dose 60 Gy) for esophageal cancer, revealed substantial late toxicities, including pericarditis in 22 (20%) and pleural effusions in 20 (18%) patients (12,13).

Mediastinal irradiation causes inflammation and progressive fibrosis of all the structures of the heart, particularly the pericardium. The approximate incidence of radiation-induced heart disease is 10% to 30% by 5 to 10 years posttreatment, although asymptomatic cardiac abnormalities are present in a much higher percentage of patients (4). Possible presentations of radiation-related damage to the cardiovascular system include pericardial disease, valvular dysfunction, coronary artery disease, arrhythmias, myocardial fibrosis with diastolic dysfunction, and carotid artery stenosis (14). Therefore, patients may present cardiac effusions many years after mediastinal RT, secondary to radiation-induced cardiomyopathy or ischemic heart disease. In addition, pleural effusion may accompany radiation-induced pericardial disease such as pericardial tamponade, constrictive pericarditis, or effusive–constrictive pericarditis. In a series of 81 patients with HD stage IA–IIA who received either extended-field (34%) or involved-field (66%) mediastinal RT (doses from 36 to 40 Gy), 9 (11%) patients presented late pulmonary toxicity and another 9 late cardiac events (myocardial infarction 3, heart failure 2, valvular sclerosis 2, restrictive cardiomyopathy 1, and pericarditis 1) over a 15-year follow-up (15).

There are a few reports of pleural effusions appearing from 1.5 to 35 years after completion of mediastinal RT, mostly for HD (2,16–21). Porcel and Tarragona (2) described a patient who developed bilateral massive pleural and pericardial effusions 16 years after receiving mantle-field RT at 40 Gy for HD (Fig. 1). The pleural fluid was an exudate with lymphocytic predominance, as found in other reports (16,17,20). Autopsy revealed severe mediastinal fibrosis as well as diffused thickening of the pericardial and pleural membranes. Mechanisms for development of these late pleural effusions include constrictive or effusive–constrictive pericarditis, superior vena cava obstruction, and impaired pleural or mediastinal lymphatic drainage, all secondary to radiation-induced fibrosis of the

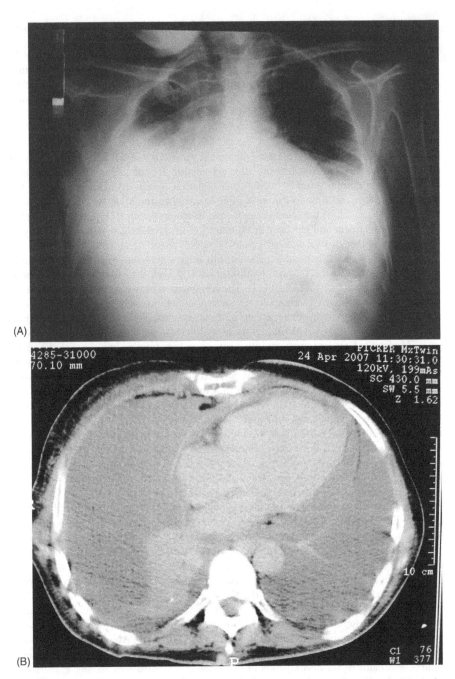

(A)

(B)

Figure 1   Chest radiography (**A**) and CT scan (**B**) of a patient with a history of radiotherapy for Hodgkin's disease showing massive pleural and pericardial effusions. *Source*: From Ref. 2.

mediastinal structures. It should be noted that when the pleural effusion is secondary to constrictive pericarditis, its biochemical characteristics may occasionally fulfill criteria for transudate (22). Because the diagnosis of radiation-induced pleural effusion is one of exclusion, other causes such as recurrent lymphoma, second neoplasms, or thyroid dysfunctions should be considered and properly investigated.

The optimal management of pleural effusion induced by RT is unclear. The treatment of radiation-associated pleuritis is usually rewarding. Symptomatic patients can be started on nonsteroidal anti-inflammatory drugs, while glucocorticoids should be reserved for those individuals who do not respond to nonsteroidal agents. Therapeutic thoracocentesis, pleurodesis with doxycycline (500 mg in 50–100 mL of saline) through a chest catheter, or thoracoscopic talc pleurodesis should be considered in massive or recurrent effusions (23). Notably, catheter insertion thorough a thick fibrotic parietal pleural may be difficult. Anecdotally, a patient with delayed radiation-induced pleuropericardial effusions, unresponsive to steroids and nonsteroidal anti-inflammatory drugs, improved with oral doxycycline (100 mg twice a day) (20). Likewise, pericarditis radiation without tamponade may be treated conservatively or by pericardiocentesis for diagnostic purposes, or if hemodynamic compromise or tamponade occurs. Pericardial constriction, which may happen in up to 20% of patients, requires pericardiectomy. However, the operative mortality is high (20%) and the postoperative five-year survival rate is very low (1%), mostly due to myocardial fibrosis (24).

More important than treatment is prevention of the adverse effects of RT. The use of modern techniques for irradiating the mediastinum has reduced the dose administered to nontumor critical structures and, therefore, the incidence rates of pleuropulmonary and cardiac toxicities. For example, mantle (extended-field) RT at >40 Gy is no longer recommended for the treatment of HD. Instead, patients with early-stage HD should receive an adriamycin, bleomycin, vinblastine, dacarbazine (ABVD) chemotherapy regimen and involved-field RT at a dose of 20 Gy (25).

Chylothorax

About a dozen chylothoraces due to RT have been reported in the literature (26–34). The diagnosis is easily made by observing the milky appearance of the fluid or, if pleural fluid does not look like a typical chyle, by analyzing its lipid content. Chylothorax is generally a delayed complication of RT, with one case occurring 23 years after mantle irradiation for HD (28). The mediastinal fibrosis and resulting occlusion of the thoracic lymph vessels or, less often, a tear in the thoracic duct (33) may explain this complication. Management does not differ from other nontraumatic chylothoraces.

Pleural Thickening

In a series of 30 consecutive early-stage breast cancer patients (T1-2 N0 M0) treated with a hypofractioned RT schedule (42.5 Gy in 16 fractions), pleural thickening was documented in 6 (20%) patients by high-resolution CT, six months after radiation (35).

Pneumothorax

The reported frequency of pneumothorax in patients with lymphoma who had received mantle RT (>30 Gy) is about 2% (36). Pneumothorax develops from one month to more than two years after chest RT, and most patients have underlying radiation-induced fibrosis of the lung (37). Among 10 patients with spontaneous pneumothoraces described by Pezner et al. (36), half had concurrent severe parenchymal pulmonary disease, including chemo- and RT-induced fibrosis. In these cases, the pneumothorax required chest drainage and tended to be bilateral and/or recurrent. Pneumothoraces in irradiated patients may result from the spontaneous or radiation-induced rupture of necrotic neoplastic tissue into the pleural space, or from the formation and rupturing of subpleural blebs and thin-walled cavities in the irradiated lung (38).

Mesothelioma

Radiation exposure has long been known to be potentially carcinogenic. In the English literature, malignant mesothelioma has been reported in about 30 patients who had received RT for previous nonpleural malignancies, particularly HD, and Wilms and breast tumors (39). Mesothelioma occurred after a latency period of 7 to 40 years. The association between mesothelioma and RT has primarily been based on case reports and animal studies.

In the first retrospective cohort study that investigated the risk of mesothelioma after radiation exposure for breast cancer and HD, no elevation in risk was found (40). The study was based on the available data at that time from the National Cancer Institute's Surveillance, Epidemiology and End Results (SEER) database. Six cases of malignant mesothelioma were observed among almost 250,000 women with breast carcinoma: two cases occurred in women who had received RT, whereas four cases occurred in women who did not receive RT. There were no cases of pleural mesothelioma among nearly 7000 HD patients treated with RT. Nevertheless, the study had several methodological limitations, and two further investigations that used updated SEER data through 2001 reported statistically significant increases in malignant mesothelioma associated with supradiaphragmatic radiation for testicular cancer and non–Hodgkin lymphoma (41,42).

A recent update of the SEER database identified 26 patients with mesothelioma as second primaries among 122,882 lymphoma survivors (43). There was a statistically significant increase in mesothelioma among men with HD who received RT (4 cases of 5610 radiated HD vs. 1 case of 6566 nonradiated HD). For non–Hodgkin lymphoma, there was a nonsignificant excess of mesothelioma among men and women following RT. The average time from the diagnosis of lymphoma to the diagnosis of mesothelioma was 16 years for HD and 7 years for non–Hodgkin lymphoma, a time period shorter than that reported with asbestos exposure. Finally, a multivariate modeling approach applied to a cohort of 18,862, 5-year survivors of HD showed a 20-fold increase in the relative risk for malignant mesothelioma (44). Taken together, these findings suggest that RT may be a factor for developing mesothelioma.

B. Radiosurgery for Lung Tumors

Stereotactic radiosurgery with real-time tumor-motion tracking is an alternative to external-beam RT for medically inoperable patients with lung cancer. Treatment of peripheral lung tumors using radiosurgery requires the implantation of three to six transthoracically placed CT-guided fiducials (45). Fiducial markers are gold seeds that are implanted in and/or around a tissue tumor to act as radiological landmarks and to define the target tumor position with millimeter precision. Approximately one week after fiducial placement, the planned treatment with a frameless and image-guided device that has a lineal accelerator mounted on a robotic arm (commercially known as CyberKnife) will ensue (45). The CyberKnife can administer radiation to a tumor from different trajectories while minimizing doses to adjacent normal tissue.

Placement of fiducial markers using a percutaneous approach with CT guidance is very similar to a CT-guided lung biopsy and, therefore, is associated with a high risk of iatrogenic pneumothorax. Transthoracic fiducial placement has a reported pneumothorax rate of 10% to 33% (46–49). For example, pneumothorax, either during or immediately following fiducial placement, occurred in 16 (33%) out of 48 patients with primary or metastatic lung neoplasms treated using an image-guided robotic radiosurgery system (49). Tube thoracostomy was necessary in 6 (37%) pneumothoraces. Whereas the performance of a concomitant core needle biopsy at the time of fiducial placement was associated with pneumothorax rates of 64% compared to 26% without biopsies, the number of fiducial placed did not influence pneumothorax rate (49). As a rule, small pneumothoraces, if stable in size, do not need further treatment. For pneumothoraces greater than 20% to 30%, aspiration, which can be done while the patient is still on the CT table, or placement of a chest tube is indicated.

C. Endobronchial Brachytherapy

Endobronchial brachytherapy is an established modality for symptom palliation in patients with airway obstruction by primary or secondary malignant tumors, particularly in advanced non–small-cell lung cancer. It refers to the placement, by using a flexible fiberoptic bronchoscope, of a catheter loaded with a radioactive source within, or in close proximity to, a malignancy in order to provide local RT (50).

In general, the treatment is well tolerated, but potential, and fortunately unusual, severe complications include hemoptysis and fistulas secondary to massive tumor shrinkage and bronchial wall necrosis. A study evaluated 81 patients treated with endobronchial brachytherapy (iridium-192 delivered in a dose of 30 Gy) for recurrent endobronchial lung cancer (51). Three (3.7%) patients developed pneumothorax that resolved with chest tube placement. In a second series of 189 patients with lung cancer who received a total of 30 Gy from iridium-192, 32 (17%) exhibited significant delayed (>2 months) side effects consisting of massive hemoptysis (13 cases), bronchial stenosis (12 cases), soft-tissue necrosis (8 cases), fistula (3 cases), and pneumothorax (1 case) (52). Finally, in a more recent experience of 288 high–dose-rate endobronchial brachytherapy sessions (total dose 20 Gy) carried out on 81 patients with malignant endobronchial tumors, only 4 (5%) complications were reported and none involved the pleural space (53). Pneumothoraces, as well as other early complications, are due primarily to bronchoscopy and catheter insertion. When the radioactive seeds are placed into the lung tumor through CT rather than bronchoscopy, the incidence of iatrogenic pneumothorax increases: 30% in a preliminary experience of 20 patients by Brach et al. (54).

III. Pleural Involvement Following Tumor RFA

RFA involves the local application of radiofrequency thermal energy to achieve necrosis of liver or lung tumors (55,56). RFA with modern thermocouple-tipped multiprobe arrays effectively ablates tumors thorough passing of alternating high-frequency current, which generates temperatures up to 90 °C in target tissues. As the temperature within the tissue becomes elevated beyond 60 °C, instantaneous protein coagulation with irreversible damage of key intracellular enzymes ensues, resulting in a region of coagulative necrosis surrounding the electrode. RFA can be applied percutaneously, during open surgery or, less frequently, during laparoscopy or thoracoscopy. The needle electrode is introduced into the tumor under the guidance of CT, MRI, or ultrasonography.

A. Liver Tumors

RFA has been used to treat both hepatocellular carcinoma and hepatic metastases (55). In general, the procedure is indicated in patients with unresectable liver tumors due to multifocal disease, poor liver function, and/or proximity of the tumor to major intrahepatic vasculature.

Although RFA may be performed safely in most patients, vascular, biliary, and extrahepatic complications related to mechanical or thermal damage may be observed. Recently, a multicenter survey has analyzed the frequency of complications that resulted from 3891 RFAs in 2614 patients with hepatocellular carcinoma (57). RFA was performed percutaneously in 2542 patients, laparoscopically in 23, and operatively in 49. Among 207 (7.9%) complications, there were 60 (2.3%) pleural effusions, 5 (0.19%) hemothoraces, and 4 (0.15%) pneumothoraces, which yielded an overall pleural complication rate of 2.6%. Chest drainage was necessary in seven patients. A previous review of the literature recorded a lesser incidence of pleural complications: 10 (0.3%) pneumothoraces, 7 (0.2%) pleural effusions, and 5 (0.14%) hemothoraces among 3670 patients who underwent RFA of liver tumors (58). Pleural involvement usually occurs within 24 hours of the ablative procedure, and can be attributed to the transpulmonary approach to highly located liver tumors (pneumothorax), inadvertent lesions of the intercostal vessels by the electrode (hemothorax), or diaphragmatic and/or pleural irritation or injury (pleural effusion).

B. Lung Tumors

Unlike the low incidence of pleural complications after RFA of liver tumors, pneumothorax and/or pleural effusions are encountered in nearly 60% of patients after RFA of lung tumors (Fig. 2). When data from five studies are combined (59–63), the proportion of 1003 lung RFA procedures performed percutaneously under CT guidance presenting the following pleural complications was: pneumothorax 47%, chest tube placement for pneumothorax 13%, pleural effusion 12%, and chest tube placement for pleural effusion 1.6%.

Several studies have specifically addressed the risk factors for pneumothorax and/or pleural effusion associated with RFA of lung tumors. In one study, emphysema, the only factor influencing the incidence of pneumothorax, was present in 23.7% of sessions that resulted in pneumothorax, as compared to 6.6% of those without this complication (60). In addition to emphysema, the absence of previous lung surgery was found in another study to be a risk factor for developing pneumothorax (62). A potential explanation is that a history of previous surgery causing pleural adhesions may preclude the occurrence of pneumothorax. According to a third study, the length of the electrode trajectory through aerated lung was the single most important factor for developing pneumothorax (64). Finally, in the most detailed investigation (59), the following variables, in decreasing order of weight, were found to increase the risk of pneumothorax: treatment of multiple tumors, length of the aerated lung traversed by the electrode, absence of previous pulmonary surgery, location of the tumor in the middle or lower lobe, and male sex. Among the patients with iatrogenic pneumothorax, this study showed that no previous history of pulmonary surgery, the use of an internally cooled cluster electrode and involvement of the upper lobe increased the risk of chest tube placement (59). Finally, risk factors for

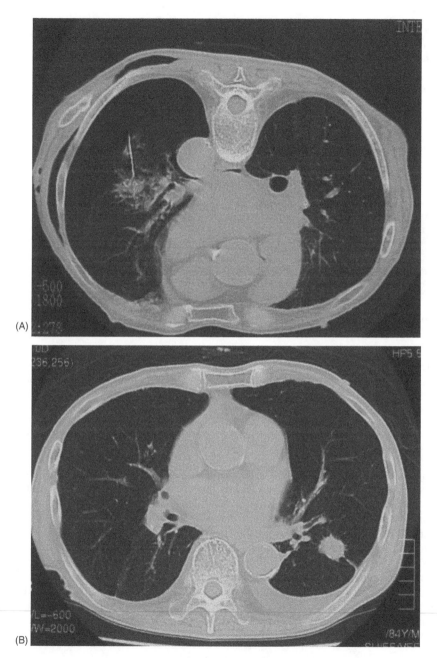

Figure 2 (A) CT showing pneumothorax and subcutaneous emphysema after RFA for recurrent lung cancer. (B) A CT scan obtained 1 month after the procedure also showed a pleural effusion. (C) The follow-up CT scan at 5 months demonstrated spontaneous resolution of the pleural effusion and decreased tumor size. *Source*: Courtesy of Dr. T. Okuma, Department of Radiology, Osaka City University Graduate School of Medicine, Osaka, Japan. (*Continued*)

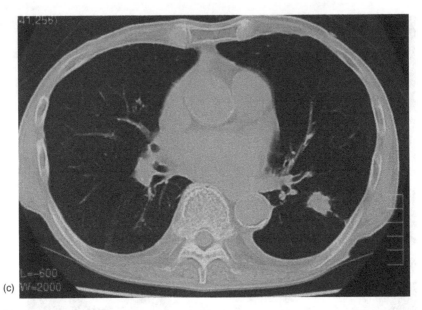

Figure 2 (*Continued*)

developing pleural effusion included the use of an internally cooled cluster electrode instead of a multitined expandable electrode, a decreased length of the aerated lung traversed by the electrode, and a decreased distance to the nearest pleura (59). These results support the notion that pneumothorax after RFA is mainly associated with the insertion of the needle, whereas pleural effusion is caused by pleurisy brought on by the heat conducted to the pleura (65).

IV. Conclusions

Pleural effusion, as a complication of RT, can be produced by radiation pleuritis (early effusions) or result from mediastinal fibrosis that causes lymphatic obstruction and/or constrictive pericarditis (late effusions). In the differential diagnosis of these effusions, recurrent or second tumors, as well as radiation-induced heart failure, should be considered. Treatment is supportive, yet sometimes a pleurodesis procedure needs to be performed. Less-common pleural complications of RT include chylothorax, pneumothorax and, possibly, mesothelioma. Refinements in RT techniques have allowed for a considerable reduction of the risks of pleuropulmonary and cardiac toxicities.

For patients with seemingly unresectable liver or lung tumors, percutaneous RFA under CT guidance has become recognized as a leading and minimally invasive therapy. Pneumothoraces and pleural effusions, sometimes requiring aspiration or tube thoracostomy, are common complications of thermal ablation.

Acknowledgment

I would like to thank Dr. Moisés Mira from the Department of Radiation Oncology (Arnau de Vilanova University Hospital, Lleida, Spain) for his contributive and helpful remarks in writing this book chapter.

References

1. Halperin EC, Perez CA, Brady LW, eds. Principles and Practice of Radiation Oncology. Philadelphia, Pennsylvania: Lippincott Williams & Wilkins, 2008.
2. Porcel JM, Tarragona J. Pleural effusion as late complication of radiotherapy for Hodgkin's disease. Int Pleural Newsl 2007; 5(4):20 [Available at: http://www.musc.edu/pleuralnews/IPN/].
3. Decadt B, Siriwardena AK. Radiofrequency ablation of liver tumours: Systematic review. Lancet Oncol 2004; 5:550–560.
4. Carver JR, Shapiro CL, Ng A, et al. American Society of Clinical Oncology clinical evidence review on the ongoing care of adult cancer survivors: Cardiac and pulmonary late effects. J Clin Oncol 2007; 25:3991–4008.
5. Abratt RP, Morgan GW, Silvestri G, et al. Pulmonary complications of radiation therapy. Clin Chest Med 2004; 25:167–177.
6. Bachman AL, Macken K. Pleural effusions following supervoltage radiation for breast carcinoma. Radiology 1959; 72:699–709.
7. Hietala SO, Hahn P. Pulmonary radiation reaction in the treatment of carcinoma of the breast. Radiography 1976; 42:225–230.
8. Fentanes de Torres E, Guevara E. Pleuritis by radiation: Reports of two cases. Acta Cytol 1981; 25:427–429.
9. Wojno KJ, Olson JL, Sherman ME. Cytopathology of pleural effusions after radiotherapy. Acta Cytol 1994; 38:1–8.
10. Järvenpää R, Holli K, Pitkänen M, et al. Radiological pulmonary findings after breast cancer irradiation: A prospective study. Acta Oncol 2006; 45:16–22.
11. Zimmermann FB, Geinitz H, Schill S, et al. Stereotactic hypofractionated radiotherapy in stage I (T1-2 N0 M0) non-small-cell lung cancer (NSCLC). Acta Oncol 2006; 45:796–801.
12. Kumekawa Y, Kaneko K, Ito H, et al. Late toxicity in complete response cases after definitive chemoradiotherapy for esophageal squamous cell carcinoma. J Gastroenterol 2006; 41:425–432.
13. Ishikura S, Nihei K, Ohtsu A, et al. Long-term toxicity after definitive chemoradiotherapy for squamous cell carcinoma of the thoracic esophagus. J Clin Oncol 2003; 21:2697–2702.
14. Senkus-Konefka E, Jassem J. Cardiovascular effects of breast cancer radiotherapy. Cancer Treat Rev 2007; 33:578–593.
15. Brusamolino E, Baio A, Orlandi E, et al. Long-term events in adult patients with clinical stage IA–IIA nonbulky Hodgkin's lymphoma treated with four cycles of doxorubicin, bleomycin, vinblastine, and dacarbazine and adjuvant radiotherapy: A single-institution 15-year follow-up. Clin Cancer Res 2006; 12:6487–6493.
16. Rodríguez-García JL, Fraile G, Moreno MA, et al. Recurrent massive pleural effusion as a late complication of radiotherapy in Hodgkin's disease. Chest 1991; 100:1165–1166.
17. Morrone N, Gama e Silva Volpe VL, Dourado AM, et al. Bilateral pleural effusion due to mediastinal fibrosis induced by radiotherapy. Chest 1993; 104:1276–1278.
18. Yamamoto N, Noda Y, Miyashita Y. A case of refractory bilateral pleural effusion due to post-irradiation constrictive pericarditis. Respirology 2002; 7:365–368.
19. Camus P. Drug-induced pleural diseases. In: Bouros D, ed. Pleural Disease. New York: Marcel Dekker, 2004:317–352.
20. Fragoulis KN, Handrinou E, Papadopoulos V, et al. Delayed effusive pericarditis and recurrent pleural effusion after radiation treatment for Hodgkin's disease responsive to per os doxycycline. Eur J Haematol 2006; 76:176–179.
21. Shigematsu N, Kitamura N, Saikawa Y, et al. Death related to pleural and pericardial effusions following chemoradiotherapy in a patient with advanced cancers of the esophagus and stomach. Keio J Med 2007; 56:124–129.
22. Light RW, ed. Pleural Diseases, 5th ed. Philadelphia, PA: Lippincott Williams & Wilkins, 2007.
23. Alexandrakis MG, Passam FH, Kyriakou DS, et al. Pleural effusions in hematologic malignancies. Chest 2004; 125:1546–1555.

24. Maisch B, Seferović PM, Ristić AD, et al. Guidelines on the diagnosis and management of pericardial diseases executive summary: The task force on the diagnosis and management of pericardial diseases of the European society of cardiology. Eur Heart J 2004; 25:587–610.

25. Hoppe RT. Hodgkin's lymphoma: The role of radiation in the modern combined strategies of treatment. Hematol Oncol Clin North Am 2007; 21:915–927.

26. Chang PY, Chao TY, Dai MS. Early occurrence of chylothorax related to thoracic irradiation and concomitant chemotherapy. Clin Oncol (R Coll Radiol) 2005; 17:291.

27. Thomson AH, Sivalingham S, Rajesh PB, et al. Chylothorax after radiotherapy in oesophageal carcinoma. Lancet Oncol 2003; 4:703–704.

28. McWilliams A, Gabbay E. Chylothorax occurring 23 years post-irradiation: Literature review and management strategies. Respirology 2000; 5:301–303.

29. Lee YC, Tribe AE, Musk AW. Chylothorax from radiation-induced mediastinal fibrosis. Aust N Z J Med 1998; 28:667–668.

30. Promisloff RA, Hogue DJ. Chylothorax: The result of previous radiation therapy? J Am Osteopath Assoc 1997; 97:164–166.

31. Neelakandan B, Neelakandhan KS. Delayed chylothorax after irradiation. Ann Thorac Surg 1996; 61:277.

32. Van Renterghem DM, Pauwels RA. Chylothorax and pleural effusion as late complications of thoracic irradiation. Chest 1995; 108:886–887.

33. Zoetmulder F, Rutgers E, Baas P. Thoracoscopic ligation of a thoracic duct leakage. Chest 1994; 106:1233–1234.

34. Van Renterghem D, Hamers J, De Schryver A, et al. Chylothorax after mantle field irradiation for Hodgkin's disease. Respiration 1985; 48:188–189.

35. Plataniotis GA, Theofanopoulou ME, Sotiriadou K, et al. High resolution computed tomography findings on the lung of early breast-cancer patients treated by postoperative breast irradiation with a hypofractionated radiotherapy schedule. Indian J Cancer 2005; 42:191–196.

36. Pezner RD, Horak DA, Sayegh HO, et al. Spontaneous pneumothorax in patients irradiated for Hodgkin's disease and other malignant lymphomas. Int J Radiat Oncol Biol Phys 1990; 18:193–198.

37. Rowinsky EK, Abeloff MD, Wharam MD. Spontaneous pneumothorax following thoracic irradiation. Chest 1985; 88:703–708.

38. Okada M, Ebe K, Matsumoto T, et al. Ipsilateral spontaneous pneumothorax after rapid development of large thin-walled cavities in two patients who had undergone radiation therapy for lung cancer. AJR Am J Roentgenol 1998; 170:932–934.

39. Witherby SM, Butnor KJ, Grunberg SM. Malignant mesothelioma following thoracic radiotherapy for lung cancer. Lung Cancer 2007; 57:410–413.

40. Neugut AI, Ahsan H, Antman KH. Incidence of malignant pleural mesothelioma after thoracic radiotherapy. Cancer 1997; 80:948–950.

41. Travis LB, Fosså SD, Schonfeld SJ, et al. Second cancers among 40,576 testicular cancer patients: Focus on long-term survivors. J Natl Cancer Inst 2005; 97:1354–1365.

42. Tward JD, Wendland MM, Shrieve DC, et al. The risk of secondary malignancies over 30 years after the treatment of non-Hodgkin lymphoma. Cancer 2006; 107:108–115.

43. Teta MJ, Lau E, Sceurman BK, et al. Therapeutic radiation for lymphoma: Risk of malignant mesothelioma. Cancer 2007; 109:1432–1438.

44. Hodgson DC, Gilbert ES, Dores GM, et al. Long-term solid cancer risk among 5-year survivors of Hodgkin's lymphoma. J Clin Oncol 2007; 25:1489–1497.

45. Hara W, Soltys SG, Gibbs IC. CyberKnife robotic radiosurgery system for tumor treatment. Expert Rev Anticancer Ther 2007; 7:1507–1515.

46. Muacevic A, Drexler C, Wowra B, et al. Technical description, phantom accuracy, and clinical feasibility for single-session lung radiosurgery using robotic image-guided real-time respiratory tumor tracking. Technol Cancer Res Treat 2007; 6:321–328.

47. Pennathur A, Luketich JD, Burton S, et al. Stereotactic radiosurgery for the treatment of lung neoplasm: Initial experience. Ann Thorac Surg 2007; 83:1820–1825.

48. Collins BT, Erickson K, Reichner CA, et al. Radical stereotactic radiosurgery with real-time tumor motion tracking in the treatment of small peripheral lung tumors. Radiat Oncol 2007; 2:39.

49. Yousefi S, Collins BT, Reichner CA, et al. Complications of thoracic computed tomography-guided fiducial placement for the purpose of stereotactic body radiation therapy. Clin Lung Cancer 2007; 8:252–256.

50. Klopp AH, Eapen GA, Komaki RR. Endobronchial brachytherapy: An effective option for palliation of malignant bronchial obstruction. Clin Lung Cancer 2006; 8:203–207.

51. Delclos ME, Komaki R, Morice RC, et al. Endobronchial brachytherapy with high-dose-rate remote afterloading for recurrent endobronchial lesions. Radiology 1996; 201:279–282.

52. Taulelle M, Chauvet B, Vincent P, et al. High dose rate endobronchial brachytherapy: Results and complications in 189 patients. Eur Respir J 1998; 11:162–168.

53. Escobar-Sacristán JA, Granda-Orive JI, Gutiérrez-Jiménez T, et al. Endobronchial brachytherapy in the treatment of malignant lung tumours. Eur Respir J 2004; 24:348–352.

54. Brach B, Buhler C, Hayman MH, et al. Percutaneous computed tomography-guided fine needle brachytherapy of pulmonary malignancies. Chest 1994; 106:268–274.

55. Lencioni R, Crocetti L. Radiofrequency ablation of liver cancer. Tech Vasc Interv Radiol 2007; 10:38–46.

56. Abbas G, Schuchert MJ, Pennathur A, et al. Ablative treatments for lung tumors: Radiofrequency ablation, stereotactic radiosurgery, and microwave ablation. Thorac Surg Clin 2007; 17:261–271.

57. Kasugai H, Osaki Y, Oka H, et al. Severe complications of radiofrequency ablation therapy for hepatocellular carcinoma: An analysis of 3,891 ablations in 2,614 patients. Oncology 2007; 72(Suppl. 1):72–75.

58. Mulier S, Mulier P, Ni Y, et al. Complications of radiofrequency coagulation of liver tumours. Br J Surg 2002; 89:1206–1222.

59. Hiraki T, Tajiri N, Mimura H, et al. Pneumothorax, pleural effusion, and chest tube placement after radiofrequency ablation of lung tumors: Incidence and risk factors. Radiology 2006; 241:275–283.

60. Yamagami T, Kato T, Hirota T, et al. Pneumothorax as a complication of percutaneous radiofrequency ablation for lung neoplasms. J Vasc Interv Radiol 2006; 17:1625–1629.

61. Sano Y, Kanazawa S, Gobara H, et al. Feasibility of percutaneous radiofrequency ablation for intrathoracic malignancies: A large single-center experience. Cancer 2007; 109:1397–1405.

62. Okuma T, Matsuoka T, Yamamoto A, et al. Frequency and risk factors of various complications after computed tomography-guided radiofrequency ablation of lung tumors. Cardiovasc Intervent Radiol 2008; 31:122–130.

63. Nomura M, Yamakado K, Nomoto Y, et al. Complications after lung radiofrequency ablation: Risk factors for lung inflammation. Br J Radiol 2008; 81:244–249.

64. Gillams AR, Lees WR. Analysis of the factors associated with radiofrequency ablation-induced pneumothorax. Clin Radiol 2007; 62:639–644.

65. Tajiri N, Hiraki T, Mimura H, et al. Measurement of pleural temperature during radiofrequency ablation of lung tumors to investigate its relationship to occurrence of pneumothorax or pleural effusion. Cardiovasc Intervent Radiol 2008; 31:581–586.

45
Iatrogenic and Rare Pleural Effusions

GEORGIOS KOULIATSIS
University Hospital of Alexandroupolis, Alexandroupolis, Greece
DEMOSTHENES BOUROS
Democritus University of Thrace Medical School, and University
Hospital of Alexandroupolis, Alexandroupolis, Greece

I.   Iatrogenic Pleural Effusions

In some cases, diagnostic or therapeutic interventional techniques or even physicians themselves are responsible for the accumulation of pleural fluid. Several causes of iatrogenic pleural effusions are listed in Table 1. In this chapter, pleural effusions due to central venous catheter or nasogastric tube misplacement, translumbar aortography, or rupture of mammary prosthesis are discussed. Other causes are discussed in other chapters of this book.

A.   Vascular Erosion by Central Venous Catheters

Percutaneous insertion of indwelling central venous catheters is widely used as an important therapeutic procedure in a wide range of medical problems (1). Complications are still rather common, although insertion techniques and catheter designs have been improved over time. Well-described complications, such as pneumothorax, infection, and thrombosis, have been reported in up to 11% of cases (2–4). A major complication of central venous catheterization that is not well recognized is vascular erosion and resultant pleural effusion, sometimes with delayed catheter migration. The incidence of this complication appears to be approximately 0.4% to 1.0% of catheter placements (1), but it may be higher considering that some cases remain unrecognized. The diagnosis should be suspected if new cardiopulmonary symptoms, enlarging pleural effusions or mediastinal widening appear after the insertion of a central venous catheter. Roentgenographic detection of extravasation of radiocontrast after injection of intravenous contrast material or thoracocentesis demonstration of either milky fluid in patients receiving intravenous fat emulsions or a pleural fluid/serum glucose ratio greater than 1 confirms the presence of erosion. Inability to withdraw blood from the catheter supports the possibility of catheter perforation, but free-flowing return does not exclude the diagnosis (5). Curvature of the distal part of the catheter has also been proposed as a possible sign of vascular perforation (6). Large-bore or left-sided central venous catheter placement increases the risk of this complication (7).

Duntley et al. reviewed 34 reports describing 61 patients with catheter-induced vascular erosion and hydrothorax (1). The median time from catheter insertion to vascular perforation was two days (range 1–60 days), although 50% of erosions occurred in the first

Table 1 Iatrogenic Causes of Pleural Effusion

Vascular erosion by central venous catheters
Perforation of pleura with a nasogastric tube
Translumbar aortography
After mammaplasty
Secondary to pharmaceutical agents
Radiation therapy
Endoscopic esophageal sclerotherapy
Ovarian hyperstimulation syndrome
Fluid overload
Coronary artery bypass surgery
Abdominal surgery

two days of catheter placement. The route of catheterization was left-sided in 74% and right-sided in 26%. Pleural effusions were present in 79% of patients at presentation, being unilateral on either side of the catheter insertion site in 69% of patients and bilateral in 31%. Pleural fluid volume was usually large, occupying one-third to one-half of a hemithorax. Pleural fluid was described as clear, milky, serous, serosanguineous, or hemorrhagic. Milky pleural fluid is diagnostic in patients receiving intravenous fat emulsions without other causes of chylothorax (8). When hyperosmolar hyperalimentation fluids, such as TPN, drain into the pleural cavity, tension hydrothorax may develop, leading to serious and acute problems (9). In a review by Duntley et al., however, glucose concentrations in the pleural fluid were relatively low compared with the infused solutions, since normal pleura rapidly uptakes or presents a negligible barrier for glucose transit into serum (1). All patients who had blood glucose concentrations measured had a pleural fluid-to-serum glucose ratio greater than 1, suggesting the value of this ratio in detecting central venous catheter erosion. Although always in the transudative range, protein concentration may vary depending on the protein content of infused fluids, the infusion rate, the degree of pleural inflammation and altered permeability induced by hyperosmolar solutions, and the presence of pleural hemorrhage. Progressive mediastinal widening was also a characteristic roentgenographic finding.

The onset of signs and symptoms of hydrothorax may present a delay from 0 to 60 days. Symptoms may appear suddenly with rapid progression or as a nonspecific discomfort with an indolent evolution. Dyspnea was present in 82% of the neurologically alert patients, chest pain in 46%, cough in 2%, whereas 10% of the patients were asymptomatic. An uncommon manifestation of extravascular migration of a central venous catheter is Horner's syndrome (10).

Delays in diagnosis ranged from 0 to 11 days, and attribution of symptoms and roentgenographic findings to other cardiopulmonary abnormalities was common. Misdiagnosis or delayed diagnosis contributed to patient morbidity and mortality. There was 12% mortality directly attributable to venous perforation (1).

Walshe et al. (11) reviewed prospectively collected intravenous nutrition service audit records of 1499 patients (2992 catheters) over a 14-year period and reported five erosions, representing an incidence of 0.17% per catheter. One of the patients died. Symptoms and signs included dyspnea ($n = 5$), chest pain ($n = 2$), and pleural effusion

($n = 5$). Diagnosis was delayed by a mean of 1.6 days. Three erosions occurred in left subclavian catheters ($n = 583$) and two in left internal jugular catheters ($n = 453$). None occurred in right-sided catheters ($n = 1956$). Older age was a statistically significant risk factor. There was no significantly greater risk of vascular erosion in subclavian than internal jugular catheters.

Early detection of catheter erosion is important because the catheter should be removed immediately. Diagnosis requires a high level of suspicion for this rare but nevertheless possible complication and close observation for clinical findings compatible with extravascular catheter migration. Observation is warranted if the effusion is small, but therapeutic thoracocentesis should be performed in patients with serious respiratory compromise. Hemothorax requires the insertion of a chest tube, and if bleeding persists, exploratory thoracotomy may be necessary.

B. Perforation of Pleura with a Nasogastric Tube

Enteral tube feeding is an attractive alternative to intravenous alimentation for nutritional support. Small-bore, silicone nasoenteric feeding tubes are increasingly utilized in the critically ill patients to provide nutritional support. The metallic-weighted tips and stiffening-introducing stylets create the potential for misplacement with potentially serious consequences, changing the spectrum of complications seen with previously used larger nasogastric tubes. Although perforation of the esophagus by a nasogastric tube or an intracranial tube has only been reported sporadically, malpositioning of nasogastric tubes in the tracheobronchial tree appears to be more common (12–19). All pleuropulmonary complications are the result of inadvertent passage of tubes into the tracheobronchial tree with eventual perforation into the lung and pleural space. Guide wires used to aid passage may contribute to this complication (17,18). In a report by Bankier et al., the incidence of abnormal tube positioning in the tracheobronchial tree during an 11-month period in intensive care unit, patients who received nasogastric tubes was 0.8% (14/1700) (12). In 4 of these 14 patients, the nasogastric tubes perforated the bronchial tree and the pleura. All four patients suffered subsequent pneumothoraces that had to be drained by chest tubes. None of these patients had alimentary feeding over the malpositioned nasogastric tube. In all patients, supine or semi-erect frontal chest radiographs accurately demonstrated that the nasogastric tube was malpositioned in the tracheobronchial tree. Sabga et al. reported a case of inadvertent administration of activated charcoal in water into the right lung and pleural cavity of a 51-year-old man treated for a salicylate overdose due to misplacement of the nasogastric tube (15). A mild chemical pneumonitis and a sterile empyema developed. Charcoal-stained fluid drained through a thoracostomy tube for eight weeks. Major underlying factors favoring tube malpositioning include depressed sensorium, impaired gag reflex, recent endotracheal intubation, decreased laryngeal sensitivity, and neuromuscular blocking drugs (12,14). The presence of cuffed tracheostomy or endotracheal tubes does not prevent this occurrence (16). The traditional criteria for proper tube placement, like insufflation of air with sounds heard over the region of the stomach or aspiration of fluid, are suboptimal in critically ill patients. Therefore, institution of nasogastric tubes should be performed according to strict guidelines, which include radiographic confirmation of desired position (20), especially before feedings are initiated, limited and supervised use of stylets, and a need for special precautions in patients who are obtunded or receiving intubated respiratory assistance (12,15–18).

C. Translumbar Aortography

A hemorrhagic pleural effusion may also complicate translumbar aortography resulting from blood leakage from the aorta in the pleural space (21). Therapeutic thoracocentesis is indicated in this case. Surgical intervention is not necessary because usually the leak stops spontaneously. Moreover, irritation of the pleural space from extravasated contrast medium may lead to an exudative effusion.

D. Mammaplasty-Induced Pleural Effusion

There are three case reports of rupture of a silicone bag mammary prosthesis leading to silicone migration to the pleura and the development of a pleural effusion (22–24). Hirmand et al. present a case of silicone particles found in the pleural space of a patient 20 years after bilateral augmentation mammaplasty with silicone gel implants (22). When the patient experienced pain in the upper back, a ruptured left implant was found and a left pleural effusion developed subsequently. Analysis of the pleural effusion fluid by scanning electron microscopy suggested the presence of silicone. In the case described by Stevens et al., an oily layer was observed on the top of the aspirated pleural fluid from a patient with a ruptured implant, which was consistent with the presence of silicone gel in the aspirate (23). The findings of the pleural biopsy in this patient were suggestive of a foreign body reaction. In both cases, the effusion did not recur after thoracocentesis and further pulmonary complications or other symptoms have not developed.

II. Yellow Nail Syndrome

The yellow nail syndrome, first described in 1964 by Samman and White in 13 patients, consists of a triad of yellow nails, lymphedema, and respiratory tract illness, which is rarely present at initial presentation. Pleural effusion is usually a late manifestation and does not regress spontaneously. Respiratory manifestations include pleural effusions, bronchiectasis, recurrent pneumonias, bronchitis, or sinusitis.

It is considered to be a rare clinical condition. Until 1986, only 97 cases of this syndrome had been reported (25) and approximately a dozen ever since. Women are afflicted about twice as often as men, and the age of onset varies from birth to the eighth decade, with the median age being 40 years (25,26). In a review of 96 patients, yellow nails were the presenting manifestation in 37% and lymphedema in 34% (27,28). Yellow nails were present in 89% of the cases, lymphedema in 80%, and pleural effusion in 36% of all cases (25). Patients may develop pericardial effusion (29–32) or chylous ascites and intestinal lymphangiectasia (27,29,33). There are reports of prenatal manifestation of this disorder as nonimmune fetal hydrops with patients' mothers having yellow nail syndrome (28,34).

An autosomal dominant transmission of the disorder has been shown from previous reports (28,35), and new cases of familial yellow nail syndrome are reported until nowadays (36). In a recent report by Hoque et al. on 11 cases of yellow nail syndrome, only one of the patients had a positive family history, suggesting that yellow nail syndrome may not be primarily a genetic disease as it is currently classified (37). The etiology of the syndrome remains obscure, but the pathogenesis seems to involve a congenital defect of the lymphatics. In most patients, lymphangiograms of the lower extremity demonstrate hypoplasia of at least some lymphatic vessels and impaired lymphatic flow (26). Edema can be pitting or nonpitting and may be confined to the fingertips.

There seems to be an association of the syndrome with recent lower respiratory tract infections, chronic pulmonary infections, and chronic sinus infections (38,39). There is a hypothesis that lower respiratory tract infections or pleural inflammation cause further damage to already impaired but adequate lymphatic vessels (40). The lymphatic drainage becomes insufficient and a pleural effusion develops. Histological study of the pleura in a patient with the syndrome showed that it was thickened with fibrosis and chronic inflammatory infiltrates. The lymphatic capillaries in the visceral pleura were dilated (41). Lewis et al. reported that a biopsy of the parietal pleura revealed abnormally dilated lymphatics, neogenesis of lymphatic channels, and edematous tissues in some areas (42). Runyon et al. measured the pleural fluid turnover by radioiodized albumin to trace the efflux of fluid by lymphatics (43). The pleural lymphatic flow was low in comparison to previous estimates in a variety of other conditions. However, Mambretti-Zumwalt et al. reported that the albumin turnover rate in the pleural fluid is not greatly decreased in patients with this syndrome (44).

Affected nails are thickened, excessively curved along both axes, very slow growing with yellowish-gray hue. Cuticle and lunula are usually absent, and onycholysis is frequently evident (27). Women frequently cover their unsightly nails with opaque nail polish, which may obscure the finding from the unwary clinician (45).

Pleural effusions are usually recurrent after a thoracocentesis, are bilateral in 50% of cases, and vary in size (26,46). The pleural fluid is exudative with $\geq$200 nucleated cells per cubic millimeter, predominantly lymphocytic (>80%) (26,47). The glucose is equivalent to serum, and the pH approximates 7.40. There have been cases of the syndrome complicated by an empyema (48,49) and cases associated with cancer and immunodeficiency disease (50–52). However, no direct relationship has been found between the syndrome and malignancies, immunological disorders, endocrine abnormalities, or connective tissue disease.

There is no specific causative treatment for the syndrome. Following thoracocentesis, fluid typically recurs over a few days to several months. Chemical pleurodesis, open pleural abrasion, pleurectomy, or pleuroperitoneal shunting may be applied to control the symptomatic pleural effusion (42,53–56). Octreotide and OK-432 have been reported to be used with success for pleurodesis in recent case reports (57,58). The new oral antifungal drugs may be of value in the treatment of the yellow nail syndrome (45). Some improvement has also been described with the use of decongestive physiotherapy (59). Local steroid injections and oral vitamin E have been reported to be successful in treating the yellow nails. Spontaneous partial or complete recovery of nail abnormalities occurs in 30% of patients, who may experience occasional relapses. Lymphedema and pleural effusions are persistent, and spontaneous full recovery has not been reported.

III. Uremia

Uremic pleuritis has been recognized as a complication of uremia since 1836 (60). Hopps and Wissler reported an incidence of fibrinous pleuritis as high as 20% in patients who died of uremia (61). This pleuritis can become evident as pleuritic chest pain with pleural rubs (62), pleural effusion (62–69), or pulmonary restriction (64,66,70,71). Uremia-associated serosal injury may allow transudation of fluid into the pleural space, but the specific pathogenesis of uremic pleural effusion is not clear (67). The mechanism of pleural effusion and restrictive fibrosis is considered to be similar to that of hemorrhagic and constrictive pericarditis seen in uremia.

The incidence of uremic pleural effusion in patients receiving long-term hemodialysis is reported to be 1% to 58% (63,66,72). There has not been found a relationship between the level of uremia and the development of a pleural effusion (63). Patients may be asymptomatic or may present with fever (15–50%), chest pain (30–31%), cough (35%), and dyspnea (20%) (63,65,68). Up to 88% of patients may also have cardiomegaly (65). Pleural effusions are bilateral in 50% of patients (65,69) and may be massive (63,69).

Uremic patients have increased susceptibility to many causes of pleural effusion. Uremic pleural effusion should be considered when common etiologies of effusions such as volume overload, congestive heart failure, infection, and malignancy have been excluded (66,67).

Pleural effusions are common in patients receiving long-term hemodialysis. Coskun et al. reported pleural effusion as a thoracic CT finding in 51% of 117 uremic patients (73). Jarratt and Sahn found 21% incidence of pleural effusions in adult hospitalized patients receiving long-term hemodialysis (65). Pleural effusions resulted from heart failure in 46% patients and nonheart failure causes in 54% patients. Uremic pleurisy (16%), parapneumonic effusion (15%), and atelectasis (11%) accounted for most of the noncardiac failure causes.

Pleural fluid neopterin levels can be used to differentiate uremic pleural effusions from other causes of effusion (74). In a study of 93 patients, neopterin levels were strikingly elevated in patients with uremic pleural effusion compared to tuberculous, malignant, parapneumonic, and other kinds of effusions (74).

A uremic pleural effusion is characterized as a necrotizing fibrinous exudate that is often hemorrhagic with a paucity of nucleated cells that are predominantly lymphocytes (63–69). In a series of eight patients with uremic pleuritis, the mean pleural fluid pH was 7.37 ± 0.03, the number of nucleated cells was $1231 \pm 379/\mu L$ with $22 \pm 7\%$ neutrophils, the total protein was 3.9 ± 0.2 g/dL, the LDH level was 163 ± 33 IU/L, and the glucose PF/S ratio was 1.8 ± 0.1 (65). Pleural tissue obtained by open or closed biopsy showed chronic fibrosing pleuritis (63–66,68–71).

Uremic pleuritis generally responds to continued hemodialysis (63,67). In a study of 14 patients, the effusions resolved with continued dialysis in four to six weeks after thoracocentesis in 11 patients and recurred in 3 patients (63,67). The prognosis is usually good, but fatal cases have also been reported (68,69).

The fibrosing pleuritis may be severe enough to cause disabling restriction and warrant decortication (64,66,70,71). Decortication of the chest wall and the lung can be carried out safely with minimal bleeding, producing restoration of pulmonary function and clinical improvement (70,71). Surgical decortication should be considered in cases with a severe clinical course when uremic pleurisy is complicated by progressive pleural thickening and pulmonary restriction.

IV. Trapped Lung

The term "trapped lung" describes persistent atelectasis with failure of the lung to re-expand following evacuation of a chronic pleural effusion. It most commonly results from the development of a fibrous peel over the visceral pleura in the setting of chronic pleural inflammation (75). The initial pleural inflammation is usually caused due to pneumonia or hemothorax, but it may also be caused by spontaneous pneumothorax, thoracic operations including coronary artery bypass surgery (76), uremia (70,71), or collagen vascular disease. An ongoing malignant process in the pleural space may also produce a thick visceral pleural peel (75). The peel restricts expansion of the underlying lung parenchyma, generating higher negative pleural pressures within the pleural space. The negative pleural pressure in turn leads to increased pleural fluid formation despite decreased pleural fluid absorption and the development of a chronic pleural effusion. Negative initial pleural pressures and/or rapid changes in the pressures as fluid is withdrawn during thoracocentesis are suggestive of trapped lung (77,78). One characteristic of the pleural effusion with trapped lung is that the amount of fluid remains stable from one study to another and after thoracocentesis reaccumulates rapidly to its previous level (79).

Patients may exhibit dyspnea at rest or with exertion, cough, or they may be asymptomatic. Symptoms of acute pleural inflammation are absent, but the patient may give a history of fever or pleuritic chest pain in the past. Dyspnea in the setting of trapped lung is likely multifactorial and due not only to restrictive ventilatory dysfunction caused by the pleural peel, but also to physiological changes attributable to the effusion (75). These may include distention of the thoracic cavity, dysfunction of the affected hemidiaphragm, and decreased lung compliance and atelectasis. Patients with trapped lung fail to demonstrate full lung re-expansion despite complete drainage of the pleural effusion. However, they may exhibit symptomatic improvement because of partial lung re-expansion and improvement in these physiological parameters (75).

The pathognomonic radiographic sign of trapped lung is the pneumothorax ex vacuo or suction pneumothorax, a small-to-moderate–sized air collection in the pleural space after evacuation of the effusion, often seen in association with a visibly thickened visceral pleural surface (80,81).

The pleural fluid is usually borderline exudate (77). The ratio of pleural fluid-to-serum protein is about 0.5, and the ratio of the pleural fluid LDH level to the serum LDH level is about 0.6. The finding of elevated total pleural fluid protein may be related to factors other than active pleural inflammation or malignancy and does not exclude the diagnosis of trapped lung (82). The pleural fluid glucose level is normal and the pleural fluid white blood cell (WBC) count is usually less than $1000/mm^3$, with the differential WBC revealing predominantly mononuclear cells (77).

The diagnosis of trapped lung requires pleurectomy with decortication (70,71,75,76). In cases of malignant pleural effusion in patients with short-life expectancy, therapeutic options include repeated thoracocentesis, long-term thoracostomy drainage, small-bore indwelling pleural catheters, and pleuroperitoneal shunting (75,83). In asymptomatic or minimally symptomatic patients a surgical procedure is not indicated, and such patients with trapped lung syndrome should be observed.

V. Therapeutic Radiation Exposure

Radiation exposure can cause pleural effusion by two mechanisms: radiation pleuritis and systemic venous hypertension or lymphatic obstruction from mediastinal fibrosis (84). In animals, thoracic radiation causes at an early stage actinic pneumonia and a small pleural effusion. Later on lung changes regress completely and a large pleural effusion appears, probably due to lymphatic block (85). Bachman and Macken followed 200 patients treated with between 4000 and 6000 rads to the hemithorax for breast carcinoma (86). Eleven (5.5%) patients developed pleural effusions with no other obvious explanation, which were attributed to radiation. In all cases, the pleural effusion developed within six months of completing radiation therapy and concomitant radiation was also present. Most pleural effusions were small, but at least one occupied nearly 50% of the hemithorax. Hietala and Hahn performed chest roentgenograms regularly before and a long time after radiotherapy in 157 patients with breast cancer (87). Radiation-induced parenchymal changes were demonstrated in 73% of the patients and pleural effusions in about 10%. The radiation-induced pleural effusion had no special characteristics, with one exception— it occurred simultaneously with radiation-induced parenchymal infiltrates. The pleural fluid characteristics, however, have not been well described. In a study of two cases of pleuritis by radiation, pleural fluid was found to be a hemorrhagic exudate with multiple reactive mesothelial cells with vacuole formation within the cytoplasm and nuclei (88). In 4 of the 11 patients followed by Bachman and Macken, the fluid gradually disappeared spontaneously in 4 to 23 months (86). In the rest of the patients, the fluid gradually decreased in size over the follow-up period of 10 to 40 months.

The pleural effusions associated with radiation pleuritis and mediastinal fibrosis tend to occur one to two years following intensive (4000–6000 rads) mediastinal radiation (84). Mechanisms for development of pleural effusion as a late complication of radiation therapy include constrictive pericarditis (with or without tamponade), superior vena cava obstruction, and lymphatic obstruction, all complications of mediastinal fibrosis (84,89,90). Rodriguez-Garcia et al. described a patient with recurrent massive pleural effusions eight years after mediastinal therapy for Hodgkin's disease (84). The pleural fluid was a serohemorrhagic exudate without malignant cells, and thoracoscopy showed diffuse thickening of the pleura. There is a report of a patient developing bilateral pleural effusion 19 years after thoracic irradiation for Hodgkin's disease (90). The pleural liquid was an exudate with lymphocytic predominance, and thoracoscopy revealed enlarged lymphatic channels in the visceral pleura. Fragoulis et al. reported a case of effusive pericarditis and recurrent pleural effusion, which first developed 23 years after radiation treatment for the nodular sclerosis type of Hodgkin's disease that were treated successfully with per os doxycycline (91).

VI. Drowning

Pleural effusion is a common finding both in saltwater and in freshwater drowning. Morild reviewed the files from 133 cases of drowning examined at his institute in the years 1987 to 1991 (92). Increased pleural fluid was present in 71 (53.4%) of the cases. The mean amount of fluid observed was 432.8 mL, while the maximum amount was 3000 mL. According to this study, the time spent in water is correlated to the production of pleural fluid. There are drowning cases, however, in which a large volume of pleural fluid has been found although the victim had only been in the water for a short time and cases in which no increased amount of fluid is present although the body had been in the water for a considerable time. In this study, for example, one victim spent only six to seven minutes in the water but had 900 mL of pleural fluid. The reason for this is unknown. It was also found that more pleural fluid is produced in saltwater than in freshwater drowning. Yorulmaz et al. reviewed the cases of drowning at their institute from the years 1994 to 1998 (93). An attempt was made to correlate the amount of pleural fluid in bodies recovered from water with several parameters registered on the judicial files as well as autopsy findings. The number of cases with pleural fluid increase was found to be very high in saltwater drowning ($p < 0.001$). But, when the freshwater and saltwater drowning cases with pleural fluid increase were compared according to pleural fluid amount, no significant difference was detected (521 ± 340 and 768 ± 536 mL, respectively). A link was found between the time spent in water and the amount of pleural effusion. Salt water is hyperosmolar and will lead to plasma leakage out of the capillaries into the alveolar spaces, whereas in freshwater drowning, water will leak into the capillaries and cause a hemodilution. After death, the gradual breakdown of membranes and the degradation of lung surfactant phospholipids will possibly also add to the leak of fluid through the lungs into the pleural cavities. However, there must be other factors than just passive leak of fluid from the alveolar spaces that contribute to the formation of pleural fluid after drowning. An experimental study in rats (94) showed that the concentrations of sodium and chloride ions in the pleural effusion of rats that drowned in seawater were significantly greater than those rats that were drowned in freshwater. These results suggest that analysis of electrolytes in pleural effusion may be useful for determining whether drowning has occurred in seawater or in freshwater. More experimental studies are necessary in order to determine the mechanisms contributing to pleural fluid accumulation after drowning.

VII. Amyloidosis

Although amyloidosis of the respiratory tract is well recognized, pleural involvement is considered to be uncommon and has been rarely reported in the literature. However, this could be due to not considering this diagnosis in patients presenting with pleural effusions and multiorgan disease (95). Pleural biopsy specimens, which can be obtained by percutaneous needle biopsy (95–99), thoracoscopic (100,101), or open lung biopsy, require special staining with Congo red and/or crystal violet to detect amyloid deposition. This is likely to contribute to the underdiagnosis of pleural involvement in patients with systemic amyloidosis.

Pleural effusions can be large, unilateral or bilateral, and occasionally recurrent. Usually they are transudative (95–98) and the cause is most often considered to be congestive heart failure due to cardiac amyloid involvement. Opposing to that argument, Berk et al. (102,103) conducted a retrospective study comparing patients with primary systematic amyloidosis and persistent pleural effusions ($n = 35$) with patients with primary systematic amyloidosis and secondary cardiomyopathy without pleural effusion ($n = 120$). Indexes of plasma cell dyscrasia, nephrotic syndrome, thyroid function, and echocardiographic measures of left and right ventricle performance were compared between groups. When available, closed needle biopsies and autopsy specimens of parietal pleura were examined for amyloid deposits. No statistical differences were found between the group of patients with persistent pleural effusions and the group of patients with cardiomyopathy in echocardiographic measures of septal thickness, left-ventricular systolic function, or diastolic compliance. All pleural biopsies in the group ($n = 6$) revealed amyloid deposits. The authors concluded that large pleural effusions in systemic amyloidosis occur most often in primary systemic amyloidosis, predominantly resulting from direct infiltration of the parietal pleural surface, and that left-atrial hypertension from primary systemic amyloidosis cardiomyopathy contributes to but is not sufficient to form and sustain these effusions. Enhancing that argument, Hoyer et al. (104) treated four patients who presented with bilateral pleural effusions that were refractory to diuretic therapy with bevacizumab, an antivascular endothelial growth factor (VEGF) antibody. Three of the four patients had improvement in their pleural effusions, peripheral edema, and functional status. There are cases where exudative pleural effusions with pleural amyloidosis are reported (95,96,98,105,106). Other explanations for pleural effusions include nephritic syndrome and liver failure. The mechanism of the production of an exudative effusion is unknown, but it could be due to obstruction of the lymphatics in the parietal pleura by the amyloid deposition or it could be that previous diuretic treatment has changed the characteristics of the effusion (98). Macroscopic examination of the parietal pleura during thoracoscopy in a patient with primary amyloidosis and pleural involvement revealed a diffuse inflammation and light-brown deposits that were covered with nodules (101).

VIII. Milk of Calcium Pleural Collections

Milk of calcium is a colloidal suspension of calcium crystals, which can accumulate in cystic spaces such as renal, adrenal, or breast cysts producing a characteristic finding of half-moon contour on radiography. Im et al. described five patients with milk of calcium pleural collections (107). The diagnosis was based on needle aspiration in four patients and the presence of fat–calcium level on computed tomography (CT) in one. The concentration of calcium in the aspirated fluid was greater than 500 mg/dL. Four patients had a previous history of pleurisy. Homogeneous increased opacity with a double contour at the interface with the lung was a characteristic radiographic finding. CT showed that the lateral contour was the margin of the milk of calcium, and the medial contour was the margin of the thickened visceral pleura facing the lung. On CT, milk of calcium collection appeared as a homogeneous area of increased attenuation.

IX. Pleural Effusion in Electrical Injury

The most common visceral lesions associated with electrical burns are cardiac lesions. Pulmonary compromise is rare (108). However, when the entry or exit ports are the thoracic wall, pleural effusion, hemothorax, and pneumonitis may occur (108,109). The pleural fluid is an exudate that resolves gradually (109).

X. Mediastinal Cysts

The rupture into the pleural cavity of a benign cystic teratoma of the mediastinum is a rare complication that leads to pleural fluid formation (110–116). Several explanations have been given for the tendency to rupture of mediastinal teratomas, including ischemia due to tumor enlargement, infection, or erosion from the digestive enzymes derived from the tumor tissues (110,111). Choi et al. reported that out of 17 cases of surgically resected mediastinal teratomas, preoperative rupture was found in 7 (111). Pleural effusion was seen in 4 (57%) of the 7 ruptured masses—at the ipsilateral ruptured sites in 2 cases, and bilaterally in the other 2 cases. The authors assumed that the pleural effusion resulted from either spillage of internal components of a mass or from an inflammatory reaction to the extravasated contents. There are cases of pleural fluid formation following the rupture of benign mediastinal teratomas in which levels of carcinoembryonic antigen, CA-125, CA19–9, and amylase are elevated (110,112,116). Cobb et al. reported that the examination of the pleural fluid after the rupture of an anterior mediastinal benign cystic teratoma showed the presence of squamous and columnar epithelial cells, hairs, calcospherites (calcium deposits), keratinous material, and cholesterol against an inflammatory background (113). Mediastinal bronchogenic cysts presenting with serofibrinous or serosanguineous pleural fluid have also been described (117). These pleural effusions were probably related to an inflammatory reaction of the pleura to the bronchogenic cyst. Such inflammation could be due to the large size of the masses, perhaps with the onset of rupture.

XI. Whipple's Disease
Although the main manifestation of Whipple's disease is gastrointestinal, it is a systemic disorder, and pulmonary involvement is a frequent but not well-known finding (118). Involvement of the lung as a site of this disease was reported in Whipple's first description in 1907 (119). The lung and the pleura may be affected both before and after the development of diarrhea (120,121). Pleural effusion is reported less often than chronic nonproductive cough, dyspnea, and pleuritic chest pain (120). In cells from pleural effusions, *Tropheryma whippelii*–specific amplification products were found by PCR (122). In a report by Riemer et al., an exudative bilateral pleural effusion in a patient with Whipple's disease subsided after three months of antibiotic therapy (118).

XII. Syphilis
Pleural effusion is rarely formed in syphilis patients. Zaharopoulos and Wong described a case of a 68-year-old man with secondary syphilis who concomitantly suffered from left lower lobe pneumonia with associated pleuritis (123). Cytological examination of the pleural fluid was diagnostic of syphilis not only by the characteristic cytomorphology but also by demonstration of spirochetes by the May–Grunwald–Giemsa and Steiner staining methods. Cattini et al. also reported a case of pleurisy diagnosed in a patient with tertiary syphilis (124). The spirochetes were discovered in the pleuritic exudate.

References
1. Duntley P, Siever J, Korwes ML, et al. Vascular erosion by central venous catheters. Clinical features and outcome. Chest 1992; 101:1633–1638.
2. Borja AR, Masri Z, Shruck L, et al. Unusual and lethal complications of infraclavicular subclavian vein catheterization. Int Surg 1972; 57:42–45.
3. Herbst CA Jr. Indications, management, and complications of percutaneous subclavian catheters. An audit. Arch Surg 1978; 113:1421–1425.
4. Feliciano DV, Mattox KL, Graham JM, et al. Major complications of percutaneous subclavian vein catheters. Am J Surg 1979; 138:869–874.
5. Kollef MH. Fallibility of persistent blood return for confirmation of intravascular catheter placement in patients with hemorrhagic thoracic effusions. Chest 1994; 106:1906–1908.
6. Au FC, Badellino M. Significance of a curled central venous catheter tip. Chest 1988; 93:890–891.
7. Mukau L, Talamini MA, Sitzmann JV. Risk factors for central venous catheter-related vascular erosions. JPEN J Parenter Enteral Nutr 1991; 15:513–516.

8. Wolthuis A, Landewe RB, Theunissen PH, et al. Chylothorax or leakage of total parenteral nutrition? Eur Respir J 1998; 12:1233–1235.

9. Bennett MR, Chaudhry RM, Owens GR. Elevated pleural fluid glucose: A risk for tension hydrothorax. South Med J 1986; 79:1287–1289.

10. Milam MG, Sahn SA. Horner's syndrome secondary to hydromediastinum. A complication of extravascular migration of a central venous catheter. Chest 1988; 94:1093–1094.

11. Walshe C, Phelan D, Bourke J, et al. Vascular erosion by central venous catheters used for total parenteral nutrition. Intensive Care Med 2007; 33:534–537.

12. Bankier AA, Wiesmayr MN, Henk C, et al. Radiographic detection of intrabronchial malpositions of nasogastric tubes and subsequent complications in intensive care unit patients. Intensive Care Med 1997; 23:406–410.

13. Miller KS, Tomlinson JR, Sahn SA. Pleuropulmonary complications of enteral tube feedings. Two reports, review of the literature, and recommendations. Chest 1985; 88:230–233.

14. Roubenoff R, Ravich WJ. Pneumothorax due to nasogastric feeding tubes. Report of four cases, review of the literature, and recommendations for prevention. Arch Intern Med 1989; 149:184–188.

15. Sabga E, Dick A, Lertzman M, et al. Direct administration of charcoal into the lung and pleural cavity. Ann Emerg Med 1997; 30:695–697.

16. McWey RE, Curry NS, Schabel SI, et al. Complications of nasoenteric feeding tubes. Am J Surg 1988; 155:253–257.

17. Hand RW, Kempster M, Levy JH, et al. Inadvertent transbronchial insertion of narrow-bore feeding tubes into the pleural space. JAMA 1984; 251:2396–2397.

18. Schorlemmer GR, Battaglini JW. An unusual complication of naso-enteral feeding with small-diameter feeding tubes. Ann Surg 1984; 199:104–106.

19. Balogh GJ, Adler SJ, VanderWoude J, et al. Pneumothorax as a complication of feeding tube placement. AJR Am J Roentgenol 1983; 141:1275–1277.

20. O'Neil R, Krishnananthan R. Intrapleural nasogastric tube insertion. Australas Radiol 2004; 48:139–141.

21. Bilbrey GL, Hedberg CL. Hemorrhagic pleural effusion secondary to aortography. A case report. J Thorac Cardiovasc Surg 1967; 54:85–89.

22. Hirmand H, Hoffman LA, Smith JP. Silicone migration to the pleural space associated with silicone-gel augmentation mammaplasty. Ann Plast Surg 1994; 32:645–647.

23. Stevens WM, Burdon JG, Niall JF. Pleural effusion after rupture of silicone bag mammary prosthesis. Thorax 1987; 42:825–826.

24. Taupmann RE, Adler S. Silicone pleural effusion due to iatrogenic breast implant rupture. South Med J 1993; 86:570–571.

25. Nordkild P, Kromann-Andersen H, Struve-Christensen E. Yellow nail syndrome—The triad of yellow nails, lymphedema and pleural effusions. A review of the literature and a case report. Acta Med Scand 1986; 219:221–227.

26. Beer DJ, Pereira W Jr, Snider GL. Pleural effusion associated with primary lymphedema: A perspective on the yellow nail syndrome. Am Rev Respir Dis 1978; 117:595–599.

27. Duhra PM, Quigley EM, Marsh MN. Chylous ascites, intestinal lymphangiectasia and the 'yellow-nail' syndrome. Gut 1985; 26:1266–1269.

28. Govaert P, Leroy JG, Pauwels R, et al. Perinatal manifestations of maternal yellow nail syndrome. Pediatrics 1992; 89:1016–1018.

29. Malek NP, Ocran K, Tietge UJ, et al. A case of the yellow nail syndrome associated with massive chylous ascites, pleural and pericardial effusions. Z Gastroenterol 1996; 34:763–766.

30. Morandi U, Golinelli M, Brandi L, et al. "Yellow nail syndrome" associated with chronic recurrent pericardial and pleural effusions. Eur J Cardiothorac Surg 1995; 9:42–44.

31. Coche G, Chalaoui J, Jeanneret A, et al. Yellow nail syndrome. Apropos of a case. A review of the main radiologic manifestations. J Radiol 1986; 67:435–437.

32. Paradisis M, Van Asperen P. Yellow nail syndrome in infancy. J Paediatr Child Health 1997; 33:454–457.

33. Desrame J, Bechade D, Patte JH, et al. Yellow nail syndrome associated with intestinal lymphangiectasia. Gastroenterol Clin Biol 2000; 24:837–840.

34. Slee J, Nelson J, Dickinson J, et al. Yellow nail syndrome presenting as non-immune hydrops: Second case report. Am J Med Genet 2000; 93:1–4.

35. Herbert FA, Bowen PA. Hereditary late-onset lymphedema with pleural effusion and laryngeal edema. Arch Intern Med 1983; 143:913–915.

36. Razi E. Familial yellow nail syndrome. Dermatol Online J 2006; 12:15.

37. Hoque SR, Mansour S, Mortimer PS. Yellow nail syndrome: Not a genetic disorder? Eleven new cases and a review of the literature. Br J Dermatol 2007; 156:1230–1234.

38. Nakielna EM, Wilson J, Ballon HS. Yellow-nail syndrome: Report of three cases. Can Med Assoc J 1976; 115:46–48.

39. Venencie PY, Dicken CH. Yellow nail syndrome: Report of five cases. J Am Acad Dermatol 1984; 10:187–192.

40. Emerson PA. Yellow nails, lymphoedema, and pleural effusions. Thorax 1966; 21:247–253.

41. Solal-Celigny P, Cormier Y, Fournier M. The yellow nail syndrome. Light and electron microscopic aspects of the pleura. Arch Pathol Lab Med 1983; 107:183–185.

42. Lewis M, Kallenbach J, Zaltzman M, et al. Pleurectomy in the management of massive pleural effusion associated with primary lymphoedema: Demonstration of abnormal pleural lymphatics. Thorax 1983; 38:637–639.

43. Runyon BA, Forker EL, Sopko JA. Pleural-fluid kinetics in a patient with primary lymphedema, pleural effusions, and yellow nails. Am Rev Respir Dis 1979; 119:821–825.

44. Mambretti-Zumwalt J, Seidman JM, Higano N. Yellow nail syndrome: Complete triad with pleural protein turnover studies. South Med J 1980; 73:995–997.

45. Baran R. The new oral antifungal drugs in the treatment of the yellow nail syndrome. Br J Dermatol 2002; 147:189–191.

46. Hiller E, Rosenow EC III, Olsen AM. Pulmonary manifestations of the yellow nail syndrome. Chest 1972; 61:452–458.

47. D'Alessandro A, Muzi G, Monnaco A, et al. Yellow nail syndrome: Does protein leakage play a role? Eur Respir J 2001; 17:149–152.

48. Lodge JP, Hunter AM, Saunders NR. Yellow nail syndrome associated with empyema. Clin Exp Dermatol 1989; 14:328–329.

49. Angelillo VA, O'Donohue WJ Jr. Yellow nail syndrome with reduced glucose level in pleural fluid. Chest 1979; 75:83–85.

50. Levillain C, Faux N, Taillandier J, et al. Yellow-nail syndrome. Review of the literature apropos of 2 cases associated with cancer. Ann Med Interne (Paris) 1984; 135:440–443.

51. Guin JD, Elleman JH. Yellow nail syndrome. Possible association with malignancy. Arch Dermatol 1979; 115:734–735.

52. Chernosky ME, Finley VK. Yellow nail syndrome in patients with acquired immunodeficiency disease. J Am Acad Dermatol 1985; 13:731–736.

53. Moorjani N, Winter RJ, Yigsaw YA, et al. Pleural effusion in yellow nail syndrome: Treatment with bilateral pleuro-peritoneal shunts. Respiration 2004; 71:298.

54. Jiva TM, Poe RH, Kallay MC. Pleural effusion in yellow nail syndrome: Chemical pleurodesis and its outcome. Respiration 1994; 61:300–302.

55. Brofman JD, Hall JB, Scott W, et al. Yellow nails, lymphedema and pleural effusion. Treatment of chronic pleural effusion with pleuroperitoneal shunting. Chest 1990; 97:743–745.

56. Tanaka E, Matsumoto K, Shindo T, et al. Implantation of a pleurovenous shunt for massive chylothorax in a patient with yellow nail syndrome. Thorax 2005; 60:254–255.

57. Yamagishi T, Hatanaka N, Kamemura H, et al. Idiopathic yellow nail syndrome successfully treated with OK-432. Intern Med 2007; 46:1127–1130.

58. Makrilakis K, Pavlatos S, Giannikopoulos G, et al. Successful octreotide treatment of chylous pleural effusion and lymphedema in the yellow nail syndrome. Ann Intern Med 2004; 141:246–247.

59. Szolnoky G, Lakatos B, Husz S, et al. Improvement in lymphatic function and partial resolution of nails after complex decongestive physiotherapy in yellow nail syndrome. Int J Dermatol 2005; 44:501–503.

60. Bright R. Tabular view of the morbid appearance in 100 cases connected with albuminous urine, with observations. Guys Hosp Rep 1836; 1:380–400.

61. Hopps HC, Wissler RW. Uremic pneumonitis. Am J Pathol 1955; 31:261–273.

62. Nidus BD, Matalon R, Cantacuzino D, et al. Uremic pleuritis—A clinicopathological entity. N Engl J Med 1969; 281:255–256.

63. Berger HW, Rammohan G, Neff MS, et al. Uremic pleural effusion. A study in 14 patients on chronic dialysis. Ann Intern Med 1975; 82:362–364.

64. Galen MA, Steinberg SM, Lowrie EG, et al. Hemorrhagic pleural effusion in patients undergoing chronic hemodialysis. Ann Intern Med 1975; 82:359–361.

65. Jarratt MJ, Sahn SA. Pleural effusions in hospitalized patients receiving long-term hemodialysis. Chest 1995; 108:470–474.

66. Maher JF. Uremic pleuritis. Am J Kidney Dis 1987; 10:19–22.

67. Krishnan M, Choi M. A case of uremia-associated pleural effusion in a peritoneal dialysis patient. Semin Dial 2001; 14:223–227.

68. Horita Y, Noguchi M, Miyazaki M, et al. Prognosis of patients with rounded atelectasis undergoing long-term hemodialysis. Nephron 2001; 88:87–92.

69. Yoshii C, Morita S, et al. Bilateral massive pleural effusions caused by uremic pleuritis. Intern Med 2001; 40:646–649.

70. Gilbert L, Ribot S, Frankel H, et al. Fibrinous uremic pleuritis: A surgical entity. Chest 1975; 67:53–56.

71. Rodelas R, Rakowski TA, et al. Fibrosing uremic pleuritis during hemodialysis. JAMA 1980; 243:2424–2425.

72. Isoda K, Hamamoto Y. Uremic pleuritis—Clinicopathological analysis of 26 autopsy cases. Bull Osaka Med Sch 1984; 30:73–80.

73. Coskun M, Boyvat F, Bozcurt B, et al. Thoracic CT findings in long-term hemodialysis patients. Acta Radiol 1999; 40:181–186.

74. Chiang CS, Chiang CD, Lin JW, et al. Neopterin, soluble interleukin-2 receptor and adenosine deaminase levels in pleural effusions. Respiration 1994; 61:150–154.

75. Pien GW, Gant MJ, Washam CL, et al. Use of an implantable pleural catheter for trapped lung syndrome in patients with malignant pleural effusion. Chest 2001; 119:1641–1646.

76. Lee YC, Vaz MA, Ely KA, et al. Symptomatic persistent post-coronary artery bypass graft pleural effusions requiring operative treatment: Clinical and histologic features. Chest 2001; 119:795–800.

77. Light RW, Jenkinson SG, Minh VD, et al. Observations on pleural fluid pressures as fluid is withdrawn during thoracentesis. Am Rev Respir Dis 1980; 121:799–804.

78. Villena V, Lopez-Encuentra A, Pozo F, et al. Measurement of pleural pressure during therapeutic thoracentesis. Am J Respir Crit Care Med 2000; 162:1534–1538.

79. Moore PJ, Thomas PA. The trapped lung with chronic pleural space, a cause of recurring pleural effusion. Mil Med 1967; 132:998–1002.

80. Boland GW, Gazelle GS, Girard MJ, et al. Asymptomatic hydropneumothorax after therapeutic thoracentesis for malignant pleural effusions. AJR Am J Roentgenol 1998; 170:943–946.

81. Chang YC, Patz EF Jr, Goodman PC. Pneumothorax after small-bore catheter placement for malignant pleural effusions. AJR Am J Roentgenol 1996; 166:1049–1051.

82. Huggins JT, Sahn SA, Heidecker J, et al. Characteristics of trapped lung: Pleural fluid analysis, manometry, and air-contrast chest CT. Chest 2007; 131:206–213.

818 *Kouliatsis and Bouros*

83. Genc O, Petrou M, Ladas G, et al. The long-term morbidity of pleuroperitoneal shunts in the management of recurrent malignant effusions. Eur J Cardiothorac Surg 2000; 18:143–146.
84. Rodriguez-Garcia JL, Fraile G, Moreno MA, et al. Recurrent massive pleural effusion as a late complication of radiotherapy in Hodgkin's disease. Chest 1991; 100:1165–1166.
85. Down JD, Tarbell NJ. Pitfalls in the assessment of late lung damage in irradiated mice: Complications related to pleural effusion. Int J Radiat Biol 1989; 55:473–478.
86. Bachman AL, Macken K. Pleural effusions following supervoltage radiation for breast carcinoma. Radiology 1959; 72:699–709.
87. Hietala SO, Hahn P. Pulmonary radiation reaction in the treatment of carcinoma of the breast. Radiography 1976; 42:225–230.
88. Fentanes de Torres E, Guevara E. Pleuritis by radiation: Reports of two cases. Acta Cytol 1981; 25:427–429.
89. Whitcomb ME, Schwarz MI. Pleural effusion complicating intensive mediastinal radiation therapy. Am Rev Respir Dis 1971; 103:100–107.
90. Morrone N, Gama e Silva Volpe VL, Dourado AM, et al. Bilateral pleural effusion due to mediastinal fibrosis induced by radiotherapy. Chest 1993; 104:1276–1278.
91. Fragoulis KN, Handrinou E, Papadopoulos V, et al. Delayed effusive pericarditis and recurrent pleural effusion after radiation treatment for Hodgkin's disease responsive to per os doxycycline. Eur J Haematol 2006; 76:176–179.
92. Morild I. Pleural effusion in drowning. Am J Forensic Med Pathol 1995; 16:253–256.
93. Yorulmaz C, Arican N, Afacan I, et al. Pleural effusion in bodies recovered from water. Forensic Sci Int 2003; 136:16–21.
94. Inoue H, Ishida T, Tsuji A, et al. Electrolyte analysis in pleural effusion as an indicator of the drowning medium. Leg Med (Tokyo) 2005; 7:96–102.
95. Kavuru MS, Adamo JP, Ahmad M, et al. Amyloidosis and pleural disease. Chest 1990; 98:20–23.
96. Knapp MJ, Roggli VL, Kim J, et al. Pleural amyloidosis. Arch Pathol Lab Med 1988; 112:57–60.
97. Vilaseca J, Cuevas J, Fresno M, et al. Systemic amyloidosis in cystic fibrosis. Am J Dis Child 1981; 135:667.
98. Romero Candeira S, Martin Serrano C, Hernandez Blasco L. Amyloidosis and pleural disease. Chest 1991; 100:292–293.
99. Maeno T, Sando Y, Tsukagoshi M, et al. Pleural amyloidosis in a patient with intractable pleural effusion and multiple myeloma. Respirology 2000; 5:79–80.
100. Astoul P, Cheikh R, Cabanot C, et al. Pleural amyloidosis: Thoracoscopic diagnosis and physiopathological approach. Rev Mal Respir 1992; 9:629–631.
101. Bontemps F, Tillie-Leblond I, Coppin MC, et al. Pleural amyloidosis: Thoracoscopic aspects. Eur Respir J 1995; 8:1025–1027.
102. Berk JL. Pleural effusions in systemic amyloidosis. Curr Opin Pulm Med 2005; 11:324–328.
103. Berk JL, Keane J, Seldin DC, et al. Persistent pleural effusions in primary systemic amyloidosis: Etiology and prognosis. Chest 2003; 124:969–977.
104. Hoyer RJ, Leung N, Witzig TE, et al. Treatment of diuretic refractory pleural effusions with bevacizumab in four patients with primary systemic amyloidosis. Am J Hematol 2007; 82:409–413.
105. Graham DR, Ahmad D. Amyloidosis with pleural involvement. Eur Respir J 1988; 1:571–572.
106. Case records of the Massachusetts General Hospital. Weekly clinicopathological exercises; Case 48–1977. N Engl J Med 1977; 297:1221–1228.
107. Im JG, Chung JW, Han MC. Milk of calcium pleural collections: CT findings. J Comput Assist Tomogr 1993; 17:613–616.
108. Goldenberg DC, Bringel RW, Fontana C, et al. Pulmonary lesion in electric injury: Report of a case. Rev Hosp Clin Fac Med Sao Paulo 1996; 51:15–17.

109. Baxter CR. Present concepts in the management of major electrical injury. Surg Clin North Am 1970; 50:1401–1418.
110. Hiraiwa T, Hayashi T, Kaneda M, et al. Rupture of a benign mediastinal teratoma into the right pleural cavity. Ann Thorac Surg 1991; 51:110–112.
111. Choi SJ, Lee JS, Song KS, et al. Mediastinal teratoma: CT differentiation of ruptured and unruptured tumors. AJR Am J Roentgenol 1998; 171:591–594.
112. Matsubara K, Aoki M, Okumura N, et al. Spontaneous rupture of mediastinal cystic teratoma into the pleural cavity: Report of two cases and review of the literature. Pediatr Hematol Oncol 2001; 18:221–227.
113. Cobb CJ, Wynn J, Cobb SR, et al. Cytologic findings in an effusion caused by rupture of a benign cystic teratoma of the mediastinum into a serous cavity. Acta Cytol 1985; 29:1015–1020.
114. Krishnan S, Statsinger AL, et al. Eosinophilic pleural effusion with Charcot-Leyden crystals. Acta Cytol 1983; 27:529–532.
115. Robinson LA, Rikkers LF, Dobson JR. Benign mediastinal teratoma masquerading as a large multiloculated effusion. Ann Thorac Surg 1994; 58:545–548.
116. Ashour M, el-Din Hawass N, Adam KA, et al. Spontaneous intrapleural rupture of mediastinal teratoma. Respir Med 1993; 87:69–72.
117. Khalil A, Carette MF, Milleron B, et al. Bronchogenic cyst presenting as mediastinal mass with pleural effusion. Eur Respir J 1995; 8:2185–2187.
118. Riemer H, Hainz R, Stain C, et al. Severe pulmonary hypertension reversed by antibiotics in a patient with Whipple's disease. Thorax 1997; 52:1014–1015.
119. Whipple G. A hitherto undescribed disease characterized anatomically by deposits of fat and fatty acids in the intestinal mesenteric lymphatic tissues. Bull Johns Hopkins Hosp 1907; 18:382–391.
120. Symmons DP, Shepherd AN, Boardman PL, et al. Pulmonary manifestations of Whipple's disease. Q J Med 1985; 56:497–504.
121. Pollock JJ. Pleuropulmonary Whipple's disease. South Med J 1985; 78:216–217.
122. Muller C, Stain C, Burghuber O. *Tropheryma whippelii* in peripheral blood mononuclear cells and cells of pleural effusion. Lancet 1993; 341:701.
123. Zaharopoulos P, Wong J. Cytologic diagnosis of syphilitic pleuritis: A case report. Diagn Cytopathol 1997; 16:35–38.
124. Cattini GC, Greco N, Tosto L, et al. Syphilitic pleuritis. Description of a clinical case. Minerva Med 1983; 74:337–342.

Index